THE AMERICAN MEDICAL ASSOCIATION

HOME MEDICAL ENCYCLOPEDIA

THE
AMERICAN
MEDICAL
ASSOCIATION

HOME MEDICAL
ENCYCLOPEDIA

VOLUME ONE · A – H

MEDICAL EDITOR
Charles B. Clayman, MD

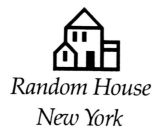

Random House
New York

Published by The Reader's Digest Association, Inc.,
with permission of Random House, Inc.

The information in this encyclopedia reflects current
medical knowledge. The recommendations and
information are appropriate in most cases; however,
they are not a substitute for medical diagnosis. For
specific information concerning your personal
medical condition, the AMA suggests that you
consult a physician.
   The names of organizations, products, or alternative
therapies appearing in this encyclopedia are given for
informational purposes only. Their inclusion does not
imply AMA endorsement, nor does the omission of any
organization, product, or alternative therapy indicate
AMA disapproval.

Library of Congress Cataloging in Publication Data

The American Medical Association home medical
   encyclopedia.

   Includes index.
   1. Medicine, Popular—Dictionaries.   I. American
Medical Association.   II. Title: Home medical
encyclopedia.
RC81.A2A522   1989   610'.3   89-10589
ISBN 0-394-58248-9 (set)
ISBN 0-394-58246-2 (v. 1)
ISBN 0-394-58247-0 (v. 2)

Manufactured in the United States of America

Computerset by M. F. Graphics Limited, England
Reproduction by Mandarin Offset Limited, Hong Kong

PREFACE

Medicine has changed a great deal in recent years. First, technological advances, such as magnetic resonance imaging, PET scanners, and endoscopes have transformed methods of diagnosis. Second, the development of new treatments—including transplants, implants, laser surgery, lithotripsy, and angioplasty—has widened the range of disorders that can be treated safely and effectively. New drugs have also extended medicine's capabilities, or made possible safer and more effective treatments than their predecessors.

However, probably the most important change has been the recognition by the medical profession that today's patients are not prepared to be merely passive recipients of medical care. Today, people want to be involved in decisions that affect their health; they want to know not only what is wrong with them, but also what the choices of treatment are, and what risks are involved. Recognizing this, most physicians now try to spend more time with patients and their families explaining the problems and options available.

This medical encyclopedia has been produced by the American Medical Association to help you understand the language of medicine. Its two volumes provide clear, illustrated explanations of how the body works and also give detailed information on all of the common diseases (and many of the less common ones). Furthermore, in contrast to many popular medical books, this encyclopedia does not expound an individual author's theory or market any "breakthrough" treatment or diet. What it does provide is a clear, systematic account of state-of-the-art, validated medical knowledge—reviewed and endorsed by expert physicians selected by the American Medical Association.

We hope you will use THE AMERICAN MEDICAL ASSOCIATION HOME MEDICAL ENCYCLOPEDIA in the best of health.

James H. Sammons, MD
Executive Vice President
American Medical Association

THE AMERICAN MEDICAL ASSOCIATION

James H. Sammons, MD · *Executive Vice President*
John T. Baker · *Vice President, Publishing*
Heidi Hough · *Director, Office of Consumer Books*
Kathy Kaye · *Managing Editor*
Brenda A. Clark · *Staff Assistant*

EDITORIAL STAFF

Charles B. Clayman, MD · *Medical Editor*
Heidi Hough · *Editor-In-Chief*
Robin Fitzpatrick Husayko · *Editor*
James Ferris · *Assistant Editor*
Julie S. Ferris · *Assistant Editor*
Brenda A. Clark · *Editorial Assistant*
Frank D. Campion · *Consulting Editor*

ACKNOWLEDGMENTS

Mary Banas
Joaquin Chang
Gary Hubler, RPh
Lynne Lamberg
Kenneth F. Lampe, PhD

Jacqueline Martin
Mary Ann McCann
William Smith
Michaela Sullivan-Fowler
Bonnie B. Wilford

Alliance for the Mentally Ill of Greater Chicago
American Dental Association
American Dietetic Association
American Osteopathic Association
American Podiatric Association
American Society of Plastic and Reconstructive Surgeons, Inc.
Mallinckrodt Institute of Radiology
National Organization for Women, Chicago Chapter
Public Health Service, US Department of Health and Human Services
University of Washington School of Medicine

Editorial Director Amy Carroll; **Managing Editor** Ruth Midgley; **Editors** Andrea Bagg, Stephen Carroll,
Robert Dinwiddie, Mary Lindsay, Ricki Ostrov, Martyn Page, Jillian Somerscales, Frances Williams,
Robert M. Youngson; **Editorial Secretary** Pat White; **Managing Art Editors** Chez Picthall, Denise Brown;
Art Editor Caroline Murray; **Designers** Tina Hill, Tracy Timson, Lydia Umney, Peter Cross, Gail Jones,
Melissa Gray, Sarah Ponder, Sandra Archer; **Picture research** Sandra Schneider; **Production** Rupert Wheeler

MEDICAL CONSULTANTS

EMERGENCY FIRST-AID TECHNIQUES

Use this quick-reference list to find illustrated first-aid boxes containing step-by-step instructions for performing emergency techniques.

SYMPTOM CHARTS

Use this quick-reference list to find question-and-answer flow charts that indicate the possible causes and significance of many common symptoms.

CONTENTS

HOW TO USE THE ENCYCLOPEDIA

This highly illustrated encyclopedia is an authoritative guide to all aspects of medicine. For swift and easy reference, encyclopedia entries are arranged alphabetically and longer entries are subdivided into sections, each with a descriptive subheading. Information within entries is presented in clear, concise language. Technical or unfamiliar medical terms are generally explained as they appear.

The main body of the encyclopedia, the **A to Z of Medicine**, contains more than 5,000 entries covering a vast range of medical and medically related topics. It is obviously impossible in a one-volume compendium to provide separate entries for every

medical term, but many additional terms and topics are discussed within relevant entries. The **Index** refers you to all such items as well as to the major entries themselves.

The encyclopedia also contains a full-color introductory section, **Medicine Today**, which gives useful information on staying healthy and describes the latest advances in diagnosis and treatment. At the back of the book, additional information on generic and brand-name drugs is contained in the **Drug Glossary.** There is also a list of telephone numbers, many of them toll free, for a wide range of **Self-help Organizations.**

HOW TO FIND THE INFORMATION YOU WANT

All entries in the **A to Z of Medicine** and in the **Index** are arranged alphabetically using the "letter-by-letter" system. In this system, any spaces or punctuation in the entry titles are ignored. *Sick building syndrome* is thus followed by *Sickle cell anemia* and then by *Sick sinus syndrome* – the fifth letter gives the order.

When the name of a topic consists of more than one word, begin by looking up what seems to be the key word. Thus, for information on general anesthesia you will find what you want under the heading *Anesthesia, general.* If the key word is not obvious, you may find it easier to turn first to the **Index,** although

many alternative topic names and common abbreviations are included as short cross-reference entries within the main part of the book.

You will also find cross-references within the entries themselves. These are indicated by italics and take several forms, which are explained in the annotated illustration below.

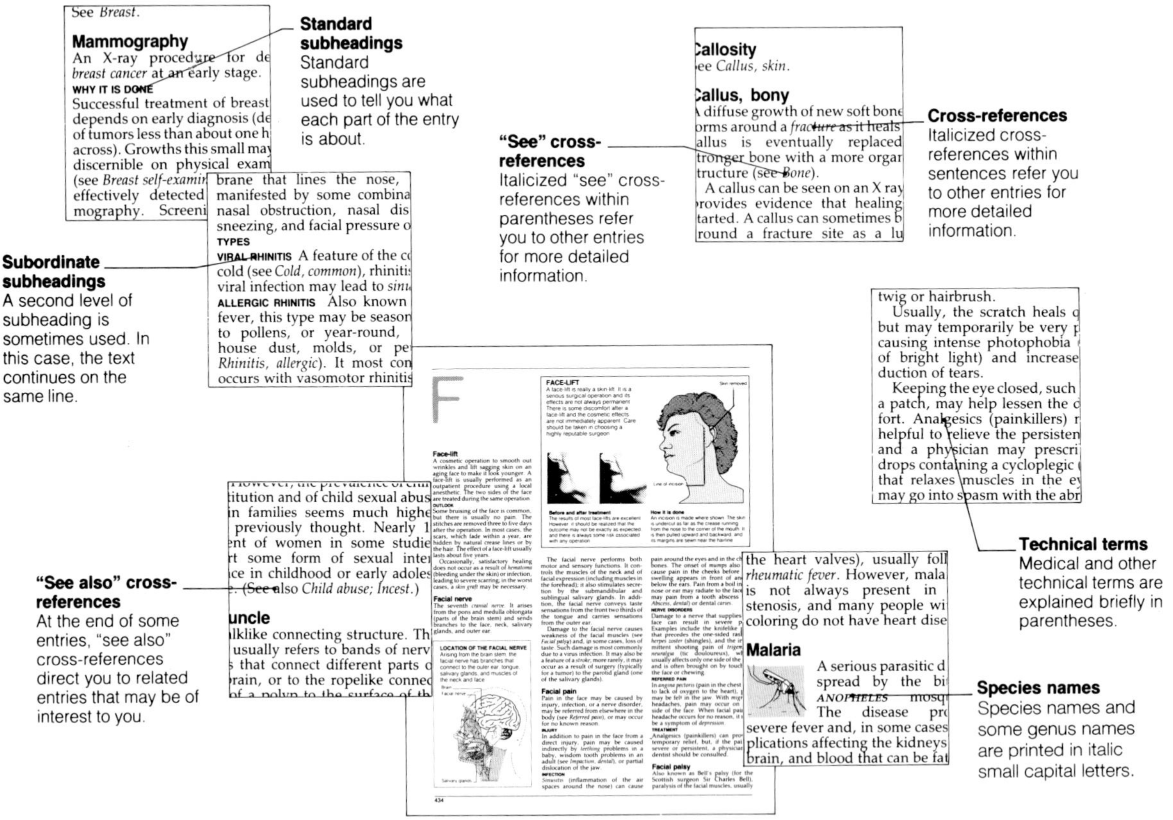

Standard subheadings
Standard subheadings are used to tell you what each part of the entry is about.

Subordinate subheadings
A second level of subheading is sometimes used. In this case, the text continues on the same line.

"See also" cross-references
At the end of some entries, "see also" cross-references direct you to related entries that may be of interest to you.

"See" cross-references
Italicized "see" cross-references within parentheses refer you to other entries for more detailed information.

Cross-references
Italicized cross-references within sentences refer you to other entries for more detailed information.

Technical terms
Medical and other technical terms are explained briefly in parentheses.

Species names
Species names and some genus names are printed in italic small capital letters.

The A to Z of Medicine contains individual entries on a wide range of physical and psychological symptoms. In general, you will find the main description of a particular symptom under its common name, if it has one. For example, *Vomiting* is the main entry and *Emesis*, the medical term for vomiting, is a short cross-reference entry. Alternative names for symptoms also appear in the **Index**.

Symptom charts

The question-and-answer symptom charts will help you understand the significance of common symptoms that have no obvious cause. Each chart singles out possible causes of the symptom, refers you to relevant entries in the encyclopedia, and suggests appropriate action, if any. Start at the top of the chart and answer "yes" or "no" to the series of carefully selected questions until you reach the box that advises you on your particular problem. For the page numbers of all symptom charts, consult page 8.

Title and description
The title of each symptom chart is followed by a brief description of the symptom in nontechnical language.

The questions
Each question is phrased so that it requires either a "yes" or "no" reply. Follow your "yes" or "no" answer to the appropriate next question and continue until you reach the box with advice on your problem.

Warning
Warning boxes draw your attention to potentially serious symptoms and give practical advice.

Cancer warning
"Cancer watch" boxes alert you to the possibility of cancer if you have certain symptoms.

CANCER WATCH
Recurrent abdominal pain (especially in people over 40) may indicate cancer, especially if the symptoms are newly developed and are accompanied by a change in eating or bowel habits. **Consult your physician without delay!**

Other information
Some symptom charts have additional boxes containing self-help advice or information directed at particular groups of people.

Emergency! Get medical help now!
This instruction indicates that the problem may be life-threatening and needs immediate medical attention. Call for an ambulance or, if you are certain that the person can be moved safely, take him or her to the nearest hospital emergency room.

Consult/call your physician without delay!
You should telephone your physician at once, either to discuss the problem over the telephone or to arrange for an early appointment at the physician's office.

Consult your physician
This instruction means that you should make an appointment to see your physician about the problem. Haste is not, however, essential.

Cross-references
When appropriate, end boxes cross-refer you to encyclopedia entries for further information.

Fever in children
...usually caused by infection ...or bacterium. However, a ...lso become feverish if ...become overheated. Do ...pirin; use an aspirin ...A raised temperature ...ild's forehead to feel hot ...increased sweating and a ...ling of being sick. Normal ...e may vary from 97 to ...37.5°C). Minor ...within this range are no ...oncern if your child seems otherwise well.
• If your baby's temperature rises above 102°F (39°C), whatever the suspected cause, call your physician at once. High temperatures can lead to seizures in some babies.

Irritation of the stomach is the most likely cause of the pain. However, there is also a possibility of an ulcer. Consult your physician.
- See • *Gastritis*
       • *Peptic ulcer*

Dull aches or cramps are often associated with menstruation. Discuss with your physician.

Discuss with your physician
You should mention the problem to your physician on your next visit, but there is no need for a special appointment.

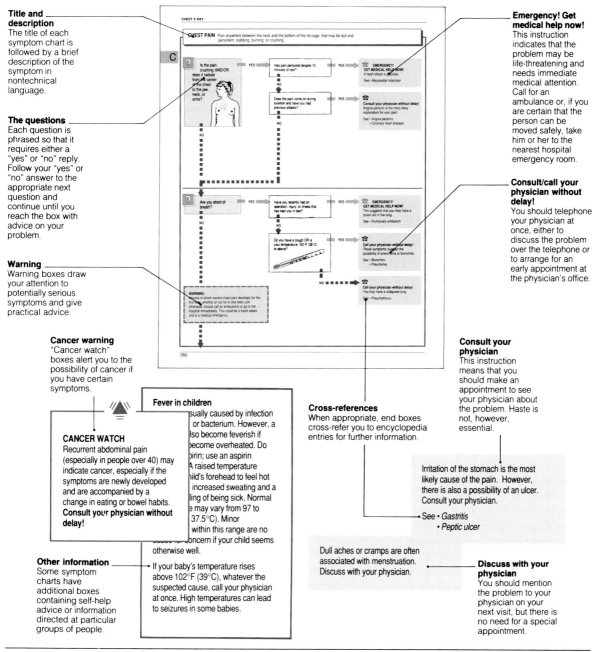

HOW TO FIND INFORMATION ON DISORDERS

The **A to Z of Medicine** contains individual entries on all major and many minor disorders. There are also general entries covering groups of disorders, such as *Genetic disorders*, or disorders that affect different parts of the body in different ways, such as *Cancer*. These group entries provide an overview and explain the basic disease processes. Specific forms, such as *Hemophilia* or *Breast cancer*, are covered in separate entries. Group entries contain cross-references to more specific entries. If you look up certain group entries in

the **Index**, you will find references to disorders in those groups.

Consult the **Index**, too, if you fail to find an entry on a specific disorder within the **A to Z of Medicine**. You may find that the disorder has another name. For example, if you look up decubitus ulcer in the **Index** you will be directed to the encyclopedia entry on *Bedsores*—decubitus ulcer and bedsore are different names for the same condition. In other cases, the **Index** will show you that a specific disorder is discussed within a more general entry. For

example, conductive deafness is included in the entry on *Deafness*.

Disorder boxes

Entries on the main organs and body parts are accompanied by boxed summaries of the various disorders that may affect them. These disorder boxes help you see at a glance the types of problems most often associated with a particular organ or body part. They also cross-refer you to entries on specific disorders and investigation techniques.

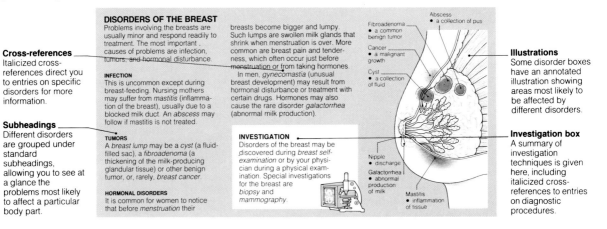

Cross-references
Italicized cross-references direct you to entries on specific disorders for more information.

Subheadings
Different disorders are grouped under standard subheadings, allowing you to see at a glance the problems most likely to affect a particular body part.

DISORDERS OF THE BREAST
Problems involving the breasts are usually minor and respond readily to treatment. The most important . causes of problems are infection, tumors, and hormonal disturbance.

INFECTION
This is uncommon except during breast-feeding. Nursing mothers may suffer from *mastitis* (inflammation of the breast), usually due to a blocked milk duct. An *abscess* may follow if mastitis is not treated.

TUMORS
A *breast lump* may be a *cyst* (a fluid-filled sac), a *fibroadenoma* (a thickening of the milk-producing glandular tissue) or other benign tumor, or, rarely, *breast cancer*.

HORMONAL DISORDERS
It is common for women to notice that before *menstruation* their

breasts become bigger and lumpy. Such lumps are swollen milk glands that shrink when menstruation is over. More common are breast pain and tenderness, which often occur just before menstruation or from taking hormones.
In men, *gynecomastia* (unusual breast development) may result from hormonal disturbance or treatment with certain drugs. Hormones may also cause the rare disorder *galactorrhea* (abnormal milk production).

INVESTIGATION
Disorders of the breast may be discovered during *breast self-examination* or by your physician during a physical examination. Special investigations for the breast are *biopsy* and *mammography*.

Abscess
● a collection of pus

Fibroadenoma
● a common benign tumor

Cancer
● a malignant growth

Cyst
● a collection of fluid

Nipple
● discharge

Galactorrhea
● abnormal production of milk

Mastitis
● inflammation of tissue

Illustrations
Some disorder boxes have an annotated illustration showing areas most likely to be affected by different disorders.

Investigation box
A summary of investigation techniques is given here, including italicized cross-references to entries on diagnostic procedures.

HOW TO FIND INFORMATION ON ANATOMY AND PHYSIOLOGY

All body systems (e.g., *Biliary system*) and major organs and body parts (e.g., *Brain* and *Coccyx*) have individual entries in the **A to Z of Medicine**. There are also entries on the senses (e.g., *Vision*) and on other body processes (e.g., *Breathing* and *Blood clotting*). Anatomy and physiology entries explain how the healthy body works and provide a background for understanding medical disorders.

Most anatomy and physiology entries are accompanied by illustrated boxes. Annotated illustrations show the main structural features of body parts, the location of different body parts in relation to each other, and, for physiology entries, the main stages in important body processes.

Medical images
Pictures obtained by specialized imaging techniques, such as X rays or scans, are used in many cases.

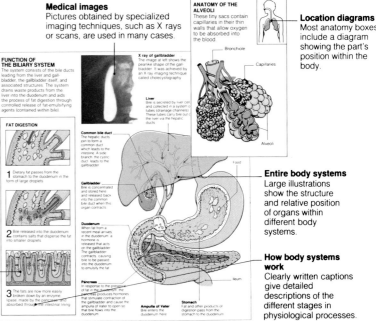

Anatomical drawings
Detailed drawings, often with cutaway sections, show the structure of body parts.

Location diagrams
Most anatomy boxes include a diagram showing the part's position within the body.

Entire body systems
Large illustrations show the structure and relative position of organs within different body systems.

How body systems work
Clearly written captions give detailed descriptions of the different stages in physiological processes.

HOW TO FIND INFORMATION ON MEDICAL TESTS

Many different tests for diagnosing or monitoring medical conditions have individual entries within the **A to Z of Medicine.** Many of these entries are illustrated by step-by-step diagrams.

More general information on tests is given in the entry headed *Tests, medical.* This entry is accompanied by a table that shows the tests used to investigate different parts of the body and directs you to individual entries within the encyclopedia. You can also find out which tests are used to investigate a particular part of the body by consulting the investigation section of the disorder box for that body part.

Entries on specific disorders in the **A to Z of Medicine** cross-refer you to entries that describe the tests used to diagnose and monitor them.

Illustrations showing techniques
Clear illustrations show a test's most important stages, including, for example, where a needle is inserted in the body or how samples are prepared for testing.

Step-by-step text
Concise captions describe the various stages in each test, including what happens to the patient and how test samples are analyzed in the laboratory.

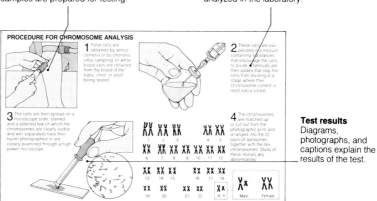

Test results
Diagrams, photographs, and captions explain the results of the test.

HOW TO FIND INFORMATION ON SURGICAL PROCEDURES

Surgical procedures are described either in individual entries or in the treatment section of disorder entries. In many cases, entries are accompanied by illustrated boxes.

Individual entries on surgical procedures are included under their generally accepted medical names. In many cases, these names are self-explanatory—*Heart-lung transplant* or *Hernia repair,* for example.

If you do not know the name of a particular procedure, look up the encyclopedia entry on the disorder for which it is a treatment, where you will find a description of, or a cross-reference to, the appropriate procedure. Alternatively, consult the **Index,** which lists some popular names. For example, if you look up *Stomach, removal of,* you will be referred to the encyclopedia entry on *Gastrectomy.*

Surgery in progress
True-to-life drawings show surgical procedures in progress and provide an accurate representation of current surgical practice.

Incision sites
A red line superimposed on a photograph of the relevant part of the body shows the position and shape of the surgeon's incision.

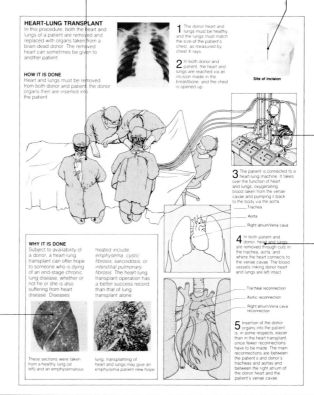

Equipment
Detailed illustrations show the workings of special equipment, such as a heart-lung machine.

Step-by-step text and illustrations
Explanatory captions and anatomically correct illustrations take you through the most important stages of surgical procedures. Large numbers show the sequence of events and help you follow the different stages.

Reasons for surgery
Different medical images – such as photographs, X rays, or scans – of diseased tissue show why operations are necessary.

HOW TO FIND INFORMATION ON DRUGS

The **A to Z of Medicine** contains individual entries on all major drug groups (from *ACE inhibitor drugs* to *Vasodilator drugs*) and on the most important generic drugs (from *Acebutolol* to *Zidovudine*). Other information on drugs can be found in general entries, such as *Drug, Drug dependence,* and *Drug poisoning.*

The **Drug Glossary** gives concise information on almost 3,000 generic and brand-name drugs, showing the generic equivalents of brand-name drugs, and identifying the drug groups to which individual drugs belong. Each glossary entry cross-refers you for more information to the **A to Z of Medicine.**

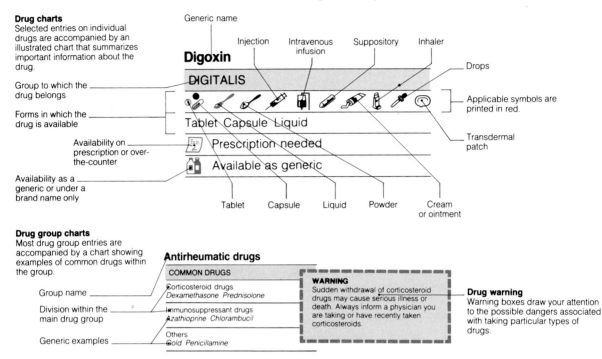

Drug charts
Selected entries on individual drugs are accompanied by an illustrated chart that summarizes important information about the drug.

Group to which the drug belongs

Forms in which the drug is available

Availability on prescription or over-the-counter

Availability as a generic or under a brand name only

Generic name

Injection   Intravenous infusion   Suppository   Inhaler

Digoxin

DIGITALIS

Tablet Capsule Liquid

Prescription needed

Available as generic

Drops

Applicable symbols are printed in red.

Transdermal patch

Tablet   Capsule   Liquid   Powder   Cream or ointment

Drug group charts
Most drug group entries are accompanied by a chart showing examples of common drugs within the group.

Group name

Division within the main drug group

Generic examples

Antirheumatic drugs

COMMON DRUGS

Corticosteroid drugs
Dexamethasone Prednisolone

Immunosuppressant drugs
Azathioprine Chlorambucil

Others
Gold Penicillamine

WARNING
Sudden withdrawal of corticosteroid drugs may cause serious illness or death. Always inform a physician you are taking or have recently taken corticosteroids.

Drug warning
Warning boxes draw your attention to the possible dangers associated with taking particular types of drugs.

HOW TO USE THE ENCYCLOPEDIA IN AN EMERGENCY

EMERGENCY FIRST-AID TECHNIQUES

Turn to page 8 for the page numbers of emergency first-aid boxes.

Lifesaving and other, less urgent, first-aid techniques are explained in easy-to-follow first-aid boxes. These boxes accompany relevant entries within the **A to Z of Medicine.** All first-aid boxes have a distinctive red border and a special heading. A list of first-aid boxes describing emergency techniques, with their page numbers, is given on page 8.

Distinctive appearance
Bold red borders and special headings make first-aid boxes easy to find.

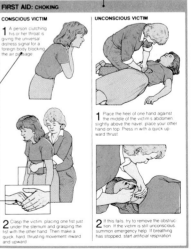

FIRST AID: CHOKING

CONSCIOUS VICTIM

1 A person clutching his or her throat is giving the universal distress signal for a foreign body blocking the air passage

2 Clasp the victim, placing one fist just under the sternum and grasping the fist with the other hand. Then make a quick, hard, thrusting movement inward and upward

UNCONSCIOUS VICTIM

1 Place the heel of one hand against the middle of the victim's abdomen slightly above the navel; place your other hand on top. Press in with a quick upward thrust

2 If this fails, try to remove the obstruction. If the victim is still unconscious, summon emergency help. If breathing has stopped, start *artificial respiration*

WARNING
Warning boxes contain essential advice and indicate when professional help should be sought.

WARNING
Frostbite is often accompanied by hypothermia, which must be treated first. Proper medical attention should be sought promptly, but first aid should be given immediately.

Step-by-step
First-aid techniques are clearly described in numbered sequences of text and illustrations.

DO NOT
- rub the affected parts
- attempt to burst blisters
- warm the affected area with direct heat
- allow the victim to walk on a frostbitten foot

DO NOT
These boxes tell you what not to do when treating an injured person.

Close-ups
More detailed illustrations show you exactly what to do.

MEDICINE
TODAY

PROGRESS IN MEDICINE

People living in developed countries today have the opportunity to be healthier than ever before. Our understanding of how the body works has broadened rapidly in the last few years, paralleled by equally dramatic improvements in medical technology. As a result of this progress, a person's chances of staying healthy into old age depend increasingly on following expert advice on a healthy life-style, making full use of preventive techniques such as vaccination and screening tests, and seeking medical advice from your physician at the first sign of illness.

This section of the encyclopedia presents an overview of recent developments in preventive health care, diagnosis, treatment, prenatal technology, and new diseases. It also discusses human potential, including the ways in which we can maximize it.

One important area of advancement in medical science is computer imaging. Computers can now provide images of the interior of the body that are based on various types of scanning techniques, such as X rays, radioactive isotopes, ultrasound, or magnetic resonance. These images—which may be two- or three-dimensional, and even colored to highlight selected features (e.g., specific tissues)—can give

physicians almost as much information as they would be able to obtain through an exploratory operation on the chest or abdomen. In some cases, such as the functional "maps" of tissue metabolism provided by PET scanning, the images provide information that cannot be obtained even by direct examination.

A second major area of advancement has been in medical treatment. As recently as the 1970s, major surgery usually required an incision large enough for the surgeon to get his or her hands into the body. Today, the emphasis in surgery is on less invasive techniques, such as extracorporeal lithotripsy, a noninvasive procedure that uses ultrasound to shatter stones in the body, and endoscopic surgery, in which a viewing tube is passed into the body through a natural orifice or through a tiny incision, directed to the target structure, and then used as a guide through which instruments are passed to enable the physician to perform the surgery. Electrocautery and the use of lasers permit bloodless surgery. As a result of these and other advances in anesthesia, the use of antibiotic drugs, and the monitoring of various body functions, medical treatment today is safer and more effective.

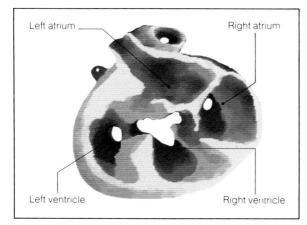

Left atrium
Right atrium
Left ventricle
Right ventricle

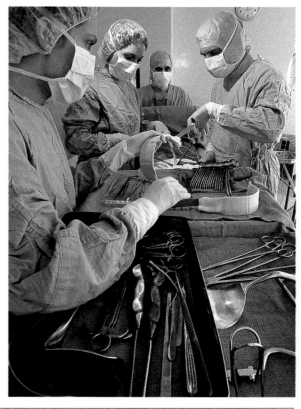

Three-dimensional magnetic resonance imaging (3-D MRI)
The image of a section through the heart showing its four chambers (above) was obtained by the recently developed technique of 3-D MRI. This technique, which is noninvasive and without known risk to the patient, gives more accurate and detailed images than could be obtained by other means. As a result, any structural abnormalities are often immediately apparent when the images are examined.

Surgery
Despite trends toward less invasive methods of treatment, conventional surgery (right) is still as important as ever. Significant growth areas include transplants, implants, and repairing damaged or obstructed blood vessels. These operations, along with the removal of cancers, will probably be performed in the future much as they are today, although there will be refinements in anesthesia and postoperative care.

STAYING HEALTHY

Today, most children in developed countries are healthier than ever before; a majority can expect to live well beyond the age of 70. These achievements are partly due to improvements in public health, such as the provision of safe water supplies and sewage disposal systems, adequate housing, and good nutrition, and partly to improvements in medical care.

The health of women today can be carefully monitored before and during pregnancy, and during the birth of the baby. After birth, the newborn infant is closely examined and, if necessary, provided with specialized care.

Throughout infancy and childhood, children are immunized against infections and given vision and hearing tests, as well as tests for physical and mental development. As a result, any problems can be detected and treated promptly.

In the US and Europe, the principal causes of death or disability in youth and middle age are preventable.

World health

Not all countries have high standards of health. In many developing countries, infant mortality is high, principally because many people do not have access to safe water, adequate food, or basic health care (see diagram, right).

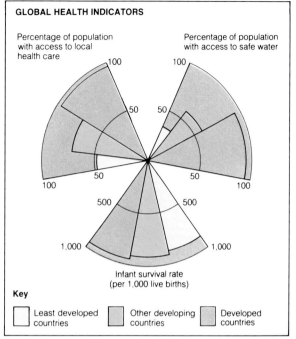

GLOBAL HEALTH INDICATORS

Percentage of population with access to local health care

Percentage of population with access to safe water

Infant survival rate (per 1,000 live births)

Key

Least developed countries

Other developing countries

Developed countries

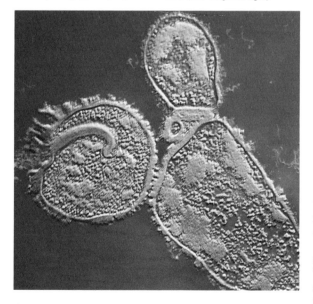

Childhood infectious diseases

The photomicrograph (above) shows the bacterium BORDETELLA PERTUSSIS, the cause of pertussis (whooping cough). In developed countries, this and other potentially serious childhood diseases (such as measles, poliomyelitis, and diphtheria) have been brought under control by immunization. In developing countries, such diseases are still common; the World Health Organization is working to combat this problem by making immunization available to all children.

In early adult life, most deaths are due to accidents or violence; other important causes include suicide, and complications of drug abuse and sexual habits (notably AIDS). In addition, the risk of developing the principal serious disorders of middle age—coronary heart disease and cancer—is reduced by following a healthy life-style and avoiding known health hazards, especially tobacco and alcohol.

Even though following a healthy life-style minimizes an individual's chance of developing life-threatening disease, people living healthy lives may still become ill, either because they have an inborn susceptibility to a disorder or simply by chance. As understanding of the genetic basis of disease improves, screening tests for familial inherited disorders will become wider ranging.

Physicians strongly advise people to become aware of the regular manner in which their bodies function. This includes monitoring bowel habits, appetite, and sleep patterns. When a change in body function is noted, advice should be sought promptly from your physician. Early attention to any illness aids treatment and promotes cure.

Avoiding premature death is not the only benefit to be gained from following a healthy life-style. The quality of life can also improve: the body's natural aging processes are slowed, and physical and mental vigor are retained for much longer.

PERSONAL HEALTH CARE

An individual's health is determined partly by inheritance and partly by external factors. Health and longevity tend to run in families, so a person whose grandparents lived beyond the age of 80 is likely to do the same. However, this is not always the case. Even the intrinsically healthiest body can be damaged by neglect or external factors, especially by unwise use of drugs, including tobacco and alcohol. With the AIDS epidemic still spreading, avoidance of illicit intravenous drugs and sexual promiscuity and adherence to "safe" sex practices are essential for the maintenance of good health.

For many people, however, these "do nots" are less important than three positive keys to a healthy lifestyle: a sound, balanced diet, a positive attitude, and regular, vigorous exercise.

Diet and exercise

For most of history, diseases associated with diet were due to vitamin or mineral deficiencies, or simply to prolonged semi-starvation. In developed countries today, however, the main dietary threat to health is caused by excess: many people overeat, and almost everybody consumes too much saturated fat. Research has shown that variations around the world in the rates of heart disease and some cancers are primarily due to differences in diet. Most Americans consume too much dairy fat, animal fat, and sugar but consume insufficient vegetables and grains. Asian people tend to eat more fish, grains, vegetables, and fruit and so have a healthier diet.

However, over the past few years, a dramatic improvement in our understanding of food and diet has taken place and the dietary habits of many people in the US and Europe have begun to improve. A growing number of people now eat larger amounts of vegetables, fruit, and cereals and have substituted unsaturated fats and oils for dairy fats. In addition, the consumption of fatty meats has declined. According to researchers, these changes have contributed to a significant decrease in the incidence of heart disease in people in many—but not all—developed countries. Nevertheless, many people in the US and other developed countries continue to eat

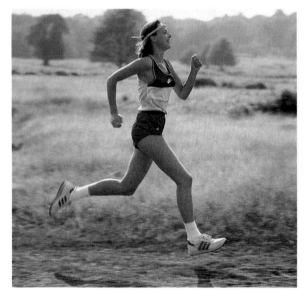

Health and exercise
Physical exercise, such as running (above), can reduce the risk of coronary heart disease, but only if it is vigorous enough to stimulate the heart and is performed three or more times a week for at least 20 minutes each session.

Types of exercise
The table (right) compares the value of various activities for improving three main aspects of health and fitness—heart and lung efficiency, joint suppleness, and muscle power. The average calorie consumption rate of each activity is also given.

THE FITNESS VALUES OF VARIOUS ACTIVITIES

Activity	Calories consumed in 20 minutes of activity	Value in improving heart and lung fitness	Value in improving joint suppleness	Value in improving muscle power
Easy walking	60	□	□	□
Light housework	90	□	□□	□□
Light gardening (weeding, etc.)	90	□	□□	□□
Golf (flat course)	90	□	□□	□
Brisk walking	100	□□	□	□□
Badminton	115	□□	□□□	□□
Gymnastics	140	□□	□□□□	□□
Heavy gardening (digging, etc.)	140	□□	□□□	□□□□
Dancing	160	□□	□□□	□
Easy jogging	160	□□□	□	□□
Tennis	160	□□□	□□□	□□
Skiing (downhill)	160	□□□	□□□	□□
Skiing (cross-country)	180	□□□□	□□□	□□
Football	180	□□□	□□	□□□
Racquetball or handball	200	□□□	□□□	□□
Brisk jogging	210	□□□□	□□	□□
Bicycling	220	□□□□	□□	□□□
Swimming	240	□□□□	□□□□	□□□□

Key

- Calories consumed in 20 minutes of activity
- Value in improving heart and lung fitness
- Value in improving joint suppleness
- Value in improving muscle power

□□□□ Excellent
□□□ Good
□□ Fair
□ Minimal

RECOMMENDED DAILY ALLOWANCES (RDAs) OF SELECTED VITAMINS

	Birth to 6 months	6 months to 1 year	1 to 3 years	4 to 6 years	7 to 10 years	11 to 14 years	15 to 18 years	19 to 22 years	23 to 50 years	51 + years	Extra needed pregnancy	Extra needed breast-feeding
Folic acid (mcg)	30	45	100	200	300	400	400	400	400	400	400	100
Niacin (mg)	6.0	8.0	9.0	11	16	M 18 F 15	M 18 F 14	M 19 F 14	M 18 F 13	M 16 F 13	2.0	5.0
Pyridoxine (mg)	0.3	0.6	0.9	1.3	1.6	1.8	2.0	M 2.2 F 2.0	M 2.2 F 2.0	M 2.2 F 2.0	0.6	0.5
Riboflavin (mg)	0.4	0.6	0.8	1.0	1.4	M 1.6 F 1.3	M 1.7 F 1.3	M 1.7 F 1.3	M 1.6 F 1.2	M 1.4 F 1.2	0.3	0.5
Thiamine (mg)	0.3	0.5	0.7	0.9	1.2	M 1.4 F 1.1	M 1.4 F 1.1	M 1.5 F 1.1	M 1.4 F 1.0	M 1.2 F 1.0	0.4	0.5
Vitamin A (mcg) 1	420	400	400	500	700	M 1,000 F 800	M 1,000 F 800	M 1,000 F 800	M 1,000 F 800	M 1,000 F 800	200	400
Vitamin B$_{12}$ (mcg)	0.5	1.5	2.0	2.5	3.0	3.0	3.0	3.0	3.0	3.0	1.0	1.0
Vitamin C (mg)	35	35	45	45	45	M 50 F 60	60	60	60	60	20	40
Vitamin D (mcg) 2	10	10	10	10	10	10	10	7.5	5.0	5.0	5.0	5.0
Vitamin E (mg) 3	3.0	3.0	5.0	6.0	7.0	8.0	M 10 F 8.0	M 10 F 8.0	M 10 F 8.0	M 10 F 8.0	2.0	3.0

1 RDA expressed in mcg of retinol (a form of vitamin A). 1 mcg of retinol (a unit called a retinol equivalent, or RE) equals 6 mcg of beta-carotene (another form of vitamin A).

2 RDA expressed in mcg of cholecalciferol (one of the forms of vitamin D). 10 mcg of cholecalciferol equals 400 international units (IU) of vitamin D.

3 RDA expressed in mg of alpha-tocopherol (one of the forms of vitamin E). 1 mg of alpha-tocopherol equals 1 alpha-tocopherol equivalent (1 alpha-TE).

RECOMMENDED DAILY ALLOWANCES (RDAs) OF SELECTED MINERALS

	Birth to 6 months	6 months to 1 year	1 to 3 years	4 to 6 years	7 to 10 years	11 to 14 years	15 to 18 years	19 to 22 years	23 to 50 years	51 + years	Extra needed pregnancy	Extra needed breast-feeding
Calcium (mg)	360	540	800	800	800	1,200	1,200	800	800	800	400	400
Iodine (mcg)	40	50	70	90	120	150	150	150	150	150	25	50
Iron (mg)	10	15	15	10	10	18	18	M 10 F 18	M 10 F 18	10	30-60	A
Magnesium (mg)	50	70	150	200	250	M 350 F 300	M 400 F 300	M 350 F 300	M 350 F 300	M 350 F 300	150	150
Phosphorus (mg)	240	360	800	800	800	1,200	1,200	800	800	800	400	400
Zinc (mg)	3.0	5.0	10	10	10	15	15	15	15	15	5.0	10

A Iron requirements while breast-feeding are approximately the same as those for nonpregnant women, but additional iron may be recommended for two to three months after the birth to replenish iron stores depleted by pregnancy.

UNITS
mg = milligrams (thousandths of a gram)
mcg = micrograms (millionths of a gram)

Vitamins and minerals
The tables (above) give recommended daily allowances (RDAs) of vitamins and minerals for which amounts have been established; when different, the RDAs for males and females are denoted by M and F.

an unhealthy diet, so diet-related diseases continue to be a major problem.

While food is the body's energy source, people who engage in little exercise can easily become overweight by eating more than they "burn off" in physical activity. Regular exercise (at least three times a week) keeps the heart, lungs, muscles, and bones in good health and slows down the aging process. A person who is in good physical condition at the age of 60 can achieve up to 80 percent of the level of physical exertion that he or she could achieve in the mid-20s. Regular exercise improves the circulation in the heart and muscles and provides increased stamina. Exercise as simple as regular, brisk walking also maintains the density of bones, thus reducing the risk of developing osteoporosis ("thinning" and weakening of the bones) and fractures. A person who exercises regularly is less likely than a person who does not exercise sufficiently to have a heart attack or to die from a heart attack if one occurs.

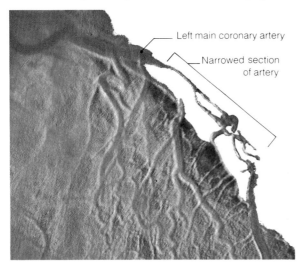

Left main coronary artery

Narrowed section of artery

Diet and atherosclerosis

The colored angiogram of the heart (left) shows narrowing of a coronary artery, a cause of coronary heart disease. Such narrowing can critically reduce the heart's blood supply during exertion; the narrowed section may even become blocked by a blood clot, causing a heart attack. The narrowing of coronary, and other, arteries is usually due to atherosclerosis, the deposition of fatty plaques in the arteries (see diagram below). The risk of athero-sclerosis is linked closely to the amount of cholesterol in the blood, which, in turn, is linked to the dietary intake of fats.

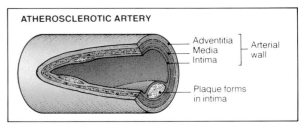

ATHEROSCLEROTIC ARTERY

Adventitia
Media
Intima

Arterial wall

Plaque forms in intima

Smoking and drinking

The full extent of the damage to health caused by smoking tobacco and drinking alcohol is gradually being revealed with continuing research. It has become apparent that many people drink regularly and heavily without being recognized as the alcoholics they have become.

Alcohol is a major contributing factor in traffic accidents and drownings. It plays an important role in domestic violence, sexual assaults, and other violent crimes. Furthermore, there is growing evidence that young people who drink heavily are more likely to experiment with other addictive drugs. Alcohol is a significant cause of ill health. Regular heavy drinking can damage the liver (eventually leading to cirrhosis), heart, stomach, and esophagus. It also leads to brain damage, resulting in impairment of motor and

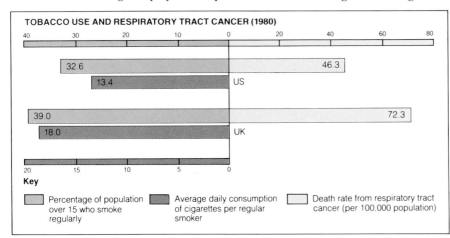

TOBACCO USE AND RESPIRATORY TRACT CANCER (1980)

US: 32.6, 13.4, 46.3
UK: 39.0, 18.0, 72.3

Key

- Percentage of population over 15 who smoke regularly
- Average daily consumption of cigarettes per regular smoker
- Death rate from respiratory tract cancer (per 100,000 population)

Tobacco smoking and mortality

It is now well established that smoking can cause cancer; it is also known that, the more a person smokes, the greater the risk. The relationship between smoking and deaths from respiratory tract cancer is shown in the chart (left). In the US in 1980, 32.6 percent of adults smoked, averaging 13.4 cigarettes per person per day; the death rate from respiratory cancer was 46.3 per 100,000 people. In the UK in 1980, 39 percent of adults smoked, averaging 18 cigarettes per person per day; the death rate from respiratory cancer was 72.3 per 100,000 people.

intellectual capabilities. Drinking during pregnancy can damage the unborn child, causing the mother to give birth to a physically and intellectually maldeveloped baby.

The adverse effects of tobacco are almost as extensive and destructive as those of alcohol. The link between smoking and lung cancer is well known. Moreover, smokers face a substantially greater risk of premature death from coronary heart disease.

It has been demonstrated that people who smoke suffer more angina (chest pain due to inadequate blood supply to the heart muscle) as well as a more recently described phenomenon in which the heart muscle is deprived of oxygen without any angina. This latter, "silent" form of coronary heart disease could be a major factor in the sudden death that can occur with this disease.

Smoking has also become the primary cause of chronic bronchitis and emphysema. It has been linked with ulcers of the stomach and duodenum, and cancers of the cervix and bladder. Smoking during pregnancy, like drinking during pregnancy, damages the developing fetus.

Although smoking is a hazard to the health of smokers themselves, it is also a threat to the health of nonsmokers, particularly children. Recent research has demonstrated that nonsmokers who are exposed to tobacco smoke—as may occur in a household with both smokers and nonsmokers—face an increased risk of respiratory disorders such as bronchitis and lung cancer.

Smoking and emphysema

Although not all smokers get lung cancer, most do develop chronic bronchitis and emphysema. In emphysema, continual irritation by smoke causes progressive damage to the lung tissue. The alveoli (the tiny air sacs across which oxygen and carbon dioxide interchange occurs) first burst and then merge to form fewer, larger sacs with less surface area (see diagrams below). As a result, the working volume of the lungs is progressively reduced, causing breathlessness.

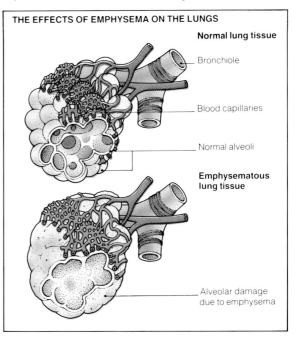

THE EFFECTS OF EMPHYSEMA ON THE LUNGS

Normal lung tissue
- Bronchiole
- Blood capillaries
- Normal alveoli

Emphysematous lung tissue
- Alveolar damage due to emphysema

HEALTHY TISSUE

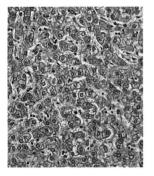

CIRRHOTIC TISSUE

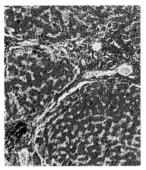

Effects of alcohol on the liver

The photomicrographs above show healthy liver tissue (left) and liver tissue damaged by alcoholic cirrhosis (right). In the healthy liver, the cells are arranged regularly; in the cirrhotic liver, the regular cell arrangement is disrupted by fibrous scar tissue (the blue areas in the photomicrograph). The scar tissue develops as a result of destruction of liver cells by alcohol. The liver attempts to compensate by growing new cells, but in some areas the damage is so great that nonfunctioning scar tissue develops instead. With continued alcohol use, increasing amounts of scar tissue are formed; eventually it affects so much of the liver that normal liver function cannot be maintained.

Alcohol and mortality

There is a close link between alcohol and death from cirrhosis. In 1980, average intake in the US was about 660 glasses of beer (or equivalent) per person; cirrhosis deaths were 13.6 per 100,000 people. This compares with 1,025 glasses of beer (or equivalent) per person and 28.5 cirrhosis-caused deaths per 100,000 people in France.

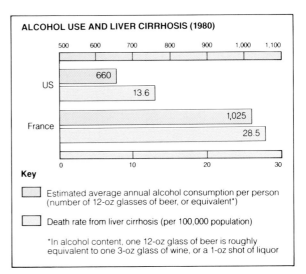

ALCOHOL USE AND LIVER CIRRHOSIS (1980)

US: 660 / 13.6

France: 1,025 / 28.5

Key

☐ Estimated average annual alcohol consumption per person (number of 12-oz glasses of beer, or equivalent*)

☐ Death rate from liver cirrhosis (per 100,000 population)

*In alcohol content, one 12-oz glass of beer is roughly equivalent to one 3-oz glass of wine, or a 1-oz shot of liquor

PREVENTIVE MEDICINE

Many common and serious diseases cause no symptoms in their early stages. This is particularly true of cancer, which often does not produce symptoms until it is beginning to or has already spread to other areas of the body. However, many of these tumors can be detected by simple, reliable tests. Treatment can then arrest or minimize the progress of the disease. Periodic screening tests for cancer become important after age 40, particularly among people in high-risk groups.

Regular check-ups

The most important medical check-ups are for weight and blood pressure. Both tend to increase with age, but a sustained rise above a normal range for a particular age increases the risk of disorders such as heart and kidney disease and stroke, and may warrant treatment. A physical examination should also include checking the eyes, ears, throat, and skin, and an assessment of the condition of all major organ systems of the body (cardiovascular-respiratory, gastrointestinal, genitourinary, musculoskeletal, and neurological). For women who have been sexually active, a cervical smear (Pap test) is included. In addition, middle-aged women should have a mammogram, every two years for those over 40 and annually after the age of 50. A dental examination should also be performed at least once a year.

During a routine check-up, the physician may ask questions designed to screen for a variety of disorders. He or she may also inquire about your life-style, including your diet, sleeping patterns, sexual activity, exercise program, alcohol and tobacco consumption, and whether you use any other addictive drugs.

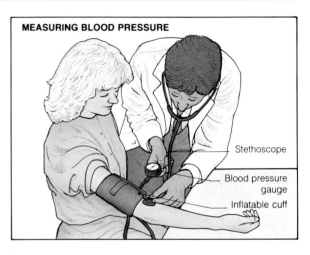

MEASURING BLOOD PRESSURE

Stethoscope

Blood pressure gauge

Inflatable cuff

Blood pressure
Blood pressure is measured by using an inflatable cuff attached to a pressure gauge, and a stethoscope to listen for sounds of blood flow that indicate maximum (systolic) and minimum (diastolic) pressure. A healthy young adult has a blood pressure of about 110/75, which rises to about 130/90 by age 60.

Screening high-risk groups

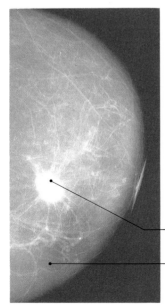

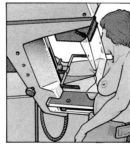

Procedure for mammography

Abnormal growth in breast (cancer, tumor, or cyst)

Normal breast tissue

The medical tests outlined above apply to all adults, irrespective of their medical history. Other specialized tests are recommended for people from families in which a particular disease is prevalent. For example, if a blood relative has had a heart attack before 50, you should tell your physician, who may want to measure the levels of lipids (LDL, HDL, and total cholesterol and triglycerides) in your blood. Coronary heart disease in early middle age almost always indicates an inherited disorder associated with raised lipid levels in the blood, but is a condition that can be treated by a combination of diet and drugs. Similarly, if your mother, father, sister, or brother has had bowel cancer, you should consult your physician about

Mammography
This procedure uses low-dose X rays to image the breasts in screening for cancer (see diagram, left). The mammogram (far left) shows a white area toward the center of the image; such "shadows" may indicate a cancer, but in most cases the cause is a noncancerous tumor or cyst. When a mammogram reveals an abnormality, a sample of the abnormal tissue may be taken for microscopic examination.

when to have regular tests for the presence of blood in your feces and a proctosigmoidoscopic examination. Detection of bowel cancer in its early stages usually enables surgery to be performed with an excellent prospect of a cure.

People who have worked in certain industries have an increased risk of developing some forms of cancer. Workers who have been in regular contact with amine dyes should make sure they have regular tests for bladder cancer.

Other high-risk groups, such as middle-aged men with vague chest discomfort or those about to embark on an exercise program, may be advised to have an exercise stress test to assess the condition of the heart. Liver function tests may be recommended to detect any early evidence of liver damage associated with alcohol consumption. In addition, people who have spent a long period in tropical countries may be advised to undergo special screening tests for tropical diseases.

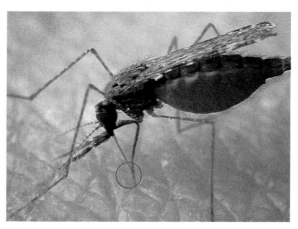

ECG TREADMILL STRESS TEST

Electrodes

ECG machine

Treadmill

Electrocardiography (ECG)

The ECG treadmill stress test (right) is a widely used test for evaluating chest pain. Electrodes are taped to the chest and connected to the ECG machine, which makes a continuous recording of the heart's electrical activity while the patient walks on a treadmill. The walking speed is then increased to the maximum the patient can tolerate. If the ECG trace remains normal during maximum exertion, it is unlikely that the person has a serious heart disorder.

Immunization and preventive drug treatment

Until as recently as the 1940s, deaths in infancy from infectious diseases, such as diphtheria, measles, and pertussis (whooping cough), were relatively common, even in some developed countries. Today, however, vaccines are available against many potentially fatal diseases, and most children in developed countries are routinely immunized against not only diphtheria, measles, and pertussis, but also against typhoid, poliomyelitis, tetanus, rubella, and mumps. Vaccines are also available against tuberculosis and some types of meningitis.

People planning to travel to a foreign country should ensure that their immunizations are current and should also be immunized against any other diseases (such as cholera, yellow fever, and hepatitis) that may exist in the region to be visited. A vaccine has yet to be developed against malaria, one of the most common tropical diseases. However, prophylactic treatment with an antimalarial drug such as chloroquine can help protect against the disease. Development of drug-resistant forms of malaria in some parts of the world requires the traveler to discuss plans with his or her physician. It is also advisable to take other preventive measures, including using insect repellents, wearing protective clothing, and sleeping under a mosquito net.

Preventing malaria

Malaria is caused by infection with protozoal parasites called plasmodia. The parasites enter the body by passing down through the proboscis (circled in the photograph above) of female *ANOPHELES* mosquitoes while they suck blood. Travelers to malarial regions can protect themselves against the disease by taking preventive antimalarial drugs (beginning a few days before entering a malarious area), which affect the parasites in the liver before they can cause symptoms. In recent years, control of malaria has become more difficult, partly because the parasites have developed resistance to certain antimalarial drugs, and partly because the mosquitoes have become resistant to many insecticides.

DIAGNOSING DISEASE

Accurate diagnosis of disease is one of the most important aspects of medicine. Without knowing the identity of a disorder, a physician can only relieve symptoms, such as pain or fever. Indeed, medicine consisted largely of a collection of remedies for specific symptoms and injuries until the fifth century BC, when the Greek physician Hippocrates (c.460-c.377 BC) attempted to identify and describe the course of a disease along with its symptoms.

A diagnosis enables the physician to make a prognosis—an estimate of the outcome of a certain disorder. The concepts of diagnosis and prognosis led physicians to identify diseases from the medical history, the patient's account of the illness. The history remains an essential element in diagnosis. It should be followed by a systematic physical examination in which the physician looks for further signs that can help confirm the underlying cause of the disorder.

Despite these developments, diagnosis remained mostly guesswork until the 17th century, when anatomists and pathologists began to study the body's structure and the changes in organs and tissues that were caused by specific diseases. The invention and development of the microscope led to a greater understanding of the body's structure and function, and to understanding how organs and tissues are affected by disease. The 19th century brought another major advance in the history of diagnosis with the discovery that microorganisms (e.g., bacteria and fungi) can cause disease. This discovery led to the development of the germ theory of disease by, among others, the French microbiologist and chemist Louis Pasteur (1822-1895) and the German bacteriologist Robert Koch (1843-1910). The germ theory of disease is generally regarded as one of the greatest achievements of medical and biological science.

Today, physicians still rely heavily on the patient's medical history to arrive at a diagnosis. Success in making a diagnosis is augmented by the physical examination and by myriad biochemical, immunological, and microbiological tests. Physicians also have access to the interior of the patient's body in ways previously unimagined. Modern techniques such as ultrasound, endoscopy, body scanning (such as CT scanning and magnetic resonance imaging), and biopsy provide detailed, accurate information

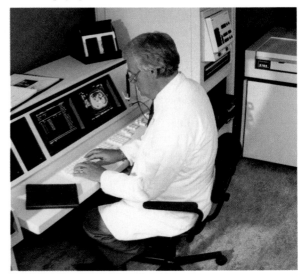

Computers and diagnosis
Many diagnostic scanning techniques, such as CT scanning and MRI, use computers to image the body (above). Computers can enhance scanning images to highlight specific features.

Diagnosing communicable diseases
Because of rapid air transport, a person with a rare infectious disease may develop the first symptoms anywhere in the world. When physicians suspect such an illness, the patient is treated in strict isolation and samples are cultured in a high-security environment (such as the one shown at left) to determine the causative microorganism.

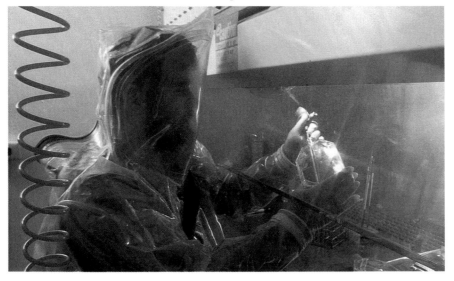

about internal organs with only minimal risk and discomfort to the patient.

Many advances in diagnosis would not have been possible without developments in other disciplines. For example, most modern scanning techniques depended on the development of the computer to process the information. These and other major landmarks in the history of diagnosis are listed in the chart below.

Medical thermometer
The Italian physician Sanctorius (1561-1636) devised the first medical thermometer in 1612 (right). An adaptation of Galileo's air thermometer, it consisted of a globe-shaped top that was placed in the mouth, a coil graduated with glass beads, and a bulbous bottom immersed in a bowl of water.

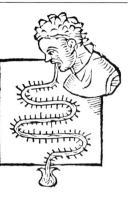

LANDMARKS IN DIAGNOSIS

Date	Development
c.400 BC	**Disease concept.** Introduced by Greek physician Hippocrates.
1612	**Medical thermometer.** Devised by Italian physician Sanctorius.
c.1660	**Light microscope.** Single-lens microscope developed by Dutch naturalist Antonj van Leeuwenhoek, who discovered microorganisms with it. A practicable compound microscope was not developed until the 19th century.
1810	**Stethoscope.** Invented by French physician René Laennec.
1850-1900	**Germ theory of disease.** Proposed by French scientist Louis Pasteur and developed by German bacteriologist Robert Koch.
1895	**X rays.** Discovered by German physicist Wilhelm Roentgen. He also produced the first X-ray picture of the body.
1905	**X-ray contrast medium.** First demonstrated (in retrograde pyelography) by Jean Athanese Sicard in Paris.
1906	**Electrocardiograph (ECG).** Invented by Dutch physiologist Willem Einthoven.
c.1932	**Transmission electron microscope (TEM).** Constructed by German scientists Max Knoll and Ernst Ruska.
1938	**Cardiac catheterization.** First performed by George Peter Robb and Israel Steinberg in New York.
1957	**Fiberoptic endoscopy.** Pioneered by South African-born physician Basil Hirschowitz at the University of Michigan.
1973	**CT scanner.** Invented by British engineer Godfrey Hounsfield of EMI Laboratories, England, and South African-born physicist Allan Cormack of Tufts University, Massachusetts.
1975	**Monoclonal antibodies.** Large-scale production method developed by Argentinean-born scientist César Milstein at the Medical Research Council Laboratories, England.
1976	**Chorionic villus sampling.** Developed by Chinese gynecologists as an aid to the early diagnosis of genetic disorders.
1981	**MRI scanner.** Developed by scientists at Thorn-EMI Laboratories, England, and Nottingham University, England.
1985	**PET scanner.** Developed by scientists at the University of California.

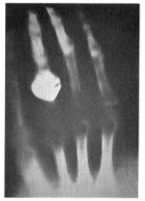

X rays
Shortly after his discovery of X rays in 1895, the German physicist Wilhelm Roentgen (1845-1923) made the first X-ray picture of the human body (above). The picture shows his wife's hand, with the ring she was wearing.

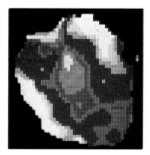

PET scanning
This technique, developed in 1985, enables the functioning of organs to be studied. For example, the image of a normal heart (above) shows the left ventricle pumping blood into the aorta; the image has been computer-colored so that the areas containing the greatest amounts of blood are shown in purple and gray.

MODERN DIAGNOSTIC TECHNIQUES

In the 19th century, physicians usually had to wait until an autopsy had been performed on a patient before they could determine whether or not their diagnosis had been correct. Today, the body's internal organs can be studied during life with minimal risk or no risk to the patient. Physicians use imaging techniques, including X rays, ultrasound, CT scanning, radioisotope scanning, and MRI (magnetic resonance imaging); endoscopy (using a fiberoptic tube to view directly the interior of hollow organs such as the lungs, stomach, bladder, or some joints); and biopsy (examination under a microscope of a small sample of tissue that has been removed from an organ by surgery, by a needle, or via an endoscope).

X rays

A type of electromagnetic radiation with extremely short wavelengths, X rays are invisible and cause no sensation when passed through tissue (although they may damage the skin and internal organs and may cause cancer many years later). When X rays pass through the body, they are absorbed more by dense structures, such as bone, than by softer tissues. Thus, when an X-ray beam is focused onto photographic film behind the patient, shadows of variable intensity are cast on the film, producing the X-ray image.

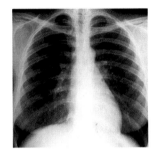

Chest X rays
Because the lungs are full of air, they offer little resistance to X rays. A radiograph of the chest (left) gives a clear picture of the ribs, heart, and major blood vessels. A "shadow on the lungs" may be caused by an area of infection (such as from tuberculosis), a tumor, or an inhaled foreign body.

Digital subtraction angiography

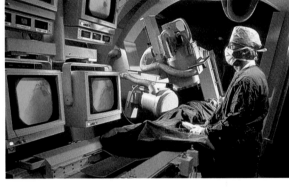

Because many organs have a relatively uniform consistency, their structure does not show up on conventional X rays. One solution is angiography—injecting a radiopaque dye into blood vessels to make them visible on X rays. In digital subtraction angiography, images before and after injection of the dye are computer-processed to remove confusing detail and produce a clear image.

Digital cardiac imaging
Digital subtraction angiography can be used to visualize the coronary arteries. The digital cardiac imaging unit (left) has four screens to monitor the introduction of radiopaque dye and to display the arteries (seen here on three of the screens).

CT scanning

Conventional X rays and angiograms are essentially shadow photographs, but CT scanning uses X rays in a completely different way. Multiple beams of X rays are passed through the part of the body being examined, and their degree of absorption is recorded by sensors. The scanner moves around the patient, emitting and recording X-ray beams from every point on the circle. The resulting data are then analyzed by a computer, which uses the variations in absorption of the X rays to construct an image.

CT scan through the trunk
The CT scan (right) shows a cross section through the trunk of the body at the level of the kidneys. The image has been colored by computer to make the internal structures (the most important of which are labeled) more clearly visible.

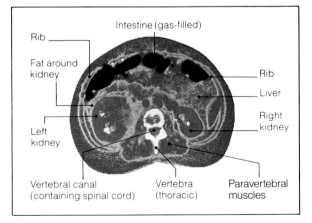

Rib

Intestine (gas-filled)

Fat around kidney

Rib

Liver

Right kidney

Left kidney

Vertebral canal (containing spinal cord)

Vertebra (thoracic)

Paravertebral muscles

Three-dimensional bone imaging
Conventional CT and MRI scanners provide physicians with a computer-generated cross-sectional image that corresponds to a slice through the body (as shown at the bottom of the previous page). However, a surgeon treating a patient with a badly damaged bone or joint sometimes requires more information than can be provided by such an image. In this situation, a powerful computer may be used to generate a three-dimensional image, such as the one shown of a damaged shoulder joint (right), which reveals that the shoulder blade has been broken into several fragments. Such images give surgeons vital information for planning treatment, enabling them to "see" precise details of the damage before undertaking an operation to repair it. Furthermore, because the operation can be planned in advance in great detail, it can be performed more quickly. Three-dimensional imaging is especially valuable for visualizing injuries of the hip, shoulder, rib cage, and skull.

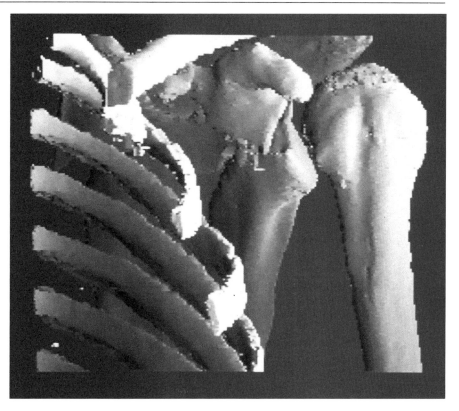

Radionuclide scanning

In conventional radiography and CT scanning, the images produced depend on physical differences (notably in density) among body structures. Imaging by radionuclide scanning utilizes another approach. In this technique, radioactive chemicals are introduced into the body; the radiation emitted by the organs or tissues, which take up the chemicals, is detected and analyzed by an instrument known as a gamma camera. The amount of radiation emitted by a part of the body depends mainly on the level of metabolic activity of its constituent cells. Thus, cells that are dividing rapidly (which occurs within cancerous tissue) show up in some cases as "hot spots" on radionuclide scans.

The substances used in radionuclide scanning are usually either radioactive forms of elements that are normally found in the body, such as iodine, or synthetic radioactive elements, such as technetium. The substance may be swallowed by the patient or injected into the bloodstream; the radiation emitted is then measured by scanning the part of the body being investigated (or, in some cases, the whole body) with a gamma camera. The levels of radiation involved in this technique are very low, usually considerably lower than those to which the body is exposed in a series of conventional X rays.

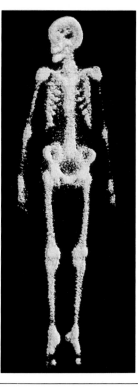

Radionuclide bone scanning
The radionuclide bone scan (left) shows a front view of the complete skeleton of a healthy person. Bone scanning is an essential step in assessing treatment for some types of cancer, such as breast cancer, because it can reveal whether or not the cancer has spread beyond its primary site and developed secondary growths (metastases) in the bones. If such growths are present— indicated by bright "hot spots" on a bone scan—then removal of all the cancer cells by surgery alone is not usually possible. In this situation, surgery is usually confined to simple removal of the primary tumor; cytotoxic drug therapy is carried out to eradicate the secondary growths. In cancer of the prostate, where spread to the skeleton is common, estrogens (female sex hormones) are given to men for pain relief.

MRI

Unlike X-ray radiography, CT scanning, and radionuclide imaging, MRI (magnetic resonance imaging) does not employ potentially harmful ionizing radiation. Instead, it exploits the natural behavior of the protons (nuclei) of hydrogen atoms when they are subjected to a very strong magnetic field and radio waves. As a result of this stimulation, the protons emit radio signals, which are detected and computer-processed to generate an image. The most abundant sources of protons in the body are the hydrogen atoms in water molecules; an MRI scan therefore reflects differences in the water content of tissues.

Superficially, MRI scans look like CT scans. However, CT scans usually show little differentiation in soft tissues; MRI scans show more of the detailed structure because of differences in water content within these tissues. For example, white and gray matter in the brain are relatively poorly differentiated in CT scans, while they are distinct and well-defined in MRI scans.

NORMAL CHEST SCAN

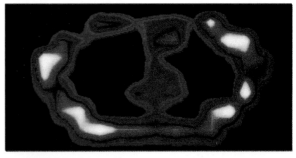

ABNORMAL CHEST SCAN

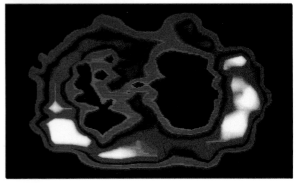

Diagnostic MRI scanning
The two MRI scans (right) show cross sections through the chest. The upper scan, which reveals a healthy chest, shows the lungs (the large black areas in the center) and ribs (the crescent-shaped red-yellow areas toward the edge). In comparison, the lower scan shows a tumor in the left lung. The tumor is indicated by the increased amount of blue in the image of that lung and by the lung's small size.

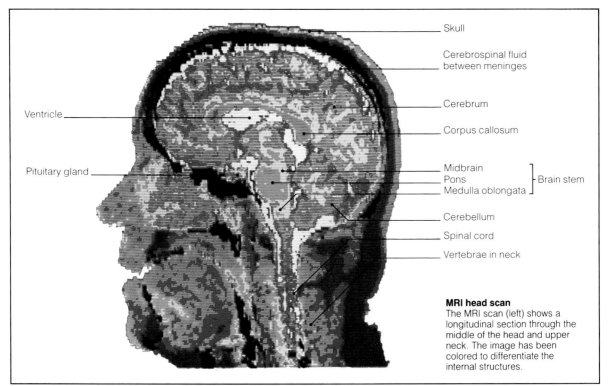

Ventricle

Pituitary gland

Skull

Cerebrospinal fluid between meninges

Cerebrum

Corpus callosum

Midbrain
Pons
Medulla oblongata } Brain stem

Cerebellum

Spinal cord

Vertebrae in neck

MRI head scan
The MRI scan (left) shows a longitudinal section through the middle of the head and upper neck. The image has been colored to differentiate the internal structures.

HOW MRI WORKS

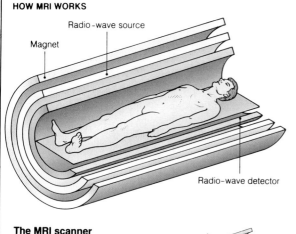

Radio-wave source

Magnet

Radio-wave detector

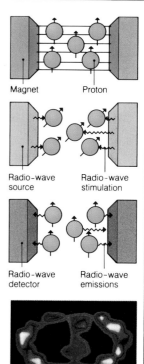

Magnet   Proton

Radio-wave   Radio-wave
source   stimulation

Radio-wave   Radio-wave
detector   emissions

The MRI scanner

An MRI scanner consists of a massive electromagnet, a radio-wave emitter, and a radio-wave detector. These instruments are arranged around a central tunnel in which the patient lies, and are connected to a computer and display screen. The electromagnet is extremely powerful. It is able to create a magnetic field up to about 60,000 times that of the Earth's magnetic field.

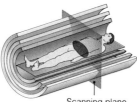

Scanning plane

Scanning plane

When the patient is inside the machine, it is set up to scan a plane ("slice") of the body.

The scanning process

Scanning begins when a plane of the body has been selected for imaging. First, the electromagnet is turned on. Normally, the protons (nuclei) of the body's hydrogen atoms point randomly in different directions, but under the influence of the scanner's powerful magnetic field they align themselves in the same direction (diagram, top right). Next, the radio-wave source emits a powerful pulse of radio waves, the effect of which is to knock the protons out of alignment (diagram, middle right). However, milliseconds later, the protons realign themselves, emitting faint radio signals as they do so; these signals are picked up by the scanner's radio-wave detector (diagram, bottom right). A computer then processes the radio signals to produce an image of the plane of the body being scanned, such as the "slice" through the chest shown in the photograph (bottom right). Computer software enables three-dimensional images to be derived from MRI.

PET scanning

PET (positron emission tomography) scanning is a development of radionuclide scanning and resembles it in many ways. Both techniques use a radioactive substance introduced into the body to produce an image that reflects the level of activity of tissues. However, radionuclide scanning usually produces an image analogous to a conventional X-ray picture; PET scanning gives a cross-sectional image that is analogous to a CT scan.

In PET scanning, a substance that takes part in metabolic biochemical processes is labeled with a radioisotope to make it radioactive; it is then injected into the bloodstream. The substance is taken up by the most metabolically active areas of tissue. In the tissue, the substance emits positrons. The positrons, in turn, release photons, which are then detected by an array of sensors around the patient. The sensors are linked to a computer, which calculates the origins of the photons to construct an image of the distribution of the substance within the tissues.

PET scanning is currently being utilized for investigating brain tumors, locating the origin of epileptic activity, and studying the brain function in various mental illnesses. It is anticipated that PET scanning will be used for other organs.

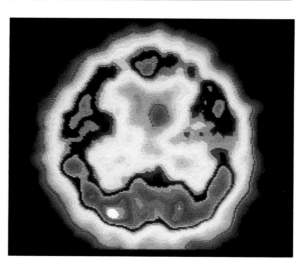

PET brain scanning

The PET scan (above) of a section through a normal brain has been colored to show levels of protein synthesis (high levels are indicated by pink, red, and orange, intermediate levels by yellow and green, and low levels by blue). In this scan, methionine (an essential amino acid) was used to show protein synthesis. Other brain functions can be imaged by using different substances—such as radioactively labeled glucose to show carbohydrate metabolism.

Biochemical analysis

Body fluids contain thousands of different chemicals. A healthy body maintains the concentration of each substance within clearly defined normal limits. However, in disease, the level of a body chemical may be abnormally high or low; detecting this abnormality by biochemical analysis can help in diagnosis.

A physician may order biochemical tests on samples of blood, urine, and other body fluids, such as spinal fluid, saliva, or sweat, when confirming a diagnosis. These tests may be part of a diagnostic investigation in which the chemical constituents of body fluids are checked primarily to confirm an illness that the physician suspects may exist based on the patient's description of his or her symptoms. The tests may also be used to assess the function of a particular organ, such as the liver or kidneys.

In recent years, the automation of equipment used for analysis has made biochemical testing faster and more accurate. New analytical techniques have been developed that make it possible to measure infinitesimal amounts of substances, such as hormones, in a person's body fluids.

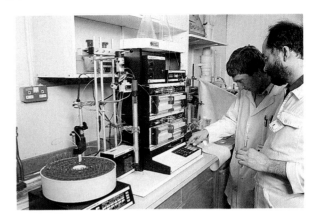

Protein analysis
Fast protein liquid chromatography (above) is one of the many laboratory techniques that provides physicians with rapid, accurate measurement of substances in the blood and other body fluids. This technique is used to separate the individual protein constituents of a complex mixture so that they can be identified and quantified by, for example, measuring differences in their molecular sizes, electrical charges, and motility.

Diagnostic ultrasound

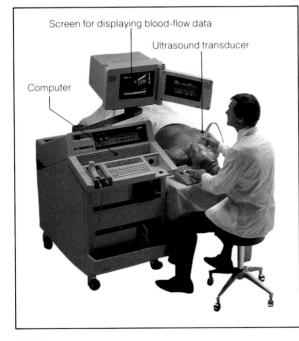

Screen for displaying blood-flow data

Ultrasound transducer

Computer

Angiodynography
This noninvasive ultrasound technique utilizes the Doppler effect to investigate blood flow. The photograph (above) shows the technique being used to examine blood flow through the neck. The physician places a transducer (an ultrasound emitter and detector) against the patient's neck; a computer processes ultrasound echo data to produce an image of the blood flow on a display unit.

The diagnostic use of ultrasound is based on the principle of sonar, in which sound waves are used to locate underwater objects by their echoes. In diagnostic ultrasound, a device called a transducer is placed on the skin and transmits inaudible high-frequency sound waves into the body, where they are reflected by the internal structures. The transducer detects these echoes, which are converted to numerical data and then displayed directly on a screen or analyzed by computer to produce an image of the structures.

In contrast to X rays, which are potentially harmful, ultrasound is thought to be completely safe—a belief based on 30 years' use on hundreds of millions of patients with no evidence of any ill effects. Ultrasound is especially useful in obstetrics because it enables the physician to examine the fetus at no known risk to either the woman or her developing child.

A modification of the basic ultrasound technique makes use of the Doppler effect (the change in pitch that occurs when a sound source is moving relative to the detector) to give information about the rate of blood flow through blood vessels. This procedure, known as angiodynography, enables the physician to detect narrowing of blood vessels or turbulence in the flow of blood.

Another ultrasound procedure, known as echocardiography, provides information about the heart, including the structure and flexibility of heart valves, the condition of the heart muscle, and the flow of blood within the heart.

Biopsy

Biopsy, the examination of a sample of tissue removed from a living patient (in contrast to necropsy, the examination of tissue after death), is a valuable aid in establishing a precise diagnosis. Samples of muscle, liver, kidney, lung, and other tissues may be removed safely and simply by passing a needle through the skin and into the target organ or tissue, sometimes using ultrasound, CT scanning, or fluoroscopy to help guide the needle. Tumors and cysts in organs such as the breast, ovary, testis, or thyroid can be sampled in the same way. Once obtained, the tissue sample may be examined under a microscope and subjected to a variety of biochemical tests, thereby yielding a diagnosis that is accurate.

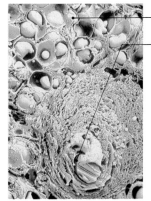

— Normal ovarian tissue

— Malignant teratoma

Ovarian biopsy sample
Tissue samples removed by biopsy may be examined under a light microscope or, occasionally, under a scanning electron microscope. The scanning electron micrograph (left) of a sample of ovarian tissue shows a malignant teratoma (a type of ovarian cancer) invading the tissue of the ovary.

Endoscopic investigation

Early endoscopes were simply rigid or partially rigid tubes, sometimes with complex lens systems and interior lighting, and were of limited use. In the late 1950s, the introduction of fiberoptics enabled endoscopes to be completely flexible, thereby greatly increasing their versatility. Today, many specialized endoscopes are available, enabling physicians to view directly virtually any structure in the body, including the digestive tract, nasal sinuses, lungs, bladder, abdominal cavity, and joints. In addition, many endoscopes can be fitted with attachments that enable samples of tissue to be taken for biopsy or surgical procedures to be carried out.

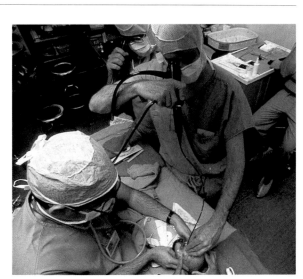

Bronchoscopy
Using a bronchoscope, a type of endoscope designed for looking at the lungs, physicians examine an infant who has breathing difficulty (right). During this procedure, fluid and debris may also be removed from the air passages.

Genetic analysis

Recent advances in genetics have allowed the genetic defects responsible for certain inherited disorders to be identified and detected. When there is a family history of an inherited disorder, such as muscular dystrophy or Down's syndrome, or when a couple has had a child with such a disorder, tests may be performed early in pregnancy to discover whether or not the fetus has the genetic defect. The tests involve removing cells from the membranes or fluid around the fetus, culturing the cells, and then analyzing their gene content by examining the chromosomes under a microscope. As a result of genetic analysis and elective termination of pregnancy, the frequency of some inherited disorders has been reduced. Parents at risk of having a baby with an inherited defect may (with genetic counseling and prenatal testing) be able to reassure themselves about the fetus's health.

GENE MAP

Sickle-cell anemia;
beta-thalassemia;
methemoglobinemia;
polycythemia vera

Acute intermittent
porphyria

Gene mapping
Every normal cell in the body contains 46 chromosomes (except the sex cells—eggs and sperm—which have only 23 each). Each chromosome carries several thousand genes; geneticists are now able to pinpoint the locations of many of the individual genes that, when defective, cause inherited disorders. For example, the gene map (left) of chromosome 11 shows the locations of gene defects responsible for the inherited blood disorders sickle cell anemia, beta-thalassemia, methemoglobinemia, and polycythemia vera, and the metabolic disorder acute intermittent porphyria.

TREATING DISEASE

Until well into this century, most of the advances in medical science focused on understanding the nature of diseases rather than their treatment. The exception was surgery, which had made considerable progress since the introduction of general anesthesia in the 1840s, antiseptic procedures in the 1870s, and blood transfusions in the early 1900s. Physicians, however, had at their disposal few effective drugs with which to work, and they could do little to cure, or even slow the progress of, most diseases.

The situation changed dramatically in the 1930s with the introduction of antibacterial drugs, advances in the production of synthetic drugs, and the development of drugs that act on the body's metabolic processes. Thereafter, progress was (and still is) rapid, as scientists developed an ever wider range of effective drugs and improved methods of drug production. Important landmarks in the development of treatment methods are listed in the accompanying charts on this page and the next.

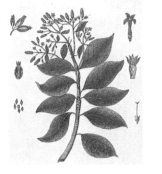

Drugs from plants
Traditionally, plants were the source of many useful drugs, including the antimalarial drug quinine, from the bark of the CINCHONA tree (called Jesuits' bark, shown above), the painkiller morphine, from poppies, and the heart drug digitalis, from the foxglove plant.

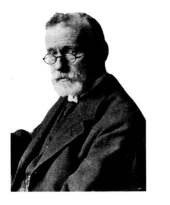

Paul Ehrlich (1854-1915)
A German bacteriologist and pioneer of chemotherapy, Ehrlich introduced (in 1911) salvarsan, the first drug to be prepared for treating the cause of a specific disease—in this case, syphilis.

LANDMARKS IN DRUG DEVELOPMENT

Date	Development
1666	**Quinine.** British physician Thomas Sydenham popularized use of Jesuits' bark (containing quinine) for treating malaria.
1785	**Digitalis.** Use of digitalis to treat heart failure described by British physician William Withering.
1796	**Smallpox vaccination.** The first vaccination to be performed, by British physician Edward Jenner. The first true vaccine (consisting of weakened microorganisms)—against chicken cholera—was developed in 1880 by French scientist Louis Pasteur.
1805	**Morphine.** Extracted from opium and used to relieve pain by German pharmacist Friedrich Sertürner.
1899	**Aspirin.** Developed as a drug by German scientist Felix Hoffmann.
1911	**Salvarsan.** Introduced by Paul Ehrlich to treat syphilis.
1928	**Penicillin.** Antibacterial action first recognized by British bacteriologist Alexander Fleming. It was produced as a drug in 1940, by Australian-born British pathologist Howard Florey, and German-born British biochemist Ernst Chain.
1935	**Sulfonamides.** Antibacterial action discovered by German pharmacologist Gerhard Domagk.
1951	**Oral contraceptive.** Developed by American physicians Gregory Pincus and John Rock, and the Austrian-born American chemist Carl Djerassi.
1959	**Librium (chlordiazepoxide).** The first benzodiazepine minor tranquilizer, introduced by Swiss pharmaceutical company Hoffmann-LaRoche.
1962	**Nethalide (pronethalol).** The first beta-blocking heart drug, developed by scientists at Imperial Chemical Industries, England.
1984	**Genetically engineered human insulin.** Developed by scientists at Genentech, California.
1986	**Zidovudine (originally called AZT).** Introduced for treating AIDS after development by scientists at Burroughs Wellcome Research Laboratories, North Carolina.

LANDMARKS IN SURGERY

Date	Development
1545	**Basic surgical principles.** Established by French surgeon Ambroise Paré.
1842	**General anesthesia.** First operation using general anesthesia performed by American surgeon Crawford Long, who used ether. In 1845, American dentist Horace Wells used nitrous oxide ("laughing gas") as an anesthetic. In 1847, British obstetrician James Simpson introduced chloroform anesthesia.
1870	**Antiseptic surgery.** Pioneered by British surgeon Joseph Lister, who used a carbolic acid (phenol) spray during surgery to help prevent infection.
1901	**Blood groups.** ABO blood groups discovered by Austrian pathologist Karl Landsteiner, so establishing the basis for safe transfusions.
1951	**Coronary artery bypass graft.** First attempted by Canadian surgeon Arthur Vineberg at the Royal Victoria Hospital, Montreal, Canada.
1955	**Kidney transplant.** First successful kidney transplant (between identical twins) performed by team of American surgeons—led by Joseph Murray—of the Harvard Medical School, Massachusetts.
1967	**Heart transplant.** First human heart transplant performed by South African surgeon Christiaan Barnard at the Groote Schuur Hospital, Capetown, South Africa.
1976	**Coronary angioplasty.** Introduced by Swiss surgeon Andreas Grüntzig at the University Hospital, Zurich, Switzerland.
1987	**Fetal tissue transplant.** First transplant of fetal brain tissue into brains of patients with Parkinson's disease performed by research groups in Mexico, the US, and Europe.

LANDMARKS IN OTHER FORMS OF TREATMENT

Date	Development
c.1270	**Eyeglasses.** Thought to have been invented in Italy. Contact lenses were invented in 1887, by Swiss optician Eugen Frick.
1817	**Dental plate.** Introduced by American dentist Anthony Plantson.
1891	**Baby incubator.** Introduced by French physician Alexandre Lion.
1901	**Hearing aid (electric).** Developed by American inventor Miller Reese Hutchinson. The first truly miniature hearing aid introduced in 1952 by the Sonotone Corporation.
1945	**Kidney dialysis machine.** Developed by Dutch surgeon Willem Kolff to treat patients with renal failure.
1978	**"Test-tube baby."** The first (Louise Brown) born in England as a result of in vitro fertilization (IVF) techniques developed by British gynecologist Patrick Steptoe and embryologist Robert Edwards.
1979	**Shock-wave lithotripsy.** Pioneered by researchers at the University Hospital, Munich, West Germany.

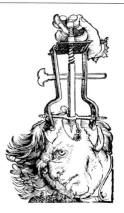

Early surgery
Boring a hole in the skull to relieve pressure on the brain (above) dates from prehistoric times. Moreover, archaeological evidence suggests that some patients survived this early form of surgery.

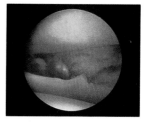

Anesthesia and surgery
A successful surgical operation (above) relies to a great degree on anesthesia. Introduced in the 1840s, anesthetics not only free the patient from pain and restless agitation, but also give the surgeon more time to perform the operation.

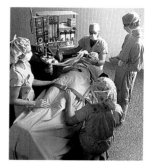

Endoscopic surgery
A view through an endoscope of a damaged knee joint is shown in the photograph (above). Endoscopes enable surgeons to directly examine, and perform operations on, internal body structures.

MODERN SURGICAL TREATMENT

Until about the 1940s, most surgery consisted of excision—cutting out abnormal tissue or structures that were diseased or damaged. The primary exception was orthopedics, in which surgeons were attempting to encourage the healing of bones by employing rods, pins, and immobilization. Since then, surgery has been transformed by technological advances such as the operating microscope, the laser scalpel, and the endoscope. Today, many operations emphasize repair or replacement rather than excision.

Transplant surgery

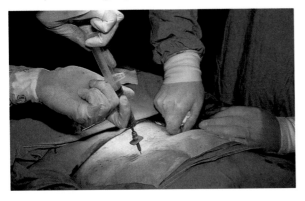

Experience with skin grafting in World War II demonstrated that the body's immune system attacks tissue from another person (causing rejection) in the same way that it attacks microorganisms. Therefore, when transplant surgery began in the 1950s, there were two challenges—the technical task of replacing a diseased organ with a healthy one, and preventing the rejection of the transplanted organ. Because drugs that prevent rejection also suppress the immune system, they lower the body's resistance to infection. Consequently, many early transplant recipients survived the operation but died from infection. Gradually, the technical problems were overcome, first with kidney transplants and later with heart and liver transplants. Improved immunosuppressant drugs were then developed, notably cyclosporine. As a result, the success rate for transplants is generally high. The primary problem today is the lack of available organ donors. Another technical and ethical problem that is currently the subject of much discussion is the use of fetal tissue and organs for transplantation.

Bone marrow transplants
These transplants replace malignant or defective marrow. A syringe is used to suck out healthy marrow from the donor's hipbone (shown above). This marrow is then injected into the recipient's bloodstream, which carries it to the bones. Drugs that suppress the immune system are given to prevent rejection of the transplanted marrow, but they make the recipient vulnerable to infection. Thus the patient must remain in an isolation unit until the new marrow "takes."

Surgical implants

There are four main problems in replacing a part of the body with an artificial implant. First, the implant must be sufficiently inert so as not to provoke the immune system to reject it. Second, it must also be tough enough to last for many years. Third, a means must be found to secure the implant in position. Fourth, scrupulous operative techniques are necessary to prevent infection. Today, these problems have largely been solved, and most implants are successful; hip joint replacements last for 10 years or more in 70 to 80 percent of cases. Furthermore, a wide range of implants is now available—joints, heart valves, lenses for the eye, sections of blood vessels, and replacements for parts of the skull.

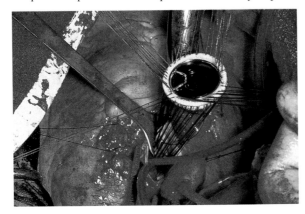

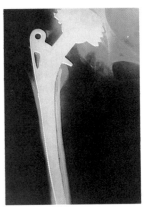

Heart valve implants
Damaged heart valves may be replaced by synthetic substitutes (or by valves from a pig or a cadaver). The photograph (left) shows a synthetic heart valve being sewn in place.

Hip joint replacement
The colored X ray (right) shows an artificial hip joint in place. Replacing the hip joint—which is usually done when it has been damaged by arthritis—is one of the most successful types of implant surgery.

Microsurgery

In microsurgery, surgeons use a specially designed microscope, tiny instruments, and delicate sutures (stitches) to perform operations on minute structures, such as small nerves or blood vessels. One of the major advantages of microsurgery is that more of the tiny blood vessels and nerves can be preserved, minimizing damage to the tissues being repaired and thus reducing the amount of scar tissue formed.

Today, microsurgical techniques are used in many operations on the eye or ear. These techniques are also used in operations that involve the joining of blood vessels, such as in reconstructive surgery when the tiny arteries and veins of skin and muscle flaps are sewn together. Microsurgery has also enabled surgeons to reattach severed fingers, toes, complete limbs, and even the two sections of a vas deferens separated in a vasectomy.

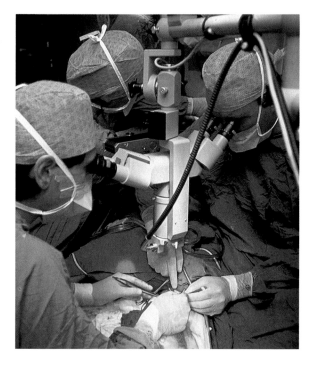

Microsurgical operations
In the photograph (right), two surgeons perform a delicate microsurgical operation. Each is looking into a binocular eyepiece of an operating microscope, which is used to magnify the structures being operated on (such as tiny blood vessels). The surgical instruments are also magnified so that the surgeons can achieve the extreme precision necessary for the operation to be successful.

Laser surgery

A laser produces a narrow beam of intense energy that surgeons can use as a "light knife" to cut through tissue (while simultaneously cauterizing blood vessels), usually without causing damage beyond the target area. Lasers are used in many operations on the eye, especially those on the retina, and are also used to seal bleeding arteries in peptic ulcers, to destroy tumors, and to remove some skin blemishes.

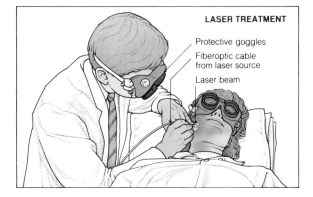

LASER TREATMENT

Protective goggles

Fiberoptic cable from laser source

Laser beam

Removing skin blemishes
Lasers are effective at removing certain skin blemishes, such as birthmarks that are due to excessive growth of blood vessels in the skin. In such treatment (shown right), the physician and patient wear goggles to protect their eyes.

Endoscopic surgery

Endoscopes are used not only for diagnosis, but also for performing certain surgical procedures. Special attachments such as scissors or a wire loop snare may be fitted to remove tumors, and sharp-toothed forceps may be used to grasp and remove foreign bodies. Other operations for which endoscopes are used include shattering stones in the urinary tract and repairing torn cartilages in joints.

Endoscopic surgery is generally safer and easier to perform than conventional surgery that requires an incision. It also causes less tissue damage, producing less discomfort and a quicker recovery for the patient.

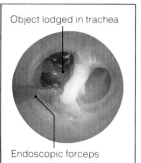

Object lodged in trachea

Endoscopic forceps

Removing foreign objects
The photograph (left), taken through an endoscope (a fiberoptic viewing tube), shows the removal of an inhaled object (the top of a martini stirrer) from the windpipe of a young child. The forceps that are being used to grasp the object have been passed through a special channel in the endoscope. The forceps are operated by remote manipulation.

DRUG TREATMENT

The medicinal herbs and plants that provide physicians with drugs have been identified over thousands of years. More recently, advances in drug production have helped pharmacologists and biochemists develop an immense range of new synthetic drugs.

Before any substance is approved for use as a drug, it is tested for effectiveness and safety. Only after satisfactory evidence has been made available to the Food and Drug Administration can a drug be approved for marketing.

Drugs from natural sources

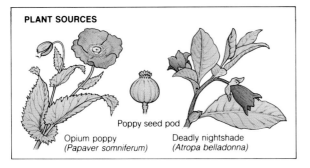

PLANT SOURCES

Poppy seed pod

Opium poppy
(Papaver somniferum)

Deadly nightshade
(Atropa belladonna)

In medicine, most drugs that were originally derived from plants have now been replaced by pure preparations of the active ingredients. For example, some of the refined derivatives of opium include morphine sulfate, codeine, and papaverine. Plants continue to be a valuable source of new substances that might prove to be effective drugs.

Drugs from plants
Morphine and atropine were once obtained directly from seed pods of the opium poppy and from deadly nightshade, respectively. Today, purified forms are available.

Antibacterials and antibiotics

The first drugs effective against bacterial infections were the chemical-based antibacterials salvarsan (introduced in 1911) and the sulfonamides (developed in the 1930s). Antibiotics (originally derived from molds or fungi, rather than chemicals) were introduced in the 1940s, when penicillin became available as a drug (although its antibacterial activity was recognized in 1928). Since then, numerous other antibacterials and antibiotics have been discovered; physicians today have a wide range of effective drugs from which to choose.

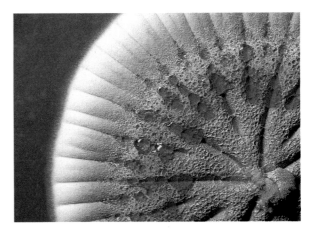

Penicillin
The photograph (right) shows a culture of the mold PENICILLIUM NOTATUM. This species was an early source of the antibiotic penicillin; today, synthetic forms of the drug are usually used.

Vaccines

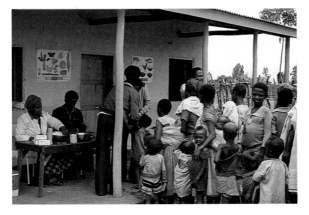

Vaccination dates from 1796, when Edward Jenner inoculated against smallpox, but vaccines against other potentially lethal diseases were not developed until this century. Today, vaccines are available to give protection against measles, mumps, diphtheria, poliomyelitis, tetanus, pertussis, rubella, and other, less common, diseases such as hepatitis, typhoid, typhus, rabies, cholera, and yellow fever.

Vaccination in developing countries
Many infectious diseases (such as measles) that have been brought under control in developed countries remain a major cause of death in developing countries. To reduce such deaths, a variety of international agencies run mass vaccination programs (left).

Synthetic drugs

Many drugs that were originally derived from natural sources are now produced synthetically in the laboratory. Such production ensures that the drugs are of consistent potency (drug extracts from natural sources tend to vary in strength) and that they are available when required.

Furthermore, recent advances in our understanding of the functioning of the body have made it possible to "tailor-make" drugs for specific purposes, rather than relying solely on synthetic analogues of natural substances. For example, propranolol was developed specifically to block the action of the natural hormones epinephrine and norepinephrine on the heart and blood vessels. This blocking effect is useful in treating some cases of high blood pressure, angina, or abnormal heart rhythms. Cimetidine was tailor-made to treat ulcers by reducing the stomach's acid-secreting response to histamine.

Drugs may also be synthesized to supplement hormones or other body chemicals that are produced in insufficient amounts due to disease. One example is the synthetic drug levodopa, which is given to counteract the deficiency of the natural chemical dopamine that occurs in Parkinson's disease. Drugs developed in this purposeful way to meet particular needs may be further modified chemically to increase their potency and duration of action, or to reduce possible adverse effects.

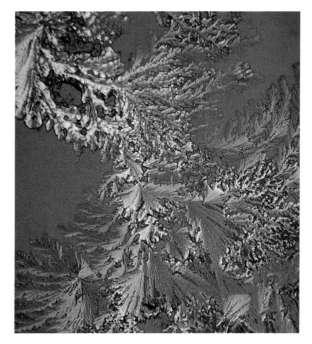

Synthetic hormones
Many hormones that are used therapeutically are produced synthetically. Epinephrine (shown in a polarized light photomicrograph, above) is used to counteract cardiac arrest and control bleeding in surgery.

Genetically engineered drugs

This recently developed technique for modifying the genetic structure of living organisms could revolutionize medicine. However, much more research is needed to explore its full potential. To date, its principal medical use has been to produce human forms of hormones and other natural body chemicals that can be used to treat certain metabolic disorders. One example is the use of genetically engineered human insulin to treat diabetes mellitus (cattle insulin was once used, but it is not well tolerated by some people with diabetes). Other substances produced by genetic engineering include human growth hormone (used to treat pituitary dwarfism), factor VIII (used to treat hemophilia), and erythropoietin (used to treat some forms of anemia).

Although technically difficult to achieve, producing a human hormone (or other body chemical) by genetic engineering is simple in theory. The gene that instructs human cells to produce the hormone is identified, isolated, and inserted into the genetic material of a microorganism such as a bacterium or yeast. The microorganism is then cultured in large vats so that it multiplies and produces large amounts of the hormone for commercial purposes.

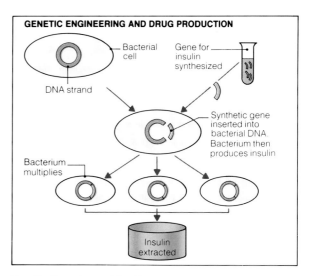

GENETIC ENGINEERING AND DRUG PRODUCTION

Bacterial cell

DNA strand

Gene for insulin synthesized

Synthetic gene inserted into bacterial DNA. Bacterium then produces insulin

Bacterium multiplies

Insulin extracted

Genetically engineered insulin
Genetic engineering can force bacteria to produce human insulin. The insulin gene is obtained (by removing it from human DNA, then purifying it) and spliced into the DNA of a bacterium, causing it to produce human insulin. The bacterium is then cultured for large-scale insulin extraction.

OTHER METHODS OF TREATMENT

Drug treatment and surgery are still the primary divisions of medical care, but technological advances have become so specialized in recent years that some types of treatment have become separate branches of medicine. Examples include the various forms of intensive care (e.g., medical, coronary, surgical, and neurosurgical). These newer forms of treatment often require specialized medical and nursing staff.

Intensive care

Some patients require continuous monitoring of their body functions—heart rate and rhythm, breathing rate, blood pressure—so that any deterioration in their condition can be detected and treated immediately. Many patients who are seriously ill also must be given fluids, nutrition, and medication intravenously, and some may require a ventilator to help them breathe. Monitoring of a patient's condition is best provided in an intensive-care unit (or, for a patient who has had or is suspected of having a myocardial infarction, a coronary-care unit), which has the necessary equipment and is staffed around the clock by specially trained hospital personnel.

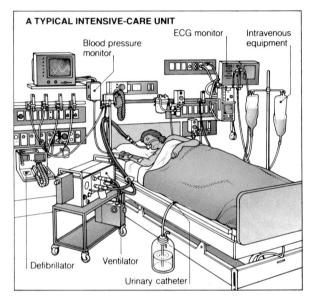

A TYPICAL INTENSIVE-CARE UNIT

Blood pressure monitor · ECG monitor · Intravenous equipment · Defibrillator · Ventilator · Urinary catheter

Intensive-care facilities

An intensive-care unit contains all the equipment needed to continuously monitor vital body functions and to maintain a stable condition in the patient. Such units are also equipped to deal with any medical crises that may arise, such as ventricular fibrillation (rapid, random beating of the lower heart chamber), which may require a defibrillator to restore a normal heart beat.

Radiation therapy

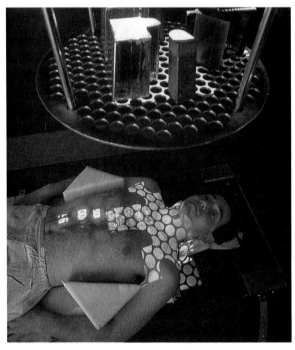

The use of X rays and implants of radium (a naturally radioactive substance) to treat cancers dates from the turn of this century. Today, X rays are still used in radiation therapy (also known as radiation oncology), but the range of treatment has been greatly expanded to include other forms or sources of radiation (e.g., neutron beams or radioactive varieties of substances such as iodine or yttrium). It is now also possible to focus radiation beams more accurately, thereby concentrating them on the tumor and minimizing damage to surrounding healthy tissue.

Radiation may be used alone to treat some tumors—such as basal cell carcinoma and certain tumors of the pituitary gland—but it is more often used in combination with surgery, chemotherapy, or both. The choice between radiation and surgery may depend on the stage of the tumor. In some cases, the results of surgery or radiation are the same.

X-ray therapy

The photograph (left) shows a patient about to receive X-ray therapy to treat cancer. The illuminated disks are the areas that will be irradiated; the pattern is determined by the arrangement of lead blocks on the metal platform (which shields the lungs from excessive radiation) below the source of the X rays.

Dialysis

A person whose kidneys fail will die within a few days unless impurities that accumulate in the blood are removed, either by a kidney dialysis machine or by peritoneal dialysis.

In hemodialysis, a dialysis machine removes impurities by filtering the patient's blood through a semipermeable membrane immersed in a special dialysis solution. The procedure takes a few hours and the patient visits a dialysis unit for each treatment. In peritoneal dialysis, the patient's abdominal cavity lining is used to filter impurities from the blood into the dialysis solution (which is passed in and out of the abdomen through a tube).

Dialysis may be necessary for only a few days if kidney failure is temporary, but it is also effective as a long-term treatment for permanent kidney failure. In most of the latter cases, the best remedy for the patient's condition is a kidney transplant.

Lithotripsy

Lithotripsy is a noninvasive procedure in which ultrasound is used to pulverize stones in the body. This technique seems likely to replace surgery as the treatment for certain kidney stones and is currently under investigation in the treatment of gallstones that cause symptoms. In lithotripsy, repeated pulses of high-energy ultrasound waves are focused on a stone to break it down into tiny particles that can be passed out of the body via the urine (with kidney stones) or via the feces (with gallstones).

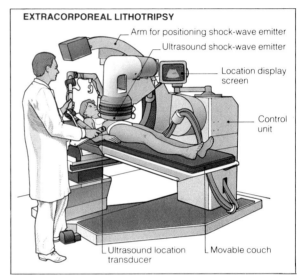

EXTRACORPOREAL LITHOTRIPSY
- Arm for positioning shock-wave emitter
- Ultrasound shock-wave emitter
- Location display screen
- Control unit
- Movable couch
- Ultrasound location transducer

Shock-wave treatment of stones
Kidney stones or gallstones may be treated by extracorporeal lithotripsy. This technique involves focusing ultrasound shock waves on a stone until it breaks into tiny fragments that can be passed out of the body. The patient lies on a couch or in a water bath. The physician pinpoints the position of the stone with a fluoroscope or an ultrasound location transducer, and the patient and shock-wave emitter are placed in position for treatment. The stone is then subjected to shock waves until it is pulverized.

Incubator

Babies born prematurely are small and have internal organs that have not fully matured. Additionally, many basic reflexes and physiological functions, such as those that regulate body temperature, are not fully developed. For this reason, a newborn weighing less than 3.5 pounds is usually placed in an incubator, where the temperature, humidity, oxygen, and the baby's vital functions can be monitored.

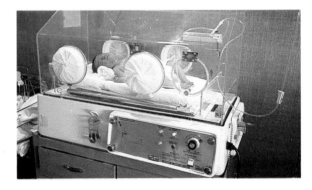

Caring for premature babies
Improved neonatal care has increased the survival rate of premature babies. Today, babies weighing as little as 1.5 pounds can often be kept alive until they reach a safe size.

Psychiatric treatment

In earlier days, people with mental disorders were incarcerated in remote mental asylums. Today, most individuals are treated in units within general hospitals or in community settings. In addition, new drugs can sometimes transform the outlook for patients with severe mental disorders such as schizophrenia. Drug therapy—often combined with psychotherapy—now enables many people to resume varying degrees of activity within the community. There have also been developments in psychotherapy; the types now available include traditional, Freudian-based psychoanalysis, group therapy, and counseling.

PRENATAL TECHNOLOGY

Since the turn of the century, improvements in medical care have resulted in a dramatic decline in infant and childhood mortality in developed countries. Currently, infant mortality is more of a socioeconomic problem. The greatest difficulties are encountered with teenage pregnancies, which are associated with little or no prenatal care. Infants born today in developed countries have a 98 percent chance of growing up healthily. There has also been much progress in prenatal medicine as the understanding of genetics, fertility, pregnancy, and embryonic development has increased. As a result, prospective parents can now be counseled on such matters as the likelihood of their children having a genetic disorder or, if there is a problem with fertility, how to maximize the chance of conception.

PROCEDURES BEFORE CONCEPTION

To maximize the chance of having a successful pregnancy and a healthy baby, a couple should examine their health habits before pregnancy occurs. Both partners—but especially the woman—should eat a balanced diet and should avoid alcohol, tobacco, and all drugs except those taken in consultation with a physician. Women with metabolic disorders, such as diabetes mellitus, should ensure that their condition is controlled. Advice should be sought if either partner is aware of a disorder that runs in his or her family.

Genetic counseling

About one child in 50 is born with a physical, metabolic, or mental defect. Many of these defects are due to an abnormality in one or more of the genes inherited from the parents. In some cases, the parents are unaware that one (or, rarely, both) of them carries a defective gene. Occasionally, the defect is a new one that is caused by a genetic mutation occurring during the formation of the sperm or ovum. Sometimes, however, a couple planning a family know that one or more of their relatives have had children with a genetic disorder. In such cases, the couple should seek genetic counseling before their first pregnancy. The counselor can often perform tests to determine if there is a risk of a genetic disorder being passed on to the children and, if that is a possibility, may be able to quantify the risk involved. This allows the couple to make an informed decision as to whether they wish to continue with the pregnancy.

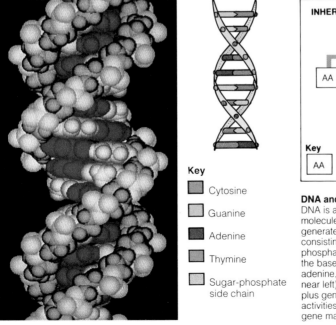

Key
- ▨ Cytosine
- ☐ Guanine
- ▨ Adenine
- ▨ Thymine
- ☐ Sugar-phosphate side chain

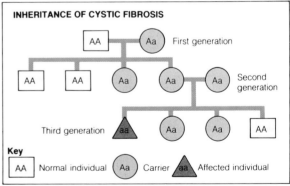

INHERITANCE OF CYSTIC FIBROSIS

First generation: AA — Aa

Second generation: AA, AA, Aa, Aa, Aa

Third generation: aa, Aa, Aa, AA

Key
- AA Normal individual
- Aa Carrier
- ▲aa Affected individual

DNA and genetic disorders
DNA is a large, double-helix molecule (see computer-generated model, far left) consisting of two sugar-phosphate side chains linked by the bases cytosine, guanine, adenine, and thymine (diagram, near left). It carries the 50,000-plus genes that control cellular activities. Thus, a defective gene may disrupt cellular function and lead to a heritable disorder, such as cystic fibrosis (see diagram, above). People with the faulty gene (**a**) in a single dose (**Aa**) are carriers of cystic fibrosis but do not suffer from the disorder; a double dose (**aa**) is necessary for the disease to develop.

Treating infertility

Approximately one in every 10 couples finds it difficult to have children. In about 40 percent of such cases, the man is subfertile or infertile; in another 40 percent, the woman has a fertility disorder. In the remaining 20 percent, both partners have some degree of infertility. Methods employed to improve the likelihood of pregnancy include microsurgery to repair damaged fallopian tubes in women or to reverse vasectomy in men; drugs or hormones to stimulate ovulation in women or improve male fertility; and in vitro fertilization ("test-tube baby") techniques, although the success rate for this procedure remains low.

Viability
The photomicrograph (right) shows a six-day-old fertilized ovum surrounded by remains of sperm (in pink). Even though the ovum has been fertilized, it will not necessarily develop into a fetus; about half of all pregnancies probably terminate naturally within the first month due to a genetic or developmental fault.

PRENATAL DIAGNOSIS

Major developmental or genetic defects occur in more than one in 50 pregnancies. Some result in stillbirths; in others, the baby is born alive. Advances in prenatal diagnosis have made it possible to identify certain major defects early in pregnancy. For some cases in which the fetus has a serious disorder of the brain and/or spinal cord (e.g., anencephaly or spina bifida), treatment is not possible. The same is true for chromosomal defects, such as the one that produces Down's syndrome. In other cases, including certain defects of the fetal heart or kidney, or blood disorders such as hemolytic disease of the newborn, early diagnosis enables treatment to be given even before the baby is born. Early diagnosis also alerts the obstetrician and pediatrician to the need for specialized care of the baby immediately after birth.

Ultrasound scanning

Ultrasound scanning is part of the care given to many pregnant women. The scanning technique, which uses the echoes of high-pitched sound waves to construct an image of the fetus, is considered harmless and causes no discomfort. The ultrasound image enables the obstetrician to identify multiple pregnancies, to measure the size of the fetus (enabling its age to be assessed), and to detect certain physical and developmental defects (such as anencephaly, spina bifida, or some congenital heart abnormalities) early in the pregnancy.

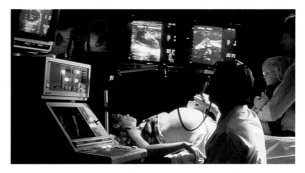

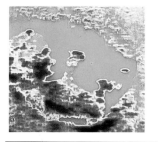
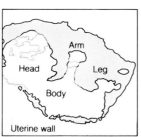

Fetal ultrasonography
A fetus can be imaged by ultrasound as early as the 12th week of pregnancy. The procedure (shown in the photograph above) usually takes about 15 minutes, and the woman is conscious throughout. It involves passing a transducer (a device that emits and receives ultrasound pulses) over the woman's abdomen; a computer then processes the ultrasound data to produce an image, which is displayed on one or more screens. An example of a fetal ultrasound image—of a 12-week-old fetus—is shown (far left), with a diagram to help interpret the image (left).

Fetoscopy

Ultrasound provides relatively clear images of a developing fetus, but in some cases it is necessary to examine the fetus directly or to carry out minor procedures on him or her. These procedures can be performed by fetoscopy, in which a fetoscope (a type of endoscope, or fiberoptic viewing tube) is passed into the woman's uterus through a small incision in her abdomen.

The direct access that fetoscopy gives allows any external fetal abnormalities, such as spinal column defects, facial clefts, or limb defects, to be assessed; it also enables samples of skin or blood to be taken from the fetus for tests. By attaching special instruments to the fetoscope, the physician can perform a variety of procedures, such as transfusing blood into the fetus to treat anemia. The fetoscope also allows some types of disorders (such as obstruction of the urinary tract) to be surgically corrected.

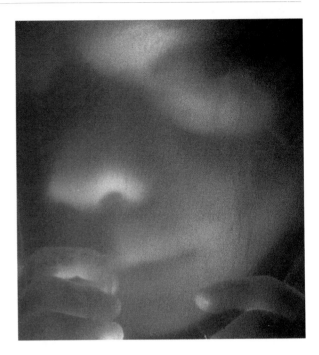

Viewing the fetus
The view of a fetus (right) was obtained using a fetoscope (fiberoptic viewing tube). The procedure carries a small risk of inducing miscarriage, so it is performed only when an obstetrician needs more information or access than is possible with other methods.

Amniocentesis and chorionic villus sampling

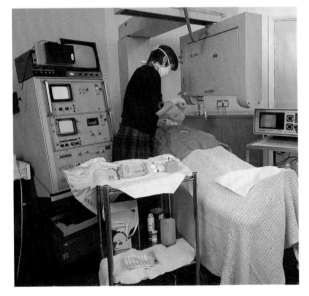

Performing amniocentesis
The photograph (above) shows a woman undergoing amniocentesis to remove a sample of amniotic fluid for analysis. Before the fluid is removed, an ultrasound scan is performed to determine the positions of the fetus and placenta. A local anesthetic is then usually applied to a small area of the abdomen, and a hollow needle is inserted through the abdominal wall and into the uterus, taking care to avoid the fetus and placenta. About half an ounce of fluid is sucked out by a syringe attached to the needle.

Amniocentesis and chorionic villus sampling can be used to diagnose certain fetal abnormalities early enough in pregnancy for elective abortion to remain a feasible option. However, because these procedures carry a small risk of inducing miscarriage, they are recommended only when there are good medical reasons for doing so, such as when the woman is older than 35 or when there is a family history of a chromosomal abnormality.

Amniocentesis involves removing and testing a sample of the amniotic fluid that surrounds the fetus. The procedure cannot be done before about the 16th to 18th week of pregnancy because there is not enough amniotic fluid before this time.

The amniotic fluid contains fetal cells, which are cultured to provide chromosomes for a karyotype analysis (a preparation of the chromosomes suitable for identifying chromosomal abnormalities). It may take two to three weeks to culture a chromosome sample, which means that results are not usually available until the 18th to 20th week of pregnancy. The amniotic fluid also contains various chemicals, the levels of which may be measured to test for other, nonchromosomal disorders of the fetus. For example, raised levels of alpha-fetoprotein may indicate a neural tube defect, such as spina bifida.

Chorionic villus sampling is another method of diagnosing fetal abnormalities due to chromosomal defects. Unlike amniocentesis, it is not suitable for detecting nonchromosomal abnormalities. In chorionic villus sampling, a small sample of tissue from the fetal side of the placenta is removed; the cells in the sample (which are genetically identical to those of the fetus) then undergo chromosomal analysis, which can usually be done immediately. Chorionic sampling can be done as early as eight to nine weeks into pregnancy (or later, if necessary). It thus gives results earlier than amniocentesis and permits a safer elective abortion if this course of action is chosen.

Chromosomal analysis
The set of chromosomes (right) from fetal cells has three rather than the normal two chromosomes in number 21. This genetic abnormality causes Down's syndrome.

PRENATAL TREATMENT

While advances in examining the fetus have been used to diagnose extremely severe defects, these same techniques have opened up possibilities for treating certain fetal disorders. The best-known example is treatment of hemolytic disease of the newborn due to Rh incompatibility.

This disorder occurs if the woman's blood is Rh negative and she is carrying a baby whose blood is Rh positive and she has previously been sensitized to Rh-positive blood. The woman can be sensitized through miscarriage, elective abortion, amniocentesis, a previous full-term pregnancy, or a blood transfusion of Rh-positive blood. In each situation except the last, Rh-positive blood has passed from the fetus to the Rh-negative woman. During subsequent pregnancies, the woman produces antibodies directed against the fetus's Rh-positive blood cells because her immune system recognizes the Rh-positive blood cells as "foreign." The fetal blood cells are destroyed by the maternal antibodies, resulting in the development of profound anemia.

If the fetus is found to be severely anemic before he or she is mature enough to be delivered safely (about 30 weeks' gestation), one or more blood transfusions are given via a fetoscope (fiberoptic viewing tube). The blood is transfused into one of the blood vessels in the umbilical cord. Alternatively, blood may be injected directly into the heart of the fetus via a needle passed through the mother's abdominal wall and into the uterus. This technique is called intracardiac transfusion and relies on accurate visualization of the fetus with ultrasound scanning. Although these measures carry some risk of inducing a miscarriage, the risk is usually justified because the ultimate outlook is excellent if the fetus can be kept alive long enough for birth to be feasible.

Sometimes, ultrasound tests show the presence of a defect in the fetus's urinary system, causing obstruction and pressure on the kidneys. In these circumstances, a fetoscope may be used to perform a simple operation to relieve the pressure and thus limit any damage to the kidneys.

Hemolytic disease (anemia) of the newborn
This disease typically occurs when a woman with Rhesus (Rh)-negative blood carries a baby with Rh-positive blood (see diagram, right). The first such pregnancy is usually normal. In subsequent pregnancies in which the fetus is Rh positive, maternal antibodies destroy fetal red blood cells, causing potentially fatal anemia. This anemia may be treated by fetal blood transfusions or prevented by injecting a woman who has Rh-negative blood with anti-D serum after childbirth. The serum prevents the woman's immune system from developing antibodies against Rh-positive blood.

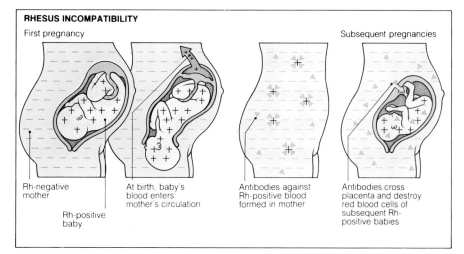

RHESUS INCOMPATIBILITY

First pregnancy

Subsequent pregnancies

Rh-negative mother

Rh-positive baby

At birth, baby's blood enters mother's circulation

Antibodies against Rh-positive blood formed in mother

Antibodies cross placenta and destroy red blood cells of subsequent Rh-positive babies

NEW DISEASES

In general, any disease is most dangerous to a human society upon first exposure; within a few generations, natural selection encourages the survival of individuals who have some natural resistance. When Europeans began colonial expansion in the 15th century, they brought new diseases (such as smallpox and measles) to the colonized lands; these diseases killed millions of indigenous inhabitants. The colonizers themselves were killed by diseases that they encountered for the first time.

EMERGENCE OF NEW DISEASES

New diseases in this century have been of three main types: those caused by microorganisms that have only recently infected humans, such as AIDS, Marburg disease, and Lassa fever; diseases that have existed for a long time but which have been identified only recently, including legionnaires' disease and campylobacter food poisoning; and conditions associated with contemporary industrial society, such as asbestosis, liver disease in smelters, drug addiction, and radiation-linked disorders.

AIDS

First recognized in 1982 as a distinct illness in young homosexual men, AIDS is now seen as having some features in common with other viral diseases, such as hepatitis B. Human immunodeficiency virus (HIV), the causative agent of AIDS, may be transmitted by sexual contact (heterosexual or between male homosexuals), blood-to-blood contact, or from a pregnant woman to her unborn child. Infection with HIV follows an unpredictable and, as yet, not completely mapped course. Some of those infected develop full-blown AIDS and die within a short time; others remain in apparent good health (but are infectious) for many years.

Scientists have learned a great deal about AIDS since it was first recognized, but they still have not found a cure or a vaccine, although treatment with

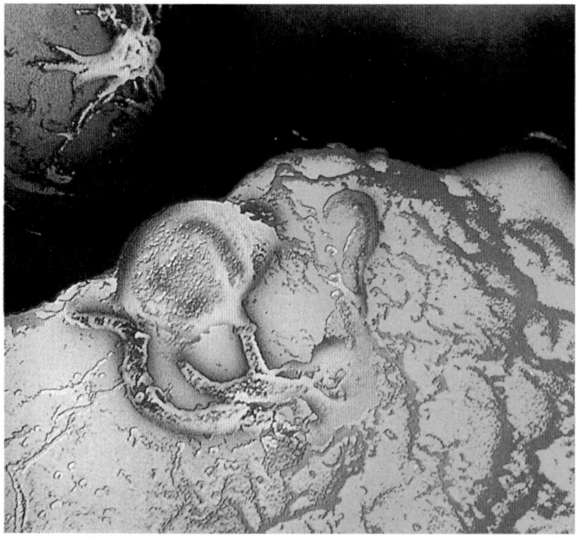

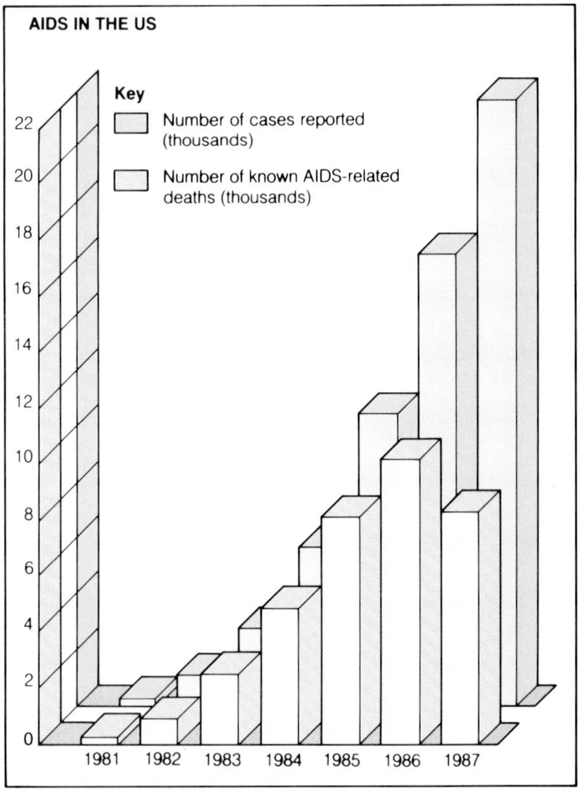
AIDS IN THE US
Key
Number of cases reported (thousands)
Number of known AIDS-related deaths (thousands)
22
20
18
16
14
12
10
8
6
4
2
0
1981
1982
1983
1984
1985
1986
1987

Incidence of AIDS in the US
The photomicrograph at left shows the virus (orange) budding from an infected lymphocyte (blue). Infection with HIV may last for years without causing symptoms, and it is not yet known whether full-blown AIDS develops in all of those infected. Also, recently developed treatment can slow the progress of AIDS, with the result that, although the number of cases increased annually between 1981 and 1987, the number of AIDS-related deaths fell in 1987 (see chart, above).

certain antiviral drugs (such as zidovudine) does slow the progression of HIV infection. Educational programs have advocated following "safe" sex practices and, for intravenous drug users, ensuring that needles and syringes are sterile, in the hope that it may control or reduce the risk of infection. However, any forecast regarding the control of AIDS relies on assumptions about public awareness and changes in behavior, and on how soon medical prevention and treatment of the disease is achieved.

Other new diseases

In developed countries, good nutrition, safe drinking water, proper sanitation, and immunization have conquered most of the previously fatal diseases, such as typhoid and diphtheria. However, many people today live and work in large, air-conditioned buildings, a modern environment that exposes them to disorders that were previously unknown, such as legionnaires' disease. In addition, windowless rooms, certain food additives, and agricultural chemicals can cause disorders that may initially puzzle physicians because their features do not correspond to any of the classic disease patterns.

Genuinely new infectious diseases are rare—AIDS is the best known example, but others include Marburg disease (a potentially fatal viral infection transmitted to humans from certain species of monkey) and Lassa fever (a serious viral infection that is acquired from a type of rat). More commonly, a new disease is identified and subsequently discovered to have existed for some time. For example, once the cause of legionnaires' disease had been identified as a bacterium, research revealed that outbreaks of the disease had occurred over the previous 40 years—

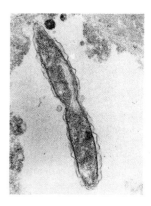

Legionnaires' disease
LEGIONELLA PNEUMOPHILA (right), one of the bacteria that causes legionnaires' disease (a form of pneumonia), was discovered after the 1976 outbreak of the disease among members of an American Legion convention. The bacterium thrives in warm, moist conditions; infection occurs by inhaling contaminated water droplets, usually from poorly maintained air-conditioning systems. Person-to-person transmission has not been demonstrated.

much earlier than the 1976 outbreak at an American Legion convention in Philadelphia that gave the disease its name. Similarly, Lyme disease (an infection that causes skin disorders and arthritis) was first recognized in 1975 in Lyme, Connecticut, but is now thought to have been in existence before that time. As time passes, it is believed that other unreported illnesses will be revealed and proved to have been present unrecognized for years.

Radiation and disease

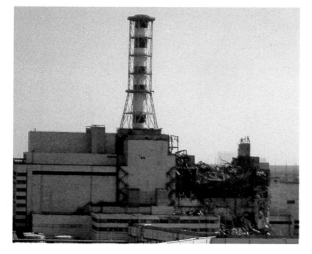

Chernobyl aftermath
The explosion at Chernobyl in 1986 destroyed a nuclear reactor (to the right in the photograph, above) and released a radioactive cloud that spread across much of Europe. Experts have calculated that, outside the immediate disaster area, a person exposed to radioactive fallout received about as much radiation as that from a chest X ray.

In recent years, events such as the catastrophes at Three Mile Island in 1979 and Chernobyl in 1986 have focused public attention on the hazards of radiation. However, the principal existing sources of radiation for the average person in the Western hemisphere are medical X rays and radioactive chemicals used in medicine, which together account for more than 90 percent of the radiation to which most people are exposed. The remaining 10 percent comes from natural sources of radiation, such as certain rocks and cosmic rays. Exposure to excessive amounts of radiation produces an acute illness that is fatal within a few weeks from the time of exposure. Therapeutic radiation may be accompanied by an acute form of radiation sickness that gets better within weeks.

Advances in medical technology have enabled conventional X rays to be replaced in many circumstances by nonhazardous imaging methods, such as ultrasound, MRI, and endoscopy. Moreover, the use of computers has enabled far lower doses of radiation to be employed in the different medical imaging procedures that do rely on radiation—such as CT scanning and PET scanning.

HUMAN POTENTIAL

Humans are an adaptable species, able to survive under a wide range of environmental conditions and physical and psychological stresses. One of the hallmarks of the human species is the ability not only to adapt to different conditions but also to modify existing conditions to suit human requirements. Much of this survival ability is a result of our species' ability to think, solve problems, and communicate. This allows us to construct a knowledge base that is passed from one generation to the next.

BIOLOGICAL LIMITS

All creatures have a natural lifespan—that is, the age at which death occurs due to natural degeneration of the vital organ system. For humans, the average lifespan seems to be about 87 years, and the maximum lifespan is thought to be about 115 years. Improvements in nutrition and health care have gradually increased the proportion of people that live to an advanced age, but it seems unlikely that further such improvements will increase the maximum lifespan. This is because maximum lifespan, like maximum height or maximum intelligence, is determined genetically. Improving living conditions can therefore be expected to increase only the proportion of people that nears the maximum lifespan, rather than increasing the maximum lifespan itself.

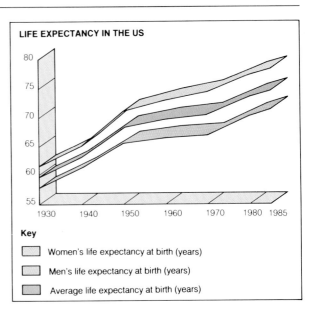

LIFE EXPECTANCY IN THE US

Key
- Women's life expectancy at birth (years)
- Men's life expectancy at birth (years)
- Average life expectancy at birth (years)

Life expectancy
The increase in life expectancy over recent decades (see chart, right) is mainly due to fewer people dying prematurely from disease, rather than to an increase in maximum lifespan. The gender difference in life expectancy is probably due to more men than women smoking earlier in this century.

Environmental constraints

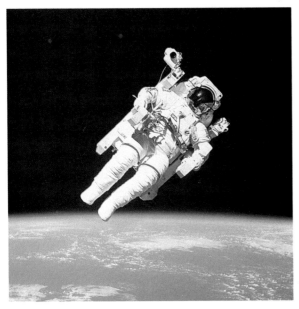

Although humans now inhabit almost every region of the Earth, the environmental conditions that are compatible with basic human life (that is, without the benefits of modern technology) are quite restricted. In general, vital basic activities such as farming and hunting require average temperatures of between about 15°F and 105°F, and average annual rainfall of some 15 to 20 inches—although some primitive peoples survive in areas with climatic extremes outside these limits. The development of modern technology also means that life in extreme environments is relatively easily sustainable.

Another environmental constraint is altitude. The higher a place is above sea level, the "thinner" the air,

Hazards of space
Modern technology has enabled humans to survive in environments to which they are not biologically adapted, such as deep space. However, technology has not yet overcome all of the problems of space travel. High levels of radiation, the adverse effects of weightlessness on bones, muscles, and the cardiovascular system, and the psychological stress of long journeys are still health hazards for astronauts.

and the faster a person must breathe to get enough oxygen into the blood. People who are born and live at high altitudes—such as those in the Andes and Himalayas—become acclimatized to thin air, but visitors from low altitudes may become acutely or fatally ill if they ascend quickly to altitudes over about 10,000 feet. A person with a respiratory disorder may have difficulty breathing even at 5,000 feet. Sustained human life seems impossible above about 20,000 feet. Mountaineers who have spent long periods above this altitude have found that their health progressively deteriorated—even though they were fully

acclimatized. Such deterioration is due to a progressive increase in the red blood cell count and a rise in the pressure of blood in the lungs.

There has been no evidence that moderate acceleration or speed is harmful to health. With specially designed acceleration couches, the human body is able to withstand the extreme g-forces that occur during a spacecraft launch. The degree to which health may deteriorate during prolonged periods in outer space—as a consequence of high levels of radiation and the adverse effects of weightlessness—is not yet fully known.

Physical constraints

In this century, athletic records have been broken repeatedly, an achievement that is due to several factors. First, the physical size and conditioning of young people increased until about the 1960s in most Western countries; this process has now virtually ceased, although it is continuing in some developing countries. Second, more young people today have access to sporting facilities, so the pool of talent has been enlarged. Finally, training and coaching methods have improved, as has the intensity of training undertaken by many athletes. However, despite these changes and the ever greater efforts made by athletes, breaking records in many sports is becoming increasingly difficult. Competitive efforts to extend physical limits and sports records have resulted in the unfair and physically dangerous practice of body building through the use of anabolic steroid drugs.

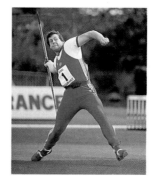
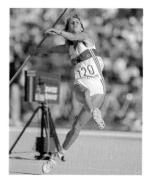

Physical sporting requirements
In javelin throwing (above) size and physical strength are advantageous. Thus, top men and women throwers tend to be tall, heavy, and muscular. However, on average, men are larger and stronger than women, which may explain why they consistently outperform women in the sport (see chart, below left).

Sex differences and sporting achievements
Because of their greater size and muscle bulk, men have a natural physical advantage over women in strength sports. This advantage is shown by world records for javelin throwing (see chart, near right), in which there has been a continual improvement in the performances of men and women, but no reduction in the performance difference between the sexes. Conversely, in stamina sports, size and muscle bulk are generally not advantageous. As a result, the performance difference between men and women has steadily decreased in many such events, such as the marathon (see chart, far right). Whether or not women will ever match—or even better—men in these sports remains open to question. Women do outperform men in many sports that are predominantly skill dependent, such as horse jumping.

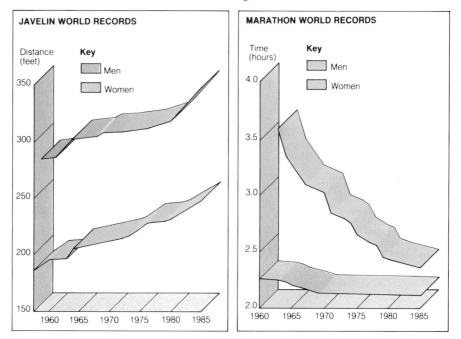

JAVELIN WORLD RECORDS

Distance (feet)

Key
Men
Women

350

300

250

200

150

1960 1965 1970 1975 1980 1985

MARATHON WORLD RECORDS

Time (hours)

Key
Men
Women

4.0

3.5

3.0

2.5

2.0

1960 1965 1970 1975 1980 1985

OPTIMIZING HUMAN POTENTIAL

Good nutrition and living conditions, absence of disease, a healthy, progressive mental attitude on the part of the parents, and a stable family relationship all contribute to a child's development. As a result, children who suffer physical and/or emotional deprivation tend not to develop to the full potential allowed by their genes and are thus, in a sense, victims of their environment.

With continuing economic growth, better nutrition, and improved prevention of childhood diseases, each generation, ideally, should include a greater proportion of children who achieve their full genetic potential for physical and mental development. However, measurements of these features in successive generations have revealed a gradual slowing of the rate of improvement in most Western countries, which raises the question of whether the natural limits of development are being reached.

Genetic modifications

Many diseases are due to genetic defects. In some cases, such a "defect" has advantages. For example, it is theorized that the gene responsible for sickle cell disease gives some protection against malaria because the malaria parasite does not invade the distorted sickle cell. Thus the person with sickle cells is not vulnerable to malaria but is at risk of dying from sickle cell disease. However, most genetic defects do not have beneficial effects, so it is desirable to eliminate them. In communities that have a high incidence of a particular genetic disorder, screening of young adults may enable carriers to be identified or affected pregnancies to be terminated; this approach has reduced the incidence of Tay-Sachs disease (a brain disorder) in some Jewish communities.

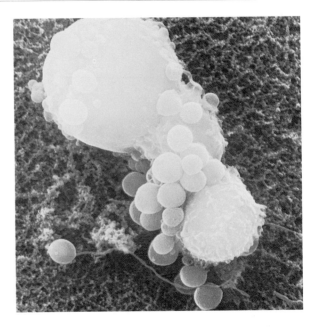

Modifying the body's defenses
The body's defenses against cancer—T-lymphocyte cells, which are shown attacking a cancer in the electron micrograph (right)—are relatively inefficient. In the future, it may be possible to improve these defenses by using genetic engineering, although much research is still needed.

Environment and development

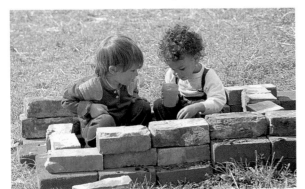

Maximizing development
Children who have plenty of mental stimulation seem to develop more rapidly than those raised in a boring environment. Some scientists also believe that maximizing mental development in early life leads to an overall increase in mental abilities.

By the age of 5 years, a child's brain is 80 percent of its adult size. The brain's rapid physical growth is paralleled by equally rapid development of mental abilities and physical coordination. By the age of 5, most children can speak fluently; have an understanding of time; can write several letters of the alphabet; and can walk, run, and jump.

Just as optimum physical growth requires good nutrition, so optimum mental development requires an intellectually stimulating environment. Children thrive best in a secure setting with plenty of contact with adults and other children, a wide range of toys and other objects to play with, and encouragement to explore, investigate, and learn as part of play. Children born in the 1970s and 1980s have scored better on intelligence tests than those born earlier, probably in part as a result of improvements in both their physical and mental environments.

THE A TO Z
OF MEDICINE

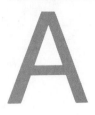

Abdomen

The area of the body between the lower border of the ribs and the upper border of the thighs. The contents of the abdominal cavity, separated from the *thorax* (chest) by the *diaphragm*, include organs of the *digestive system* and *urinary system*. The *pelvis* (the bones surrounding the lower part of the abdomen) contains the organs of the *reproductive system*.

STRUCTURE

The abdominal wall is made up of muscle, and of layers of skin, connective tissue, and fat of varying thickness. The *peritoneum*, a thin, two-layered membrane, lines the abdominal cavity and covers the stomach, intestine, and other organs.

The abdomen is protected from behind by the spinal column and lower ribs. It is vulnerable in the front, where the internal organs are covered only by the abdominal wall.

Abdomen, acute

The medical term for persistent, severe abdominal pain of sudden onset, usually associated with rigidity, guarding (voluntary contracting of the abdominal muscles), vomiting, and fever. Acute abdomen is purely a working diagnosis and usually requires urgent medical investigation. The precise cause of the abdominal pain is diagnosed by careful physician assessment and backed up by specialized tests and X rays. Occasionally, a *laparotomy* (surgical exploration of the abdomen) or a *laparoscopy* (internal examination of the abdomen using a viewing tube) is necessary.

CAUSES AND TREATMENT

The most common cause of acute abdomen is *peritonitis* (inflammation of the membrane that lines the abdomen). Inflammation of any structure in the abdomen may lead to peritonitis—for example, *salpingitis* (inflammation of the fallopian tubes); intestinal disorders, such as an inflamed appendix (see *Appendicitis*), *Crohn's disease*, or *diverticular disease*; or a perforated *peptic ulcer*. Abdominal injury may also be the cause.

Other possible causes of acute abdomen include urinary disorders, such as a stone in the ureter (see *Calculus, urinary tract*), a stone in the duct that drains the gallbladder (see *Gallstones*); and disorders that stretch the outer covering of the liver (such as *hepatitis*) or of the kidneys.

All of these conditions produce similar symptoms. The muscular wall of the abdomen goes into spasm and becomes rigid, and pain is generally first felt near the site of inflammation; later, it tends to become generalized or may temporarily disappear if an abscess ruptures.

Treatment depends on the underlying cause, but, with prompt diagnosis, the prospects for successful treatment are excellent.

Abdominal pain

Discomfort in the abdominal cavity, between the upper border of the thighs and the lower border of the ribs. Accompanying symptoms may include belching, nausea, vomiting, rumbling and gurgling noises, and flatulence (gas).

CAUSES

Minor degrees of abdominal pain are experienced by everybody at some time, and often the cause is easily recognized—for example, overeating, eating too much spicy food, or drinking too much alcohol. Abdominal discomfort may also occur with *diarrhea* or *constipation*.

Many women experience pelvic or lower abdominal pain during part of their menstrual cycles. The pain may occur before or during a period, or around the time of ovulation. Occasionally, this pain is due to a gynecological disorder such as *endometriosis* (fragments of uterine lining that have developed in other regions of the abdomen).

A common cause of pain very low in the abdomen is a urinary infection, especially in women, causing *cystitis* (inflammation of the bladder).

Abdominal pain can have a psychological origin. For example, it may result from anxiety, such as that felt by a child starting a new school or an adult changing jobs.

Spasm, or stretching, of internal organs can result in a wavelike pain known as colic. Intestinal colic, often associated with swelling of the abdomen and flatulence, can occur when the muscles lining the intestine go into spasm (as, for example, in *irritable bowel syndrome*). Colic may also develop as the result of blockage of the gallbladder, bile duct, or urinary tract, usually by a stone. It can also occur in an *ectopic pregnancy*, in which the fetus develops not in the uterus but in one of the fallopian tubes.

LOCATION OF THE ABDOMEN

The abdomen is bounded by the lower ribs at the top and the pelvis below. The illustration shows the position of the abdominal organs in an adult woman.

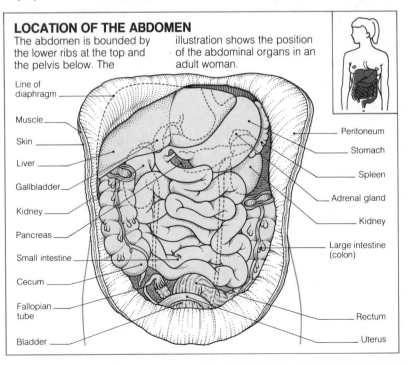

Line of diaphragm

Muscle

Skin

Liver

Gallbladder

Kidney

Pancreas

Small intestine

Cecum

Fallopian tube

Bladder

Peritoneum

Stomach

Spleen

Adrenal gland

Kidney

Large intestine (colon)

Rectum

Uterus

ABDOMINAL PAIN General or localized pain between the bottom of the rib cage and the groin that has occurred within the last 24 hours. See also Recurrent abdominal pain chart.

A

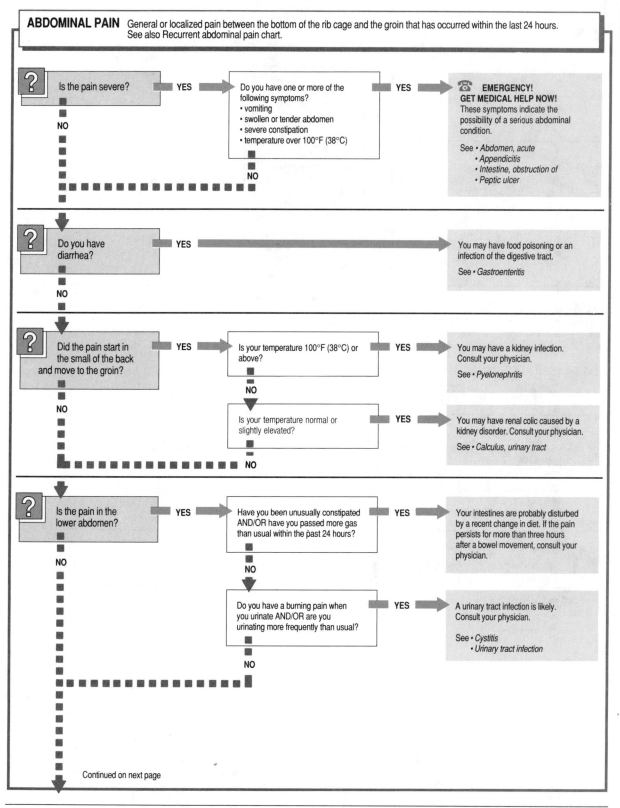

Is the pain severe? — **YES** →

Do you have one or more of the following symptoms?
• vomiting
• swollen or tender abdomen
• severe constipation
• temperature over 100°F (38°C)

— **YES** →

☎ **EMERGENCY!**
GET MEDICAL HELP NOW!
These symptoms indicate the possibility of a serious abdominal condition.

See • *Abdomen, acute*
• *Appendicitis*
• *Intestine, obstruction of*
• *Peptic ulcer*

NO

NO

Do you have diarrhea? — **YES** →

You may have food poisoning or an infection of the digestive tract.

See • *Gastroenteritis*

NO

Did the pain start in the small of the back and move to the groin? — **YES** →

Is your temperature 100°F (38°C) or above? — **YES** →

You may have a kidney infection. Consult your physician.

See • *Pyelonephritis*

NO

Is your temperature normal or slightly elevated? — **YES** →

You may have renal colic caused by a kidney disorder. Consult your physician.

See • *Calculus, urinary tract*

NO

NO

Is the pain in the lower abdomen? — **YES** →

Have you been unusually constipated AND/OR have you passed more gas than usual within the past 24 hours? — **YES** →

Your intestines are probably disturbed by a recent change in diet. If the pain persists for more than three hours after a bowel movement, consult your physician.

NO

Do you have a burning pain when you urinate AND/OR are you urinating more frequently than usual? — **YES** →

A urinary tract infection is likely. Consult your physician.

See • *Cystitis*
• *Urinary tract infection*

NO

NO

Continued on next page

A

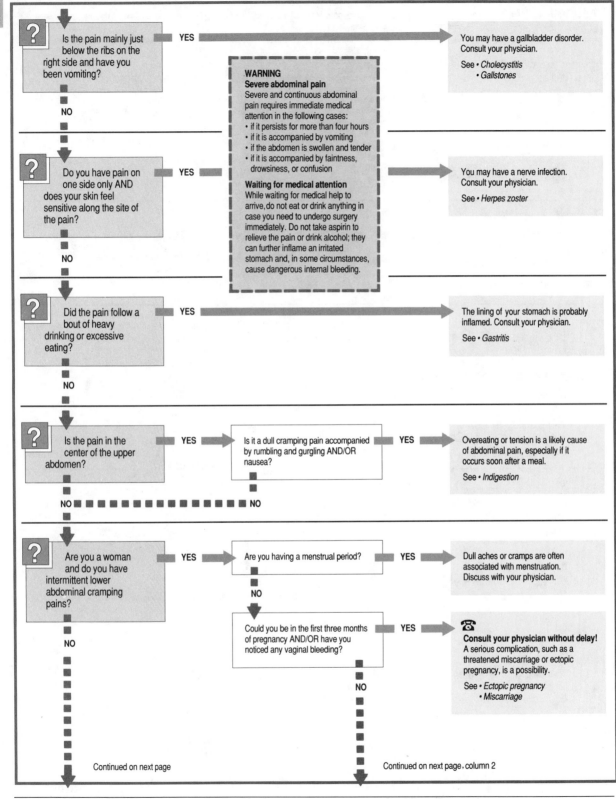

? Is the pain mainly just below the ribs on the right side and have you been vomiting?

→ **YES** → You may have a gallbladder disorder. Consult your physician.

See • *Cholecystitis*
      • *Gallstones*

NO

WARNING
Severe abdominal pain
Severe and continuous abdominal pain requires immediate medical attention in the following cases:
• if it persists for more than four hours
• if it is accompanied by vomiting
• if the abdomen is swollen and tender
• if it is accompanied by faintness, drowsiness, or confusion

Waiting for medical attention
While waiting for medical help to arrive, do not eat or drink anything in case you need to undergo surgery immediately. Do not take aspirin to relieve the pain or drink alcohol; they can further inflame an irritated stomach and, in some circumstances, cause dangerous internal bleeding.

? Do you have pain on one side only AND does your skin feel sensitive along the site of the pain?

→ **YES** → You may have a nerve infection. Consult your physician.

See • *Herpes zoster*

NO

? Did the pain follow a bout of heavy drinking or excessive eating?

→ **YES** → The lining of your stomach is probably inflamed. Consult your physician.

See • *Gastritis*

NO

? Is the pain in the center of the upper abdomen?

→ **YES** → Is it a dull cramping pain accompanied by rumbling and gurgling AND/OR nausea?

→ **YES** → Overeating or tension is a likely cause of abdominal pain, especially if it occurs soon after a meal.

See • *Indigestion*

NO ▪▪▪▪▪▪▪▪▪▪▪▪▪ **NO**

? Are you a woman and do you have intermittent lower abdominal cramping pains?

→ **YES** → Are you having a menstrual period?

→ **YES** → Dull aches or cramps are often associated with menstruation. Discuss with your physician.

NO

Could you be in the first three months of pregnancy AND/OR have you noticed any vaginal bleeding?

→ **YES** → ☎
Consult your physician without delay!
A serious complication, such as a threatened miscarriage or ectopic pregnancy, is a possibility.

See • *Ectopic pregnancy*
      • *Miscarriage*

NO

NO

Continued on next page

Continued on next page, column 2

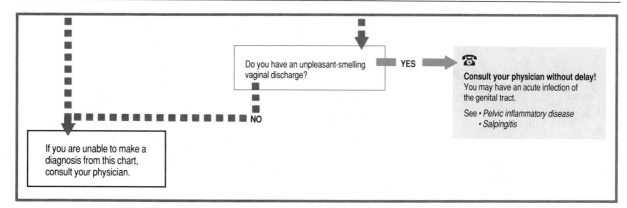

Do you have an unpleasant-smelling vaginal discharge?

YES →

☎

Consult your physician without delay!
You may have an acute infection of the genital tract.

See • *Pelvic inflammatory disease*
     • *Salpingitis*

NO

If you are unable to make a diagnosis from this chart, consult your physician.

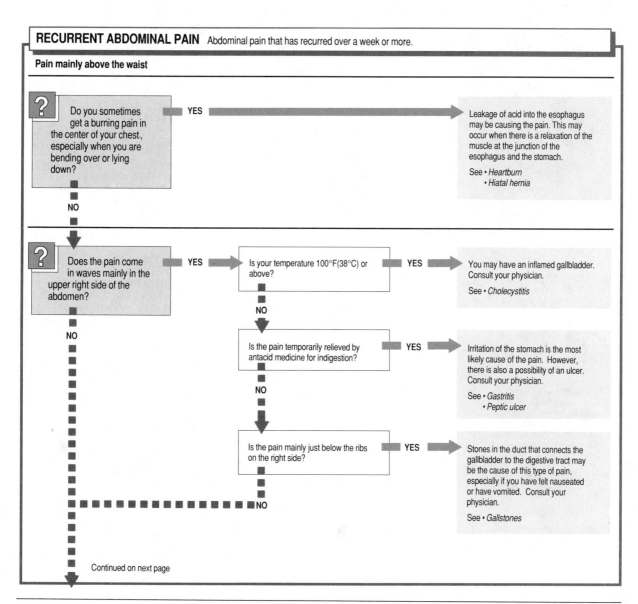

RECURRENT ABDOMINAL PAIN   Abdominal pain that has recurred over a week or more.

Pain mainly above the waist

? Do you sometimes get a burning pain in the center of your chest, especially when you are bending over or lying down?

YES →

Leakage of acid into the esophagus may be causing the pain. This may occur when there is a relaxation of the muscle at the junction of the esophagus and the stomach.

See • *Heartburn*
     • *Hiatal hernia*

NO

? Does the pain come in waves mainly in the upper right side of the abdomen?

YES → Is your temperature 100°F(38°C) or above?   **YES** →

You may have an inflamed gallbladder. Consult your physician.

See • *Cholecystitis*

NO

Is the pain temporarily relieved by antacid medicine for indigestion?   **YES** →

Irritation of the stomach is the most likely cause of the pain. However, there is also a possibility of an ulcer. Consult your physician.

See • *Gastritis*
     • *Peptic ulcer*

NO

Is the pain mainly just below the ribs on the right side?   **YES** →

Stones in the duct that connects the gallbladder to the digestive tract may be the cause of this type of pain, especially if you have felt nauseated or have vomited. Consult your physician.

See • *Gallstones*

NO

NO

Continued on next page

A

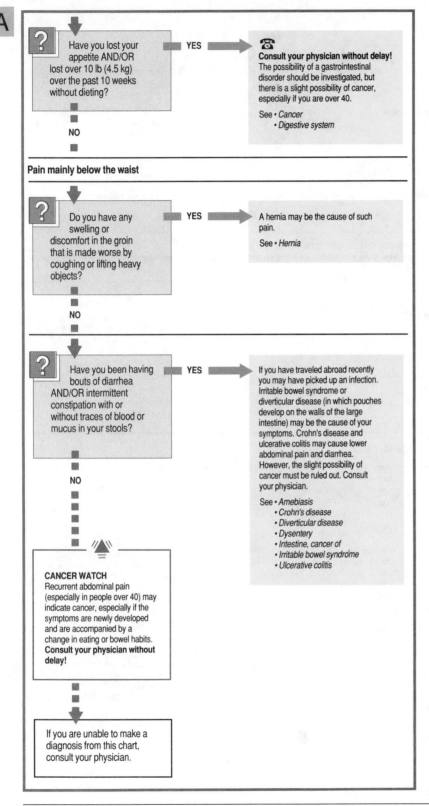

Have you lost your appetite AND/OR lost over 10 lb (4.5 kg) over the past 10 weeks without dieting?

YES →

☎ **Consult your physician without delay!**
The possibility of a gastrointestinal disorder should be investigated, but there is a slight possibility of cancer, especially if you are over 40.

See • Cancer
• Digestive system

NO

Pain mainly below the waist

Do you have any swelling or discomfort in the groin that is made worse by coughing or lifting heavy objects?

YES →

A hernia may be the cause of such pain.

See • Hernia

NO

Have you been having bouts of diarrhea AND/OR intermittent constipation with or without traces of blood or mucus in your stools?

YES →

If you have traveled abroad recently you may have picked up an infection. Irritable bowel syndrome or diverticular disease (in which pouches develop on the walls of the large intestine) may be the cause of your symptoms. Crohn's disease and ulcerative colitis may cause lower abdominal pain and diarrhea. However, the slight possibility of cancer must be ruled out. Consult your physician.

See • Amebiasis
• Crohn's disease
• Diverticular disease
• Dysentery
• Intestine, cancer of
• Irritable bowel syndrome
• Ulcerative colitis

NO

CANCER WATCH
Recurrent abdominal pain (especially in people over 40) may indicate cancer, especially if the symptoms are newly developed and are accompanied by a change in eating or bowel habits. **Consult your physician without delay!**

If you are unable to make a diagnosis from this chart, consult your physician.

An increase in the amount of acid formed in the stomach may be associated with the development of a *peptic ulcer*, which produces a recurrent gnawing pain temporarily relieved by food, milk, or antacids.

Another possible cause of abdominal pain is infection, such as *pyelonephritis* (infection of the kidneys) or *pelvic inflammatory disease* (infection of the uterus and fallopian tubes). Pain may also be due to *ischemia* (lack of blood supply), as occurs, for instance, when a *volvulus* (twisting of the intestine) obstructs blood vessels or when a clot forms in one of the intestinal blood vessels.

Tumors affecting any of the abdominal organs can cause pain by stretching the lining of the organ, by pressing on surrounding structures, or by ulcerating, perforating, or rupturing.

In rare cases, disorders of organs outside the abdomen can cause abdominal pain. For example, right lower lobe pneumonia may produce pain in the upper right abdomen that mimics acute appendicitis.

TREATMENT
Abdominal pain can sometimes be relieved by simple measures, such as drinking milk, applying a heating pad to the affected area, or taking an antacid (to neutralize excess stomach acid), an antispasmodic, or an analgesic (painkiller). If none of these methods alleviates the pain, or if the pain is severe or recurs, a physician should be consulted.

Severe pain with sweating, paleness, or dizziness sometimes indicates a serious disorder that may require immediate surgical attention. Urgent attention is also necessary if the pain is accompanied by persistent vomiting, by vomiting of blood (which may appear brown), by passing of blood-stained or black feces, or by feeling weak or faint.

Similarly, prompt medical attention should be obtained if abdominal pain lasts for more than about six hours or is not relieved by vomiting.

Abdominal pain accompanied by weight loss without dieting or by a change in bowel habits—sudden constipation or attacks of diarrhea—may indicate a serious disorder and should be investigated by a physician.

INVESTIGATION
The physician makes a diagnosis based on the patient's detailed description of the pain and its relationship to eating, urinating, and bowel movements, along with a thorough physical examination of the person.

DIAGNOSING ABDOMINAL PAIN

The physician conducts a physical examination and listens to the patient's description of the pain. More investigations, such as blood tests or X rays, may be carried out. If the diagnosis is still in doubt, gastroscopy, laparoscopy, or colonoscopy may be performed.

Gallbladder pain
A crampy or steady pain under the right ribs and often accompanied by vomiting and fever.

Kidney pain
An intermittent pain that may begin in the flank and radiate to the groin.

Appendicitis pain
This pain starts around the navel and settles in the body's lower right side.

Menstrual pain
Cramping pain occurring at the beginning of a monthly period; it usually begins during the teenage years.

Peptic ulcer pain
This pain often occurs in a precise place (usually below the sternum where the ribs meet) and may be temporarily relieved by eating.

Gas
Excess in the digestive system can cause an uncomfortable, distended feeling.

Pelvic organ inflammation
A diffuse, burning pain that extends over the lower abdomen, usually accompanied by vaginal discharge.

Ovarian pain
A pain deep within the pelvis that may be provoked by sexual intercourse.

If there is any doubt about the diagnosis, further investigations may be carried out. The investigations may include a urine test, blood tests, X rays, and *ultrasound scanning*.

If the cause still cannot be diagnosed after such tests, endoscopic examination (looking into a body cavity with a viewing tube) may be necessary. This may take the form of *gastroscopy* (inspecting the stomach and duodenum), *colonoscopy* (inspecting the large intestine), or laparoscopy (inspecting the contents of the abdominal cavity). In some cases, the diagnosis can be confirmed only by an exploratory operation on the abdomen, known as a *laparotomy*.

Abdominal swelling

Distention of the abdomen due to a number of causes. Abdominal swelling is the natural result of *obesity* and of enlargement of the uterus during pregnancy, generally noticeable after about 12 weeks.

Some causes of abdominal swelling are harmless. Gas in the stomach or intestine may cause uncomfortable bloating distention of the whole abdomen. Many women experience lower abdominal distention due to temporary water retention just before a menstrual period.

Other causes may be more serious. For instance, *ascites* (accumulation of fluid in the abdomen) may be a symptom of underlying *cancer*, *heart* disease, *kidney* disease, or *liver* disease; the swelling may also be caused by *intestinal obstruction* or an *ovarian cyst*.

INVESTIGATION AND TREATMENT
Diagnosis of the underlying cause may involve abdominal X rays or *ultrasound scanning* to look for abnormalities in the size or shape of the internal organs or for signs of intestinal obstruction. If ascites is present, some of the fluid may be drained for examination. Occasionally, a *laparotomy* (surgical exploration of the abdomen) or *laparoscopy* (internal examination of the abdomen using a flexible viewing tube) may also be necessary. (See chart, next page.)

Abdominal X ray

An X-ray examination of the abdominal contents. An abdominal X ray is usually one of the first steps in the investigation of suspected abdominal disease (after the physician takes a careful medical history and performs a physical examination).

Because organs are not completely opaque to X rays, only the outlines are visible. The radiologist can see, however, whether any organ is abnormally enlarged and is able to spot swallowed foreign bodies within the digestive tract. Useful information is also gained by studying patterns of fluid and gas. Distended loops of bowel containing collections of fluid often indicate an obstruction (see *Intestine, obstruction of*); gas found outside the intestine indicates intestinal *perforation*.

Calcium, which is opaque to X rays, is present in most kidney stones (see *Calculus, urinary tract*) and also in some *gallstones*; they can sometimes be detected on an abdominal X ray. Some aortic *aneurysms* contain calcium and therefore are visible.

Abdominal X rays often need to be followed by other procedures that give more detail, such as *endoscopy*, *ultrasound scanning*, *CT scanning*, *barium X-ray examinations*, or *intravenous pyelography*.

Abducent nerve

The sixth *cranial nerve*. The abducent nerve supplies just one muscle of each eye, the lateral rectus muscle, which is responsible for moving the eye outward. The abducent nerve originates in the pons (part of the *brain stem*) and emerges from the brain immediately below it. From this point, it extends through the skull, eventually entering the back of the eye socket through a gap between the skull bones.

As a result of its long path inside the skull, the abducent nerve is often damaged in fractures of the base of the skull, or by a disorder such as a tumor that distorts the brain. Such damage may give rise to *double vision* and a convergent *strabismus*.

Abduction

Movement of a limb away from the central line of the body, or of a digit away from the axis of a limb. Muscles that carry out this movement are called abductors. (See also *Adduction*.)

A

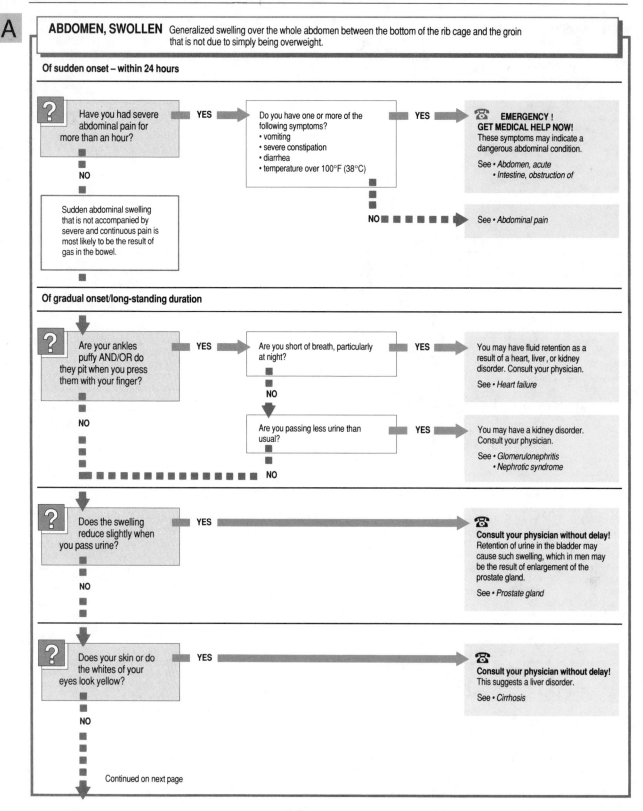

ABDOMEN, SWOLLEN
Generalized swelling over the whole abdomen between the bottom of the rib cage and the groin that is not due to simply being overweight.

Of sudden onset – within 24 hours

? Have you had severe abdominal pain for more than an hour?

YES ▶ Do you have one or more of the following symptoms?
• vomiting
• severe constipation
• diarrhea
• temperature over 100°F (38°C)

YES ▶ ☎ **EMERGENCY !**
GET MEDICAL HELP NOW!
These symptoms may indicate a dangerous abdominal condition.

See • *Abdomen, acute*
• *Intestine, obstruction of*

NO

Sudden abdominal swelling that is not accompanied by severe and continuous pain is most likely to be the result of gas in the bowel.

NO ▶ See • *Abdominal pain*

Of gradual onset/long-standing duration

? Are your ankles puffy AND/OR do they pit when you press them with your finger?

YES ▶ Are you short of breath, particularly at night?

YES ▶ You may have fluid retention as a result of a heart, liver, or kidney disorder. Consult your physician.

See • *Heart failure*

NO

Are you passing less urine than usual?

YES ▶ You may have a kidney disorder. Consult your physician.

See • *Glomerulonephritis*
• *Nephrotic syndrome*

NO

NO

? Does the swelling reduce slightly when you pass urine?

YES ▶ ☎

Consult your physician without delay!
Retention of urine in the bladder may cause such swelling, which in men may be the result of enlargement of the prostate gland.

See • *Prostate gland*

NO

? Does your skin or do the whites of your eyes look yellow?

YES ▶ ☎

Consult your physician without delay!
This suggests a liver disorder.

See • *Cirrhosis*

NO

Continued on next page

A

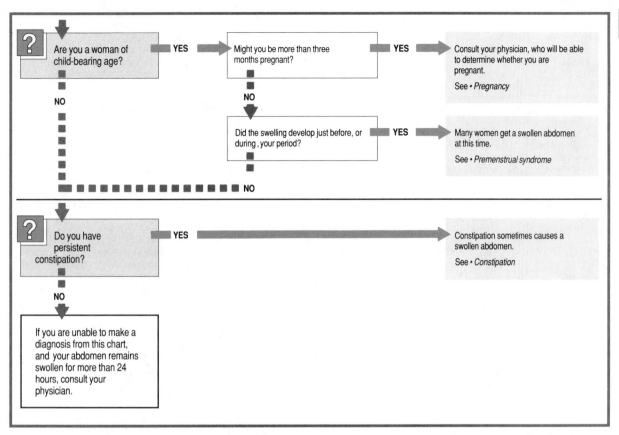

Are you a woman of child-bearing age? — **YES** → Might you be more than three months pregnant? — **YES** → Consult your physician, who will be able to determine whether you are pregnant.
See • *Pregnancy*

NO

NO → Did the swelling develop just before, or during , your period? — **YES** → Many women get a swollen abdomen at this time.
See • *Premenstrual syndrome*

NO

Do you have persistent constipation? — **YES** → Constipation sometimes causes a swollen abdomen.
See • *Constipation*

NO

If you are unable to make a diagnosis from this chart, and your abdomen remains swollen for more than 24 hours, consult your physician.

Ablation

The removal of dead or diseased tissue by excision (cutting away with a sharp instrument), freezing (see *Cryosurgery*), *radiation therapy*, burning (see *Diathermy*), or *laser treatment*. Ablation of the thyroid gland is achieved with radioactive iodine isotopes.

Abnormality

A physical deformity or malformation, a behavioral or mental problem, an alteration in function of a tissue or an organ, or a variation from normal in cells or tissues.

Abortifacient

An agent that causes *abortion*. Various substances have been claimed to cause abortion, such as large amounts of castor oil or gin, but none of these is effective. In medical practice, derivatives of local hormones called *prostaglandins* are used to induce abortion; they cause softening and widening of the cervix (neck of the uterus) and muscular contractions of the uterus. They are usually administered in the form of suppositories, placed high in the vagina, or by intravenous infusion.

Abortion

In medical terminology, the word abortion denotes either spontaneous abortion (see *Miscarriage*) or medically induced termination of pregnancy (see *Abortion, elective*).

Abortion, elective

Medically induced termination of pregnancy. Up to the 12th week of pregnancy, an elective abortion in the US is a private matter between a woman and her physician. After the 12th week, state laws may regulate abortion in ways that are related to maternal health. After the 24th week of pregnancy, state laws may regulate and even prohibit abortion except in cases where the life or health of the woman is threatened. An abortion is described as a therapeutic abortion if it is carried out to save the life or health of the mother.

MEDICAL REASONS FOR ABORTION

A physician may recommend an abortion for conditions affecting either the woman or the fetus. In the woman, examples of conditions that may worsen during pregnancy and possibly become life-threatening include

severe heart disease, chronic kidney disease, and cancer, especially of the breast or cervix.

Fetal conditions, revealed by *ultrasound scanning*, *amniocentesis*, or *chorionic villus sampling*, include severe developmental defects incompatible with normal life (such as *anencephaly*) and serious *chromosomal abnormalities* (such as *Down's syndrome*). Termination may also be recommended if the woman contracts *rubella* (German measles) during the early stages of pregnancy; this virus can severely damage the baby, especially his or her eyes, ears, and heart. Certain other infections in the woman may also damage the fetus. Termination is recommended if the mother has been infected by the *AIDS* virus because it can be transmitted to the baby.

HOW IT IS DONE

EARLY ABORTION Vacuum suction techniques are the simplest and safest means of terminating an early pregnancy. Within two weeks of a missed period, before pregnancy has been confirmed, *menstrual extraction* (an office-based suction procedure) can be carried out. However, vacuum suction curettage is the most commonly used method. It is performed between the seventh and 12th week of pregnancy at a clinic or in a hospital outpatient department.

The procedure may be performed with either a general or a local anesthetic. If local anesthesia (paracervical block) is used, it may be supplemented by an intravenous narcotic or tranquilizer. The cervix is dilated with curved metal rods, and a narrow plastic tube is then inserted into the uterus. The outer end of the tube is connected to a suction machine, which sucks out the fetal and placental tissue into a vacuum bottle. After this procedure, which usually takes less than 10 minutes, the gynecologist scrapes the lining of the uterus with a curet (a spoonlike instrument) to make sure that no placental tissue has been left behind. The tissue is analyzed in a laboratory to confirm that a pregnancy existed and that the tissue appears complete, since an *ectopic pregnancy* or abdominal pregnancy would require more surgery.

Recovery is fast, although strenuous activity should be avoided for several days. There is usually some bleeding, and sometimes mild cramps, for up to a week. A normal period starts four to six weeks after the termination. Sexual intercourse can be resumed after two or three weeks.

LATE ABORTION Between 12 and 15 weeks, either the suction procedure used in early abortion or the evacuation procedure described below may be recommended, depending on the facilities available. After the 15th week, it is normally considered safer to perform an abortion by causing the uterus to contract so that the fetus is expelled, as in natural labor. Contractions are induced by introducing saline solution or, more commonly, a *prostaglandin* hormone into the uterus. This may be done either by injection directly through the woman's abdomen into the amniotic fluid or by infusion, via the cervix, into the gap between the amniotic sac (the membrane that surrounds the fetus) and the uterine wall. Alternatively, a vaginal suppository containing prostaglandin may be placed high in the vagina.

It usually takes about 12 hours for the fetus to be expelled, during which time the woman is given analgesics (painkillers). She remains in the hospital for 24 to 48 hours after completion of the termination to be monitored for complications.

COMPLICATIONS
If termination is performed in a well-equipped clinic or hospital by a qualified gynecologist, complications are few. Infection, resulting in a condition called septic abortion, or serious bleeding occurs in fewer than 1 percent of cases. Mortality is less than one per 100,000 when abortion is performed before the 13th week, rising to three per 100,000 after the 13th week. (For comparison, maternal mortality for full-term pregnancy is nine per 100,000.) Multiple terminations may increase the risk of miscarriage in subsequent pregnancies, although there is little evidence that a single termination has any effect on future fertility.

Illegal abortions, although rare in the US, are common worldwide; they carry a high risk of complications, including perforation of the uterus, septic abortion, and severe bleeding. Infertility or death often result.

Abrasion, dental
The wearing away of enamel, often accompanied by the wearing away of dentin (the layer beneath the enamel) and cementum (the bonelike tissue that covers the tooth root), usually through overvigorous brushing. The areas most commonly affected are the root surface and the front surfaces of the canine and premolar teeth where they emerge from the gum. The depressions produced by abrasion are often sensitive to very cold or hot food and may require use of a desensitizing dentifrice and/or protection with a *bonding* agent or *filling*.

Abreaction
The process of becoming consciously aware of repressed thoughts and feelings. In Freudian theory, abreaction ideally occurs via *catharsis*, the open expression of emotions associated with the forgotten memories. The term abreaction is sometimes used interchangeably with catharsis but, in its strictest sense, is the result of catharsis. Abreaction is an important part of *psychotherapy* and is more easily achieved when a recent, specific traumatic event is the source of the patient's symptoms.

Abscess
A collection of pus formed as a result of infection by microorganisms, usually bacteria. The pus is formed from destroyed tissue cells, from leukocytes (white blood cells) that have been carried to the area to fight infection, and from dead and live

microorganisms. The abscess may enlarge or subside, depending on whether the microorganisms or leukocytes gain the upper hand. Usually, a protective lining (pyogenic membrane) gradually forms around the abscess.

TYPES
Abscesses may develop in any organ and in the soft tissues beneath the skin in any area. Common sites include the breast (see *Mastitis*) and gums (see *Abscess, dental*). Rarer sites include the liver (see *Liver abscess*) and the brain (see *Brain abscess*).

Common sites for abscesses under the skin include the axilla (armpit) and the groin; these two areas have a large number of lymph glands that are responsible for fighting infection. A collar-button abscess is one in which a small abscess cavity under the skin connects via a sinus (channel) to a much larger one in deeper tissues.

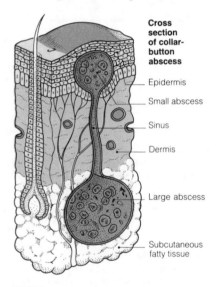

Cross section of collar-button abscess

Epidermis

Small abscess

Sinus

Dermis

Large abscess

Subcutaneous fatty tissue

CAUSES
Common bacteria, such as staphylococci, are the most common cause, although the bacillus responsible for tuberculosis is an important abscess-forming type. Fungal infections sometimes cause abscesses, while amebae (single-celled animal parasites) are an important cause of liver abscesses (see *Amebiasis*). The infection usually reaches an organ via the bloodstream or penetrates tissues under the skin via an infected wound or bite.

SYMPTOMS AND SIGNS
Symptoms of discomfort or pain depend mainly on the site of the abscess, though most larger ones, since they are a source of infection

within the body, cause fever (sometimes with chills), sweating, and malaise. Abscesses close to the skin usually cause inflammation with redness, increased skin temperature, and tenderness. Tuberculous abscesses are the exception; hence their description as cold abscesses.

DIAGNOSIS

The presence of an abscess within an organ may be apparent from symptoms and signs. Occasionally the diagnosis is confirmed by imaging techniques, such as *CT scanning*, *MRI*, or *radionuclide scanning* (using radioactively labeled white blood cells or the element gallium, which becomes concentrated in regions where pus has recently formed).

TREATMENT

Antibiotics are usually prescribed to treat a bacterial infection, antifungal drugs to treat fungi, and antiamebic drugs to treat amebiasis. However, the lining of the abscess cavity tends to reduce the amount of drug that can penetrate the source of infection from the bloodstream. The cavity itself therefore requires draining by making a cut in the lining and providing an escape route for the pus, either through a drainage tube (see *Drain, surgical*) or by leaving the cavity open to the skin.

OUTLOOK

Many abscesses subside after drainage alone; others subside after drainage and drug treatment. Occasionally, their presence within a vital organ, such as the liver or brain, damages enough surrounding tissue to cause some permanent loss of normal function.

Abscess, dental

A pus-filled sac in the tissue around the root of a tooth.

CAUSE

An abscess may occur when bacteria invade the pulp (the nerves and blood vessels that fill the central cavity of the tooth), causing the pulp to die. This most commonly happens as a result of dental *caries*, which destroy the tooth's enamel and dentin, allowing bacteria to reach the pulp. Bacteria can also gain access to the pulp when a tooth is injured. Bacteria enter either directly through a fracture or along damaged blood vessels. The infection in the pulp spreads into the surrounding tissue to form an abscess.

Abscesses can also result from *periodontal disease*, in which bacteria accumulate in the deep pockets that form between the teeth and gums.

SYMPTOMS AND SIGNS

The affected tooth aches or throbs and biting or chewing is usually extremely painful. The gum around the tooth is tender and may be red and swollen. An untreated abscess eventually erodes a sinus (small channel) through the jawbone to the gum surface, where it forms a gumboil (swelling). The gumboil may burst, discharging foul-tasting pus into the mouth, which usually lessens the pain. As the abscess spreads through surrounding tissues and bone, the glands in the neck and the side of the face may become swollen. Eventually, symptoms of infection, such as headache and fever, may develop.

TREATMENT

It is always best to try first to save the tooth. To do this, the abscess is drained by drilling through the crown of the tooth and into the pulp cavity to allow the pus to escape. The pulp cavity is then carefully cleaned and disinfected. An antibiotic may be prescribed if the infection has spread beyond the tooth. When the infection has cleared, the cavity is filled with dental cement (see *Root canal treatment*), sealed, and crowned.

When an abscess is caused by diseased pulp and the infection cannot be cleared with endodontic treatment, it is necessary to extract the tooth. However, this is a last resort. Extraction removes the source of infection and drains the abscess. Antibiotics are usually prescribed to clear any residual infection.

An abscess in a periodontal pocket can usually be treated by passing a probe into the pocket and gently scraping away infected material; sometimes it is necessary to make a small incision in the pocket to reach the abscess. If there is loss of bony support and periodontal ligament attachment due to severe periodontal disease, a dental *extraction* may need to be performed.

Absence

In medical terminology, a temporary loss or impairment of consciousness that occurs in some forms of *epilepsy*, typically petit mal seizures.

Acanthosis nigricans

A rare, untreatable condition characterized by thickened dark patches of skin in the groin, armpits, neck, and other skin folds. It may occur in young people as a genetic, inherited disorder, or as the result of an endocrine disorder, such as Cushing's

syndrome. It is also seen in people with carcinomas (malignant tumors) of the lung and other organs. The affected skin, which is thickened, rough, and may itch, is gray to black.

Pseudoacanthosis nigricans is a much more common condition, usually seen in dark-complexioned people who are overweight. In this form, the skin in fold areas, such as the groin, armpits, or neck, is both thicker and darker than the surrounding skin; there is usually excessive sweating in these areas. The condition may improve with dieting.

Access to care

A phrase used to describe a nation's medical system. Access refers both to the geographic accessibility of physicians and facilities, and the financial accessibility of medical services (i.e., the availability of funding provided individually, governmentally, charitably, or by insurance that would enable a person to pay for available needed medical care).

The degree of access in a medical system affects its cost; various attempts have been made to control costs through the regulation of access. Cost-sharing devices (making the patient financially responsible for a share of the fee or service) are regarded as a means of controlling access and, ultimately, overall costs.

Accident-prone

A tendency to have numerous mishaps as a result of some personality trait. Many psychologists doubt that the concept is valid, even though studies have shown that accidents are not distributed evenly among the population according to the laws of chance. A small group of people do seem to have more accidents, but this group changes constantly from study to study and no psychological test can isolate it.

Accidents may be slightly more common in aggressive and nonconforming men. However, emotional stress is probably the most important factor. Cycles of accidents seem to occur in the months after stressful "life events" regardless of the personality of the person involved.

Accidents

In people 1 to 37 years old, accidents are now the leading cause of death in the US. Accidental injuries, burns, drownings, and poisonings account for more than half of all deaths in youths aged 15 to 24 and for a quarter

A

CAUSES AND INCIDENCE OF ACCIDENTAL DEATH

In young people (up to 37 years), accidents are the leading cause of death. Burns, drownings, poisonings, and motor vehicle accidents are the most common causes. The very young and the very old are at greatest risk in their homes. The age groups in between tend to be victims of accidents elsewhere.

FIVE MOST COMMON CAUSES OF ACCIDENTAL DEATH BY AGE (Rates per 100,000 in each age group)

Age	0–1	1–4	5–14	15–24	25–44	45–64	65–74	75+	All ages
Most common cause	Choking 6.1	Motor vehicle 8.0	Motor vehicle 6.7	Motor vehicle 37.0	Motor vehicle 21.4	Motor vehicle 15.4	Motor vehicle 17.4	Falls 65.7	Motor vehicle 19.7
2nd	Motor vehicle 5.7	Drowning 4.8	Drowning 2.1	Drowning 4.2	Drowning 2.6 and Poison 2.6	Falls 4.0	Falls 10.1	Motor vehicle 25.2	Falls 5.2
3rd	Suffocation 4.5	Fires, burns 4.7	Fires, burns 1.4	Firearms 1.3		Fires, burns 2.3	Fires, burns 4.0	Choking 10.6	Drowning 2.7
4th	Fires, burns 3.8	Choking 0.9	Firearms 0.7	Poison 1.2	Falls 1.4 and Fires, burns 1.4	Drowning 1.9	Medical complications 3.9	Medical complications 9.0	Fires, burns 2.2
5th	Drowning 2.5	Falls 0.6	Falls 0.3	Fires, burns 1.1		Poison 1.5	Choking 3.6	Fires, burns 8.1	Poison 1.5

Accident mortality by age
Certain accidents are more common than others among different age groups. The very young are most likely to die from choking on bits of food or small objects, while the elderly are more likely to die as a result of falling in the home.

Incidence of fatal accidents by age
Among all age groups from infancy through the early 40s, accidents are the single most important cause of death.

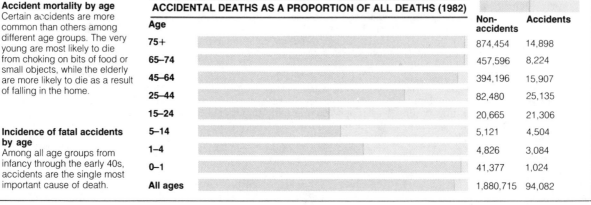

ACCIDENTAL DEATHS AS A PROPORTION OF ALL DEATHS (1982)

Age		Non-accidents	Accidents
75+		874,454	14,898
65–74		457,596	8,224
45–64		394,196	15,907
25–44		82,480	25,135
15–24		20,665	21,306
5–14		5,121	4,504
1–4		4,826	3,084
0–1		41,377	1,024
All ages		1,880,715	94,082

of all deaths in those aged 25 to 44. Accidents also cause much long-term physical and mental handicap; for every accident resulting in death, there are almost 10 that cause either major or minor disability.

Motor vehicle accidents are the most common cause of accidental death, accounting for 50 percent of the total. Nevertheless, the number of vehicle-related deaths has decreased in recent years. The introduction of lower speed limits in 1973 contributed to a steady decline in death rates (taking into account miles driven and number of cars owned). In the last few years there has been a decline in the actual number of deaths. This may be due in part to the raising of the drinking age in many states. Alcohol is an important factor in at least half of all fatal motor vehicle accidents. Another factor may be the introduction of mandatory seat belt laws in a growing number of states.

The home appears to be the most dangerous place for both the elderly and the very young. Falls are the second leading cause of death overall; in the elderly, they take first place. Twice as many people 75 years and older die from falls as from motor vehicle accidents. Most of these falls take place in the home while the victim is going about his or her everyday activities. Young people usually suffer only a bruise when they fall, but, in the elderly, bones are much more brittle and more than one third of the falls in those over 74 years old result in fracture of the spine, hipbone (femur), or wrist. Death often follows as a result of complications associated with the fracture.

Up to the age of 1 year, the most important cause of accidental death is choking on a morsel of food or an object placed in the mouth. Death from smothering by bedclothes, plastic bags, or other material is another major home hazard for infants.

THE MECHANISM OF ACCOMMODATION

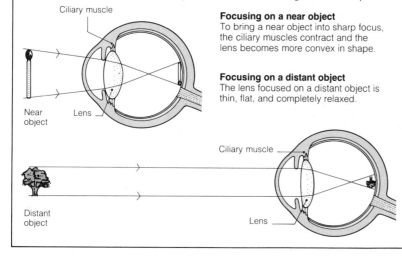

In a normal, healthy eye, light reflected from a near object is brought into focus on the retina by a process called accommodation. Focusing is achieved by an automatic change in lens shape.

Focusing on a near object
To bring a near object into sharp focus, the ciliary muscles contract and the lens becomes more convex in shape.

Focusing on a distant object
The lens focused on a distant object is thin, flat, and completely relaxed.

The young and the old are also particularly vulnerable to death from burns or asphyxiation as a result of house fires. One third of these victims are under 4 or over 75.

The third leading cause of accidental death is drowning. Eighty percent of the victims are male and most are under 45. Drowning most often occurs when victims are swimming or playing in water. However, it can also result from boating accidents or from falling into water near docks, bridges, or shores. At home, most drownings occur in the family's or a friend's swimming pool. For the very young, the bathtub is also a hazard.

For those 25 to 44, poisoning is almost as common a cause of death as drowning. In many cases, it is due to drug overdose, and suicide may be suspected. If it cannot be proved, the death is classified as accidental.

Accidents at work resulting in death have steadily decreased since the beginning of the century; they now account for less than 2 percent of all accidental deaths.

Accommodation
Adjustment, especially the process by which the eye adjusts itself to focus on near objects. At rest, the eye is focused for distant vision, with the lens relatively thin and flat. To make it possible to focus on a nearer object, the ciliary muscle of the eye contracts, allowing the elastic lens to become thicker and more convex.

With age, the lens loses its elasticity and, as a result, accommodation becomes increasingly difficult. This results in a form of farsightedness called *presbyopia*.

Accreditation
A device traditionally used by medical organizations to maintain and upgrade the standards of medical care through the granting or withholding of approval for teaching institutions, hospitals, and their programs.

Early in this century, the process became more effective as the states began to require graduation from an "accredited" medical school as a condition of licensure. In the very early part of this century, the *American Medical Association* led in the evaluation of medical schools; it was joined later in the accreditation of medical schools by the Association of American Medical Colleges. The American College of Surgeons began the early monitoring of the medical capabilities of hospitals. The accreditation process continues, but the various accrediting bodies now have a broader base, including a wider variety of organizations.

Acebutolol
A *beta-blocker* commonly used in the treatment of *hypertension* (high blood pressure), *angina pectoris* (chest pain due to impaired blood supply to heart muscle), and certain types of *arrhythmia* (irregular heart beat).

ACE inhibitor drugs

COMMON DRUGS

Captopril Enalapril

A group of *vasodilator drugs* introduced in 1981. ACE inhibitors (angiotensin-converting enzyme inhibitors) are used to treat *hypertension* (high blood pressure) and *heart failure* (reduced pumping efficiency), usually when other drugs have been ineffective. They are sometimes prescribed with other drugs such as *diuretic drugs* or *beta-blocker drugs*.

HOW THEY WORK
ACE inhibitors block the action of the enzyme that converts angiotensin (a protein present in the blood) from an inactive form, angiotensin I, to an active form, angiotensin II, which constricts (narrows) blood vessels. By reducing production of angiotensin II, ACE inhibitors reduce constriction of blood vessels, making it easier for blood to flow through them, and thus reducing blood pressure.

POSSIBLE ADVERSE EFFECTS
These include nausea, loss of taste, headache, dizziness, and a dry cough. The first dose may reduce blood pressure so dramatically that the patient collapses; treatment is therefore often started in the hospital.

Acetaminophen

ANALGESIC

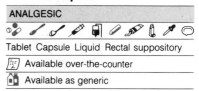

Tablet Capsule Liquid Rectal suppository

Available over-the-counter

Available as generic

A drug widely used since 1955 as an *analgesic* (painkiller). Acetaminophen is used to treat mild pain (for example, headache or toothache) and to reduce fever. Unlike *aspirin*, it does not cause stomach irritation or bleeding and so is particularly useful in the treatment of people who suffer from *peptic ulcer* or who cannot tolerate aspirin. Acetaminophen may also be used with safety to treat children. It was first introduced in the US in liquid form for infants and children. Acetaminophen does not have an anti-inflammatory effect, however, and so is less effective than aspirin as a treatment for joint pain in *arthritis*.

POSSIBLE ADVERSE EFFECTS
Taken in normal doses, nausea or a rash rarely occur. An overdose of acetaminophen may permanently damage the liver and can be fatal.

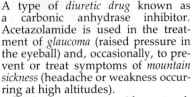

Acetazolamide

A type of *diuretic drug* known as a carbonic anhydrase inhibitor. Acetazolamide is used in the treatment of *glaucoma* (raised pressure in the eyeball) and, occasionally, to prevent or treat symptoms of *mountain sickness* (headache or weakness occurring at high altitudes).

During treatment with acetazolamide, adverse effects may include lethargy, nausea, diarrhea, weight loss, and impotence.

Acetic acid

The colorless, pungent, organic (carbon-containing) acid that gives vinegar its characteristic sour taste. In medicine, acetic acid is an ingredient of antiseptic jellies that are used to restore the acidity of the vagina in some types of vaginal infections.

Acetohexamide

An oral *hypoglycemic drug* used to treat non-insulin-dependent *diabetes mellitus*. Acetohexamide stimulates the secretion of *insulin*, a hormone that lowers the blood glucose level by increasing glucose absorption by cells.

Acetylcholine

A type of *neurotransmitter* (a chemical that transmits messages between nerve cells or between nerve and muscle cells). Acetylcholine (sometimes abbreviated to ACh) is the neurotransmitter at all nerve-muscle junctions as well as at many other sites in the nervous system. The actions of acetylcholine are called cholinergic actions; these actions are blocked by *anticholinergic drugs*.

Acetylcysteine

A *mucolytic drug* used in the treatment of chronic *bronchitis* and as an antidote for *acetaminophen* overdose.

HOW IT WORKS

Inhaled by *nebulizer*, acetylcysteine makes the mucus in sputum less sticky and therefore easier to cough up. To be effective as an antidote to acetaminophen poisoning, acetylcysteine must be taken by mouth within a few hours of the overdose; it works by reducing the amount of toxic substances produced during the breakdown of acetaminophen, thus reducing the risk of liver damage.

POSSIBLE ADVERSE EFFECTS

In rare cases, vomiting, rash, or increased breathing difficulty may occur when acetylcysteine is taken by nebulizer. Vomiting is common when this drug is taken by mouth.

Achalasia

A condition in which the muscles in the wall of the *esophagus* and the sphincter (valve) between the esophagus and stomach fail to relax after swallowing to permit food to enter the stomach.

Food normally stimulates the muscles in the wall of the esophagus to begin a series of contractions that pushes food toward the stomach. In achalasia, the sphincter does not relax to allow food to pass from the esophagus to the stomach, and the lowest part of the esophagus becomes narrowed and blocked with food.

INCIDENCE AND CAUSE

This rare condition can occur at any age, but is unusual before the age of 15. The underlying cause is unknown.

SYMPTOMS AND SIGNS

Symptoms include difficulty and pain with swallowing and pain in the lower chest and upper abdomen. Regurgitated food that may have been swallowed a day or two earlier may cause a foul taste and bad breath. The ability to swallow gradually deteriorates until there is difficulty swallowing liquids as well as solids.

DIAGNOSIS

A barium swallow (a type of *barium X-ray examination*) will show abnormal, ineffective movement of the esophageal wall and varying degrees of dilatation of the esophagus, as well as narrowing at the lowest end of the esophagus and failure of the sphincter to open after swallowing. *Gastroscopy*, in which a narrow viewing tube is passed down the esophagus, is used to check for *cancer* of the lowest end of the esophagus.

In achalasia, the pressure in the area of the lower esophageal sphincter is markedly elevated; pressure recordings taken while the patient swallows reveal that the esophageal sphincter is incompletely relaxed.

TREATMENT

Drug therapy may rarely help the symptoms of achalasia by relaxing the muscles at the lower end of the esophagus. If drug treatment fails, or if the symptoms worsen, it is possible to widen the esophagus for prolonged periods by passing a slender rubber bag down it and filling the bag with air or water to stretch the muscles (see *Esophageal dilatation*).

There is a surgical procedure that cuts some of the muscles at the stomach entrance to widen the passageway for food. Swallowing may return to normal, but the person may experience *acid reflux*.

Achilles tendon

The tendon that pulls up the back of the heel. It is formed from the calf muscles (the gastrocnemius, soleus, and plantar muscles) and attached to the *calcaneus* (heel bone). The tendon is named for the legendary Greek hero Achilles, who was vulnerable only in the heel.

Minor injuries to the tendon are common. They are usually due to overexercise, faulty running technique, or wearing incorrect footwear (particularly sport shoes with "tendon protectors"). All of these can cause inflammation of the tendon (*tendinitis*) and tearing of the tendon fibers. These conditions usually clear up with rest and physical therapy.

Violent stretching of the Achilles tendon can cause it to rupture. In such cases, surgical repair of the tendon may be necessary.

LOCATION OF THE ACHILLES TENDON
The tendon runs from the base of the calf to the calcaneus.

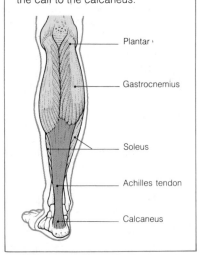

Plantar

Gastrocnemius

Soleus

Achilles tendon

Calcaneus

Achlorhydria

Absence of stomach acid secretions. This may be due to chronic atrophic *gastritis* or to an absence or malfunction of parietal, acid-producing cells in the internal lining of the stomach.

About one in every 20 normal people has achlorhydria without symptoms. Achlorhydria in itself is no cause for concern. It is, however, a feature of pernicious anemia, a blood disorder caused by defective absorption of vitamin B_{12} from the stomach (see *Anemia, megaloblastic*) and is present with some stomach cancers.

Achondroplasia

A rare disorder of bone growth, present from birth and leading to *short stature* (once called dwarfism). The affected bones are mainly the long bones of the arms and legs. The cartilage that links each bone to its epiphysis (growing area at its tip) is converted to bone too early, thus preventing further limb growth. Most other bones are able to grow normally.

Affected individuals have short, strong limbs, a well-developed trunk, and a head of normal size except for a somewhat protruding forehead.

INCIDENCE AND CAUSES

In the US and Europe, about two to three persons per 100,000 are achondroplastic. The condition is caused by a gene defect of the dominant variety (see *Genetic disorders*), although exactly how the gene defect leads to the disorder of bone growth is not known.

The children of achondroplastics each have a 50 percent chance of inheriting the defective gene and also of being achondroplastic. However, the parents of most achondroplastics are of normal stature. In these cases, the abnormality has arisen from a new gene defect, or *mutation*.

SYMPTOMS AND OUTLOOK

Achondroplasia is usually obvious at birth or during the first year of life, when there is already a noticeable stunting of the limbs relative to the size of the head. Growth of the limb bones slows and stops during childhood, and no treatment is available to alter the outlook. Intelligence and sexual development are not affected. Life span is close to normal.

Acid

Chemically, an acid is defined as a donor of hydrogen ions (atoms of hydrogen with a positive electrical charge). A wide variety of substances are acids. They include corrosive, mineral acids, such as sulfuric acid (used in automobile batteries) and hydrochloric acid (produced by the stomach lining), and organic acids, such as acetic acid (found in vinegar) and citric acid (found in lemon juice).

When mixed with, or dissolved in, water, acid molecules dissociate (split up) to release their constituent ions; all acids release hydrogen as the positive ion (positively charged ions are called cations, negatively charged ones are called anions). In addition, many acids react with some metals to release hydrogen gas. (See also *Acid-base balance; Alkali; Burns.*)

Acid-base balance

A combination of mechanisms that ensures that the body's fluids are neither too *acid* nor too alkaline (*alkalis* are also called bases). The body functions healthily only when its fluids are close to chemical neutrality.

Body metabolism involves the conversion of sugars and fats into energy, a process that uses oxygen and produces carbon dioxide (which forms carbonic acid when dissolved in water) and organic acids such as lactic and pyruvic acids. This produces fluctuations in the acidity and alkalinity of the blood and other body fluids.

To maintain normal acid-base balance, the body has three mechanisms: buffers, breathing, and the activities of the kidneys. Buffers are substances in the blood that tend to neutralize acid or alkaline wastes. Rapid breathing increases the rate at which carbon dioxide is eliminated from the blood, thereby making it less acid; conversely, slow breathing allows the blood to become more acid. The kidneys help maintain a constant acidity level in the blood by regulating the amounts of acid or alkaline wastes in the urine.

Disturbances of the acid-base balance result in *acidosis* (excessive blood acidity) or *alkalosis* (excessive blood alkalinity).

Acidosis

A disturbance of the body's *acid-base balance* in which there is an accumulation of acid or loss of alkali (base). There are two types of acidosis: metabolic and respiratory.

CAUSES

In metabolic acidosis, an increased amount of acid may be produced. Ketoacidosis, a form of metabolic acidosis, occurs in uncontrolled *diabetes mellitus* and, to a lesser degree, in starvation. Metabolic acidosis may also be caused by bicarbonate loss through severe diarrhea. In kidney failure there is insufficient excretion of acid in the urine. An overdose of aspirin, which is acidic itself and also causes an increase in acids produced by the process of cell metabolism, is a fairly common cause of metabolic acidosis.

Respiratory acidosis occurs when breathing fails to remove enough carbon dioxide from the lungs, which causes increased blood acidity because the excess carbon dioxide remains in the blood, where it dissolves to form carbonic acid. Impaired breathing leading to respira-

tory acidosis may be due to conditions such as *bronchitis*, bronchial *asthma*, or *airway obstruction*.

Acid reflux

Regurgitation of acidic fluid from the stomach into the *esophagus* (the tube connecting the throat with the stomach). It is associated with heartburn (a burning pain in the chest), and often leads to *esophagitis* (inflammation of the esophagus).

Mild acid reflux is common and of no serious significance. It may occur in pregnancy and often affects people who are overweight.

Acid reflux is attributed to inefficiency of the muscular valve at the lower end of the esophagus, which permits regurgitation of the acidic fluid. Repeated episodes of discomfort may indicate the presence of a *hiatal hernia*, a weakness in the diaphragm that permits part of the stomach to protrude into the chest.

Acne

A chronic skin disorder caused by inflammation of the hair follicles and the sebaceous glands.

TYPES

The most common type of acne is acne vulgaris, which mainly affects adolescents. Tropical acne affects young whites on unaccustomed exposure to hot, humid environments. Infantile acne, a rare condition affecting male infants, is associated with subsequent severe acne vulgaris in the teen years. Chemical acne is caused by exposure to certain chemicals and oils and results in acne in unusual sites, such as the legs. Chloracne is a form of acne caused by exposure to chlorinated hydrocarbon chemicals; many cases occurred following a severe explosion at a factory in Seveso, Italy, in 1976.

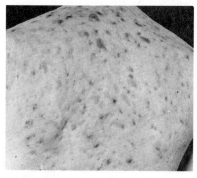

Severe acne
An example of cystic acne, with widespread scarring across the back. Few cases are as extensive as this.

INCIDENCE

Acne almost always begins during puberty, although it may develop later in life; most adolescent boys and many girls have some acne.

CAUSE

Acne spots are caused by the obstruction of the follicle by sebum (the oily substance secreted by the sebaceous glands in the skin). When a plug of sebum becomes trapped in the follicle, bacteria multiply and the follicle becomes inflamed. The cause of the change in sebum at puberty is uncertain but it seems to be linked with increased levels of *androgen hormones* (male sex hormones). There may also be a genetic factor, since acne can run in families.

Some drugs may bring on or aggravate existing acne (for example, corticosteroids and androgens, which increase oil production by the skin). Other drugs that can aggravate acne include barbiturates, isoniazid, rifampin, bromides, and iodides.

Oil and grease may also cause acne. The natural oil from the scalp may cause acne around the hairline. Regular contact with mineral or cooking oil, as in restaurant kitchens, can make the condition worse. Cosmetics with oily bases are also associated with an increased tendency to acne.

SYMPTOMS

Acne occurs in areas that have a high concentration of sebaceous glands, mainly the face, center of the chest, upper back, shoulders, and around the neck. The most common acne spots are comedones (blackheads), milia (whiteheads), pustules, nodules (firm swellings below the skin), and cysts (larger firm swellings in the skin). As each spot heals, others tend to appear. The healing spots often fade to a pink mark that usually disappears altogether, although some spots, particularly the cystic ones, may leave scars. Acne scars often appear as small, depressed pits. Occasionally, as with other scars, keloids (overgrowths of scar tissue) may form.

PREVENTION

There are many myths about the prevention of acne, particularly relating to diet. There is no evidence that diet plays any part in causing acne. For example, there is little point in avoiding sweets such as chocolate. Although washing affected areas does not prevent acne, it may keep it from spreading. The skin should be washed twice daily; more frequent washing is unnecessary, since washing simply removes surface oil.

TREATMENT

There is no instant cure for acne, although many treatments are available to relieve it. Topical (applied to the skin) treatments act by unblocking the pores and removing the sebum. They also help to promote healing. Topical applications that are most often used include benzoyl peroxide, retinoic acid, antibiotic lotions, and sulfur-containing creams. Ultraviolet light is often beneficial in treating acne. Exposure to natural sunlight is helpful, and artificial ultraviolet light may be used to treat more severe cases. The spots should not be picked or squeezed; this can worsen the condition and can lead to scarring.

If topical treatment has failed, long-term therapy with oral antibiotics often helps. The antibiotics are prescribed regularly for up to six months at a time. They have an effect not only on the bacteria in the skin but may also have a direct effect on inflammatory cells in acne lesions, as well as on sebum production.

A recent development in the treatment of acne is the use of retinoid drugs. These drugs are prescribed only for severe acne when antibiotics and other measures have not helped. Retinoid drugs reduce oil production and have a drying effect on the skin, but must be taken cautiously because they may cause liver damage and other serious problems.

Acne cysts can often be treated by intralesional therapy (direct injection of a drug into the acne spots), which also helps to reduce scarring. In cases of severe, extensive scarring, *derm-abrasion* (removal of the top layer of affected skin) can help improve the cosmetic appearance.

OUTLOOK

Acne improves slowly over a period of time, often clearing up by the end of the teenage years. With modern treatment, no one should have severe, scarring acne.

Acoustic nerve

Also called the auditory nerve, the acoustic nerve is the part of the *vestibulocochlear nerve* (the eighth *cranial nerve*) concerned with hearing.

Acoustic neuroma

A rare, benign tumor arising from supporting cells that surround the eighth cranial (auditory or acoustic) nerve, usually within the internal auditory meatus (the canal in the skull through which the nerve emerges into the inner ear).

INCIDENCE AND CAUSES

Acoustic neuromas constitute about 5 to 7 percent of primary *brain tumors*. They most commonly occur in people between the ages of 40 and 60 and are slightly more common in women than in men. In the US, about four to five cases per million population per year are diagnosed. Usually the cause is unknown. In some cases, however, tumors simultaneously affect the nerves on both sides of the head and may be part of a widespread *neurofibromatosis*, a disease characterized by changes in the nervous system, skin, and bones.

SYMPTOMS AND DIAGNOSIS

Acoustic neuroma can cause *deafness*, *tinnitus* (noises in the ear), loss of balance, and pain in the affected ear. As the tumor enlarges, it may compress the brain stem and cerebellum, causing *ataxia* (loss of coordination). As it expands, it presses on the fifth cranial nerve, causing pain in the face, or on the sixth cranial nerve, causing double vision.

Diagnosis is made by *hearing tests* and tests of balance, such as the *caloric test* or *electronystagmography*, followed by X rays or *CT scanning* to visualize the internal auditory meatus.

TREATMENT

The tumor is treated by surgical removal. Before the operation, a CT scan or MRI is used to show the location of the tumor and its approximate size, so that the surgeon can decide on the best route for removal. The results of surgery depend on the size of the tumor; in many cases, hearing can be preserved with no damage to the acoustic nerve. Occasionally, numbness and weakness of part of the face result from unavoidable damage to other surrounding nerves.

Acrocyanosis

A condition in which the hands and feet turn blue, may become cold, and sweat excessively. Acrocyanosis is caused by spasm in small blood vessels and is usually aggravated by cold weather.

Acrocyanosis is distantly related to a more serious circulatory disorder, *Raynaud's disease*, in which the skin of the fingers and toes may be damaged by chronically reduced blood flow.

Acrodermatitis enteropathica

A rare, inherited disease in which the skin of the fingers and toes, and the anal, mouth, and scalp area of infants, is reddened, ulcerated, and covered with pustules.

Acrodermatitis enteropathica is caused by an inability to absorb enough zinc from food. The addition of zinc supplements to the diet leads to quick improvement.

Acromegaly

A rare disease characterized externally by abnormal enlargement of the skull, jaw, hands, and feet.

CAUSE AND SYMPTOMS

Acromegaly is caused by excessive secretion of *growth hormone* from the anterior pituitary gland at the base of the brain and is the result of a benign tumor (see *Pituitary tumors*).

If such a tumor develops in a person within the first 10 years of life, the result is *gigantism* (in which growth is accelerated) and not acromegaly. More commonly, the tumor develops after growth in the long bones of the limbs has stopped. This leads to acromegaly, although it may take several years before the symptoms and signs appear.

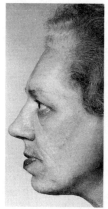

Appearance of acromegaly
The woman in profile at left shows many of the typical features of acromegaly—including lengthening of the face, enlargement of the jaw and nose, and general coarsening of the facial features.

Symptoms and signs of acromegaly include enlargement of the hands and feet, coarsening of the facial features, enlargement of the ears and nose, a jutting jaw, and a long face. Sufferers may notice a gradual increase in ring, shoe, glove, and hat size, and deepening or huskiness of the voice. Other possible symptoms are those common to any tumor in the brain, such as headache and visual disturbances.

DIAGNOSIS AND TREATMENT

If acromegaly appears to be developing in a person, the level of growth hormone in the blood is measured before and after a quantity of glucose has been administered. Glucose usually suppresses growth hormone secretion; if it has no effect on the blood level of the hormone, this confirms uncontrolled secretion of the hormone by the pituitary gland. *CT scanning* or *MRI* may reveal a tumor or overgrowth of the pituitary gland.

In some cases the drug bromocriptine may cause the pituitary tumor to regress; alternatively, the tumor may be treated by *radiation therapy* or removed surgically.

Acromioclavicular joint

The joint between the outer end of the clavicle (collarbone) and the acromion (the bony prominence at the top of the shoulder blade).

INJURIES TO THE JOINT

Injuries to the joint are rare. They are usually due to a fall on the shoulder and may result in subluxation (partial dislocation with the bones still in contact) or, rarely, dislocation (complete displacement of the bones).

In subluxation, the synovium (joint lining) and the ligaments around it are stretched and bruised, the joint is swollen, and the bones are felt to be slightly out of alignment. In dislocation, the ligaments are torn, the swelling is greater, and the bone deformity is pronounced. In both subluxation and dislocation, the joint is painful and tender, and movement of the shoulder is restricted.

Subluxation is treated by resting the arm and shoulder in a sling. If the pain and tenderness persist, an injection of a corticosteroid and a local anesthetic into the joint often helps.

Dislocation requires a strapping around the clavicle and elbow to pull the outer end of the clavicle back into position. The strapping is usually left on for three weeks.

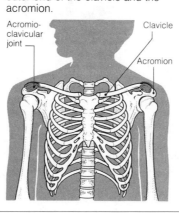

LOCATION OF THE ACROMIOCLAVICULAR JOINT
The joint lies at the junction of the outer end of the clavicle and the acromion.

Acromio-clavicular joint

Clavicle

Acromion

Osteoarthritis (degeneration of the joint), which makes shoulder movement painful, can develop if the joint suffers repeated injuries.

Acroparesthesia

A medical term used to describe tingling in the fingers or toes (see *Pins and needles sensation*).

ACTH

The commonly used abbreviation for adrenocorticotropic hormone (also called corticotropin), which is produced by the anterior part of the *pituitary gland* and stimulates the adrenal cortex (outer layer of the *adrenal glands*) to release various *corticosteroid hormones*. ACTH is also necessary for the maintenance and growth of the cells of the adrenal cortex.

ACTIONS

ACTH stimulates the adrenal cortex to increase production of the hormones *hydrocortisone* (cortisol), *aldosterone*, and *androgen hormones*. Most important of these is its stimulation of hydrocortisone production.

ACTH production is partly controlled by the *hypothalamus* (an area in the center of the brain) and partly by the level of hydrocortisone in the blood. When ACTH levels are too high, hydrocortisone production is increased; this, in turn, suppresses the release of ACTH from the pituitary gland. If ACTH levels are too low, the hypothalamus releases its hormones, stimulating the pituitary gland to increase ACTH production. This action stimulates the adrenal cortex to form hydrocortisone.

ACTH levels increase in response to stress, emotion, injury, infection, burns, surgery, and a decrease in blood pressure.

DISORDERS

A tumor of the pituitary gland can cause excessive ACTH production which, in turn, leads to overproduction of hydrocortisone by the adrenal cortex, resulting in *Cushing's syndrome*. Insufficient ACTH production due, for example, to hypopituitarism (underactivity of the pituitary gland), is rare. When it does occur, it causes *adrenal failure*.

MEDICAL USES

ACTH is used to treat inflammatory disorders such as *arthritis*, *ulcerative colitis*, and some types of *hepatitis*. It has also been employed to induce remissions in *multiple sclerosis* but its efficacy is uncertain. ACTH is also used to diagnose disorders of the adrenal glands.

A

Acting out

Impulsive actions that reflect unconscious wishes. The term is most often used by psychotherapists to describe behavior during analysis when the patient "acts out" rather than reports fantasies, wishes, or beliefs. Acting out can also occur outside of psychoanalysis as a reaction to frustrations encountered in everyday life. In this case it usually takes the form of antisocial, aggressive behavior that may be directed toward oneself or others. Typical behavior includes wrist-cutting, stealing, or impulsively starting new relationships; these activities cannot, however, always be explained in terms of acting out.

Actinic

Pertaining to changes caused by the ultraviolet rays in sunlight, as in actinic *dermatitis* (inflammation of the skin) and actinic *keratosis* (roughness and thickening of the skin), both of which are caused by overexposure, especially in the Southwest.

Actinomycosis

An infection caused by *ACTINOMYCES ISRAELII* or related actinomycete bacteria. These bacteria resemble fungi and cause diseases of the mouth and jaw, pelvis, and chest.

TYPES

The most common form of the disease affects the mouth and jaw. A painful swelling appears, usually on the jaw. Small openings later develop on the skin of the face and discharge pus and characteristic yellow granules. Poor oral hygiene may contribute to this form of the infection.

Another form of actinomycosis, affecting the pelvis, occurs in women and may cause lower abdominal pain, fever, and bleeding between menstrual periods. This form of the infection has been associated with the use of *IUDs* that do not contain copper. Rare forms of actinomycosis affect the appendix or lung.

DIAGNOSIS AND TREATMENT

A diagnosis of actinomycosis is usually confirmed by the presence of the granules. Treatment with large doses of penicillin is usually successful, although, in severe infections, medication may need to be continued for several months.

Acuity, visual

See *Visual acuity.*

Acupressure

A derivative of *acupuncture* in which pressure instead of a needle is applied to meridians (set points on the body).

Acupuncture

A branch of Chinese medicine in which needles are inserted into a patient's skin as therapy for various disorders or to induce anesthesia.

Traditional Chinese medicine holds that the Chi (life force) flows through the body along meridians (channels); blockage in one or more of these meridians is believed to cause ill health. Acupuncturists aim to restore health by inserting needles at appropriate sites, known as acupuncture points, on the affected meridians.

A cautious view is taken of acupuncture by orthodox medical practitioners, but some use it to complement other treatments.

HOW IT WORKS

Research suggests that acupuncture causes the release within the central nervous system of morphinelike substances, *endorphins*, which act as natural analgesics (painkillers). It has also been suggested that acupuncture may work by inducing a form of hypnosis or because insertion of the needles stimulates peripheral nerves, acting as a distraction from or a counterirritant to the original pain.

WHY IT IS DONE

Acupuncture has been used successfully as an anesthetic for dental procedures and surgical operations, and also during labor and delivery (including cesarean sections). Some practitioners use acupuncture to reduce pain after operations and also to relieve chronically painful conditions, such as arthritis, that are not responding to standard treatments.

It is claimed to be particularly effective for conditions of the muscles, bones, joints, eyes, heart, and the digestive, respiratory, and nervous systems; it is also claimed to help treat addiction, depression, and anxiety.

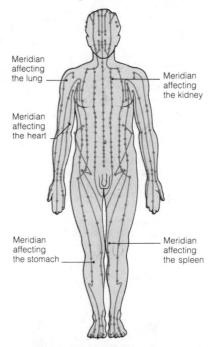

Meridian affecting the lung

Meridian affecting the kidney

Meridian affecting the heart

Meridian affecting the stomach

Meridian affecting the spleen

Acupuncture meridian lines

There are 14 major acupuncture meridians, each considered to affect a particular part of the body. Each meridian contains numerous acupuncture points (sites at which needles may be inserted).

HOW IT IS DONE

The traditional Chinese physician recognizes that accurate diagnosis is essential so that the acupuncturist knows which acupuncture points to use. Diagnosis in traditional Chinese medicine is made by examination of the patient's 12 pulses (six in each wrist). Each pulse is believed to give information about the health of a particular body region.

The precise disorder being treated or the degree of anesthesia required determines the temperature of the needle used, the angle of insertion, whether needles are twisted or vibrated while inserted, the speed of insertion and withdrawal, and the length of time the needles remain in position. Some practitioners pass a mild current through the needle to act as a stimulant in unblocking the meridian; others inject homeopathic remedies into the acupuncture point.

RISKS

Currently there are few legal checks on acupuncturists in the US and no formal qualification is necessary to practice. Infection is a possible risk but good practitioners avoid this with scrupulous sterilization techniques. It is rare that a blood vessel, body cavity, or organ is punctured.

Some people find that they experience a temporary exacerbation of their symptoms immediately following acupuncture treatment. Others experience lightheadedness, drowsiness, or exhilaration, although these feelings disappear soon after the treatment session has ended.

Acute

A term used to describe a disorder or symptom that comes on suddenly. Acute conditions may or may not be severe, and they are usually of short duration. (See also *Chronic*.)

Acyclovir

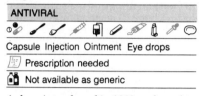

ANTIVIRAL

Capsule Injection Ointment Eye drops

Prescription needed

Not available as generic

A drug introduced in 1982 and used in the treatment of the virus that causes *herpes simplex* infections. Acyclovir is also used in the treatment of *herpes zoster* (shingles). Acyclovir also has some effect against *cytomegalovirus* and *Epstein-Barr virus* infections. To be effective, acyclovir must be prescribed soon after infection; it does not prevent attacks from recurring but does reduce their severity.

POSSIBLE ADVERSE EFFECTS
Adverse effects are uncommon. Acyclovir ointment may cause skin irritation or rash. Taken by mouth, acyclovir may cause headache, dizziness, nausea, or vomiting. In rare cases, acyclovir injections can cause kidney damage.

Adam's apple

A projection at the front of the neck, just beneath the skin, that is formed by a prominence on the thyroid cartilage, part of the larynx (voice box). It enlarges in males at puberty.

Addiction

Physiological and psychological dependence on and craving for a chemical substance (see *Alcohol dependence*; *Drug dependence*).

Addison's disease

A rare disorder in which symptoms are caused by a deficiency of the corticosteroid hormones *hydrocortisone* and *aldosterone*, normally produced by the adrenal cortex (part of the adrenal glands). The disease is named for the English physician Thomas Addison (1793-1860). It was invariably fatal before hormone treatment became available in the 1950s.

CAUSES
Addison's disease can be caused by any disease process that destroys the adrenal cortices. The most common cause is an *autoimmune disorder*, in which a person's immune system produces antibodies that attack the adrenal glands. *Tuberculosis* of the adrenal glands, once the main cause, is now very rare.

In addition to the deficient production of aldosterone and hydrocortisone, excessive amounts of ACTH and other hormones are poured out by the pituitary gland. Included among these hormones is one that increases the synthesis of melanin pigment in the skin.

SYMPTOMS AND DIAGNOSIS
Addison's disease generally has a slow onset and chronic course, with symptoms developing gradually over months or years. However, acute episodes, called Addisonian crises, can also occur; they are brought on by infection, injury, or other stresses. During these crises, the adrenal glands cannot increase their production of aldosterone and hydrocortisone, which normally help the body to cope with stress.

The symptoms of Addisonian crises are mainly due to aldosterone deficiency (which leads to excessive loss of sodium and water in the urine), extreme muscle weakness, dehydration, *hypotension* (low blood pressure), confusion, and coma.

Symptoms of the chronic form of Addison's disease include tiredness, weakness, vague abdominal pain, and weight loss. A more specific symptom is darkening of the skin in the creases of the palms and pressure areas of the

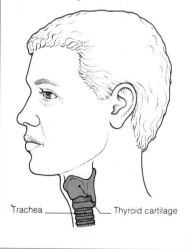

LOCATION OF THE ADAM'S APPLE
This projection at the front of the neck, beneath the skin, is formed by a prominence on the thyroid cartilage.

Trachea   Thyroid cartilage

body, and most particularly in the mouth. The darkening is caused by excessive production by the pituitary of the hormone that stimulates melanin production.

Diagnosis is generally made if the patient fails to respond to an injection of ACTH, which normally stimulates the secretion of hydrocortisone.

TREATMENT
Treatment of acute Addisonian crises involves monitoring blood pressure and heart rate during the rapid infusion of saline, and supplementary doses of hydrocortisone and fludrocortisone to correct the sodium deficiency and dehydration. Long-term treatment of the disease requires replacement of the deficient hormones with *corticosteroid drugs*.

Because patients with Addison's disease cannot increase their output of corticosteroid hormones in response to stress, they are at risk during stressful situations such as infection, surgery, or injury. Their physicians must instruct them in the use of increased doses of corticosteroid drugs at such times so that the body mechanisms that fight infection and promote healing are not impaired.

Adduction

Movement of a limb toward the central line of the body, or of a digit toward the axis of a limb. Muscles that carry out this movement are often called adductors. The opposite movement is called *abduction*.

Adenitis

Inflammation of a gland, particularly of a lymph gland. Cervical adenitis (swollen, tender lymph glands in the neck) occurs in certain infections (especially *tonsillitis*) caused by streptococcal bacteria, and in infectious *mononucleosis*. In the past, adenitis was often due to scrofula (tuberculosis infection of the cervical lymph nodes).

Mesenteric lymphadenitis is inflammation of the lymph glands in the peritoneum (the membrane that encloses the intestines) caused by a viral infection. The symptoms of mesenteric lymphadenitis—mainly abdominal pain and tenderness—may mimic those of appendicitis and may require an exploratory operation to confirm a diagnosis.

Treatment of adenitis may include the use of analgesics (painkillers), hot compresses, or a heating pad, and, if a bacterial infection is suspected, antibiotic drugs. The inflammation usually subsides within a few days.

Adenocarcinoma

The technical name for a malignant tumor, or cancer, of a gland or glandular tissue, or a tumor of which the gland-derived cells form glandlike structures. An adenocarcinoma arises from epithelium, the layer of cells that lines the inside of an organ.

Cancers of the colon (the main part of the large intestine), breast, pancreas, and kidney are usually adenocarcinomas, as are a proportion of cancers of the cervix, esophagus, salivary glands, and many other organs. (See *Intestine, cancer of; Pancreas, cancer of; Kidney cancer.*)

Adenoidectomy

Surgical removal of the *adenoids*, usually performed on a child with abnormally large adenoids that are causing recurrent infections of the middle ear or air sinuses. The operation is often performed in conjunction with *tonsillectomy*.

Adenoidectomy is generally an operation with minimal aftereffects. The patient usually can begin to eat normally the following day.

Adenoids

Two swellings at the back of the nose, above the tonsils, made up of *lymph nodes* (tissues that contain lymphocytes, which are white cells that help fight infection). These nodes form part of the body's defense against upper respiratory tract infections; they tend to enlarge during early childhood, a time when infections of this type are common.

DISORDERS
In most children, adenoids shrink after the age of about 5 years, disappearing altogether by puberty. In some children, however, they become even larger and obstruct the passage from the nose to the throat, causing snoring, breathing through the mouth, and a characteristically nasal voice. They can also block the eustachian tube (which connects the middle ear to the throat), causing infection and deafness.

Obstruction to the flow of secretions behind the nose can result in rhinitis (infection of the nose), which can spread to the middle ear (see *Otitis media*) and the air sinuses behind the nose (see *Sinusitis*).

DIAGNOSIS AND TREATMENT To discover whether ear, nose, and throat infections are being caused by abnormally enlarged adenoids, the physician usually inspects the back of the throat using a mirror with a light attached. Infections usually respond to antibiotics; if infections recur frequently, *adenoidectomy* (surgical removal of the adenoids) may be advised.

Adenoma

A benign, noncancerous tumor arising from the epithelium (cell layer lining the inner surface) of any gland, forming a benign glandlike tumor or cyst.

Adenomas of endocrine glands (those that secrete hormones directly into the bloodstream), such as the pituitary, thyroid, and adrenal glands and pancreas, can cause disease resulting from excessive hormone production. Pituitary adenomas, for example, can result in *acromegaly* or *Cushing's syndrome*.

Adenomatosis

An abnormal condition of glands in which they are affected either by *hyperplasia* (overgrowth) or by the development of numerous *adenomas* (benign tumors).

Adenomatosis may simultaneously affect two or more different endocrine glands, such as the adrenal, parathyroid, and pituitary glands and pancreas. (See also *Adrenal tumors; Parathyroid tumors.*)

ADH

The abbreviation for antidiuretic hormone (also called vasopressin), which is released from the posterior part of the *pituitary gland* and acts on the kidneys to increase their reabsorption of water into the blood.

ACTIONS
ADH reduces the amount of water lost in the urine and helps control the body's overall water balance. Water is continually being taken into the body in food and drink and is also produced by the chemical reactions in cells. Conversely, water is continually being lost in urine, sweat, feces, and in the breath as water vapor. ADH helps maintain the optimum amount of water in the body.

ADH production is controlled by the *hypothalamus* (an area in the center of the brain), which detects changes in the concentration and volume of the blood. If the blood concentration increases (i.e., contains less water), the hypothalamus stimulates the pituitary gland to release more ADH. If the blood is too dilute, less ADH is produced and, as a result, more water is lost from the body in the urine.

DISORDERS
Various factors can affect ADH production and thus disturb the body's water balance. For example, alcohol reduces ADH production by direct action on the brain, resulting in temporarily increased production of urine. This may also occur in *diabetes insipidus*, a disorder in which there is either insufficient production of ADH in the pituitary gland or, rarely, failure of the kidneys to respond to ADH.

The reverse effect, water retention, may result from temporarily increased ADH production after a major operation or accident. Water retention may also be caused by the secretion of ADH by some tumors, especially of the lung.

DRUG THERAPY
Synthetic ADH is given via the nose or by injection to treat diabetes insipidus. High intravenous doses cause narrowing of blood vessels and may stop bleeding from *esophageal varices*. Adverse effects include abdominal cramps, nausea, headache, drowsiness, and confusion.

Adhesion

Fibrous tissue within the body that joins normally unconnected parts. Although sometimes present from birth, adhesions are usually scar tissue formed after inflammation.

The most common site of adhesions is the abdomen, where they often form after *peritonitis* (inflammation of the abdominal lining), or following surgery as part of the natural healing

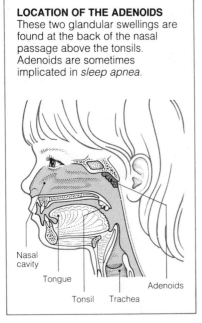

LOCATION OF THE ADENOIDS
These two glandular swellings are found at the back of the nasal passage above the tonsils. Adenoids are sometimes implicated in *sleep apnea*.

Nasal cavity

Tongue

Adenoids

Tonsil   Trachea

process. Abdominal adhesions infrequently bind together loops of intestine, resulting in intestinal obstruction (see *Intestine, obstruction of*). In such cases, an operation is usually required to cut the fibrous tissue and free the intestinal loops.

Adipose tissue

A layer of fat just beneath the skin and around various internal organs. After puberty, the distribution of superficial adipose tissue differs in males and females. Adipose tissue makes up a larger proportion of total body weight in women than it does in men.

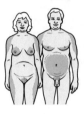

Distribution of adipose tissue
In adult males, adipose tissue accumulates around the shoulders, waist, and abdomen; in women, it accumulates on the breasts, hips, and thighs.

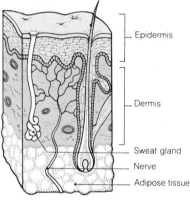

Epidermis

Dermis

Sweat gland

Nerve

Adipose tissue

FUNCTIONS AND DISORDERS

Adipose tissue is built up from fat deposited as a result of excess food intake, thus acting as an energy store; excessive amounts of adipose tissue produce *obesity*. The tissue acts as an insulator against loss of body heat, particularly in babies. Adipose tissue helps absorb shock in areas subject to sudden or frequent pressure, such as the buttocks and feet. It also surrounds and cushions the heart, kidneys, and other internal organs.

Adjuvant

A substance that enhances the action of another substance in the body. The term is usually used to describe an ingredient added to a *vaccine* to increase the production of antibodies by the immune system, therefore enhancing the vaccine's efficiency in conferring immunity. Adjuvant

chemotherapy is the addition of treatment with cytotoxic (anticancer) drugs to the surgical removal of a tumor.

Adlerian theory

A discipline of psychology set forth by the Austrian psychiatrist Alfred Adler (1870-1937).

Adolescence

The period between childhood and adulthood. Broadly speaking, adolescence corresponds to the teen years. A complex stage of personality development and psychological upheaval, adolescence overlaps with, but is not the same as, *puberty*. Puberty is the period of hormonally regulated development when the secondary sex characteristics appear, marking the onset of physical and sexual maturity.

FEATURES

Adolescence is a time of much change for the individual and for the adolescent's family. The adolescent must come to terms with the body's physical changes and with the fact that family and society no longer expect or tolerate childish behavior. During adolescence, the adult's self-identity is formed. This involves achieving independence and emotional separation from parents, understanding adult sexual roles, and learning to use increased aggressive drive. Adolescence is also a time of forming attitudes and opinions.

Adolescents would like to be independent but many must still rely on adults for emotional and financial support. Parental conflicts often arise when adolescents demand increased independence before their parents consider them ready for it.

During the process of achieving an adult identity, the adolescent ceases to define himself or herself only in terms of the adults who are at home and at school, which is what a child does. He or she may seek other figures (such as pop stars) as role models or leaders and may rebel against parental standards and family. Adolescents experiment with views and opinions, with allegiances to peer groups and gangs, and with political movements. They may adopt outrageous fashions of dress, appearance, and behavior.

Sexual experimentation occurs in fantasy and in reality, alone and with others. Gender identity may be questioned; this may be the time that a person first realizes that he or she is homosexual. Often during adolescence, homosexual behavior occurs temporarily. Coming to terms with

sexual drives may be influenced by the adolescent's perception of his or her parents' relationship.

PROBLEMS

Common patterns of adolescent behavior include moodiness, loss of interest in school, fluctuating school performance, and, in extreme cases, truancy. Adolescents worry tremendously about their physical appearance, acne, their changing body shape, and whether they are physically attractive. They may feel nervous, depressed, and withdrawn, and may become painfully shy and lacking in confidence. Often they feel very unsure of their personal identity, suffering a so-called "identity crisis." There may be a strong sense of alienation from parents, who may feel they can no longer talk to their children.

Some adolescents are overassertive and strive prematurely for independence. Rebellion against parents is often exaggerated in adolescents who were overdependent on, or overprotected by, their parents during childhood (such as those with a chronic physical illness). Childhood deprivation that has resulted in weak *bonding* between child and parents can also lead to extreme rebelliousness. On the other hand, a teenager who remains too dependent may remain stuck in adolescence and not grow enough to make his or her own decisions or to form new relationships outside the family.

Aggressive drives that are not controlled and used constructively can lead to outbursts of bad temper or other undesirable behavior. Delinquency is common in adolescents from all backgrounds, but is usually a transient phase if dealt with by a mixture of firmness and understanding.

Adolescents (and children who are younger) may become involved in drug abuse for experimentation, for kicks, or commonly because of peer group pressure. Those youngsters who take drugs to relieve anxiety or depression are more likely to become dependent. Recently, solvent abuse (glue sniffing) has become widespread, particularly among boys.

A high proportion of adolescents with serious or prolonged psychological and behavioral problems, particularly drug abuse and delinquency, are from disturbed or deprived home environments where there is poverty, marital disharmony, alcoholism, or psychiatric disturbance in the parents. Unsocial behavior is also more likely in adolescents who have had

A

behavioral problems (see *Behavioral problems in children*).

Adolescents are often referred for specialized advice because parents or teachers are worried about their behavior. Only a small percentage of those referred need psychiatric medicines and/or hospitalization. Most have temporary problems that resolve on their own. Psychological problems underlie the development of *anorexia nervosa*. Major psychotic illnesses—*schizophrenia* and *manic-depressive illness*—are almost never seen before adolescence, although "identity crisis" may mimic psychosis temporarily. Love problems and family problems can provoke suicidal attempts in disturbed adolescents.

Maintaining communication with their offspring is highly important but not always easy for parents. Parents should give practical help on problems such as acne and diet and never laugh off or underestimate seemingly minor problems; this may undermine the adolescent's confidence. The most valuable support a parent can give the adolescent is encouraging self-confidence. Confidence will provide a firm foundation for coping with the increasing pressures and responsibilities of adult life.

ADP
Abbreviation for adenosine diphosphate, the chemical that takes up energy released during biochemical reactions to form *ATP* (adenosine triphosphate), the main energy-carrying chemical in the body. When ATP releases its energy, ADP is reconstituted. (See also *Metabolism*.)

Adrenal failure
Insufficient production of hormones by the adrenal cortex. It can be acute (of sudden onset) or chronic (of more gradual onset). When chronic adrenal failure is due to a disease or damage to the adrenal gland itself, it is called *Addison's disease*. It can, however, also result from reduced stimulation of the adrenal cortex by *ACTH*, a hormone produced by the pituitary gland (see *Adrenal glands* disorders box).

Adrenal glands
A pair of endocrine glands (glands that secrete hormones directly into the bloodstream). Small and triangular, they sit on top of the kidneys.

Each adrenal gland can be divided, anatomically and functionally, into two distinct organs. The outer region is the adrenal cortex. It secretes *cor-*

ANATOMY OF THE ADRENAL GLANDS
Also sometimes called the suprarenal glands, the adrenal glands are situated on top of the kidneys. Each one is divided into two regions: the adrenal cortex (which secretes hormones that affect the metabolism) and the adrenal medulla (which is part of the sympathetic nervous system).

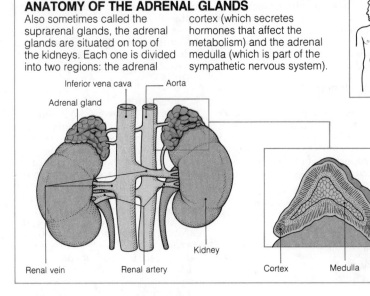

ticosteroid hormones that have important effects on the body's *metabolism* (the way in which energy stores and food are used), on chemicals in the blood, and on characteristics such as hairiness and body shape.

The smaller, inner region of the gland is the adrenal medulla, which is part of the *sympathetic nervous system*, the body's first line of response and defense against physical and emotional stresses.

FEEDBACK MECHANISM
The rate at which many glands produce hormones is influenced by other hormones, especially those secreted by the pituitary gland and the hypothalamus. If too much hormone is produced, negative feedback mechanisms act on the hypothalamus and pituitary so that they produce less of their stimulating hormones; thus reducing the target gland's activity. If too little hormone is produced, the feedback weakens, leading to increased production of the stimulating hormones.

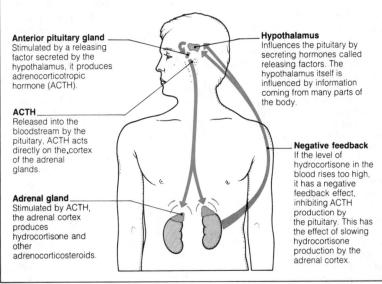

Anterior pituitary gland
Stimulated by a releasing factor secreted by the hypothalamus, it produces adrenocorticotropic hormone (ACTH).

ACTH
Released into the bloodstream by the pituitary, ACTH acts directly on the cortex of the adrenal glands.

Adrenal gland
Stimulated by ACTH, the adrenal cortex produces hydrocortisone and other adrenocorticosteroids.

Hypothalamus
Influences the pituitary by secreting hormones called releasing factors. The hypothalamus itself is influenced by information coming from many parts of the body.

Negative feedback
If the level of hydrocortisone in the blood rises too high, it has a negative feedback effect, inhibiting ACTH production by the pituitary. This has the effect of slowing hydrocortisone production by the adrenal cortex.

DISORDERS OF THE ADRENAL GLANDS

Excessive or deficient production of hormones by the adrenal glands can occur in a variety of ways. These disorders are uncommon, but may be serious. Disturbed hormone production by the adrenal cortex is more common than disturbance of the adrenal medulla.

CONGENITAL DEFECTS

Congenital *adrenal hyperplasia* affects about one newborn baby in 10,000. The adrenal cortex is unable to synthesize sufficient hydrocortisone and (sometimes) aldosterone, and the baby is ill or fails to thrive. As a side effect of the reduced hydrocortisone production, the glands are stimulated to produce androgens (male sex hormones) in excess; this can cause masculinization of female babies.

TUMORS

Growths in the adrenal glands are rare and generally lead to excess hormone production. Excess secretion of aldosterone causes *aldosteronism*, a condition characterized by thirst and high blood pressure. Excess secretion of hydrocortisone causes *Cushing's syndrome*, which is characterized by muscle-wasting and obesity of the trunk. Androgens may also be produced to excess, causing masculinization in females.

Tumors of the adrenal medulla include *pheochromocytoma* and *neuroblastoma*. Excess epinephrine and norepinephrine are secreted, causing a rise in blood pressure.

AUTOIMMUNE DISORDERS

Deficient production of hormones by the adrenal cortex is called *adrenal failure*; if due to disease of the adrenal glands themselves, it is called *Addison's disease*. The most common cause of Addison's disease is an autoimmune process (in which the body's immune system attacks its own tissues). Addison's disease can take a chronic course, characterized by weakness, weight loss, and skin darkening, or an acute form (Addisonian crisis or acute adrenal failure), in which the patient may become confused and comatose.

INFECTION

Destruction of the adrenal glands by *tuberculosis* was once a major cause of Addison's disease; it is now uncommon compared with autoimmune causes. The onset of infection or other acute illness can precipitate acute adrenal failure in someone with Addison's disease.

IMPAIRED BLOOD SUPPLY

Loss or obstruction of the blood supply to the adrenals, sometimes as a result of arterial disease, is another possible cause of Addison's disease or acute adrenal failure.

OTHER DISORDERS

In many cases disturbed activity of the adrenals is caused not by disease of the glands, but by an increase or decrease in the blood level of hormones that influences their activity.

Hydrocortisone production by the adrenal cortex is controlled by the secretion of *ACTH* (adrenocorticotropic hormone) by the pituitary gland. A tumor or other disorder of the pituitary, or tumors elsewhere in the body, can cause excess ACTH secretion, leading to too much hydrocortisone being produced by the adrenals and, hence, leading to Cushing's syndrome. Pituitary disease is, in fact, the most common cause of Cushing's syndrome.

Destruction or removal of the pituitary has the opposite effect, stopping ACTH secretion, preventing stimulation of the adrenal cortex, and leading to adrenal failure.

INVESTIGATION

Suspected disturbance of adrenal function is investigated by measurement of the levels of hormones such as hydrocortisone, aldosterone, epinephrine, and ACTH in the blood plasma and/or urine.

Tests may also be carried out to measure the effects of an injected substance that would normally modify the production of a hormone. Such tests can help localize the underlying cause of the disorder—for example, to distinguish Cushing's syndrome due to an adrenal tumor from that due to pituitary disease.

If disease of the adrenal glands themselves is suspected, the glands may be imaged by such techniques as *CT scanning*, *arteriography*, *radionuclide scanning*, or intravenous *pyelography* (which is more likely to show any downward displacement of the kidney by an adrenal gland tumor). If a tumor or overgrowth of a gland is present, it will usually be detectable by one of these techniques.

THE ADRENAL CORTEX

The adrenal cortex is made up of three distinct zones, visible under a microscope. The outermost zone secretes the hormone *aldosterone*, which inhibits the amount of sodium excreted in the urine, maintaining blood volume and blood pressure.

The inner and middle zones together secrete the hormones *hydrocortisone* (also called cortisol) and corticosterone, as well as small amounts of *androgen hormones* (hormones that stimulate the development of male sex characteristics). Hydrocortisone is the most important human corticosteroid, controlling the body's use of fats, proteins, and carbohydrates. Hydrocortisone and corticosterone also have the effect of suppressing inflammatory reactions in the body and also, to some extent, the activities of the *immune system*.

Like the other endocrine glands, the adrenal cortices secrete hormones directly into the blood; the amount is governed by other hormones made in the hypothalamus and pituitary.

The rate of hydrocortisone secretion, controlled by the release of *ACTH* (adrenocorticotropic hormone) by the pituitary gland, varies throughout the 24-hour cycle, being minimal at midnight, rising to a peak at around 6:00 AM, and then falling slowly during the day.

Emotion, stress, and injury are potent stimulators of ACTH and hydrocortisone release; without hydrocortisone, the body is unable to recover properly from stress.

THE ADRENAL MEDULLA

The adrenal medulla is closely related to nervous tissue and secretes the hormones *epinephrine* and *norepinephrine* in response to stimulation by sympathetic nerves. These nerves are most active at times of stress.

A

The release of these hormones into the circulation produces effects similar to sympathetic nerve stimulation. The heart rate and force of contraction increases so that more blood can be pumped around the body, and the airways of the lungs are widened to make breathing easier. The hormones constrict blood vessels in the intestines, kidneys, and liver, and widen blood vessels supplying the skeletal muscles. Consequently, more blood is supplied to the active muscles and less to the internal organs.

Adrenal hyperplasia, congenital

A rare disorder, present at birth, caused by the deficient production of the hormones *hydrocortisone* and *aldosterone* by the adrenal glands and overproduction of *androgen hormones* (male sex hormones).

CAUSES

Most cases result from a gene defect (see *Genetic disorders*), causing lack of an enzyme required by the adrenal cortex to make hydrocortisone. Instead, the materials normally used to make hydrocortisone are channeled into manufacturing androgens, which are produced to excess.

The disorder affects about one in 10,000 babies and is the most common cause of ambiguous genitals at birth.

SYMPTOMS

Symptoms, which vary considerably in severity, are caused by excess androgens and the deficiency of hydrocortisone and aldosterone.

In the most severe forms, a female infant is born with what appears to be a penis and scrotum. Within a few days, vomiting and dehydration occur. Similar symptoms occur in male babies except that the genitals appear normal.

In less severe cases, a considerable delay may occur before the syndrome is recognized. In girls, the clitoris may enlarge to form what appears to be a small penis, and other male characteristics develop, such as deepening of the voice and absence of menstruation at puberty. In boys, puberty may occur early. Untreated, the condition causes infertility in both sexes.

DIAGNOSIS AND TREATMENT

The diagnosis is suggested by the signs and symptoms at birth or later in childhood or adolescence and is confirmed by the measurement of corticosteroid hormones in the blood and urine. *Ultrasound scanning* will show the adrenals to be enlarged but with no tumor present.

Treatment consists of replacing the missing hormones. If the condition is recognized and treatment started early, normal sexual development and fertility usually follow. (See also *Hermaphroditism; Sex determination*.)

Adrenaline
See *Epinephrine*.

Adrenal tumors
Rare malignant or benign tumors within the adrenal gland that usually secrete hormones to excess.

Aldosterone-secreting and hydrocortisone-secreting tumors of the adrenal cortex cause, respectively, primary *aldosteronism* (also called Conn's syndrome) and *Cushing's syndrome*.

Excess secretion of epinephrine and norepinephrine from the adrenal medulla may be caused by two types of adrenal tumors—*neuroblastoma* or *pheochromocytoma*. The tumors cause *hypertension* (high blood pressure) and sweating attacks.

Surgical removal of a tumor, or even a whole adrenal gland, often results in cure of the conditions caused by the excess hormone secretion. (See also *Adrenal glands* disorders box.)

Adrenocorticotropic hormone
See *ACTH*.

Adrenogenital syndrome
See *Adrenal hyperplasia, congenital*.

Aerobic
Requiring oxygen to live and grow. Humans and almost all other forms of life are dependent on oxygen for "burning" foods to produce energy (see *Metabolism*). Because of this dependence, they are described as obligate aerobes. In contrast, many bacteria have fundamentally different metabolisms and thrive without oxygen (some of them are even killed by it); such microorganisms are described as *anaerobic*. There are also some bacteria and yeasts (called facultative aerobes) that flourish in oxygen but can also live without it.

Aerobics
Exercise in which the body is able to meet the muscles' increased demand for oxygen continuously during increased activity. Aerobic means "requiring air to live."

Oxygen is necessary to release energy from the body's stores of fat, glycogen (starchy storage material), and sugars. In aerobic exercises, a constant supply reaches the muscles.

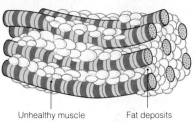

Unexercised muscle

Unhealthy muscle   Fat deposits

Exercised muscle

Healthy muscle

Good flow of oxygen

Benefits of aerobic exercise
Regular aerobic exercise improves the condition of the muscles. The supply of blood-carrying oxygen to the muscles is increased and the cells' capacity to use oxygen is consequently enhanced.

During aerobic exercises, such as swimming, jogging, and cycling, the rate at which oxygen reaches the muscles keeps pace with the rate at which it is used up. Because of this continual replenishment, the activity can be sustained for long periods. In contrast, anaerobic exercises rely on a different series of biochemical reactions to obtain energy from the stores of sugar and fat in muscle. The waste products of anaerobic exercise are acidic and, as they accumulate in muscles, the muscles become fatigued. Brief high-intensity exercises are anaerobic and can be performed for only short periods.

BENEFITS OF AEROBIC EXERCISE

To benefit your health, aerobic exercises should involve the large muscles of the trunk, upper body, and legs and need to be performed continuously for 20 minutes at least three times a week.

When performed regularly, aerobic exercises improve stamina and endurance. They encourage the growth of capillaries (small blood vessels), thus improving the supply of blood to the cells. They also increase the size and number of mitochondria (the energy-producing part of muscle cells), thus improving the cells' capacity to use oxygen and increasing the amount of oxygen that the body can use in a given time.

The condition of the heart is also improved as the body becomes more fit. The heart rate becomes slower during both exercise and rest, the heart muscle becomes thicker and stronger, and the stroke volume (the amount of blood pumped with each beat) is increased. As a result of these changes, the heart must do less work to achieve the same level of efficiency.

For all-around fitness, which includes strength and suppleness, other types of exercise should be performed as well as aerobics. (See also *Exercise; Fitness.*)

Aerodontalgia

Sudden pain in a tooth brought on by a change in surrounding air pressure. Flying at a high altitude in a lowered atmospheric pressure can cause a pocket of air within the dental pulp chamber to expand and irritate the nerve in the root. Common sources of aerodontalgia are improperly fitted fillings, inadequately filled root canals, and the presence of pulpitis (inflammation of the pulp).

Aerophagia

Excessive swallowing of air. This can occur during rapid eating or drinking or it can be caused by anxiety. It may also be a deliberate action to relieve indigestion by inducing belching. After *laryngectomy* (surgical removal of the larynx), voluntary aerophagia is used to produce esophageal speech.

Affect

Inner feelings at a particular moment; mood. This Freudian term is sometimes used to describe the mood as perceived by another person. Normal affect varies according to personality and setting. A person whose responses to events seem flat—so that nothing excites, nothing angers—is said to have a shallow, flattened, or reduced affect; this characteristic may be a sign of a mental disorder (see *Affective disorders*).

Affective disorders

Mental illnesses dominated by a disturbance of affect (mood). Affective disorders include various degrees of *mania* (elation and excitement) and *depression*, as well as *manic-depressive illness* (swings of mood between the two). The disorders may be psychotic (involving loss of contact with reality) or neurotic (involving no loss of contact with reality) and are sometimes the result of another physical or psychiatric illness.

Affinity

The attraction between chemicals that causes them to bind together, as, for example, between an *antigen* (a protein that stimulates the body to produce antibodies against it) and an antibody (see *Immune response*). The term is also used in microbiology to describe a physical similarity between organisms (e.g., viruses); it is used in psychology to describe an attraction between two people.

Aflatoxin

 A poisonous substance produced by *ASPERGILLUS FLAVUS* molds, which contaminates stored foods, especially grains, peanuts, and cassava. Aflatoxin has been found to cause liver cancer in laboratory animals and is believed to be one of the factors responsible for the high incidence of this cancer in tropical Africa and Asia.

Afterbirth

Common name for the *placenta*, the structure that provides the link between the circulations of the woman and fetus.

Afterpains

Contractions of the uterus that continue after childbirth. Afterpains are normal and indicate that the uterus is shrinking as it should. They are common during the first few days after delivery and are particularly painful during breast-feeding. Afterpains disappear after a few days but may require analgesics (painkillers).

Agar

An extract of certain seaweeds with properties similar to those of gelatin. Its full name is agar-agar. It is sold to soften and give bulk to feces in cases of constipation, and to relieve indigestion and heartburn because of its bland, soothing properties. It is also used as a gelling agent in media for growing bacterial *cultures*.

Age

Of medical significance in diagnosis and in determining treatment, age is usually measured chronologically (in terms of the period of time since birth). However, age can also be measured in terms of physical, mental, or developmental maturity.

PHYSICAL AGE

Physical age can be measured even before birth. The age of a fetus is measured in terms of gestational age. Estimation of gestational age is important in neonatal pediatrics for identifying those babies who are too small for their gestational age and who may have problems because of their low birth weight. Gestational age can be assessed from the date of the woman's last menstrual period and by the size of her pregnant uterus. More accurate determination is made by measuring the size of the fetus by *ultrasound scanning*. The gestational age of a newborn baby can be estimated to within about two weeks by physical examination.

Children vary greatly in the rate at which they develop and grow, but their physical age is a measure of maturity that provides a common scale of development that can be used throughout the long period of growth. In adults, physical age is difficult to assess other than through physical appearance. Physical age can be estimated after death by the state of certain organs, particularly by the amount of atheroma (fatty deposits) lining the arteries.

The most useful measure of physical development in children is bone age. Bone age measures how much the bones of a body area have matured, as seen on an X ray. Measures such as height and weight are less useful as age standards because they vary greatly among individuals of the same chronological age. In contrast, all healthy individuals reach the same adult level of skeletal maturity and each bone passes through the same sequence of changes of shape as it grows.

Assessment of bone age is particularly useful in investigating delayed puberty or *short stature* in children. A prediction of the final adult height can be made by the physician if the chronological age, bone age, and current height are known.

Dental age is another, though less useful, measure of physical maturity. It can be assessed by counting the number of teeth that have erupted (see *Eruption of teeth*), and by comparing the amount of dental calcification (as seen on X rays) with standard values in much the same way as bone age is measured.

MENTAL AND DEVELOPMENTAL AGE

Mental age is assessed by comparing scores achieved in intelligence or achievement tests with standard scores for different chronological ages (see *Intelligence tests*).

A young child's age can be expressed in terms of developmental level. Patterns of normal development have been described for children from birth to the age of 5 years in the fields of speech, vision, hearing, and motor skills (principally walking and delicate hand-eye coordination). Specific tasks in these fields are achieved at certain ages (see *Child development*).

Agenesis

The complete or partial absence at birth of an organ or component of the body, caused by failure of development in the embryo.

Agent

Any substance or force capable of bringing about a biological, chemical, or physical change. An agent can also be a person acting on behalf of someone else. (See also *Reagent*.)

Agent Orange

A preparation of the toxic chemical dioxin, used as a defoliant in the Vietnam War (see *Defoliant poisoning*).

Age spots

Blemishes that appear on the skin with increasing age. Most common are seborrheic warts, which are brown or yellow, slightly raised spots that can occur at any site and sometimes get caught on clothing. Also common in the elderly are freckles, keratoses (small, wartlike blemishes caused by overexposure to the sun), and De Morgan's spots (cherry angiomas), which are red, pinpoint blemishes that occur on the trunk.

Treatment is usually unnecessary for any of these age spots apart from keratoses, which may progress to skin cancer. Freezing the keratoses with liquid nitrogen is the usual treatment; they may also be removed surgically using a local anesthetic.

Most spots are harmless but any unexplained blemish, or one that grows rapidly or bleeds, should be seen by your physician because of the possibility of skin cancer.

Ageusia

Lack or impairment of the sense of taste (see *Taste, loss of*).

Aggregation

The clumping of blood cells. Aggregation of platelets (small, sticky blood particles) takes place when a blood vessel is damaged, forming the first stage of *blood clotting* and thus helping to plug the injured vessel. Aggregation, however, can also have adverse effects. It con-

tributes to the formation of atheroma (the fatty substance that accumulates inside arteries and causes *atherosclerosis*) and thrombi (blood clots), which can cause *thrombosis*.

In the treatment of disorders in which thrombosis plays a part—coronary heart disease, for example—drugs such as aspirin, dipyridamole, or sulfinpyrazone may be prescribed to reduce aggregation.

Aggression

A general term for a wide variety of acts of hostility that are outside the range of normal social behavior.

CAUSES

Among animals, aggression serves to protect the species by way of self-defense and in defense of food, territory, and the young. In humans, there seem to be other factors, perhaps based on the needs of prehistoric survival. Some see it as resulting from frustration, lack of affection, and the attitudes of parents; others consider it part of the creative urge.

EEG studies show changes in brain-wave patterns in people who are continuously aggressive. Aggression centers (for example, the amygdaloid area) have been described. Brain disease (such as a tumor) or head injury may sometimes result in aggressive behavior. Even so, such outbursts do seem to be related to events; the person does not start fights for no reason at all, but rather over-reacts aggressively to problems.

Androgens, the male sex hormones, seem to promote aggression, whereas estrogen, the female sex hormone, actively suppresses it. Age is another factor, since aggression is more common in adolescence and the early 20s, but becomes increasingly rare the older people get. People truly do seem to mellow with age.

Psychiatric conditions associated with aggressive outbursts are *schizophrenia* (especially the catatonic and paranoid types), *antisocial personality disorder*, *mania*, and abuse of amphetamines or alcohol. *Temporal lobe epilepsy*, *hypoglycemia*, and *confusion* due to physical illness are other, less common, medical causes. *Dementia*, whether associated with *Alzheimer's disease* or *alcohol dependence*, may remove control of aggression.

Aging

The physical and mental changes that occur in a person over time. The aging process is sometimes seen as bringing with it only frailty and increased

vulnerability to disease and injury, but many societies value their old people for their wisdom and experience and recognize other virtues that often come with age (e.g., patience and acceptance).

BIOLOGICAL AGING

All animals have a finite life span, and the maximum for humans seems to have changed little since biblical times. Very few people live beyond 100 years, and the average life span in the absence of disease seems to be about 85 years.

Gerontologists have yet to agree on the biological processes that underlie aging. Among the many theories are the "worn template" concept—that every time cells divide, the copying mechanism is more likely to introduce errors; the accumulated toxins theory, according to which the body is gradually poisoned by the accumulation of chemicals it cannot excrete; and the immune surveillance theory, which postulates that there is a progressive decline in the immune system's ability to detect and destroy microorganisms and developing tumors.

Aging is associated with degenerative changes in various organs and tissues, such as the skin, bones, joints, blood vessels, and nervous tissue (see chart). These changes may be accelerated by factors such as smoking, excessive alcohol consumption, poor diet, insufficient exercise, and excessive exposure of the skin to strong sunlight.

Nevertheless, the provocative evidence of 90 year olds who have smoked and drunk alcohol all their lives shows that an important factor determining life expectancy is genetic. Just as a person's height is determined by the interaction of his or her diet with the genetic potential inherited from the parents, so life span depends to a large extent on heredity.

NORMAL CHANGES

As people age, they discover that their physical performance declines, although not by as much as is often believed. A 60 year old who has always exercised regularly may retain some 80 percent of the physical strength and stamina that he or she had at the age of 25. However, the natural decline in lung function limits exertion past the age of about 60. Wound healing and resistance to infection also decline.

Sexual activity past the age of 60 is variable. Prolonged abstinence tends to lead to loss of libido and potency, whereas those who have remained

THE PRACTICAL EFFECTS OF AGING

In the body, aging is associated with loss of elasticity in the skin, blood vessels, and tendons. There is also progressive decline in the functioning of organs such as the lungs, kidneys, and liver. Mechanical wear and tear causes cumulative damage to certain organ systems. Brain cells, specialized kidney units, and many other body structures are never replaced after they have reached maturity.

Hip joint in young person
The X ray shows the rounded head of the thigh bone (femur) separated by cartilage from the surrounding hip socket.

Hip joint in elderly person
This X ray of an osteoarthritic hip shows almost complete degeneration and disappearance of the cartilage in the joint.

EFFECTS OF AGING

Organ or tissue	Natural effects	Accelerated by
Skin	Loss of elastic tissue causes skin to sag and wrinkle. Weakened blood capillaries cause skin to bruise more easily.	Exposure to sun; smoking.
Brain and nervous system	Loss of nerve cells leads to reduction in ability to memorize or to learn new skills. Reaction time of nerves increases, making responses slower.	Excessive consumption of alcohol and other drugs; repeated head trauma (for example, from boxing).
Senses	Some loss of acuity in all senses, mainly due to loss of nerve cells.	Overexposure to loud noise; smoking.
Lungs	Loss of elasticity with age, so that breathing is less efficient.	Air pollution; smoking; lack of exercise.
Heart	Becomes less efficient at pumping, causing reduced tolerance to exercise.	Excessive use of alcohol and cigarettes; a fatty diet.
Circulation	Arteries harden, causing poor blood circulation and higher blood pressure.	Lack of exercise; smoking; poor diet.
Joints	Pressure on intervertebral disks causes height loss; wear on hip and knee joints reduces mobility.	Athletic injuries; being overweight.
Muscles	Loss of muscle bulk and strength.	Lack of exercise; starvation.
Liver	Becomes less efficient in processing toxic substances in the blood.	Damage from alcohol consumption and virus infections.

Young skin
The outer skin layer has an appreciable thickness. The deeper layers contain numerous collagen fibers, which give the skin elasticity.

Elastic fibers

Older skin
The outer layer has become thinned, wrinkled, and prone to injury. There are fewer elastic fibers in the deeper layers.

sexually active often find little, if any, decline in their sex life.

As with physical performance, certain of our mental abilities inevitably deteriorate with age. Most people over 60 experience "benign forgetfulness," finding greater difficulty in such things as recalling names or telephone numbers. Many people find this change frightening, but, in fact, about 80 percent of people older than 80 are not demented.

AGING AND SOCIETY

In the twentieth century there have been dramatic changes in the age structure of Western societies because infant and childhood mortality has declined markedly. Today, few adults under the age of 50 die from natural causes (accidental death is now much more frequent in young adults than death from disease). The result has been a substantial increase in the proportion of people who live beyond the age of 65; the proportion living to beyond 75 continues to increase. However, today about one third of people older than 75 have some disability that restricts their daily lives in some way; improvements in preventive medicine are likely to bring about a decrease in this proportion in the future.

Agitation

Restless inability to keep still, usually due to underlying anxiety or tension. Agitated people may pace up and down, pluck at clothes or sheets, wring their hands, and start tasks without completing them. Because they cannot relax or concentrate, agitated people constantly repeat such aimless activities.

Agitation is usually caused by worry over a particular situation—a father anxiously awaiting the birth of his child, for example. Persistent agitation is also seen in *anxiety disorders*, especially when there is an underlying physical cause such as alcohol withdrawal. Depressive illness (see *Depression*) in older people is usually accompanied by severe agitation. Phenothiazines, antidepressants, and other drugs may also be a cause of the agitation.

A

Agnosia

An inability to recognize objects despite adequate sensory information about them reaching the brain via the eyes or ears or through touch. For an object to be recognized, the sensory information about it must be interpreted, which involves recall of memorized information about similar objects. Agnosia is caused by damage to areas of the brain involved in these interpretative and memory recall functions. The most common causes of such brain damage are *stroke* and *head injury*.

TYPES AND SYMPTOMS

Agnosia is usually associated with just one of the main sensations: vision, hearing, or touch. For example, an object may be recognizable by hearing and sight but not by touch. Some people, after a stroke that damages the right cerebral hemisphere, may seem unaware of any disability in their affected left limbs. This is called anosognosia or sensory inattention.

TACTILE AGNOSIA is an inability to recognize by touch alone objects that are placed in the hands, despite adequate sensation in the fingers.

VISUAL AGNOSIA is an inability to recognize and name objects despite normal vision. Affected people may be able to describe the color, shape, and size of an object but cannot name what they see or indicate its use.

AUDITORY AGNOSIA is an inability to recognize familiar sounds despite normal hearing.

OUTLOOK

There is no specific treatment for agnosia but some of the lost interpretative ability may return over time.

Agoraphobia

Fear of going into open spaces and of entering shops, restaurants, or other public places. The condition often overlaps with *claustrophobia* (fear of enclosed spaces), another *phobia*.

The thought of visiting a public place or mixing with many other people fills sufferers with such dread that they avoid going out as much as possible. Sufferers fabricate any of a number of excuses for their friends and family to remain at home. If they do venture out, they may have a *panic attack*, which leads to further restriction of their activities. Eventually, agoraphobics become completely housebound. People seek psychiatric treatment for agoraphobia more often than for any other phobia and are usually successfully treated by psychotherapy and antidepressants.

Agraphia

Loss of or reduced ability to write, despite normal function of hand and arm muscles, caused by damage to parts of the cerebrum (the main mass of the brain) concerned with writing.

CAUSES

Writing depends on a complex sequence of mental processes, including the selection of words, recall from memory of how these words are spelled, formulation and execution of the hand movements required, and visual checking that written words match their representation in the brain. These processes probably take place in a number of connected brain areas. Agraphia may be caused by damage to various parts of these areas (usually within the left cerebral hemisphere) and can be of different types and severity. The most common reasons for such damage are head injury, *stroke*, and *brain tumors*.

Agraphia rarely occurs on its own. It is often accompanied by *alexia* (loss of the ability to read) or may be part of an expressive *aphasia* (general disturbance in the expression of language).

TREATMENT AND OUTLOOK

There is no specific treatment for agraphia. Over time, following a stroke or other event that has caused brain damage, some of the lost writing skills may return.

Ague

An outdated term for malaria or other diseases causing fever in which the sufferer alternately feels excessively hot and shiveringly cold.

AIDS

A deficiency of the *immune system* due to infection with *HIV* (human immunodeficiency virus). In its present form, AIDS (acquired immune deficiency syndrome) appears to be new to the human population. As yet, there is no curative treatment and no vaccine for AIDS, but the symptoms and complications variably respond to antibiotics, antiviral agents, radiation therapy, and anticancer drugs.

INCIDENCE

AIDS is not present in all individuals who are infected with HIV. The proportion of those infected whose condition progresses to AIDS has varied widely in different countries and in different risk groups. Every year, AIDS will develop in between 1 and 5 percent of people infected with HIV, but there is some evidence that in a few infected people (less than 1 percent) both the virus and the antibodies eventually disappear from the blood, suggesting that the body has fought off the infection.

Once AIDS has been diagnosed, the condition is considered fatal. By the end of the 1980s, close to 100,000 men, women, and children in the US had been diagnosed as having AIDS and about half of them had died.

The main risk groups are homosexual or bisexual men and people who inject themselves with drugs using unsterile needles and syringes. Many hemophiliacs also became infected in the early 1980s as a result of receiving infected blood products, but this route of infection is now closed by better screening of blood and treatment of blood products. Other risk groups include heterosexual contacts of infected individuals, children of infected women, and people who have received infected transfusions.

HISTORY

In 1981, the Centers for Disease Control (CDC) in Atlanta, Georgia, was alerted to reports of cases of a rare lung infection in previously healthy homosexual men in Los Angeles and then in New York. Infection was found to be with *PNEUMOCYSTIS CARINII*, a protozoan organism that had previously caused pneumonia only in patients with suppressed immune defenses.

Later, cases of a rare tumor (*Kaposi's sarcoma*) were reported in young homosexual men. Kaposi's sarcoma was recognized as a slow-growing skin tumor previously seen in Africa and also in the US, where it mainly affected elderly men. In the AIDS cases, the tumor behaved much more aggressively and was found in parts of the body besides the skin.

Soon it appeared that there was a rapidly increasing epidemic of conditions associated with depression of the immune system—most being *opportunistic infections* (i.e., infections that do not usually affect people with efficient immune defenses).

These conditions were observed not only in male homosexuals, but also in intravenous drug users and hemophiliacs, suggesting that transmission was related to blood as well as to sexual activity. An infective cause seemed likely and, in 1984, French and American researchers identified the responsible virus. It was named LAV (lymphadenopathy-associated virus) by the French and HTLV III (human T-cell lymphotropic virus, strain III) by the Americans. In 1986, the virus was renamed HIV.

CAUSES AND PREVENTION OF AIDS

AIDS is caused by the human immunodeficiency virus (HIV) (right), which consists of some nucleic acid (genetic material) inside two protective shells and an outer envelope. Full-blown AIDS develops in only some people infected with HIV.

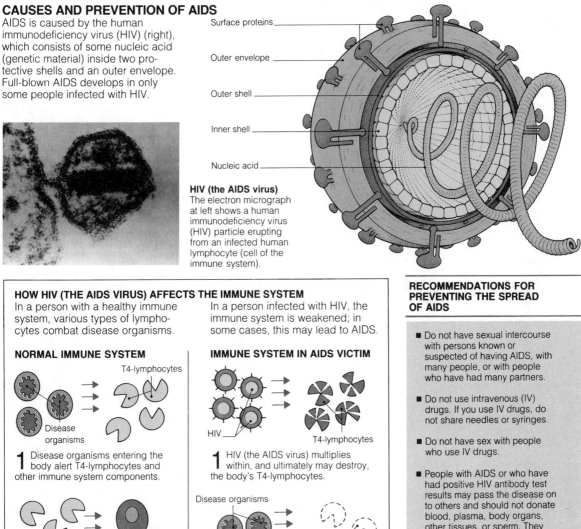

Surface proteins
Outer envelope
Outer shell
Inner shell
Nucleic acid

HIV (the AIDS virus)
The electron micrograph at left shows a human immunodeficiency virus (HIV) particle erupting from an infected human lymphocyte (cell of the immune system).

HOW HIV (THE AIDS VIRUS) AFFECTS THE IMMUNE SYSTEM

In a person with a healthy immune system, various types of lymphocytes combat disease organisms.

In a person infected with HIV, the immune system is weakened; in some cases, this may lead to AIDS.

NORMAL IMMUNE SYSTEM

T4-lymphocytes
Disease organisms

1 Disease organisms entering the body alert T4-lymphocytes and other immune system components.

T4-lymphocytes
Other lymphocytes

2 The T4-lymphocytes help regulate the response of other lymphocytes (cells of the immune system).

Other lymphocytes
Disease organisms

3 These lymphocytes then counterattack and destroy the disease organisms by various mechanisms.

IMMUNE SYSTEM IN AIDS VICTIM

HIV
T4-lymphocytes

1 HIV (the AIDS virus) multiplies within, and ultimately may destroy, the body's T4-lymphocytes.

Disease organisms
Destroyed T4-lymphocytes

2 When disease organisms invade, immune responses may fail, due to absence of the vital T4-lymphocytes.

Disease organisms

3 The disease organisms may then overwhelm the immune system and lead to the features of AIDS.

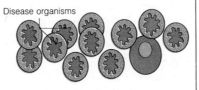
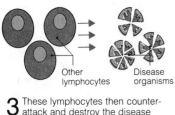
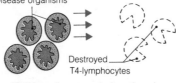

RECOMMENDATIONS FOR PREVENTING THE SPREAD OF AIDS

- Do not have sexual intercourse with persons known or suspected of having AIDS, with many people, or with people who have had many partners.

- Do not use intravenous (IV) drugs. If you use IV drugs, do not share needles or syringes.

- Do not have sex with people who use IV drugs.

- People with AIDS or who have had positive HIV antibody test results may pass the disease on to others and should not donate blood, plasma, body organs, other tissues, or sperm. They should not exchange body fluids during sexual activity.

- There is a risk of infecting (or being infected by) others through sexual intercourse, sharing needles, and, possibly, exposure of others to saliva through oral-genital contact or "wet" kissing. The effectiveness of condoms in preventing infection with HIV is not proved, but their consistent use may reduce transmission, since exchange of body fluids is known to increase risk.

- Toothbrushes, razors, or other implements that could become contaminated with blood should not be shared.

A

HOW AIDS HAS BEEN CONTRACTED IN THE US

Cases (%)

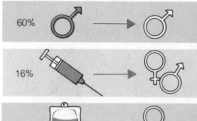

60%

Male homosexual activity
This has accounted for the most cases.

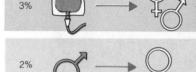

16%

Needle-sharing by drug abusers
The number of cases is increasing in this second largest group of AIDS victims.

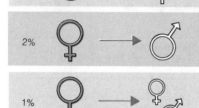

3%

Received infected blood or blood product transfusions
This is no longer a significant mechanism of transmission in the US.

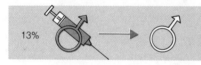

2%

Male-to-female sexual transmission
In the US, this has accounted for relatively few AIDS cases, but the percentage from this cause is rising.

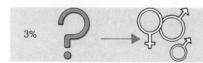

2%

Female-to-male sexual transmission
Again, this has accounted for relatively few AIDS cases, but the percentage from this cause is rising.

1%

Mother-to-child via placenta
A baby born to a woman who has AIDS or who has tested positively for HIV antibodies has a high risk of being infected.

13%

Multiple risk factors
This group consists of victims with more than one risk factor—mainly homosexual males who have also shared needles.

3%

Other/unknown
This group, many of them hospital workers, contracted AIDS by another means (e.g., needle injury) or by unknown means.

NO-RISK ACTIVITIES

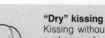

Touching
AIDS virus cannot be transmitted by social contact such as shaking hands.

"Dry" kissing
Kissing without exchange of saliva poses no risk of virus transmission.

Embracing
There is no risk of transmitting the virus by embracing or cuddling.

Sharing utensils
The virus cannot be transmitted by sharing a glass or cutlery.

Giving blood
Only sterile needles are used for taking blood from donors in the US.

Other contact
The virus cannot be caught from toilet seats or other objects.

THE EFFECTS OF THE VIRUS

The virus infects a cell known as the T4 or T-helper lymphocyte, which is crucial for the regulation of the immune mechanisms. The infected cell may die or the virus may remain dormant in the cell, with the possibility of reactivation later. Many infected individuals have no sign of disease; they are "asymptomatic carriers." Or they have vague complaints, such as weight loss, fevers, sweats, or unexplained diarrhea. People in this group have been referred to as having AIDS-related complex (ARC).

In its most severe form, HIV infection interferes with the immune system to make the individual susceptible to a variety of infections and cancers, such as Kaposi's sarcoma and lymphoid tumors (see *Lymphoma*).

METHODS OF TRANSMISSION

HIV has been isolated from blood, semen, saliva, tears, nervous system tissue, breast milk, and female genital tract secretions. However, only semen and blood have been proved to transmit infection.

The major methods of transmission are sexual contact (penis to anus, vagina, or mouth), blood to blood (through transfusions or needle sharing in addicts), and from woman to fetus. Other rare methods are through accidental needle injury, artificial insemination by donated semen, and kidney transplantation.

"Casual" or household spread does not occur. The infection is not spread by touching or hugging, by breathing the same air, or by sharing cutlery or crockery. Heterosexual transmission

does occur. By the late 1980s, this mode of transmission accounted for approximately 4 percent of all known cases in the US. In Africa, AIDS affects men and women equally; heterosexual transmission plays a more important role for unknown reasons.

SYMPTOMS AND SIGNS

Individuals infected with the virus may have no symptoms; others experience a short-lived illness, sometimes resembling infectious *mononucleosis*, when they first become infected. Medical examination of patients without symptoms may reveal abnormalities, most commonly lymph gland enlargement.

Minor features of HIV infection include skin disorders such as seborrheic *dermatitis* (skin inflammation particularly affecting the face). More severe features include marked weight loss, diarrhea, fever, and oral *candidiasis* (thrush).

Other infections that are more common or more severe in HIV-infected patients include *herpes simplex* infections, *shingles*, *tuberculosis*, salmonellosis, and shigellosis. HIV may also affect the brain, causing a variety of neurological disorders including dementia.

The features of full-blown AIDS include cancers, such as Kaposi's sarcoma and lymphoma of the brain, and infections, such as *pneumocystis pneumonia*, severe *cytomegalovirus* infection, *toxoplasmosis*, diarrhea caused by CRYPTOSPORIDIUM or ISOSPORA, candidiasis, disseminated *strongyloidiasis*, *cryptococcosis*, and chronic herpes simplex.

DIAGNOSIS
HIV infection may be suspected in someone with lymph gland enlargement or unexplained weight loss if the person is in a high-risk group.

Confirmation of HIV infection involves testing a blood sample for the presence of antibodies to HIV. Testing for the virus itself is more difficult. A positive HIV antibody test result indicates exposure to the virus; most antibody-positive individuals are virus carriers. Any positive reaction is rechecked by other tests for full confirmation. A negative test result may occur in someone who has very recently come into contact with the virus; a negative result should be followed by repeated testing after six months if the individual is at risk.

Diagnosis of full-blown AIDS is based on positive results for the HIV antibody test and Western blot (a confirmatory test), along with observation of the characteristic infections and tumors.

PREVENTION OF INFECTION
Until a cure or vaccine is found, prevention is the most important measure against AIDS. Risks can be reduced by practicing *"safe"* sex.

Anyone who feels that he or she may have been exposed to the virus can request a blood test, although it is wise to obtain counseling first on the advisability of the test and implications of the result. A person who knows that he or she has been infected should alter his or her sexual life-style to avoid transmitting the virus. An uninfected person should also adopt safe sex procedures to avoid becoming infected.

Safe sex techniques involve reducing the number of sex partners;

ideally sex should be restricted to partners whose sexual histories are known. Unprotected anal and vaginal intercourse should be avoided. Hugging, mutual masturbation, and "dry" kissing are safe. Saliva may contain the virus but is unlikely to be important in transmission; the risk of "wet" kissing with saliva exchange is unknown. If penile penetration occurs, a condom should be worn. Spermicidal jellies seem to inactivate the virus and should be used as lubricants. The risk of oral sex is not fully known, but ejaculation into the mouth should be avoided.

Intravenous drug users should avoid sharing needles to prevent spread of infection; their sexual partners may also be at risk.

In Africa, prostitutes show a high rate of infection. Although rates are much lower in the US, prostitutes are a potential means of spread. They should be encouraged to require use of condoms to protect themselves and their clients.

There is a small risk to hospital and other health workers when handling infected blood products or needles. The risk of transmission by needles in hospitals has, however, been lower than expected; it is minimized if care is taken with all procedures involving sharp instruments, including careful disposal of contaminated materials.

People in risk groups are advised against donating blood and semen. All donated blood, organs, and semen are screened for HIV antibodies.

TREATMENT
There is no cure for AIDS. Supportive treatment is available only for its complications. Pneumocystis pneumonia is treated with antibiotics (such as pentamidine or trimethoprim-sulfamethoxazole), but troublesome side effects often occur and the infection often recurs. Treatment of Kaposi's sarcoma by radiation therapy or anticancer drugs is rarely curative.

Several antiviral drugs, such as zidovudine (AZT) and acyclovir, are being used to treat patients with AIDS and those with HIV infection. Zidovudine has serious side effects, but it does slow the progression of HIV infection. Full assessment will come only after more patients have been treated for long periods.

OUTLOOK
Research is continuing on other methods of attacking the virus or halting its effects. In laboratory tests, several drugs have inhibited an enzyme essential for viral multiplica-

tion, but these drugs have failed in clinical trials or have been drastically limited by severe side effects.

While research into drug treatment for AIDS continues, the failure of medical science to achieve curative treatment for other viral infections makes anything approaching a cure unlikely in the near future.

Medical prevention is possible if a vaccine against HIV can be developed. A successful vaccine has been developed against feline leukemia virus, which bears similarities to HIV, so the technology for vaccine development is available and work is progressing with this intent.

AIDS-related complex
A combination of weight loss, fever, and enlarged lymph nodes in a person who has been infected with *HIV* (the *AIDS* virus), but does not actually have AIDS itself. Many people with AIDS-related complex (ARC) will eventually have the features of AIDS.

Air
The colorless, odorless mixture of gases that forms the Earth's atmosphere. Air consists of 78 percent *nitrogen*, 21 percent *oxygen*, small quantities of *carbon dioxide* and other gases, and some water vapor.

The balance among the various atmospheric gases is maintained largely by the mutual needs of animals and plants. Animals use oxygen and produce carbon dioxide as a waste product; plants use carbon dioxide and release oxygen in a process called photosynthesis. The level of carbon dioxide in the atmosphere is gradually increasing as a result of extensive deforestation and the large-scale burning of fossil fuels. This disturbance of the atmospheric balance is causing concern among scientists because of its potentially disastrous consequences for all life on this planet. (See also *Pollution*.)

Air conditioning
Any system that controls the purity, humidity, and temperature of the air in a building. Air conditioning is essential to the sanitation of hospitals, but is also important in maintaining hygienic conditions in hotels, offices, and other large buildings.

WHY IT IS USED
Air conditioning acts both on the air already in rooms and on air drawn in from outside, filtering out dust, pollen, smoke, bad smells, and excess moisture, and either cooling or heat-

ing the air to keep it at a comfortable temperature. In this way, air conditioning helps prevent heat disorders, such as *prickly heat*, headaches, nasal congestion, and chest disorders. By bringing in air from outside, which has been filtered and exposed to the antiseptic effect of ultraviolet light, air conditioning also reduces the risk of airborne infections and of allergies.

Hospital sterile units, used for nursing high-risk patients, have air conditioning units fitted with special bacterial filters that minimize the risk of spreading infection.

DISORDERS

Despite its generally beneficial effects, air conditioning may be responsible for certain disorders. For example, some outbreaks of *legionnaires' disease* (a type of pneumonia) have been linked to contaminated air conditioning systems; and humidifier fever (a lung disease that causes fever, coughing, and breathing difficulty) is thought to be caused by the spread of infectious microorganisms (usually fungi) by air conditioning. Air conditioning has also been blamed for some cases of *sick building syndrome*, which is attributed to the physical working environment; it produces headache, irritability, and loss of energy.

Air embolism

Blockage of a small artery by an air bubble brought to the site of obstruction by the flow of blood.

An air *embolism* is a rare event. The air usually has entered the blood circulation via a vein in the course of an injury or an accident during a surgical procedure. It can also occur as a result of a pressure accident (as can occur when scuba diving or flying), causing rupture of lung tissues and escape of the air bubbles.

Air pollution

See *Pollution*.

Air swallowing

See *Aerophagia*

Airway

Collective term for the passages from the openings of the mouth and nose to the alveoli (air sacs in the lungs) through which air enters and leaves the lungs. The airway is made up of the nasal passages, oral cavity, upper part of the pharynx (throat), larynx (voice box), trachea (windpipe), bronchi (main airways in the lungs), and bronchioles (airways off the bronchi that end with the alveoli).

The term airway is also applied to an *endotracheal tube*, the artificial airway inserted into the trachea in a person who is under general anesthesia, and to the incision through the neck and into the trachea made in a *tracheostomy* operation. (See *Respiratory system*.)

Airway obstruction

Narrowing or blockage of the respiratory passages. The obstruction may be due to a foreign body, such as a piece of food, that becomes lodged in part of the upper airway and may result in *choking*. Certain diseases or disorders, such as *diphtheria*, affect the airway and can cause obstruction. Additionally, a spasm of the muscular walls of the airway, as occurs in *bronchospasm* (a feature of *asthma* and *bronchitis*), results in *breathing difficulty*. (See also *Artificial respiration*; *Lung* disorders box.)

Akathisia

An inability to sit still, occurring occasionally as a side effect of an *antipsychotic drug* used to treat mental disorders such as schizophrenia and depression. Less commonly, akathisia occurs as a complication of *Parkinson's disease* or as a manifestation of *hysteria*.

Akinesia

Complete or almost complete loss of movement. Akinesia may be due to paralysis (loss of power) in a group of muscles caused by damage to the nerves that supply them (for example, after a *stroke*). It may also occur in the presence of normal power but with rigidity (stiffness) of muscles (for example, in *Parkinson's disease*).

Albinism

A congenital condition (present from birth) characterized by a lack of the pigment melanin that gives color to the skin, hair, and eyes. Although rare, albinism occurs in all races. Affected individuals (albinos) suffer visual problems and a tendency to have skin cancers.

TYPES

In oculocutaneous albinism (the most common type), the hair, skin, and eyes are all affected. There are at least two main forms. In the more severe form, the skin and hair are snowy white throughout life (although the tips of the hairs may turn slightly yellow with age). In the less severe type, the skin and hair are white at birth but darken slightly with age, and numerous freckles develop on sun-exposed skin parts. In both forms, the

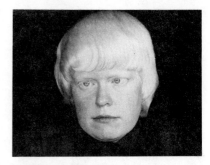

Appearance of albinism
The condition is caused by lack of melanin pigment in the skin, hair, and eyes.

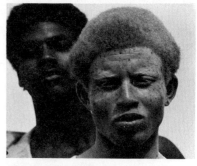

Albinism in an African boy
Albinism is found in people of all races, although it occurs only rarely.

eyes are affected by *photophobia* (intolerance to bright light), *nystagmus* (abnormal flickering movements), and, frequently, *strabismus* (squint) and *myopia* (nearsightedness).

Other rare types of albinism affect only the skin and hair or the eyes.

CAUSES AND INCIDENCE

The gene defects responsible for the two main forms of oculocutaneous albinism show an autosomal recessive pattern of inheritance (see *Genetic disorders*). In most cases, the parents have normal skin coloring; they are carriers of the gene defect in a hidden form. If a normally pigmented couple has an albino child, any subsequent children generally have a one in four chance of also being affected.

The overall prevalence of oculocutaneous albinism is low in the US and Europe—less than five people per 100,000 are affected. The prevalence is much higher in certain parts of the world (for example, about 20 persons per 100,000 are affected in southern Nigeria).

COMPLICATIONS AND TREATMENT

SKIN The most serious complication of oculocutaneous albinism derives from the lack of melanin, which normally protects the skin against harmful radiation in sunlight. The skin cannot tan, ages prematurely, and is prone to cancers on sun-exposed areas (see *Skin cancer*).

EYES The visual problems of albinos, such as photophobia and nystagmus, can cause great difficulties, particularly with reading at school. Expert assessment and treatment should be sought at an early age; glasses are usually needed, preferably tinted to help reduce photophobia.

Albumin

The most abundant protein in the body. Albumin is made in the liver from amino acids that have been absorbed from digested protein in the small intestine.

Albumin has several important functions. It helps retain substances (such as calcium, some hormones, and certain drugs) in the circulation by binding to them and thereby preventing their being filtered out by the kidneys and excreted in the urine. Albumin is also important in regulating the movement of water between tissues and the bloodstream by *osmosis* (the attraction of water to an area with a higher concentration of salts or proteins). See also *Albuminuria*.

Albuminuria

The presence of the protein *albumin* in the urine; a type of *proteinuria*. Normally, the glomerulus (filtering part of the kidney) does not allow albumin to pass through it and into the urine, so albuminuria usually indicates a failure of the kidney's filtering mechanism. Such a failure may be due to a kidney disorder, such as *glomerulonephritis* or *nephrotic syndrome*, or it may be a sign that the kidneys have been damaged by *hypertension* (high blood pressure).

Albumin in the urine can be detected by a simple test, providing a valuable preliminary screening for kidney disease.

Albuterol

A *bronchodilator drug* used in the treatment of *asthma*, chronic *bronchitis*, and *emphysema* (a lung disorder). Albuterol relaxes the muscles in the bronchi and in the wall of the uterus. It is currently under investigation for use in the prevention of premature labor.

Alcohol

A colorless liquid produced from the fermentation of carbohydrates by yeast. Also known as ethanol or ethyl alcohol, alcohol is the active constituent of alcoholic drinks such as beer, wine, and spirits. In medicine, alcohol is used as an antiseptic and a solvent. *Methanol*, also known as methyl alcohol or wood alcohol, is a related substance obtained from distilling wood and is highly poisonous.

Alcohol is used by most adults in developed countries, where the number of women and young drinkers has greatly increased in recent years. Recently its use has become common in developing countries as well.

Any society where alcohol is freely used and available is invariably afflicted by the problems of acute alcohol intoxication (drunkenness), *alcohol dependence* (habitual, compulsive, long-term heavy drinking), and *alcohol-related disorders* including liver disorders, heart disease, *hypertension*, *neuropathy*, and *Wernicke-Korsakoff syndrome*. Alcohol is also an important factor in vehicular and industrial accidents, domestic violence, marriage breakdown, child abuse, and other types of crime.

EFFECTS

The effect of alcohol on the *central nervous system* (the brain and spinal cord) is as a depressant, decreasing its activity and thus reducing anxiety, tension, and inhibitions. Taken in moderate amounts, it gives the drinker a feeling of relaxation and confidence that may enable him or her to socialize more easily. However, any feeling of heightened mental and physical efficiency is illusory. Tests have shown that even a low level of alcohol in the blood slows reactions. The more alcohol drunk, the more concentration and judgment are impaired. At the same time, the drinker's confidence is increased—a potentially lethal combination while driving. If excessive amounts are drunk, poisoning or intoxication results, with effects ranging from euphoria to unconsciousness (see *Alcohol intoxication*).

In addition to significantly altering mood and behavior, alcohol has various other effects on the body. As a result of peripheral *vasodilation* (widening of the small blood vessels), the face becomes flushed and the drinker feels warm, although in fact a greater amount of body heat is lost. Small amounts of alcohol increase the flow of gastric juices and therefore stimulate the appetite and aid digestion—although large amounts over a long period can cause erosive *gastritis* (inflammation of the stomach lining with superficial, surface ulcers) and hematemesis (vomiting blood).

The quantity of urine passed increases (over and above that expected from the intake of drink), because the production of *ADH* (antidiuretic hormone) is inhibited. Heavy drinkers thus often become dehydrated; great thirst, a dry tongue, and a hangover may be associated with the effects of alcohol.

Finally, the effects of alcohol on sexual behavior are as summarized by William Shakespeare: "It provokes the desire but it takes away the performance."

TOLERANCE

Habitual drinkers acquire a tolerance to alcohol. This means that, to obtain the same effects, they gradually must increase the amount they drink. The liver breaks down alcohol at a faster rate, necessitating a greater intake to achieve the same level in the blood. At the same time, nerve cells in the brain become less and less responsive to a given amount of alcohol. Paradoxically, however, after years of drinking, many alcoholics experience a reduced tolerance.

Alcohol dependence

An illness characterized by habitual, compulsive, long-term, heavy consumption of alcohol and the development of withdrawal symptoms when drinking has stopped suddenly. The description "alcohol dependence" is generally preferred medically to "alcoholism," but the terms are virtually synonymous.

INCIDENCE

The incidence of alcohol dependence has been rising throughout the world for many years. Statistics on the extent of the problem are difficult to quote with any certainty. Rough estimates indicate there are approximately five million alcohol-dependent persons in the US (one in 50 of the population) and another seven million who have some trouble controlling their consumption of alcohol.

CAUSES

There is no single cause of alcohol dependence. Three causative factors interact in the development of the illness: personality, environment, and the addictive nature of the agent (i.e., the drug alcohol). Thus, if all other factors (such as the availability of alcohol) are equal, then inadequate, insecure, or immature personalities are more at risk than more emotionally mature individuals.

Inherited, genetic factors probably play a part in causing dependence in some cases but it is now widely

A

ALCOHOL AND THE BODY

Alcohol is a drug and, even in small amounts, its effects on the body are noticeable. Problems arise when people fail to take into account the effects of alcohol on tasks requiring coordination (such as driving), when they become intoxicated, or when they become dependent on the drug. Alcohol dependence can cause early death and is a major factor in crime, marital breakdown, child abuse, accidents, and absenteeism. Prolonged heavy drinking that stops short of dependence still may cause a wide variety of diseases, such as *cirrhosis* of the liver and *cardiomyopathy*.

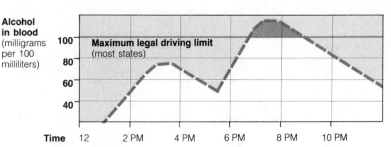

Alcohol in blood (milligrams per 100 milliliters)

Maximum legal driving limit (most states)

Time 12   2 PM   4 PM   6 PM   8 PM   10 PM

Cumulative effects of alcohol

It takes some time for the body to eliminate even small amounts of alcohol. For instance, if a person has two drinks at lunchtime and then has one or two more drinks early in the evening, his or her cumulative blood alcohol level could be over the legal limit for driving even though several hours have passed.

EFFECTS OF INCREASING BLOOD ALCOHOL LEVELS

Concentration (milligrams per 100 milliliters)	Observable effects
30–50 150–200	Flushed face, euphoria, talkativeness, increased social confidence
50–150 200–350	Disturbed thinking and coordination, irritability, reduced self control, irresponsible talk and behavior
150–250 350–500	Marked confusion, unsteady gait, slurred speech, unpredictable shows of emotion and aggression
250–400 500–700	Extreme confusion and disorientation, difficulty remaining upright, drowsiness, delayed or incoherent reaction to questions progressing to coma (a state of deep unconsciousness from which the person cannot be aroused)
400–500 700+	Risk of death due to arrest of breathing (although habitual drinkers may survive even such high levels)

☐ Occasional social drinker

☐ Alcoholic/problem drinker

Alcohol levels in different drinks

Alcoholic drinks come in many forms and contain varying levels of pure alcohol. It can be very difficult to estimate alcohol intake because the strengths of drinks vary. The standard measures shown here contain approximately equal amounts of pure alcohol.

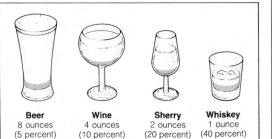

Beer
 8 ounces
 (5 percent)

Wine
 4 ounces
 (10 percent)

Sherry
 2 ounces
 (20 percent)

Whiskey
 1 ounce
 (40 percent)

LONG-TERM EFFECTS ON THE BODY

Persistent heavy drinking eventually damages body tissues; the main effects are shown below.

Liver

The liver is the main organ responsible for metabolizing alcohol from the blood; it manifests many of the long-term effects of heavy drinking. These effects include fatty liver, hepatitis, cirrhosis, and liver cancer.

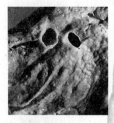

Cirrhotic liver

In this condition, commonly caused by heavy drinking, bands of scar tissue form in the liver, impairing its function.

Brain and nervous system
 Alcohol depresses the central nervous system. Prolonged alcohol abuse permanently impairs brain and nerve function.

Skin
 Alcohol causes facial flushing, which becomes constant in heavy drinkers.

Heart and circulation
 Prolonged heavy drinking can cause coronary heart disease, hypertension, heart failure, and stroke.

Digestive system
 Irritation from large amounts of alcohol can cause gastritis and ulcers.

Urinary system
 Alcohol acts as a diuretic, increasing urine output. Prolonged heavy drinking can cause renal failure.

Reproductive system
 Alcohol increases sexual confidence, but high levels cause impotence.

DEATHS FROM ALCOHOL-RELATED CAUSES IN THE US (1980–1983)

Cause	Deaths	1980	1981	1982	1983
Alcoholic cirrhosis of liver		9,166	8,567	7,893	7,571
Alcohol dependence		4,350	4,207	3,914	4,002
Alcoholic liver damage		1,812	1,782	1,752	1,753
Alcoholic fatty liver		1,166	951	961	1,027
Alcohol abuse		889	771	768	835
Acute alcoholic hepatitis		794	785	687	725
Alcoholic cardiomyopathy		650	647	664	711
Alcohol psychosis		454	453	389	346
Toxic effects of alcohol		385	384	412	341
Total		19,666	18,547	17,440	17,311

This table lists deaths that are known to be wholly attributed to a specific alcohol-related cause. Many other causes are omitted because they are only partly related to alcohol consumption. The most obvious omissions are fatalities suffered as a result of motor vehicle accidents. Alcohol also often contributes to accidents in the home.

believed that any person, irrespective of environment, genetic background, or personality, can become alcoholic if he or she drinks heavily for a prolonged period.

Environmental factors are important, especially the ready availability, affordability, and widespread social acceptance of alcohol in the individual's national culture and among the people he or she associates with at work and during leisure hours. Thus alcoholism is much more common in certain countries, occupations, and social groups than in others.

Stress is another important factor. Many formerly moderate drinkers begin to drink excessively at times of bereavement. Women may turn to drink when their adolescent children leave home. Hormonal factors may also play a role in heavy drinking among women.

Once social and/or psychological factors have induced heavy drinking, the discovery that taking alcohol in the morning relieves the withdrawal symptoms induced by the previous night's drinking tends to accelerate the development of dependence.

DEVELOPMENT OF DEPENDENCE
The development of alcohol dependence can be divided into four main stages, which merge imperceptibly. The time scale of these changes may be from five to 25 years, although the average is about 10 years.

In the first phase, tolerance (being able to drink more alcohol before experiencing its ill effects) develops in the heavy social drinker. Entering the second phase, the drinker experiences memory lapses relating to events occurring during the drinking episodes. The third phase is characterized by loss, or lack, of control over alcohol; the drinker can no longer be certain of discontinuing drinking whenever he or she wants to. The final phase starts with prolonged binges of intoxication, with the drinker suffering observable mental or physical, complications.

Some people halt their consumption, temporarily or permanently, during one of the first three phases.

SYMPTOMS AND EFFECTS
BEHAVIORAL SYMPTOMS are varied and can include any combination of the following: furtive behavior (such as hiding bottles); aggressive or grandiose behavior; personality changes (such as irritability, jealousy, uncontrolled anger, selfishness); frequent change of jobs; constant promises to self and others to give up drinking; changes in drinking pattern (for example, switching to early-morning drinking, or changing from beer to spirits); neglect of food intake and personal appearance; and lengthy periods of intoxication.

PHYSICAL SYMPTOMS can also be varied. The drinker may exhibit any of the following: nausea, vomiting, or shaking in the morning; abdominal pain; cramps; numbness or tingling; weakness in the legs and hands; irregular pulse; redness and enlarged capillaries in the face; unsteadiness; confusion; poor memory; and incontinence. After sudden withdrawal of alcohol, the dependent person may experience *delirium tremens* (severe shakes, hallucinations, and convulsions).

In addition, alcohol-dependent persons are more susceptible than others to a wide variety of specific physical and mental diseases and disorders (see *Alcohol-related disorders*).

Combinations of physical, mental, personality, and often financial stresses lead to difficulties at work and at home for the alcoholic. Often, the person's marriage suffers. Suicide threats and attempts may occur.

ALCOHOL AND PREGNANCY
The damage that alcohol can cause a fetus has been recognized only recently. Drinking more than two drinks per day (for example, two 1-ounce glasses of spirits, two 4-ounce glasses of wine, or two 8-ounce glasses of beer) increases the chance of *fetal alcohol syndrome*. This disorder consists of facial abnormalities such as *cleft lip and palate*, heart defects, abnormal limb development, and lower-than-average intelligence. This level of drinking also increases the risk of miscarriage. Occasional binge drinking may cause the same effects even if the mother drinks little otherwise. Because a proportion of the alcohol from any drink reaches the baby, there is a risk that drinking even small amounts may disrupt normal development (causing, for example, low birth weight).

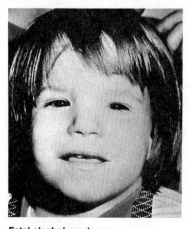

Fetal alcohol syndrome
An affected baby is abnormally short, has small eyes and a small jaw, and may have heart defects or a cleft lip and palate. He or she may suck poorly, sleep badly, and be irritable.

A

PREVENTION

Steps for avoiding the development of alcohol dependence include the following: keep to safe limits of alcohol intake as recommended by medical authorities; drink slowly instead of gulping; and never drink for relief of anxiety, tension, or depression, or on an empty stomach. No person should ever feel embarrassed about refusing an alcoholic drink.

TREATMENT

Many alcoholics require detoxification (medical help in getting over their physical withdrawal symptoms when they stop drinking). Detoxification is followed by long-term treatment. No single form of treatment is best for all alcoholics. Sometimes psychological, social, and physical treatments may be combined.

PSYCHOLOGICAL TREATMENTS involve *psychotherapy* and are now commonly and more reasonably carried out in groups (see *Group therapy*). There are various types of group therapy, using different techniques.

SOCIAL TREATMENTS include help with problems at work and, in particular, the inclusion of family members in the treatment process.

PHYSICAL TREATMENT is needed only by some alcoholics. It generally includes the use of disulfiram, a drug that sensitizes the drinker to alcohol so that he or she is afraid to drink because of unpleasant symptoms.

Alcoholics are strongly advised to use the self-help fellowship of organizations (i.e., *Alcoholics Anonymous*), where the alcoholic greatly benefits from meeting fellow sufferers who share their experiences.

Alcoholics Anonymous

A worldwide fellowship of people who readily admit to being alcoholics and who help each other stay sober. Alcoholics Anonymous (AA) was started in 1935 in the US and now consists of an estimated 67,000 local groups and over 1.5 million members in 92 countries. In the US alone there are more than 1 million members, with at least one group in all but the smallest towns and several groups in large cities. Contact addresses can be found in telephone directories.

Membership is open to anyone who has a drinking problem and has a desire to become and/or to continue to stay sober. There is no membership fee; the organization relies on voluntary contributions from members. Members are of all races, nationalities, and occupations, and range from

people whose health, careers, and relationships were totally destroyed by alcoholism to those who sought help at a much earlier stage of the illness. AA is not affiliated with any sect, political party, institution, or other organization. It has a policy of cooperation with other organizations that fight alcoholism.

Local AA meetings are of two types. At open meetings, which anyone (including members' families) can attend, speakers describe their lives as alcoholics and the effect AA has had in helping them refrain from drinking. At closed meetings, which only members can attend, new members are invited to describe their drinking problems and their difficulties abstaining. Other members who have had the same experiences suggest methods of staying sober and ways in which other problems can be surmounted. A program of recovery is suggested. Many members find that helping other alcoholics is the best way to remain sober themselves.

Members of AA do not reveal the names of other members to people outside AA. The fellowship does not keep membership records, monitor or attempt to control its members, engage or sponsor research on alcoholism, dispense drugs or psychiatric treatment, or provide detoxification, nursing, social services, or vocational counseling.

Alcohol intoxication

The common condition, also known as drunkenness, that results from drinking an excessive amount of alcohol over a relatively short period (usually about 30 minutes to several hours). Alcohol causes acute poisoning if taken in sufficiently large amounts. It depresses the activity of the central nervous system (the brain and spinal cord), leading to loss of normal mental and physical control. In extreme cases, a person who drinks a large amount of alcohol over a short period may lose consciousness and even die.

SYMPTOMS

The effects of a large alcohol intake depend on many factors, including physical and mental state, body size, social situation, and acquired tolerance (see *Alcohol*). Thus, a person may become "jocose, lachrymose, bellicose, or comatose" (cheerful, tearful, argumentative, or unconscious). There are wide individual variations. The important factor, however, is the blood alcohol level (see chart).

TREATMENT

For intoxication that stops short of coma, no treatment is required. Recovery takes place naturally as the alcohol in the person's body is gradually broken down.

If a drinker lapses into a coma, medical attention should be sought, particularly if the person is known or suspected to be diabetic or to have been taking another drug, whether prescribed by a physician (such as a sedative) or illicit (such as cocaine) in addition to alcohol. The person's clothing should be loosened and the mouth and back of the throat checked to make sure there is no obstruction to breathing. No attempt should be made to make the person drink water or make him or her vomit. If breathing stops, *artificial respiration* should be carried out until breathing restarts or medical help arrives.

For the chronic mental, physical, and social effects of long-term heavy drinking, see *Alcohol dependence* and *Alcohol-related disorders*.

Alcoholism

See *Alcohol dependence*.

Alcohol-related disorders

Apart from the many health and social problems that may result from *alcohol dependence*, and the high accident rate associated with *alcohol intoxication*, people who consume large quantities of alcohol are susceptible to numerous physical and mental disorders.

Alcohol consumption can lead to tissue damage and disease by any, or a combination, of three main mechanisms. First, alcohol or its breakdown products from metabolism can have a direct toxic or irritant effect on cells and tissues. Second, many alcoholics eat little or no nutritious food—alcohol satisfies their calorie requirements and at the same time reduces appetite through an irritant effect on the stomach. However, it provides no protein, vitamins, or minerals. Consequently, chronic alcoholics are prone to diseases caused by nutritional deficiency, particularly deficiency of *vitamin B_1* (thiamine).

Third, a continual high level of alcohol in the blood and tissues can cause wide-ranging disturbances in body chemistry. These disturbances can lead to *hypoglycemia* (reduced glucose in the blood) and *hyperlipidemia* (increased fat), which may contribute to malfunction and disease of such organs as the heart, liver, and blood vessels.

ALCOHOL-RELATED DISORDERS

Cancer	High alcohol consumption increases the risk of cancers of the mouth, tongue, pharynx (back of the throat), larynx (voice box), and esophagus, probably due to irritant action. In each of these cancers, alcohol	consumption along with smoking produces a much higher total risk of cancer than the sum of their separate risks. The risk of *liver cancer,* along with most types of liver disease, is also higher among alcoholics.
Liver damage and disease	Liver diseases caused by a high alcohol consumption include *fatty liver,* alcoholic *hepatitis, cirrhosis,* and liver cancer. They develop in sequence over a period of years. It is thought that a breakdown product of alcohol (acetaldehyde) has a toxic effect on liver cells and is the main cause of these diseases, although nutritional deficiency may also play some part.	The risk of alcoholic hepatitis and cirrhosis developing increases in proportion to the amount of alcohol consumed and the number of years of high consumption; liver cancer develops in about one in five sufferers of cirrhosis. However, about one third of heavy drinkers never get liver disease and in another third, only a fatty liver develops.
Nervous system disorders	Thiamine (vitamin B_1) deficiency, also known as *beriberi* (which disturbs nerve functioning), may develop in alcoholics. The effect of severe deficiency on the brain produces *Wernicke's encephalopathy,* with symptoms such as confusion, disturbances of speech and gait, and eventual coma. *Korsakoff's*	*psychosis* may also occur. The effect on the peripheral nervous system (nerve pathways outside the brain and spinal cord) produces polyneuropathy, with symptoms such as pain, cramps, numbness, tingling, and weakness in the legs and hands. Injections of thiamine and resumption of a normal diet can produce a dramatic cure.
Heart and circulatory disorders	Severe thiamine deficiency in alcoholics can cause *heart failure* (reduced pumping efficiency of the heart), usually combined with *edema* (fluid collection in the tissues). A high alcohol consumption also	increases the risk of coronary heart disease, of *hypertension* (high blood pressure) and of suffering a *stroke.* Heavy drinkers of certain beers risk *cardiomyopathy.*
Other physical disorders	Other physical diseases and disorders associated with a high alcohol consumption include *gastritis, pancreatitis,* and *peptic ulcer,* all probably linked	to an irritant action of alcohol. Heavy drinking during pregnancy carries a risk of the baby being born with *fetal alcohol syndrome.*
Psychiatric illnesses	Alcoholics are more likely than others to suffer from *anxiety* and *depression* (frequently related to financial, work, or family problems) and from paranoia. They are also more likely to	have *dementia* (irreversible mental deterioration) develop. The incidence of *suicide* attempts and actual suicide is also higher among alcoholics.

Alcohol, rubbing

A liquid preparation, consisting mainly of ethyl alcohol, that has a soothing and hardening effect when applied to the skin. It is widely used before injections as an *antiseptic* and may also be used to prevent bedsores and to protect the soles of the feet before a long walk or run.

Aldosterone

A hormone secreted by the adrenal cortex (part of the adrenal gland) that is important in the control of blood pressure and the regulation of sodium and potassium concentration.

Aldosterone acts on the kidney to decrease the amount of sodium lost in the urine; the sodium is reabsorbed from urine before it leaves the kidney and replaced in the urine by potassium. The sodium carries with it, increasing the blood volume and raising the blood pressure.

The production of aldosterone is stimulated mainly by the action of *angiotensin* II, a chemical produced by the enzyme renin released by the kidneys. Its production is stimulated by the action of *ACTH,* produced by the pituitary gland.

Aldosteronism

A disorder caused by the excessive production of the hormone *aldosterone.* It can be caused by a tumor of the adrenal gland (called Conn's syndrome) or by a disorder that has reduced the flow of blood through the kidney, which leads to overproduction of *renin* and angiotensin, and, in turn, to excessive aldosterone production. *Heart failure* and *cirrhosis* of the liver can cause reduced blood flow through the kidney.

SYMPTOMS

Symptoms are directly related to the actions of aldosterone. Too much sodium is retained in the body, leading to elevated blood pressure; at the same time, excess potassium is lost in the urine. The low potassium level causes tiredness and muscle weakness and impairs kidney function, leading to overproduction of urine and thirst due to fluid loss.

DIAGNOSIS AND TREATMENT

The diagnosis is suggested by a combination of *hypertension,* a raised level of sodium in the blood, and a low level of potassium.

Treatment in all cases includes restriction of salt in the diet and use of the diuretic drug spironolactone. This drug blocks the action of aldosterone on the kidneys, leading to increased loss of sodium from the body, lowered blood pressure, and reduced loss of potassium. With Conn's syndrome, the tumor may be surgically removed.

Alexia

Word blindness; the inability to recognize and name written words, thus severely disrupting the ability to read in a person who was previously literate. The disability is caused by damage (e.g., by a *stroke*) to part of the cerebrum and is a much more severe reading disability than *dyslexia.*

Alienation

Feeling like a stranger, even when among familiar people or places, and being unable to identify with a cul-

A

ture, family, or peer group. Alienated people feel unhappy and uncertain and may turn to unusual religions or alternative life-styles in their search for the meaning of life.

Deprived groups such as immigrants or the poor may feel distanced from the society in which they live as a result of cultural differences, language difficulties, or financial problems. Alienation is also a common feeling among adolescents, made worse by parental neglect or friction, and is sometimes an early symptom of *schizophrenia* or part of a *personality disorder*. Feelings of alienation are thought to be a contributing cause of suicide, attempted suicide, and inner-city violence.

Alignment, dental
The movement of teeth by braces or fixed *orthodontic appliances* to correct *malocclusion* (incorrect bite).

Alimentary tract
The tubelike structure that extends from the mouth to the anus (see *Digestive system*). It is also known as the alimentary canal.

Alkali
Also known as a base, an alkali is chemically defined as a donor of hydroxyl ions (an atom of hydrogen linked to an atom of oxygen and having an overall negative electrical charge). Alkalis include a variety of substances, some of which are corrosive. Examples of alkalis include caustic soda (sodium hydroxide); lime (calcium oxide); various bicarbonates, such as bicarbonate of soda; and *antacids*, such as aluminum hydroxide, used to neutralize stomach acid in the treatment of peptic ulcers. (See also *Acid; Acid-base balance; Burns.*)

Alkaloids
A group of nitrogen-containing substances isolated from plants for use as a drug (for example, *morphine, codeine,* and *nicotine*) or as a poison (for example, strychnine).

Alkalosis
A disturbance of the body's *acid-base balance* in which there is an accumulation of alkali (base) or loss of acid.

CAUSES
There are two types of alkalosis: metabolic and respiratory. In the former, the increase in alkalinity may be caused by taking too much antacid or by losing a large amount of stomach acid as a result of severe vomiting.

Respiratory alkalosis is caused by a reduction in the level of carbon dioxide in the blood (carbon dioxide dissolves in the blood to form carbonic acid). This reduction is caused by *hyperventilation* (deep, fast breathing), which may occur during a panic attack or at high altitudes as a result of lack of oxygen. (See also *Acidosis.*)

Allergist
A physician who diagnoses and treats any form of *allergy*. The allergist conducts tests to determine the agents to which a person is allergic. Once the offending agent or agents have been identified, the allergist can recommend ways to avoid exposure, may attempt to build up the patient's immunity through inoculations of tiny amounts of the allergen, and may put the patient on a regimen of medication to control the reactions.

Allergy
A collection of disease symptoms caused by exposure of the skin to a chemical, of the respiratory system to particles of dust or pollen, or of the stomach and intestines to a particular food, which in the majority of people causes no symptoms.

Allergies are inappropriate or exaggerated reactions of the *immune system* and occur only on second or subsequent exposures to the offending agent, after the first contact has sensitized the body. Many common illnesses, such as *asthma* and allergic *rhinitis* (hay fever), are caused by allergic reactions.

TYPES AND CAUSES
The function of the immune system is to recognize *antigens* (foreign proteins) contained on the surfaces of microorganisms (such as viruses and bacteria) and to form *antibodies* (also called immunoglobulins) and sensitized white blood cells (called *lymphocytes*) that will interact with these antigens when next encountered, leading to destruction of the microorganisms.

In allergies, a similar process occurs, except that the immune system forms antibodies or sensitized lymphocytes against harmless substances—because these allergens (as they are called) are misidentified as potentially harmful antigens.

The inappropriate or exaggerated reactions seen in allergies are termed *hypersensitivity* reactions and can have any of four different mechanisms (termed Types I through IV hypersensitivity reactions). Most well-known

allergies are caused by the Type I variety (also known as anaphylactic or immediate hypersensitivity).

TYPE I HYPERSENSITIVITY REACTIONS Common allergens that can cause Type I reactions include flowers, grasses, and tree pollens, animal dander (tiny particles of skin and hair), house dust, house-dust mites, yeasts, certain drugs and foods, and constituents of bee and wasp venom. Of the food allergens, the most common are milk, eggs, shellfish, dried fruits, nuts, and certain food dyes.

These allergens provoke the immune system to produce specific antibodies, belonging to a type called immunoglobulin E (IgE), which coat cells (called mast cells or basophils) present in the skin and the lining of the stomach, lungs, and upper respiratory airways. When the allergen is encountered for the second time, it binds to the IgE antibodies and causes granules in the mast cells to release several different chemicals, which are responsible for the symptoms of the allergy.

Among the chemicals released is histamine, which causes blood vessels to widen, fluids to leak into tissues, and muscles to go into spasm. Symptoms may be restricted to the skin (itchy swelling or rash), upper airways (inflammation or mucus secretion, sneezing in hay fever, and spasm and narrowing of the airways in asthma), eyes (inflammation), or stomach and intestines (vomiting and diarrhea). Or the symptoms may affect several organs, especially when the allergies are to injected drugs, insect venom, or some foods. Particular illnesses associated with Type I reactions include asthma, hay fever, *urticaria* (hives), *angioedema, anaphylactic shock* (a severe, generalized allergic reaction), possibly atopic *eczema*, and many types of food allergy producing immediate symptoms.

TYPES II THROUGH IV HYPERSENSITIVITY REACTIONS These reactions have different mechanisms from Type I reactions (see *Hypersensitivity*) and are less often implicated in allergies. However, Type III reactions are responsible for a type of lung disease called allergic *alveolitis* (which includes *farmers' lung*) and for the skin swellings that occur after booster vaccinations. Type IV reactions are responsible for contact *dermatitis* (a rash caused by contact with substances such as nickel, elastic, detergents, and cosmetics).

It is not known why certain individuals and not others get allergies,

ALLERGY AND THE BODY

An allergy is an inappropriate response (causing troublesome symptoms) to substances that, in most people, cause no response. The response is mainly to harmless substances that come in contact with the skin, respiratory airways, or the eye's surface. In diagnosing an allergy, the individual's medical history is important. The physician needs to know whether the symptoms vary according to the time of day or the season, and whether there are any pets or other likely sources of allergens in the home.

THE MOST COMMON ALLERGENS

Airborne		Foods	
	Grass pollens		Dairy products
	Tree pollens		Eggs
	Spores from molds		Strawberries
	House-dust mites		Fish and shellfish
	Animal dander		Cereals

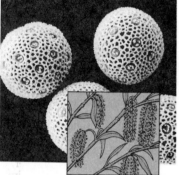

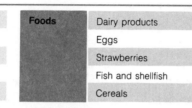

Animal dander
It is often assumed that allergy results from contact with animal hair. In fact, allergy is caused by flakes of dead skin (dander).

Feathers
Bedding containing feathers may produce an allergic reaction. Instead, use pillows and quilts containing synthetic stuffing.

Mites in house dust
Fragments of mites and their feces in house dust may cause an allergic reaction. Keeping the house dust-free helps.

Pollen
Airborne pollen from plants (especially from grasses and trees) may trigger an allergic reaction; symptoms appear during the warmer months. The most common reaction is allergic rhinitis (hay fever), which occurs when pollen is breathed in and irritates the nasal lining.

DIAGNOSING SKIN ALLERGY

Tests are performed to identify specific reactions to allergens. Small amounts of various substances are applied to the skin. A wheal indicates sensitivity to a particular allergen.

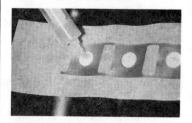

Conducting a patch test
Three different allergens are put on a patch (above left) and taped to the skin.

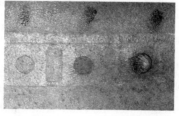

Results are (above right): no reaction; mild inflammation; severe contact dermatitis.

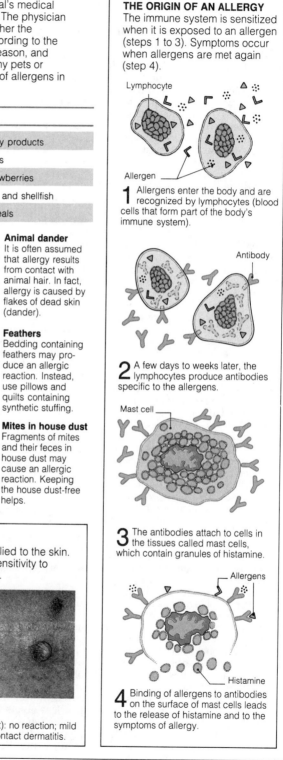

THE ORIGIN OF AN ALLERGY

The immune system is sensitized when it is exposed to an allergen (steps 1 to 3). Symptoms occur when allergens are met again (step 4).

Lymphocyte

Allergen

1 Allergens enter the body and are recognized by lymphocytes (blood cells that form part of the body's immune system).

Antibody

2 A few days to weeks later, the lymphocytes produce antibodies specific to the allergens.

Mast cell

3 The antibodies attach to cells in the tissues called mast cells, which contain granules of histamine.

Allergens

Histamine

4 Binding of allergens to antibodies on the surface of mast cells leads to the release of histamine and to the symptoms of allergy.

A

although about one person in eight seems to have an inherited predisposition to have allergies (see *Atopy*).

Certain mild deficiencies of the immune system are associated with allergy. Environmental conditions are sometimes involved; a child living in a house with a cat or dog may slowly become sensitized to the pet and an allergic reaction such as hives or asthma may develop. Exposure to some viruses may precipitate or increase allergic responses. Emotional factors are also thought to contribute to allergic diseases such as asthma.

TREATMENT

Immunotherapy can be valuable for people who suffer allergic reactions to insect venom, house-dust mites, and some pollens. Gradually increasing doses of the allergen are given to promote the formation of antibodies that will then block future adverse reactions. The therapy is effective in about two thirds of the cases, but usually requires two to three years of treatment. It can produce mild side effects, such as itching, swelling, or rashes; occasionally, more serious side effects occur, such as bronchospasm or anaphylactic shock. Low-dosage, long-acting methods of desensitization are being researched.

Drug treatment for allergic reactions includes the use of *antihistamine drugs*, which relieve the symptoms (the itching produced by an insect bite, for example). Most available antihistamine drugs are sedative, which is particularly useful in treating the itching due to eczema because they permit the sufferer to sleep more soundly. Several of the newer antihistamines do not cause drowsiness.

Other drugs, such as cromolyn sodium and *corticosteroid drugs*, can be taken regularly to prevent symptoms from developing. Corticosteroid creams are useful for treating eczema, but prolonged use on the same area can damage the skin. In severe allergic diseases, such as asthma, the use of oral corticosteroids may be necessary.

Whenever possible, the most effective treatment for allergy of any kind is avoidance of the relevant allergen. For example, anyone with an allergy to eggs should avoid eating eggs or any dishes containing eggs as an ingredient, and should check the recipes of dishes consumed in restaurants or at parties. If pollen is the allergen, it may be harder to avoid; measures such as keeping car windows closed while driving and closing bedroom windows at night afford some protection.

Allopathy

A term that describes conventional medicine as practiced by a graduate of a medical school or college granting the MD degree. (See also *Homeopathy*.)

Allopurinol

A treatment for *gout* that works by reducing *hyperuricemia* (raised levels of uric acid in the blood). Allopurinol does not relieve pain in acute attacks but does reduce their frequency.

POSSIBLE ADVERSE EFFECTS

These include itching, rash, and nausea. Occasionally, during the first few months of treatment, allopurinol increases the frequency of gout attacks. *Colchicine* may be prescribed to counteract this effect.

Alopecia

Loss or absence of *hair*, which is usually noticeable only on the scalp but which may occur at any hair-bearing site on the body.

TYPES

HEREDITARY ALOPECIA This includes male pattern baldness, the most common form of alopecia. Normal hair is lost initially from the temples and crown, where it is replaced by fine, downy hair. The affected area gradually becomes wider as the line of normal hair recedes. This pattern of hair loss is inherited; it usually affects men, although young women and women who have passed the menopause are occasionally affected.

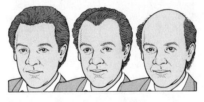

Stages in male pattern baldness
In this common form of alopecia, the man loses hair first from the temples and from the crown; the bald area then gradually widens.

Other hereditary forms of hair loss are rare. They may be due to an absence of hair roots or to abnormalities of the hair shaft, causing it to snap under the normal effects of sun, wind, shampooing, and combing.

GENERALIZED ALOPECIA In this rare form of alopecia, the hair falls out in large amounts, leaving a nearly invisible covering over the entire scalp. Such hair loss occurs because all the hairs simultaneously enter the resting phase and then fall out about three months later. Regrowth occurs when the cause is corrected.

Causes include various forms of stress, such as an operation, fever, prolonged illness, or *chemotherapy*.

LOCALIZED ALOPECIA This may be due to permanent damage to the skin—for example, by burns or *radiation therapy*. Another common cause of hair loss is trauma to the hair roots. Trauma may be due to excessive pulling of the hair to produce a particular hairstyle or, rarely, to a nervous disorder in which sufferers pull out their hair.

Fungal infection of the scalp (see *Tinea*) may cause a localized hair loss due to breakage of weakened hair shafts. Other skin diseases, such as *lichen planus, lupus erythematosus,* and *skin tumors,* may also be responsible. The bald skin always looks abnormal in conditions such as these and hair stubble can usually be seen in the affected area.

Alopecia areata is a disorder characterized by localized areas of hair loss in which the bald skin looks and feels normal. The cause is unknown.

Alopecia universalis is a rare, permanent form of alopecia areata that causes all the hair on the scalp and the body to be lost, including the eyelashes and eyebrows.

Wigs and toupees are often used to disguise alopecia affecting the scalp. *Hair transplants* are sometimes successful as a permanent method of replacing the lost hair.

Alpha-fetoprotein

A protein produced in the liver and gastrointestinal tract of the fetus and by some abnormal tissues in adults.

ALPHA-FETOPROTEIN IN PREGNANCY

Alpha-fetoprotein (AFP) is excreted in the fetal urine into the *amniotic fluid* (in which the fetus floats in the uterus); the fluid is then swallowed by the fetus, which introduces AFP into the fetal digestive system. Most of the AFP is broken down in the fetal intestine, but some passes from the fetus' circulation. AFP can be measured in the maternal blood from the second quarter of pregnancy onward, peaking between weeks 15 and 20 and then slowly decreasing.

Raised levels of AFP are found in some cases of fetal abnormality and occasionally when the fetus is normal. In *neural tube defects* (such as *spina bifida* or *anencephaly*), excess AFP may leak into the amniotic fluid. AFP levels are also raised in certain kidney abnormalities and can result from impaired breakdown in the intestine if the fetus cannot swallow properly because of malformation of the esophagus.

AFP levels are also raised in multiple *pregnancy* and in threatened or actual *miscarriage*. They may misleadingly appear to be raised when there has been an error in the calculation of gestation dates. AFP levels may be unusually low in pregnancies in which a baby has *Down's syndrome*.

TESTING AFP LEVELS IN PREGNANCY Ideally, pregnant women should be offered prenatal screening by measurement of blood AFP and *ultrasound scanning* at about 16 weeks. Scanning accurately dates the pregnancy, may show multiple pregnancy, and may show certain fetal abnormalities. If the blood AFP level is raised, the test is repeated one week later. If the second result is also raised, the woman may be carrying a baby with a neural tube defect. An ultrasound scan may strengthen or confirm the suspicion. *Amniocentesis* (removal of a small amount of the fluid surrounding the fetus) may be performed, and further measurements of AFP may be made on the sample. If the level is significantly raised, the chances that the woman is carrying an affected baby are high; a termination of pregnancy (see *Abortion, elective*) may then be considered.

About 10 percent of cases of neural tube defect are missed during screening because AFP levels are not significantly raised in every case. Conversely, in about five cases per 1,000 in which both amniotic fluid and blood levels of AFP are raised, the fetus is normal.

AFP IN ADULTS
In adults, AFP is produced in certain abnormal tissues. Levels are commonly raised in patients with hepatoma (see *Liver cancer*) and in those with malignant *teratoma* of the testes or ovaries. Some patients with cancer of the pancreas, stomach, and lung also have raised levels. Because it is present in abnormal quantities in some cancers, AFP is known as a "tumor marker." However, AFP levels are also raised in some benign conditions, including viral and alcoholic *hepatitis* and in *cirrhosis*.

AFP levels can be used to monitor the treatment of hepatomas and teratomas; increasing levels after surgery or chemotherapy are a useful indicator of tumor recurrence.

Alpha-tocopherol
The most potent of the tocopherols, an alcohol that is the main active constituent of *vitamin E*. It is fat-soluble and occurs in many foods. Deficiency of alpha-tocopherol is rare.

Alprazolam
A member of the family of *benzodiazepine drugs* used to treat *anxiety*, *panic attacks*, and *phobias*.

Alprostadil
A *prostaglandin drug* given to newborn infants who have certain types of congenital *heart disease* (such as *tetralogy of Fallot*, in which blood flow to the lungs is impaired). Alprostadil keeps open the ductus arteriosus—which normally closes after birth—and thus provides an alternative route for blood to reach the lungs. The ductus arteriosus links the aorta (the main artery carrying blood to the body) to the pulmonary artery (which takes blood to the lungs). Alprostadil, which is given by *intravenous infusion*, is used as a temporary measure until heart surgery can be performed.

Alprostadil also improves blood flow in general and is currently under investigation as a treatment for *Raynaud's disease* (a circulatory disorder affecting the hands and feet).

ALS
Amyotrophic lateral sclerosis (see *Motor neuron disease*).

Alternative medicine
Any medical system based on a theory of disease or its treatment that is incompatible with the orthodox science of medicine as it is taught in medical schools. Complementary medicine, by contrast, is the use by orthodox physicians of treatment techniques, such as *acupuncture* or manipulation, that are not generally included among orthodox therapies. In complementary medicine these alternative techniques are used empirically, that is, they are used in circumstances in which experience has suggested they may be effective, although the mechanism of their action may be unknown or uncertain.

Every society has its *folk medicine* and traditional healers who use methods and beliefs handed down through the generations. In some cultures, such as in China (see *Chinese medicine*), textbooks of traditional medicine date back several thousands of years. Some systems, such as acupuncture and *acupressure*, are based on theories of disease that emphasize internal balances.

Many cultures contain traditions of *herbal medicine*, plant-based remedies for common complaints. Some plants have properties recognized by orthodox medicine.

European folk medicine, based on the four humors described by the ancient Greeks and on ordinary herbal medicine, was transformed by the scientific discoveries of the eighteenth and nineteenth centuries.

The early nineteenth century brought the development and flourishing of many new alternative systems, including *chiropractic*, *homeopathy*, and *naturopathy*. The popularity of these alternative practices declined from the 1930s to 1950s with the successes of orthodox medicine—notably vaccines, antibiotics, diuretics, antidepressants, and advances in anesthesia and surgery. In the last decade, however, a small but increasing number of people have questioned the ability of orthodox medicine to provide all the answers. Numerous new and rediscovered disciplines, such as *aroma therapy* and naturopathy, have won a following without conclusive scientific confirmation.

Many alternative practitioners are sympathetic listeners who give sensible advice backed by treatments that have, at the very least, a powerful placebo effect. The opposition by orthodox physicians to alternative therapies is based on the principle that the first step in the treatment of any disorder is accurate diagnosis, which itself requires extensive medical knowledge. Treatment of symptoms without knowing their cause may be disastrous if an underlying remediable but progressive condition has not been recognized. Some herbal remedies, although based on natural ingredients, may cause adverse reactions in some people and might also be dangerous if taken at the same time as conventional medicines.

Altitude sickness
See *Mountain sickness*.

Aluminum
A light metallic element that is abundant in various minerals, such as bauxite. Aluminum is also found in relatively low concentrations in the body, though it is not known to have any useful function and is almost certainly harmful.

Sources of ingested aluminum include antacids, cooking utensils and foil, antiperspirants, some baking powders, and food additives such as potassium alum (used to whiten flour) and aluminum calcium silicate (used to keep table salt running freely). Most of the aluminum that is taken into the body is excreted. The remainder is stored in the lungs, brain, liver, and thyroid gland.

ADVERSE EFFECTS
Industrial processes in which aluminum aerosols are used (i.e., aluminum processing, pottery making, and explosives manufacturing) are associated with various lung diseases, including *fibrosis* of the lungs and *emphysema*.

Aluminum hydroxide is widely used in *antacids* for the treatment of peptic ulcers and acid indigestion; prolonged use can cause weakness, tiredness, and loss of appetite. Some people get an allergic reaction to the aluminum chloride contained in *antiperspirants*, resulting in *dermatitis* (itchy, inflamed skin).

Aluminum-induced *dementia* (a form of mental disorder) has developed in some patients undergoing *dialysis* (artificial purification of the blood, used to treat kidney failure) due to the aluminum content of the water used. However, the condition can be prevented by adequate monitoring procedures. There is no convincing evidence linking aluminum with *Alzheimer's disease*.

Alveolectomy
See *Alveoloplasty*.

Alveolitis
Inflammation of the alveoli (tiny air sacs) in the lungs, with thickening of their walls. Alveolitis reduces the elasticity of the lungs during breathing and reduces the efficiency of transfer of gases between the lungs and the surrounding blood vessels.

CAUSES
There are a number of causes of alveolitis. The most common is an allergic reaction to an inhaled dust of animal or plant origin, often containing fungal spores. This allergic alveolitis may be related to occupation. Examples include *farmers' lung* (caused by spores from moldy hay), *bagassosis* (spores from moldy bagasse, a material used in cardboard manufacture), and bird breeders' lung (caused by particles from bird droppings).

Fibrosing alveolitis may be an *autoimmune disorder*, in which the body's defenses produce antibodies against its own tissues, in this case the lung tissues. The exact cause of this disorder is unknown, although in some cases it occurs with other autoimmune disorders such as systemic *lupus erythematosus* or *rheumatoid arthritis*.

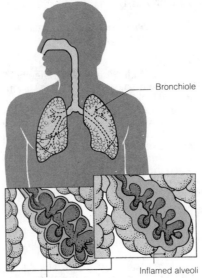
Bronchiole

Inflamed alveoli

Normal alveoli

Signs of alveolitis
The alveoli become inflamed and their walls thicken, causing the lungs to become less elastic and less efficient.

Radiation alveolitis is inflammation caused by exposure to radiation, usually as a rare complication of *radiation therapy* treatment for lung or breast cancer.

SYMPTOMS AND DIAGNOSIS
Alveolitis usually causes a dry cough and breathing difficulty on exertion.

A chest X ray usually shows mottled shadowing across the lungs. Blood tests may be performed to show specific antibodies to an allergen or as evidence of an autoimmune disorder. *Pulmonary function tests* will demonstrate reduced lung capacity without obstruction to airflow through the bronchi. A lung *biopsy* may be performed to examine an area of damaged lung tissue under the microscope and may be the only way to make a conclusive diagnosis.

TREATMENT AND OUTLOOK
The conditions of some people with alveolitis show improvement on a course of *corticosteroid drugs*. In fibrosing alveolitis, a low dose of corticosteroids may be continued indefinitely as a maintenance treatment; in other types, the benefit of corticosteroids will apply only to a short course.

If the cause of allergic alveolitis is recognized and avoided before any damage occurs, there is often no permanent disability. In fibrosing alveolitis, however, the lung damage

progresses despite treatment, causing increasing breathing difficulty and, sometimes, respiratory failure. (See also *Hypersensitivity*; *Pneumonitis*.)

Alveoloplasty
Dental surgery to remove protuberances and to smooth out other uneven areas from tooth-bearing bone in the jaw prior to fitting dentures. Alveoloplasty is carried out on people whose alveolar ridge underlying the gums would not otherwise be even enough for dentures to be fitted easily or worn comfortably.

HOW IT IS DONE
Minor alveoloplasty may require only local anesthesia but in most cases the patient is given a general anesthetic. An incision is made in the gum, which is peeled back to expose the uneven bone. The bone is either reshaped with large bone forceps or filed down to the required shape. The gum is then replaced and stitched together.

Some bruising and swelling of the mouth may occur, just as it sometimes does after a tooth is extracted. The gum usually heals within two weeks.

Alveolus, dental
The bony cavity or socket that supports each tooth in the jaw.

Alveolus, pulmonary
One of a group of minute, balloonlike sacs at the end of a bronchiole (one of the many small air passages in the

ANATOMY OF THE ALVEOLI
These tiny sacs contain capillaries in their thin walls that allow oxygen to be absorbed into the blood.

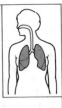

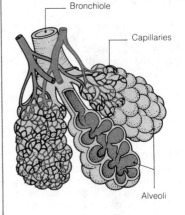
Bronchiole

Capillaries

Alveoli

lungs). Inhaled oxygen is absorbed into the bloodstream by capillaries in the thin wall of each alveolus, and carbon dioxide passes the other way (from the blood into the lungs) to be breathed out. There are about 300 million alveoli in each lung.

Alzheimer's disease

A progressive condition in which nerve cells degenerate in the brain and the brain substance shrinks. Alzheimer's disease is the single most common cause of *dementia*. Although originally classified as a "presenile" dementia, Alzheimer's disease is now known to be responsible for 75 percent of dementia cases in those over 65 years old. Because of the increasing numbers of elderly citizens, interest and research into the causes and treatment of Alzheimer's disease have greatly expanded in recent years. The progress of the disease (which, in most cases, represents several years of intellectual and personal decline until death) cannot be arrested.

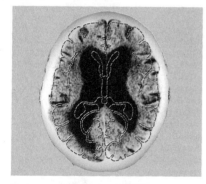

Brain scan in Alzheimer's disease
The volume of the brain substance (gray area) has shrunk markedly. Its normal outline is shown by the dotted line.

CAUSES

The cause of Alzheimer's disease is unknown, although a number of theories have been proposed, ranging from the effects of a chronic infection to those of toxic poisoning by a metal such as aluminum. There is known to be a reduced level of *acetylcholine* and other brain chemicals in people with Alzheimer's disease. A genetic factor is also a possibility; the disease is more common in those with *Down's syndrome*, and 15 percent of the victims of Alzheimer's disease have a family history of the disease, occasionally with a dominant pattern of inheritance (in which children with one affected parent have a 50 percent chance of inheriting the disease).

INCIDENCE

Onset is rare before the age of 60, but thereafter increases steadily with age. Up to 30 percent of people over the age of 85 are affected.

SYMPTOMS AND SIGNS

The features of the disease vary among individuals, but there are three broad stages. At first the patient notices his or her increasing forgetfulness and may try to compensate by writing lists or by soliciting the help of others. Problems with memory often cause the patient to feel anxious and depressed, but these symptoms frequently go unnoticed.

Forgetfulness gradually shades into a second phase of severe memory loss, particularly for recent events. Victims may remember long-ago events, such as their schooldays and young adulthood, but they are unable to recall yesterday's visitors or what they saw on television. They also become disoriented as to time or place, losing their way even on familiar streets; their concentration and ability to calculate numbers declines and *dysphasia* (inability to find the right word) is noticeable. Anxiety increases, mood changes are sudden and unpredictable, and personality changes soon become apparent.

In the third stage, patients become severely disoriented and confused. They may also suffer from symptoms of *psychosis*, such as *hallucinations* and paranoid *delusions*. Symptoms are worsened by the patient's disorientation and memory losses and are usually most severe at night. Signs of nervous system disease begin to emerge, such as primitive *reflexes* (involuntary actions that occur normally in newborn babies) and incontinence of urine and feces. Some patients become demanding, unpleasant, and sometimes violent, and lose all awareness of social norms. Some become docile and somewhat helpless. They neglect personal hygiene and may wander purposelessly. Eventually the burden for caring relatives becomes impossible, and full-time hospital care and nursing are often inevitable. Once the patient is bedridden the complications of bedsores, feeding problems, and pneumonia make life expectancy very short.

DIAGNOSIS

Alzheimer's disease can be definitely diagnosed only by examination of the brain, either by brain *biopsy* or after death. Not only is the brain shrunken in size, but under the microscope it is possible to observe a loss of nerve cells, specks of brain debris, and tangles of nerves resembling pieces of unwound string.

In the absence of any absolute diagnostic test for the disease during life, the diagnosis is a clinical one. An *EEG* (recording of brain-wave patterns) will show increasingly slow waves, but will add nothing by itself to that which is clinically apparent. *CT scanning* and *MRI* of the brain show evidence of reduced cerebral size. Mental status tests indicate a decrease in the person's intellectual ability.

Some 10 percent of people with symptoms of dementia have a reversible disease (such as *hypothyroidism*, pernicious anemia or vitamin B_{12} deficiency, a tumor, or subdural *hematoma*). Routine investigations should be carried out to ensure that any treatable diseases are noted. It is also not uncommon for the elderly to have a depressive pseudodementia, in which the patient appears to be demented but is actually suffering from the effects of *depression*.

TREATMENT

There is no specific treatment for the disease itself apart from the provision of suitable nursing and social care for both victim and relatives. Keeping the victim well nourished, exercised, and occupied helps alleviate anxiety and personal distress, especially in the earlier stages when the person is still sufficiently aware of his or her condition. Tranquilizing medication can often improve difficult behavior and help the patient sleep.

Counseling of victims' families can help to prevent problems, such as physical abuse of the afflicted person, and can minimize disruption of family life. Provision of suitable day-care facilities (where patients stay temporarily to give families a break), personal care facilities (where patients live in a structured environment until inpatient care is necessary), and inpatient care for advanced cases all can help ease the burden on families.

OUTLOOK

With the increasing numbers of elderly people, the pressure on public health care services is becoming intense. Ideally, care is best provided at home, but this may be impossible. Although efforts are being made to expand facilities, a shortage of suitable places exists for elderly people with dementia. Research into drug therapy is continuing.

AMA

See *American Medical Association*.

A

Amalgam, dental

A material used to fill teeth, consisting of an alloy of mercury with one or more other metals. Amalgam is soft enough to be easily workable by the dentist but sets rapidly (within 24 hours) into a hard, strong solid; it is thus ideal for use as a filling, especially for back teeth (see *Filling, dental*).

Amantadine

An *antiviral drug* used in the prevention and treatment of *influenza* A. Amantadine more recently has been used to help relieve symptoms of *Parkinson's disease*.

Amaurosis fugax

Brief loss of vision, lasting for periods of seconds to minutes, usually caused by the temporary blockage of small blood vessels in the eye by tiny *emboli* (particles of solid matter such as cholesterol crystals and particles of clotted blood). These emboli are carried in the bloodstream from diseased carotid arteries in the neck or, rarely, from the heart. Sufferers typically experience a loss or dimming of vision, in one eye only, that is like a shade being pulled down or up.

Attacks may be infrequent or may occur many times a day. This symptom should never be ignored since it is a clear warning that the person is at increased risk of *stroke* or *coronary heart disease*. Medical investigation, with special attention to the state of the arteries, is urgently needed.

Amaurotic familial idiocy

A term covering a range of rare inherited disorders, of which the best known is *Tay-Sachs disease*. In these conditions, the nervous system suffers progressive degeneration and atrophy, with early involvement of the optic nerves and retinas, leading to blindness. Brain involvement causes mental deterioration. The conditions are incurable but are exceedingly uncommon. They may be diagnosed early in pregnancy and termination of the pregnancy may be considered.

Ambidexterity

The ability to perform manual skills, such as writing or using cutlery, equally well with either hand because there is no definite *handedness* (preference for using one hand). Ambidexterity is an uncommon and often familial trait.

Amblyopia

A permanent visual acuity defect in which there is usually no structural abnormality in the eye. In many cases there is now known to be a failure in the linkup of nerve connections in the visual pathway between the retina and the brain. The term is also sometimes applied to toxic or nutritional causes of decreased visual acuity, as in tobacco-alcohol amblyopia.

If normal vision is to develop during infancy and childhood, it is essential that clear, corresponding visual images are formed on both retinas so that compatible nerve impulses pass from the eyes to the brain. If no images are received, normal vision cannot develop. If images from the two eyes are very different, one will be suppressed to avoid double vision, and normal vision may not develop in one of the eyes.

CAUSES
The most common cause of amblyopia is *strabismus* (squint) in very young children, in which only one eye points at a selected object while the different image from the other eye is suppressed. Failure to form normal retinal images may also result from congenital *cataract* (opacity of the internal lens of the eye at birth), and severe, or unequal, focusing errors in a young child, such as when one eye is normal and the other eye has an uncorrected large *astigmatism*, causing a blurred retinal image. Toxic and nutritional amblyopia may result from damage to the retina and/or optic nerve.

TREATMENT AND OUTLOOK
It is important to treat amblyopia at an early age; after the age of 8, amblyopia usually cannot be remedied. For amblyopia due to strabismus, patching (covering up the good eye to force the deviating eye to function properly) is the usual treatment. Glasses and/or surgery to place the deviating eyes in the correct position may be necessary. Glasses may also be necessary to correct severe focusing errors. Congenital cataracts may be removed.

Ambulance

A vehicle for conveying sick, injured, or disabled people. There are two types of ambulance: nonemergency ambulances (medi-cars or vans) and emergency ambulances.

A medi-car or van is designed for people traveling to outpatient departments at hospitals and to day-care clinics. The van usually has eight to 10 seats and an elevator for moving wheelchairs.

The emergency ambulance responds to 911 calls, taking accident victims and severely ill people to the hospital. In addition to stretchers, it contains many items useful in emergency situations, including oxygen, intravenous fluids, ECG equipment, a cardioversion unit with paddles (to treat heart attack victims), analgesics, splints, and dressings.

Ambulatory care

Medical care given without the patient being admitted to a hospital.

Ambulatory surgery

Surgery done without the patient being admitted to a hospital. Ambulatory surgery may, however, be performed in the outpatient section of a hospital. It is also performed in physicians' offices, or in outpatient surgical centers specially designed for cases in which an overnight stay in a hospital is not necessary.

Amebiasis

An infection caused by a tiny animal parasite, *ENTAMOEBA HISTOLYTICA*, which lives in the human large intestine. The infection is characterized by persistent moderate to severe diarrhea and, occasionally, the development of abscesses in the liver or, more rarely, in the brain.

INCIDENCE
Amebiasis is prevalent in poor countries where standards of public hygiene and sanitation are low. Although it can be acquired anywhere, most cases in the US and other developed countries occur among travelers who have recently returned from developing countries in the tropics or subtropics.

About 5,000 to 10,000 cases are diagnosed per year in the US, leading to about 20 deaths annually.

CAUSES
ENTAMOEBA HISTOLYTICA is an ameba, a type of single-celled animal that multiplies by simple division and moves around in the intestine, scavenging for small morsels of food and bacteria. The life cycle of this organism, and method by which it is spread from one person to another, is shown in the diagram.

Many people (few in the US) carry *ENTAMOEBA HISTOLYTICA* in their intestines and excrete amebic cysts but have no symptoms, probably because the strain of amebae they carry is harmless. Other strains, for unknown reasons, invade the intestinal wall,

THE CYCLE OF AMEBIASIS

The parasite ENTAMOEBA HISTOLYTICA lives in the large intestine, where it multiplies; sometimes protective cysts develop. Passed out in feces, the cysts can survive long periods before the next host acquires them.

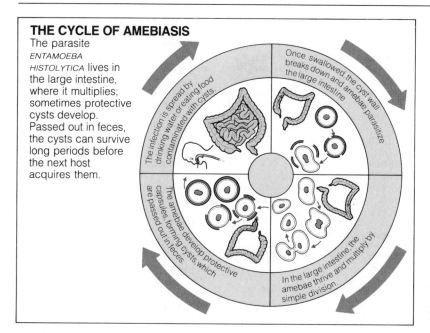

The infection is spread by drinking water or eating food contaminated with cysts.

Once swallowed the cyst breaks down and amebae parasitize the large intestine

In the large intestine, the amebae thrive and multiply by simple division.

The amebae develop protective capsules, forming cysts which are passed out in feces

causing bleeding and mucus secretion into the intestines and diarrhea—an illness called amebic dysentery. Ulcers are formed in the intestinal wall and sometimes the amebae gain access to the bloodstream, by which they travel to the liver to form abscesses. Brain infection is rare.

PREVENTION

Travelers to countries where sanitary standards are low can reduce their chances of acquiring amebiasis by drinking only water that has been bottled or boiled (water-purifying tablets are ineffective against amebic cysts) and by not eating uncooked vegetables (especially lettuce) or unpeeled fruit.

SYMPTOMS

The diarrhea caused by amebiasis may vary from two or more rather loose stools per day, accompanied by rumbling pains in the stomach, to full-blown dysentery, with high fever and the frequent passage of watery, bloody diarrhea.

The symptoms of amebic liver abscess are shaking chills, fever, weight loss, and painful enlargement of the liver. Abscesses may develop in people who have never had digestive tract symptoms.

TREATMENT

Treatment of all forms of amebiasis is with drugs such as metronidazole or iodoquinol, which effectively kill the parasite within a few weeks, leading to full recovery. Occasionally, it is necessary to drain a liver abscess.

Amebic dysentery

See *Amebiasis*.

Amebicides

A group of drugs used to treat *amebiasis* (an infection caused by amebae). Some amebicides (for example, iodoquinol) act only on amebae in the intestine. Others, such as *chloroquine* and *metronidazole*, also destroy amebae in other tissues, such as the liver.

Amelogenesis imperfecta

An inherited condition of the teeth in which the enamel is either abnormally thin or deficient in calcium. Affected teeth may be pitted and discolored (see *Discolored teeth*), and, depending on the type of imperfection, may be more susceptible to dental *caries*.

Amenorrhea

Absence of menstrual periods. Primary amenorrhea is defined as failure to start menstruating by the age of 16. Secondary amenorrhea is the temporary or permanent cessation of periods in a woman who has menstruated regularly in the past.

PRIMARY AMENORRHEA The main cause of primary amenorrhea is a delay in the onset of puberty. A delay of this type may be natural, or, in rare cases, it may result from a disorder of the *endocrine system*. This may be the direct result of a *pituitary tumor*; the indirect result of other hormonal disorders, such as *hypothyroidism* (underactivity

of the thyroid gland), an *adrenal tumor*, or *adrenal hyperplasia*; or it may occur for no known reason. A rare cause of delayed puberty is *Turner's syndrome*, in which one female sex chromosome is missing.

In some cases, menstruation fails to take place because the vagina or uterus has been absent from birth, or because there is no perforation in the hymen (the membrane across the opening of the vagina) to allow the menstrual blood to escape.

SECONDARY AMENORRHEA The most common cause of secondary amenorrhea is pregnancy.

Periods may temporarily cease after a woman has stopped taking the birth-control pill. This temporary cessation of menstrual flow usually lasts for only six to eight weeks, but it may persist for a year or longer. Secondary amenorrhea can also be the result of interference with the release of hormones due to emotional stress, depression, *anorexia nervosa*, or drugs.

Rarely, periods may stop as a result of the same disorders of the endocrine system that can cause primary amenorrhea. Another possible cause of secondary amenorrhea is a disorder of the *ovary*, such as *polycystic ovary* or a tumor of the ovary (see *Ovary, cancer of*).

Amenorrhea occurs permanently after the *menopause* or after a *hysterectomy* (surgical removal of the uterus).

INVESTIGATION

Investigation of amenorrhea usually includes a physical examination, blood tests to measure hormone levels, *laparoscopy* to inspect the ovaries, *CT scanning* of the skull to exclude the possibility of a pituitary tumor, and *ultrasound scanning* of the abdomen and pelvis to exclude an adrenal gland or ovarian tumor.

TREATMENT

Some women with either primary or secondary amenorrhea may choose not to have treatment, but in every case the cause should be identified. If an *ovarian cyst* or tumor is the cause, it requires removal. Anorexia nervosa, too, needs treatment because of its long-term threat to health. If a woman with amenorrhea wants treatment and the cause is related to the endocrine system, ovulation can usually be induced by treatment with *clomiphene* or *gonadotropin hormones*.

American Medical Association

The largest physician organization in American medicine, with approximately 279,000 members (1986) and an annual budget of approximately $133 million. Its members, nearly all of whom pay annual dues of $375, tend to be physicians engaged in patient care. Although the AMA is a federation of state and county medical societies, it provides representation in its policy-making body for many other medical groups, such as medical specialty societies, hospital and staff physicians, the deans of medical schools, residents, medical students, and physicians in the armed services, the Veterans Administration, and the US Public Health Service.

The house of delegates meets twice a year to debate issues, make policy, take positions, and elect officers. Officers include a president, who serves a one-year term, and a board of trustees, which makes policy decisions between the meetings of the house. An executive vice-president serves as a chief executive, overseeing a staff of more than 1,000 employees, most of them based at AMA headquarters in Chicago.

Ametropia

Optical defect of the eye that alters *refraction*. (See *Hyperopia*; *Myopia*; *Astigmatism*; *Presbyopia*.)

Amiloride

A potassium-sparing *diuretic drug*. Combined with loop or thiazide diuretic drugs, amiloride is used in the treatment of *hypertension* and *edema* due to *heart failure* or to *cirrhosis* of the liver.

Amino acids

A group of chemical compounds that forms the basic structural units of all *proteins*. Each amino acid molecule consists of nitrogenous amino and acidic carboxyl groups of atoms linked to a variable chain or ring of carbon atoms.

Individual amino acid molecules are linked together—by chemical bonds, called *peptide* bonds, between the amino and carboxyl groups—to form short chains of molecules called *polypeptides*. Hundreds of polypeptides are, in turn, linked together—also by peptide bonds—to form a protein molecule. What differentiates one protein from another is the arrangement of the amino acids.

There are 20 different amino acids that make up all the proteins in humans. Of these, 12 can be made by the body; they are known as nonessential amino acids, because they do not need to be obtained from the diet. The other eight, the essential amino acids, cannot be made by the body and must be obtained from the diet.

The 20 amino acids that make up proteins also occur free within cells and in body fluids. In addition, there are more than 200 other amino acids that are not found in proteins but which play an important part in chemical reactions within cells.

Aminoglutethimide

An *anticancer drug* that, in 1987, was under investigation as a treatment for certain types of breast cancer and for endocrine gland tumors.

Aminophylline

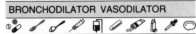

BRONCHODILATOR VASODILATOR			
Tablet	Liquid	Injection	Rectal suppository
Prescription needed			
Available as generic			

A drug used in the treatment of *asthma*, chronic *bronchitis*, and other respiratory disorders.

HOW IT WORKS
Aminophylline relieves breathing difficulty by widening the bronchi in the lungs. It also increases the production of urine and dilates (widens) blood vessels, which improves blood flow from the heart.

POSSIBLE ADVERSE EFFECTS
Unless the dose is carefully controlled, adverse effects, such as nausea, vomiting, headache, dizziness, and palpitations, may occur. During long-term treatment, blood tests may be carried out to monitor the level of aminophylline in the body.

Aminosalicylic acid

A drug existing in three distinct chemical forms. Para-aminosalicylic acid is an *antibacterial drug* used with other drugs to treat *tuberculosis*. Two forms (4-aminosalicylic acid and 5-aminosalicylic acid) are under investigation for use in the treatment of inflammatory bowel diseases such as *ulcerative colitis*.

Amitriptyline

An *antidepressant drug*, amitriptyline also has a sedative effect; it is useful in the treatment of *depression* accompanied by *anxiety* or *insomnia*.

Possible adverse effects include dry mouth, blurred vision, dizziness, drowsiness, and hot flashes, all of which may disappear if the dosage is reduced. Amitriptyline usually takes between two and six weeks to become fully effective.

Ammonia

A colorless, pungent gas that dissolves in water to form an alkaline solution (see *Alkali*). Ammonia consists of one nitrogen atom linked to three hydrogen atoms. Although it is poisonous, ammonia is produced by the body; it plays a valuable role in maintaining the *acid-base balance*.

In severe liver damage, the capacity of the liver to convert ammonia to *urea* is diminished. This leads to a high level of ammonia in the blood, which is thought to be a cause of the impairment of consciousness that occurs with liver failure.

Amnesia

Loss of the ability to memorize information and/or to recall information stored in memory. Memory can be divided into short-term and long-term: in the former, material is retained for seconds or minutes only, in the latter, it is retained indefinitely. In most amnesic conditions, the storage of information in long-term memory and/or the recall of such information is impaired.

CAUSES
Amnesia is caused by damage or disease of brain regions concerned with memory functions. Possible causes of such damage include head injuries (including concussion), degenerative disorders such as *Alzheimer's disease* and other forms of *dementia*, infections such as *encephalitis*, thiamine deficiency in alcoholics leading to *Wernicke-Korsakoff syndrome*, and also *brain tumors*, *strokes*, and *subarachnoid hemorrhage*. Amnesia can also occur in some forms of psychiatric illness (in which there is no apparent physical damage).

With many types of amnesia, the patient has a gap in memory extending back for some time from the moment of onset of the brain damage. This is called retrograde amnesia and is principally a deficit of recall. Usually the memory gap gradually shrinks over time. A patient may additionally (or alternatively) be unable to store new information in the period following damage to the brain. The resultant gap in memory, called an anterograde amnesia, extends from the moment of onset of the amnesia to the time when long-term memory resumes (if it ever does). This gap in the memory is usually permanent.

Amniocentesis

A diagnostic procedure in which a small amount of *amniotic fluid* is withdrawn from the amniotic sac, the membrane that surrounds the fetus in the uterus.

WHY IT IS DONE

The amniotic fluid contains cells and chemicals from the fetus that can be analyzed to detect fetal abnormalities, such as *Down's syndrome*, which is a chromosomal abnormality. Amniocentesis can also help detect other chromosomal abnormalities, sex-linked disorders (such as *hemophilia*), metabolic diseases (such as *Tay-Sachs disease*), or developmental disorders (such as *spina bifida*). It is also used to assess fetal disorders such as *hemolytic disease of the newborn* and *respiratory distress syndrome*.

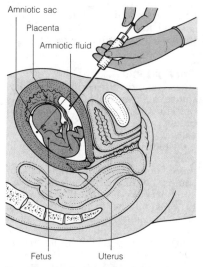

Procedure for amniocentesis
A needle is introduced through the abdomen and uterine wall into the amniotic sac; a sample of amniotic fluid is then drawn.

HOW IT IS DONE

Genetic amniocentesis is usually performed between the sixteenth and eighteenth week of gestation. *Ultrasound scanning* is used to estimate the age and position of the fetus, the placental site, and the amount of amniotic fluid. A needle is then inserted through the abdomen and uterine wall into the amniotic sac, avoiding the fetus and placenta. A syringe is attached to the needle and about 20 to 30 ml of fluid is removed.

A local anesthetic is occasionally used. The woman can usually go home soon after the procedure but is advised to rest for 24 hours.

RESULTS

The amniotic fluid may be analyzed biochemically and a chromosome *culture* performed to test for fetal abnormalities such as Down's syndrome and spina bifida.

Chromosome cultures take up to four weeks, so any results may not be available until about 20 weeks' gestation. The sex of the fetus is also determined by the chromosome analysis and the woman should indicate whether or not she wishes to receive this information.

COMPLICATIONS

There is a slight increased incidence of threatened miscarriage and early rupture of the membranes after amniocentesis (older studies show a risk of 1 to 2 percent; more recent studies show a risk of about 0.5 percent). For these reasons, amniocentesis is usually recommended only for women over the age of 35 (who are more likely to have a child with Down's syndrome) or when there are other compelling medical reasons, such as a family history of a chromosomal abnormality. (See also *Chorionic villus sampling*.)

Amnion

The membranous sac that surrounds the *embryo* and fills with watery *amniotic fluid* as pregnancy advances. The outside of the amnion is covered by another membrane called the chorion.

Amnioscopy

Another name for *fetoscopy*, direct observation of the fetus and amniotic fluid by means of an *endoscope* (viewing tube) passed through the pregnant woman's abdomen into the uterus.

Amniotic fluid

The clear fluid or "waters" that surround the fetus in the uterus throughout pregnancy. The fluid is contained within the amniotic sac (a thin membrane).

The fetus floats in the amniotic fluid and, in the early months of pregnancy, can move about freely while still remaining attached by the umbilical cord to the placenta (the organ that nourishes the fetus during pregnancy). The amniotic fluid cushions the fetus against pressure from internal organs and protects it from any injury from the mother's movements.

The fluid is produced by the cells that line the amniotic sac and is constantly circulated. It is swallowed by the fetus, absorbed into its bloodstream, then excreted by the fetal kidneys as urine. Amniotic fluid

is 99 percent water. The remainder consists of dilute concentrations of the substances found in blood plasma, along with cells and *lipids* (fats) that have flaked off from the fetus.

Amniotic fluid appears during the first week after conception and gradually increases in volume until the tenth week, when the increase becomes very rapid. By 35 weeks' gestation the volume of fluid is about 2 pints. Thereafter it slowly declines until it is just over 1 pint at term.

In a small number of women, excessive fluid is formed; this is known as *hydramnios* or polyhydramnios. Less frequently, insufficient amniotic fluid is formed (a condition called *oligohydramnios*).

Amniotomy

Artificial rupture of the amniotic membranes (breaking of the waters) performed for *induction of labor*.

Amoxapine

A tricyclic *antidepressant drug*. Amoxapine has a weaker sedative effect than many antidepressant drugs and is used when they have caused daytime drowsiness. Amoxapine may cause dry mouth and constipation before the dosage is adjusted.

Amoxicillin

A *penicillin*-type *antibiotic drug* used to treat a wide variety of infections, including *bronchitis, cystitis, gonorrhea*, and ear and skin infections.

An allergic reaction to amoxicillin may cause a blotchy rash and, rarely, fever, swelling of the mouth, itching, and breathing difficulty.

Amphetamine drugs

COMMON DRUGS

Dextroamphetamine Methamphetamine

A group of *stimulant* drugs that has an *appetite suppressant* effect.

In the past, amphetamine drugs were commonly prescribed to treat *obesity*; this use has been largely abandoned today because of dependence problems and abuse.

Amphetamines are now used mainly in the treatment of *narcolepsy* (abnormal daytime sleepiness).

HOW THEY WORK

Amphetamine drugs stimulate the secretion of *neurotransmitters* (chemicals released by nerve endings), such as *norepinephrine*, which increase nerve activity in the brain and make a person wakeful and alert.

A

POSSIBLE ADVERSE EFFECTS

Taken in high doses, amphetamines can cause tremor, sweating, palpitations, anxiety, and sleeping difficulties. Delusions, hallucinations, high blood pressure, and, rarely, seizures may also occur. Prolonged use may cause *tolerance* and physical dependence (see *Drug dependence*).

ABUSE

Amphetamines are abused for their stimulant effects; their manufacture and distribution are governed by the Controlled Substance Act.

Amphotericin B

A drug used to treat fungal infections. Minor infections of the eyes, ears, or skin are treated with drops, lotions, or creams. Life-threatening infections, such as *cryptococcosis* and *histoplasmosis* are treated with injections.

Adverse effects are likely only when amphotericin B is given by injection; these include vomiting, fever, headache, and, rarely, seizures.

Ampicillin

A *penicillin*-type *antibiotic drug* used to treat infections including *cystitis*, *bronchitis*, and ear infections. Ampicillin is also useful in the treatment of *gonorrhea*, *typhoid fever*, and *biliary system* infections.

Some people have an allergic reaction to ampicillin. This may cause rash, diarrhea, and, rarely, fever, swelling of the mouth and tongue, itching, and breathing difficulty.

Amputation

Surgical removal of part or all of a limb, usually to prevent *gangrene* (death and decay of tissues) or infection. Until the introduction of antibiotics in the early 1940s, amputation was a common operation, especially in wartime; it was the only means of preventing gangrene when an open fracture (one in which the broken bone is exposed) became infected.

WHY IT IS DONE

Today, the use of antibiotics to treat infected wounds means that amputation is restricted mainly to severe cases of arterial disease. Eighty-five percent of the 25,000 amputations performed in the US each year are carried out on patients with *peripheral vascular disease*, in which a combination of *atherosclerosis* and *thrombosis* may completely block the blood supply to a limb, causing gangrene.

Amputation may be performed to prevent the spread of bone cancer or malignant *melanoma* (a skin cancer).

HOW IT IS DONE

Before the operation, the surgeon decides where on the limb to operate; the tissue at the amputation site must be healthy if the wound is to heal rapidly. Investigative techniques used at this stage include *angiography* (injection into an artery of a solution visible on X ray) and *thermography* (recordings of surface temperatures of the body with a heat-sensitive camera).

During the operation, skin and muscle are cut below the level at which the bone is to be severed to create flaps that will later provide a fleshy stump. Blood vessels are tied off, the bone is sawed through, the area is washed with saline, and the flaps of skin and muscle are stitched over the sawed end of bone to form a smooth and rounded stump.

While amputating, the surgeon tries to ensure that nerves are severed well above the stump, reducing the risk of pressure pain when a prosthesis (see *Limb, artificial*) is fitted. But, despite every precaution, a painful *neuroma* (a benign tumor of nerve tissue) sometimes develops in the stump.

In an amputation at the ankle (Syme's amputation), the tough skin of the heel pad is retained to cover the stump. The patient can then place weight on the stump without necessarily having to use a prosthesis.

Amputations below the knee are now more satisfactory than before. Newer techniques for shaping the stump make it easier to fit a prosthesis, and new prostheses, attached by suction rather than straps, are easier to put on and take off.

RECOVERY PERIOD

As the wound heals, bandaging and plaster casts are used to mold the stump to a shape suitable for accepting a prosthesis. The stump is usually swollen for about six weeks after the operation and a permanent prosthesis can be fitted only after it has settled down to a stable size. The patient is usually helped to move around using a temporary prosthesis during this period to avoid becoming unaccustomed to walking.

For some time after an amputation, some patients have the unpleasant sensation that the amputated limb is still present—a phenomenon known as "phantom limb."

OUTLOOK

The prospect of a person who has had a leg amputation remaining mobile afterward depends on several factors: age, attitude, general health, the amount of limb lost, and whether the pressure of a prosthesis on the stump causes pain. Some healthy people lead almost as active lives as they did before, but many older people become confined to *wheelchairs*.

Amputation, congenital

Absence of the lower part of a limb from birth (see *Limb defects*).

Amputation, traumatic

Loss of a finger, toe, or limb through injury. (See also *Microsurgery*.)

Amyl nitrite

A *nitrate drug* once prescribed to relieve *angina pectoris* (chest pain due to impaired blood supply to the heart muscle). Because amyl nitrite frequently causes adverse effects (including headache, hot flashes, palpitations, and restlessness) it has been largely superseded by other drugs.

Amyl nitrite is sometimes abused for its effect of intensifying pleasure during orgasm.

Amyloidosis

An uncommon disease in which a substance called amyloid, which contains protein and starch, accumulates in tissues and organs.

CAUSES

Amyloidosis may occur for no known reason, when it is called primary; more commonly, it is a complication of some other disease, when it is called secondary. Conditions that may lead to amyloidosis include *rheumatoid arthritis*, *multiple myeloma* (a cancer of bone marrow), and *tuberculosis* or a pyogenic (pus-generating) process such as chronic osteomyelitis. Exactly why amyloid is deposited in any of these circumstances is not known.

SYMPTOMS AND SIGNS

Amyloid may accumulate in any organ. The symptoms and signs of amyloidosis vary, depending on which part of the body is involved. The liver, kidney, tongue, spleen, and heart are often affected. The organs become enlarged and may have a rubbery consistency and a waxy, pink or gray appearance if examined.

Accumulation of amyloid in the heart may result in *arrhythmias* (disturbances of the heart beat) and *heart failure* (reduced pumping efficiency). If the stomach and intestines are affected, symptoms such as diarrhea may develop and the lining of these organs may become ulcerated. The joints may be affected.

Primary amyloidosis is often characterized by deposits of amyloid in the skin. Slightly raised, waxy spots appear, usually clustered around the armpits, groin, face, and neck.

Some forms of amyloidosis are inherited. These forms of the disease tend to involve the nervous system. Symptoms include peripheral *neuropathy*, postural *hypotension*, urinary or fecal *incontinence*, and reduced *sweating*. Death may result from *renal failure* caused by deposits of amyloid in the kidneys.

DIAGNOSIS AND TREATMENT

Diagnosis depends on microscopic examination of a *biopsy* sample of tissue from the affected organ.

There is no treatment, but secondary amyloidosis may be arrested or even reversed when the underlying disorder is treated.

Amyotrophic lateral sclerosis

See *Motor neuron disease.*

Amyotrophy

Shrinkage or wasting away of a muscle, caused by a reduction in the size of its constituent contractile fibers and leading to weakness. It is usually due to poor nutrition, reduced use of the muscle (as when a limb is immobilized for a long period), or disturbance to the muscle's blood or nerve supply, as can occur in *diabetes mellitus* or *poliomyelitis*.

Anabolic steroids

See *Steroids, anabolic.*

Anaerobic

Capable of living and growing without oxygen. Many important bacteria are anaerobes and thrive in the intestinal canal or in tissue with a poor supply of oxygenated blood. These species can cause various diseases, including *food poisoning*, *tetanus*, *gangrene*, and a form of diarrhea (pseudomembranous enterocolitis).

Some human body cells are capable of limited anaerobic activity. For example, when muscular exertion is so strenuous that oxygen is used faster than the blood circulation can supply it, the muscle cells can temporarily work anaerobically. When this happens, lactic acid is produced as waste (instead of the carbon dioxide from *aerobic* activity). Compensation for this anaerobic activity (converting the lactic acid to glucose) requires oxygen, which explains why we need to continue to breathe rapidly after vigorous exertion. The deficit of oxygen that builds up in the muscles during exercise is known as the oxygen debt.

Anal dilatation

A procedure for enlarging the anus. Anal dilatation is used to treat conditions in which the anus becomes too tight, such as *anal stenosis* and *anal fissure*. It is also used as a treatment for *hemorrhoids*. Anal dilatation can be performed using general anesthetic by a surgeon, using fingers or an anal dilator, or by the patient, using a dilator and lubricating jelly.

Anal discharge

The loss of mucus, blood, or pus from the anus. *Hemorrhoids*, *anal fissures* (tears in the anal margin), and *proctitis* (inflammation of the rectum) all can cause anal discharge. The production of mucus from the anus tends to irritate the surrounding skin and may cause pruritus ani (*itching* of the anus). Anal discharge can be temporarily relieved by warm, shallow baths.

Analeptic drugs

Drugs that stimulate breathing, used in the treatment of *apnea* (absent breathing) in a newborn infant. Analeptics, which include doxapram and nikethamide, are occasionally used to treat *respiratory failure* caused by a drug overdose and to hasten recovery from a general anesthetic. Analeptics work by stimulating the respiratory center, a group of nerve endings in the brain stem that control the rate and volume of breathing.

Anal fissure

A fairly common anal disorder caused by an elongated ulcer that extends upward into the anal canal from the anal sphincter. The fissure probably originates from a tear in the lining of the anus caused by the passage of hard, dry feces.

SYMPTOMS

There is usually pain during defecation and the muscles of the anus may go into spasm. There may be a small amount of bright red blood on the feces or the toilet paper.

TREATMENT

The tear often heals naturally in the course of a few days, although spasm of the anal muscles may delay healing. Treatment of recurrent or persistent fissures usually includes *anal dilatation* (a procedure to enlarge the anus) and a high-fiber diet, including whole-grain products, fruits, vegetables, and plenty of fluids, to soften the feces. Fissures usually heal within a few days after such treatment, but, if this treatment is unsuccessful, surgery to remove the fissure may be necessary.

Anal fistula

An abnormal channel connecting the inside of the anal canal with the skin surrounding the anus.

CAUSES

A fistula is occasionally an indication of *Crohn's disease*, *colitis*, or *cancer* of the large intestine. However, in most cases it results from an abscess (which develops for unknown reasons in the anal wall) that discharges pus both into the anus and out onto the surrounding skin.

A fistula is treated surgically by opening the channel, removing the fistulous lining, and draining the abscess of thin pus. The operation is performed using a general anesthetic.

Analgesia

Loss of pain sensation. Analgesia differs from *anesthesia* (loss of all sensation) in that the person's sensitivity to touch is still preserved. (See also *Analgesic drugs.*)

Analgesic drugs

COMMON DRUGS

Nonnarcotic
Acetaminophen Aspirin Sodium salicylate

Narcotic
Codeine Meperidine Morphine Pentazocine Propoxyphene

> **WARNING**
> Over-the-counter (nonnarcotic) analgesics should be used only for 48 hours before seeking medical advice. If pain persists, becomes more severe, recurs, or differs from pain previously experienced, consult your physician.

Drugs that relieve pain. The two main types of analgesics are nonnarcotic (most of which contain *aspirin*, aspirinlike substances, or *acetaminophen*) and narcotic (which are related to *morphine*).

WHY THEY ARE USED

Nonnarcotic analgesics are useful in the treatment of mild or moderate pain (for example, headache or toothache). For more severe pain, a preparation combining one of the weaker narcotic analgesics (such as *codeine*) with a nonnarcotic analgesic (such as aspirin) is usually prescribed. The most potent narcotic analgesic drugs are used only when other preparations would be ineffective.

HOW THEY WORK

When body tissues are damaged (for example, by injury, infection, or

A

HOW ANALGESICS WORK

When tissue is damaged (for example, by injury, inflammation, or infection) the body produces prostaglandins. These substances combine with opiate receptors (specific sites on the surface of cells in the brain and spinal cord). As a result, a signal is passed along a series of nerve cells to the brain, where the signal is interpreted as pain by brain cells. Analgesics (except for acetaminophen) work either by preventing the production of prostaglandins or by blocking pain impulses in the brain and spinal cord. Acetaminophen works by blocking the pain impulses in the brain itself. This action prevents the perception of pain.

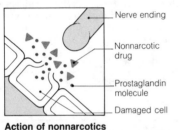

Action of nonnarcotics
Nonnarcotic drugs block the production of prostaglandins (the chemical released in response to tissue damage). This action prevents stimulation of the nerve endings so that no pain signal passes on to the brain. As a result, these drugs provide pain relief.

Action of narcotics
When tissue damage occurs, the body produces prostaglandins, chemicals that trigger the transmission of pain signals (above). Normally, the pain signal is transmitted between brain cells, but narcotic drugs (below) combine with opiate receptors to prevent the signals from actually reaching the brain.

inflammation), they produce *prostaglandins*, chemicals that trigger the transmission of pain signals to the brain. Nonnarcotic analgesics (except acetaminophen) work by preventing prostaglandin production. Acetaminophen blocks the pain impulses in the brain itself, thereby preventing the perception of pain.

Narcotic analgesics act in a similar way to *endorphins* (substances formed within the body that relieve pain). They block pain impulses at specific sites (called opiate receptors) in the brain and spinal cord.

POSSIBLE ADVERSE EFFECTS

Adverse effects are uncommon with acetaminophen. Aspirin may irritate the stomach lining and cause nausea, pain, and, occasionally, a peptic ulcer. Nausea, vomiting, drowsiness, constipation, and breathing difficulties may occur with narcotic analgesic drugs. The stronger types may also produce euphoria.

ABUSE

The euphoric effects produced by some narcotic analgesics have led to their abuse. In most cases, long-term abuse causes *tolerance* and physical dependence (see *Drug dependence*). Both the manufacture and the distribution of strong narcotic analgesics are governed by the Controlled Substance Act.

Anal stenosis

A tightness of the anus, sometimes referred to as anal stricture, which makes it too small to allow the normal passage of feces. This often leads to constipation and pain during defecation. Anal stenosis can be a congenital abnormality. It may also be caused by a number of conditions in which scarring has occurred, such as *anal fissure*, *colitis*, or cancer of the anus. It sometimes occurs after surgery on the anus—for example, to treat *hemorrhoids*. It is treated by *anal dilatation* (a

procedure to enlarge the anus), which in some cases may be performed by the patient.

Anal stricture

See *Anal stenosis*.

Analysis, psychological

See *Psychoanalysis*.

Analysis, scientific

Determination of the identity of a substance or of the individual chemical constituents of a mixture. Analysis may be qualitative, as in determining whether or not a particular substance is present, or it may be quantitative, that is, measuring the amount or concentration of one or more constituents. (See also *Assay*.)

Anaphylactic shock

A rare, severe, frightening, and life-threatening allergic reaction. It is a Type I hypersensitivity reaction (see *Allergy*) that occurs only rarely in people in whom an extreme sensitivity to a particular substance (or allergen) has developed. The reaction occurs most commonly after an *insect sting* or as a reaction to an injected drug—for example, penicillin, anti-tetanus serum, a local anesthetic, or during *immunotherapy* for an allergy. Less commonly, the reaction occurs after a particular food or drug has been taken by mouth.

Entry of the allergen into the bloodstream provokes the release of massive amounts of histamine and other chemicals with effects on body tissues. The blood vessels widen, with a sudden severe lowering of blood pressure. Other symptoms include an itchy, raised rash (hives), bronchospasm (constriction of the airways in the lungs), pain in the abdomen, swelling of the tongue or throat, and diarrhea.

FIRST AID AND TREATMENT

If a person becomes severely ill or collapses soon after an insect sting or an injection, medical help should be summoned immediately.

The victim should be laid down and the legs raised to improve blood flow to the heart and brain. An injection of *epinephrine* is often lifesaving and must be given as soon as possible.

People who have suffered previous severe reactions to insect stings, drugs, or foods should carry a preloaded syringe of epinephrine, so that they can inject themselves (if still conscious) or can have the dose administered promptly by someone familiar with the method of injection. Otherwise, medical help should be awaited. If the person's breathing or heart beat stops, measures should be employed to restart them (see *Cardiopulmonary resuscitation*).

Apart from epinephrine, medical treatment administered by a physician may include *antihistamine drugs* and *corticosteroid drugs*.

Individuals who have suffered anaphylactic reactions to insect venom may respond to a course of immunotherapy, although this procedure itself carries a risk of repetition of the anaphylaxis and should be carried out only by a physician with a supply of epinephrine and other emergency medications at hand.

Anastomosis

A natural or artificial connection in the body; a communication between two tubular cavities or blood vessels that may or may not normally be joined.

A natural anastomosis usually takes the form of two blood vessels joining (see *Arteriovenous fistula*). Surgical anastomosis is used to treat various disorders. For example, if an artery is blocked by *thrombosis* (clot) or *atheroma* (fat deposits), an operation may be performed to remove the blockage and directly hook up the two ends of the vessel. Alternatively, an operation to bypass the blockage may be performed by joining a synthetic substitute or a section of a vein from the patient to the artery above and below the obstruction. Or, the internal mammary artery in the chest wall may be joined beyond the narrowing directly to a coronary artery.

Another common use of surgical anastomosis is to treat intestinal obstruction; a section of intestine is cut out and the healthy ends joined. To bypass this same area, two openings are made in a loop of the intestine (one either side of the defective area) and the openings joined.

Anatomy

The structure of the body of any living thing, and the scientific study of it. The science of human anatomy dates back to ancient Egyptian times and, together with *physiology* (the functioning of the body), forms the foundation of all medicine. The primary source of information for anatomists is dissection of human corpses.

The ancient Greek physician Galen produced many medical treatises containing some anatomical descriptions that are still in use today, but his work is also full of gross errors. It was not until 1543 that the first accurate, comprehensive anatomical text, "De Humani Corporis Fabrica" ("On the structure of the human body"), was produced by the Flemish scientist Andreas Vesalius.

BRANCHES OF ANATOMY

Anatomy as a scientific study today is subdivided into many branches. They include comparative anatomy (the study of the differences between human and animal bodies), surgical anatomy (the practical knowledge required by surgeons, especially recognition of the surface markings of internal organs and the pattern of blood vessels within them), *embryology* (the study of structural changes that occur during the development of the embryo and fetus), systematic anatomy (the study of the structure of particular body systems, such as the urinary system), and *cytology* and *histology* (the microscopic study of, respectively, cells and tissues).

DESCRIPTIVE TERMS

In textbook descriptions of human anatomy, the body is assumed to be standing upright, with the arms hanging down and the palms facing forward. The body is divided by the median (or sagittal) plane into right and left halves, and by the coronal plane into front (anterior or ventral) and rear (posterior or dorsal) halves.

Every anatomical structure is scientifically named in Latin, but today many anatomists prefer to use simpler terms when they exist. For example, the main blood vessel in the thigh is usually called the femoral artery rather than the arteria femoralis.

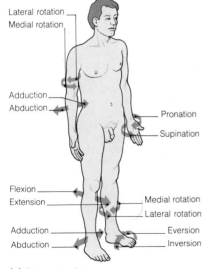

Joint movements
Flexion bends and extension straightens a joint; abduction moves a body part away from, adduction toward, the median plane. Rotations are movements around a long axis.

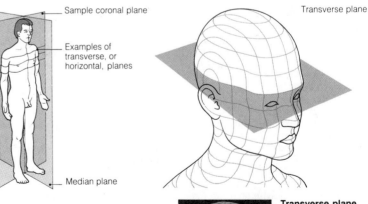

Planes through the body
Different body movements and sections through the body may be described by reference to various planes. The median plane divides the body evenly into right and left halves. Coronal planes are vertical planes at right angles to the median plane; the coronal plane most often referred to divides the body into front and back halves. Transverse planes are horizontal slices through the body.

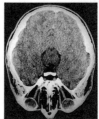

Transverse plane through head
Computerized tomographic (CT), MRI, and other scans of the head are often taken in one or a series of transverse planes. One such scan is shown at left.

Ancylostomiasis

See *Hookworm infestation*.

Androgen drugs

A group of drugs that has effects similar to the *androgen hormones*; one of the most important of these hormones developed as a drug is *testosterone*.

Androgen drugs are used in the treatment of male *hypogonadism* (underactivity of the testes) to stimulate the development of sexual characteristics, such as growth of facial and pubic hair, enlargement of the genitals, and deepening of the voice. This treatment improves libido and potency but does not increase the production of sperm.

Androgen drugs are also used to stimulate production of new blood cells by the bone marrow in aplastic *anemia*. They also may occasionally be used in the treatment of certain types of *breast cancer*.

Androgen drugs are commonly used by athletes and bodybuilders wishing to increase muscle bulk and strength, but this practice is condemned by physicians due to doubts concerning the drugs' benefits and the risk of adverse effects.

POSSIBLE ADVERSE EFFECTS

Adverse effects include fluid retention, weight gain, increased levels of cholesterol in the blood, and, rarely, liver damage. When taken by women the drugs can cause deepening of the voice and other male characteristics. Because androgen drugs affect sexual development of babies, they are not prescribed during pregnancy or breast-feeding. They are prescribed with caution during adolescence because they may prematurely halt the growth of the long bones.

Androgen hormones

A group of hormones that causes *virilization* (the development of male secondary sexual characteristics), such as the growth of facial hair, deepening of the voice, and increase in muscle bulk.

FORMATION

Androgens are produced by specialized cells in the testes in males and in the adrenal glands in both sexes. The ovaries secrete very small quantities of androgens until the menopause. The most active androgen is *testosterone*, which is produced in the testes. Androgens produced by the adrenal glands are less active than testicular androgens, and have no significant masculinizing effects unless produced to excess.

The production of androgens by the testes is controlled by certain pituitary hormones, called *gonadotropins*. Adrenal androgens are controlled by *ACTH*, another pituitary hormone.

EFFECTS

Androgens stimulate the appearance of male secondary sexual characteristics at puberty, including enlargement of the penis and growth of facial and body hair. Androgens have what is called an anabolic effect, that is, they raise the rate of protein synthesis and lower the rate at which it is broken down. This increases muscle bulk, especially in the chest and shoulders, and accelerates growth, especially during early puberty. At the end of puberty, androgens cause the long bones to stop growing.

Androgens also promote aggression, a characteristically male trait. They stimulate sebum secretion, which, if excessive, causes *acne*. In early adult life, androgens promote male-pattern baldness. Absence of androgens protects against male-pattern baldness.

ANDROGEN DEFICIENCY

Adult males may be deficient in androgens if their *testes* are diseased or if the pituitary gland fails to secrete gonadotropins. Such men are termed "hypogonadal." Results of androgen deficiency include decreased body hair and beard growth, smooth skin, a high-pitched voice, reduced sexual drive and performance, underdeveloped genitalia, and lack of muscle development.

ANDROGEN EXCESS

Overproduction of androgens may be the result of adrenal disorders (see *Adrenal tumors*; *Adrenal hyperplasia, congenital*), of testicular tumors (see *Testis, cancer of*), or, rarely, of androgen-secreting ovarian tumors (see *Ovary, cancer of*).

In adult males, excess androgens accentuate male physical characteristics. In boys, they cause premature sexual development. Initially they increase bone growth but adult height is reduced because they cause the long bones to stop growing.

In females, excess androgens cause virilization, that is, the development of masculine features such as increase in body hair, deepening of the voice, enlargement of the clitoris, and *amenorrhea* (absence of menstruation).

Anemia

A condition in which the concentration of the oxygen-carrying pigment *hemoglobin* in the blood is below normal. Hemoglobin molecules are carried inside red *blood cells* and function to transport oxygen from the lungs to the tissues. Under normal circumstances, stable hemoglobin concentrations in the blood are maintained by a strict balance between red cell production in the bone marrow and red cell destruction in the spleen. Anemia may result if this balance is lost.

By far the most common form of anemia worldwide is due to a deficiency of iron, an essential component of hemoglobin. However, there are numerous other causes of anemia, which is not a disease itself but a feature of many different diseases and disorders.

TYPES AND CAUSES

Red blood cells are formed in the bone marrow over a period of about five days from less specialized cells called stem cells. During this time, the cells change their appearance and accumulate hemoglobin. The red cells released from the bone marrow into the blood are called reticulocytes. Over a few days reticulocytes mature into adult red blood cells. The adult cells circulate in the bloodstream for about 120 days; they age and are eventually trapped in small blood vessels (mainly in the spleen) and destroyed. Some cell components, including iron, are recycled for use in new cells.

The various forms of anemia can be classified into those caused by decreased or defective production of red cells by the bone marrow and those caused by decreased survival of the red cells in the blood (see illustrated box on types and causes).

SYMPTOMS

The symptoms common to all forms of anemia result from the reduced oxygen-carrying capacity of the blood. Their severity depends on how low the hemoglobin concentration in the blood is. Normal blood hemoglobin concentrations are between 14 to 16 g/100 ml for men and 12 to 14 g/100 ml for women. Concentrations below 10 g/100 ml can cause headaches, tiredness, and lethargy. Concentrations below 8 g/100 ml can cause breathing difficulty on exercise, dizziness due to reduced oxygen reaching the brain, *angina pectoris* due to reduced oxygen supply to the heart muscle, and palpitations as the heart works harder to compensate. General signs include pallor, although this is not a reliable indicator of the severity of the anemia. Symptoms also depend upon the speed of development of an anemia. The slowly developing form is toler-

A

TYPES AND CAUSES OF ANEMIA

Anemia results either from reduced or defective production or from an excessively high rate of destruction of oxygen-carrying red blood cells.

Four of the main types are shown below, but anemia can have many other causes (such as various forms of leukemia).

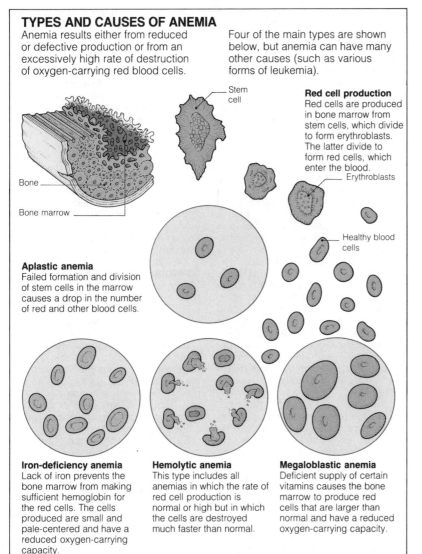

Stem cell

Red cell production
Red cells are produced in bone marrow from stem cells, which divide to form erythroblasts. The latter divide to form red cells, which enter the blood.

Erythroblasts

Bone

Bone marrow

Healthy blood cells

Aplastic anemia
Failed formation and division of stem cells in the marrow causes a drop in the number of red and other blood cells.

Iron-deficiency anemia
Lack of iron prevents the bone marrow from making sufficient hemoglobin for the red cells. The cells produced are small and pale-centered and have a reduced oxygen-carrying capacity.

Hemolytic anemia
This type includes all anemias in which the rate of red cell production is normal or high but in which the cells are destroyed much faster than normal.

Megaloblastic anemia
Deficient supply of certain vitamins causes the bone marrow to produce red cells that are larger than normal and have a reduced oxygen-carrying capacity.

bone marrow biopsy and measurement of the levels of substances such as folic acid, bilirubin, and vitamin B_{12} in the blood. Sometimes, more investigations must be carried out to establish the exact cause.

Treatment is aimed at correcting, modifying, or diminishing the mechanism or process that is leading to defective red cell production or reduced red cell survival. Treatment tends to be more straightforward for anemias caused by deficiencies (iron deficiency and megaloblastic anemias) than for those caused by inherited disorders or other disease processes (thalassemia and many types of hemolytic anemia).

Anemia, aplastic

A rare but important type of *anemia* in which the red cells, white blood cells, and platelet cells in the blood are reduced in number. Aplastic anemia is caused by failure to produce stem cells, the earliest form of all blood cells, in the *bone marrow*.

CAUSES AND INCIDENCE

Treatment of cancer with *radiation therapy* or *anticancer drugs* can interfere with the marrow's cell-producing capacity, as can certain viral infections and other drugs. In these cases, the bone marrow usually recovers and resumes normal production of cells once the cause is removed.

Long-term exposure to the fumes of benzene (a constituent of gasoline) or insecticides has been implicated as a cause of more persistent aplastic anemia, while a moderate to high dose of nuclear radiation (from radioactive fallout or nuclear explosions) is another recognized cause. In some people, aplastic anemia develops for no known reason—a condition that is known as primary or idiopathic aplastic anemia.

Aplastic anemia is most common around the age of 30.

SYMPTOMS

A low level of red blood cells may result in symptoms common to all types of anemia. Deficiency of white cells increases susceptibility to infections, while deficiency of platelets may lead to bruising easily, bleeding gums, or nosebleeds.

DIAGNOSIS

The disorder is usually suspected from the results of a blood test, particularly a *blood count*, and is confirmed by a *bone marrow biopsy*, in which a small sample of marrow is removed and examined for the presence or absence of blood-forming cells.

ated well until it becomes advanced; the sudden development of anemia causes immediate symptoms depending on the degree of blood loss.

Other symptoms may occur with particular forms of anemia. For example, some degree of *jaundice* occurs in most types of hemolytic anemia, because the high rate of destruction of red cells leads to increased bilirubin in the blood.

DIAGNOSIS

Anemia is diagnosed from the patient's symptoms and by the measurement of a low level of hemoglobin in the blood. To establish the type and cause of the anemia, a sample of blood is first examined

under the microscope, the numbers of different types of blood cells are counted, and their appearance is noted (see *Blood count; Blood smear*). A low proportion of reticulocytes suggests that the cause is decreased production of red cells; a high proportion of reticulocytes suggests that cells are being destroyed at a high rate. The size of the red cells—whether small, normal, or large—provides further clues. With some specific forms—for example, *sickle-cell anemia* (a type of hemolytic anemia)—some of the red cells have an abnormal shape.

Other investigations that may help the diagnosis include examination of cells in the bone marrow by means of a

A

TREATMENT

When aplastic anemia is due to infection or treatment for cancer, transfusions of red cells and platelets are given until the marrow returns to its normal state.

In persistent aplastic anemia, *bone marrow transplantation* may be carried out if a suitable donor is available. The donor must be someone whose tissue type closely matches that of the patient genetically (usually a brother or a sister).

OUTLOOK

Recovery usually occurs in mild forms of the disease. However, without bone marrow transplantation, severe aplastic anemia frequently is fatal.

Anemia, hemolytic

A form of *anemia* (reduced level of the oxygen-carrying pigment *hemoglobin* in blood) caused by the premature destruction of red cells in the bloodstream—a process known as hemolysis. Bone marrow has the capacity to increase red cell production approximately sixfold over normal rates. Anemia results only if the shortening of the red cell life span is sufficiently severe to overcome the marrow's reserve capacity.

TYPES AND CAUSES

Hemolytic anemias can be classified according to whether the cause of the problem is inside the red cell, in which case it is usually an inherited condition, or outside the cell, in which case it is usually acquired later in life.

RED CELL DEFECTS Hemolysis due to disorders within the red cell results from an abnormal rigidity of the cell membrane (the envelope that surrounds the cell). This causes the cell to become trapped at an early stage of its life span in the smaller blood vessels (usually of the spleen) and eventually be destroyed by macrophages (types of white blood cell).

The abnormal rigidity may result from an inherited defect of the cell membrane (as in hereditary *spherocytosis*), from a defect of the hemoglobin within the cell (as in *sickle-cell anemia*), or from a defect of one of the cell's enzymes. There are only two chemical processes occurring in red cells that are essential to their survival—one that provides energy and one that helps protect the cell from chemical damage. The last process is of great importance; a deficiency of one of the enzymes that catalyzes the process, called glucose-6-phosphate dehydrogenase, is a common cause of hemolytic anemia. A variety of it is

very common among blacks in the US and results from exposure to many types of drugs, including antibiotics and antimalarials (see *G6PD deficiency*). Another variety, in which hemolysis occurs after eating a certain type of bean, is most common in Greece (see *Favism*).

DEFECTS OUTSIDE THE RED CELL Hemolytic anemias resulting from defects outside the red cell fall into three main groups. First are disorders in which red cells are destroyed by mechanical buffeting (for example, when the lining of the blood vessels is abnormal, when the blood flows past artificial surfaces such as replacement heart valves, or in conditions in which a blood clot has formed inside the blood vessel). In all these conditions the otherwise normal red cell is physically disrupted by mechanical forces.

A second group of conditions is one in which red cells are destroyed by antibodies produced by the *immune system* and directed against the red cells. These immune hemolytic anemias may occur if foreign blood cells enter the bloodstream, as during an incompatible blood transfusion, or if the immune system becomes defective and fails to recognize the body's own red cells. This is a type of *autoimmune disorder*. Commonly, the reaction is triggered by a drug such as methyldopa. In *hemolytic disease of the newborn*, the baby's red cells are destroyed by antibodies produced by the mother.

In a third group of conditions, the red cells are destroyed by microorganisms in the blood. By far the most important cause is *malaria*.

SYMPTOMS AND DIAGNOSIS

People with hemolytic anemia may have symptoms common to all types of anemia (such as pallor, headaches, fatigue, and shortness of breath on exertion) or symptoms specifically due to the hemolysis (such as *jaundice*, caused by an excessive concentration in the blood of bile pigments formed from red cell destruction).

The diagnosis of hemolytic anemia depends on microscopic examination of the blood (see *Blood smear*), which often shows abnormally large numbers of immature red cells and, with some specific types, red cells that are abnormally shaped. The patient's racial background and medical history may also help establish the diagnosis.

TREATMENT

Some inherited causes of hemolytic anemia can be controlled by removing the main site of destruction of the red

cells—the spleen (see *Splenectomy*). Others, such as G6PD deficiency and favism, are largely preventable through avoidance of the drugs or foods that precipitate hemolysis.

Treatment of hemolysis caused by mechanical buffeting of red cells relies on reducing the disruptive forces. Those caused by immune or autoimmune processes can often be controlled through the use of *immunosuppressant drugs*.

More specific treatments may be required in particular cases—for example, the use of antimalarial drugs in hemolysis caused by malaria. Transfusions of red blood cells, or exchange transfusions of whole blood, are sometimes required for emergency treatment of severe life-threatening anemia.

Anemia, iron-deficiency

The most common form of *anemia* (a reduced level of the oxygen-carrying pigment *hemoglobin* in the blood); it is caused by a deficiency of iron, an essential constituent of hemoglobin.

Iron-deficiency anemia develops if insufficient iron is available to the bone marrow, where hemoglobin is manufactured and packaged into red blood cells. Anemia occurs when iron loss, along with any extra demand for iron required for growth, exceeds iron gained from the diet.

Small losses of hemoglobin and iron occur normally from the body through occasional minor bleeding; in women of childbearing age, these losses are much greater due to menstrual blood loss. Small amounts of iron are also shed in skin cells as they peel off from the body surface and tiny amounts are lost when red blood cells are destroyed at the end of their life span (most of the iron is efficiently repackaged into new red cells).

Because of their menstrual blood losses, women of childbearing age tend to have low, or no, built-up stores of iron and thus tend to become anemic more quickly in the event that iron losses exceed iron intake. The advent of pregnancy stops the menstrual losses but is replaced by an even greater drain on iron stores (from the baby); hence, pregnant women are at particular risk.

CAUSES

INCREASED LOSSES The main cause of iron-deficiency anemia is loss of iron at a greater rate than normal as a result of bleeding that is abnormally heavy or persistent. It may be caused by disease or by particularly heavy periods (see *Menorrhagia*). The diseases most commonly responsible for persistent bleeding are those of the digestive tract, such as erosive *gastritis*, *peptic ulcer*, *stomach cancer*, *inflammatory bowel disease*, and sometimes *hemorrhoids*. Prolonged treatment with aspirin and aspirinlike *nonsteroidal anti-inflammatory drugs* (NSAID) can cause gastrointestinal bleeding. In some countries, *hookworm infestation* of the digestive tract is an important cause.

Blood lost from the lower part of the intestine and from the rectum is bright red and usually noticed when feces are passed. If the bleeding is in the stomach or upper intestine, it is invisible; when it is excessive, it usually makes the feces black.

Bleeding may also take place in urinary tract disorders (such as *kidney tumors* or *bladder tumors*, *cystitis*, and *prostatitis*), when it colors the urine.

INSUFFICIENT INTAKE The second most common cause of iron deficiency is poor absorption of iron from the diet, usually as the result of surgical removal of part or all of the stomach (see *Gastrectomy*) but also sometimes due to *celiac sprue*, a digestive disorder of the small intestine.

The third possible, and the least common, cause is a diet that does not provide enough iron. Those most affected are old people who live alone and who eat a generally poor diet, and children and pregnant women, because of their extra needs. Women should be sure to have an iron-rich diet and may be prescribed iron tablets during pregnancy.

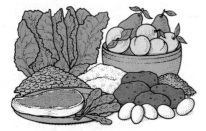

Foods containing iron
Foods such as fruit, whole-grain bread, beans, lean meat, and green vegetables are good sources of iron that help prevent iron-deficiency anemia.

SYMPTOMS
The symptoms are those of the underlying cause (for example, symptoms accompanying a peptic ulcer that bled), along with those common to all forms of anemia—fatigue and headaches, sometimes a sore mouth or tongue, brittle nails, and, in severe cases, breathlessness and pain in the center of the chest.

DIAGNOSIS AND TREATMENT
The diagnosis is made from the measurement of a low level of hemoglobin in the blood and from a *blood smear* test that usually shows the red blood cells to be smaller than normal. When the cause is not clear, investigations such as fecal analysis (for evidence of blood) and *barium X-ray examination* (to find digestive tract disorders) are carried out.

Treatment is for the underlying cause, along with a course of iron tablets or injections (or syrup for children) to build up the depleted iron stores and correct the anemia.

Anemia, megaloblastic

An important type of *anemia* (reduced level of the oxygen-carrying pigment *hemoglobin* in blood), caused by a deficiency of vitamin B_{12} or another vitamin, folic acid. Either of these deficiencies seriously interferes with the production of red blood cells in the bone marrow; the red blood cells that are formed are enlarged and deformed and are known as macrocytes.

CAUSES
VITAMIN B_{12} DEFICIENCY Vitamin B_{12} is found only in food of animal origin, such as meat, fish, and dairy products. It is absorbed from the small intestine after first combining with a chemical called intrinsic factor, produced by the stomach lining. In most diets, there is much more vitamin B_{12} than the body requires; the excess is stored in the liver, where it can last for a few years. If a person on a normal diet acquires a vitamin B_{12} deficiency, it is due not to lack of the vitamin but to an inability to absorb it.

The most common cause of such a deficiency is called pernicious anemia; it is caused by failure of the stomach lining to produce intrinsic factor, usually because of an *autoimmune disorder*, in which antibodies are produced that block the production of intrinsic factor. Pernicious anemia has a tendency to run in families, to start in middle age, and to affect women more than men. It is sometimes associated with other disorders, such as *diabetes mellitus* or *myxedema*. Total gastrectomy (removal of the stomach) prevents intrinsic factor production by removing its source.

Other causes of malabsorption of the vitamin include removal of part of the small intestine (where vitamin B_{12} is absorbed) and *Crohn's disease*.

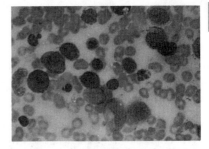

Bone marrow in megaloblastic anemia
In this microscopic view, some of the large cells are abnormal red cell precursors (megaloblasts).

In a minority of cases, vitamin B_{12} deficiency is the result of a vegan diet, which excludes eggs and dairy products as well as meat and fish.

FOLIC ACID DEFICIENCY Present to some extent in many foods, folic acid is found mainly in green vegetables and liver. However, unlike vitamin B_{12}, it is not stored in the body in large amounts; therefore, a constant supply is needed (and pregnant women require supplements). For this reason, the usual cause of deficiency is a poor diet. The disorder is most common in the poor and in old people living by themselves. It may also occur in people with alcohol dependence.

Deficiency can also be caused by anything that interferes with the absorption of folic acid from the small intestine (e.g., disorders such as *Crohn's disease* and *celiac sprue* or removal of part of the small intestine).

SYMPTOMS
Many people with mild megaloblastic anemia have no symptoms. In others, symptoms may include any or all of the following: tiredness, headaches, a sore mouth and tongue, weight loss, and, in pernicious anemia, *jaundice*, shown by a slight yellow tint to the skin. In severe cases there may also be breathlessness, chest pain, and sometimes loss of balance and tingling in the feet due to damage to the nervous system from lack of the vitamins.

DIAGNOSIS
The anemia is usually first suspected following *blood tests* that show a low level of hemoglobin, a preponderance of large red blood cells, and low levels of either vitamin B_{12} or folic acid or both. The disease is confirmed if a *bone marrow biopsy* (removal of a small sample of marrow for analysis) reveals the presence of large numbers of megaloblasts. Tests may also be carried out to discover an underlying cause in cases where it is not clear.

Pernicious anemia is sometimes diagnosed by a special test, the Schilling test, in which the absorption of vitamin B_{12} into the bloodstream is measured with the vitamin first unbound and then bound to intrinsic factor. If the vitamin is found to be absorbed only when bound to intrinsic factor, it confirms the cause as pernicious anemia.

TREATMENT

When megaloblastic anemia is due to poor diet, it can be remedied by adopting a normal diet and taking a short course of vitamin B_{12} injections or folic acid tablets.

In cases when the deficiency is due to inability to absorb the vitamin, it can sometimes be remedied by treating the underlying cause, but often the power of absorption is lost permanently. A lifelong course of replacement injections or tablets of vitamin B_{12} or folic acid is then required.

Anemia, pernicious

One of the main types of anemia caused by vitamin B_{12} deficiency. See *Anemia, megaloblastic.*

Anencephaly

Absence at birth of the brain, cranial vault (top of the skull), and spinal cord. Most affected infants are stillborn or survive only a few hours. Anencephaly is detectable early in pregnancy by measurement of *alphafetoprotein*, by *ultrasound scanning*, and by *amniocentesis*; if anencephaly is detected, termination of the pregnancy may be considered.

Anencephaly is due to a failure in development of the neural tube, the nerve tissue in the embryo that eventually develops into the spinal cord and brain. Maldevelopment of the neural tube may also result in *spina bifida* and *hydrocephalus*. These abnormalities are collectively known as *neural tube defects* and seem likely to have similar causes. Anencephaly occurs in about five in every 1,000 pregnancies, but only in about one third of these does the pregnancy continue to term.

Anesthesia

Literally, the absence of all sensation. It may occur in an area of the body after nerve tissues are damaged by injury or disease. Rarely, anesthesia may be a result of extreme arousal, as in the case of boxers or soldiers who do not notice painful blows or wounds. Psychological factors may be responsible for numbness, particularly in the hand or foot (see *Conversion disorder*). Anesthesia is also induced artificially to abolish pain during surgical procedures and childbirth.

Two types of anesthesia are used for medical purposes. Under local anesthesia (see *Anesthesia, local*), the patient remains conscious and sensation is abolished in only part of the body. This is usually accomplished by injection of drugs that temporarily interrupt the nerve supply from the region to be anesthetized. Local anesthetics can also be given in the form of eye drops, sprays, skin creams, and suppositories. It may be possible to produce local pain relief by using *acupuncture*; this technique is widely used in China, but is rarely used by Western practitioners, who have less success with it.

Using general anesthesia (see *Anesthesia, general*), the patient is rendered unconscious and maintained in this state by being given a combination of drugs that are either injected intravenously or inhaled. These drugs affect all parts of the body but have their main sites of action in the brain and spinal cord.

Anesthesia, dental

Loss of sensation induced in a patient to prevent pain during dental treatment or dental surgery. Most dental procedures are carried out using local anesthesia; general anesthesia is usually reserved for surgical procedures and special cases.

LOCAL ANESTHESIA

For minor restorative work, such as fillings, some patients and dentists choose no anesthesia; otherwise, a local anesthetic (for example, lidocaine or procaine) is injected into the gum at the site that is being treated. Sometimes it is not possible to inject directly into the area to be treated because the gum is painfully inflamed or because there is a risk of spreading an infection in the gum. In these cases, the anesthetic is injected into or around the nerve a short distance away from the site of operation, a procedure known as a peripheral *nerve block*. Topical anesthetics on the gums are often used in conjunction with injected anesthetics.

SEDATION

In addition to receiving a local anesthetic, a patient who is abnormally anxious, agitated, or uncooperative may need to be calmed by sedation. To sedate the patient, an antianxiety agent is given orally or intravenously, or through inhalation. These antianxiety agents include tranquilizers, nitrous oxide (laughing gas), and barbiturates.

GENERAL ANESTHESIA

The most common use for general anesthesia is in surgical procedures such as periodontal (gum) surgery and multiple tooth extractions. General anesthesia is also used for young children, for people who are allergic to local anesthetics or who have extremely sensitive teeth, and for those who are unable to cooperate due to, for example, a mental disorder or physical handicap.

For relatively short dental surgery, general anesthesia is given by an injection of a barbiturate, such as methohexital or thiopental, into a vein, with a mixture of nitrous oxide and oxygen being given during surgery to maintain anesthesia.

For longer or more complicated procedures, general anesthesia is carried out as it is for other surgery (see *Anesthesia, general*).

Anesthesia, general

Loss of sensation and consciousness induced in a patient, most often to prevent pain and discomfort during surgery. The state of general anesthesia is produced and maintained by an *anesthesiologist*, who gives combinations of drugs by injection, inhalation, or both. The anesthesiologist is also responsible for the preanesthetic assessment of patients, their safety during surgery, and their recovery during the postanesthetic period.

HISTORY

Until the middle of the nineteenth century, pain relief during surgery relied on natural substances such as alcohol, opium, and cannabis. However, the relief obtained was often inadequate and short-lived. It was not until the 1840s that solutions began to be found to the problem of inducing unconsciousness in a manner that was safe, easily maintained for long periods, and reversible. *Ether* was first demonstrated successfully in Boston in 1846, where a tooth was extracted without pain while the patient was breathing ether. Soon after, the anesthetic properties of chloroform and nitrous oxide were discovered, heralding a new era in surgery.

WHY IT IS DONE

The primary objectives of general anesthesia are to abolish pain, awareness, muscle tone, and cardiovascular reflexes in the patient to make conditions suitable for surgery or diagnostic procedures and easier for the patient.

TECHNIQUES FOR GENERAL ANESTHESIA

The main phases in the administration of a general anesthetic are induction (bringing on unconsciousness), maintenance, and emergence (returning the patient to consciousness). Some of the main stages are shown below. Often, to allow surgical manipulation, a muscle relaxant must be given in addition to anesthetic gases or injections. Because the relaxant temporarily paralyzes the breathing muscles, the patient's lungs must be ventilated artificially.

DRUGS USED IN GENERAL ANESTHESIA

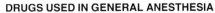

Type	Action	Examples
Drugs given as premedication	Relax patient, abolish pain, reduce saliva and mucus formation	Diazepam, morphine, atropine
Induction agents	Induce unconsciousness	Thiopental sodium
Anesthetic gases and volatile agents	Induce and/or maintain unconsciousness	Nitrous oxide, halothane, enflurane, isoflurane
Analgesics	Abolish pain	Morphine, fentanyl
Muscle relaxants	Relax muscles	Pancuronium, vecuronium
Reversal agents	Reverse muscle relaxation	Neostigmine

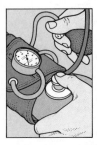

1 Before the operation, the anesthesiologist talks to and examines the patient and assesses his or her fitness for anesthesia and surgery. He or she also answers the patient's questions.

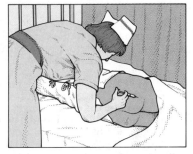

2 Before the operation, premedication may be given. It may include a drug that relieves pain or anxiety and one that prevents excessive salivation.

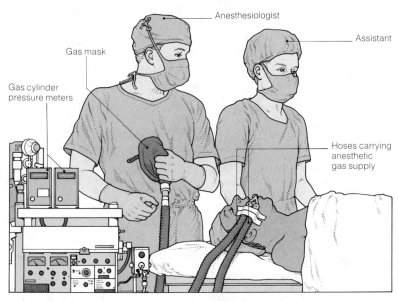

Anesthesiologist

Assistant

Gas mask

Gas cylinder pressure meters

Hoses carrying anesthetic gas supply

6 While surgery is in progress, the patient is kept at a level of anesthesia deep enough to be unaware of the operation. The composition of the gas mixture, and the patient's heart rate, breathing, blood pressure, temperature, blood oxygenation, and exhaled carbon dioxide are continuously monitored.

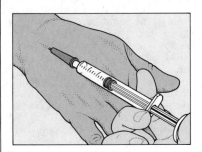

3 The induction agent is usually given via a cannula inserted into a vein. The cannula is left in position so that other drugs can be given rapidly if needed.

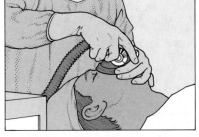

4 Sometimes, anesthesia is induced or maintained with gases delivered by mask. If no muscle relaxant is used, the patient may be able to continue breathing naturally.

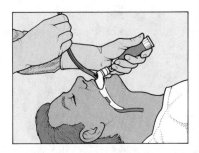

5 In other cases, a breathing tube is inserted for delivery of the anesthetic gases. If a muscle relaxant is used, artificial ventilation is necessary.

COMPLICATIONS

The likelihood of any complications occurring depends on the preoperative condition of the patient, the anesthetic technique used, and the nature of the operation performed.

General anesthesia is associated with many possible complications necessitating the administration of several powerful drugs. Complications include *hypotension* (low blood pressure), cardiac *arrhythmia* (irregular heart beat), *myocardial infarction* (heart attack), inhibited respiration, *airway obstruction*, life-threatening febrile (feverish) reactions, allergic reactions, nausea, vomiting and *aspiration* (inhaling vomit into the lungs), *hypoxia*, physical injury (such as chipped teeth, muscle cramps, and brain damage), and death.

AWARENESS DURING ANESTHESIA It is possible, though rare with modern anesthetic techniques, for patients to remain aware of events during surgery but, because of muscle relaxants, to be unable to signal this distressed state to the anesthesiologist. The concentrations of anesthetic agents required to produce adequate anesthesia in the majority of patients are well documented. In addition, the anesthesiologist can detect an inadequate level of anesthesia by noting physical signs, such as increased sweating, tearing, and salivation, and irregular breathing, changes in muscle tone, spontaneous eye movements, and increases in the patient's heart rate and blood pressure.

Anesthesia, local

Loss of sensation induced in a limited region of a person's body to prevent pain during examinations, diagnostic procedures, treatments, and surgical operations. Local anesthesia is produced by the administration of drugs that temporarily interrupt the action of pain-carrying nerve fibers.

HOW IT IS DONE

For minor surgical procedures, such as stitching of small wounds, local anesthesia is usually produced by direct injection into the area to be treated. When it is necessary to anesthetize a large area, or when local injection would not penetrate deeply enough into body tissues, a *nerve block* may be used. For a nerve block, nerves at a point remote from the area to be treated are injected (i.e., the palm of the hand may be anesthetized by injecting points near the elbow, which blocks the ulnar and median nerves). This is known as regional anesthesia.

LOCAL ANESTHETICS

Drug	Common uses	How taken	Action
Benzocaine	To treat skin irritation, toothache, teething pains, hemorrhoids	Cream, ointment, spray, gel, liquid	Rapid action, short duration
Bupivacaine	As a nerve block (e.g., epidural anesthesia)	Injection	Medium action, long duration
Cocaine	Formerly used for minor surgical procedures on eye, ear, nose, and throat	Liquid, spray	Rapid action, short duration
Lidocaine	To treat skin irritation, relief of pain during dental treatment, nerve blocks (e.g., epidural anesthesia)	Cream, ointment, spray, injection	Rapid action, medium duration
Procaine	For relief of pain before surgical and dental treatment	Injection	Slow action, short duration
Tetracaine	For anal irritation, relief of pain during dental treatment and throat examinations, minor surgical procedures on the eye	Cream, ointment, spray, liquid, eye drops	Rapid action, medium to long duration

Nerves can also be blocked as they branch off from the spinal cord, as in *epidural anesthesia*, which is widely used during childbirth, and spinal anesthesia (see *Spinal block*), which is used mainly for surgery of the lower limbs and lower abdomen.

Some parts of the body that are permeable to local anesthetic drugs can be anesthetized by applying an anesthetic drug directly to the area. The throat, larynx, and respiratory passages can be sprayed before *bronchoscopy*, and the urethra can be numbed with a gel for performing *catheterization* or *cystoscopy*. A cream has been developed that is rubbed onto the skin so that injections will be painless. Other applications include lozenges for sore throats, and ointments or rectal suppositories for relieving hemorrhoids.

For some procedures, particularly if the patient is anxious, a sedative is given with the local anesthetic.

COMPLICATIONS

Patients can have adverse reactions to the anesthetic drug if the dose is too high or has been absorbed too rapidly. Such reactions include dizziness, loss of consciousness, seizures, and cardiac arrest. In rare cases, people have an allergic reaction to the drug itself. During major (epidural and spinal) blocks, reduced activity of the blocked sympathetic nervous system may result in hypotension and reduced blood flow to the brain and heart. Infections at the site of injection range from inconsequential to life-threatening (e.g., meningitis). Certain local anesthetics may cause long-term nerve damage.

Anesthesiologist

A specialist who administers the drugs that "put you to sleep" during an operation. Anesthesiologists also assess the condition of a patient's heart, lungs, and circulation before he or she is sent into the operating room. They decide what type and how much anesthesia is needed, determine the patient's position on the operating table, watch for signs of trouble, and decide what actions should be taken if an emergency develops. An anesthesiologist is also responsible for monitoring the progress of the waking patient and watching for any developing complications in the recovery room after surgery. In many institutions the anesthesiologist is responsible for respiration therapy.

Aneurysm

Ballooning of an artery due to the pressure of blood flowing through a weakened area. The weakening may be due to disease, injury, or a congenital defect in the artery wall.

TYPES

Some of the common types, sites, and shapes of aneurysm are shown in the illustrated box.

A dissecting aneurysm, usually associated with atherosclerosis, is a condition in which a longitudinal, blood-filled split forms within the lining of the wall of an artery—usually the aorta—and spreads so that extensive areas of the vessel are weakened. There is usually severe pain and the vessel may rupture. When the aneurysm is located in the arch or ascending aorta and dissects into the pericardium (membrane surrounding the heart), the pressure of the blood around the heart may be fatal because it prevents the heart from beating. If an abdominal aorta ruptures, it hemorrhages behind the peritoneum (outside the abdominal cavity).

The heart wall may also develop an aneurysmal swelling after weakening of the muscle from *myocardial infarction* (heart attack). Such aneurysms seldom rupture but they often interfere with the efficient pumping action of the heart.

A traumatic aneurysm is one caused by mechanical injury that weakens the blood vessel wall.

CAUSES

There are several reasons why aneurysms form. One is congenital weakness of the muscular middle layer of an artery; normal blood pressure causes dilation (ballooning) of the blood vessel wall at the weak point. *Marfan's syndrome*, a condition in which the middle layer of the wall of the aorta is defective, often leads to aneurysm just above the heart. The arterial wall can also be weakened by inflammation, as in *periarteritis nodosa*.

The great majority of aneurysms of the aorta—usually in the lower part of the vessel—are caused by atherosclerotic (see *Atherosclerosis*) weakening of a segment of the wall. Aneurysm of the ascending aorta once commonly resulted from untreated *syphilis* but this is now rare. Aneurysms of smaller vessels (mycotic aneurysms) may occur in septicemia as a result of local infection of the wall of the artery.

SYMPTOMS AND SIGNS

Symptoms vary according to the type, size, and location of the swelling.

TYPES OF ANEURYSM

An aneurysm forms when pressure from the blood flow causes a weakened artery wall to distend or forces blood through a fissure.

Aneurysms can form anywhere in the body, although the most common sites are the aorta and the arteries supplying the brain.

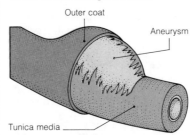

Common aneurysm
This type forms when the tunica media, the artery's middle wall, is weakened; the strong force of the blood flow distends the wall of the artery.

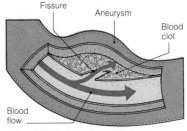

Dissecting aneurysm
This type occurs when there is a fissure in the internal wall of the artery; blood forced through the fissure forms a swelling.

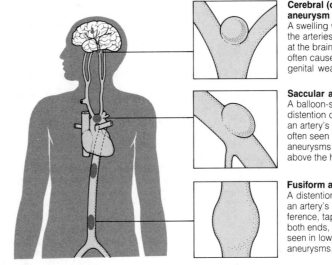

Cerebral (or berry) aneurysm
A swelling where the arteries branch at the brain's base, often caused by congenital weakness.

Saccular aneurysm
A balloon-shaped distention of part of an artery's wall, often seen in aortic aneurysms just above the heart.

Fusiform aneurysm
A distention around an artery's circumference, tapered at both ends, often seen in lower aortic aneurysms.

Cerebral aneurysms may persist for many years without causing symptoms, but the close proximity of so many important neurological structures makes them very dangerous. Sudden enlargement and bursting of a berry aneurysm produces obvious symptoms and signs, such as paralysis of eye movement, drooping of the lid, dilation of the pupil, neck rigidity, severe headache, and unconsciousness (symptoms similar to those of a stroke).

Pressure from an aneurysm on surrounding structures may cause damage, especially within the confined space of the skull.

Aneurysms may rupture, sometimes causing fatal blood loss, or, in the case of cerebral aneurysms, severe damage to the brain structure (see *Subarachnoid hemorrhage*).

Aneurysms of the thoracic (chest) part of the aorta are usually accompanied by hoarseness (due to pressure on the esophagus or a nerve controlling a vocal chord), difficult swallowing, and chest pain that may be mistaken for myocardial infarction (heart attack). Abdominal aortic aneurysm is sometimes visible as a throbbing swelling and may also cause backache.

DIAGNOSIS

X rays will sometimes reveal an aneurysm in a larger blood vessel, but *angiography* provides more detailed information. In the case of cerebral aneurysms, valuable information may be obtained from *CT scanning* or *MRI*.

TREATMENT AND OUTLOOK

This varies with the site of the aneurysm and the age and health of the patient. Nonurgent surgery for aortic aneurysms of the chest offers an 80 to 90 percent chance of survival; emergency surgery carries a high risk. A ruptured aneurysm in the chest always requires surgery, but the outlook is poor. Ruptured or enlarged aneurysms require urgent surgery (see *Arterial reconstructive surgery*). If cerebral aneurysm causes symptoms, surgery is recommended if possible.

Angel dust

One of the common names for phencyclidine, an illicit drug taken for its hallucinogenic properties. Adverse effects of the drug include respiratory depression, agitation, muscle rigidity, vomiting, and convulsions; several deaths have also been reported.

Angiitis

See *Vasculitis*.

Angina

A term that describes a strangling or oppressive heaviness or pain. Angina has become synonymous with the heart disorder *angina pectoris* (chest pain caused by lack of oxygen to the heart muscle, usually a result of poor blood supply). Other types of angina include abdominal angina (abdominal pain after eating caused by poor blood supply to the intestines) and Vincent's angina, pain caused by inflammation of the mouth (see *Vincent's disease*).

Angina pectoris

Pain in the chest and arms or jaw due to a lack of oxygen to the heart muscle, usually when the demand for oxygen is increased during exercise and at times of stress.

CAUSES

Inadequate blood supply to the heart is usually due to *coronary heart disease*, in which the coronary arteries are narrowed by *atherosclerosis* (fat deposits on the walls of the arteries). Other causes include coronary artery spasm, in which the blood vessels narrow suddenly for a short time but return to normal with no permanent obstruction, *aortic stenosis* (narrowing of the aortic valve), and *arrhythmias* (abnormal heart rhythm).

Rare causes of angina pectoris include severe *anemia*, which reduces the oxygen-carrying efficiency of the blood, and *polycythemia* (increased numbers of red blood cells), which thickens the blood, causing it to slow

its flow through the heart muscle. *Thyrotoxicosis* (excessive production of thyroid hormones) can precipitate angina pectoris by making the heart work much harder and faster than its blood supply will permit.

INCIDENCE

This very common condition may occur at any time in men. It is common in men in their fifties, but has been known to occur after the age of 30; in women it usually starts later in life.

SYMPTOMS

The chest pain varies from mild to severe and is often described as a sensation of pressure on the chest. It usually starts in the center of the chest but can spread to the throat, upper jaw, back, and arms (usually the left one) or between the shoulder blades.

The pain usually comes on when the heart is working harder and requires more oxygen—for example, during exercise, when under stress, in extremes of temperature, or during milder exercise soon after a meal. Typically the pain develops at the same point in daily activities—for example, the third flight of stairs on the climb to the office, or halfway up the hill to the stores—and is relieved by a short rest.

Other symptoms may include nausea, sweating, dizziness, and breathing difficulty. These symptoms are usually characteristic of angina pectoris, but somewhat similar symptoms can be caused by *esophagitis* (inflammation of the esophagus), spasm of the esophagus, arthritis in the upper spine or rib cage, or a pulled muscle in the chest wall.

A prolonged and usually more severe attack of angina pectoris may be due to *myocardial infarction* (heart attack), in which the heart muscle is permanently damaged.

DIAGNOSIS

Angina pectoris cannot be diagnosed with certainty by a physical examination; more tests are necessary. Tests usually include an ECG (measurement of the electrical activity in the heart) while the patient is at rest and a *cardiac stress test* (an ECG performed while the patient is exercising enough to cause chest pain—for example, while walking on a treadmill). The resting ECG will show no signs of the angina (unless it is occurring), but may show former heart damage.

Blood tests may be performed to look for an underlying cause, such as *anemia* or *hyperlipidemia* (abnormally high levels of fat in the blood, which can cause *atherosclerosis*).

TREATMENT

Initial treatment attempts to control the symptoms. It is important to stop smoking; nicotine and carbon monoxide contribute to the progressive development of coronary heart disease and make the symptoms worse. Overweight people should lose weight to reduce stress on the heart during exercise.

Attacks of angina pectoris may be prevented and treated by *nitrates* (nitroglycerin), which increase the flow of blood through the heart muscle and improve blood flow around the body. If nitrates are not effective, or are causing severe headaches due to an increased blood flow through the brain, other drugs may be used, including *beta-blockers* and *calcium channel blockers*.

If *hypertension* (high blood pressure) is found during examination, it is treated with antihypertensive drugs to reduce the work of the heart in pumping out blood. Other specific causes can also be treated—for example, arrhythmias with antiarrhythmic drugs and hyperlipidemia with a low-fat diet and/or drugs.

Drug treatment can control the symptoms of angina pectoris for many years but it cannot cure the disorder. If attacks become more severe, more frequent, or more prolonged, despite drug treatment, and if there is angiographic evidence of advanced narrowing of vessels, then *coronary artery bypass* surgery or *angioplasty* may be performed to reestablish blood flow to the heart muscle.

OUTLOOK

The effect of angina pectoris on lifestyle depends on the severity of the underlying disease and the effectiveness of drug treatment or surgery. Some people are able to lead a normal life apart from some restriction on strenuous exercise. Others are severely disabled and can do very little for themselves.

Angioedema

An allergic reaction, also known as angioneurotic edema. It is similar to *urticaria* (hives) and characterized by large, well-defined swellings, of sudden onset, in the skin, larynx (voice box), and other areas. These swellings may last several hours or days if they are left untreated.

INCIDENCE AND CAUSES

Angioedema primarily affects young people (especially those in their twenties) and those with a general tendency toward allergies (see *Atopy*).

The most common cause is a sudden allergic reaction to a food, such as eggs, strawberries, or seafood. Less commonly, it results from allergy to a drug (such as penicillin), a reaction to an insect sting or bite, or from infection, emotional stress, or exposure to animals, molds, pollens, or cold conditions. There is also a hereditary form of the disease.

SYMPTOMS
Angioedema may cause very sudden difficulty breathing, speaking, and swallowing accompanied by obvious swelling of the lips, face, and neck.

Angioedema of the throat and the larynx may be life-threatening because it can block the airway, causing *asphyxia* (suffocation). If the gastrointestinal tract is involved, colic, nausea, and vomiting may occur.

TREATMENT
Severe cases are treated with injections of *epinephrine* and may require intubation (passage of a breathing tube via the mouth into the windpipe) or *tracheostomy* (surgical creation of a breathing hole in the windpipe) to prevent suffocation. *Corticosteroid drugs* may also be prescribed to be taken intravenously or by mouth. In less severe cases, *antihistamine drugs* often relieve symptoms.

Angiography
A procedure that enables blood vessels to be seen on film after the vessels have been filled with a contrast medium (a substance that is opaque to X rays).

WHY IT IS DONE
Angiography is used to detect diseases that alter the appearance of the blood vessel channel. These diseases include *aneurysms* (weakening of the blood vessel wall and ballooning of the vessel itself), and narrowing or blockage from *atheroma* (fatty deposits) or from a thrombus or embolus (clot). Angiography is also used to detect changes in the pattern of blood vessels that lead to tumors and to organs that have been injured. By noting the abnormal arrangement of blood vessels, the physician can evaluate the extent of disease and plan treatment accordingly.

TYPES
Carotid angiography is sometimes performed on patients suffering from *transient ischemic attacks* (symptoms of *stroke* lasting less than 24 hours) to see whether there is a blockage or substantial narrowing in one of the carotid arteries (in the neck), which supply blood to the brain. Cerebral

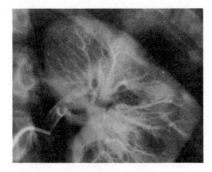

Angiogram of a normal kidney
Contrast medium is passed through the catheter into the kidney's arterial system and a series of X-ray pictures is taken.

angiography is used to demonstrate the presence of an aneurysm within the brain or to help visualize a brain tumor prior to surgery. Angiography of the coronary arteries, often combined with cardiac *catheterization*, is carried out to identify the sites of narrowing or blockage in arteries, which may be treated by *coronary artery bypass* or balloon *angioplasty*.

HOW IT IS DONE
Contrast medium is usually injected into the vessel to be examined through a fine catheter (flexible plastic tube) inserted into the femoral artery at the groin, the brachial artery just over the elbow, or the carotid arteries that run up the neck.

To insert the catheter, the skin and tissues around the artery are numbed with local anesthetic and then a needle is inserted through the skin into the artery. A long, thin wire with a soft tip is inserted through the needle, the needle is removed, and the catheter is then threaded over the wire into the blood vessel. Under X-ray control, the tip of the catheter is further guided into the vessel to be examined and contrast medium is injected. A rapid sequence (or movie) of X-ray pictures is taken so that the flow along the vessels can be studied.

Angiography can take from as little as a few minutes to as long as two or three hours.

DIGITAL SUBTRACTION ANGIOGRAPHY
This type of angiography uses computer techniques to process images and subtract, or remove, unwanted background information, leaving only an image of the blood vessels being studied. This technique makes it possible to use a much smaller amount of contrast medium (sometimes injected intravenously), which makes the procedure somewhat safer; in

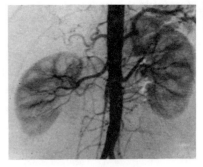

Digital subtraction angiography
Here, the normal kidneys are revealed more clearly because the computer eliminates unwanted information.

some cases, it removes the need for direct injection of contrast medium into vessels not accessible by catheter. However, the detail provided is not always as good as in conventional angiography.

RISKS
The contrast medium usually produces a sensation of warmth lasting a few seconds; it may be felt to a greater degree in the part of the body that has been injected. Allergy to the contrast medium is a more serious side effect, but with new contrast agents the risk of a severe reaction is less than one in 80,000 examinations.

Damage to blood vessels can occur at the site of puncture, anywhere along the vessel during passage of the catheter, or at the site of injection.

With digital subtraction angiography, the risks are considerably reduced because the catheter does not need to be passed as far into the blood vessels, thus lessening the possibility of damage or blockage.

OUTLOOK
Angiographic techniques have, in the last few years, been adapted to allow not only diagnosis, but certain types of treatment that, in some cases, eliminate the need for surgery. For example, small balloons can be inflated at the tip of a catheter to expand a narrowed or blocked segment of artery (balloon angioplasty), foreign material can be injected to reduce or shut off blood supply to a tumor (see *Embolism, therapeutic*), and medication to control bleeding or treat tumors can be infused directly into the blood supply to individual organs.

Angioma
A benign tumor made up of blood vessels (see *Hemangioma*) or lymph vessels (lymphangioma).

A

Angioplasty, balloon

A technique for treating stenosis (narrowing) or occlusion (blockage) of a blood vessel or heart valve by introducing a balloon into the constricted area to widen it.

WHY IT IS DONE

Balloon angioplasty is used in the treatment of *peripheral vascular disease* to increase or restore the flow of blood through a significantly narrowed artery in a limb; it is also used in the treatment of stenosis of the coronary arteries (see *Coronary heart disease*).

COMPLICATIONS

There is a slight risk of damaging the artery or valve during this procedure and immediate surgery may be required. Prolonged interruption of blood supply to an area of the heart, when the balloon is inflated, can lead to *myocardial infarction* (heart attack). The mortality for balloon angioplasty is about the same as for a coronary artery bypass graft.

RESULTS

In the US, coronary balloon angioplasty is successful in improving the condition of about two thirds of the patients treated with it. In three quarters of these cases the improvement continues after a year; in the remainder, stenosis recurs in the affected vessel, but angioplasty may be repeated successfully.

Angioplasty of peripheral vessels is most successful in treating the iliac and femoral arteries, particularly when the area of stenosis or occlusion is small. After five years, 85 to 90 percent of iliac arteries treated by angioplasty remain free of stenosis. For femoral arteries, the success rate is 50 to 70 percent after two years.

Angiotensin

The name of two related proteins involved in regulating blood pressure. The first of these, angiotensin I, is itself inactive and is converted to the second, active form, angiotensin II, by the action of a converting enzyme. Angiotensin II causes narrowing of the small blood vessels in tissues, resulting in an increase in blood pressure. It also stimulates the release from the adrenal cortex (the outer part of the *adrenal glands*) of the hormone *aldosterone*, which also causes an increase in blood pressure.

Certain kidney disorders can increase the production of angiotensin II, causing *hypertension* (high blood pressure). Whatever the cause of the hypertension, it may be treated with drugs that are known as

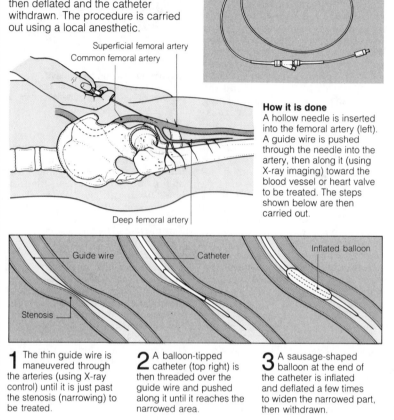

PROCEDURE FOR BALLOON ANGIOPLASTY

A blockage or narrowing of a blood vessel may be treated by introducing a balloon catheter into the area and then inflating the balloon to stretch the constricted part. The balloon is then deflated and the catheter withdrawn. The procedure is carried out using a local anesthetic.

BALLOON CATHETER

Superficial femoral artery
Common femoral artery

Deep femoral artery

How it is done

A hollow needle is inserted into the femoral artery (left). A guide wire is pushed through the needle into the artery, then along it (using X-ray imaging) toward the blood vessel or heart valve to be treated. The steps shown below are then carried out.

Guide wire   Catheter   Inflated balloon

Stenosis

1 The thin guide wire is maneuvered through the arteries (using X-ray control) until it is just past the stenosis (narrowing) to be treated.

2 A balloon-tipped catheter (top right) is then threaded over the guide wire and pushed along it until it reaches the narrowed area.

3 A sausage-shaped balloon at the end of the catheter is inflated and deflated a few times to widen the narrowed part, then withdrawn.

ACE inhibitors (angiotensin-converting enzyme inhibitors), which reduce angiotensin II formation.

Animal experimentation

The use of living animals in research and safety testing to provide information about biological science and to increase knowledge about human physiology or behavior. Animal experimentation is most prolific in developed countries, where medical standards are high and there is intense concern for public health and safety.

The species most extensively used in animal experimentation are rats and mice, which are bred for laboratory research. Less than 1 percent of experiments involve cats, dogs, farm animals, nonhuman primates, frogs, fish, and birds.

LEGISLATIVE CONTROLS

Animal experimentation is controlled by law in most countries but the controls vary in their stringency. Governments must balance pressures for very tight controls against the weight of medical and scientific opinion, which maintains that animal experiments are indispensable to health and safety.

TYPES OF EXPERIMENTS

The experiments for which animals are used fall into several groups. One group consists of experiments to test the safety of nonmedical substances, such as pesticides, cleaning chemicals, and cosmetics, before they are released for public use.

Another group includes the many medical experiments in which a condition in an animal corresponds to a human disease. This provides the potential for testing new treatments to discover cures for the disease in the animal and therefore in humans.

Other experiments are performed to discover new drugs and medical procedures or to develop new substances for use in the environment.

ETHICAL OBJECTIONS
Campaigners for animal rights point out that animals suffer in many of these experiments. Sometimes the suffering is an implicit part of the research, as in research to study the mechanism of pain or to create models of painful conditions on which to test analgesics (painkillers). Some of the conditions or effects being studied necessarily cause illness, stress, or pain, such as infecting animals with disease or studying the irritant or poisonous effects of chemicals.

Two safety tests, often required by law, have received considerable criticism from protest groups and scientists alike. One test is the LD50 test, which measures acute toxicity (short-term poisonous effects) by estimating the dose that would kill 50 percent of the animals in a test group. The other test is the Draize test, which measures irritant damage of chemicals and substances to eyes and skin.

BENEFITS
Experiments on animals have contributed greatly to the advancement of science and have specifically produced benefits to humanity by virtue of new medical and surgical treatments. In the past 30 years, smallpox has been eradicated and the incidence of polio and other infections has been reduced enormously as a result of vaccines produced after such testing.

Antibiotics developed using animal experiments have also prolonged and saved many lives. It has been estimated that the reduction in infant mortality as a result of antibiotics has alone saved half a million lives. Drugs for the treatment of noninfectious disorders, such as arthritis, diabetes, and hypertension (high blood pressure), are also the result of animal-based research. Surgical treatments may also be developed in animals; the success of transplant operations and microsurgery techniques are notable recent advances.

ALTERNATIVES
Alternatives to animal experiments have been developed and are used whenever possible. Laboratory tests using cultured cells or tissues have replaced many experiments that once involved animals. Other alternatives involve the use of simple organisms,

such as bacteria or yeasts, or the computerized or mathematical modeling of an experiment.

New techniques have also led in some cases to the replacement of animals as a source of vaccines and hormones. Cell culture techniques have now almost replaced the use of animals in vaccine production, while genetically engineered bacteria and yeasts are increasingly used to produce substances, such as insulin, that were once derived only from animals.

However, even with these newer methods, it is dangerous—and illegal—not to undertake confirmatory studies on animals before releasing the drug or vaccine in question.

Animals, diseases from
See *Zoonoses*.

Anisometropia
Unequal focusing power in the two eyes, usually due to a difference in size and/or shape in the eyes. For example, one eye may be normal and the other myopic (nearsighted) or hyperopic (farsighted), or there may be astigmatism in one eye.

Significant anisometropia may cause visual discomfort. Although glasses may give clear vision in each eye, if significant anisometropia exists, the images on the retinas will be of different sizes, which can be disturbing. There is no entirely satisfactory remedy, but contact lenses minimize the effect. Full correction may not be prescribed in severe cases because the resulting perception of differences in image size could cause discomfort.

Ankle joint
The hinge joint between the talus (uppermost bone in the foot) and tibia (shin). The talus fits between the two bony protuberances on either side of the ankle. Strong ligaments on each side of the joint provide support and prevent overmovement. The ankle allows upward and downward movements of the foot. Other movements, such as tilting and rotation, take place around joints in the foot itself.

DISORDERS
An ankle *sprain* is one of the most common of all injuries. It usually results from the foot twisting over onto its outside edge, which produces overstretching and bruising of the ligaments on the outside of the ankle. Very severe sprains may cause extensive tearing of the ligaments, which requires surgical repair.

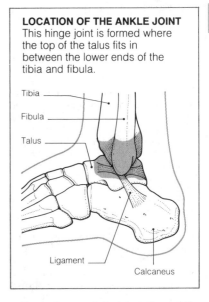

LOCATION OF THE ANKLE JOINT
This hinge joint is formed where the top of the talus fits in between the lower ends of the tibia and fibula.

Tibia

Fibula

Talus

Ligament

Calcaneus

Excessive or violent twisting of the ankle can cause a combined fracture and dislocation (called *Pott's fracture*), in which the fibula (outer of the two bones of the lower leg) breaks above the ankle, and either the tibia breaks or the ligaments tear, resulting in dislocation of the ankle.

Ankylosing spondylitis
An inflammatory disease affecting joints between the vertebrae of the spine and the sacroiliac joints (joints between the spine and the pelvis).

CAUSES
In most cases the cause of this condition remains unknown. A related disorder is preceded either by *colitis* (inflammation of the intestine) or *psoriasis* (a skin disease).

INCIDENCE
Ankylosing spondylitis affects less than 1 percent of the population, is more common in men than women, and has its onset between the ages of 20 and 40 years. It also seems to run in families. A genetic marker or tissue type (HLA-B27) is found much more often in people with this condition than in the rest of the population.

SYMPTOMS
Ankylosing spondylitis usually starts with discomfort in the lower back and hips, with pain and stiffness worse after resting. Typically, exercise helps reduce the stiffness.

Other symptoms include pain in the chest (from the joints between the spine and the ribs), loss of appetite, tiredness, and, occasionally, redness and pain in the eyes due to *iritis*

A

(inflammation of the iris). In about one fifth of patients, other joints may be inflamed—for example, the hips, knees, and ankles. Inflammation of tissues around the heel can cause pain and tenderness.

In time, the inflammation in the spine can lead to *ankylosis* (permanent stiffness and limitation of motion) and *kyphosis* (curvature of the spine). Movement is restricted and expansion of the chest is often limited.

DIAGNOSIS

Back pain and stiffness that is worse in the morning and relieved by exercise is suggestive of this condition. Other causes of back pain are usually mechanical and improve with resting.

Blood tests can be performed to measure inflammation and to indicate the presence of the HLA-B27 antigen on white blood cells. At the onset, X rays of the back may be normal, but later in the disease ankylosis is shown by loss of space between joints and bony outgrowths.

TREATMENT

There is no curative treatment but symptoms may be reduced by a program of heat, massage, and supervised exercise. Regular daily exercise (such as swimming) is essential to keep the back muscles strong. To prevent curvature of the spine, patients are taught breathing exercises and exercises to improve posture; they are also advised to lie facedown during the night. Anti-inflammatory drugs may be prescribed to reduce the pain and stiffness.

OUTLOOK

The inflammatory process tends to become less active with age. With treatment, most people suffer only minor deformity of the spine and are able to lead a normal life.

Ankylosis

Complete loss of movement in a joint caused by degeneration and fusion of the bony surfaces. This may be due to injury, infection, or inflammation. Ankylosis may also occur as a result of a surgical fusion of a diseased joint to correct deformity or to alleviate persistent pain.

Anodontia

Failure of some or all of the teeth to develop. Anodontia may be due to congenital absence of tooth buds or may be the result of damage to developing tooth buds caused by infection or systemic disease. Both primary and permanent teeth, or permanent teeth only, may be affected.

If only a few teeth are missing, a *bridge* can fill the gap; if all the teeth are missing, a *denture* is needed.

Anomaly

A deviation from what is accepted as normal, especially as a result of a birth defect such as a limb malformation.

Anorexia

The medical term for loss of appetite (see *Appetite, loss of*).

Anorexia nervosa

An eating disorder characterized by intense fear of being fat, by severe weight loss, and, in time, by *amenorrhea* (absence of monthly periods). Sufferers have a distorted body image and "see" themselves as fat even when they are of normal weight or even emaciated. Anorexia nervosa primarily affects teenage and young adult women and occasionally young men. Popularly known as the "slimming disease," it is difficult to treat and sometimes fatal.

CAUSES

There is much debate as to the causes of anorexia nervosa. Many anorectics seem to be part of very close, constricted families, having a special relationship with one of the parents. Anorectics are often highly conforming people and anxious to please, even obsessional in their habits. As their bodies change with puberty, anorectics try to take control over their lives by dieting stubbornly. It seems as if they do not wish to grow up and are trying to keep their childhood shapes. The exercise of control also helps anorectics compensate for a general sense of ineffectiveness.

Others have suggested that anorexia is a true *phobia* about putting on weight, which leads to a special fear of eating foods containing fats or carbohydrates. Hormonal changes related to weight loss and amenorrhea have led some physicians to regard anorexia as a physical illness caused by a disorder of the *hypothalamus* (part of the midbrain concerned with hunger, thirst, and sexual development). It is likely that these changes are secondary to the starvation.

Changes in fashion may also be a contributing factor; the disorder seems to have increased in the last 30 years, during which slimness has become closely identified with beauty. In the US and Europe, most women diet at some time, especially models, athletes, and dancers, all of whom are more prone to the disorder. About one

in 100 young, middle-class women have anorexic symptoms, although the figure is five times greater in the "at-risk" groups.

Some physicians see anorexia merely as a symptom rather than a separate disease, citing *depression, personality disorder,* or even *schizophrenia* as the real cause. However, despite the numerous cases of anorexia, it is frequently difficult to identify any such underlying cause.

SYMPTOMS AND SIGNS

The most obvious sign is emaciation (extreme thinness), with one third or more of the body's weight being lost. Starvation causes certain biochemical disorders and the balance of sex hormones is disrupted; amenorrhea develops as a result of these changes. A number of other physical changes and characteristic behavior patterns occur. They may indicate a person is suffering from anorexia.

FEATURES OF ANOREXIA NERVOSA

Weight loss

Overactivity and obsessive exercising

Tiredness and weakness

Lanugo (babylike) hair on body, thinning of hair on head

Extreme choosiness over food

Binge eating

Induced vomiting

Use of laxatives to promote weight loss

The anorectic often feels intensely hungry, although hunger pains are denied. Food and weight dominate the anorectic's thinking to an extreme degree; drug and alcohol abuse occasionally occur.

TREATMENT

The characteristic stubbornness and ability of anorectics to cause discord between health care professionals and family members has shown that anorectics are usually best treated in the hospital by a team experienced in managing the disorder.

Treatment is usually based on a closely controlled refeeding program, combined with individual *psychotherapy* or with *family therapy*. Unless a strict watch is kept on feeding, patients tend to hide or secretly throw away food. Often, a system of rewards

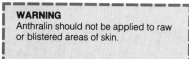

is organized, so that for every pound of weight gained the anorectic is allowed more privileges, such as having visitors or watching a favorite TV show.

Drugs may be needed if there is a clear depressive or other illness. Chlorpromazine is often helpful in the early stages to calm patients and promote weight gain. Once they have achieved a more normal weight, patients may need to continue psychotherapy for months or years.

OUTLOOK

Relapses are common whenever there is the slightest stress and about half of hospital patients still have symptoms for many years. Five to 10 percent of patients treated for anorexia nervosa in a hospital later die from starvation or suicide.

Anorgasmia

Inability to achieve orgasm (see *Psychosexual dysfunction*).

Anosmia

Loss of *smell*.

Anoxia

A medical term that means literally a complete absence of oxygen within a body tissue—for example, the brain or a muscle. Anoxia causes a disruption of cell *metabolism* (chemical activity) and cell death unless corrected within a few minutes.

Anoxia is a very rare occurrence, whereas *hypoxia* (the reduction of oxygen supply to a tissue) is a more common disorder.

Antacid drugs

COMMON DRUGS

*Aluminum hydroxide Magnesium hydroxide
Sodium bicarbonate*

WARNING
Antacid drugs should not be taken regularly except under medical supervision as they may suppress the symptoms of a more serious disorder or provoke serious complications.

A group of drugs taken to relieve the symptoms of *indigestion, heartburn, esophagitis* (inflammation of the esophagus), *acid reflux* (regurgitation of stomach acids into the esophagus), and *peptic ulcer*.

TYPES

Antacid drugs usually contain compounds of *magnesium* or *aluminum*, which have a long-lasting effect, or

sodium bicarbonate, which produces a rapid, short-lived effect. Some antacid drugs also contain dimethicone (to relieve flatulence), alginate (to help prevent heartburn), or a local anesthetic (used in esophagitis to numb pain).

HOW THEY WORK

Antacid drugs neutralize stomach acids, an action that helps prevent or relieve inflammation and pain in the digestive system. Antacid drugs also give the stomach lining time to heal when it has been damaged by a peptic ulcer and is sensitive to normal amounts of stomach acid.

POSSIBLE ADVERSE EFFECTS

Since aluminum may cause constipation, and diarrhea may occur with magnesium, these ingredients are often given together to avoid these effects. A person taking sodium bicarbonate may experience fluid retention and, because this substance combines with acid to produce gas, bloating and belching. Antacid drugs should not be taken with other medication without the advice of a physician because they interfere with the absorption of other drugs.

Antepartum hemorrhage

Vaginal bleeding after the beginning of the third trimester of pregnancy.

CAUSES AND INCIDENCE

Antepartum hemorrhage is most commonly due to a defective placenta, the organ in the uterus that sustains the developing fetus. The placental problem may be *placenta previa* (a low-lying placenta), in which the placenta is close to the birth canal, a placental abruption (detachment of part of the placenta from the wall of the uterus), or bleeding from the edge of a normally sited placenta. Bleeding can also be caused by *cervical erosion* or lesions of the cervix or vagina.

Antepartum hemorrhage occurs in about 3 percent of all pregnancies.

SYMPTOMS

The bleeding is often painless but, when the placenta has become partly separated from the uterus, there may be abdominal pain.

INVESTIGATION AND TREATMENT

The physician may be able to ascertain whether the fetus is alive by listening for a heart beat and the woman will be admitted to the hospital. There, the fetus' heart beat will be monitored and the position of the placenta will be located by *ultrasound scanning* (not by a physical examination, which could damage a low-lying placenta).

If bleeding is not heavy, it is necessary only to keep a careful watch on

the condition of the woman and baby. In cases of severe bleeding, the woman is given an *intravenous infusion* and sometimes blood transfusions. When bleeding is severe the baby may be starved of oxygen, in which case immediate delivery is essential, sometimes by *cesarean section*.

When delivery is not necessary, the woman usually stays in the hospital for at least 48 hours. If the woman is felt to be at risk of more bleeding, which could endanger her or the baby, she sometimes stays in the hospital until delivery. Otherwise, if the bleeding has stopped and the conditions of woman and baby are considered satisfactory, the woman is allowed to go home—though her condition is carefully monitored for the remaining weeks of the pregnancy.

COMPLICATIONS

Because of good obstetric care, mortality of women and babies today is low. Death of the baby is more likely than maternal death; it is caused by lack of oxygen or by prematurity if bleeding triggers labor.

Anterior

Relating to the front of the body. In human *anatomy*, the term is synonymous with *ventral*.

Anthracosis

A medical term for coal workers' *pneumoconiosis*, a lung disease of workers in the coal industry caused by inhalation over many years of small amounts of coal dust. It is likely that all people living in large industrial cities have a mild form of anthracosis.

Anthralin

WARNING
Anthralin should not be applied to raw or blistered areas of skin.

A drug used to treat *psoriasis* (a skin disorder caused by excessive skin cell production). Anthralin, which is prescribed as an ointment or a cream, works by slowing the rate at which skin cells multiply. This effect is sometimes boosted by ultraviolet light treatment (see *Phototherapy*).

POSSIBLE ADVERSE EFFECTS

Skin inflammation causing redness and irritation is a common reaction; it may be relieved by the application of a *corticosteroid drug*. The skin around patches of psoriasis can be protected from inflammation by applying petroleum jelly.

Anthralin may stain clothing and, temporarily, the skin and hair. It is therefore advisable to wear gloves and old clothes when applying the drug.

Anthrax

A serious bacterial infection of livestock, occasionally spread to people. The most common type of human infection—in the skin—is readily treatable. Anthrax is rare today, mainly due to widespread vaccination of livestock, but some serious epidemics have occurred in animals and humans in some developing countries, usually due to lapse of control programs.

CAUSES AND INCIDENCE

Anthrax is caused by a bacterium, *BACILLUS ANTHRACIS*. It produces spores that can survive dormant for many years in soil and animal products but are capable of reactivation. Animals become infected by grazing on contaminated land.

People may become infected by handling materials from animals that have died of anthrax, by inhaling spores contained in these materials, or by eating infected meat.

In the US, human cases of anthrax are extremely rare. There was one case in 1980 and six cases in 1978.

SYMPTOMS AND TREATMENT

The most common site of human anthrax infection is the skin; the bacterium enters via a scratch or sore when contaminated animal material is handled. A raised, itchy, area develops at the site of entry, progressing to a large blister and finally to a black scab, with swelling of the surrounding tissues.

If infected meat is eaten, the symptoms are those of severe *gastroenteritis*, with fever, diarrhea, and vomiting. If anthrax spores are inhaled, the result may be a severe form of *pneumonia*. Anthrax is curable in its early stages with penicillin.

Antianxiety drugs

A group of drugs used to relieve symptoms of *anxiety*. Benzodiazepines and *beta-blockers* are the two main types of antianxiety drugs. Other drugs used to treat anxiety include *antidepressant drugs* and, rarely, *barbiturate drugs*.

WHY THEY ARE USED

Antianxiety drugs are used to provide temporary relief from anxiety when it limits a person's ability to cope with everyday life. In most cases, the underlying disorder is best treated by *counseling* or *psychotherapy*.

Antianxiety drugs are sometimes used to calm a person before surgical treatment (see *Premedication*) or before a public performance.

HOW THEY WORK

Benzodiazepines promote mental and physical relaxation by reducing nerve activity in the brain. Beta-blockers work by reducing the physical symptoms of anxiety, such as shaking and palpitations.

POSSIBLE ADVERSE EFFECTS

Long-term drug treatment with benzodiazepines should be ended gradually due to a risk of physical dependence (see *Drug dependence*).

Antiarrhythmic drugs

A group of drugs used to treat different types of *arrhythmia* (irregular heart beat). Antiarrhythmic drugs include *beta-blockers*, *calcium channel blocker drugs*, *digitalis drugs*, and *disopyramide*. The choice of drug depends on the type of arrhythmia.

WHY THEY ARE USED

An arrhythmia can reduce the pumping efficiency of the heart, causing breathlessness, dizziness, and chest pain. Antiarrhythmic drugs relieve these symptoms and, in some cases, restore normal heart beat.

HOW THEY WORK

The heart's pumping action is governed by electrical impulses. Some antiarrhythmic drugs work by altering these impulses within or on their way to the heart. Others affect the response of the heart muscle to the impulses received.

Antibacterial drugs

A group of drugs used to treat infections caused by *bacteria*. Antibacterial drugs share the actions of *antibiotic drugs* but, unlike antibiotics, have always been produced synthetically.

The largest group of antibacterial drugs are the *sulfonamide drugs*, used mainly for the treatment of *urinary tract infection*.

Antibiotic drugs

COMMON DRUGS
Aminoglycosides *Gentamicin Streptomycin*
Cephalosporins *Cefaclor Cephalexin*
Penicillins *Amoxicillin Penicillin V*
Tetracyclines *Doxycycline Oxytetracycline*
Others *Erythromycin Neomycin*

> **WARNING**
> You must inform your physician of any previous allergic reaction to an antibiotic drug. Always complete a course of antibiotics or the infection may return.

A group of drugs used to treat infection caused by *bacteria*. Originally derived from molds and fungi, antibiotic drugs are now made synthetically.

HOW ANTIBIOTICS WORK

Antibiotic drugs are either bactericidal (killing bacteria) or bacteriostatic (halting bacterial growth, allowing the immune system to cope with the infection). Penicillin drugs and cephalosporin drugs are bactericidal; these drugs work by disrupting bacterial cell walls.

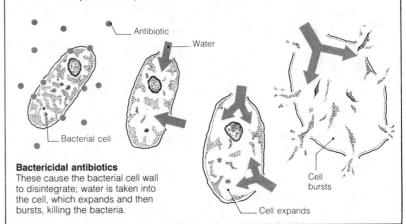

Bactericidal antibiotics
These cause the bacterial cell wall to disintegrate; water is taken into the cell, which expands and then bursts, killing the bacteria.

Antibiotic
Water
Bacterial cell
Cell bursts
Cell expands

TYPES

Some antibiotic drugs are effective against only certain types of bacteria. Others, known as broad-spectrum antibiotics, are effective against a wide range of bacteria. The choice of antibiotic drug depends on both the type of bacteria and the site of the infection. This choice is most effectively made by growing a culture of the bacteria and checking its sensitivity to various types of antibiotic.

More than one antibiotic drug may be prescribed to increase the efficiency of treatment and to reduce the risk of antibiotic resistance.

WHY THEY ARE USED

Antibiotic drugs help fight infection either when the body has been invaded by harmful bacteria or when bacteria present within the body multiply uncontrollably. They also prevent infection in cases when the *immune system* is impaired or when there is a risk of *endocarditis* (inflammation of the lining of the heart).

ANTIBIOTIC RESISTANCE

Some bacteria develop resistance to a previously effective antibiotic drug. Resistance may occur if a type of bacteria develops a method of growth that is not disrupted by the effects of the drug or if it begins to produce an enzyme that breaks down or inactivates the drug.

Resistance is most likely to develop if a person fails to take an antibiotic drug as directed or during long-term treatment. Some powerful antibiotic drugs are available to treat severe infections resistant to the commonly prescribed antibiotic drugs.

POSSIBLE ADVERSE EFFECTS

Apart from side effects typical of each specific group, most antibiotic drugs can cause nausea, diarrhea, or a rash. Antibiotic drugs may kill bacteria naturally present in the body and fungi may grow in their place, causing oral, intestinal, or vaginal *candidiasis* (thrush). Some people occasionally experience a severe allergic reaction, causing facial swelling, itching, or breathing difficulty.

Antibody

A protein that is manufactured by lymphocytes (a type of white blood cell) to neutralize an *antigen* (foreign protein) in the body. Bacteria, viruses, and other microorganisms commonly contain many antigens; antibodies formed against these antigens help the body neutralize or destroy the invading microorganisms. Antibodies may also be formed in response to *vac-*

cines, thereby giving immunity against some infections. Antibodies are also known as *immunoglobulins*.

In some cases, inappropriate or excessive formation of antibodies leads to illness. The body's response to certain substances may lead to *allergy*, as in *asthma* or *eczema*. Antibodies against antigens in skin grafts or organ transplants may result in rejection. In some disorders, antibodies are formed against the body's own tissues, resulting in an *autoimmune disorder*, such as some forms of *arthritis* and the *collagen diseases*. (See also *Immune response*.)

Antibody, monoclonal

An artificially produced *antibody* that neutralizes only one specific *antigen* (foreign protein).

Monoclonal antibodies are produced in the laboratory by stimulating the growth of large numbers of antibody-producing clones. (A clone is a group of cells that is genetically identical, or an individual member of such a group.) In effect, this cloning process enables antibodies to be tailor-made so that they will react with a particular antigen.

Monoclonal antibodies are used in the diagnosis and treatment of some forms of cancer.

Anticancer drugs

COMMON DRUGS

Cytotoxic
Azathioprine Chlorambucil
Cyclophosphamide Doxorubicin Fluorouracil
Melphalan Mercaptopurine Methotrexate

Sex hormone-related
Aminoglutethimide Diethylstilbestrol Ethinyl
estradiol Medroxyprogesterone Megestrol
Nandrolone Tamoxifen

Drugs used to treat *cancer*. They are particularly useful in the treatment of *lymphomas, leukemias,* and cancer affecting the ovary and testis. These drugs are sometimes used after surgery or *radiation therapy*.

TYPES

Most anticancer drugs are cytotoxic drugs (drugs that kill or damage cells). Others are synthetic forms of sex hormones and substances related to these hormones (e.g., *androgen drugs, estrogen drugs*, and *progesterone drugs*).

Anticancer drugs are often prescribed in combination to maximize their effects. The choice of drugs depends on the type of cancer, its stage of development, and the general health of the patient.

HOW THEY WORK

All anticancer drugs kill cancer cells by preventing them from growing and dividing. Some cytotoxic drugs work by damaging the cells' *DNA*. Others block the chemical processes in the cell necessary for growth.

Sex hormones stimulate the growth of certain cancers (for example, estrogen stimulates some types of breast cancer). Substances related to these hormones may inhibit growth by blocking their stimulatory effect. The growth of other cancers is sometimes disrupted by a synthetic sex hormone given in high doses. Cancer of the prostate gland, for example, may be treated with *diethylstilbestrol* (DES), an estrogen drug.

POSSIBLE ADVERSE EFFECTS

In the early stages of treatment, nausea, vomiting, and diarrhea may occur and be sufficiently serious to make hospitalization necessary.

Anticancer drugs may alter the rate at which noncancerous cells grow and divide. This effect may cause alopecia (hair loss) and reduce the number of blood cells produced by the bone marrow, causing *anemia*, increased susceptibility to infection, and/or abnormal bleeding. Regular blood tests are usually carried out to monitor blood cell production.

To minimize adverse effects, anticancer drugs are usually given in short courses with time between each course to enable noncancerous cells to recover from the drugs' effects.

Anticholinergic drugs

COMMON DRUGS

Atropine Benztropine Diphenhydramine
Orphenadrine Procyclidine Propantheline
Scopolamine

A group of drugs that blocks the effects of *acetylcholine*, a chemical released from nerve endings in the parasympathetic division of the *autonomic nervous system*. Acetylcholine triggers activity in a number of reactive cells. For example, it stimulates muscle contraction, increases secretions in the mouth and lungs, and slows the heart beat.

WHY THEY ARE USED

Anticholinergic drugs are used in the treatment of *irritable bowel syndrome* and certain types of urinary *incontinence* (see also *Antispasmodic drugs*). They are given in the treatment of *Parkinson's disease, asthma*, and bradycardia (abnormally slow heart beat) and are also used before an examina-

A

A

HOW ANTICHOLINERGICS WORK

Acetylcholine combines with a receptor on the cell's surface. This interaction stimulates activity in that cell (e.g., contraction of a muscle fiber or secretion of a fluid). Anticholinergic drugs block the stimulatory action of acetylcholine by combining with the acetylcholine receptors. This action produces, for example, muscle relaxation (e.g., in the bladder, intestine, and bronchi) and dries up secretions in the mouth and lungs. Anticholinergic drugs are used to treat asthma.

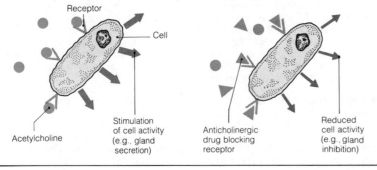

Receptor

Cell

Stimulation of cell activity (e.g., gland secretion)

Acetylcholine

Anticholinergic drug blocking receptor

Reduced cell activity (e.g., gland inhibition)

tion of or surgical procedure on the eye. Anticholinergic drugs are also helpful as a *premedication* before general *anesthesia* and in the treatment of *motion sickness*.

POSSIBLE ADVERSE EFFECTS

Anticholinergic drugs may cause dry mouth, blurred vision, abnormal retention of urine, and confusion.

Anticoagulant drugs

COMMON DRUGS

Dicumarol Heparin Warfarin

> **WARNING**
> Many drugs, such as aspirin and alcohol, may increase the risk of an anticoagulant drug causing abnormal bleeding. Always consult your physician before taking any other drug during anticoagulant treatment.

A group of drugs used to treat and prevent abnormal *blood clotting*. They are used to treat *thrombosis*, and may be used to prevent and treat *stroke* or *transient ischemic attack*. Anticoagulant drugs are also prescribed to prevent the development of abnormal blood clotting after major surgery (especially heart valve replacement) or during hemodialysis (see *Dialysis*).

HOW THEY WORK

Heparin increases the effect of antithrombin III, an enzyme that blocks the activity of other enzymes—known as coagulation factors—that are needed for blood to clot. This drug is given by injection and begins to work within a few hours.

Other anticoagulant drugs are taken by mouth and begin to act within a day. They work by reducing the production of some coagulation factors.

By disrupting the blood clotting mechanism, anticoagulant drugs prevent an abnormal blood clot from forming. When a blood clot already exists, anticoagulant drugs stop it from enlarging and reduce the risk of an *embolus* breaking off and blocking another blood vessel. Unlike *thrombolytic drugs*, they do not dissolve blood clots that have already formed.

POSSIBLE ADVERSE EFFECTS

Anticoagulant drugs in high doses may cause abnormal bleeding in different parts of the body. As a result, regular *blood clotting tests* are carried out to monitor treatment.

Anticonvulsant drugs

COMMON DRUGS

Carbamazepine Clonazepam Diazepam Ethosuximide Phenobarbital Phenytoin Primidone Valproic acid

> **WARNING**
> Never suddenly stop taking an anticonvulsant drug after long-term treatment; the dose should be reduced gradually or symptoms may return.

A group of drugs used in the treatment of *seizures* (see also *Epilepsy*). Anticonvulsant drugs are taken on a regular basis to reduce the frequency and severity of seizures and as an emergency treatment to stop a prolonged seizure. Anticonvulsant drugs are also given to prevent seizures following a serious head injury or some types of brain surgery; they may be given to a child with a high fever who has a history of febrile seizures (see *Seizure, febrile*).

The choice of drug is largely determined by the type of seizure. In long-term treatment of certain types of seizure, more than one anticonvulsant drug may be needed. Even in people taking regular anticonvulsant medication, an occasional seizure may occur. The frequency with which these seizures occur determines, in part, whether the dose of a medication is increased, another drug added, or the entire drug program is changed.

HOW THEY WORK

Seizures are caused by an abnormally high level of electrical activity in the brain. Anticonvulsant drugs have an inhibitory effect that neutralizes this excessive electrical activity and the spread of this activity throughout areas of the brain.

POSSIBLE ADVERSE EFFECTS

These include reduced concentration, impaired memory, poor coordination, and fatigue. Such effects are usually monitored by regular blood tests.

Antidepressant drugs

COMMON DRUGS

Tricyclics
Amitriptyline Amoxapine Doxepin Imipramine

Monoamine oxidase inhibitors (MAOIs)
Isocarboxazid Phenelzine

Others
Lithium Maprotiline Trazodone

> **WARNING**
> Food and drink containing tyramine (e.g., cheese and red wine) and certain drugs may produce a potentially fatal rise in blood pressure if taken during treatment with an MAOI. Always tell your physician if you are taking an MAOI.

Drugs used in the treatment of *depression*. Antidepressant drugs are prescribed when depression lasts longer than a few days, causing symptoms such as lethargy, loss of appetite or sex drive, or a feeling of despair. The two main types are tricyclic antidepressant drugs and monoamine oxidase inhibitors.

HOW THEY WORK

Some antidepressant drugs trigger the release of chemicals in the brain that stimulate nerve activity. Others, notably tricyclic antidepressants and monoamine oxidase inhibitors, prolong the active life of these chemicals after their release. Antidepressant drugs usually take at least ten days to have any beneficial effect and up to eight weeks to become fully effective.

POSSIBLE ADVERSE EFFECTS

Most antidepressant drugs can cause dryness of the mouth, blurred vision, dizziness, drowsiness, constipation, and difficulty with urination; these symptoms often improve as treatment continues. An antidepressant drug overdose may cause abnormal heart rhythm, seizures, coma, and, occasionally, death.

Antidiarrheal drugs

COMMON DRUGS

Narcotics
Codeine Diphenoxylate with atropine Loperamide

Bulking agents
Kaolin Methylcellulose Psyllium

> **WARNING**
> Do not take antidiarrheal drugs regularly except under medical supervision because they may mask a serious underlying disorder.

A group of drugs used to treat *diarrhea*; they are either *narcotic* substances or bulking agents.

WHY THEY ARE USED

Antidiarrheal drugs may be recommended if diarrhea persists for more than 24 to 48 hours. They are often prescribed while the cause of persistent diarrhea is being investigated, especially if the diarrhea is severe and debilitating. Antidiarrheal drugs are given to help regulate bowel action in people with a *colostomy* or *ileostomy*.

HOW THEY WORK

Narcotic antidiarrheal drugs affect the muscles in the wall of the intestine. This action slows the passage of the feces and allows more time for water to be absorbed into the bloodstream. As a result, both the fluidity and frequency of bowel movements are reduced. Bulking agents (such as fiber in the diet) absorb water from the feces, making them more solid.

POSSIBLE ADVERSE EFFECTS

Antidiarrheal drugs may cause constipation. If diarrhea is caused by an infection, these drugs may delay recovery by slowing the elimination of the microorganisms. Prolonged use of a narcotic antidiarrheal may cause

physical dependence (see *Drug dependence*), producing nausea, abdominal pain, and diarrhea if the drug is suddenly stopped. Bowel obstruction may result if bulking agents are used without sufficient water. Obstruction of the bowel may also occur if a narrowing exists in the bowel.

Antidiuretic hormone
See *ADH*.

Antidote

A substance that neutralizes or counteracts the effects of a poison. The antidote for acid is alkali, and vice versa. A chemical antidote works by combining with a poison to form an innocuous substance, or in some way blocking or diverting the action of the poison. A mechanical antidote prevents the absorption of poison.

Antiemetic drugs

COMMON DRUGS

Anticholinergics
Scopolamine

Antihistamines
Dimenhydrinate Meclizine Promethazine

Phenothiazine antipsychotics
Fluphenazine Perphenazine Prochlorperazine Promazine

Others
Dronabinol Metoclopramide

> **WARNING**
> An antiemetic drug should not be taken regularly except under medical supervision as it may mask a serious underlying disorder.

A group of drugs used to treat *nausea* and *vomiting* caused by *motion sickness, vertigo, Meniere's disease, radiation therapy,* or certain drugs (especially *anticancer drugs*). Some antiemetic drugs are also used to treat severe vomiting during pregnancy.

Drugs from this group are seldom prescribed to treat food poisoning because it is believed that vomiting enables the body to rid itself of harmful substances.

HOW THEY WORK

Some antiemetic drugs reduce nerve activity at the base of the brain and thereby suppress the vomiting reflex. Antihistamine drugs and also anticholinergic drugs reduce the vomiting associated with vertigo by suppressing nerve activity in the balance center in the inner ear. Other antiemetic drugs prevent vomiting by

relaxing the muscles in the lower part of the stomach. This action enables the stomach contents to pass into the small intestine.

POSSIBLE ADVERSE EFFECTS

Many antiemetic drugs cause drowsiness. Some must not be taken during pregnancy because they may damage the developing fetus.

Antifreeze poisoning

Most antifreeze contains ethylene glycol or methanol (methyl alcohol), both of which are poisonous when drunk. Antifreeze poisoning is rare. Most of the 50 or so deaths each year in the US occur in alcoholics (who use antifreeze as a substitute for alcoholic drinks); some people commit suicide by this method.

SYMPTOMS AND TREATMENT

Drinking small amounts of antifreeze initially produces the same effects as alcohol intoxication. When a large amount has been ingested, vomiting, stupor, seizures, and coma occur successively within a few hours; within 24 to 36 hours, acute *renal failure* occurs. If the antifreeze contains methanol, blindness may also result.

Any person believed to have drunk antifreeze needs immediate medical help. Until help arrives, the person, if conscious, should be given a small amount of alcohol (approximately two shots of liquor), which reduces the rate at which antifreeze is metabolized and becomes toxic in the body.

Hospital treatment may include gastric *lavage* (pumping out the stomach) and giving *diuretic drugs,* alcohol, and bicarbonate (by drip into a vein) to correct excess acidity in the body fluids.

Antifungal drugs

COMMON DRUGS

Amphotericin B Ciclopirox Clotrimazole Econazole Griseofulvin Ketoconazole Miconazole Nystatin Tolnaftate

A group of drugs prescribed to treat infections caused by *fungi.* Antifungal drugs are commonly used to treat different types of *tinea,* including tinea pedis (athlete's foot), tinea cruris (jock itch), and tinea capitis (scalp ringworm). They are also used to treat *candidiasis* (thrush) and rare fungal infections (such as *cryptococcosis*) that affect internal organs.

Antifungal preparations are available as tablets, lozenges, suspensions, creams, injections, and vaginal suppositories.

HOW THEY WORK

Antifungal drugs damage the cell walls of fungi, causing chemicals essential for normal function and growth to escape. The fungal cells are unable to survive without these chemicals and die.

POSSIBLE ADVERSE EFFECTS

Preparations applied to the skin, scalp, mouth, or vagina may occasionally increase irritation. Antifungal drugs given by mouth or injection may cause more serious side effects, including damage to the kidney or to the liver.

Antigen

A substance that can trigger an *immune response*, resulting in production of an *antibody* as part of the body's defense against infection and disease. Many antigens are foreign proteins (those not found naturally in the body); they include microorganisms, toxins, and tissues from another person used in organ transplantation.

Antihelmintic drugs

COMMON DRUGS

Niclosamide Niridazole Piperazine Praziquantel Pyrantel Thiabendazole

A group of drugs used in the treatment of *worm infestations*. The body's *immune system* does not deal with worms effectively and, as a result, persistent infestations are common. Antihelmintic drugs eliminate worms from the body and prevent the complications (such as *anemia*, vitamin deficiency, or intestinal obstruction) that occur when worm infestation persists. Different types of antihelmintic drugs are used to treat infestation by different types of worms.

HOW THEY WORK

Antihelmintic drugs either kill or paralyze worms. These drugs cause intestinal worms to pass out of the body in the feces by preventing them from gripping onto the intestinal walls. To hasten this process, laxatives are occasionally prescribed with antihelmintic drugs.

Antihelmintic drugs kill worms in other tissues by making them more vulnerable to attack by the immune system. Once these worms have been killed, they may require surgical removal along with any cysts that the worms have caused.

POSSIBLE ADVERSE EFFECTS

Adverse effects include nausea, vomiting, abdominal pain, headache, dizziness, and rash.

Antihistamine drugs

COMMON DRUGS

Chlorpheniramine Diphenhydramine Promethazine Terfenadine Trimeprazine Triprolidine

WARNING

Do not drive or operate potentially dangerous machinery while taking an antihistamine drug until you are certain that the treatment is not causing dizziness or drowsiness or impairing your coordination.

A group of drugs that blocks the effects of *histamine*, a chemical released during an allergic reaction (see *Allergy*).

WHY THEY ARE USED

Antihistamine drugs are used in the treatment of *urticaria* (hives) and other rashes to relieve itching, swelling, and redness. Drugs of this type are also used in the treatment of allergic *rhinitis* (hay fever) to relieve sneezing and a runny nose.

Antihistamine drugs are sometimes included in *cough remedies* and *cold remedies* because they dry up nasal secretions and suppress the nerve centers in the brain that trigger the cough reflex.

Antihistamine drugs are also used as *antiemetic drugs* because they suppress the vomiting reflex.

Because most antihistamine drugs have a sedative effect, they are sometimes used to induce sleep, especially when itching keeps the sufferer awake at night.

Antihistamine drugs may be given by injection in an emergency to aid in treating *anaphylactic shock* (a severe allergic reaction).

HOW THEY WORK

Antihistamine drugs block the effect of histamine on tissues such as the skin, eyes, and nose. Without drug treatment, histamine would dilate (widen) small blood vessels, resulting in redness and swelling of the surrounding tissue due to leakage of fluid from the circulation. Antihistamines also prevent histamine from irritating nerve fibers, which would otherwise cause itching, and prevent it from stimulating nerve activity in parts of the brain.

POSSIBLE ADVERSE EFFECTS

Most antihistamines cause drowsiness and dizziness. Other possible side effects include loss of appetite, nausea, dry mouth, blurred vision, and difficulty passing urine.

Antihypertensive drugs

COMMON DRUGS

ACE inhibitors
Captopril Enalapril

Beta-blockers
Atenolol Metoprolol

Calcium channel blockers
Nifedipine Verapamil

Diuretic drugs
Chlorthalidone Hydrochlorothiazide

Vasodilator drugs
Hydralazine Minoxidil Prazosin

Others
Clonidine Methyldopa

WARNING

Never stop taking antihypertensive drugs suddenly as this may cause a dramatic rise in blood pressure with serious results.

A group of drugs used in the treatment of *hypertension* (high blood pressure) to prevent complications such as *stroke*, *myocardial infarction* (heart attack), *heart failure* (reduced pumping efficiency), and kidney damage. Antihypertensive drugs are also used to relieve symptoms, such as tiredness and dizziness, caused by hypertension.

HOW THEY WORK

Beta-blockers reduce the force of the heart beat, thereby lowering the pressure of blood flow into the circulation. *Diuretic drugs* increase the amount of salts and water excreted in the urine, but the way in which they lower the blood pressure is not entirely clear. Other types of antihypertensive drugs cause the blood vessels to dilate (widen), which allows the blood to circulate more easily throughout the body.

POSSIBLE ADVERSE EFFECTS

Apart from side effects typical of specific groups, all antihypertensive drugs may cause dizziness and fainting by lowering the blood pressure too much.

Anti-inflammatory drugs

Drugs that reduce the symptoms and signs of *inflammation*. (See *Nonsteroidal anti-inflammatory drugs*; *Corticosteroid drugs*; *Analgesics*.)

Antiperspirant

COMMON DRUGS

Aluminum chloride Aluminum chlorohydrate

A drug applied to the skin in the form of a lotion, cream, or spray to reduce excessive sweating.

WHY IT IS USED

An antiperspirant is used to prevent the accumulation of sweat, which usually occurs under the arms. When sweat remains on the skin, it creates a moist environment in which bacteria can thrive. The bacteria break down the chemicals in the sweat, causing body odor.

High concentrations of antiperspirants are sometimes prescribed to treat *hyperhidrosis* (abnormally profuse sweating). Results of this treatment are variable.

HOW IT WORKS

An antiperspirant reduces the production of sweat by the sweat glands and blocks the ducts that drain sweat onto the surface of the skin.

POSSIBLE ADVERSE EFFECTS

Antiperspirants may cause skin irritation and a burning or stinging sensation. Such effects are more common when high concentrations are used. If the irritation persists when a lower dose is used, treatment should be stopped to prevent *dermatitis*. (See also *Deodorants*.)

Antipsychotic drugs

COMMON DRUGS

Phenothiazines
Chlorpromazine Fluphenazine
Perphenazine Thioridazine Trifluoperazine

Others
Haloperidol Lithium Thiothixene

A group of drugs used to treat *psychoses* (mental disorders involving loss of contact with reality), particularly *schizophrenia* and *manic-depressive illness*. Antipsychotic drugs enable many people suffering from mental illness to live relatively normal lives outside mental institutions.

Antipsychotic drugs are also used to calm or sedate people with other mental disorders (such as *dementia*) who have become highly agitated or aggressive.

Antipsychotic drugs include *phenothiazine drugs* and various other drugs, including *lithium*, which is used specifically to treat the symptoms of *mania* (abnormal elation and overactivity).

HOW THEY WORK

Most antipsychotic drugs block the action of dopamine, a *neurotransmitter* acting on the brain. Lithium is thought to reduce the release of *norepinephrine*, another neurotransmitter.

POSSIBLE ADVERSE EFFECTS

Most antipsychotic drugs can cause drowsiness, lethargy, *dyskinesia* (jerky movements of the mouth, face, and tongue), and *parkinsonism* (a disorder with symptoms similar to those of *Parkinson's disease*). Other possible side effects include dry mouth, blurred vision, and difficulty passing urine. Lithium may cause nausea, diarrhea, tremor, rash, weight gain, and muscle weakness.

Antipyretic drugs

Drugs that reduce fever, such as *aspirin* and *acetaminophen*.

Antirheumatic drugs

COMMON DRUGS

Corticosteroid drugs
Dexamethasone Prednisolone

Immunosuppressant drugs
Azathioprine Chlorambucil

Others
Gold Penicillamine

A group of drugs used in the treatment of *rheumatoid arthritis* and types of arthritis caused by other *autoimmune disorders* (disorders in which the body's immune system attacks its own tissues)—for example, systemic *lupus erythematosus*. Antirheumatic drugs are prescribed when *nonsteroidal antiinflammatory drugs* (NSAIDs) fail to relieve joint pain and stiffness or when the disease is causing progressive deformity and disability.

HOW THEY WORK

Antirheumatic drugs limit the damage caused by the immune system by suppressing either the production or activity of white blood cells. Each type of drug works in a different way, but all antirheumatics damp down the inflammation caused by the autoimmune reaction and prevent or slow down the degeneration of the cartilage that lines joints.

The effectiveness of each type of antirheumatic drug varies according to the individual. Beneficial effects may not appear for several weeks.

POSSIBLE ADVERSE EFFECTS

All antirheumatic drugs may cause serious adverse effects. For example, gold and penicillamine may cause kidney damage, chloroquine may damage the eyes, and *immunosuppressant drugs* may cause blood disorders. Regular medical examinations, including blood and urine tests, are carried out during treatment to monitor toxic effects.

Antiseptics

Chemicals applied to the skin to destroy bacteria and other microorganisms and thus prevent *sepsis* (infection). Antisepsis (the use of antiseptics to prevent infection) is not the same as asepsis, which is the creation of a germ-free environment (see *Aseptic technique*). Antiseptics are milder than *disinfectants*, which decontaminate inanimate objects but are too strong to be used on the body.

Antiseptic fluids are generally used for bathing wounds, whereas creams are applied to wounds before they are dressed. Among the more commonly used antiseptics are iodine, hydrogen peroxide, and thimerosal.

Antiserum

A preparation containing antibodies that combine with specific *antigens* (foreign proteins), usually components of microorganisms (such as viruses or bacteria). Such antibody-antigen interaction leads to the inactivation or destruction of the microorganisms. Antiserum samples are prepared from the blood of animals or humans who have been injected with killed, or live but harmless, strains of particular viruses or bacteria—in other words, people who have already been immunized against these organisms.

Antiserum is usually used, along with *immunization*, as an emergency treatment when someone has been exposed to a dangerous infection such as *lassa fever* and has not previously been immunized against the infection. The antiserum helps to provide some immediate protection against the infective microorganisms while full immunity is developing.

Such measures are not as effective in preventing disease as earlier (preexposure) immunization.

Antisocial personality disorder

Failure to conform to social norms of behavior. The category of antisocial personality is relatively new and was devised to provide clear guidelines for diagnosing psychiatric illness. In the past, people displaying antisocial behavior were classified in a number of ways, such as "sociopaths" or "psychopaths," but it was argued that these labels described character traits rather than specific illnesses causing a change in personality or behavior.

DIAGNOSIS

For a person to be diagnosed as suffering from this type of disorder, the antisocial behavior must have started

A

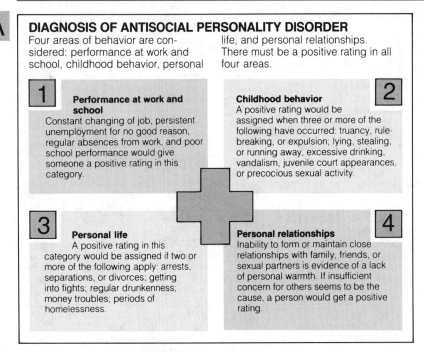

DIAGNOSIS OF ANTISOCIAL PERSONALITY DISORDER

Four areas of behavior are considered: performance at work and school, childhood behavior, personal life, and personal relationships. There must be a positive rating in all four areas.

1 Performance at work and school
Constant changing of job, persistent unemployment for no good reason, regular absences from work, and poor school performance would give someone a positive rating in this category.

2 Childhood behavior
A positive rating would be assigned when three or more of the following have occurred: truancy, rule-breaking, or expulsion; lying, stealing, or running away; excessive drinking, vandalism, juvenile court appearances, or precocious sexual activity.

3 Personal life
A positive rating in this category would be assigned if two or more of the following apply: arrests, separations, or divorces; getting into fights; regular drunkenness; money troubles; periods of homelessness.

4 Personal relationships
Inability to form or maintain close relationships with family, friends, or sexual partners is evidence of a lack of personal warmth. If insufficient concern for others seems to be the cause, a person would get a positive rating.

before the age of 15 and must not be a result of mental handicap or obvious illness. Since there must be evidence of persistent disturbance over a period of time, the term cannot be used to describe anyone under 18 years old.

TREATMENT
Given such categories, it is clear that behavior is being judged. The aim of treatment is to alter behavior; this may include residence in *therapeutic communities*, *behavior therapy*, various forms of *psychotherapy*, and participation in community help programs. There is a clear overlap with legal punishment, since criminal activity is common, but the debate as to whether people with this disorder are "bad" or "mad" remains unsolved.

Antispasmodic drugs

COMMON DRUGS

Belladonna Dicyclomine

A group of drugs that relaxes spasm in smooth (involuntary) muscle in the wall of the intestine or bladder. Antispasmodic drugs are used in the treatment of *irritable bowel syndrome* and *irritable bladder*.

Antispasmodic drugs may have an anticholinergic action (that is, they work by blocking the action of *acetylcholine*, a chemical that is released from nerve endings that stimulates muscle contraction).

Adverse effects of antispasmodic drugs include dry mouth, blurred vision, and difficulty passing urine. (See also *Anticholinergic drugs*.)

Antitoxin

Any of a variety of commercially prepared substances, each of which contains *antibodies* that can combine and neutralize the effect of a specific toxin released into the bloodstream by bacteria (such as those that cause *tetanus* and *diphtheria*).

Antitoxins are prepared by inoculating animals, usually horses, with specific toxins that provoke the animal's immune system to produce antibodies that will neutralize the toxins. Extracts of the animal's blood are used as the antitoxin.

Antitoxins are usually administered by injection into a muscle, under the supervision of a physician. Occasionally, an antitoxin may cause an allergic reaction; rarely, it causes an *anaphylactic shock* (severe allergic reaction) requiring emergency treatment.

Antitussive drugs

Drugs that prevent or relieve *cough*. (See *Cough remedies*.)

Antivenin

 A specific treatment for snake, scorpion, spider, or other venomous animal bites. Antivenin is prepared by inoculating animals, usually horses, with small but increasing amounts of venom from a particular poisonous animal. This provokes the production of *antibodies* that will neutralize the poisons in the venom. A preparation containing these antibodies or antivenins can then be produced from samples of the horse's blood.

In the US, commercial antivenins are available against all types of pit viper (rattlesnakes, cottonmouth, and copperhead) and for coral snake bites. Antivenins for treating the bites of snakes originating outside the US and various scorpions, spiders, fish, and jellyfish can be obtained from zoos and veterinarians.

Antiviral drugs

COMMON DRUGS

Acyclovir Amantadine Idoxuridine Trifluridine Zidovudine

A group of drugs used in the treatment of infection by a *virus*. Drugs that kill viruses have proved difficult to develop because viruses live only within body cells and there is a danger that antiviral drugs will damage the host cell as well as the virus. To date, no drugs have been developed that can effectively eradicate viruses and cure the illnesses that they cause.

Immunization is at present more important than drug treatment in fighting serious viral infections. However, some drugs have already proved successful in treating a few viral infections, particularly those caused by *herpes* viruses. Antiviral drugs reduce the severity of these infections but may not eliminate them completely, so attacks may recur. Other antiviral drugs are currently being developed and used (e.g., to treat AIDS).

HOW THEY WORK
Most antiviral drugs destroy viruses by disrupting chemical processes necessary for viruses to grow and multiply within cells. Some antiviral drugs prevent viruses from actually penetrating cells.

POSSIBLE ADVERSE EFFECTS
Antiviral drugs against AIDS carry a high risk of causing anemia due to bone marrow damage. Most other antiviral drugs rarely cause side effects. Antiviral creams and ointments may irritate the skin, causing redness. Antiviral drugs given by mouth or injection can cause nausea and dizziness, and, rarely, in long-term treatment, kidney damage.

Antral irrigation

Irrigation of the antrum (also called the maxillary sinus), one of the nasal sinuses, to diagnose and treat persistent *sinusitis*.

WHY IT IS USED

Antral irrigation is used when sinusitus persists after an adequate course of medical therapy, consisting mostly of antibiotics and decongestants, and sometimes dental consultation. Antral irrigation allows a firm diagnosis of infection to be made and sometimes cures the infection.

The normal drainage channel from the antrum into the nose is usually at least partially blocked in chronic sinusitis, so that infected material builds up within the cavity. Antral irrigation creates a temporary opening that allows the contents to be flushed out through the natural opening.

HOW IT IS DONE

A cannula (hollow, flexible tube) is inserted into the antrum, guided by a trocar (sharp, pointed rod). The trocar enters through the nose or under the upper lip. The trocar is withdrawn, leaving the cannula in place. A syringe is then attached to the cannula and the contents of the sinus are sucked out and sent to the laboratory for bacteriological culture to identify the organism responsible for the infection and to test sensitivity to antibiotics.

A large syringe filled with warm saline is attached to the cannula and the antrum is thoroughly washed out by injecting the solution into the cavity and having it flow out through the natural sinus opening. This is repeated until the fluid is clear.

RESULTS

Unless the sinusitis has been present for so long that permanent damage to the mucosa (lining of the sinus) has occurred, antral irrigation may be curative. If the infection fails to resolve after several weeks, and an irrigation confirms that the antrum is still infected, more surgery to enlarge the drainage channel may be required.

Anuria

Complete cessation of urine production by the kidneys; the extreme of oliguria (reduced urine production).

Failure to pass urine is an indication of a serious problem in the urinary tract because, even when a person is severely dehydrated, some urine is produced. Much more common than anuria as a cause of failure to urinate is a complete blockage to the flow of urine—due, for example, to an enlarged *prostate gland*, *bladder tumor*, or urinary tract calculus (stone). True anuria may be due to oxygen depletion as a result of reduced blood flow through the kidneys, as occurs in *shock*, or to severe kidney damage, resulting in acute *renal failure* or tubular necrosis.

Anuria requires urgent investigation to establish the cause and may require dialysis. Untreated, it leads to *uremia* (excess waste products in the blood) and death.

Anus

The canal at the end of the alimentary tract through which feces are expelled from the body. About 1.5 inches (4 cm) long, the anus is an extension of the

STRUCTURE OF THE ANUS

A canal at the end of the alimentary tract, with internal and external sphincters to open and close the orifice.

Rectum

Internal sphincter muscle

External sphincter muscle

rectum as it passes backward and downward through the pelvic floor. The orifice at the end of the anal

DISORDERS OF THE ANUS

Most anal disorders are minor. Many are aggravated by constipation and may be helped by regular toilet habits, an increased intake of fluids, whole-grain products, fruits, and vegetables to soften the feces, and the use of glycerin suppositories.

CONGENITAL DEFECTS

Imperforate anus is an uncommon birth defect in which the anus is sealed. This abnormality is detected and operated on at birth (see *Anus, imperforate*).

In *anal stenosis*, the anus is too narrow to allow the normal passage of feces. This is sometimes a congenital abnormality, but can also result from scarring after surgery for some other anal disorder.

INJURY

Anal fissures originate from small tears in the lining of the anus, usually as a result of straining to pass hard, dry feces.

TUMORS

Cancer of the skin around the anus is rare (see *Anus, cancer of*).

OTHER DISORDERS

Hemorrhoids are enlarged blood vessels under the lining of the anus and may cause bleeding during defecation, itching, and pain.

An *anal fistula* is an abnormal tunnel connecting the inside of the anal canal to the skin surrounding the anus. These fistulas usually result from an abscess in the wall of the anus.

Pruritus ani (itching of the anus) may result from an anal fistula, hemorrhoids, or pinworm infestation. It may also be an isolated symptom.

INVESTIGATION

Investigation of anal disorders is usually by visual inspection, sometimes including *proctoscopy* (use of an internal viewing tube), and digital examination (feeling with a finger). Sometimes a biopsy (specimen of tissue for analysis) or swab may be taken for bacteriological culture.

A

canal is only open during defecation—at other times it is kept closed by the muscles of the anal sphincter. These muscles are arranged in two layers, the internal sphincter, which cannot be controlled voluntarily, and the external sphincter, which can be relaxed at will for defecation. (See also *Digestive system*.)

Anus, cancer of

A rare cancer of the skin of the anus that is not usually related to the cells occurring in cancer of the intestine.

In the early stages of anal cancer there may be a swelling at the outside of the anus as well as some bleeding and discomfort. Surgical removal of the cancer is the usual treatment.

Anus, imperforate

A rare congenital abnormality, detected and treated at birth, in which the anal opening appears to be covered over.

TYPES

The two main types of imperforate anus, high and low, depend on whether or not the bowel ends above or below the pelvic floor. In the high type, the anal canal fails to develop and there is no connection between the rectum and the anus. Many of the normal anal structures, such as the muscles, are missing and the disorder is associated with other abnormalities, especially of the urinary organs. The low type may have only a skin covering at the anal opening.

TREATMENT

Treatment for high imperforate anus involves major surgery to open up the end of the rectum and join it to the anus. This operation is usually successful and the long-term outlook is good. In some cases, a *colostomy* may be needed.

Treatment for low imperforate anus usually involves surgical removal of the skin over the anus. *Anal dilatation* (enlargement of the anus) may be needed for several months afterward.

Anxiety

An unpleasant emotional state ranging from mild unease to intense fear. The anxious person usually feels a sense of impending doom, although there is no obvious threat, and has certain physical and psychological symptoms. A certain amount of anxiety is normal and serves to improve our performance. However, anxiety becomes a symptom when it starts to inhibit thought and disrupt normal activities of daily life.

SYMPTOMS AND SIGNS

The most common symptoms relate to the chest. They include palpitations (awareness of a more forceful or faster heart beat), throbbing or stabbing pains, a feeling of tightness and inability to take in enough air, and a tendency to sigh or overbreathe (see *Hyperventilation*).

Tension of the muscles leads to headaches, spasms in the neck, back pains, grasping too tightly, and an inability to relax. Restlessness, tremor of the hands, and a sense of tiredness are also common.

Gastrointestinal symptoms include dryness of the mouth, a feeling of distention, diarrhea, nausea, changes in appetite, constant belching, and difficulty swallowing. Some sufferers may actually vomit or have severe pain mimicking serious illness.

There are also certain, socially obvious symptoms, such as sweating, blushing, and pallor, or the constant need to urinate or defecate. Dizziness, hyperventilation (deep and fast breathing), sighing, yawning, belching, and the light-headedness that results occur especially in public and are related to fears. Paresthesia (a pins and needles sensation) and a fixed spasm of the arms can result from hyperventilation, which prevents the muscles from functioning by depriving them of carbon dioxide.

People with anxiety usually have a constant feeling that something bad is going to happen. They may fear that they have a chronic or dangerous illness—which is reinforced by the physical symptoms outlined above—or that the health or safety of family and friends is in danger. Fear of losing control is also common. This fear leads to increasing dependence on others, irritability, a sense of fatigue, and a state of being easily frustrated. Inability to relax may lead to difficulty getting to sleep and constant waking during the night. Frightening dreams often occur.

A particularly strange yet common symptom is that of *depersonalization* (the sense of being cut off from oneself) or the related *derealization* (the sense of being cut off from the world). These symptoms can begin suddenly and last for a long time, leading people to fear they are going mad.

CAUSES

Three different areas of research have contributed theories for the cause of anxiety. Physiological measures show that anxious individuals have a raised level of *arousal* in the central nervous system, so that they react more excitedly and adapt more slowly to events. This feeling also leads to physical symptoms, such as palpitations, which themselves are unpleasant and reinforce the anxiety.

Psychoanalytical ideas derive from Freud, who coined the term "anxiety neurosis" and believed that anxiety stems from repressed unresolved childhood experiences. Originally, anxiety was thought to be due to unsatisfied sexual needs, but the importance of *bonding* and child-parent separations has now led to theories based on the fear of losing loved objects. Unconscious conflict can also lead to anxiety.

Behavioral psychologists describe anxiety as a learned response to, for example, pain or mental discomfort. The anxiety initially serves to drive people to improved learning and performance, but eventually becomes a habit that is brought on by the slightest difficulty. It thus impairs performance and thought, though people become so deeply conditioned that they cannot control it.

ANXIETY AND ILLNESS

Symptoms of anxiety usually result from an *anxiety disorder*, or are part of another psychological disorder, such as *hypochondriasis*, *depression*, or a type of *psychosexual disorder*. However, because the symptoms of anxiety mimic the symptoms of so many other diseases, the physician tries to avoid reinforcing the patient's anxiety, which can lead to numerous unnecessary consultations and treatments—including surgery. People with anxiety disorders ideally are referred for psychotherapy to determine the real causes of their fears.

Anxiety disorders

A group of mental illnesses in which symptoms of anxiety are the main feature. Anxiety disorders include a number of specific syndromes, though there is considerable overlap among them and boundaries are not always clear.

Anxiety disorders are common, affecting roughly 4 percent of the population, mainly younger adults; the disorders occur equally in men and women and heredity is a contributing factor. Symptoms tend to vary during the course of the illness.

TYPES

Generalized anxiety disorder (the traditional "anxiety neurosis") is diagnosed if the patient has had at least one definite period of anxiety, accompanied by at least one physical or psychological symptom that impairs normal activity. *Panic disorders* are characterized by sudden, intense attacks of panic (extreme, unreasonable fear and anxiety), while *phobias* are dominated by irrational fears that lead to avoidance of certain situations or objects, such as open spaces or spiders. *Posttraumatic stress disorder* is associated with a serious specific event, such as rape, and symptoms include reliving the event in dreams and a general feeling of numbness and lack of involvement. The main features of *obsessive-compulsive behavior* are recurrent and persistent thoughts and ritualized, repetitive behavior.

TREATMENT
Treatment of anxiety disorders is most effective when there is an identifiable and justified reason for stress. Treatment is more successful in people who have stable, underlying personalities. Reassurance, *counseling*, and *psychotherapy* are used, as are *antianxiety drugs* (especially *benzodiazepine drugs*).

Aorta
The main *artery* of the body. The aorta arises directly from the left ventricle (lower chamber of the heart) and supplies oxygenated blood to all other arteries except the pulmonary artery (which carries deoxygenated blood from the heart to the lungs).

DISORDERS
Like other arteries, the aorta can become narrowed as a result of *atherosclerosis* (fat deposits on the walls), which often causes *hypertension* (high blood pressure). There are also specific aortic disorders, notably *coarctation of the aorta* (in which the aorta is abnormally narrow at birth) and *aortitis* (inflammation of the wall of the aorta), a rare condition associated with untreated *syphilis* and *ankylosing spondylitis* (inflammation of the joints of the spine).

Both aortitis and atherosclerosis can cause an aortic *aneurysm* (a balloonlike swelling of the vessel wall), which may require surgery to correct impaired blood flow and to remove the risk of rupture and fatal blood loss. (See also *Arteries, disorders of; Circulatory system*.)

Aortic insufficiency
Leakage of blood through the aortic valve, resulting in a backflow of blood into the left ventricle (lower chamber of the heart).

CAUSES
Failure of the aortic valve to close correctly may be due to a congenital abnormality. Another cause of aortic insufficiency is *aortitis* (inflammation of the aorta), which occurs in some people who have bacterial *endocarditis* of the aortic valve (in which the bac-

teria destroy the valve leaflets). This condition can occur in intravenous drug users. Aortic insufficiency is also found in untreated *syphilis, ankylosing spondylitis* (inflammation of joints in the spine), and *Marfan's syndrome* (a congenital disorder of connective tissues). *Rheumatic fever* was once a common cause of aortic incompetence but this infection has become very rare. Atherosclerosis is associated with both aortic insufficiency and *aortic stenosis*.

SYMPTOMS AND SIGNS
Aortic insufficiency may not cause any symptoms. It is sometimes found during a routine medical examination; the physician hears a murmur (abnormal heart sound) over the front of the chest wall to the left of the breastbone.

The heart compensates for the backflow of blood into the left ventricle by working harder, until the combination of hypertrophy (muscle thickening) and dilation (ballooning) of the left ventricle wall leads to *heart failure* (reduced pumping efficiency); this results in breathing difficulty and *edema* (fluid retention).

DIAGNOSIS
A *chest X ray* may show white patches of calcium in the area of the aortic valve, an enlarged heart, and dilation of the aorta.

An *ECG* (measurement of the electrical activity of the heart) may show evidence of thickening of and strain on the left ventricle.

Echocardiography (imaging heart structures by measuring the pattern of deflection of sound waves from them) will show the diameter of the valve opening and the diameter of the aortic ring, a thickening of the wall of the left ventricle, and reduced movement of the aortic valve. Doppler echocardiography shows the blood flow across the valve.

A cardiac catheter (flexible tube inserted into the heart through blood vessels) can be used to demonstrate the degree of insufficiency; a radiopaque dye is injected into the heart through the catheter and X-ray pictures taken (see *Catheterization, cardiac*). The information provided by preoperative catheterization studies is not substantially different from that provided by the aforementioned noninvasive studies (those not requiring penetration within the body).

TREATMENT
Heart failure resulting from aortic insufficiency can be treated with diuretics to remove retained fluid from the lungs. Heart valve surgery to

---

LOCATION AND STRUCTURE OF THE AORTA
From its origin at the left ventricle, the aorta passes upward, curves behind the heart, and runs downward, passing through the thorax (chest) and into the abdomen, where it terminates by dividing into two common iliac arteries. The aorta is thick-walled and large in diameter (about 1 inch, or 2.5 cm, at its origin) to cope with the high pressure and large volume of blood that passes through it. The thick walls of the aorta have an elastic quality that helps even out the peaks and troughs of pressure that occur with each heart beat.

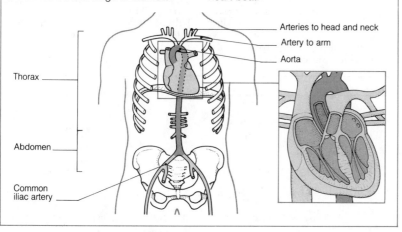

Thorax

Abdomen

Common iliac artery

Arteries to head and neck

Artery to arm

Aorta

A

replace the damaged valve may not be required for many years from the time of diagnosis; it is considered when symptoms develop or substantial changes in the valve occur.

Aortic stenosis

Narrowing of the aortic valve opening, causing obstruction of blood flow into the circulation. This makes the heart work harder and causes the muscle in the wall of the left ventricle (lower chamber) to thicken.

CAUSES

The most common cause is deposition of calcium on the aortic valve, usually associated with *atherosclerosis*. Aortic stenosis may also be due to a rare congenital abnormality. Another cause is *cardiomyopathy* (heart muscle disease in which thickening of the heart muscle may lead to narrowing of the aortic valve). In the past, *rheumatic fever* was a common cause of heart valve damage; today it is rare.

SYMPTOMS AND SIGNS

Aortic stenosis may not cause any symptoms. It is sometimes found during a routine medical examination; the physician hears a murmur (abnormal heart sound) over the front of the chest wall to the right of the breastbone and sometimes up into the neck. Symptoms, when they do occur, include fainting attacks, lack of energy, chest pain on exertion (*angina pectoris*), and breathing difficulty. Other signs include a weak pulse felt at the wrist and *cardiomegaly* (heart enlargement) at a late stage.

DIAGNOSIS

A *chest X ray* may show white patches of calcium in the area of the aortic valve. The heart may also appear enlarged on an X ray.

An *ECG* (measurement of the electrical activity of the heart) may show evidence of thickening of and strain on the left ventricle.

Echocardiography (imaging heart structures by measuring the pattern of deflection of sound waves from them)

usually reveals the diameter of the valve opening and thickness of the valve leaflets, abnormal movement within the aortic valve, and thickening of the left ventricle walls. *Doppler* studies can confirm and quantitate the reduced flow across the valve.

A cardiac catheter (a flexible tube inserted into the heart through blood vessels) can be fitted with a pressure-measuring device to measure the degree of aortic stenosis; the difference in pressure on either side of the valve reflects the severity of the stenosis. The information provided by preoperative catheterization studies is not substantially different from that provided by the aforementioned *noninvasive* studies (those not requiring penetration within the body).

TREATMENT

Before developments in *heart valve surgery*, the outlook for people with aortic stenosis was gloomy; once symptoms developed, the predicted life span was only a year or so. Now, provided that valve replacement is done before irremediable damage to the left ventricle, the outlook is good.

Aortitis

Inflammation of the aorta, the large artery that carries blood from the heart to supply all parts of the body except the lungs. It is a rare condition occurring in people with *arteritis* (inflammation of arteries) or untreated *syphilis* and in some people with *ankylosing spondylitis* (inflammation of joints of the spine).

Aortitis may cause part of the aorta to widen and its walls to become thinner. This may then lead to the formation of an *aneurysm* (a swelling of the artery), which may burst and cause severe, sometimes fatal, blood loss. Aortitis may also damage the ring surrounding the aortic valve, leading to *aortic insufficiency*. This allows regurgitation of blood back to the heart, which can cause *heart failure*.

Aortography

A procedure that allows the aorta and its branches to be seen on X-ray film after injection with contrast medium (a substance opaque to X rays).

WHY IT IS DONE

Aortography is used to detect aortic *aneurysm* (weakening of the wall and ballooning of the vessel) and to investigate *peripheral vascular disease* before surgery.

HOW IT IS DONE

Contrast medium is usually injected into the aorta through a fine catheter (flexible plastic tube) inserted into the femoral artery at the groin or the brachial artery just inside of the elbow (see *Angiography*). In people with severe arterial disease, the major arteries may be blocked and the contrast medium may have to be injected directly into the lumbar aorta through a hollow needle.

COMPLICATIONS

There is a small risk of allergic reaction to the contrast medium. Damage to a vessel during puncture or catheterization can also occur.

Aperient

A mild laxative. (See *Laxative drugs*.)

Apgar score

A system devised by Virginia Apgar, an American anesthesiologist, to assess the condition of a newborn baby. Five features are scored at one minute and at five minutes after birth. The features are respiratory effort, heart rate, color, muscle tone, and motor reactions. The most important features are the infant's attempts to breathe and the infant's heart rate. In general, if these two are satisfactory, the other features are as well. Each feature is scored from 0 to 2, making a total of 10 possible points. A low total score of 0 to 3, which will occur if the baby does not breathe or if the heart rate is too slow, means the child needs urgent resuscitation. A score of 7 to 10 indicates a well baby.

APGAR CHART

Sign	0	1	2
Color	Blue, pale	Body pink; extremities blue	Completely pink
Respiratory effort	Absent	Weak cry; irregular breathing	Good strong cry; regular breathing
Muscle tone	Limp	Bending of some limbs	Active motion; limbs well-flexed
Reflex irritability	No response	Grimace (response to stimulation)	Cry
Heart rate	Absent	Slow (below 100 beats per minute)	Over 100 beats per minute

All too often anxious parents attach undue importance to the Apgar score. The score was originally intended to try to quantitate the enormous changes a newborn goes through in the first few minutes of life and help direct appropriate care. Certainly a very low score (0 to 4) means emergency care is needed. However, middle scores (5 to 7) do not indicate a damaged baby or some lack in the pre-natal care.

Aphakia

The absence of the crystalline lens from the eye. Aphakia occurs if the lens has been surgically removed, as in *cataract surgery*, or if it has been destroyed by a penetrating injury and subsequently absorbed into the aqueous humor (the fluid within the eyeball). Removal of cataracts produces aphakia in both eyes.

Aphakia causes severe loss of focus-ing in the affected eye or eyes and requires correction by lens implants, contact lenses, or glasses.

Aphasia

A disturbance of previously acquired language skills caused by cerebral dys-function; aphasia affects the ability to speak and write, and/or the ability to comprehend and read. Strictly, aphasia is a complete absence (and dysphasia a disturbance) of these communication and comprehension skills, but the distinction between the two terms is not useful.

The difficulty with speech expres-sion in aphasia is different from that caused by disease or damage to the parts of the body involved in the mechanics of speech (see *Dysarthria*; *Dysphonia*). The comprehension difficulties are not due to defective hearing or sight.

Related disabilities that may occur as a feature of aphasia or, more rarely, by themselves, are *alexia* (word blind-ness) and *agraphia* (writing difficulty).

CAUSES

A *stroke* or a *head injury* is the most common cause of brain damage lead-ing to aphasia.

Language function within the brain lies in the dominant cerebral hemisphere (see *Cerebrum*). Two par-ticular areas in the dominant hemisphere, called Broca's and Wer-nicke's areas (named after their discoverers) and the pathways con-necting the two, are known to be important in language skills. Damage to these areas is the most common cause of aphasia.

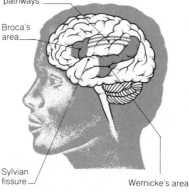

Linking pathways

Broca's area

Sylvian fissure

Wernicke's area

Language function and the brain
Damage to two particular areas (and the path-ways between them) in the dominant cerebral hemisphere results in aphasia.

TYPES AND SYMPTOMS

BROCA'S (EXPRESSIVE) APHASIA Damage to Broca's area causes difficulty in the expression of language. Speech is nonfluent, slow, labored, with loss of normal rhythm. The few words uttered do tend to be meaningful.

WERNICKE'S (RECEPTIVE) APHASIA Damage to Wernicke's area causes difficulty in comprehension. Speech is fluent but, because of the impaired comprehen-sion, its content is disturbed, with many errors in word selection and grammar, indicating that "internal speech" is impaired. Writing is also impaired and spoken or written com-mands are not understood.

GLOBAL APHASIA In global aphasia there is a total or near total inability to speak, write, or understand spoken or written words. This is usually caused by widespread damage to the domi-nant cerebral hemisphere.

NOMINAL APHASIA This is restricted to a difficulty in naming objects or in find-ing words, although the person may be able to choose the correct name from several offered. Nominal aphasia may be caused by generalized cerebral dysfunction or damage to specific language areas.

TREATMENT AND OUTLOOK

Some recovery from aphasia is usual after a stroke or head injury, although the more severe the aphasia, the less the chances of recovery. *Speech therapy* is the main treatment. (See also *Speech*; *Speech disorders*.)

Apheresis

Also called pheresis, a procedure in which blood is withdrawn from a donor and then reinfused after selected components, such as plate-lets, white blood cells, or plasma, have been separated and removed. (See also *Blood donation*.)

Aphonia

Total loss of the voice, usually sudden in onset and caused by emotional stress. A physician examining the larynx (voice box) would see that the vocal cords fail to meet as normal when the patient tries to speak, though they come together when the person coughs. Otherwise, there is no detectable abnormality in the larynx.

There is no treatment other than reassurance and *psychotherapy*. The sufferer's voice usually returns as sud-denly as it disappeared.

Disease or damage to the larynx, as, for example, in *laryngitis* (inflamma-tion of the larynx) or following surgery to remove a laryngeal cancer, normally causes only partial loss of voice pro-duction, known as *dysphonia*.

Aphrodisiacs

Substances thought to stimulate erotic desire and enhance sexual perfor-mance. Aphrodisiacs are named for Aphrodite, the ancient Greek goddess of love.

Various substances have been used as "love potions" over the centuries—honey, ginseng, ginger, strychnine, rhinoceros horn, and oysters, among many others. In fact, no substance has a proven aphrodisiac effect, although virtually anything may produce the desired results if the person taking it believes strongly enough that it will work. Alcohol can encourage sexual desire; it is a mental depressant and usually removes inhibitions. How-ever, a high level of alcohol in the blood can impair sexual performance.

Probably the best known "aphrodisiac" is Spanish fly, which consists of powdered, dried beetles of the species LYTTA VESICATORIA. The substance's active ingredient, cantharidin, irritates the lining of the bladder and urethra (the tube between the bladder and outside) and may, in some cases, cause *priapism* (persistent erection). Spanish fly is potentially dangerous; some men have died as a result of using it.

Other substances used for their pur-ported aphrodisiac effects include marijuana, yohimbine (a chemical obtained from the bark of the West African yohimbe tree), and amyl nitrite (a drug once used to treat angina). There is no scientific evidence that any of these is effective, and amyl nitrite may reduce blood pressure to dangerously low levels.

The male sex hormone *testosterone* is sometimes regarded as a sexual stimulant but, in normal men, it actually reduces sperm production. However, in men who have a testosterone deficiency, the hormone may restore both libido and potency.

Aplasia

Incomplete or reduced growth and development of any organ or tissue. For example, in bone marrow aplasia, the rate of cell division in the bone marrow is considerably reduced, leading to reduced formation of blood cells of one or all types (see *Anemia, aplastic*). A number of birth defects—for example, the presence of one or more stunted limbs (see *Phocomelia*)—are due to incomplete organ formation during prenatal development.

Aplastic anemia

See *Anemia, aplastic*.

Apnea

Cessation of breathing either temporarily (for a few seconds to a minute or two) or for a prolonged period, which is life-threatening.

CAUSES

Breathing is an automatic process controlled by the respiratory center in the brain stem. The respiratory center sends nerve impulses to the muscles in the chest that regulate lung expansion and contraction.

Prolonged apnea can occur if the brain stem is damaged by a *stroke*, by a *transient ischemic attack* (symptoms of stroke lasting less than 24 hours), or by a head injury. Prolonged apnea can also occur as an effect of certain drugs or as the result of *airway obstruction*, usually by food, drink, vomit, or a small inhaled object.

Deliberate temporary apnea occurs in *breath-holding attacks* and in underwater swimmers. Nondeliberate temporary apnea can also occur, usually during sleep (see *Sleep apnea*).

Another type of apnea occurs in *Cheyne-Stokes respiration*, which is characterized by cycles of deep, rapid breathing alternating with episodes of breath stoppage.

Apnea requires investigation and treatment of the underlying cause. Treatment may be aimed at relieving any airway obstruction. It may also include the use of respiratory stimulants if the respiratory center in the brain stem is affected.

Apocrine gland

A gland that discharges cellular material in addition to the fluid it secretes. The term is usually applied to the type of *sweat glands* that occur only in hairy areas of the body and appear after puberty.

Aponeurosis

A wide sheet of tough, fibrous tissue that acts as a tendon (i.e., attaches a muscle to a bone or a joint).

Apoplexy

An outdated term for a *stroke* (interruption of blood flow within the brain), resulting in sudden loss of consciousness, paralysis, or loss of sensation. The usual cause of apoplexy is rupture of a brain artery or blockage by a clot.

Apothecary

An obsolete term for a *pharmacist*.

Appendectomy

Surgical removal of the appendix to treat acute *appendicitis*.

WHY IT IS DONE

Appendectomy is carried out to prevent the inflamed appendix from bursting and causing *peritonitis* (inflammation of the abdominal lining) or an abdominal abscess.

Acute appendicitis is often difficult to diagnose and, sometimes, because of the dangerous complications that can develop from the condition, a *laparotomy* (an exploratory operation on the abdomen) is performed even when appendicitis is only suspected. In this case, the appendix, which has no apparent useful function in humans, is removed even if it is normal to prevent the possibility of appendicitis in the future.

HOW IT IS DONE

If there is time before the operation, the patient is started on a course of antibiotics to prevent the operative wound from becoming infected, an ever-present risk in appendectomy. Next, the physician makes a small incision in the abdomen (see box).

If the appendix has burst, the abdominal cavity in the area is washed out with saline (salt solution) and a plastic drainage tube is inserted into the infected area through another small incision to drain off pus.

Appendectomy may take from 10 minutes to more than an hour to perform, depending on the problems and complications involved.

COMPLICATIONS

Infection is the most common postoperative complication of appendectomy. The infection frequently involves the wound in the abdominal wall; it may also involve localized peritonitis or abscess at the site of appendix removal.

PERFORMING AN APPENDECTOMY

The patient is given a general anesthetic. A small incision is made in the lower right abdomen, above the groin, revealing the cecum (the chamber that links the small and large intestine), to which the appendix is attached.

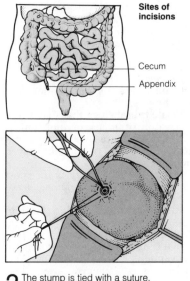

Sites of incisions

Cecum

Appendix

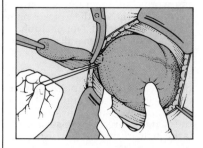

1 The appendix is carefully and gently brought to the surface of the draped abdomen, clamped, tied off at the base (where it joins the cecum), and cut off.

2 The stump is tied with a suture, sometimes touched with phenol, inverted, and tucked into the cecum with a suture to prevent fluid from leaking into the abdomen.

RECOVERY PERIOD

Following an uncomplicated appendectomy, the patient is usually able to drink and eat light food within 24 hours of the operation. If a drainage tube has been inserted, it is removed after about 48 hours; the wound seals itself. Normally, the patient can go home after two or three days. Stitches are removed seven to 10 days after the operation (an outpatient procedure). Normal physical activities can usually be resumed after two or three weeks. If there are complications, recovery may take much longer.

Appendicitis

Acute inflammation of the appendix, which is a common cause of abdominal pain and *peritonitis* (inflammation of the lining of the abdominal cavity) in children and young adults.

CAUSES

The cause is not always known, but appendicitis is sometimes due to obstruction of the appendix by a lump of feces or, occasionally, by worms in *pinworm infestation*. The closed end of the appendix beyond the obstruction becomes inflamed, swollen, and infected. This may lead to *gangrene* (tissue death) of the appendix wall, which may perforate (burst).

INCIDENCE

Appendicitis affects about 200 per 100,000 people per year in the US. Although anyone can get appendicitis, it is rare in the very young and the very old. It is the most common abdominal surgical emergency in the Western world but is comparatively rare in developing countries.

SYMPTOMS

The first symptom is usually vague discomfort just above and around the navel. Within a few hours this gradually develops into a sharper, more localized pain. This pain is usually most intense in the lower right-hand side of the abdomen. If the appendix descends behind the cecum over the brim of the pelvis, appendicitis may cause little abdominal pain, but severe pain on rectal examination. If it impinges on the ureter, there may be bloody urine passed.

The pain and abdominal tenderness characteristic of appendicitis are usually accompanied by a slight fever, loss of appetite, nausea, vomiting, a coated tongue, and foul breath, sometimes preceded by constipation. Anyone who has sudden abdominal pain and other symptoms of appendicitis should consult a physician without delay.

DIAGNOSIS

Diagnosis can sometimes be difficult because the symptoms of appendicitis are similar to those of many other abdominal disorders. Nonspecific abdominal pain (also called mesenteric adenitis), which is common in childhood and often follows a viral respiratory tract infection, has symptoms and signs that resemble those of appendicitis. Disorders of the right fallopian tube and ovary, *Crohn's disease*, and right-sided *pyelonephritis* (inflammation of the kidney) can also mimic appendicitis. Sometimes a *laparotomy* (surgical investigation of the abdomen) is necessary to confirm or exclude the diagnosis.

COMPLICATIONS

If treatment is delayed, the inflamed appendix may perforate, releasing its contents into the abdomen. This causes peritonitis. In some cases, the omentum (fold of peritoneum covering the intestines) envelops the inflamed appendix; this prevents the spread of infection and results in a localized abscess around the appendix. Peritonitis or an abscess causes a high swinging fever (sometimes with chills) as well as increasing pain that recurs hours or a day or so following the abrupt cessation of pain (which occurs when the appendix ruptures) and tenderness in the abdomen.

TREATMENT

The usual treatment is *appendectomy* (surgical removal of the appendix). If an abscess of the appendix is suspected, drainage of the abscess and an appendectomy may be delayed until the infection has been reduced by large doses of antibiotics.

Appendix

A narrow, small, finger-shaped tube branching off the large intestine that has no known function. In adults it is usually about 3.5 inches (9 cm) long, with a thick wall, narrow cavity, and a lining similar to that of the intestine. It contains a large amount of lymphoid tissue, which provides a defense against local infection.

The appendix projects out of the first part of the colon at the lower right-hand side of the abdomen. It may lie behind the cecum (the first part of the large intestine), but in some people descends over the brim of the pelvis, lies below the cecum, or lies in front of or behind the ileum (part of the small intestine). Its varying position partly determines the set of symptoms produced by acute *appendicitis* (inflammation of the appendix).

Appetite

A desire for food; a pleasant sensation felt in anticipation of eating, as opposed to *hunger*, a disagreeable feeling caused by the need for food.

Appetite, which is regulated by two parts of the brain (the hypothalamus and the cerebral cortex), is learned by enjoying a variety of foods that smell, taste, and look good. Ideally, it combines with hunger to ensure that the correct amount of a wide range of foods is eaten to promote health, to produce growth in children, and to maintain a proper weight in adults.

Appetite may be lost as a result of various disorders, both physical and psychological (see *Appetite, loss of*).

Appetite, loss of

Known medically as anorexia, loss of appetite is usually temporary and due to an emotional upset or minor feverish illness. Persistent loss of appetite may be a symptom of a more serious underlying physical or psychological disorder and requires investigation by a physician.

CAUSES

In adolescents and young adults, loss of appetite may be due to *anorexia nervosa* (rejection of food due to psychological causes), or to abuse of drugs, particularly the abuse of

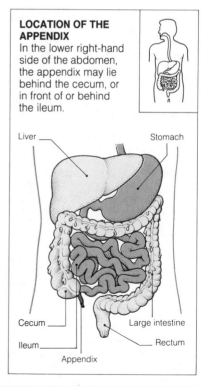

LOCATION OF THE APPENDIX
In the lower right-hand side of the abdomen, the appendix may lie behind the cecum, or in front of or behind the ileum.

Liver
Stomach
Cecum
Ileum
Large intestine
Rectum
Appendix

A

amphetamine drugs. Depression or anxiety can cause loss of appetite at any age.

Among possible physical causes are a *stroke, brain tumor,* or a brain injury that has damaged the hypothalamus or cerebral cortex, the parts of the brain that control appetite. Other physical causes include intestinal disorders, such as *gastritis* (inflammation of the stomach lining, common in alcoholics), a stomach tumor (see *Stomach cancer*) or a *gastric ulcer,* and liver disorders, such as *hepatitis.* Many infectious diseases, notably *influenza,* also cause loss of appetite.

Between the ages of about 2 and 4, some children go through a phase of refusing food. If there are no other symptoms, this period of food refusal should be regarded as a normal part of child development.

For a person who is otherwise healthy, a period of two or three days without food is not harmful, provided that plenty of nonalcoholic fluids are taken. However, if there are other health problems, particularly *diabetes mellitus,* or if regular medication is being taken, a physician should always be consulted.

All cases of loss of appetite that last for more than a few days should be investigated by a physician. Appetite generally returns to normal once any underlying illness has been treated. (See also *Appetite stimulants.*)

Appetite stimulants

There are no known drugs that safely and effectively stimulate the appetite. Lost appetite usually returns when an underlying illness subsides. A variety of drugs (including alcohol and elixirs containing small quantities of iron, quinine, and strychnine) have been prescribed, without benefit.

Appetite suppressants

COMMON DRUGS
Diethylpropion Fenfluramine Mazindol Phenmetrazine Phentermine Phenylpropanolamine

A group of drugs that reduces the desire to eat food. Appetite suppressants may be used in the treatment of *obesity,* along with advice on diet and exercise. These drugs are thought to suppress appetite by affecting the *hypothalamus* (part of the brain).

POSSIBLE ADVERSE EFFECTS
Adverse effects include dry mouth, dizziness, palpitations, nervousness, restlessness, and difficulty getting to sleep. Symptoms usually disappear after a few days of treatment.

Taking an appetite suppressant regularly for more than six weeks may lead to dependence (see *Drug dependence*). Newer appetite suppressants are less addictive than the *amphetamine drugs* that used to be prescribed.

Apraxia

An inability to carry out purposeful movements despite normal muscle power and coordination. Apraxia is caused by damage to nerve tracts within the cerebrum (the main mass of the brain) that translate the idea for a movement into an actual movement. People with apraxia usually know what they want to do but appear to have lost the ability to recall from memory the sequence of actions necessary to achieve the movement. The damage to the cerebrum may be caused by a direct *head injury,* infection, *stroke,* or *brain tumor.*

TYPES AND SYMPTOMS
Various forms of apraxia are known, each related to damage within different parts of the brain. A person with ideomotor apraxia is unable to carry out a spoken command to make a particular movement—for example, to lick his or her lips—but at another time can be observed making precisely the same movement unconsciously.

Agraphia (difficulty writing) and expressive *aphasia* (severe difficulty speaking) are special forms of apraxia.

TREATMENT AND OUTLOOK
Recovery from events such as a stroke or head injury, and from accompanying syndromes such as apraxia, is highly variable. Usually some deficit remains and it may require considerable effort and patience for the person to relearn lost skills.

APUD cell tumor

A growth, sometimes called an apudoma, composed of cells that produce various hormones. These cells—amine precursor uptake and decarboxylation (APUD) cells—are similar, even though they occur in different parts of the body.

Some tumors of the thyroid glands, pancreas, and lungs are APUD cell tumors, as are a *carcinoid* tumor and *pheochromocytoma* (an adrenal tumor).

Arachnodactyly

Long, thin, spiderlike fingers and toes that sometimes occur spontaneously but are characteristic of *Marfan's syndrome,* an inherited connective tissue disease.

Arachnoiditis

An uncommon condition characterized by chronic inflammation and thickening of the arachnoid mater, the middle of the three meninges (membranes that cover and protect the brain and spinal cord).

Arachnoiditis may develop up to several years after an episode of *meningitis* (infection of the meninges) or *subarachnoid hemorrhage* (bleeding beneath the arachnoid). It may be a feature of diseases and disorders such as *syphilis* or *ankylosing spondylitis,* or may result from trauma or procedures such as *myelography* (injection of radiopaque dye into the spinal canal followed by X rays). Usually, however, no cause is found.

The signs and symptoms vary with the extent of the disorder. It may cause headache, epileptic seizures, blindness, or slowly progressive spastic paralysis (difficulties with movements due to increased muscle tension) affecting both legs or all four limbs. There is no effective treatment.

ARC

Abbreviation for *AIDS-related complex.* (See also *AIDS.*)

Arcus senilis

A gray-white ring in the cornea, at the front of the eye, that occurs almost invariably during old age. The ring overlies the outer rim of the iris and is encircled by a narrow zone of unaffected cornea. Arcus senilis is caused by degeneration of fatty material within the cornea.

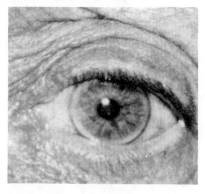

Arcus senilis
The arcus senilis is the lighter ring that overlies the edge of the iris (the colored part of the eye).

Arcus senilis develops gradually during adult life, usually starting in the lower part of the cornea, then appearing in the upper part, before affecting the sides to form a complete ring. It never spreads to the center, does not affect eyesight, and is not believed to be related to health.

A similar phenomenon in the young is called arcus juvenilis; this condition may be associated with the metabolic disorder *hyperlipidemia*.

Aroma therapy

 A range of treatments using aromatic oils extracted from plants. Many ancient civilizations, particularly the Chinese, documented the use of essential oils in treating different disorders. Recently, interest in aroma therapy has been rekindled along with other alternative therapies (see *Alternative medicine*). Practitioners claim that the treatment can be used for a range of disorders, but that it is particularly effective in *psychosomatic* and stress-related disorders.

The patient describes his or her symptoms to the therapist, who chooses the most appropriate oil or oils from a prepared range. The oil is applied in small quantities through massage or is inhaled or incorporated into creams or lotions. Very occasionally the oil is taken internally.

There is no conclusive scientific evidence that the benefits achieved are greater than those achieved by the power of suggestion.

Arousal

The awakening of a person from unconsciousness or semiconsciousness. Physicians test the depth of unconsciousness in a patient who may be suffering, for example, from concussion, a drug overdose, or alcohol intoxication with reference to the amount of stimulus required for arousal. Stimuli used include speech, a pinprick, and pressure on the Achilles tendon, which lies at the back of the ankle.

The term arousal is also used to describe any state of heightened awareness, such as that caused by sexual stimulation or fear.

Arousal is regulated by the reticular formation within the *brain stem*.

Arrhenoblastoma

A rare tumor of the ovary, also called andreoblastoma, that occurs in young women. Although the tumor is benign, it secretes androgens (male sex hormones) that cause *virilization* (the development of male sex characteristics). Treatment is by surgical removal of the affected ovary.

Arrhythmia, cardiac

An abnormality of the rhythm or rate of the *heart beat*. Arrhythmia is caused by a disturbance in the electrical impulses to the heart (see box).

TYPES
Arrhythmias can be divided into two main groups: the tachycardias, in which the rate is faster than normal (greater than 100 beats per minute), and the bradycardias, in which the rate is slower than normal (fewer than 60 beats per minute). The rhythm may be regular, as in the normal heart beat, with each beat of the atria being followed by one beat of the ventricles, or it may be irregular. The beat may originate at the sinus node or some other area of the heart.

TACHYCARDIAS In *sinus tachycardia*, the rate is raised (100 to 160 beats per minute), the rhythm is regular, and the beat originates in the sinoatrial node. *Supraventricular tachycardia* is faster (with a rate of 120 to 200 beats per minute), the rhythm is regular, and the beat may arise anywhere in the conducting tissue above the ventricles. When rapid, irregular heart beats (120 to 200 per minute) originate in the ventricles, it is called *ventricular tachycardia*.

In *atrial flutter*, the atria beat regularly and very rapidly (200 to 400 beats per minute), but not every impulse reaches the ventricles, which beat at a rate of about 100 to 200 beats per minute. Totally uncoordinated beating of the atria at about 300 to 500 beats per minute is called *atrial fibrillation* and produces completely irregular ventricular beats. Any isolated irregular beat is called an *ectopic beat* (which does not necessarily indicate the presence of an abnormality).

BRADYCARDIAS A slow, regular beat is called *sinus bradycardia*. In *heart block*, the conduction of electrical impulses through the heart muscle is partially or completely blocked, leading to slow, irregular beating. Periods of bradycardia alternate with periods of tachycardia due to a fault in impulse generation (see *Sick sinus syndrome*).

CAUSES
A common cause of arrhythmia is *coronary heart disease*. In this condition, vessels supplying blood to the heart

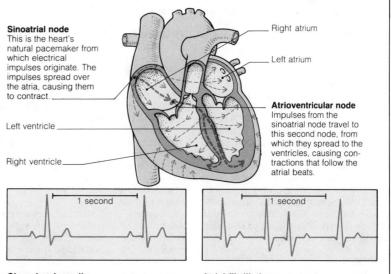

CARDIAC ARRHYTHMIA
Any disorder that interferes with the generation or transmission of impulses through the heart's electrical conducting system (below) can lead to a disturbance of cardiac rate or rhythm. These ECG recordings show two kinds of arrhythmia: sinus bradycardia and atrial fibrillation.

Sinoatrial node
This is the heart's natural pacemaker from which electrical impulses originate. The impulses spread over the atria, causing them to contract.

Left ventricle

Right ventricle

Right atrium

Left atrium

Atrioventricular node
Impulses from the sinoatrial node travel to this second node, from which they spread to the ventricles, causing contractions that follow the atrial beats.

1 second

1 second

Sinus bradycardia
The heart rate is slow but the rhythm normal, with each atrial beat (small rise) followed by a ventricular beat (spike). Sinus bradycardia is common in athletes, but can also be caused by hypothyroidism.

Atrial fibrillation
The atria beat rapidly and irregularly. Ventricular beats (spikes) do not follow each atrial beat and are irregularly spaced. This arrhythmia is common in the elderly and people with hyperthyroidism.

A

are narrowed by *atheroma* (fatty deposits) and are unable to supply sufficient blood to the conducting tissue, which becomes damaged. Arrhythmias due to coronary heart disease come on more frequently after a *myocardial infarction* (heart attack).

Sinus tachycardia may be a normal response to exercise or stress; likewise, sinus bradycardia often occurs in healthy athletes.

Caffeine and other drugs can cause tachycardia in some individuals. Amitriptyline and other antidepressants can cause serious cardiac arrhythmias if taken in high doses.

SYMPTOMS
Sudden onset of tachycardia can cause palpitations, with the individual becoming aware of an abnormally fast heart beat. Any sudden arrhythmia can cause faintness or dizziness due to reduction of blood flow to the brain. If a bradycardia reduces the flow of blood to the lungs, breathing difficulty may occur. If there is underlying heart disease, arrhythmia may lead to *angina pectoris* (chest pain due to reduced blood supply) or *heart failure* (reduced pumping efficiency).

DIAGNOSIS
The physician makes a preliminary assessment by feeling the patient's pulse and listening to the heart.

The type of arrhythmia is confirmed by an *ECG*, which shows the pattern of electrical activity within heart muscle. In some cases, if the arrhythmia is intermittent, it may be necessary to make continuous ECG recordings for 24 hours using a portable monitor.

TREATMENT
There are many different drugs that can be used to treat arrhythmias (see *Antiarrhythmic drugs*). When an arrhythmia occurs suddenly after a myocardial infarction, *defibrillation* (administration of an electric shock to the heart) may be required.

Artificial *pacemakers* can be used to stimulate heart beat in cases of heart block. Pacemakers usually consist of a small generating unit implanted under the skin of the chest wall that passes electrical impulses to the heart by means of electrodes.

Arsenic

A metallic element that occurs naturally in its pure form and as various chemical compounds. The term arsenic is popularly used to refer to the poisonous trioxide. Arsenic is present in trace amounts in water and many foods and, as a result, most people have minute quantities in their bodies, particularly in their hair and in their skin.

POISONING
Arsenic has been used intentionally to murder, but most poisoning occurs industrially or through accidental ingestion, particularly in rural areas, where arsenic is an important constituent of some pesticides.

Arsenic poisoning may be acute or chronic. Acute poisoning primarily affects the lining of the intestine, producing painful symptoms of sudden onset. The victim experiences nausea, vomiting (sometimes with blood stains), diarrhea, excessive sweating, and burning of the throat, followed by collapse and death if untreated.

Chronic poisoning is usually first noticeable as weakness, tiredness, scaly skin, *keratosis* (changes in skin pigmentation), and swelling of the lining of the mouth. *Neuropathy* (degeneration of nerves) then sets in, which produces tingling, then numbness in the hands and feet.

INVESTIGATION AND TREATMENT
Arsenic poisoning, once suspected, may be confirmed by urine analysis. Treatment of acute poisoning includes gastric *lavage* (pumping out the stomach), replacement of lost fluids, treatment of shock and pain, and administration of dimercaprol, a drug that helps to remove the poison from the body. Chronic poisoning is also treated with dimercaprol.

Arterial reconstructive surgery

Operation to repair arteries that are narrowed, blocked, or weakened.

WHY IT IS DONE
Arterial reconstructive surgery is most often performed to repair arteries narrowed or blocked by *atheroma* (fatty deposits) in arterial disease. It is also used to repair *aneurysms* (balloonlike swellings at areas of weakness) that may be congenital or may be due to *atherosclerosis*. Arteries that have been damaged by injury can also be repaired surgically.

HOW IT IS DONE
A narrowed or blocked section of artery can be bypassed by sewing in a length of vein—usually taken from the patient's leg—above and below the constricted area. This technique is most often used for coronary arteries (see *Coronary artery bypass*).

For damaged arteries elsewhere in the body, it is more common to cut out the affected section and replace it with an artificial tube or a section of vein taken from another part of the body.

OUTLOOK
Arterial reconstructive surgery is generally successful, depending on the age and health of the patient. Aortic reconstruction carries an operative death rate of up to 5 percent; untreated, larger aortic aneurysms may eventually rupture, however, and the risks of emergency surgery are much higher. (See also *Angiography*; *Angioplasty, balloon*; *Endarterectomy*.)

Arteries, disorders of

Disorders of the arteries may take the form of abnormal narrowing (which reduces blood flow and may cause tissue damage), complete obstruction (which may cause tissue death), or abnormal widening and thinning of an artery wall (which may cause rupture of the blood vessel).

TYPES

ATHEROSCLEROSIS Affecting most adults to some extent, atherosclerosis (fat deposits on the artery walls) is the most common arterial disease. It can involve arteries throughout the body, including the brain (see *Cerebrovascular disease*), the heart (see *Coronary heart disease*), and the legs (see *Peripheral vascular disease*). It is the main type of *arteriosclerosis*, a group of disorders that causes thickening and loss of elasticity of artery walls.

HYPERTENSION High blood pressure is another common cause of thickening and narrowing of arteries. It predisposes people to coronary heart disease and increases the risk of having a *stroke* as well as *renal failure*.

ARTERITIS This is a group of disorders in which inflammation of artery walls causes narrowing and sometimes blockage (see *Arteritis*).

THROMBOSIS A thrombus (blood clot) may form within an artery, causing partial or complete obstruction of the blood flow. Thrombosis usually occurs in areas already damaged by atherosclerosis or aneurysm.

EMBOLISM Obstruction of an artery by an embolus (usually a fragment of thrombus that has broken off from a larger vessel or the wall of the heart, although it may consist of fat particles from a bone fracture or an air bubble from decompression sickness).

ANEURYSM Thinning and swelling of an artery wall, this may occur in arteries damaged by atherosclerosis or as a congenital defect. In the aorta, an aneurysm may be due to *aortitis* (inflammation of the aorta wall), which may be part of a generalized arteritis or, rarely today, due to untreated syphilis.

RAYNAUD'S DISEASE This is a disorder involving intermittent spasm of small arteries in the hands and feet, usually due to cold. This obstruction of blood flow causes a change in skin color, numbness, and a pins and needles sensation. Occasionally, if the obstruction lasts, skin damage with the formation of an ischemic ulcer (see *Ischemia*) may result.

TREATMENT
Embolism and thrombosis of arteries may be treated with thrombolytic drugs (tissue plasminogen activator or streptokinase) that will dissolve the clot, and then may be prevented with *anticoagulant drugs* or by surgery to remove the obstruction (see *Embolectomy*). The various forms of arteritis (except those caused by syphilis) often respond to treatment with corticosteroid drugs. Aneurysms and arterial damage may sometimes be repaired surgically (see *Arterial reconstructive surgery*).

Arteriography
Another name for *angiography*.

Arteriole
A blood vessel that branches off an *artery* to link it to a *capillary*. Arterioles are intermediate in size and structure between arteries and capillaries. However, arterioles have proportionately more smooth muscle in their walls; their nerve supply allows the arterioles to be constricted or dilated to meet variations in the blood-flow needs of the tissues they supply.

Arteriopathy
Any abnormal condition or disorder of an artery. (See *Arteries, disorders of*.)

Arterioplasty
Surgical repair of an artery (see *Arterial reconstructive surgery*).

Arteriosclerosis
A group of disorders that causes thickening and loss of elasticity of artery walls. *Atherosclerosis* is the most common type of arteriosclerosis. Different types include medial arteriosclerosis (in which muscle and elastic fibers from the lining of large and medium-sized arteries are replaced by fibrous tissue) and Monckeberg's arteriosclerosis (in which there are deposits of calcium within the lining of the arteries).

Arteriovenous fistula
An abnormal communication or malformation between an artery and a vein that may occur congenitally or as a result of injury or infection. It can also be created surgically to provide an easy route of access into the bloodstream. The technique is useful in performing *dialysis*.

If the fistula is close to the skin surface, it may cause a small pulsating swelling. If several fistulas are present in the lungs, they can impair the uptake of oxygen into the blood, cause *cyanosis* (blue skin color), cause breathing difficulty on exertion, and sometimes cause *hemoptysis* (coughing up blood).

If an isolated fistula is causing symptoms, it is usually cut away, the channel restored, and the ends of the blood vessels sutured (stitched). If there are large numbers of fistulas, surgery is not practicable. Some arteriovenous malformations in inaccessible areas of the brain are treated with proton-beam radiation (see *Radiation therapy*).

Arteritis
Inflammation of the artery wall, causing narrowing or complete obstruction of the affected arteries, reduced blood flow, and, in some cases, thrombosis (blood clot formation) and damage to tissues.

Buerger's disease includes an arteritis that affects the limbs, causing pain, numbness, and, in severe cases, *gangrene* (death of tissue).

Periarteritis nodosa, an *autoimmune disorder* (in which the body's defense mechanism against disease attacks its own tissues), can affect arteries in any part of the body, causing symptoms such as abdominal and testicular pain, chest pain, breathing difficulty, and tender lumps under the skin.

Temporal arteritis affects arteries in the scalp over the temples, causing headache and scalp tenderness; if the retinal artery is affected, there is a risk of permanent blindness.

A very rare type of arteritis is Takayasu's arteritis. The cause is unknown but thought to be autoimmune (the body's defense mechanisms attacking its own tissues—in this case, the artery walls). Takayasu's arteritis usually affects young women and involves the arteries that branch from the first part of the aorta into the neck and arms.

Artery
A blood vessel that carries blood away from the heart. Systemic arteries carry blood from the left ventricle (lower chamber) of the heart, through the *aorta* (the largest artery in the body), to all parts of the body except the lungs. The pulmonary arteries carry blood from the right ventricle of the heart to the lungs. Pulmonary arteries are shorter, thinner-walled, and contain blood under a lower pressure than systemic arteries.

STRUCTURE AND FUNCTION
Arteries are pliable tubes with thick walls that enable them to withstand the high blood pressure to which they are subjected every time that the heart muscle beats.

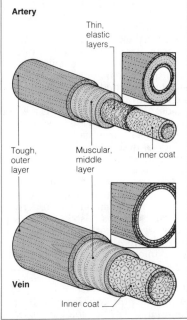

STRUCTURE OF AN ARTERY
An artery's walls consist of three layers: a smooth, inner lining, a thick, muscular, elastic, middle layer, and a tough, fibrous, outer covering. Veins have thinner walls and most contain valves.

Artery — Thin, elastic layers; Tough, outer layer; Muscular, middle layer; Inner coat

Vein — Inner coat

The structure of arteries helps even out the peaks and troughs of blood pressure caused by the heart beat, so that the blood is flowing at a relatively constant pressure by the time it reaches the smaller blood vessels. These smaller blood vessels include the *arterioles*, which branch directly off the artery. The arterioles connect to the even smaller *capillaries*. (See also *Arteries, disorders of*.)

Arthralgia
A term meaning pain in the joints. (See *Joint*; *Arthritis*.)

A

Arthritis

Inflammation of a joint; characterized by pain, swelling, stiffness, and redness. Arthritis is not a single disorder but the name of joint disease from a number of causes. The arthritis may involve one joint or many, and can vary in severity from a mild ache and stiffness to severe pain and, later, joint deformity.

TYPES AND CAUSES

OSTEOARTHRITIS Also known as degenerative arthritis, this is the most common type of arthritis. It results from wear and tear on the joints, evolves in middle age, and most commonly troubles older people.

RHEUMATOID ARTHRITIS The most severe type of inflammatory joint disease, this is an *autoimmune disorder* in which the body's *immune system* acts against and damages joints and surrounding soft tissues. Many joints—most commonly those in the hands, feet, and arms—become extremely painful, stiff, and deformed.

STILL'S DISEASE Juvenile rheumatoid arthritis; it is most common in children under the age of 4. It usually clears up after a few years but even then may stunt growth and leave the child with permanent deformities.

SERONEGATIVE ARTHRITIS This is a group of disorders that causes symptoms and signs of arthritis in a number of joints, although blood test results for rheumatoid arthritis are negative. It can be associated with skin disorders (such as *psoriasis*), inflammatory intestinal disorders (such as *Crohn's disease*), or autoimmune disorders.

INFECTIVE ARTHRITIS Also known as septic or pyogenic arthritis, this is joint disease caused by the invasion of bacteria into the joint from a nearby

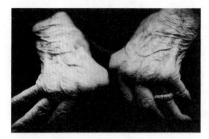

Arthritis in the hands
Severely deformed joints in the hands of an elderly woman who is suffering from rheumatoid arthritis.

infected wound or from *bacteremia* (infection in the bloodstream). The infected joint usually becomes hot as well as painful and swollen.

Arthritis may also occur as a complication of an infection elsewhere in the body, such as *chickenpox, rubella* (German measles), *mumps, rheumatic fever,* or *gonorrhea*; it may also be a complication of *nonspecific urethritis,* in which case the joint inflammation forms part of *Reiter's syndrome.*

ANKYLOSING SPONDYLITIS In this arthritis of the spine, the joints linking the vertebrae become inflamed and the vertebrae fuse. The arthritis may spread to other joints, often the hips.

GOUT This disorder is associated with a form of arthritis in which uric acid (one of the body's waste products) accumulates in joints in the form of crystals, causing inflammation. It usually affects one joint at a time.

DIAGNOSIS

The diagnosis is made from the patient's symptoms and signs. To discover the cause, fluid may be withdrawn through a needle from an affected joint. This fluid may then be

examined microscopically for the presence of microorganisms, or uric acid or other crystals. Sometimes a *culture* is made from the fluid so that it can be analyzed for any infection.

X rays may be carried out to reveal the type and extent of damage to joints. *Blood tests* can reveal the presence of proteins typical of rheumatoid arthritis, a high level of uric acid indicative of gout, or sometimes a high *ESR* (erythrocyte sedimentation rate), indicating inflammation.

TREATMENT

There are specific treatments for the different types of arthritis—for example, *antibiotic drugs* for septic arthritis, *anti-inflammatory drugs* for treating rheumatoid arthritis and osteoarthritis, and allopurinol for gout. Many other drugs are used to treat different forms of arthritis, but none seems able to effect a cure.

In a severe attack of arthritis affecting several joints, a few days' bed rest will help settle the inflammation; individual joints can be splinted to reduce the pain, and heat and supervised exercises help keep the deformity in the joints to a minimum. Obese people with arthritis in weight-bearing joints should lose weight.

Diseased joints that have become extremely painful, unstable, or deformed may require *arthroplasty* (replacement of the joint with an artificial substitute) or *arthrodesis* (fusion of the bones in the joint).

OUTLOOK

Arthritis has many forms and varies widely in its effects. Only a few sufferers become severely disabled. Most are able to lead productive lives, although activity may need to be altered to preserve joint function.

Arthrodesis

A surgical procedure in which the two bones in a diseased joint are fused to prevent the joint from moving.

WHY IT IS DONE

If pain and deformity in a diseased joint are so severe that they cannot be relieved by drugs, splinting, and physical therapy (as can occur in *rheumatoid arthritis*), or if a joint has become unstable, usually as the result of an injury, some form of surgery is required. In most cases, the operation of first choice is *arthroplasty* (reconstruction of a diseased joint using artificial replacements), since this procedure retains movement in the joint. When arthroplasty is not feasible or fails, arthrodesis is used.

HOW IT IS DONE

A local anesthetic may be all that is required for a small joint, such as a finger. Otherwise, general anesthetic is used. The technique of the operation varies according to the joint being treated, but in most cases cartilage (smooth, shock-absorbing tissue) is removed from the ends of the two bones, along with a surface layer of bone from each. The two ends are then joined so that, when fresh bone cells grow, the ends will fuse. The bones may need to be kept in position with plates, rods, or screws; a *bone graft* may also be carried out.

In arthrodesis of the knee or ankle, additional immobilization of the joint—by transfixing it with pins

inserted through the skin—may be necessary to keep the area stable until healing is complete.

RECOVERY PERIOD

Complete union of the bones can take up to six months but is usually much quicker. In some cases the bones fail to fuse, but often this is irrelevant because fibrous tissue fills the gap between them and is strong enough to provide the same effect and strength as bone fusion.

OUTLOOK

One advantage of arthrodesis over arthroplasty is that, once performed, it needs no regular surveillance or further care; the patient can be reasonably certain that the problem with the joint has been solved permanently.

Arthrography

A diagnostic technique for examining the interior of a damaged joint by injecting into it a radiopaque solution (one visible on X ray). The procedure is gradually being replaced by *ultrasound scanning* and *arthroscopy*.

Arthrogryposis

See *Contracture*.

Arthropathy

A medical term for *joint* disease.

Arthroplasty

Replacement of a joint or part of a joint by metal or plastic components. *Hip replacements* were the first operations of this type to be introduced and are still the most successful and often performed. Replacement of other joints, including the knee (see *Knee joint replacement*), finger (see *Finger joint replacement*), shoulder, and elbow, is also routine.

The first attempts to replace part of a damaged hip joint with a man-made substitute were made in the 1930s. In the 1960s, hip replacement operations were revolutionized by developments on three fronts. First, metal and plastic materials were developed that were strong enough to allow a good level of activity while being to some extent self-lubricating; second, cement was used to help fix the artificial joint to the bones; and third, the risk of infection in the joint—a very serious complication—was virtually eliminated by performing the surgery in an operating room in which the air is filtered and all members of the surgical team wear all-enveloping clothing.

These principles have now been applied to the full range of replacement joints. Engineers and orthopedic surgeons are still developing and improving replacements for the knee and shoulder, which are more complex than the hip.

Arthroscopy

Inspection through an *endoscope* (a flexible viewing tube) of the interior of a joint, usually for the purpose of diagnosing a condition affecting that joint. Arthroscopy has rapidly become one of the most frequently performed procedures in orthopedic surgery, thanks to the development of modern lens systems and brighter lighting by means of fiberoptics.

WHY IT IS DONE

Arthroscopy is most frequently used to inspect the inside of the knee joint. Many conditions affecting the knee do

HOW ARTHROSCOPY IS DONE

The procedure is usually performed using a general anesthetic, but sometimes a *nerve block* is used. The joint is distended by injecting air or a saline solution; the instrument is inserted into the joint through a small skin incision. While watching through the endoscope, the surgeon can probe or lift structures to check for damage.

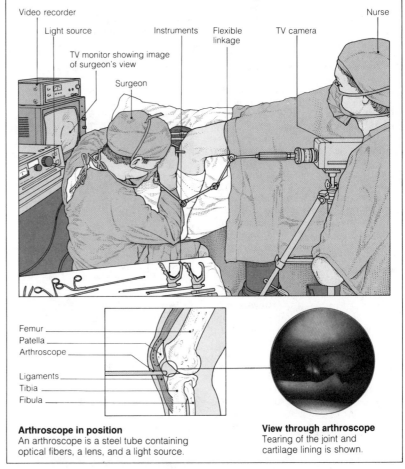

Arthroscope in position
An arthroscope is a steel tube containing optical fibers, a lens, and a light source.

View through arthroscope
Tearing of the joint and cartilage lining is shown.

not show up on X rays and are difficult to diagnose on the basis of symptoms alone. Arthroscopy allows the surgeon to see the surfaces of the bones that come into contact in the joint, the ligaments and cartilages within the joint, and the synovial membrane that lines the internal surface of the joint capsule. Specimens of these structures can be removed for examination and analysis.

A new and exciting development is the application of arthroscopic surgery techniques. Instruments that fold down as they are passed through a channel in the arthroscope enable surgeons to carry out some procedures that formerly necessitated opening up the knee. Procedures include removal of damaged cartilage, repair of torn cartilage and ligaments, and shaving or drilling the surface of the patella (kneecap). Arthroscopic surgery substantially reduces the time a patient needs to stay in the hospital, and the time an athlete is unable to participate in his or her sport.

Artificial insemination

The introduction of semen into the cervix (opening of the uterus) by means of an instrument instead of through sexual intercourse, with the aim of inducing conception and pregnancy. Artificial insemination was first carried out in the US in 1866. About 10,000 babies are born here annually as a result of the procedure.

TYPES

There are two principal types of artificial insemination. AIH (artificial insemination using the husband's semen) is the use of semen from the woman's permanent sexual partner. It is usually employed for couples who are unable to have intercourse, either because of psychosexual difficulties, such as impotence, or because of physical injury or deformity. Occasionally, it may be used when the husband has a low sperm count or a low volume of ejaculate or if the acid in the woman's vagina creates a hostile environment for the sperm. It is also used when semen has been stored from a man who is to undergo medical treatment (such as chemotherapy or radiation therapy) that may make him sterile. AID (artificial insemination using a donor's semen) is the use of semen from an anonymous male donor. It is available to couples if the man is infertile, has a genetic disease, or may be a carrier of such a disease. It may also be used by a woman who wants children but has no male partner.

HOW IT IS DONE

Both AID and AIH are carried out at centers that are specially staffed and equipped to obtain and store semen from donors, to carry out the insemination, and to give counseling before and after the procedure.

Donors must be in good health and are usually screened for as many physical and mental disorders as possible. However, there is no safeguard against the use of sperm from a carrier of a genetic disease.

Fresh semen is usually used for AIH. For AID, the semen is frozen in liquid nitrogen and then stored; before it is used it is tested to exclude the presence of any infection-causing microorganisms. The viruses causing *hepatitis B* and *AIDS* have been transmitted through AID. As a result, all stored semen is placed in quarantine until the donor has been tested for antibodies to these viruses and until test results have been negative on two occasions three months apart.

Insemination is carried out by injecting semen into the cervix with a small syringe. Two or three inseminations are carried out during the two to four optimum days for conception in the woman's menstrual cycle and, unless pregnancy occurs, they are repeated for up to five more cycles.

RESULTS

When fresh semen is used, the success rate of artificial insemination in bringing about pregnancy over a six-month period is 60 to 70 percent. With frozen semen, the success rate is 55 percent.

Artificial kidney

Common name for the machine used in renal *dialysis*.

Artificial respiration

Forced introduction of air into the lungs of someone who has stopped breathing (see *Respiratory arrest*) or of someone whose breathing is inadequate. Artificial respiration may be administered by the mouth-to-mouth or mouth-to-nose method. It may also be given by the use of ventilating equipment administered by skilled technicians (see *Ventilation*).

WHY IT IS DONE

Artificial respiration should be started as soon as possible after someone has stopped breathing; delay in breathing for more than six minutes can cause death. When someone has stopped breathing there is no rise-and-fall movement of the chest or abdomen, the face becomes blue-gray, and no exhaled breath can be felt. When there is no breathing, it is likely that the

---

FIRST AID: ARTIFICIAL RESPIRATION

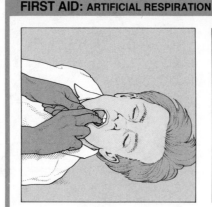

1 If possible, send for medical help, but start resuscitation immediately—do not waste time loosening clothing around the neck unless there is obvious strangulation. Lay the victim on his or her back on a firm, rigid surface. Quickly clear the mouth and airway of any foreign material with your fingers.

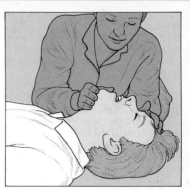

2 If there does not appear to be any neck injury, gently tilt the victim's head backward and maintain it in the midline by placing one hand under the back of the neck and lifting upward. Place the heel of the other hand on the victim's forehead and press downward so that the chin is elevated.

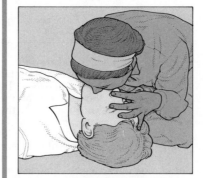

3 Using the hand that is placed on the victim's forehead, pinch the victim's nostrils, using your thumb and index finger. Take a deep breath. Place your open mouth tightly around the victim's open mouth and blow air from your lungs into the victim's lungs. Stop blowing when the victim's chest is expanded.

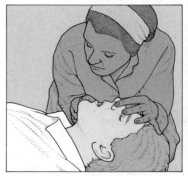

4 Remove your mouth and turn your head toward the victim's chest. Listen for air leaving his or her lungs and watch the chest fall. Give four quick breaths, taking a deep breath between each one. Continue at the rate of 12 breaths per minute, until you see the victim beginning to breathe on his or her own.

heart has stopped beating. If no pulse can be felt in the wrist or neck, cardiac compressions should be carried out in conjunction with artificial respiration (see *Cardiopulmonary resuscitation*).

When breathing is weak or shallow, movements of the chest are minimal and hardly any breath can be felt. If breathing is not restored, the brain is deprived of oxygen; permanent brain damage or death can result.

HOW IT IS DONE

MOUTH-TO-MOUTH RESUSCITATION This is the simplest and most effective method of introducing air into the victim's lungs (see illustrated box). The method is safe to use on a person whose breathing is weak, shallow, or labored. Time your exhalations with the victim's inhalations.

MOUTH-TO-NOSE RESUSCITATION If the victim has a facial injury, it may be difficult for you to breathe into his or her mouth. In such cases, follow steps 1 and 2 shown in the box, left. Remove your hand from the back of the victim's neck and close his or her mouth by lifting the chin. Take a deep breath and seal your mouth around the victim's nose. Blow strongly into the nose. Remove your mouth and hold the victim's mouth open with your hand, so that air can escape. Repeat as for mouth-to-mouth resuscitation every five seconds.

RESUSCITATION OF BABIES AND CHILDREN The method of resuscitating a baby or young child is basically the same as the method of resuscitating an adult, except that you will find it easier to seal your mouth over both the mouth and nose of the child. Do not tip the child's head back very far, because a child's neck and airway are more fragile than an adult's. Blow gentle breaths of air into the lungs, one breath every two to three seconds (20 to 30 breaths per minute) until the child's chest starts to rise.

Artificial sweeteners

Synthetic substitutes for sugar used by people on reducing diets, by diabetics, and by the food industry.

Saccharin is 500 to 600 times sweeter than cane sugar (though it has a sour aftertaste) and has no calories. Saccharin has been associated with bladder cancer in animal experiments but the risk of it causing cancer in humans is negligible. (Cyclamate, another artificial sweetener, was banned in the late 1960s after it had been proved to cause cancer in animals.)

Aspartame is about 200 times sweeter than sugar—although its sweetness

is destroyed by prolonged heating—and is virtually calorie free. It has no known adverse effects when taken in normal quantities but in excess may cause neurological disorders.

Although saccharin and aspartame are often recommended for use in reducing diets, they are of questionable value because they do nothing to reduce the craving for sweet foods.

Sorbitol, which occurs naturally in certain fruits, is another sugar substitute. It is used by diabetics but its high caloric value (about 140 Calories per ounce) makes it unsuitable for use in reducing diets. One problem with using sorbitol is that its poor absorption from the intestine into the bloodstream may cause diarrhea by pulling fluid into the bowel channel.

Asbestosis

A chronic lung disease caused by inhaling fibers of asbestos, a heat-resistant and insulating material. Those affected are mainly workers employed in the mining of asbestos, the manufacture of asbestos products, or in the building industry. Asbestosis is probably the single most important work-related lung disease.

CAUSES AND INCIDENCE

Asbestos fibers penetrate and irritate the outer parts of the lung, causing inflammation and, over the years, *pulmonary fibrosis* (thickening and scarring of the lung tissue). An extended period (20 years or more) may elapse between exposure to the dust and onset of the disease.

In the US, it is estimated that more than one million people have been exposed to significant levels of asbestos fibers. Fewer than 10 new cases of asbestosis are diagnosed per 100,000 population each year; the incidence is higher in areas where there has been a heavy concentration of asbestos-related industry.

PREVENTION

Recently there has been a far greater awareness of the dangers of working with asbestos and workers are regularly screened by *chest X rays*. If the X-ray films show any shadows on the lungs, the person is advised to stop working with asbestos, even if there are no symptoms.

SYMPTOMS AND COMPLICATIONS

Breathlessness is the main symptom; it becomes increasingly severe as the disease develops. There may also be a dry cough and a feeling of tightness in the chest. Eventually, *respiratory failure* develops.

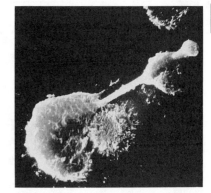

Asbestos fiber in lung
The term asbestos refers to any of a group of fibrous minerals that can cause lung disease.

Asbestosis sufferers have a higher-than-average risk of acquiring *tuberculosis* and *lung cancer*, particularly if they smoke cigarettes. Exposure to asbestos may also be a predisposing factor in the development of lung cancer (without asbestosis) and of *mesothelioma* (a tumor of the lung covering), especially in smokers.

DIAGNOSIS AND TREATMENT

Along with chest X rays, *pulmonary function tests* are used in diagnosis to measure breathing efficiency. Once asbestosis has developed, there is no effective treatment; the disease usually causes disability and death.

OUTLOOK

Since the middle 1970s, asbestos has been replaced, wherever possible, by other materials, such as glass fiber. Along with rigorous screening, this should produce a reduction in the incidence of the disease.

Ascariasis

A worm infestation, common worldwide and especially in the tropics. The parasite responsible, *ASCARIS LUMBRICOIDES*, is a pale, cylindrical, tapered roundworm, between six and 15 inches in length in adult form, which lives in the small intestine of its human host. One or several worms may be present, but symptoms usually occur only in people with heavy worm infestations.

INCIDENCE AND CAUSES

Ascariasis affects up to 80 to 90 percent of the population in poorer countries, where children living in rural areas are prone to heavy infestations. In developed countries, such as the US, about 1 percent of the population may have a light infestation at any one time, although few people are aware of the presence of worms.

A

LIFE CYCLE OF THE ASCARIASIS WORM

The person becomes infested by swallowing the eggs. They hatch into larvae in the intestine, then travel via the wall of the intestine and the blood to the lungs, up the windpipe, and are swallowed back to the small intestine. There they become adult worms.

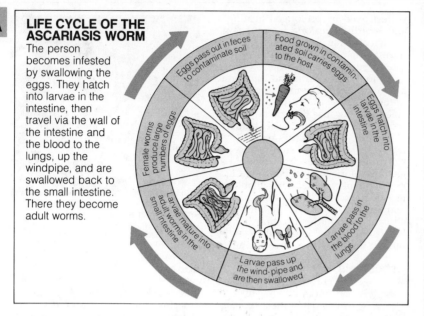

Eggs pass out in feces to contaminate soil

Food grown in contaminated soil carries eggs to the host

Eggs hatch into larvae in intestine

Larvae pass in the blood to the lungs

Larvae pass up the wind-pipe and are then swallowed

Larvae mature into adult worms in the small intestine

Female worms produce large numbers of eggs

The life cycle of the worm and the mechanism by which the infestation is acquired are shown above.

In some dry, windy climates, air-borne eggs may be swallowed after being blown into the mouth.

SYMPTOMS

Light infestations may cause either no symptoms or occasional nausea, abdominal pain, and irregular bowel movements. A worm may be passed via the rectum or vomited.

A heavy load of worms may compete with the host for food, leading to malnutrition and anemia, which in children can retard growth.

DIAGNOSIS AND TREATMENT

Ascariasis is diagnosed by finding the worm's eggs in a person's feces during microscopic examination.

The infection is treated with *antihelmintic drugs*, such as piperazine, which is highly effective in a single dose. The worms are passed via the rectum some days after the drug is taken. The patient usually makes a complete recovery.

Ascites

An excess of fluid in the peritoneal cavity—the space between the two layers of membrane, or peritoneum, that line the inside of the abdominal wall and the outside of the abdominal organs. A few gallons of fluid may be present, which causes distention.

CAUSES

Ascites may occur in any condition that causes generalized *edema* (excessive accumulation of fluid in the body

tissues). The most important of these conditions are congestive *heart failure*, *nephrotic syndrome*, and liver *cirrhosis*.

Ascites may occur in *cancer* if metastases (secondary growths) from lung, breast, or intestinal tumors are deposited on the surface of the peritoneum. Ascites also occurs in cases of *tuberculosis* infecting the abdomen, a rare disease today.

SYMPTOMS AND TREATMENT

In addition to abdominal swelling and discomfort, ascites may cause difficulty breathing due to pressure on and immobilization of the diaphragm, the sheet of muscle that separates the thorax (chest) and the abdomen.

Ascites is detected during physical examination. Diagnosis of the cause involves the physician performing a careful history and physical examination and removing and analyzing a sample of ascitic fluid via a sterile needle inserted through the abdominal wall. The fluid is examined under the microscope for malignant cells. Its color, turbidity (opacity), and chemical composition also help identify whether the cause is due to inflammation or a condition such as cirrhosis.

Treatment depends on the precise cause of the ascites, but in many cases includes bed rest, and fluid and salt (sodium) restriction. Alcohol is eliminated when liver disease is implicated. *Diuretic drugs*, particularly spironolactone, may be prescribed.

If the ascites causes discomfort or breathing difficulty, fluid can be drained from the peritoneal cavity.

Ascorbic acid

The chemical name for *vitamin C*.

Aseptic technique

The creation of a germ-free environment, mainly by the use of *sterilization*, to protect a patient from infection. Aseptic sterilization is distinct from antisepsis, which is the destruction of germs by chemicals (*antiseptics*).

WHY IT IS DONE

Aseptic technique is needed for any procedure in which there is a danger of introducing infection into the body. The patient can be contaminated from four main sources: other people, instruments, the patient himself or herself, and the air. To prevent such contamination, aseptic technique is used for surgery in an operating room as well as for minor office procedures, such as inserting a urinary catheter or stitching a wound. Aseptic technique is also needed when caring for patients with suppressed immune systems (such as those being treated for leukemia) and for those who have reduced natural defenses against infection (see *Isolation*).

HOW IT IS DONE

All people who come in contact with the patient must scrub their hands and wear presterilized gowns and disposable gloves and masks. Instruments are sterilized beforehand in an *autoclave* and placed on a cart covered with sterile material.

The area of the patient that is to be operated on is cleaned with antiseptic solutions of iodine or hexachlorophene, and the surrounding skin is covered with sterile drapes. In addition, before operations on the intestine, the bowel is cleared by giving laxatives and sometimes enemas to prevent any contamination of the abdominal area by feces.

Throughout the procedure, care is taken to place used, possibly contaminated, instruments well away from sterile instruments and dressings.

In an operating room it is important to keep the air and the room scrupulously clean. The windows remain closed and the only air that enters the room is through a special ventilation system that purifies the air and maintains it at a certain humidity.

Aspergillosis

Infection caused by aspergillus, a fungus found in old buildings or decaying plant matter. It is an occasionally fatal, *opportunistic infection* (one caused by organisms that are usually harmless to healthy people but that produce illness in those whose resistance is reduced.

Aspermia

Failure to produce or ejaculate sperm. (See *Ejaculation, disorders of.*)

Asphyxia

The medical term for suffocation. Asphyxia may be due to obstruction of a large airway, usually by a foreign body (see *Choking*), to a lack or falling levels of oxygen in the surrounding air (as occurs when a closed plastic bag is put over the head), or to poisoning with a gas such as carbon monoxide that interferes with the uptake of oxygen into the bloodstream.

The person initially breathes more rapidly and strongly to try to overcome the lack of oxygen in the blood. There is also an increase in heart rate and blood pressure.

TREATMENT

First-aid treatment consists of *artificial respiration* after first moving the person into the open air and clearing the airway of any obstruction. Untreated asphyxia causes death.

Aspiration

The withdrawal of fluid or tissue from the body by suction. The term also refers to the act of breathing in a foreign body, usually food or drink.

Aspiration *biopsy* is the removal of tissue or fluid for examination by suction through a needle attached to a syringe. The procedure is used mainly to obtain cells from a fluid-filled cavity (such as a breast cyst); from the bone marrow (see *Bone marrow biopsy*); or from internal organs, when a narrow needle is guided to the site of the biopsy by *CT scanning* or *ultrasound scanning*. The cells obtained are examined under a microscope, particularly for any evidence of cancer.

Aspiration pneumonia is inflammation of the lungs that results from inhalation of foreign material; this material could be vomit inhaled during induction of anesthesia or during a coma, or infected secretions from the nose or throat.

Aspirin

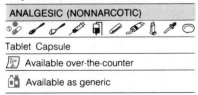

ANALGESIC (NONNARCOTIC)

Tablet Capsule

Available over-the-counter

Available as generic

WARNING
Never take aspirin regularly for more than two days except under medical supervision; it may mask the symptoms of a serious disorder.

An *analgesic drug* (painkiller) that has been used for more than 80 years to treat disorders such as headache, menstrual pain, and muscle ache. Because aspirin has an anti-inflammatory action, it is particularly useful in treating joint pain and stiffness caused by *osteoarthritis* and other types of arthritis. Aspirin also reduces fever and is therefore included in a number of *cold remedies*.

In small doses it reduces the stickiness of platelets (blood particles involved in clotting). This has led to its use in preventing *thrombosis* (abnormal blood clots) in some individuals at risk of having a *stroke* or *myocardial infarction* (heart attack).

HOW IT WORKS

Aspirin reduces the production of certain *prostaglandins* (hormonelike chemicals) that can be responsible for inflammation, pain, fever, or clumping of platelets.

POSSIBLE ADVERSE EFFECTS

In children there is a slight risk of *Reye's syndrome* (a rare brain and liver disorder). Aspirin should not be given to children except under close medical supervision; acetaminophen should be used instead.

Aspirin may cause irritation of the stomach lining, resulting in indigestion or nausea. These side effects may be reduced by taking the drug with food or by taking a coated tablet that does not release the drug until it reaches the intestine. Prolonged use of aspirin may cause bleeding from the stomach due to *gastric erosion* (disruption of the surface lining of the stomach) or *peptic ulcer* (a deeper penetration of the wall of the stomach or duodenum).

Assay

Analysis of a substance to determine its presence or effects. A qualitative assay determines only whether or not a substance is present, whereas a quantitative assay determines the actual amount present.

Biological assays (called bioassays) are concerned mainly with measuring the response of an animal or specific organ to a drug or hormone. They are used, for example, to assess the side effects of a particular drug. (See also *Immunoassay*.)

Assignment

One way in which a physician is reimbursed for services to patients enrolled in Medicare. If a physician wishes to receive direct payment from Medicare and is willing to allow that organization to determine the amount of payment, he or she may elect assignment. The patient agrees to have Medicare benefits assigned to the physician. By assignment, the patient and physician effectively agree to accept Medicare's determination of a "reasonable charge" for the services rendered. Medicare reimburses the physician directly for the services, but pays only 80 percent of the "reasonable charge" as determined by a formula. The physician may bill the patient for the remaining 20 percent.

As an alternative, the physician may refuse assignment and bill a Medicare patient for a fee the physician determines himself or herself. The patient may submit the bill to Medicare (through the insurance company that handles Medicare's billing locally) and expect as reimbursement 80 percent of Medicare's predetermined "reasonable charge."

Astereognosis

An inability to recognize objects by touch when they are placed in one hand—even though there is no defect of sensation in the fingers or any difficulty holding the object. Testing for astereognosis is part of any detailed examination of the central nervous system. Astereognosis is either left-sided or right-sided; tactile recognition is normal on the other side. If both sides are affected, the condition is called tactile *agnosia*.

Both astereognosis and tactile agnosia are caused by disease or damage to parts of the cerebrum (the main mass of the brain) concerned with recognition by touch.

Asthenia

A term meaning loss of strength and energy (see *Weakness*).

Asthenia, neurocirculatory

See *Cardiac neurosis*.

Asthma

Recurrent attacks of breathlessness, characteristically accompanied by wheezing when breathing out and varying in severity from day to day and from hour to hour. The illness frequently starts in childhood and tends to clear up or become less severe in early adulthood.

A

LIVING WITH ASTHMA

Breathlessness and wheezing in asthma is caused by narrowing of the bronchioles (small airways in the lungs). Breathing is most difficult and wheezing most pronounced when the sufferer is breathing out because the lungs collapse to expel air. This causes further narrowing of the bronchioles. Inflammation of the linings of these bronchioles causes an increased production of sputum (phlegm), which makes the obstruction worse. A dry cough often develops as the sufferer attempts to clear the airways.

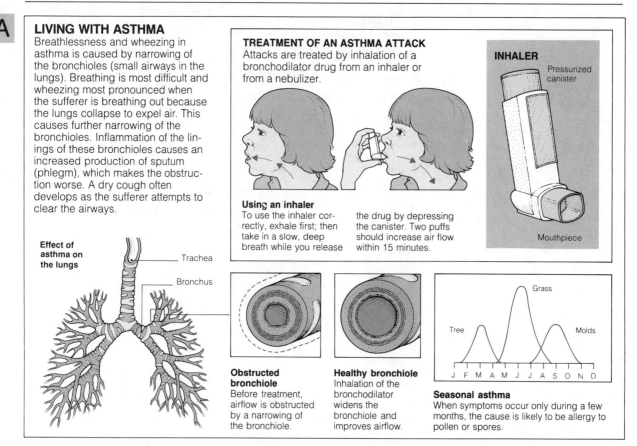

Effect of asthma on the lungs

Trachea

Bronchus

TREATMENT OF AN ASTHMA ATTACK
Attacks are treated by inhalation of a bronchodilator drug from an inhaler or from a nebulizer.

Using an inhaler
To use the inhaler correctly, exhale first; then take in a slow, deep breath while you release the drug by depressing the canister. Two puffs should increase air flow within 15 minutes.

INHALER

Pressurized canister

Mouthpiece

Obstructed bronchiole
Before treatment, airflow is obstructed by a narrowing of the bronchiole.

Healthy bronchiole
Inhalation of the bronchodilator widens the bronchiole and improves airflow.

Grass

Tree

Molds

J F M A M J J A S O N D

Seasonal asthma
When symptoms occur only during a few months, the cause is likely to be allergy to pollen or spores.

The familiar form of asthma is more correctly called bronchial asthma; this use of the full name distinguishes it from a condition associated with wheezing caused by heart failure (see *Asthma, cardiac*).

Although asthma frequently begins early in life (most people have their first attack before the age of 5), it can develop at any age.

CAUSES
Asthma is of two main types: extrinsic, in which an allergy (usually to something inhaled) triggers an attack, and intrinsic, in which there is no apparent external cause.

The most common allergens responsible for asthma are pollens, which often also cause allergic *rhinitis* (hay fever). Other common allergens include house dust, house-dust mites, animal fur, dander, or feathers. Extrinsic asthma may also be triggered by a respiratory infection (such as a cough, cold, or bronchitis), by exercise (especially in cold air), by tobacco smoke or other air pollutants, and by allergy to a particular food or drug (most commonly aspirin).

Intrinsic asthma tends to develop later in life than extrinsic asthma, with the first attack often following a respiratory tract infection. Emotional factors, such as stress or anxiety, may precipitate attacks.

PREVALENCE
About one in 20 of the overall population is asthmatic but the prevalence among children is much greater—about one in 10.

Heredity is a major factor in the development of extrinsic asthma. Asthma seems to be becoming more common in the US and other developed countries.

SYMPTOMS
Asthmatic attacks vary greatly in their severity, ranging from a slight breathlessness to respiratory failure. Attacks may be most frequent in the early morning.

The main symptoms are breathlessness, wheezing, a dry cough sometimes brought on by exercise, and a feeling of tightness in the chest.

During a severe attack, breathing becomes increasingly difficult, causing sweating, rapid heart beat, and

great distress and anxiety. The sufferer cannot lie down or sleep, may be unable to speak, breathes rapidly, and wheezes loudly.

In a very severe attack, the low amount of oxygen in the blood may cause *cyanosis* (blue-purple discoloration) of the face, particularly the lips, and the skin may become pale and clammy. Such attacks may be fatal. In 1979, more than 1,800 people died as a direct result of an asthma attack; an additional 4,400 people died of asthmatic complications.

PREVENTION
Although there is no cure for asthma, attacks can be prevented to a large extent. For sufferers of extrinsic asthma, tests are available to discover whether any of the common allergens is responsible for triggering attacks; if a specific cause is discovered, steps can be taken to avoid it. For example, if pollen is the cause, the person will need to avoid gardens, parks, and the countryside during the pollen season. If the house-dust mite is responsible, mattresses (in which the mites flourish) should be enclosed in airtight

plastic covers and the home should be kept as free of dust as possible.

Immunotherapy (a course of injections of the allergen) can be performed but has a limited success rate. Much more successful in preventing attacks are prophylactic (preventive) drugs, such as cromolyn sodium and inhaled *corticosteroid drugs*. To be effective, they must be taken several times daily, usually through an inhaler.

TREATMENT
Once an attack has started, a prophylactic drug has limited effects and a *bronchodilator* (a drug that relaxes and widens the airways), such as albuterol, must be used. Most asthmatic people learn to administer the drug themselves with a hand-held plastic inhaler (see illustration).

An inhaler loses its effectiveness after a certain period (the date is marked on the container), so it is essential for the asthmatic person to renew his or her supply regularly. Oral theophylline preparations are also used preventively for their bronchodilating properties.

EMERGENCY PROCEDURE
Most attacks of asthma either pass naturally or can be controlled by use of a bronchodilator. In some cases, however, an attack may be so severe that it fails to respond to the recommended dose of the drug. In this case, the dose should be repeated. If it has no effect, a physician should be seen or the person taken to the hospital.

Emergency treatment at home or in the hospital may include the administration of oxygen, a corticosteroid, and a bronchodilator through a nebulizer or an intravenous injection of aminophylline. If these measures are ineffective (which is rare), the patient requires a *ventilator*, which forces air or oxygen under pressure into the lungs.

OUTLOOK
More than half of affected children grow out of asthma completely by the age of 21. In a large proportion of the remainder, attacks become decreasingly severe as they grow older. With modern drug treatment, even people who suffer repeated attacks as adults can expect to live a normal life. In most cases, quality of life need not be impaired (demonstrated by the success of world-class athletes who have had asthma).

Asthma, cardiac
Difficulty breathing caused by fluid collection in the lungs that causes bronchospasm and wheezing. This response is usually due to reduced pumping efficiency of the left side of the heart (see *Heart failure*), causing congestion and increased pressure within the blood circulation through the lungs and fluid collection.

Although cardiac asthma has a different cause from the more familiar bronchial asthma, the two conditions have similar symptoms, including wheezing and breathing difficulty. A chest X ray may show fluid in the lungs. Treatment is primarily for heart failure but may include use of bronchodilator drugs.

Astigmatism
A condition in which the front surface of the cornea of the eye is not truly spherical. Although the eye is perfectly healthy, the corneal surface has discrepancies in the curvature, so that magnification in one direction is greater than in others.

A minor degree of astigmatism is normal and glasses are not necessary to correct it. More severe astigmatism causes blurring of lines set at a particular angle. A person with astigmatism might see horizontal lines clearly but vertical lines blurred, or the blurring may occur in an oblique meridian.

TREATMENT
Ordinary "spherical" eyeglass lenses cannot correct astigmatism. Lenses are needed that have no optical power in the normal meridian but appropriate curvature in the others. These cylindrical lenses must be framed at a precise angle.

Hard contact lenses bridge over the anomalous corneal curve and present a perfect spherical surface for focusing; they give excellent vision in astigmatism. Ordinary soft lenses tend to mold to the astigmatic curve, but special "toric" soft lenses are available to treat this condition.

Astringent:
Astringent

COMMON DRUGS

Aluminum acetate Potassium permanganate Silver nitrate Zinc sulfate

A substance that causes tissue to dry and shrink by reducing its ability to absorb water. Astringents are widely used in *antiperspirants* and skin tonics. They are also used to promote healing of broken or inflamed skin. Astringent drugs are used to treat *otitis externa* (inflammation of the ear canal) and watering of the eye due to minor irritation. Astringents may cause burning or stinging when applied.

Astrocytoma
A type of malignant *brain tumor*. Astrocytomas are the most common type of *glioma*, a tumor arising from the glial (supporting) cells within the nervous system, and are composed of cells called astrocytes.

Astrocytomas most commonly develop within the cerebrum (the main mass of the brain). Although all types are very serious, they are classified in four grades (I through IV) according to their rate of growth and malignancy. A grade I astrocytoma is a slow-growing tumor that may spread widely throughout the brain but may be present for many years before causing symptoms. A grade IV astrocytoma is a very fast-growing tumor that causes rapid development of disabling symptoms.

Symptoms are similar to those seen with other types of brain tumor. Diagnosis is made after the physician performs a history, physical examination, *CT scanning* or *MRI* and, often, *angiography*. Few astrocytomas can be completely surgically removed.

Asylum
An outdated term for an institution that provides care for those who are mentally ill.

Asymptomatic
A medical term that means without *symptoms*—those indications of illness noticed by the patient (as distinct from *signs*, which are observed by the physician). Examples of conditions that may be asymptomatic include *hypertension* (high blood pressure), which is usually discovered during a routine blood pressure test, and *diabetes mellitus*, which is often diagnosed from a blood or urine test. Most disorders are asymptomatic in their early stages. In the case of cancer, much effort has been made to devise screening tests to detect tumors at the asymptomatic stage.

Asystole
A term meaning absence of the heart beat (see *Cardiac arrest*).

Ataxia
Incoordination and clumsiness, affecting balance and gait, limb or eye movements, and/or speech.
CAUSES
Ataxia may be caused by damage to the *cerebellum* (part of the brain concerned with coordination) or to the nerve pathways that carry information to and from the cerebellum.

Possible causes include injury to the brain or to the spinal cord. In adults, ataxia may be caused by drug or alcohol intoxication (the most common cause), by a *stroke* or *brain tumor* affecting the cerebellum or brain stem, by a disease of the balance organ in the ear, or by *multiple sclerosis* or other types of nervous system degeneration. In rare cases, it is a result of untreated *syphilis*. In children, causes of ataxia include acute infection, brain tumors, and the inherited condition *Friedreich's ataxia*.

SYMPTOMS

Symptoms depend on the site of damage within the nervous system, although an awkward gait is common to most forms. The typical ataxic gait is lurching and unsteady, like a drunk, with the feet widely placed. If the damage is to nerves that carry sensory information from joints and muscles to the cerebellum, sensory ataxia results. In such cases, the person's unsteadiness is much worse when the eyes are closed. Damage to parts of the brain stem concerned with the control of eye movements often cause *nystagmus* (jerky eye movements).

Damage to the cerebellum itself usually causes *dysarthria* (slurred speech) as well as an unsteady gait. Sometimes, if damage is confined to one side of the cerebellum, incoordination is confined to the limbs on the same side and is often accompanied by a tremor in the limbs during purposeful movements. When walking, the person often has a tendency to veer or fall toward the affected side. Other features may include decomposition of complex actions into their component parts, producing jerky, puppetlike movements, and "overshoot" when attempts are made to touch or pick up objects.

DIAGNOSIS AND TREATMENT

Discovery of the cause of ataxia may be helped by *CT scanning* or *MRI*. Treatment depends on the cause.

Atelectasis

Collapse of part or all of a lung caused by obstruction of the bronchus (the main air passage through the lung) or the bronchioles (smaller air passages). When this happens, air already in the lung cannot be breathed out and, instead, is absorbed into the blood, leading to the collapse of all or part of the lung. After collapsing, the lung loses its elasticity and cannot take in air; consequently, the blood passing through it can no longer absorb oxygen or dispose of carbon dioxide.

In an adult, atelectasis is usually not life-threatening, since unaffected parts of the lung (or, if the whole lung has collapsed, the other lung) expand to compensate for the loss of function in the collapsed area. However, when a lung collapses in a newborn baby—as the result of mucus blocking the bronchus—the baby's life is at risk. (For lung collapse caused by a perforation in the pleura, the outer covering of the lung, see *Pneumothorax*.)

CAUSES AND INCIDENCE

The bronchus is usually obstructed by one of four mechanisms. First, secretions of mucus in the bronchus or bronchioles may accumulate and cause blockage. This can happen after an abdominal or chest operation that has made the dispersal of mucus by coughing difficult due to pain; as a possible complication of general anesthesia; in a baby at birth; in *asthma*; or in certain infections, such as *pertussis* (whooping cough) in children or chronic *bronchitis* in adults.

Second, an accidentally inhaled *foreign body*, such as a peanut, may stick in the bronchus; this is more common in children than in adults. Third, a benign or malignant *tumor* in the lung may press on the bronchus. Fourth, enlarged lymph glands (which occur in *tuberculosis*, other lung infections, or some forms of *cancer*) may exert pressure on the airway.

SYMPTOMS, DIAGNOSIS, AND TREATMENT

The main symptom is breathing difficulty. There may also be a cough and chest pain, depending on the underlying cause.

The condition is diagnosed when the physician carefully examines the chest and takes *chest X rays*. Treatment is directed to deal with the cause of the blockage. If the cause is an accumulation of mucus, chest clapping, deep breathing, coughing, and *postural drainage* will be used.

Once the obstruction has been removed, the collapsed lung usually reinflates gradually, although some areas of it may be permanently damaged or scarred.

Atenolol

A *beta-blocker* commonly used in the treatment of *hypertension* (high blood pressure), *angina pectoris* (chest pain due to impaired blood supply to heart muscle), and certain types of *arrhythmia* (irregular heart beat).

Atheroma

Fatty deposits on the inner lining of an artery that can cause *atherosclerosis*.

Atherosclerosis

A disease of the arterial wall in which the inner layer thickens, causing narrowing of the channel and thus impairing blood flow.

The narrowing is due to the formation of *plaques* (raised patches) in the inner lining of the arteries. These plaques consist of low-density lipoproteins (see *Fats and oils*), decaying muscle cells, fibrous tissue, clumps of blood platelets, *cholesterol*, and sometimes calcium; they tend to form in regions of turbulent blood flow and are found most often in people with high concentrations of cholesterol in the bloodstream. The number and thickness of plaques increase with age, causing loss of the smooth lining of the blood vessels and encouraging the formation of thrombi (blood clots). Sometimes fragments of thrombi break off and form *emboli*, which travel through the bloodstream and block smaller vessels.

INCIDENCE

Atherosclerosis is responsible for more deaths in the US than any other single condition. Atherosclerotic heart disease involving the coronary arteries is the most common single cause of death, accounting for one third of all deaths (see *Coronary heart disease*); atherosclerotic interference with blood supply to the brain (causing stroke) is the third most common cause of death after cancer. Atherosclerosis also causes a great deal of serious illness by reducing the blood flow in other major arteries, such as those to the kidneys, the legs, and the intestines.

CAUSES

Certain risk factors increase the probability that atherosclerosis will develop. These risk factors are cigarette smoking, *hypertension* (high blood pressure), male gender, obesity, physical inactivity, a high serum cholesterol level, family history of arterial disease, and, possibly, an anxious or aggressive personality.

The risk of atherosclerosis increases with age, probably in part because of the length of time it takes for the plaques to develop. The influence of gender can be illustrated if men are compared with premenopausal women. In the group aged 35 to 44, coronary heart disease kills six times as many men as women.

PREVENTION

Modifications of the risk factors, especially early in adult life, can markedly reduce the probability that atherosclerosis will develop or will at

ARTERIAL DEGENERATION IN ATHEROSCLEROSIS

Atherosclerosis is narrowing of the arteries caused by plaques on their inner linings. These plaques are composed mainly of fats deposited from the bloodstream. They disrupt the normal flow of blood through the affected artery. Men are affected earlier than women because premenopausal women are protected by natural estrogen hormones.

RISK FACTORS

Cigarette smoking

Hypertension

Male gender

Obesity

Physical inactivity

Diabetes mellitus

Heredity

Aggressive personality

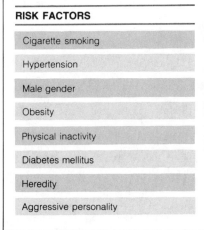

X ray showing atherosclerosis
The leg arteries shown here appear as bright channels. One is narrowed at a point corresponding to the dark gap.

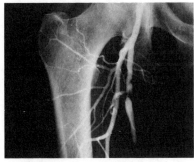

Direction of blood flow

Normal artery

Atheromatous plaque

Atherosclerotic artery
A deposit of atheromatous plaque disrupts normal blood flow through the artery at the point where it branches. This occurs because of the greater level of turbulence in this area.

---

least delay its manifestations. Smoking should be stopped, blood pressure checked regularly, and hypertension treated. Diet should be low in saturated fat and obesity avoided. If cholesterol levels remain high despite diet therapy, drug therapy for this condition may be warranted. Meticulous control of diabetes is important. Regular exercise is of great value in maintaining the health and efficiency of the heart and circulation.

SYMPTOMS
Unfortunately, atherosclerosis produces no symptoms until the damage to the arteries is severe enough to restrict blood flow. Restriction of blood flow to heart muscle due to atherosclerosis can cause *angina pectoris*. Restriction of blood flow to the muscles of the legs causes intermittent *claudication* (pains in the legs brought on by walking and relieved by rest). Narrowing of the arteries supplying blood to the brain may cause *transient ischemic attacks* (symptoms and signs of a *stroke* lasting less than 24 hours) and episodes of dizziness.

DIAGNOSIS
A general medical history and examination will reveal a great deal about the health of the circulation, but special investigation may be necessary. The flow of blood within an artery can be demonstrated by *angiography* (X rays after injection of a radiopaque dye), or, less invasively, by *Doppler* ultrasound velocity detec-

tion, or by *plethysmography* (a technique that produces a tracing of the pulse pattern).

TREATMENT
Medication is unsatisfactory in treating atherosclerosis since the damage has already been done. *Anticoagulant drugs* have been used to try to minimize secondary clotting and embolus formation, but have little or no effect on the progress of the disease. *Vasodilator drugs* are helpful in providing symptom relief but are of no curative value.

Surgical treatment is available for those unresponsive to medical treatment or in certain high-risk situations. Balloon *angioplasty* can open up narrowed vessels and promote an improved blood supply. The blood supply to the heart muscle can be restored by a vein graft bypass (see *Coronary artery bypass*). Large atheromatous and calcified arterial obstruction can be removed by *endarterectomy*, and entire segments of diseased peripheral vessels can be replaced by woven plastic tube grafts (see *Arterial reconstructive surgery*).

Athetosis
A nervous system disorder, characterized by slow, writhing involuntary movements, most often seen in the head, face, neck, and limbs. The movements commonly include facial grimacing, with contortions of the mouth and lips. Often, the person also

has difficulty balancing and walking. In some cases the muscles are abnormally flaccid (floppy), while in others they are spastic (tight).

Very commonly athetosis is combined with *chorea* (involuntary fidgety movements)—a combination called choreoathetosis. Both conditions arise from damage to the *basal ganglia*, clusters of nerve cells deep within the brain that are concerned with the control of movements. Causes include damage to the brain prior to or around the time of birth (see *Cerebral palsy*), *encephalitis* (brain infection), degenerative disorders such as *Huntington's chorea*, or certain drugs such as phenothiazines or levodopa derivatives. If drug treatment is the cause, the abnormal movements may stop when the drug is withdrawn.

Athlete's foot
A common skin condition in which the skin between the toes becomes itchy and sore, may crack and peel away, and occasionally blisters. The fourth and fifth toe webs are most often involved. Athlete's foot is rare in young children and is associated with wearing shoes and sweating; it is rare where most people go barefoot.

CAUSES
Athlete's foot is usually caused by a dermatophyte (fungal) infection called tinea pedis. Secondary infection occurring through skin cracks is bacterial.

TREATMENT
Athlete's foot sometimes clears up without medication. Careful drying of the affected area is necessary; wearing dry cotton socks or sandals may help. Disinfecting the floors of showers and locker rooms helps control the spread of infection.

Most fungal infections respond to treatment with antifungal creams, such as tolnaftate, miconazole, or compound undecylenic acid.

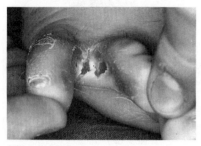

Athlete's foot
The typical appearance shows fissuring in the cleft between the fourth and fifth toes. There is usually an annoying itch.

Atony
Complete loss of tension in a muscle, so that the muscle is completely flaccid (floppy). Atony can occur in some nervous system disorders or after injury to nerves. The arm muscles may become atonic after injury to the *brachial plexus* (nerve roots in the neck passing into the arm).

Atopy
A predisposition to various allergic reactions. Atopic individuals have a tendency to suffer from one or more allergic-based disorders, such as *asthma*, *eczema*, *urticaria* (hives), and allergic *rhinitis* (hay fever).

The mechanism that causes the predisposition is not fully understood, although various theories have been proposed. There is some evidence that atopy may be caused in the first few weeks of life by the absorption into the body of abnormally high levels of *antigens* (substances foreign to the body, capable of becoming allergens). This could be due to a breakdown in the normal mechanisms by which potential allergens are prevented from penetrating surfaces, such as the lining of the intestines or the airways in the lungs; or it could be due to excessively high exposure to potential allergens—babies born during the grass pollen and house-dust mite seasons are more likely than the average person to become atopic.

There is also a distinct genetic, or inherited (familial), basis to atopy—the relatives of atopic individuals are much more likely than the average person to be atopic (even after allowance is made for bias caused by similarities of environment).

ATP
The abbreviation for adenosine triphosphate, the chief energy-carrying chemical in the body. (See also *ADP; Metabolism.*)

Atresia
The absence or closure of a body opening or canal, present at birth and caused by a failure of development while in the uterus. Examples are *biliary atresia*, in which the bile ducts between the liver and duodenum are absent; *esophageal atresia*, in which the esophagus comes to a dead end; pulmonary atresia, in which the pulmonary artery between the right side of the heart and the lungs is closed off; and anal atresia, in which the anal canal is narrowed and shut off. Most forms of atresia require surgical correction early in life.

Atrial fibrillation
A type of irregular heart beat (see *Arrhythmia, cardiac*) in which the atria (upper chambers of the heart) beat irregularly and very rapidly (300 to 500 beats per minute). Not all these beats pass through the atrioventricular node (the impulse carrier between the atria and the ventricles, the lower chambers of the heart). As a result, the ventricles beat irregularly at a rate of 80 to 160 beats per minute.

CAUSES
Atrial fibrillation can occur in almost any form of long-standing heart disease in which there is enlargement of the atria. It is common in rheumatic heart disease (see *Rheumatic fever*), *thyrotoxicosis*, and atherosclerotic heart disease.

SYMPTOMS AND SIGNS
Sudden onset of atrial fibrillation can cause *palpitations* (awareness of fast heart beat) or *angina pectoris* (chest pain due to reduced blood supply). The inefficient pumping action of the heart in *heart failure* can reduce the output of blood into the circulation by as much as 30 percent. *Embolism*, in which blood clots in the atria enter the bloodstream and become lodged in an artery, can occur. This is most serious when it affects the main artery to the lungs (*pulmonary embolism*) or an artery in the brain (*stroke*).

DIAGNOSIS
The pulse is irregular in rate and strength and does not correspond with the heart rate; many heart beats that can be heard when the chest is listened to fail to reach the wrist because the heart has contracted prematurely when only partly filled. The diagnosis of atrial fibrillation is confirmed by an *ECG*, which shows the electrical activity within the heart.

TREATMENT
The first step usually is to control the heart rate by giving *digoxin* or, in certain instances, intravenous verapamil. If the fibrillation is of recent onset, treatment is directed at remedying the cause—for example, removal of the thyroid or drug treatment for thyrotoxicosis, or replacement of heart valves damaged by rheumatic heart disease. When recent onset atrial fibrillation persists, it can often be reversed by *defibrillation* (a short electrical shock applied to the heart).

If atrial fibrillation is long-standing, or is combined with severe heart disease, the likelihood of reversing it is small. In this case, control of the heart rate with digoxin is continued and *beta-blockers* are sometimes also used. *Anticoagulant drugs* may also be given to reduce the risk of embolism.

Atrial flutter
A type of irregular heart beat (see *Arrhythmia, cardiac*) in which the atria (upper chambers of the heart) beat very rapidly at 200 to 400 beats per minute. At these rates the atrioventricular node, the conducting mechanism between the atria and the ventricles (lower chambers of the heart), is unable to respond to every beat. As a result, the ventricles beat only once to every two, three, or four beats of the atria. The condition generally occurs in people over 40 who have severe heart disease.

Some people with atrial flutter have no symptoms; others may complain of palpitations (an awareness of a fast heart beat). The condition can lead to *heart failure* (reduced pumping action of the heart) or *angina pectoris* (chest pain due to reduced blood supply).

When treatment is urgent, *defibrillation* (electric shocks delivered to the heart) is effective. For nonurgent treatment, digoxin may be prescribed by the physician.

Atrial natriuretic peptide
A substance produced in the muscular wall of the atria (upper chambers of the heart). It is released into the

bloodstream in response to an increase in atrial muscle tension caused, for example, by *heart failure* (reduced pumping action of the heart) or by some types of *hypertension* (high blood pressure).

The chemical increases the amount of sodium excreted in the urine; sodium draws water out with it, decreasing the volume of water in the circulation and helping to lower the blood pressure. Atrial natriuretic protein also lowers the blood pressure by causing blood vessels to dilate (widen) so that blood can flow more easily.

Children with congenital heart disorders causing heart failure (see *Heart disease, congenital*) have high levels of atrial natriuretic peptide. These levels fall after successful surgery to correct the abnormality.

Atrium

Either of the two (right and left) upper chambers of the *heart*.

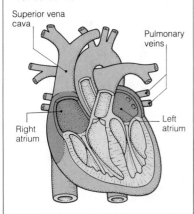

ANATOMY OF THE ATRIUM
The left atrium receives oxygenated blood from the pulmonary veins; the right atrium receives deoxygenated blood from the venae cavae.

Superior vena cava
Pulmonary veins
Right atrium
Left atrium

Atrophy

Shrinkage or wasting away of a tissue or organ due to a reduction in the size or number of its cells. Atrophy is commonly caused by disuse (such as when a limb has been immobilized in a plaster cast) or by inadequate cell nutrition due to poor blood circulation. Atrophy may also occur during prolonged serious illness, when the body needs to use up the protein reserves in the muscles. Other, less common, causes include nerve damage that partly or completely immobilizes part of the

body, and lack of a specific *enzyme* or *hormone* that stimulates growth of a cell or an organ.

Atropine

ANTICHOLINERGIC				
Tablet	Liquid	Injection	Ointment	Eye drops

Prescription needed
Available as generic

A drug used to treat *uveitis* (inflammation of the iris) and *corneal ulcer*. Atropine is also used in young children to dilate (widen) the pupil of the eye for examination.

It is given as a *premedication* before general *anesthesia* to reduce secretion from the lungs and is also used as an emergency treatment for bradycardia (abnormally slow heart beat).

Combined with an *antibacterial drug* and an *analgesic* (painkiller), atropine is occasionally prescribed for antispasmodic effects to relieve the symptoms of *urinary tract infection*.

POSSIBLE ADVERSE EFFECTS
Adverse effects include dry mouth, blurred vision, abnormal retention of urine, and, in the elderly, confusion. Atropine eye drops are rarely given to adults because they cause disturbance of vision lasting two to three weeks and may precipitate acute glaucoma in a susceptible person.

Attachment

An affectionate bond between individuals, especially between parent and child (see *Bonding*), or between a person and an object, as in the case of young children and security objects such as a blanket or a doll. The attachment gives emotional satisfaction.

The term attachment is also used to note the joining of a muscle or tendon to a bone.

Attending physician

A hospital term that refers to the physician who has the principal responsibility and authority for the care of a patient who has been admitted. Residents, who may perform a number of procedures necessary for the patient's care, do so under the direction and supervision of the attending physician.

Audiogram

A graph produced as a result of certain *hearing tests* that shows at what level of intensity (loudness) an individual can hear sounds of different frequencies.

Audiologist

A specialist in defining and treating hearing and speech-related problems. Audiologists are not physicians and thus cannot treat infections or other diseases. They conduct *hearing tests* to determine the degree of damage done to the hearing ability by injury or disease. Audiologists also can recommend *hearing aids* and train people to overcome problems related to hearing loss or speech impediments. Audiologists often test and work with children in schools.

Audiology

The study of hearing, especially of impaired hearing that cannot be corrected by drugs or surgery.

Audiometry

Measurement of the sense of hearing. The term often refers to specific *hearing tests* in which a machine is used to electronically produce sounds of a defined intensity (loudness) and frequency (pitch) and in which the hearing in each ear is measured over the full range of normally audible sounds.

Auditory nerve

Also called the acoustic nerve, the part of the *vestibulocochlear nerve* (the eighth *cranial nerve*) concerned with the sense of hearing.

Aura

A peculiar "warning" sensation that precedes or marks the onset of a *migraine* attack or a seizure in a person suffering from *epilepsy*.

An epileptic aura may be a distorted perception, such as a hallucinatory sound or smell, or a sensation of movement in part of the body. One type of attack (in people with temporal lobe epilepsy) is often preceded by a vague feeling of discomfort in the upper abdomen, sometimes accompanied by borborygmi (rumbling, gurgling bowel sounds) and followed by a sensation of fullness in the head.

A migraine attack may be preceded by a feeling of elation, unusual well-being, excessive energy, or drowsiness. The sufferer recognizes these as warning signs of an attack. Thirst or a craving for sweet foods may develop. An attack of migraine may also be heralded by flashing lights seen before the eyes, blurred or tunnel vision, or difficulty speaking. Weakness, numbness, or tingling of one half of the body may occur. As these symptoms subside, the migraine headache pain begins.

Auranofin

A *gold* preparation used as an *antirheumatic drug* in the treatment of people with *rheumatoid arthritis*. Auranofin, unlike other gold preparations, is effective when it is taken by mouth.

Auricle

Another name for the *pinna*, the external flap of the ear. The term was also once used as a synonym for *atrium* (one of the two upper chambers of the heart). Small, earlike appendages of the atria are still called auricles.

Auscultation

The procedure of listening to sounds within the body to assess the functioning of an organ or to detect the presence of disease. The sounds are heard through a stethoscope.

To listen to the heart, the physician places the stethoscope at four points on the chest, corresponding to the location of the heart valves. With the patient sitting up, in a semireclining position, or lying on his or her left side, the physician listens for any abnormality in the rate and rhythm of the heart beat and for heart *murmurs* or other abnormal *heart sounds* that may indicate a possible heart defect or *heart valve* disorder.

When listening to the lungs, the physician places the stethoscope on many different areas of the front and back of the chest. The patient breathes normally and then takes deep breaths while the physican compares the sounds of the air movement on the left and right sides. Abnormal sounds, or rales, can indicate *pneumonia*, *bronchitis*, or *pneumothorax*. Additional sounds (called crepitations) which resemble crackling or bubbling, are caused by fluid in the lungs. Wheezing sounds result from spasm of the airways, usually as a result of *asthma*. In *pleurisy*, a scratching sound can be heard, produced by inflamed areas of the lung rubbing together.

The physician also tests for vocal resonance by asking the patient to whisper something. The sound produced is louder if there is pus in the lung (e.g., as a result of pneumonia) because sound is transmitted better through this medium than through normal air-containing lung tissue.

Blood vessels near the skin surface (usually the carotid artery in the neck, abdominal aorta, and renal artery) can be listened to for bruits (sounds made by turbulent or abnormally fast blood circulation). They occur when blood vessels are narrowed by *atheroma* (fatty deposits) or widened (such as by an *aneurysm*), or when heart valves are narrowed or damaged (such as in *endocarditis*).

The abdomen is auscultated for borborygmi (very loud sounds made by the movement of air and fluid in the intestines) and abnormal bowel sounds. The former may have no significance; the latter may indicate *intestinal obstruction*.

PROCEDURE FOR AUSCULTATION

A physician's examination often includes auscultation—listening to sounds within the body using a stethoscope. Some organs make sounds during normal functioning.

Examples are the movement of fluid through the stomach and intestine, the opening and closing of heart valves, and the flow of air through the lungs and airways. However, the presence of abnormal sounds usually indicates disease of that tissue. The obstetrician listens to the baby's heart beat as part of routine examination during pregnancy.

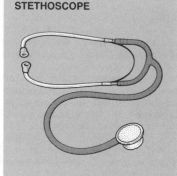

STETHOSCOPE

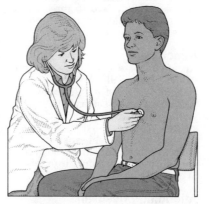

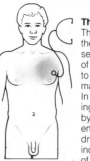

The heart
The stethoscope is usually placed at four places on the chest overlying the sites of the heart valves. The physician listens for the presence of murmurs, clicks, and extra heart sounds that indicate disease of a heart valve.

Using a stethoscope
The end is held against the skin. The diaphragm picks up most noises, while the bell detects quiet, deep noises.

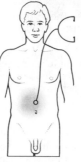

Carotid artery and abdominal aorta
The physician may listen to the flow of blood through a blood vessel that passes just beneath the skin. The presence of a bruit usually indicates abnormal narrowing or widening of an artery.

The abdomen
The physician may listen to the abdomen for the sounds made by movement of fluid through the intestine. A disorder of the intestine may cause these sounds to be absent, abnormal, or very loud.

The lungs
The physician places the stethoscope over several different areas of the chest and back to listen to sounds made during breathing. In addition to comparing the sounds made by each lung, the presence of crackles and dry or moist wheezes indicates various types of lung disease.

Autism

A condition in which children fail to form relationships with others. The term was originally used to describe active withdrawal from relationships, such as occurs in *schizophrenia*, but is not generally used in this sense today.

INCIDENCE

Autism is rare, occurring in about two to four out of every 10,000 children. Nearly three times more boys than girls are affected, and it seems more common among the higher social classes. Autism is by definition evident before the age of 30 months and is usually apparent within the first year of life.

CAUSES

The precise causes of autism are unknown, but evidence points to a physical basis. Because about one quarter of autistic children have signs of a neurological disorder and epileptic seizures develop in nearly one third in adolescence, it is likely that there is a subtle form of brain damage. The earlier theory that a lack of warmth from parents was a cause is now rejected. At the most, parents may react to the stress of coping with a disturbed child.

SYMPTOMS AND SIGNS

Often, autistic children are normal for the first few months of life before becoming increasingly unresponsive to parents or other stimuli. The first sign may be resistance to being cuddled, with the child screaming to be put down when picked up, even if hurt or tired.

The child remains aloof from parents and others and fails to form relationships. He or she avoids eye-to-eye contact, prefers to play alone, and is often indifferent to the feelings of others and to social conventions.

Extreme resistance to change of any kind is an important feature. The child reacts with severe tantrums to alteration in routine or interference with activities. Rituals develop in play and often the child becomes attached to unusual objects or collections, or obsessed with one particular topic or idea. This wish for sterile "sameness" makes it very difficult to teach the autistic child new skills.

Delay in speaking is very common. The autistic child lacks the ability to understand or copy speech or gestures and responds to sounds inappropriately. Even when speech is acquired, it is immature, unimaginative in content, and has a robotlike sound. The child often makes up words and echoes what has been said.

There may be other behavioral abnormalities, such as walking on tiptoe, flicking or twiddling fingers for hours on end, rocking, self-injury, sudden screaming fits, and *hyperactivity*. Unusual fears and difficulty learning manual tasks are also common in autistic children.

Despite all these bizarre symptoms, appearance and muscular coordination are normal. Sometimes autistic children have an isolated special skill, such as an outstanding rote memory or musical ability.

TREATMENT

There is no known effective treatment. Special schooling, support and *counseling* for parents and families, and sometimes *behavior therapy* (for example, to reduce violent self-injury) can be helpful. Medication is useful only for specific problems, such as *epilepsy* or *hyperactivity*.

OUTLOOK

Outlook depends on IQ and language ability. Only about one sixth of autistic children can lead any form of independent life; the majority need special care, sometimes in an institution.

Autoclave

Apparatus that produces steam at high pressure within a sealed chamber; the resulting high temperature of the water vapor destroys microorganisms. Autoclaving is used in hospitals as a means of sterilizing surgical equipment (see *Sterilization*).

Autoimmune disorders

Any of numerous disorders, including *rheumatoid arthritis*, insulin-dependent *diabetes mellitus*, and systemic *lupus erythematosus*, caused by a reaction of the individual's *immune system* against the organs or tissues of his or her own body.

The function of the immune system is to respond to invading microorganisms (e.g., bacteria or viruses) by producing antibodies or sensitized lymphocytes (types of white blood cell) that will recognize and destroy the invaders. Autoimmune disorders occur when these reactions unexplainably take place against the body's own cells and tissues, producing a variety of disorders.

The disease-producing processes in autoimmunity are termed *hypersensitivity* reactions; there are a variety of types. Hypersensitivity reactions also occur in *allergy*, which is a related phenomenon. Both are inappropriate responses of the immune system, except that, with allergy, the response is to substances from outside the body. People who have allergies are thought by some to be susceptible to autoimmune disorders.

CAUSES

The immune system normally distinguishes "self" from "nonself." Some lymphocytes are capable of reacting against self, but these lymphocytes are generally suppressed. Autoimmune disorders occur when there is some interruption of the normal control process, allowing lymphocytes to escape from suppression, or when there is an alteration in some body tissue so that it is no longer recognized as "self" and is consequently attacked. The exact mechanisms causing these changes are not fully understood, but bacteria, viruses, and drugs may play a role in triggering an autoimmune process in someone who already has a genetic (inherited) predisposition.

It is speculated that the inflammation (infectious or toxic) initiated by these agents somehow provokes in the body, along with the usual inflammatory response, a "sensitization" to the involved tissues.

TYPES

Autoimmune processes can have various results—for example, slow destruction of a particular type of cell or tissue, stimulation of an organ into excessive growth, or interference in its function. Organs and tissues frequently affected include the endocrine glands (such as the thyroid, pancreas, and adrenal glands), components of the blood (such as the red blood cells), and the connective tissues, skin, muscles, and joints.

Specific autoimmune disorders are frequently classified into organ-specific and non-organ-specific types. In organ-specific disorders, the autoimmune process is directed mainly against one organ. Examples (with the organ affected) include *Hashimoto's thyroiditis* (thyroid gland), pernicious *anemia* (stomach), *Addison's disease* (adrenal glands), and insulin-dependent *diabetes mellitus* (pancreas).

In non-organ-specific disorders, autoimmune activity is widely spread throughout the body. Examples include systemic *lupus erythematosus* (SLE), *rheumatoid arthritis*, and *dermatomyositis*. Some autoimmune diseases fall between the two types. Patients may experience several organ-specific or non-organ-specific diseases simultaneously. However, there is little overlap between the two ends of the spectrum.

A

FUNCTIONS OF THE AUTONOMIC NERVOUS SYSTEM

The autonomic nervous system is responsible for controlling the involuntary body functions, such as sweating, digestion, and heart rate. The system affects smooth muscles, such as those of the airways and the intestines, rather than the striated muscles, which are under the body's voluntary control.

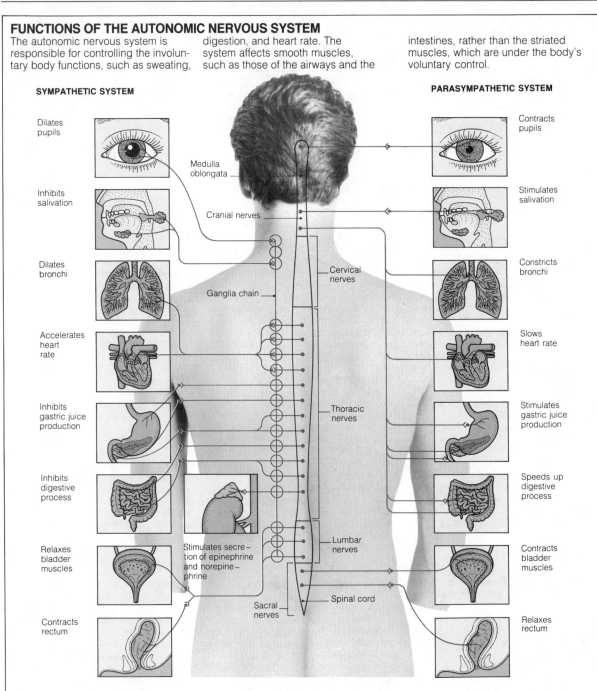

SYMPATHETIC SYSTEM

Dilates pupils

Inhibits salivation

Dilates bronchi

Accelerates heart rate

Inhibits gastric juice production

Inhibits digestive process

Relaxes bladder muscles

Contracts rectum

Medulla oblongata

Cranial nerves

Ganglia chain

Stimulates secretion of epinephrine and norepinephrine

Sacral nerves

Cervical nerves

Thoracic nerves

Lumbar nerves

Spinal cord

PARASYMPATHETIC SYSTEM

Contracts pupils

Stimulates salivation

Constricts bronchi

Slows heart rate

Stimulates gastric juice production

Speeds up digestive process

Contracts bladder muscles

Relaxes rectum

The autonomic nervous system

The autonomic nervous system is divided into two subsidiary systems: the sympathetic nervous system and the parasympathetic nervous system. The sympathetic system is the one that is primarily concerned with preparing the body for action; it dominates at times of stress or excitement. The sympathetic system stimulates functions such as heart rate and sweating, and dilates the blood vessels to the muscles so that more blood is diverted to them. Simultaneously, it subdues the activity of the digestive system. In contrast, the parasympathetic nervous system is concerned mainly with the body's everyday function of excreting waste products; this system dominates during sleep. The parasympathetic system slows the heart rate and stimulates the organs of the digestive tract. Most of the time, activity is balanced between the two systems, with neither dominating. Both of the systems play an important part in sexual arousal and orgasm in both men and women.

TREATMENT

The first principle in treating any autoimmune disorder is to correct any major deficiencies. This may involve replacing hormones, such as thyroxin or insulin, that are not being produced by a gland. Alternatively, it may involve replacing components of the blood by transfusion.

The second principle is to diminish the activity of the immune system; this necessitates a delicate balance, controlling the disorder while maintaining the body's ability to fight disease in general. The drugs most commonly used are *corticosteroid drugs*. More severe cases can be treated with other more powerful *immunosuppressant drugs* such as cyclophosphamide, methotrexate, and azathioprine, but all of these drugs can damage rapidly dividing tissues, such as the bone marrow, and so are used with caution. Drugs that act more specifically on the immune system (for example, by blocking a particular hypersensitivity reaction) are being devised.

Automatism

A state in which behavior is not controlled by the conscious mind. The individual carries out movements and activities without being aware of doing so, and later has no clear memory of what happened. The episodes, which are uncommon, start abruptly and usually last a few seconds or minutes at the most.

Automatisms are the primary symptom of psychomotor *epilepsy*; this diagnosis can be confirmed by *EEG*. Other causes include *dissociative disorders*, *hysteria*, *alcohol intoxication* or *drug abuse*, *brain disorders*, and *hypoglycemia*.

Autonomic nervous system

The part of the *nervous system* that controls the involuntary, seemingly automatic, activities of organs, blood vessels, glands, and a variety of other tissues in the body. The autonomic nervous system consists of a network of nerves divided into two parts: the *sympathetic nervous system* and the *parasympathetic nervous system*.

In general, the sympathetic nervous system heightens activity in the body—quickening the heart beat and breathing rate as if it were preparing the body for a *fight or flight response*. The parasympathetic system has the opposite effect.

The two systems act in conjunction and normally balance each other. However, during exercise or at times of stress or fear, the activity of the sympathetic system predominates, while during sleep the parasympathetic system exerts more control.

SYMPATHETIC NERVOUS SYSTEM

The sympathetic nervous system consists of two chains of nerves that pass from the spinal cord throughout the body to the organs and other structures they control. Into these tissues the nerve endings release the *neurotransmitter* chemicals *epinephrine* and *norepinephrine*. The system also stimulates the release of epinephrine from the adrenal glands into the bloodstream.

Among the most important effects produced by the neurotransmitters of the autonomic system are accelerating and strengthening the heart beat, widening the airways, dilating the blood vessels in muscles and constricting those in the skin and abdominal organs (to increase blood flow through the muscles), decreasing the activity of the digestive system, dilating the pupil of the eye, and producing the contractions in the male urethra by which sperm are ejaculated at orgasm.

PARASYMPATHETIC NERVOUS SYSTEM

The parasympathetic nervous system is composed of one chain of nerves that passes from the brain and another that leaves the lower spinal cord. The nerves are distributed to the same organs and structures that are supplied by the nerves of the sympathetic system. The parasympathetic nerves release the neurotransmitter *acetylcholine*, which has the opposite effects of those produced by epinephrine and norepinephrine. The parasympathetic nervous system also helps to produce and maintain erection of the penis in sexually aroused men.

EFFECT OF DRUGS

Certain disorders can be treated by giving drugs that affect the autonomic nervous system. *Anticholinergic drugs*, for example, block the effect of acetylcholine, which can reduce painful muscle spasms in the intestine. *Beta-blocker drugs* block the action of epinephrine and norepinephrine on the heart and thus slow the rate and force of its beat.

Autopsy

A postmortem examination of the body, sometimes required by statute, sometimes not. In instances of unnatural death or death under suspicious circumstances, states require an autopsy to be performed by the county coroner (not necessarily a physician) or the medical examiner, who is a physician with qualifications in pathology. Some states require a report to the medical examiner in the case of any death occurring outside a hospital. When the cause of death is not suspicious, but when examination of the organs after death will be useful for research or teaching, hospitals and physicians must seek the next-of-kin's permission for an autopsy.

Autosuggestion

Putting oneself into a receptive hypnotic-type state as a means of stimulating the body's ability to help itself. The idea that symptoms could be relieved merely through attitude was put forth by a Frenchman at the end of the nineteenth century. He observed that, if people accepted a physician's suggestion that a treatment would be effective, it was often enough to make it so. It was thought that people could try to make suggestions to themselves with equally effective results.

As an aid to achieving the necessary relaxed state for successful autosuggestion, the repetition of the key phrase "Every day in every way, I am getting better and better" was advocated. Although autosuggestion enjoyed only brief popularity, some techniques used today are based on its premise. For example, in one method used to control anxiety symptoms, people are taught muscular relaxation (biofeedback) techniques and then learn to summon up calming imagery or thoughts.

Aversion therapy

An outdated form of *behavior therapy* in which unpleasant stimuli, such as electric shocks, are applied to suppress unwanted behavior (e.g., alcoholism or drug addiction).

Aviation medicine

The medical specialty concerned with the physiological effects of flight and the causes and treatment of medical problems during air travel. Aviation medicine covers assessment of the fitness of passengers and crew to fly, the management of medical emergencies in the air, the consequences of special types of flight (for example, in helicopters and spacecraft), and the investigation of aircraft accidents.

EFFECTS OF REDUCED OXYGEN

Increasing altitude causes a fall in air pressure and with it a fall in the pressure of oxygen. *Hypoxia* (a seriously reduced oxygen concentra-

A

tion in the blood and tissues) is the single most serious threat to anyone who flies.

In healthy air travelers, the oxygen saturation of the blood falls from nearly 100 percent to about 60 percent at 10,000 feet. To avoid the development of hypoxia, airliners are kept at a pressure equivalent to an altitude of about 6,000 feet during flight, although the cruising altitude may be as high as 39,000 feet (even higher in a Concorde). This means that the cabin pressure is about 30 percent less than at ground level but much higher than the outside pressure. Any sudden failure of the aircraft's pressure hull leads to a rapid fall in cabin pressure, with a risk of hypoxia and *decompression sickness*. Rapid decompression in civil aircraft is extremely rare, but passengers and crew are provided with oxygen masks for use in emergencies while the aircraft descends to a safe altitude.

ANXIETY AND HYPERVENTILATION

Hypoxia or, more commonly, anxiety during flight can lead to *hyperventilation* ("overbreathing"). In this condition, increased breathing efforts lead to excess loss of carbon dioxide, which alters the acidity of the body and gives rise to symptoms such as tingling around the mouth, muscle spasms, and light-headedness. The symptoms of hyperventilation are themselves likely to increase anxiety.

Although flying can be an exhilarating experience, many people are anxious at some stage of a flight; others suffer an acute fear of flying and may need mild preflight sedation. If the symptoms of hyperventilation develop, the treatment is to rebreathe air from a paper bag held over the nose and mouth, which reduces the loss of carbon dioxide.

DECOMPRESSION SICKNESS

Aviators' decompression sickness has the same causes as the condition that affects scuba divers and deep tunnel workers (see *Decompression sickness*). It is not a risk for passengers on normal flights, except when there is a marked, rapid depressurization in the cabin or when a passenger has recently been exposed to pressure changes—in most cases due to scuba diving (which should be avoided in the 24 hours prior to a flight).

PRESSURE EFFECTS ON BODY CAVITIES

The changes in cabin pressure during a flight affect the body's gas-containing cavities, principally the middle ears, facial sinuses, lungs, and intestines. When pressure drops dur-

CONDITIONS AFFECTING PASSENGER SUITABILITY FOR AIR TRAVEL

Conditions	Comments
Have a lung disease (such as chronic bronchitis or emphysema) Have a severe anemia Have a heart condition (such as angina pectoris, heart failure, or recent heart attack)	The lowered cabin pressure (and thus the oxygen level) at higher altitudes aggravates an already impaired ability to oxygenate the blood and/or tissues and may cause severe respiratory distress or collapse. Seek your physician's advice. Flying may be possible if you are able to walk 50 yards without breathlessness or chest pain.
Have had a recent stroke	Seek your physician's advice. You may need to wait some weeks before flying.
Have had recent surgery to inner or middle ear, abdomen, chest, or brain, a recently collapsed lung, or a fractured skull	Seek your physician's advice. You may need to wait before flying to avoid damage to your hearing mechanism or from expansion of gas trapped in the chest, abdomen, or skull.
Are pregnant	No flying after 34 to 36 weeks on most airlines.
Are newborn	An infant should not fly until at least 48 hours old.
Have psychiatric disorders	May need trained escort.
Have an infectious disease, or terminal illness, or are vomiting	May be refused entry to aircraft. Check with airline.

ing ascent, the volume of gas in these cavities expands; on descent, the gas volume decreases as pressure rises.

On ascent, unless there is a catastrophic fall in pressure, air from the lungs is harmlessly released via the windpipe, air in the large intestine and stomach can also escape freely (although trapped gas in the small intestine can give rise to a feeling of fullness), and air in the middle ears and sinuses can leave via ducts linking them to the back of the nose.

It is during descent that pressure changes in the ears and sinuses may fail to keep up with cabin repressurization. Unless preventive measures are taken, this may lead to pain and, rarely, damage (see *Barotrauma*).

ACCELERATION AND DECELERATION

The accelerational forces experienced by civil aircraft passengers are mild, even during takeoff and descent, and no precautions are necessary other than the wearing of a seat belt. Military aircraft pilots, on the other hand, may experience severe accelerations, frequently in an upward direction, and must wear special suits and use a reclined seat to prevent pooling of blood in the feet, which causes immediate loss of consciousness.

OTHER EFFECTS

The problem of *motion sickness* is usually less for air than for road or sea

travelers. Affected passengers may benefit from one of the antimotion sickness preparations available.

Air travel has made possible the rapid crossing of several time zones within a short period. This can affect sleep-waking cycles, causing tiredness and reduced mental performance, often at inconvenient times of the day (see *Jet lag*).

FITNESS TO FLY

Most aircraft passengers are well able to tolerate travel in the comfort of a pressurized cabin. Those with preexisting disorders, however, are advised to seek medical advice before undertaking a journey by air, especially if the condition is likely to be made worse by even the mild hypoxia induced at normal cabin pressures.

AVIATION MEDICINE SPECIALISTS

Most large airlines have a medical department staffed by physicians, trained in aviation medicine, who are responsible for the health care of the airline staff. The physicians also give advice on the transportation of sick passengers, the provision of training and equipment to deal with illness during a flight, and the maintenance of airline hygiene.

Avoidant personality disorder

A term that describes the characteristic behavior of people whose sensitivity to criticism affects their entire lives. Such people see the most innocent behavior as "getting at" them, do not make friends easily, and have a limited social life. They have a very low opinion of themselves, constantly downgrade their personal accomplishments, and easily become anxious and depressed over their supposed shortcomings.

Unlike those with a *schizoid personality disorder*, those with avoidant personality disorder want to have a social life and are often desperate to be loved and accepted. They may also have a form of social *phobia*, avoiding situations in which they might be drawn into relationships with other people and thus risk possible humiliation or rejection.

This disorder usually extends from childhood and is said to be quite common. Long-term *psychotherapy* or *counseling* may help, as does the maturity that comes with age.

Avulsed tooth

A tooth that has become completely dislodged from its socket as the result of an accident. The tooth should be carried to the dentist immediately in a glass of milk or cool water, or in a loosely wrapped, damp cloth. The dentist will reimplant the tooth into the socket as rapidly as possible, and immobilize it with a splint (see *Reimplantation, dental*). If the tooth is reimplanted within 30 minutes of the accident, it will reattach itself to the socket in 90 percent of the cases. After 90 minutes, the success rate falls to about 70 percent.

Avulsion

The tearing away of a body structure from its point of attachment. Avulsion may be due to an injury, such as a severe ankle sprain in which the ligaments on the outside of the ankle are stretched so much that a small fragment of bone is torn from its attachment point to the two bones in the lower leg.

Alternatively, avulsion may be performed deliberately as part of a surgical procedure. In the treatment of *varicose veins*, for example, the stripping of veins from the leg is described as an avulsion.

Axilla

The medical name for the armpit.

Ayurvedism

Asiatic Indian herbal medicine (see *Indian medicine*).

Azatadine

An *antihistamine drug* used in the treatment of *urticaria* (hives) and insect bites to relieve itching, swelling, and redness of the skin. Azatadine is also given to help relieve nasal congestion in allergic *rhinitis* (hay fever).

Possible adverse effects include dry mouth and blurred vision. Azatadine has a strong sedative effect, which may cause drowsiness during the day; it is useful if persistent itching is disturbing sleep at night.

Azathioprine

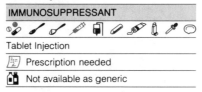

IMMUNOSUPPRESSANT
Tablet   Injection
Prescription needed
Not available as generic

A drug used in the treatment of severe *rheumatoid arthritis* and other *autoimmune disorders* (disorders in which the *immune system* attacks the body's own tissues). Azathioprine is prescribed when other treatments (for example, *corticosteroid drugs* and other *antirheumatic drugs*) fail to slow the progress of the disease or to improve symptoms. Azathioprine is also among the drugs used to prevent the rejection of a transplanted organ (see *Transplant surgery*).

HOW IT WORKS
Azathioprine reduces the efficiency of the body's immune system by preventing lymphocytes (a type of white blood cell) from multiplying. Lymphocytes destroy proteins not normally found in the body and, in autoimmune disorders, attack proteins that the immune system considers to be foreign.

POSSIBLE ADVERSE EFFECTS
Abnormal bleeding and increased susceptibility to infection may occur as a result of reduced blood cell production.

Azoospermia

The absence of sperm from semen; an important cause of *infertility* in males. Azoospermia may be congenital or may develop later in life. The condition is thought to affect about one male in 100.

CAUSES
Congenital azoospermia may be the result of a chromosomal abnormality, such as *Klinefelter's syndrome* (the presence of an extra sex chromosome); failure of the testes to descend into the scrotum; absence of the vas deferens

(the ducts that carry sperm from the testes to the seminal vesicles, the sacs where sperm is stored before ejaculation); or *cystic fibrosis*, a genetic disorder that affects the lungs and pancreas that may also cause defects of the vas deferens. *Orchitis* caused by mumps may result in azoospermia, although, more often, some abnormal sperm persist.

In some males, puberty fails to take place, usually because the pituitary gland produces an insufficient amount of *follicle-stimulating hormone* (FSH), which is necessary for sperm production. In other males, puberty occurs but the testes fail to function properly. This disorder may also cause azoospermia.

The most common cause of azoospermia in later life is *vasectomy*, the sterilization operation in which the vas deferens are cut and tied off. Another cause is blockage of the ducts, which may follow a sexually transmitted disease, tuberculosis, or surgery on the groin (usually performed to repair a hernia or to lower undescended testes in a boy).

Azoospermia can also develop because of a temporary or permanent failure of the testes to produce sperm. This can follow radiation therapy, accidental radiation, treatment with particular drugs (especially anticancer drugs and the antidiarrheal drug sulfasalazine), and prolonged exposure to heat, insecticides, or industrial chemicals. In some cases, production of sperm ceases permanently for no known reason.

DIAGNOSIS
The diagnosis is made by analyzing at least two samples of semen, given a month apart, for the presence of sperm. Other tests are carried out to discover or confirm the cause. Blood samples are analyzed for evidence of chromosomal abnormalities or measured for levels of FSH. A *biopsy* of cells from the testes that gives a normal result indicates that the cause is a blockage; X rays can reveal the site.

TREATMENT AND OUTLOOK
Injections of FSH may cause puberty to develop and surgery can sometimes unblock ducts closed by infection; most other causes of azoospermia are untreatable. Most men with azoospermia who wish to become parents must do so through *artificial insemination* by using donor sperm (AID) or adoption.

AZT

The abbreviation for azidothymidine, the former name for *zidovudine*.

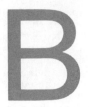

Babesiosis

An infectious disease caused by a parasitic protozoan (a type of single-celled microorganism). The disease is transmitted to humans by the bites of ticks that have picked up the protozoa from infected animals, such as rodents or horses.

Human infection is rare but cases have been reported in Europe and in the offshore islands of New England during the summer months. Avoidance of tick-infested areas and prompt removal of any attached ticks further reduces the already slim chances of infection.

Symptoms include fever and chills and closely resemble those of *malaria* (which is caused by a similar parasite). No specific treatment is available. Most patients recover without treatment, although intensive hospital care may be required in cases where infection is severe.

Babinski's sign

A reflex movement in which the big toe bends upward when the outer edge of the sole of the foot is scratched. Babinski's sign indicates damage or disease of the brain or the spinal cord.

Baby blues

A common name for a mild form of depression that is likely to occur after childbirth. It almost always disappears without treatment, but can develop into a more serious illness. (See *Postpartum depression*.)

Baby Doe case

A celebrated legal case involving the medical care of infants born with severe physical handicaps. In 1983 the Department of Health and Human Services began requiring that the maximum of resources be used to preserve life in such cases.

Traditionally, the decision to preserve the life of the severely handicapped was determined after consultation among the physician, the child's family, and, often, the family minister. Acting as one of the plaintiffs, the AMA prevailed in the Supreme Court in a challenge of the federal government's intervention in such decisions, involving as they do many difficult ethical, moral, and economic considerations.

Bacampicillin

A common penicillin-type antibiotic. (See *Penicillin drugs*.)

Bacilli

Rod-shaped *bacteria*. They are responsible for many diseases, including diphtheria, dysentery, tetanus, and tuberculosis.

Bacitracin

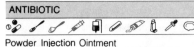

ANTIBIOTIC

Powder Injection Ointment

Ointment available over-the-counter

Available as generic

An *antibacterial drug* active against many of the bacteria that cause skin and eye infections. It is often used in combination with other antibiotics, such as neomycin and polymyxin B, that complement its antibacterial activity.

Bacitracin is usually applied to the skin as a powder or ointment and to the eye in the form of an ointment. It is not absorbed into the bloodstream when taken by mouth and is therefore given by injection when used to treat a severe infection.

Kidney damage is a possible adverse effect and bacitracin is therefore used only for severe infections that have not responded to other more common antibiotics.

Back

The area from the shoulders to the buttocks. The back is supported by the spinal column (see *Spine*), which is bound together by ligaments and supported by muscles that also control posture and movement.

Back disorders

Problems involving the back are numerous. They arise from a number of causes affecting the *spine*, and can involve disorders of bones, muscles, ligaments, tendons, nerves, and joints in the spine. These disorders can cause *back pain* with or without *sciatica*—pain in the buttock and down the back of the leg. (See also *Spine* disorders box.)

Back pain

Most people suffer from back pain at some time in their lives. In many cases it is labeled "nonspecific back pain" and no exact diagnosis is made because the pain resolves with rest and because analgesics (painkillers) are used before any tests such as X rays are performed.

CAUSES

Nonspecific back pain is one of the largest single causes of lost working days through illness in the US. People most likely to suffer from back pain are those whose jobs involve much heavy lifting and carrying, or those who spend long periods sitting in one position or bending awkwardly. Overweight people are also more prone to back pain—their backs carry a heavier load and they tend to have weaker abdominal muscles, which help provide back support.

Nonspecific back pain is thought to be due to a mechanical disorder affecting one or more structures. The disorder may be a ligament strain, a muscle tear, damage to a spinal facet joint, or a *disk prolapse*.

In addition to pain from a damaged structure, spasm of surrounding muscles will cause additional pain and tenderness over a wider area and can cause temporary *scoliosis*.

Abnormalities of a facet joint and disk prolapse can both cause *sciatica* (pain in the buttock and down the back of the leg into the foot), resulting from pressure on a sciatic nerve root as it leaves the spinal cord. Coughing, sneezing, or straining will increase the pain. Pressure on the sciatic nerve can cause "pins and needles" in that leg and weakness in muscles activated by the nerve. Rarely, pain can radiate down the femoral nerve on the front of the thigh.

Osteoarthritis in the joints of the spine can cause persistent back pain. *Ankylosing spondylitis* causes back pain and stiffness with loss of back mobility. *Coccygodynia* (pain and tenderness at the base of the spine) can occur after a fall in which the coccyx has struck the ground, during pregnancy, or for unknown reasons.

Fibrositis is a controversial term used to describe pain and tenderness in muscles usually in the back. It is often worse in cold and damp weather and is occasionally associated with feeling sick. Unlike other causes of back pain, fibrositis is not accompanied by muscle spasm or restriction of back movement. It often responds to nonsteroidal anti-inflammatory drugs.

BACKACHE Pain and/or stiffness in the back that may be continuous or intermittent.

B

Of recent origin

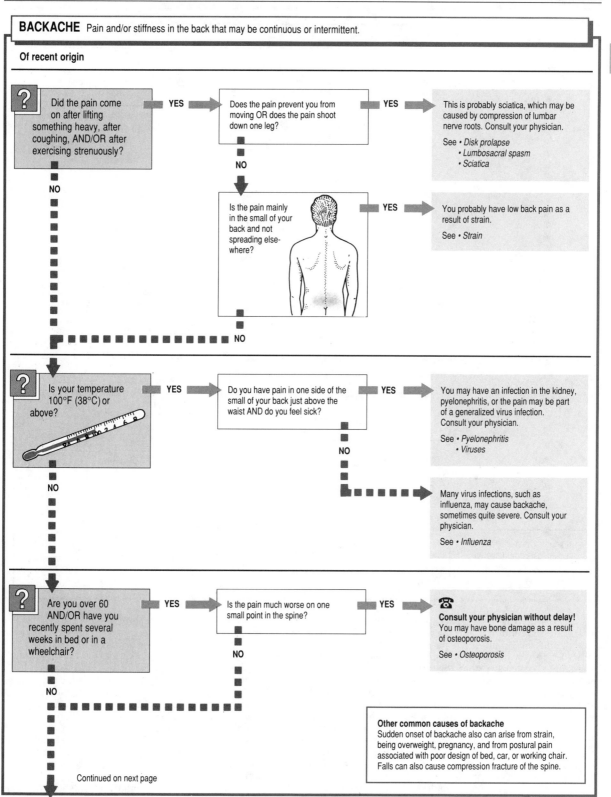

? Did the pain come on after lifting something heavy, after coughing, AND/OR after exercising strenuously? → **YES** → Does the pain prevent you from moving OR does the pain shoot down one leg? → **YES** → This is probably sciatica, which may be caused by compression of lumbar nerve roots. Consult your physician.

See • Disk prolapse
• Lumbosacral spasm
• Sciatica

NO

Is the pain mainly in the small of your back and not spreading elsewhere? → **YES** → You probably have low back pain as a result of strain.

See • Strain

NO

? Is your temperature 100°F (38°C) or above? → **YES** → Do you have pain in one side of the small of your back just above the waist AND do you feel sick? → **YES** → You may have an infection in the kidney, pyelonephritis, or the pain may be part of a generalized virus infection. Consult your physician.

See • Pyelonephritis
• Viruses

NO

Many virus infections, such as influenza, may cause backache, sometimes quite severe. Consult your physician.

See • Influenza

NO

? Are you over 60 AND/OR have you recently spent several weeks in bed or in a wheelchair? → **YES** → Is the pain much worse on one small point in the spine? → **YES** → ☎ **Consult your physician without delay!** You may have bone damage as a result of osteoporosis.

See • Osteoporosis

NO

NO

Other common causes of backache
Sudden onset of backache also can arise from strain, being overweight, pregnancy, and from postural pain associated with poor design of bed, car, or working chair. Falls can also cause compression fracture of the spine.

Continued on next page

B

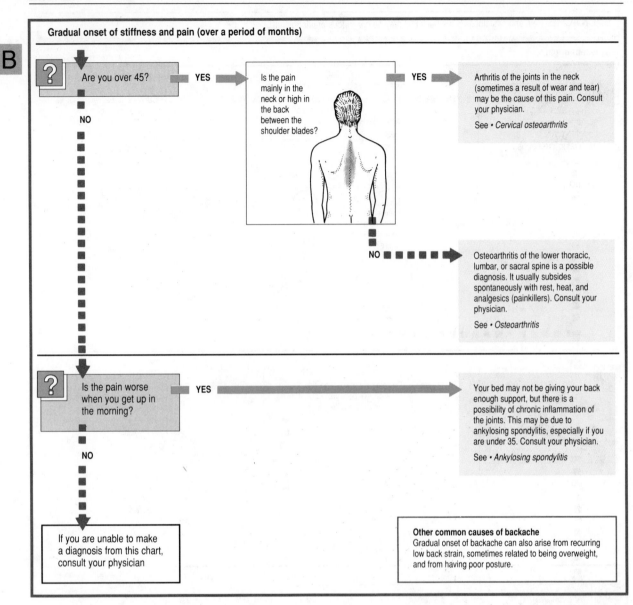

Gradual onset of stiffness and pain (over a period of months)

? Are you over 45? — **YES** →

Is the pain mainly in the neck or high in the back between the shoulder blades?

YES → Arthritis of the joints in the neck (sometimes a result of wear and tear) may be the cause of this pain. Consult your physician.

See • *Cervical osteoarthritis*

NO → Osteoarthritis of the lower thoracic, lumbar, or sacral spine is a possible diagnosis. It usually subsides spontaneously with rest, heat, and analgesics (painkillers). Consult your physician.

See • *Osteoarthritis*

NO

? Is the pain worse when you get up in the morning? — **YES** → Your bed may not be giving your back enough support, but there is a possibility of chronic inflammation of the joints. This may be due to ankylosing spondylitis, especially if you are under 35. Consult your physician.

See • *Ankylosing spondylitis*

NO

If you are unable to make a diagnosis from this chart, consult your physician

Other common causes of backache
Gradual onset of backache can also arise from recurring low back strain, sometimes related to being overweight, and from having poor posture.

Pyelonephritis can cause back pain with pain and tenderness in the loin, fever, chills, and pain when passing urine. Cancer in the spine can cause persistent back pain that disturbs sleep and is unrelieved by rest.

SELF-HELP

Back pain and sciatica may improve by resting in bed on a firm mattress or a board. Analgesics (painkillers) and the application of heat to the back can help the pain. If the pain persists, is very severe, or is associated with weakness in a leg or problems with bladder control, a physician should be consulted without delay.

INVESTIGATION

Examination of the back may show tenderness in specific areas and loss of motion of the back. Weakness or loss of sensation in the legs implies pressure on a nerve root; this requires prompt investigation.

X rays of the spine may show narrowing between the spinal disks, osteoarthritis, osteoporosis, ankylosing spondylitis, compression fracture, stress fracture, bone *metastasis*, or *spondylolisthesis* (displacement of vertebrae). X rays will not reveal ligament, muscle, facet joint, or disk damage. To reveal pressure on a nerve root (for example, due to prolapse of a disk), *myelography*, *CT scanning*, or *MRI* is performed.

TREATMENT

If a specific cause is found for back pain, treatment will be for that cause. Acute, nonspecific back pain is treated with periods of rest and use of analgesic drugs (painkillers). Chronic nonspecific back pain is more difficult to treat. Treatment may include taking aspirinlike medication, *anti-inflammatory drugs*, or *muscle-relaxant drugs*; *acupuncture* or spinal injection; or exercise, spinal *manipulation*, wearing an elastic *brace*, or spinal surgery.

BACK PAIN

Most people experience back pain some time in their lives, but in most cases it is not serious and the problem corrects itself before investigation takes place. However, some kinds of back pain can be related to a specific disorder. In the diagram below, you will find the most common sites affected by back pain.

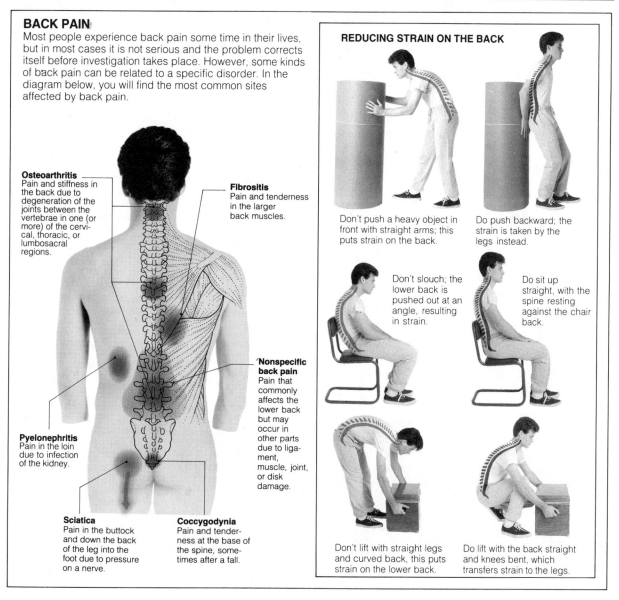

Osteoarthritis
Pain and stiffness in the back due to degeneration of the joints between the vertebrae in one (or more) of the cervical, thoracic, or lumbosacral regions.

Fibrositis
Pain and tenderness in the larger back muscles.

Pyelonephritis
Pain in the loin due to infection of the kidney.

Nonspecific back pain
Pain that commonly affects the lower back but may occur in other parts due to ligament, muscle, joint, or disk damage.

Sciatica
Pain in the buttock and down the back of the leg into the foot due to pressure on a nerve.

Coccygodynia
Pain and tenderness at the base of the spine, sometimes after a fall.

REDUCING STRAIN ON THE BACK

Don't push a heavy object in front with straight arms; this puts strain on the back.

Do push backward; the strain is taken by the legs instead.

Don't slouch; the lower back is pushed out at an angle, resulting in strain.

Do sit up straight, with the spine resting against the chair back.

Don't lift with straight legs and curved back, this puts strain on the lower back.

Do lift with the back straight and knees bent, which transfers strain to the legs.

Baclofen

MUSCLE RELAXANT

Tablet

Prescription needed

Not available as generic

A *muscle relaxant* that blocks nerve activity in the spinal cord. It relieves muscle spasm and stiffness that have been caused by brain or spinal cord injury, *stroke*, or neurological disorders such as *multiple sclerosis*. Baclofen does not cure the underlying disorder but it allows other treatment to be carried out. Often, it makes walking and performing tasks with the hands easier.

To reduce the risk of side effects such as drowsiness and muscle weakness, the dose is usually increased slowly under medical supervision until the desired effect is achieved.

Bacteremia

The presence of bacteria in the bloodstream. Bacteremia occurs for a few hours after many minor surgical operations and may also occur with infections such as tonsillitis.

In people with abnormal heart valves due to a congenital defect or previous rheumatic fever that has scarred the valves, the bacteria may cause *endocarditis*. Also, if a person's immune system has been weakened by illness or a major operation, bacteremia may lead to *septicemia* and shock.

Bacteria

A group of single-cell *microorganisms*, some of which cause disease. Commonly known as "germs," bacteria have been recognized as a cause of disease for a century now but we still do not fully understand why some

B

people become ill while others remain well when exposed to the same sources of infection. Abundant in the air, soil, and water, most bacteria are harmless to humans. Some, indeed, are beneficial, such as those that live in the intestine and help to break down food. Types of bacteria that cause disease are known as pathogens.

Bacteria were discovered in the seventeenth century, with the introduction of the microscope, but it was not until the mid-nineteenth century that the French chemist Louis Pasteur established beyond doubt that they were the cause of many diseases.

Bacteria are only one of various types of microorganisms that produce disease in man. The others are classified into eight main groups: *viruses, chlamydiae, mycoplasmas, rickettsiae, fungi, protozoa, parasites* (eggs and larvae), and *ectoparasites*.

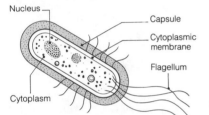

Magnified bacterium
A typical bacterial cell enlarged to approximately 20,000 times its normal size.

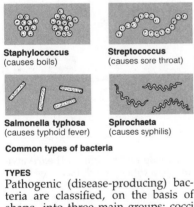

Staphylococcus
(causes boils)

Streptococcus
(causes sore throat)

Salmonella typhosa
(causes typhoid fever)

Spirochaeta
(causes syphilis)

Common types of bacteria

TYPES

Pathogenic (disease-producing) bacteria are classified, on the basis of shape, into three main groups: cocci (spherical), bacilli (rod-shaped), and spirilla (spiral-shaped).

Among the wide range of diseases that are caused by cocci are pneumonia, tonsillitis, bacterial endocarditis, meningitis, toxic shock syndrome, and various conditions affecting the skin.

Bacilli produce diseases that include leprosy, tuberculosis, dysentery (i.e., typhoid, shigellosis, campylobacter,

or salmonellosis), whooping cough, tetanus, diphtheria, legionnaires' disease, and botulism.

The third, and smallest group of bacteria, spirilla, is responsible for syphilis, yaws, leptospirosis, and Lyme disease.

GROWTH, MOVEMENT, REPRODUCTION

The bacteria that colonize the human body thrive in warm, moist conditions. Some are aerobic—that is, they require oxygen to grow and multiply—and so they are most commonly found near the surface, on the skin or in the respiratory system. Anaerobic bacteria thrive where there is no oxygen—deep within tissue, the colon, or deep wounds.

Many bacteria are naturally static and, if they move around the body, do so only on currents of air or fluid. Some, however, such as salmonella (responsible for food poisoning and typhoid) are highly motile, moving through fluid by lashing with their flagella (whiplike, filamentous tails).

Bacteria reproduce by dividing into two cells, which in turn divide, and so on. Under ideal conditions (exactly the right temperature and sufficient nourishment for all cells), this division can take place every 20 minutes, an extremely rapid rate of reproduction. After only six hours one bacterium can have multiplied to more than one quarter of a million. This very rarely happens, however, because ideal conditions rarely occur and in a healthy individual the body's *immune system* destroys the invading bacteria.

As well as dividing, some types of bacteria—such as, for example, clostridia (responsible for botulism, tetanus, pseudomembranous colitis, and anthrax)—also multiply, in a more restricted way, by each producing a spore, a single new bacterium that is protected by a tough membrane and can survive high temperatures, dryness, and lack of nourishment.

HOW BACTERIA ENTER THE BODY

Bacteria can enter through the lungs if droplets breathed, coughed, or sneezed out by an infected person are inhaled. Diseases contracted in this way include tuberculosis, diphtheria, and whooping cough.

The digestive tract can become infected if contaminated food is eaten. Bacteria may be brought to food by flies or by contaminated hands.

Microorganisms that enter the genitourinary system include those causing sexually transmitted diseases (e.g., syphilis, pelvic inflammatory disease, and gonorrhea).

Bacteria penetrate the skin in various ways: through hair follicles, as in boils; through surface cuts or abrasions, as in erysipelas; or through deep wounds, as with tetanus.

HOW BACTERIA CAUSE DISEASE

Bacteria produce poisons that are harmful to human cells. If they are present in sufficient quantity and the affected person is not immune to them, disease results. Some bacteria release poisons known as endotoxins, which can cause fever, hemorrhage, and shock. Others produce exotoxins, which account for the major damage in diseases such as diphtheria, tetanus, and toxic shock syndrome.

RESISTANCE BY THE BODY

The body's first means of preventing invasion by harmful bacteria are the substances hostile to bacteria in the skin, lining of the respiratory tract, digestive tract, and genitourinary system. The eyes are protected by an enzyme in the tears, and the stomach secretes hydrochloric acid, which kills many bacteria in food and water.

If the bacteria break through this defense, two types of white blood cell attack them: neutrophils engulf and destroy many of the bacteria, and lymphocytes produce antibodies against them. The antibodies attack the bacteria directly. After an infection, antibodies remain in the blood for a considerable time—many years in the case of smallpox, rubella (German measles), typhoid, and scarlet fever—so that any further attacks of the disease are usually prevented or are mild.

TREATMENT OF BACTERIAL DISEASE

The response of the immune system to bacterial illness is sometimes enough by itself to bring about recovery, but in many cases medical treatment is necessary. The main form of treatment is *antibiotic drugs*, either by mouth or by injection. Some, such as penicillin, destroy the invading bacteria; others, such as tetracycline, prevent them from multiplying further, permitting the immune system to overcome the invaders.

Some diseases—among them diphtheria, tetanus, botulism, and gas gangrene—are treated by the injection of an antiserum. This is a fluid taken from the blood of a horse (or, less commonly, a person) that has been given a series of immunizing injections and whose blood therefore contains antitoxin against the disease.

Superficial inflammation and infected wounds may be treated with antiseptic solutions.

PREVENTION

Immunity to certain bacterial diseases (for example, diphtheria, typhoid, whooping cough, and tetanus) can be acquired by active *immunization* (injection with weakened or killed forms of the bacteria or their poisons).

People with infections should take steps to prevent their spread; those with respiratory infections should keep away from crowded places to prevent the possibility of droplet infection, and should always use a handkerchief when coughing or sneezing. Food handlers should be meticulous about their health and personal hygiene.

Any wound should be washed with an antiseptic solution to destroy bacteria, and then covered with a clean, dry dressing.

Bactericidal

A substance that kills bacteria. (See *Antibacterial drugs*.)

Bacteriology

In medicine, this is the study of *bacteria* that cause disease. The pioneer of this science was the French chemist Louis Pasteur (1822-1895), who was the first to prove that bacteria are the cause and not the result of illness. He was followed by the German physician Robert Koch (1843-1910), who not only discovered a large number of the bacteria responsible for particular diseases but also laid down the principles for isolating and identifying disease-producing bacteria on which modern bacteriology is based.

METHODS OF IDENTIFYING BACTERIA

To discover which bacterium is causing a disease, it must be isolated. A throat swab or a specimen of urine, feces, blood, spinal fluid, sputum, or pus is first taken from an infected person. This material is then examined by one of three main methods.

STAINING The application of special stains makes it possible to look at and differentiate different bacteria under the microscope. In a sample treated with Gram's stain, for example, staphylococci, the cause of many abscesses as well as toxic shock syndrome, or streptococci would be seen to turn purple, whereas many bacteria, such as salmonella, which causes diarrhea, would turn red.

CULTURE For this method of examination, the sample material is introduced into a nutrient, where the bacteria multiply. Different antibiotics are introduced and their effects studied (see panel).

CULTURING AND TESTING BACTERIA

1 The bacteria are introduced onto a nutrient plate (i.e., agar or blood agar) and incubated at body temperature.

2 Any bacteria present multiply rapidly to form visible colonies that can be studied under the microscope and identified by different patterns of growth.

3 To test sensitivity to specific antibiotics, disks of different antibiotics are placed within the colonies of bacteria.

4 Any clear areas around each disk indicate that the bacteria are being killed by a particular antibiotic.

ANTIBODY TESTING This is done by extracting serum from the blood of an infected person and adding it to a sample of the type of bacteria suspected of causing the infection. If the suspicion is correct, antibodies against the bacteria already present in the serum will visibly clump together with the bacteria in the sample.

Bacteriostatic

A term used to describe a substance that stops the growth or multiplication of bacteria. (See *Antibacterial drugs*.)

Bacteriuria

The presence of bacteria in the urine. A small, harmless number of bacteria may be found in the urine of many healthy people, so bacteriuria is worrisome and of significance only if more than 100,000 colonies are present in each milliliter (1/30 of an ounce) of urine, or 100 bacterial colonies per milliliter if white blood cells (pus cells) are also present. This level of bacteriuria accompanies infection of the bladder, urethra, or kidneys.

Bad breath

See *Halitosis*.

Bagassosis

An occupational disease affecting the lungs of workers who handle paper and other products made from sugarcane bagasse (the fibrous residue of sugarcane after the juice has been extracted). Bagassosis is one cause of an allergic *alveolitis*, a reaction of the lungs to inhaled dust containing fungal spores.

Acute attacks usually develop four to five hours after inhalation of dust. The symptoms may include shortness of breath associated with wheezing, fever, headache, and cough; typically they last no more than 24 hours. Repeated exposure to dust may lead to permanent lung damage, chronic sickness, and weight loss. Bagassosis is a recognized industrial hazard; protective measures taken by industry have now made the disease rare.

Baker's cyst

A collection of fluid that forms a firm, walnut-sized lump behind the knee. The fluid-filled *bursa* (sac) is created by a backward "ballooning out" of the membrane covering the knee joint. Baker's cysts are caused by increased pressure within the knee due to a persistent *effusion* (secretion of fluid)—for example, in a joint affected by *rheumatoid arthritis*.

B

The cyst is usually painless and may remain for months or disappear spontaneously. Occasionally a Baker's cyst may rupture. Fluid then seeps down between the layers of the calf muscles and may cause pain and swelling.

Diagnosis may be assisted by *arthrography* (imaging of the joint with X rays after injection of radiopaque material). Treatment may consist simply of a supportive bandage, although occasionally the cyst requires surgical removal.

Balance

The ability to remain upright and move without falling over. Keeping one's balance is a complex process that relies on a constant flow of information about body position to the brain. Integration of this information and a continual flow of instructions from the brain allow various parts of the body to perform the changes needed to maintain balance.

Information about body position comes from three sources: the eyes (which give visual information about the body's position relative to its surroundings), sensory nerves in the skin, muscles, and joints (called proprioceptors, which provide information about the position and movement of the different parts of the body), and the three semicircular canals of the labyrinth in the inner ear (which detect movements and the speed of head movements). The portion of the brain called the cerebellum collates this information and instructs muscles to contract or relax.

DISORDERS
Various disorders can affect balance, particularly disorders of the inner ear, such as *labyrinthitis* (inflammation of the labyrinth) and *Meniere's disease* (abnormally high pressure of fluid in the labyrinth). In some cases, *otitis media* (inflammation of the middle ear) may also affect the inner ear and disturb balance. These disorders also cause *dizziness* or *vertigo*.

Damage to nerve tracts in the spinal cord, which carry information from proprioceptors, may occur as a result of tabes dorsalis (a complication of *syphilis*), spinal tumors, vascular disorders, or nerve degeneration due to deficiency of vitamin B_{12}. These disorders produce a distinctive, wide-based, clumsy gait.

A tumor or stroke that affects the cerebellum may cause not only clumsiness of the arms and legs, but also speech disorders and other features of impaired muscular coordination.

Balance billing
See *Assignment*.

Balanitis

Inflammation of the glans (head) of the penis and sometimes the foreskin as well. The main symptom is a painful or itchy glans, and the entire area may be red and moist. Causes include infection with bacteria or fungi, injury from a tight foreskin, or irritation by chemicals in clothing or contraceptive cream. Infection may be the result of poor hygiene, but fungal infections such as *candidiasis* (thrush) are usually contracted from a sexual partner. Uncircumcised men are more susceptible than those who are circumcised.

Washing the penis, applying a soothing cream (your physician will recommend one), and taking a course of antibiotics will relieve the symptoms. (See also *Phimosis*.)

Baldness
See *Alopecia*.

Balloon catheter

A type of *catheter* with one or more balloons, which, when inflated, keep the catheter in place or apply pressure on an organ or vessel.

USES
The oldest and simplest type, the Foley catheter, is used to drain the bladder. This catheter is passed into the bladder and water is injected into one channel to inflate the balloon, which prevents the catheter from dropping out of or being pulled out of the urethra. Urine flows out of the bladder through a second channel.

Balloon catheters are infrequently used when a blood vessel has been blocked by an *embolus* (blood clot). The end of the catheter is passed through the clot, the balloon is inflated, and, when the catheter is withdrawn, the balloon pulls the clot out with it. This is called a balloon *embolectomy*.

A type of balloon catheter with a sausage-shaped balloon is used to expand narrow arteries. In many cases this technique, known as balloon *angioplasty*, avoids the need for surgery, although narrowing of the vessel may recur.

Another use of the balloon catheter is to treat bleeding *varices* (enlarged veins in the esophagus or stomach), a life-threatening complication of some kinds of liver disease. The tube is passed down the esophagus and into the stomach, where a balloon at the tip keeps the tube in position. Another balloon higher up the tube is inflated

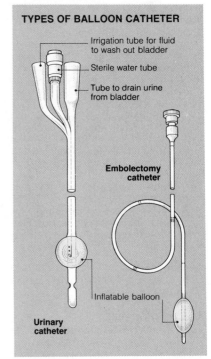

TYPES OF BALLOON CATHETER
Irrigation tube for fluid to wash out bladder
Sterile water tube
Tube to drain urine from bladder
Embolectomy catheter
Inflatable balloon
Urinary catheter

to compress the veins; this usually stops or controls the bleeding until the patient can be prepared for surgery.

Recently, balloons have been developed that can be placed by the catheter into a blood vessel, inflated with a quick-setting durable material, detached, and left in permanent position, thereby completely shutting off blood flow in that vessel. These catheters are used to control bleeding or to starve a tumor of its blood supply.

Balm

A soothing or healing medicine applied to the skin.

Bandage

A strip of fabric used to keep *dressings* in position, to apply pressure, to control bleeding, or to support a *sprain* or strain. Roller bandages are the traditional type of bandage and still the most widely used. Tubular gauze bandages are a newer type that are in many ways quicker and easier to apply than roller bandages. They are, however, more expensive and require a special applicator. Tubular gauze bandages are mainly used for small cuts, grazes, and burns on parts of the body that are awkward to bandage, such as a finger. Triangular bandages are used to make *slings* that support limbs. (See also *Wounds*.)

FIRST AID: APPLYING BANDAGES

TUBULAR BANDAGE

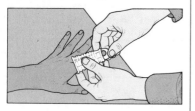

1 Cut a length of tube gauze about two and a half times the length of the finger and put it all onto the applicator. Push the applicator over the finger and hold onto the end of the gauze.

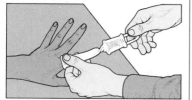

2 Still holding the gauze end on the finger, gently pull back the applicator, leaving the tube of gauze in position. Then twist it once or twice, but not more, or you may impair circulation.

3 Push the applicator back onto the finger; again, hold onto the two gauze ends, then pull it off again leaving two layers in position. Secure the ends of the gauze with tape.

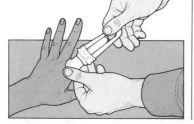

ROLLER BANDAGE

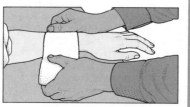

1 Place the end of the bandage on the arm and hold it firmly while you make a straight turn with the rolled end to secure it.

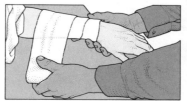

2 Work up the limb, making a series of spiral turns so that each successive turn covers two thirds of the previous one.

3 Complete the bandaging with a straight turn, cut off the spare bandage roll, and secure the end with a safety pin, adhesive tape, or bandage clip.

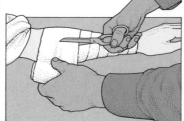

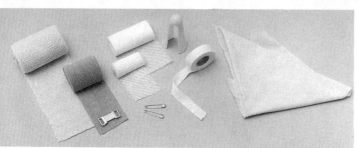

Bandaging equipment
Shown, from top left, are two crepe and two gauze roller bandages, a bandage clip, safety pins, a roll of tubular bandage and applicator, and a triangular bandage.

Barbiturates

COMMON DRUGS

Amobarbital Pentobarbital Phenobarbital Secobarbital Thiopental

> **WARNING**
> Barbiturates may be habit-forming or fatal if taken with large amounts of alcohol.

A group of *sedative drugs* that works by depressing activity within the brain. Barbiturates were formerly in wide use as antianxiety drugs, sleeping drugs, and anticonvulsants. Today, their use is strictly controlled because they are habit-forming and widely abused. Overdosage can be fatal, particularly with alcohol.

WHY THEY ARE USED
Phenobarbital is still often used in the treatment of *epilepsy* (see *Anticonvulsant drugs*), and thiopental remains a drug of choice for inducing anesthesia (see *Anesthetics, general*). However, *benzodiazepines* and other nonbarbiturate drugs have now largely replaced barbiturates in the treatment of sleeplessness and anxiety (see *Sleeping drugs; Antianxiety drugs*). Barbiturates that are used today to treat sleeplessness include amobarbital, pentobarbital, and secobarbital.

HOW THEY WORK
The sedative action of barbiturates is produced by molecules of the drug passing through the membrane walls of the nerve cells within the brain. The drug blocks the conduction of stimulatory chemical signals and reduces the ability of the cells to respond.

Barbiturates, especially phenobarbital, also reduce the sensitivity of brain cells to abnormal electrical activity. This action is beneficial in the treatment of epilepsy because it reduces the likelihood of seizures.

POSSIBLE ADVERSE EFFECTS
Adverse effects include excessive drowsiness, staggering gait, and, in some cases, excitability. The depressant effect on the brain (including suppression of the respiratory center) is dangerously increased by alcohol.

Barbiturates are likely to produce dependence if used for longer than four weeks; withdrawal effects (which may include sleeplessness, twitching, nightmares, and convulsions) may occur when regular treatment is suddenly stopped. Tolerance, in which increasingly large doses are needed to produce the same effect, often develops. (See also *Drug dependence*.)

B

Barium X-ray examinations

A group of procedures used to detect and follow the progress of some diseases of the gastrointestinal tract. Powdered barium sulfate mixed with water is passed into the part of the tract that needs to be examined and *X-ray* pictures of the area are taken. Because barium, a metallic chemical, is impervious to X rays, it provides an image of the tract on the X-ray film.

WHY THEY ARE DONE

Barium X rays are among the studies used to diagnose the cause of pain or difficulty in swallowing, abdominal pain, blood-stained vomit, bleeding from the rectum, a change in bowel habits, persistent diarrhea or con- stipation, and unexplained weight loss. In many instances they have been replaced or supplemented by *endoscopy*. Disorders that can be detected include narrowing or inflam- mation of the esophagus, disorders of the swallowing mechanism, hiatal hernia, stomach and duodenal ulcers and tumors, inflammatory bowel

---

BARIUM X-RAY PROCEDURES

BARIUM SWALLOW, MEAL, AND INTESTINAL FOLLOW-THROUGH

1 No food or drink is permitted for six to nine hours beforehand.

2 At the examina- tion, the patient swallows a glass of barium mixed with a flavored liquid, or is given a piece of bread or a cookie soaked in barium if a disorder of the swallowing mecha- nism is being investigated.

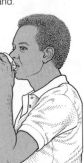

3 The X-ray technician then takes X-ray pictures. For a barium swallow, the patient stands; for a barium meal, the patient lies on the table in different posi- tions; for a barium follow-through, the patient lies on the right side and X rays are taken at intervals until the barium has progressed through the small intestine.

BARIUM SMALL-BOWEL ENEMA

1 No food or drink is permitted for nine hours beforehand.

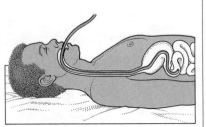

2 At the examination, the patient lies down and the X-ray technician passes a fine tube through the mouth or nose, down through the stomach and duodenum, and into the small intestine.

3 Barium is then passed down the tube directly into the small intestine.

BARIUM ENEMA

1 For successful examination, the large intestine needs to be as empty and clean as possible, since feces can obscure or simulate a polyp or tumor. For this reason the patient's intake of food and fluids is sometimes restricted for a few days before the examination, and laxatives are given.

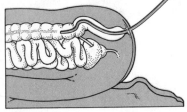

2 The patient is positioned on the X-ray table.

3 The X-ray technician introduces barium into the intestine through a tube inserted in the rectum.

X-RAY TECHNIQUES

There are two different techniques.

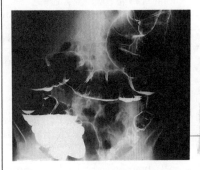

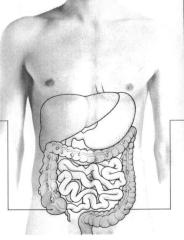

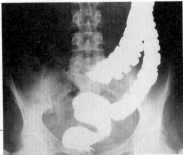

Double-contrast technique
Air, as well as barium liquid, is introduced into the tract. As a result, the barium does not fill the tract but forms only a film on its inner surface. This provides an image of small, surface abnormalities that would not be visible using the single-contrast technique.

Single-contrast technique
The section of intestine is filled with barium liquid, which provides an outline image that shows up prominent abnor- malities.

disease, diverticular disease, Crohn's disease, celiac disease, and colonic tumors and polyps.

HOW THEY ARE DONE

Barium X-ray examinations are generally carried out on an outpatient basis, and no anesthetic is required. A fluorescent screen connected to the X-ray machine enables the radiologist to follow the progress of the barium through the gastrointestinal tract, and to see the abnormalities outlined by the barium. Permanent records of the examination are provided by X-ray photographs or video recordings.

Because barium sulfate liquid dries out as water is absorbed in the colon, it often causes constipation. Patients may therefore need a fiber-rich diet, plenty to drink, and in some cases laxatives to get rid of the chemical.

TYPES OF EXAMINATION

Different types of barium X-ray examination are used to investigate the gastrointestinal tract.

BARIUM SWALLOW, BARIUM MEAL, BARIUM FOLLOW-THROUGH These types are used to investigate disorders of the upper gastrointestinal tract: barium swallow for the esophagus, barium meal for the lower esophagus, stomach, and duodenum, and barium follow-through for the small intestine.

In a barium swallow examination, the patient usually takes in enough air with the barium to facilitate double-contrast imaging. If a double-contrast barium meal examination is required, it is necessary to give carbonated barium, usually with gas-producing tablets or granules. Double-contrast is usually not possible for follow-through as it is too difficult to introduce air into this part of the tract.

Barium swallow and meal take about 10 minutes to perform; follow-through may last up to five hours.

BARIUM SMALL-BOWEL ENEMA Also known as enteroclysis, this single-contrast X-ray technique provides a more detailed examination of the small intestine than the barium follow-through because more barium reaches the area. Sedation may be necessary because the procedure, which takes 20 to 25 minutes, can cause some discomfort.

BARIUM ENEMA This barium technique is used to investigate disorders of the lower gastrointestinal tract: the large intestine and rectum. For a single-contrast image, the large intestine is filled with diluted barium liquid. For a double-contrast examination, a smaller quantity of thicker barium liquid is introduced, followed by air. The whole procedure lasts about 20 minutes, and in most cases causes only mild discomfort.

After the examination, a small amount of barium is expelled from the body immediately, and the rest is excreted later in the feces. (Procedures for all barium X rays are given in the panel, opposite.)

Barotrauma

Damage or pain mainly affecting the middle ear and facial sinuses caused by the effects of a change in atmospheric pressure. Air travelers are the largest group at risk, but scuba divers face similar problems, with an additional risk of damage to the lungs (see *Scuba-diving medicine*).

CAUSE

When an aircraft ascends to cruising height, cabin pressure is usually reduced by about one third. A "popping" sensation may be felt as air, trapped at ground level pressure in the middle ears and sinuses, escapes via the eustachian tubes and sinus ducts (which, respectively, link the middle ears and sinuses to air passages at the back of the throat).

When the aircraft descends, cabin pressure is increased again and becomes greater than the pressure within the ears and sinuses. Some pain may be felt as the eardrum is pushed inward. To ease this, air needs to be reintroduced into the middle ears and sinuses to equalize the internal and external pressures. This can be achieved by vigorous swallowing or an action similar to bearing down with the mouth closed and nose pinched—the Valsalva maneuver.

If the sinus ducts or eustachian tubes are blocked with mucus, as during a head cold, equalizing pressure in this way can be difficult or impossible. Minor damage can occur if equalization is prevented or delayed, or if the Valsalva maneuver is carried out overenthusiastically. The damage usually involves rupture of tiny blood vessels in the walls of the middle ears, or in the membranes lining the inside of the sinuses.

Changes in pressure sufficient to rupture the eardrum are unlikely during ordinary airline flights but may be suffered by scuba divers or high altitude pilots (see *Eardrum, perforated*).

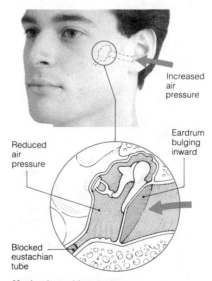

Reduced air pressure

Increased air pressure

Eardrum bulging inward

Blocked eustachian tube

Mechanism of barotrauma
The diagram above shows the location of the middle ear and pressure changes when the eustachian tube is blocked and there is an increase in surrounding air pressure.

PREVENTION

Anyone with a severe head cold should avoid flying if possible. If flying is unavoidable, a decongestant nasal spray should be used shortly before descent. Air travelers should also know how to perform the Valsalva maneuver. Infants should be breast- or bottle-fed during descent; the baby's sucking and swallowing produces the same effect as the Valsalva maneuver.

SYMPTOMS

Pain in the ears, or over the cheekbones and forehead, during aircraft descent is a warning of pressure differences. Minor pressure damage in the middle ear, called barotitis, may cause continued pain, some hearing loss, and *tinnitus* (ringing in the ears) for a few days; pressure damage within the facial sinuses, called barosinusitis, may also cause pain, and possibly a discharge of mucus or blood for a couple of days.

TREATMENT

In most cases, no treatment is necessary and symptoms wear off within hours or days. However, if an infection is present, these symptoms may become aggravated and persist for several days. If sinus pain persists or a discharge from the nose is noticed, suggesting infection, medical advice should be sought. Treatment with antibiotic drugs, decongestant drops or nasal sprays, or sometimes *antral irrigation* may be required. (See also *Ear; Sinus; Aviation medicine*.)

B

Barrier cream

A cream used to protect the skin against the effects of irritant substances and of excessive exposure to water, which may occur when the hands are washed frequently. (See also *Spermicides*.)

Barrier method

Method of preventing pregnancy by blocking the passage of sperm to the woman's uterus. (See *Contraception, barrier methods*.)

Bartholin's glands

A pair of oval, pea-sized glands whose ducts open into the vulva (the folds of flesh that surround the opening of the vagina). During sexual arousal these glands secrete a fluid that lubricates the vulval region.

DISORDERS

Infection of Bartholin's glands causes bartholinitis, in which an intensely painful red swelling forms at the opening of the ducts. Treatment is with antibiotics, analgesics (painkillers), and warm baths.

If the infection develops into an *abscess*, the gland is cut open and drained—an outpatient procedure that requires only a local anesthetic. Should abscesses recur, an operation may be performed either to convert the duct into an open pouch or to remove the gland altogether.

If an infection narrows the duct by scarring, the gland may not be able to empty, and a Bartholin's cyst, a painless swelling of the duct, may form. The cyst may become repeatedly infected, in which case the same treatment as for a recurrent abscess is needed. Even if both are removed or destroyed by infection, the other glands in the vagina are capable of secreting adequate lubricants.

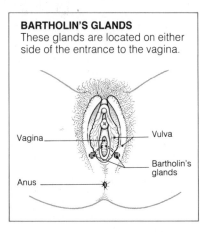

BARTHOLIN'S GLANDS
These glands are located on either side of the entrance to the vagina.

Vagina

Vulva

Bartholin's glands

Anus

Bartonellosis

A disease transmitted by the bite of a sand fly carrying the bacterium *BARTONELLA BACILLIFORMIS*. It is found only on the western slopes of the Andes.

The illness has two distinct forms. The first, Oroya fever, starts about three weeks after the bite and is characterized by fever, anemia, and joint pain. The second, milder form consists of crops of spots on the face and limbs. Treatment with antibiotics rapidly brings about a full recovery.

Avoidance, for travelers to the Andes, is through the use of insect repellents, insecticides, and protective clothing. (See *Insect bites*.)

Basal cell carcinoma

A type of skin cancer that occurs most commonly on the face or neck. The cells of the tumor closely resemble, and are possibly derived from, cells in the basal (innermost) skin layer.

INCIDENCE

Basal cell carcinoma is the most common skin cancer in the US with an overall incidence of about 150 cases per 100,000 population per year.

Fair-skinned persons over 50 are the most commonly affected (dark and black-skinned people are affected only rarely). The incidence also increases significantly in those with outdoor occupations and living in sunny climates—such as Arizona and Texas, or Queensland, Australia, where over half the white population has had a basal cell carcinoma by age 75.

CAUSE

Direct skin damage from ultraviolet radiation contained in sunlight is thought to be the cause in most cases. Dark-skinned people are protected by the higher amounts of the ultraviolet radiation-absorbing pigment, melanin, in their skin.

SYMPTOMS

Over 90 percent of basal cell carcinomas occur on the face, often at the side of an eye or on the nose, but the tumor can appear virtually anywhere on the body. It starts as a small, flat nodule and grows slowly, eventually breaking down at the center to form a shallow ulcer with raised edges.

Unless treated, the growth gradually invades and bites deeper into surrounding tissues.

Fortunately, basal cell carcinomas virtually never metastasize (spread to other parts of the body).

Diagnosis is made by microscopic examination of cells from the tumor.

PREVENTION

Individuals at risk, particularly fair-skinned people, should avoid overexposure to strong sunlight through the use of protective clothing and headgear, and sunscreen containing para-aminobenzoic acid (PABA).

TREATMENT AND OUTLOOK

The tumor can be destroyed by *radiation therapy* or removed by surgical excision, and this usually gives a complete cure. New tumors may, however, develop in people who do not take adequate preventive measures. (See also *Sunlight, adverse effects of; Squamous cell carcinoma; Melanoma, malignant*.)

Basal ganglia

Paired nerve cell clusters in the brain, deep within the *cerebrum* and upper part of the *brain stem*. They play a vital part in producing smooth, continuous muscular actions and in stopping and starting movement.

Disease or degeneration of the basal ganglia and their connections may lead to the appearance of involuntary movements, trembling, and weakness; the best known examples are *Parkinson's disease* and *chorea*.

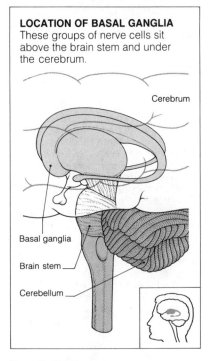

LOCATION OF BASAL GANGLIA
These groups of nerve cells sit above the brain stem and under the cerebrum.

Cerebrum

Basal ganglia

Brain stem

Cerebellum

Baseball elbow

Either of two types of injury to the elbow that can occur as a result of playing baseball.

The first and more common injury is caused by repeated overstraightening of the elbow, either when pitching or batting the ball. This results in damage to the cartilage that lines the joint. Loose flakes of cartilage may then interrupt the free movement of the elbow, friction between exposed areas of bone can cause pain on elbow movement, and the eroded bony surfaces may form into osteophytes (bony spikes) that further disrupt joint movement.

Surgery to remove flakes of cartilage and trim osteophytes can help restore joint movement, but, if the individual continues to play baseball without altering his or her pitching or batting technique, the problems will return.

The second type of injury (an avulsion fracture) results from sudden straightening of the elbow at high speed when pitching. This action can cause a piece of cartilage or bone to be torn off at the point where the tendon of the biceps muscle is attached to the joint. The injury leaves the person with weakness when bending or rotating the elbow. It is treated by stitching the end of the tendon back onto its attachment to the joint. Healing normally takes about four to eight weeks. (See also *Tennis elbow*; *Golfers' elbow*.)

Baseball finger

Injury to the fingertip caused by a heavy blow to the end of the finger that forces the tip from a straight into a bent position. The injury, also called mallet finger, can occur in any sport where a ball (e.g., a baseball, softball, football, or basketball) strikes the finger in this way.

The sudden bending of the extended finger may tear the tendon on the back of the finger, or, if the tendon doesn't "give," pull off a fragment of bone. In either case, the fingertip is left bent. Treatment is with an external splint or the insertion of a temporary wire through the bones to hold the finger straight. The injury heals over a period of two to three months.

Battered baby syndrome

Injuries to a child that suggest repeated physical assault. They often include bruises, burns, and fractures. Usually the full extent of past injuries is apparent only when the child is examined and the complete skeleton is X rayed. (See *Child abuse*.)

B cells

See *Lymphocyte*.

BCG vaccination

A vaccine that provides immunity against *tuberculosis*. BCG is prepared from an artificially weakened strain of bovine (cattle) tubercle bacilli, the microorganisms responsible for the disease. The initials BCG stand for "bacille Calmette-Guérin," after the two Frenchmen who developed the vaccine in 1906.

WHY IT IS DONE

In the US, vaccination is usually given only to people who are likely to be exposed repeatedly to tuberculosis infection and who respond negatively to a tuberculin skin test, showing they have not naturally become immune. BCG vaccination is sometimes recommended shortly after birth—for example, if someone in the family has tuberculosis.

HOW IT IS DONE

The vaccine is usually injected into the upper arm. Six to twelve weeks later a small pustule appears. This normally heals completely, leaving a small scar. The tuberculin skin test is repeated two to three months after vaccination. If it proves negative, the vaccination should be repeated.

An occasional complication is development of a chronic ulcer because the pustule fails to heal.

Beclomethasone

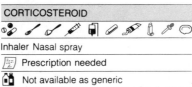

CORTICOSTEROID
Inhaler   Nasal spray
📄 Prescription needed
🔲 Not available as generic

A *corticosteroid drug* prescribed as a nasal spray to relieve the symptoms of allergic *rhinitis* and as an inhaler to treat *asthma*. Beclomethasone controls nasal symptoms by reducing inflammation and mucus production in the nose. In asthma, it helps to reduce wheezing and coughing by reducing inflammation in the bronchi. It also reduces the severity and frequency of asthma attacks. However, once an attack has started, this drug will not help relieve symptoms because it takes several hours to have any effect.

Beclomethasone is given primarily to people whose asthma does not respond to *bronchodilators* alone. Side effects may include hoarseness, throat irritation, and, rarely, fungal infections in the mouth. Irritation may be prevented by thoroughly rinsing the mouth and gargling with water after each inhalation.

Becquerel

See *Radiation* units box.

Bed bath

Method of washing a person who is confined to bed. To give a bed bath, wash and dry a small area at a time.

Bedbug

Flat, wingless, brown insect 0.20 inch (5 mm) long and 0.12 inch (3 mm) wide. Bedbugs live in furniture, especially beds, and floors during the day and emerge at night. They rarely transmit disease but their bites may become infected.

Bedpan

A metal, plastic, or fiber container into which a patient confined in bed can defecate and, if female, urinate. A *urinal* is used for male patients. In the past, bedpans and urinals were used routinely, but today, unless the patient is immobile, the use of the toilet or a bedside *commode* is considered to be less stressful.

Bed rest

A term used to describe periods spent in bed. It may be an essential part of treatment in certain illnesses, such as rheumatic fever, and for some types of injuries, such as a fractured vertebra.

Bed rest may involve various risks for the patient, among them muscle wasting, *bedsores*, weakness, depression, and calcium loss leading to bone demineralization and urinary tract *calculi* (stones). Those recovering from an operation are at special risk of developing deep vein thrombosis and, for the elderly in particular, hypostatic pneumonia is also a threat. To prevent these problems, patients today are encouraged to be physically active while in bed and are made to get out of bed sooner than in the past.

Bedridden

A term describing a person who is unable to leave bed due to illness or injury. Most likely to be confined to bed in this way are the very elderly, the terminally ill, or those paralyzed as the result of an accident.

Beds

Special beds for nursing sick or injured patients, used in hospitals and sometimes in the home.

TYPES

STANDARD HOSPITAL BED This bed is made of metal to allow it to be disinfected, mounted on wheels for

B

ease of movement, jointed to allow tilting in any direction, and adjustable in height. The higher position is used for nursing procedures; the lower position allows the patient to get in and out of bed easily. A firm mattress provides support for the patient during procedures and is generally more comfortable.

TURNING FRAMES These beds, including the Stryker frame and the Foster frame, enable patients with extensive burns, multiple injuries, pelvic and spinal fractures, or spinal cord injuries to be turned with a minimum of handling and without disturbing body alignment. The patient lies prone or supine on a canvas-covered frame. When turning is required, a second canvas is placed on top of the patient, both canvases (with the patient sandwiched between) are rotated through 180 degrees, and the top canvas is then removed.

REVOLVING CIRCULAR BED This bed is used for the same purposes as manual turning frames, but allows the patient to be placed in a variety of sitting or standing positions at any angle between vertical and horizontal. It is particularly useful in patients with spinal cord injury who may develop hypotension (fall in blood pressure) when sitting or placed upright after being immobilized in a horizontal position for a long period. Gradual rehabilitation of patients is also facilitated because they can adjust gradually from lying flat to standing upright, while remaining supported.

AIRBEDS AND WATERBEDS Beds with air- or water-filled mattresses can help prevent bedsores by providing uniform support for the patient's whole body. Airbeds are more commonly used than waterbeds because they are lighter and more comfortable for patients. A modern type of airbed, the ripplebed, has a small motor that alternately fills and empties coils inside the mattress with air, creating a rippling effect. Continuous motion stimulates the patient's circulation, which, it is claimed, helps keep the skin healthy and less prone to sores.

BALKAN FRAME This type of bed is used for the attachment of traction apparatus. It incorporates a hanging bar so that the patient can pull himself or herself up.

Bedsores

Also known as decubitus ulcers or pressure sores, these are ulcers that develop on the skin of patients who are bedridden, unconscious, or

PREVENTING BEDSORES

Once a bedsore has developed it will heal only if pressure on it is minimized, so good nursing care of a bedridden, immobile patient is crucial. The patient's position should be changed at least every two hours and it is important to wash and dry pressure areas carefully, especially if there is incontinence. Barrier creams can be used for additional protection.

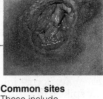

Common sites
These include the shoulders, elbows, lower back, hips and buttocks, knees, ankles, and heels.

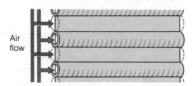

Air flow

Ripple bed mattress
A rippling effect is created by pumping air in and out of the mattress, so stimulating the circulation.

Cushions and pillows
These can be used to relieve pressure by placing them between the knees and under the shoulder.

Sheepskins
A sheepskin under the buttocks and booties under the heels relieve pressure.

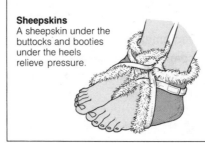

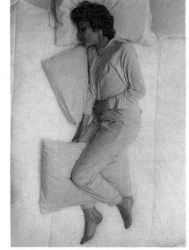

immobile. They commonly affect victims of stroke or spinal cord injuries that result in a loss of sensation. Constantly wet skin, caused by incontinence, may also be a factor.

Bedsores start as red, painful areas that become purple before the skin breaks down, developing into open sores. Once the skin is broken, they often become infected, enlarge, deepen, and are very slow to heal.

TREATMENT
Deep, chronic ulcers may require treatment with antibiotics, packing with plastic foam, and possibly *plastic surgery*. New medications for topical application to the skin are constantly being evaluated.

Bed-wetting

The common name for lack of bladder control at night. (See *Enuresis*.)

Bee stings

See *Insect stings*.

Behavioral problems in children

Behavioral problems are seen occasionally in all children; specialist management is called for when they become frequent and disrupt school and/or family life. Enuresis (bed-wetting), sleep difficulties, tantrums, feeding difficulties, truancy, disobedience, stealing, jealousy, aggressive attitudes toward siblings, and alcohol and drug abuse are all common problems. When a particular form of disturbed behavior continues for a long time or forms part of a larger pattern, it has become a cause for concern. Almost inevitably, however, stressful external events, such as moving, changing schools, peer pressure, birth of a sibling, divorce, remarriage, hospitalization, chronic disease in family or child, unemployment, or death in the family may produce periods of problem behavior.

TYPES OF PROBLEM, BY AGE

Babies up to 18 months	Sleeping and feeding difficulties, colic, crying
Toddlers and small children 1-4 years	Head-banging, tantrums, biting, breath-holding attacks, separation anxiety, poor social interaction, difficulty changing from one activity to another, toilet-training problems
Early childhood 4-8 years	Nail-biting, thumb-sucking, aggression, clinginess, anxiety about illness and death, nightmares, enuresis
Middle childhood/ adolescence 9-18 years	Lying, stealing, smoking, truancy, disobedience, aggression, low achievement in school, drug or alcohol use, running away, sexual promiscuity

MANAGEMENT
BABIES Most problems resolve themselves over a matter of months; your physician will discuss any concerns you may have. (See *Crying in infants*; *Colic, infantile*; *Feeding, infant*.)
TODDLERS Parents need to be realistic and consistent in their expectations, and should provide some room for decision sharing. Toilet-training should be delayed until a child is physically and emotionally ready; separations should be carefully planned. Parents who exercise adequate self-control provide the best model for a toddler. (See *Breath-holding attacks*; *Toilet-training*.)
EARLY CHILDHOOD Parents should reward good behavior rather than punish bad behavior, which tends to exaggerate difficulties or create new ones. Close cooperation is needed between home and playgroup/school because children often exhibit bad behavior in only one place. (See *Enuresis*; *Nightmares*; *Thumb-sucking*.)
MIDDLE CHILDHOOD/ADOLESCENCE Firm, but not punitive, parental treatment can help the child at this stage. If the child's difficulties persist and there are stressful events happening in the

family, this may be a useful time to seek professional advice. Drug or alcohol use (or suspicions of) necessitates immediate medical attention.
OUTLOOK
Parents who find a baby difficult to care for may be better able to cope with an older child. When an older child's behavior is linked to a deterioration in the family situation, improvements can be expected when circumstances improve. Whether family problems persist or are resolved, professional advice should be sought if the child's behavior continues to be difficult. Even when the family situation is satisfactory, worried parents can benefit from the reassurance that professional advice can bring.

Behaviorism
American school of psychology founded by John Broadus Watson, PhD, early this century. He argued that, because behavior, rather than experience, was all that could be observed in others, it should constitute the sole basis of psychology.

Behavior therapy
A collection of techniques for treating mental disorders based on changing abnormal behavior rather than attempting to analyze underlying causes. Behavior therapy can be effective in the treatment of phobic and obsessional disorders and certain kinds of sexual and marital problems. Behavior therapy deals with eliminating the symptom without affecting the underlying psychological cause. Often, it is not the procedure but the unspoken relationship with the therapist performing the behavior modification that is really important.

The concept of behavior modification originated with animal psychologists, but the techniques have been expanded and refined by psychiatrists in the last decade. Treatment relies on two basic ideas: that repetition of a feared experience under safe conditions will render it less threatening, and that desirable behavior can be encouraged by using a system of rewards. Aversion therapy—using punishment to discourage undesirable behavior—was used in the past, particularly in the treatment of alcoholics and drug addicts.
TYPES
EXPOSURE THERAPY Also called desensitization, this consists of exposing the patient in stages to the cause of his or her anxiety. At the same time, the patient is taught to cope

with anxiety symptoms by using relaxation techniques. The intensity of the anxiety-provoking stimulus is gradually increased until the patient is able to deal with the situation.
FLOODING Instead of being introduced to the cause of the phobia in stages, the patient is confronted with the anxiety-provoking stimuli at once, but with the support of the therapist. The patient remains in this situation until the feelings of anxiety eventually disappear.
RESPONSE PREVENTION The patient is prevented from carrying out an obsessional task. This technique is used in combination with other methods.
MODELING The therapist acts as a model for the patient, performing the anxiety-provoking activity first, so that the patient may copy.
HOW IT IS USED
TREATMENT OF PHOBIC DISORDERS This is dependent on exposure therapy. In *agoraphobia* (fear of open spaces), the patient is reassured that he or she can cope outside the house, and then the therapist accompanies him or her on a short journey, providing emotional support. The patient uses relaxation techniques to help cope with anxiety. Gradually, the distance traveled from home is increased, and the therapist withdraws from the treatment as the patient gains confidence.

Flooding techniques are especially useful in treating fears of objects. A patient who is frightened of dogs might be placed in a room with a number of dogs until the fear disappears.
TREATMENT OF OBSESSIONAL RITUALS This consists of three different aspects: prevention, exposure, and modeling. For example, a patient with a hand washing compulsion would be prevented from carrying out the washing rituals. At the same time, exposure to materials that the patient might consider contaminated is encouraged, the therapist acting as a model by touching the "contaminated" objects first.
TREATMENT OF MARITAL AND SEXUAL PROBLEMS This is based on partners rewarding each other for pleasing behavior. (See *Marital counseling*; *Sex therapy*.)

Behçet's syndrome
A rare disorder of which the most frequent symptom is recurrent mouth ulcers, which are more severe than the common (aphthous) ulcers in the mouth. Other major symptoms are ulcers on the genitals, eye inflammation, rashes, arthritis, and venous thrombosis. Less common manifestations include intestinal ulcers, arterial

B

B

aneurysms, epididymo-orchitis, and neuropsychiatric symptoms. Behçet's syndrome was first described by the Turkish dermatologist Hulusi Behçet (1889-1948).

The cause of the disorder is unknown. It is uncommon in the US, but more common in some Middle Eastern countries.

The diagnosis relies on three or more of the major characteristic symptoms being present. Treatment is difficult and may require use of *anticancer drugs* or *corticosteroid drugs*. The condition becomes chronic in many patients.

Belching
The noisy return of air from the stomach through the mouth. Swallowing air is usually a nervous habit of which the person is unaware. It also may be due to eating or drinking too much too quickly.

Each time a person belches, he or she swallows air, which makes further belching more likely. Sometimes, belching helps alleviate discomfort caused by indigestion or acid *dyspepsia*. During pregnancy, belching very briefly helps relieve nausea and heartburn, which disappear following delivery of the baby.

Belladonna

An extract of the deadly nightshade plant, containing *alkaloids* including atropine, which has been used in medicine since ancient times. Women used to apply belladonna to their eyes to dilate the pupils (the name in Italian means beautiful lady). In modern medicine belladonna alkaloids are used as *antispasmodics* in the treatment of gastrointestinal disturbances. (See *Anticholinergic drugs*.)

Bell's palsy
Another name for *facial palsy*.

Bendroflumethiazide
One of the thiazide group of *diuretics* used to treat *hypertension* (high blood pressure) and *heart failure* (reduced pumping efficiency).

Bends
A term popularly applied to all forms of *decompression sickness* suffered by divers who surface too rapidly, or sometimes more specifically to the severe bone and joint pains that are a common symptom.

The origin of the term "bends" is uncertain, but it may have referred to the diver being literally bent double in pain, or to the slight easing of pain achieved by flexing an affected joint.

Benign
The term used to describe a relatively mild form of a disease. More specifically, a benign tumor will not spread throughout the body, whereas a *malignant* tumor may.

Benoxaprofen
A *nonsteroidal anti-inflammatory drug* (NSAID) introduced in the early 1980s. It proved very effective in the treatment of arthritis. Unfortunately, in some users, it caused photosensitization (rash when exposed to sunlight). More seriously, its use was associated with a number of deaths, mainly in the elderly, from liver damage. It was therefore withdrawn from the market.

Benzodiazepine drugs
Among the best-known and most widely prescribed drugs in the world, benzodiazepines are used mainly as *tranquilizers* for the control of symptoms due to *anxiety* or *stress* and as sleeping tablets for *insomnia*.

WHY THEY ARE USED
For the regular treatment of anxiety, benzodiazepines are given for short periods to promote mental and physical relaxation. They reduce feelings of agitation and restlessness, slow mental activity, and relax the muscles.

Most benzodiazepines also have a strong sedative effect and help to relieve *insomnia*. They cause drowsiness and sleep when given in a higher dose than that used to treat anxiety.

Benzodiazepines are used in the management of alcohol withdrawal and in the control of *epilepsy*.

HOW THEY WORK
Benzodiazepines promote sleep and relieve anxiety by depressing brain function. By interfering with chemical activity in the brain and nervous system, they reduce the communication between nerve cells. This leads to a reduction in brain activity, which varies in proportion to the amount of drug taken.

POSSIBLE ADVERSE EFFECTS
Minor adverse effects include daytime drowsiness, dizziness, and forgetfulness. Benzodiazepines may also cause unsteadiness and may slow reactions, thus impairing the ability to drive or operate machinery.

The main risk of benzodiazepines is that regular users may become psychologically and physically dependent on them. For this reason, they are usually given for courses of two to three weeks or less. When benzodiazepines are stopped suddenly, withdrawal symptoms, such as excessive anxiety, nightmares, and restlessness, may occur. When they are taken for longer than two weeks, they are therefore withdrawn gradually under medical supervision.

Benzodiazepines have been abused for their sedative effect and so they are prescribed with caution.

Benzoyl peroxide
An *antiseptic* agent used in the treatment of *acne*.

Bereavement
The death of a loved relative or friend and the emotional reaction following such a loss. A bereaved person's feelings will vary in intensity according to his or her level of maturity and the nature of emotional problems or conflict in the bereaved person prior to the loss. Also involved is the nature and quality of the bereaved person's relationship with the deceased and the kind of relationship they shared before the death. The expression of grief is individual to each person, but there are recognized stages of bereavement, each one characterized by a particular attitude.

STAGES OF BEREAVEMENT
Numbness, hallucinations, and an unwillingness to recognize the death are defense mechanisms against admitting and therefore accepting the loss and associated pain. Numbness is the pervading feeling that enables the bereaved person to get through the funeral arrangements, family gatherings, and applications for pensions and insurances. It can last anywhere from three days to three months. Often, the reality of the death does not penetrate completely at this time, and many people continue to behave as if the dead person were still alive. Hallucinations, too, are a common experience among the recently bereaved. They may consist of a sense of having seen or heard the dead person, or of having been aware of his or her presence. This comforts some people but others find it disturbing.

Depression is a reaction to loss. Once the numbness wears off and the bereaved person can know and feel that a loss has occurred, he or she may be overwhelmed by feelings of anxiety, anger, and despair that can develop into a depressive illness (see *Depression*). Gastrointestinal disturbances and mental disorders are not uncommon, nor is attempted suicide, which is an abnormal expression of grief. An increase in the intake of alcohol, tranquilizers, and other drugs is common, but may cause problems. Insomnia, malaise, agitation, and tearfulness are normal.

ACCEPTANCE Gradually, but usually within two years, the bereaved person adjusts to the loss and begins to make positive plans for the future. This process can involve periods of pain and despair (sometimes mourning occurs in "waves"), alternating with ones of enthusiasm and interest; eventually, positiveness usually triumphs over despair. Research suggests, however, that the death of a spouse may increase the mortality for people in every age group, although there is little consistent information on the length of survival after widowhood. Survival may depend on whether the bereaved can develop or tries to develop other relationships.

SUPPORT AND COUNSELING
Family and friends can often provide the support a bereaved person needs, but sometimes other factors can impede the recovery process. Outside help may be required and may be given by a social worker, health visitor, clergy, or self-help group (the number of self-help groups is increasing in the US). For some people, however, the care of a psychiatrist is necessary when depression, apathy, and lethargy obstruct any chance of recovery. In these cases, specialized *counseling* and *psychotherapy* should be encouraged by family and friends. (See also *Stillbirth*.)

Beriberi
A metabolic disorder resulting from a lack of thiamine (vitamin B_1) in the diet. The illness is seen only in people who are starving or on an extremely restricted diet (such as alcoholics). Breast-fed babies can develop beriberi if their mother's milk is seriously deficient in thiamine as a result of severe dietary restriction.

CAUSES
Thiamine, found in whole-grain cereals, meat, green vegetables, potatoes, and nuts, is essential for the metabolism of carbohydrates. Without it, the brain, nerves, and muscles (including the heart muscle) cannot function properly.

INCIDENCE
Beriberi occurs among underfed populations in developing countries. The illness was once a major problem in the Far East among people subsisting on rice from which the thiamine-rich outer layer had been removed, but improved milling has led to a dramatic decline in the disorder.

In developed countries, the illness is restricted to chronic alcoholics, those living in extreme poverty, and elderly people on a very poor diet.

SYMPTOMS AND SIGNS
Two forms of the illness—"dry" and "wet" beriberi—are recognized. In dry beriberi, the thiamine deficiency mainly affects the nerves and skeletal muscles. Symptoms include numbness, a burning sensation in the legs, and wasting of the muscles. In severe cases, the patient becomes emaciated, virtually paralyzed, and bedridden.

In wet beriberi, the main problem is *heart failure* (inability of the heart to keep up with its task of pumping blood). This in turn leads to congestion of blood in the veins, and *edema* (swelling caused by fluid collection) in the legs and sometimes the trunk and face. Other symptoms include poor appetite, rapid pulse, and breathlessness. As the heart failure worsens, breathing becomes difficult and, without medical treatment, the patient will die.

DIAGNOSIS AND TREATMENT
The diagnosis is usually obvious from the symptoms and environmental factors; it can be confirmed by a test of the thiamine level in the blood.

Treatment consists of thiamine, given orally or by injection, which brings a rapid and complete cure.

Berylliosis
An occupational disease caused by the inhalation of dust or fumes containing beryllium, a metallic element that, with its compounds, is used in high-technology industries, such as nuclear energy, electronics, and aerospace.

Short exposure to high concentrations of beryllium may lead to an episode of severe *pneumonitis* (lung inflammation) characterized by coughing and breathlessness. Exposure over many years to smaller concentrations may lead to more permanent lung and liver damage. The lung changes may lead eventually to severe breathlessness after the slightest exertion.

Treatment with *corticosteroid drugs* can help alleviate the symptoms of berylliosis, but does not alter the course of the illness. The main emphasis is on preventing the disease through adequate protection against beryllium fumes.

Beta-blocker drugs

COMMON DRUGS

Cardioselective
Acebutolol Atenolol Metoprolol

Noncardioselective
Nadolol Oxprenolol Propranolol

WARNING
Do not suddenly stop taking a beta-blocker; a severe recurrence of your previous symptoms and a significant rise in blood pressure may result.

A group of drugs, also known as beta-adrenergic blocking agents, prescribed principally to treat heart disorders. They have been used since the 1960s and, although other, newer drugs have been found to treat many of the conditions for which they are effective, beta-blockers are still prescribed widely today.

WHY THEY ARE USED
Beta-blockers are used in the treatment of *angina pectoris* (chest pain due to a lack of oxygen in the heart muscle), *hypertension* (high blood pressure), and cardiac *arrhythmia* (irregular heart beat). They are sometimes given after a *myocardial infarction* (heart attack) to reduce the likelihood of further damage to the heart muscle.

Beta-blockers may also be given to prevent *migraine* attacks and to reduce the physical symptoms of *anxiety* (such as palpitations, tremor, and excessive sweating). They may be given to control symptoms of *thyrotoxicosis* (overactive thyroid gland). A beta-blocker is sometimes given in the form of eye drops in the treatment of *glaucoma* (raised fluid pressure in the eyeball) to lower the fluid pressure.

HOW THEY WORK
See explanatory box, overleaf.

POSSIBLE ADVERSE EFFECTS
By reducing heart rate and air flow to the lungs, beta-blockers may reduce an individual's capacity for strenuous exercise, although this may not be noticed if physical activity is already limited by heart problems.

Beta-blockers may worsen the symptoms of asthma, bronchitis, or other lung disease. They may also reduce blood flow to the limbs and thus aggravate peripheral vascular disease.

If long-term treatment with beta-blockers is abruptly withdrawn, there may be a sudden severe recurrence of the patient's symptoms and a significant rise in blood pressure. These problems can be avoided by gradually decreasing the dosage.

B

HOW BETA-BLOCKERS WORK

Beta-blockers block beta-receptors—specific sites on body tissues where *neurotransmitters* (chemicals released from nerve endings) bind. There are two types of beta-receptor: beta$_1$-receptors found in heart tissue and beta$_2$-receptors found in the lungs, blood vessels, and other tissues. The neurotransmitter chemicals epinephrine and norepinephrine are released from nerve endings in the *sympathetic nervous system*, the part of the involuntary nervous system that enables the body to deal with stress, anxiety, and exercise. These neurotransmitters bind to beta-receptors to increase the force and speed of the heart beat, to dilate the airways to increase air flow to the lungs, and to dilate blood vessels.

Cardioselective beta-blockers combine predominantly with beta$_1$-receptors; noncardioselective beta-blockers combine with both types.

Beta-blockers slow heart rate and reduce the force of contraction of the heart muscle. These effects can be used to slow a fast heart rate and regulate abnormal rhythms.

Beta-blockers prevent angina pectoris attacks by reducing the work performed by the heart muscle and so the heart's oxygen requirement. High blood pressure is reduced because the rate and force at which the heart pumps blood into the circulation is lowered.

The effect of blocking beta-receptors on tissues elsewhere in the body is to reduce the muscle tremor of anxiety and an overactive thyroid gland. Beta-blockers can help to reduce the frequency of migraine attacks by preventing the dilation of blood vessels surrounding the brain, which is responsible for the headache. In glaucoma they lower pressure in the eye by reducing fluid production in the eyeball.

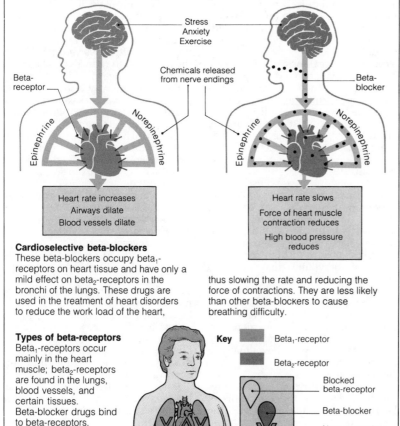

Cardioselective beta-blockers
These beta-blockers occupy beta$_1$-receptors on heart tissue and have only a mild effect on beta$_2$-receptors in the bronchi of the lungs. These drugs are used in the treatment of heart disorders to reduce the work load of the heart,

thus slowing the rate and reducing the force of contractions. They are less likely than other beta-blockers to cause breathing difficulty.

Types of beta-receptors
Beta$_1$-receptors occur mainly in the heart muscle; beta$_2$-receptors are found in the lungs, blood vessels, and certain tissues. Beta-blocker drugs bind to beta-receptors, thereby blocking neurotransmitters.

Key

- Beta$_1$-receptor
- Beta$_2$-receptor
- Blocked beta-receptor
- Beta-blocker
- Neurotransmitter

Betamethasone

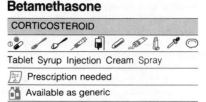

CORTICOSTEROID

Tablet Syrup Injection Cream Spray

Prescription needed

Available as generic

Betamethasone is used in the treatment of inflammation. It is used to treat *eczema* and *psoriasis* and to reduce the severity and frequency of *asthma*. To be effective as a treatment for asthma, it must be inhaled regularly. Betamethasone is also prescribed to treat allergic *rhinitis*.

As a tablet, betamethasone is used to treat severe cases of asthma and *arthritis*. It is also occasionally used to reduce cerebral edema (swelling in the brain) and, in women about to deliver prematurely, to lessen the risk to the baby of developing *respiratory distress syndrome*.

POSSIBLE ADVERSE EFFECTS
Adverse effects are unlikely to occur when betamethasone is inhaled or used as ear drops. This is because the dose that reaches the bloodstream is low. A higher dose may be absorbed when the drug is applied to the skin and for this reason it is only prescribed as a short-term treatment for skin disorders and the user is advised to apply it sparingly. Even when used with caution, betamethasone can cause thinning of the skin. It may also aggravate a skin infection and is therefore sometimes prescribed with an antibiotic if skin infection is present. Taking betamethasone tablets for a prolonged period or in high doses can cause adverse effects typical of other *corticosteroid drugs*.

Bezoar
A ball of food and mucus, vegetable fiber, hair, or other indigestible material, in the stomach. Bezoars are rare in adults except after partial *gastrectomy* (removal of part of the stomach). Trichobezoars (composed of hair) occur in children who nibble at, or pull out and swallow, their hair, or in adult patients who have severe emotional disturbances.

Bezoars can cause loss of appetite, constipation, nausea and vomiting, and abdominal pain. If they pass into the intestines they may cause an obstruction. Bezoars are diagnosed by means of a *barium X-ray examination* or *gastroscopy* (passage of a viewing tube down the digestive tract), and are removed by washing out the stomach (see *Lavage, gastric*), by use of a pincer attachment to the gastroscope, by surgery, or by use of drugs to digest the protein portion of the bezoar.

A low-fiber diet may help prevent recurrent bezoars in affected adults.

Bi-
The prefix meaning two or twice, as in bilateral (two-sided).

Bicarbonate of soda
See *Sodium bicarbonate.*

Biceps muscle
The name, meaning "two heads," given to a muscle originating at one end as two separate parts, which then fuse. The biceps in the upper arm bends the arm and rotates the forearm; the biceps muscle at the back of the thigh bends the leg and extends the thigh.

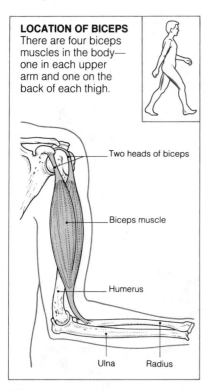

LOCATION OF BICEPS
There are four biceps muscles in the body—one in each upper arm and one on the back of each thigh.

Two heads of biceps

Biceps muscle

Humerus

Ulna   Radius

Bicuspid
The term meaning to have two cusps (curved, pointed structures) used to describe certain *heart valves* and *teeth.*

Bifocal
A term used to describe a lens with two different focal lengths. Glasses with bifocal lenses correct the eyes for both close and distant vision.

Bilateral
Affecting both sides of the body, or affecting both organs if they are paired (e.g., both ears in bilateral deafness).

Bile
A liquid secreted by the liver. It carries away waste products formed in the liver and helps break down fats in the small intestine during digestion.

The main constituents of bile, apart from waste products (such as the pigments *bilirubin* and biliverdin, which give the liquid its greenish-brown color) are *cholesterol* and bile salts. It is the bile salts that aid in the breakdown and absorption of fats.

Bile passes out of the liver via the bile ducts and is then concentrated and stored in the gallbladder until, after a meal, it is expelled and enters the small intestine by way of the common bile duct. Bile is normally excreted from the body in the feces, which it colors dark brown. (See also *Biliary system.*)

Bile duct
Any of the ducts by which bile is carried from the liver, first to the gallbladder and then to the duodenum (the first section of the small intestine).

STRUCTURE
The bile duct system starts as tiny tubular canals called canaliculi that surround the liver cells and collect the bile. Canaliculi join together to form a network of cholangioles of ever-increasing size, which emerge from the liver, on the underside, as the two hepatic ducts.

These ducts join within or just outside the liver to form the common hepatic duct and, shortly after the junction, another duct known as the cystic duct branches off to the gallbladder. This lies in a hollow on the undersurface of the liver. The continuation of the common hepatic duct past the junction with the cystic duct is known as the common bile duct. This leads directly into the duodenum. (See also *Biliary system.*)

Bile duct cancer
See *Cholangiocarcinoma.*

Bile duct obstruction
A blockage or constriction of any of the ducts that carry bile from the liver to the gallbladder and then to the duodenum (see *Biliary system*).

This results in *cholestasis* (accumulation of bile in the liver), and the development of *jaundice* due to accumulation of *bilirubin* in the blood. Prolonged obstruction over many years can lead to secondary *biliary cirrhosis*, a serious type of advanced liver disease.

CAUSES
The bile ducts can become blocked or narrowed for a variety of reasons. *Gallstones* are perhaps the most common cause. They have usually formed in the gallbladder and escaped into the common bile duct.

A tumor of the pancreas can compress the lower end of the common bile duct, and occasionally cancers of other organs may spread to the biliary system and cause obstruction. Cancer of the bile ducts, *cholangiocarcinoma*, is a very rare cause of blockage.

Other causes include trauma, including injury during gallbladder operations, *cholangitis* (inflammation of the bile ducts), and, in the Far East, the entry of various flukes or worms into the ducts.

SYMPTOMS
All patients develop "obstructive" jaundice, characterized by pale-colored feces (due to lack of the normal bilirubin content) and dark urine (excess bilirubin content) as well as the yellow skin coloration. Some patients complain of itching caused by the presence of bile salts in the skin.

Other symptoms depend on the cause of the biliary obstruction—for example, abdominal pain with gallstones or weight loss with many types of cancer.

DIAGNOSIS AND TREATMENT
Liver function tests show any blockage, which can be confirmed by *ultrasound scanning* and *cholangiography* or *ERCP.*

Treatment consists of removing the cause of the obstruction if possible—by surgery or by means of an attachment to an *endoscope* (viewing instrument) passed down the digestive tract and up the common bile duct. When the obstruction is due to cancer too advanced for surgical removal, the obstruction is usually bypassed to relieve the jaundice. A loop of intestine may then be joined to the gallbladder or biliary system above the blockage. Another possibility is to push a tube through the blockage, either from the intestinal side using an endoscope or with catheters from the liver side of the duct under X-ray viewing. The tube is left in place for bile to flow through.

Bilharziasis
An alternative name for the tropical parasitic disease *schistosomiasis.*

Biliary atresia

A rare disorder, present from birth, in which the bile ducts, either outside or inside the liver, fail to develop or have developed abnormally. As a result, bile cannot flow through the ducts to the duodenum (the first part of the small intestine) and becomes trapped in the liver (see *Cholestasis*). Unless treated, secondary *biliary cirrhosis* will develop and may prove fatal.

The main signs of biliary atresia are deepening *jaundice*, which usually appears a few days after birth and persists more than two weeks, together with the passing of dark-colored urine and pale feces.

DIAGNOSIS AND TREATMENT

If biliary atresia is suspected, blood tests and *liver biopsy* (removal and examination of a small sample of the organ) are performed. These tests rule out *hepatitis* or other causes of jaundice in the newborn infant. An operation is then performed to examine the liver and bile ducts directly. If this confirms the diagnosis of biliary atresia, surgery is done to bypass the ducts by joining a loop of small intestine directly to the liver. If the bypass operation fails, or if the jaundice recurs, a *liver transplant* is the only possible treatment.

FUNCTION OF THE BILIARY SYSTEM

The system consists of the bile ducts leading from the liver and gallbladder, the gallbladder itself, and associated structures. The system drains waste products from the liver into the duodenum and aids the process of fat digestion through controlled release of fat-emulsifying agents (contained within bile).

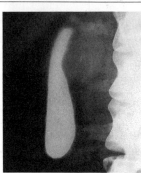

X ray of gallbladder
The image at left shows the pearlike shape of the gallbladder. It was achieved by an X-ray imaging technique called cholecystography.

Liver
Bile is secreted by liver cells and collected in a system of tubes (drainage channels). These tubes carry bile out of the liver via the hepatic ducts.

FAT DIGESTION

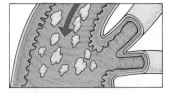

1 Dietary fat passes from the stomach to the duodenum in the form of large droplets.

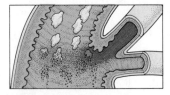

2 Bile released into the duodenum contains salts that disperse the fat into smaller droplets.

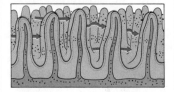

3 The fats are now more easily broken down by an enzyme, lipase, made by the pancreas, and absorbed through the intestinal lining.

Common bile duct
The hepatic ducts join to form a common duct, which leads to the intestine. A side branch, the cystic duct, leads to the gallbladder.

Gallbladder
Bile is concentrated and stored here and released back into the common bile duct when this organ contracts.

Duodenum
When fat from a recent meal arrives in the duodenum, a hormone is released that acts on the gallbladder. The gallbladder contracts, causing bile to be passed into the duodenum to emulsify the fat.

Pancreas
In response to the presence of fat in the duodenum, the pancreas produces hormones that stimulate contraction of the gallbladder and cause the ampulla of Vater to open so that bile flows into the duodenum.

Ampulla of Vater
Bile enters the duodenum here.

Stomach
Fat and other products of digestion pass from the stomach to the duodenum.

Food

Ileum

Biliary cirrhosis

An uncommon variety of liver *cirrhosis* that results from disease or defects of the bile ducts.

There are two types: primary and secondary biliary cirrhosis. Both types are characterized by *cholestasis* (accumulation of bile in the liver), which impairs liver function.

PRIMARY BILIARY CIRRHOSIS

Here, the bile ducts within the liver become inflamed and destroyed. The cause is unknown, but the disease seems to be associated with a malfunction of the *immune system*. Middle-aged women are the group most commonly affected.

The first symptom is itching, followed later by *jaundice*, an enlarged liver, and sometimes abdominal pain, fatty diarrhea, and *xanthomatosis* (the appearance of fatty deposits under the skin). *Osteoporosis* may develop. Over a number of years the patient may develop other symptoms of liver cirrhosis and *liver failure*.

The disease is diagnosed by *liver function tests*, by *liver biopsy*, and by *cholangiography* or *ERCP*. Drug treatment has been aimed mainly at relieving symptoms, such as itching, and minimizing complications. A *liver transplant*, if available, provides the only long-term cure.

SECONDARY BILIARY CIRRHOSIS

This results from prolonged *bile duct obstruction* or *biliary atresia* (absence or abnormality of the bile ducts from birth). The symptoms and signs include abdominal pain and tenderness, liver enlargement, fevers and chills, and sometimes blood abnormalities. Treatment is as for bile duct obstruction or biliary atresia.

Biliary colic

A severe pain in the upper right quadrant of the abdomen usually caused by the gallbladder's attempts to expel *gallstones* or the movement of a stone in the bile ducts. The pain, which is extremely severe and can mimic that of a heart attack, often lasts up to an hour; it may radiate to the right shoulder or penetrate through to the center of the back from the tip of the breastbone. Injections of an analgesic (painkiller) and an *antispasmodic drug* may be given to relieve the colic. Tests such as *cholecystography* or *ultrasound scanning* are usually carried out to determine whether gallstones are definitely present; if they are, *cholecystectomy* (removal of the gallbladder) may be considered.

Biliary system

The organs and ducts by which bile is formed, concentrated, and carried from the liver to the duodenum (the first part of the small intestine). It removes waste products from the liver and carries bile salts, necessary for the breakdown and absorption of fat, to the intestine.

Bile is secreted by the liver cells and collected by a system of tubes that mirror the blood supply to the organ. This network of bile-drainage channels carries the bile out of the liver by way of the hepatic ducts, which join together to form a common duct, running into the duodenum by way of a controlled opening called the ampulla of Vater. Bile does not run directly into the duodenum but is first concentrated and then stored until needed in the gallbladder, a pear-shaped reservoir lying in a hollow under the liver, to which it gains access by way of the cystic duct.

When food is eaten, the presence of fat in the duodenum causes the secretion of a hormone, which opens the ampulla of Vater and causes the gallbladder to contract, squeezing stored bile via the cystic and common bile ducts into the duodenum. Bile salts act to emulsify fat, breaking it down to a kind of milk of microscopic globules, which are easily absorbed in the small intestine.

DISORDERS

The main disorder of the gallbladder is the formation of *gallstones*, which can have multiple complications affecting the entire biliary system (see *Gallbladder* disorders box). The main disorders of the bile ducts are congenital *biliary atresia* (absence or abnormality of the bile ducts from birth) and *bile duct obstruction*, which may itself be caused by gallstones or by other causes, such as cancer. Bile duct obstruction can have important complications affecting the liver.

Biliousness

A term commonly and erroneously used to describe nausea or vomiting. More accurately, biliousness describes a condition in which bitter bile is brought up to the mouth from the stomach.

Bilirubin

The main pigment found in *bile*. It is produced by the breakdown of *hemoglobin*, the red pigment in blood cells. Bilirubin is responsible for the brown color of feces and is the pigment associated with jaundice.

Billings' method

A technique (also called mucus inspection method) in which a woman notes changes in her normal vaginal discharge to predict the time of ovulation for *contraception* or *family planning*.

Billroth's operation

A type of partial *gastrectomy* (surgical removal of the lower part of the stomach) devised by the Viennese surgeon Theodor Billroth. It was the first successful operation on the stomach and is still one of the standard operations today for the treatment of peptic ulcer and certain types of gastric tumor.

Binet's test

The first *intelligence test* that attempted to measure higher mental functions rather than more primitive abilities, such as reaction times. It was devised by Alfred Binet and Theodor Simon for French schoolchildren in 1905.

Binge-purge syndrome

A feature of the psychiatric illness *bulimia*, characterized by the ingestion of large quantities of food and their elimination by induced vomiting or through abuse of laxatives. (See also *Anorexia nervosa*.)

Bio-

A prefix that describes a relationship to life, as in biology, the science of life.

Bioavailability

The amount of a drug that enters the bloodstream and thus reaches the tissues and organs around the body, usually expressed as a percentage of the dose given. In this way, the effectiveness of various means of administration or types of preparation can be compared. For instance, intravenous administration produces 100 percent bioavailability since the drug is injected directly into the bloodstream. Drugs given by mouth have a much lower bioavailability, because only a proportion of the drug can be absorbed through the digestive system; some drugs may be broken down in the liver before reaching the general circulation.

Preparations that have the same bioavailability are said to be "bioequivalent." (See also *Drugs*.)

Biochemistry

A science that studies the chemistry of living organisms, including human beings. The human body is made up of millions of cells that require

B

nutrients and energy, and which grow, multiply, and die. The chemical processes that provide their energy, eliminate their wastes, repair damage, and lead to growth and normal and abnormal cell division are all studied by biochemists.

Life is maintained by a huge number of chemical reactions, which are carried out inside cells and are linked in a complex way. These reactions make up the body's *metabolism*, which has two main aspects. The reactions that produce energy by breaking down food, energy stores, and body structures are known as catabolism. The reactions that build up body structures and energy stores are known as anabolism. These processes are controlled largely by *hormones*—simple chemicals secreted into the bloodstream by the *endocrine glands*—and are actually carried out by *enzymes* (biological catalysts).

Some vital chemical processes occur in every cell in the body; others are confined to specialist organs. (When cells of the same type mass together they form a particular type of *tissue*, which makes up organs such as the heart.) For instance, after digestion, the chemical constituents of food are carried in the portal vein to the liver for storage and chemical manipulation. In addition to regulating the amount of fluid in the body, the kidneys control the amounts of minerals and other basic materials in the blood.

There is a constant interchange between fluids, which move in and out of the cells, and blood and urine. As a consequence, biochemists can learn about the chemical changes going on inside cells from measurements of the various minerals, gases, enzymes, hormones, and proteins contained in blood and urine. Such tests are used to make diagnoses, to screen people for disease, and to monitor the progress of a disease and its treatment. The most important biochemical tests are *blood tests*, such as *liver function tests, kidney function tests,* and parts of *urinalysis.*

Biofeedback training

A technique in which a person uses information about a normally unconscious body function, such as blood pressure, to gain conscious control over that function.

WHY IT IS USED

Biofeedback training may help in the treatment of stress-related conditions, including certain types of hypertension, anxiety, and migraine.

HOW IT IS DONE

The physician connects the patient to a recording instrument that can measure one of the unconscious body activities: blood pressure, pulse rate, body temperature, muscle tension, the amount of sweat on the skin, brain waves, or stomach acidity. The patient receives information (feedback) on the changing levels of these activities from alterations in the instrument's signals—a flashing light, a fluctuating needle, or a sound changing its tone.

After some experience, the person starts to become aware of how he or she is feeling whenever there is a change in the recording instrument's signal. Relaxation techniques may also be used to bring about a change in the signal; the instrument's response may indicate which methods of relaxation are most effective.

With time, the patient learns to change the signals by consciously controlling the body function being tested. Once acquired, control can be exercised without the instrument.

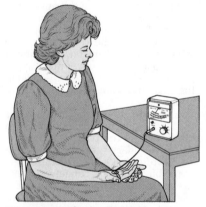

Example of biofeedback training
Here, a patient learns to relax using a device that monitors sweatiness of the palm.

Biomechanical engineering

A discipline that applies engineering principles and methods to the human body to explain how it functions and to treat disorders. Joint movements, the reaction of bone to stress, and the flow of blood are among the body activities that can be looked at in terms of these principles. Practical applications are varied and include the design of artificial joints, renal dialysis machines, and artificial heart valves.

Biopsy

A diagnostic test in which tissue or cells are removed from the body for examination under the microscope.

Most of these procedures are minor and require no sedation, but some require anesthesia. Biopsy is an accurate method of diagnosing many illnesses, including cancer.

The term "biopsy" is also commonly used by the public for the cell or tissue sample itself (although the term "biopsy specimen" is more correct).

WHY IT IS DONE

Microscopic examination of tissue (*histology*) or cells (*cytology*) usually gives a correct diagnosis. Biopsy is valuable for discovering whether a tumor is benign or malignant, since the malignant tumor usually has many features that clearly distinguish it from a benign tumor. In the case of a malignant tumor, biopsies of the surrounding tissue and the lymph nodes can be done to determine whether the cancer has spread. Another important use of biopsies is to determine the cause of unexplained infections and inflammations.

HOW IT IS DONE

SKIN OR MUSCLE BIOPSY This consists of cutting away a small piece of skin or muscle for analysis. The skin or muscle biopsy is a straightforward procedure that requires only a local anesthetic.

NEEDLE BIOPSY A needle is inserted through the skin and into the organ or tumor to be investigated. The needle may be fitted with a cutting tip to help remove a piece of tissue for microscopic examination. Aspiration biopsy is another type of needle biopsy in which the cells that are sucked from a tumor are examined cytologically. In most cases only a local anesthetic is required.

Until recently, if the target area could not be felt through the skin, or the organ was not accessible by endoscopic biopsy (see below), the physician would have to work "blindly," relying only on experience and a knowledge of anatomy, so that deep-needle biopsy was almost never done. Today, "guided" biopsy, using *ultrasound scanning* or *CT scanning* to precisely locate the tissue to be biopsied and follow the progress of the needle, makes the procedure far more accurate, safe, and productive. In addition, the recent use of very fine needles for biopsies allows for safe sampling of tumors in organs such as the salivary glands and pancreas, in which sampling with larger needles was considered dangerous.

ENDOSCOPIC BIOPSY An *endoscope* (instrument with a viewing lens) is passed into the organ to be investigated and an attachment (forceps to remove tissue and brushes to remove cells) is used to take a sample.

The procedure, which usually requires sedation, is used to take samples from the lining of accessible hollow organs, such as the colon, esophagus, stomach, and bladder.

OPEN BIOPSY This is part of an operation, usually requiring a general anesthetic, in which the surgeon opens a body cavity, such as the chest or abdomen, to reveal a diseased organ or tumor, and removes a sample. Open biopsy is carried out when neither guided nor endoscopic biopsy is possible, or when it is likely that the organ or tumor will require removal. After a tissue sample has been taken, prompt analysis of it can enable the surgeon to remove the diseased area immediately.

EXCISIONAL BIOPSY If a lump is found in the skin or an organ, such as the breast, the surgeon may remove it completely and send the whole specimen for laboratory examination. For lesions (abnormalities) discovered only through *mammography*, the abnormal area may first be identified for the surgeon with the use of injected dye or fine wire probes.

OBTAINING A RESULT

When an immediate diagnosis is essential (for example, to enable breast cancer to be operated on without delay), the tissue can be prepared for staining in a few minutes by freezing or by smearing cells onto slides to study their cytologic features. The more time-consuming, wax-embedded techniques are also carried out for later examination.

In the investigation of infections and inflammations, tissue is sometimes tested with specific antibodies, or tissue *culture* may be required.

The electron *microscope* is used with some kidney biopsies and to distinguish the cell origin of certain tumors. Special enzyme and antibody *staining* techniques are also used in certain cases as well as other histochemical stains performed directly on the fixed and wax-embedded tissues. All of these procedures prolong the time required to make an exact diagnosis but allow for greater accuracy and more precise information about prognosis of certain diseases and tumors.

Biorhythms

A term used to describe all of the physiological functions that vary in a rhythmic way (e.g., the menstrual

BIOPSY PROCEDURES

ASPIRATION BIOPSY

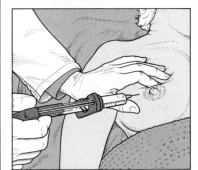

1 The area is usually first numbed with local anesthetic, although occasionally a general anesthetic is required. A needle attached to a syringe is then inserted into the cyst or tumor to be investigated and cells are sucked out to be examined cytologically.

2 Before examination, the fluid is sometimes spun at high speed in a centrifuge and a small amount is placed on a slide.

3 The cells are then fixed (preserved) and finally stained for viewing. The cytologist examines individual cells for abnormalities, paying particular attention to the size, shape, and structure of the nucleus.

Cells as seen through microscope

TISSUE BIOPSY

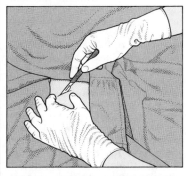

1 The area is first numbed with a local anesthetic and a section of tissue is cut away. The wound is then stitched.

2 The tissue is then embedded in wax so that it is given a firm consistency suitable for slicing. This process usually takes 24 hours.

3 The tissue is then cut into ultrathin slices and transferred to a slide. The pathologist conducts an examination, looking for distortion or alteration of tissue structure.

Tissue sample as seen through microscope

ENDOSCOPIC BIOPSY

If an area of abnormal tissue is to be removed for further examination, the forceps attachment, shown here, is passed through an endoscope to remove the piece of tissue.

Endoscope

Forceps attachment

The forceps attachment removing a tissue sample from a stomach.

cycle, which repeats itself about every 28 days in fertile women).

Most biorhythms are based on a twice-daily or circadian (24-hour) cycle. Our bodies are governed by an internal clock, itself regulated by *hormones*—chemicals secreted into the bloodstream by the *endocrine glands*. Periods of sleepiness and wakefulness are influenced by the level of melatonin, secreted by the pineal gland in the brain. Release of melatonin is stimulated by darkness and suppressed by light. When the normal regular division between night and day is distorted by air travel to a distant time zone, the body's internal clock is disrupted and the result is *jet lag* (the symptoms of which, research suggests, may be relieved by the administration of melatonin).

Cortisol, secreted by the adrenal glands, also reflects the sleeping and waking states, being low at bedtime and high during the very early morning waking hours.

The applications of biorhythms are still being explored. For example, many asthmatics feel worse in the morning due to the cyclic release of hormones. This finding has implications for the management of their condition, and research groups are studying the optimum time of day for the administration of *bronchodilators* and other drugs that interact with functions subject to body rhythms.

Bipolar disorder
An illness that varies between opposite extremes. The principal example is *manic-depressive illness*.

Birth
See *Childbirth*.

Birth canal
The passage, extending from the dilated, effaced cervix (neck of the uterus, which becomes the uterus "mouth" during labor) to the introitus (vaginal opening), through which the baby passes during *childbirth*.

Birth control
Control of the number of children born by preventing or lessening the frequency of conception. Birth control can refer to the narrow area of using natural or artificial means to prevent pregnancy. In a broader sense it refers to control of family or population size by limiting births.

Most people in the US and other developed nations regulate childbirth, so that the population growth rate has

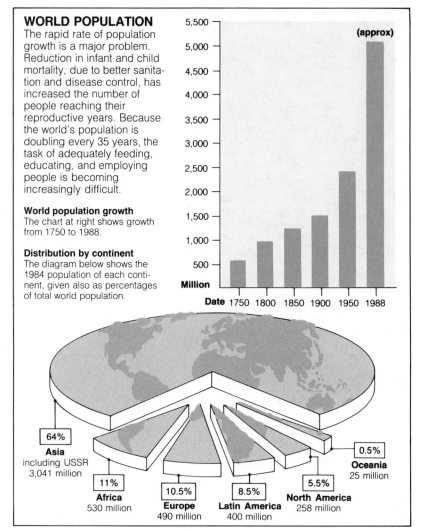

WORLD POPULATION
The rapid rate of population growth is a major problem. Reduction in infant and child mortality, due to better sanitation and disease control, has increased the number of people reaching their reproductive years. Because the world's population is doubling every 35 years, the task of adequately feeding, educating, and employing people is becoming increasingly difficult.

World population growth
The chart at right shows growth from 1750 to 1988.

Distribution by continent
The diagram below shows the 1984 population of each continent, given also as percentages of total world population.

64%
Asia
including USSR
3,041 million

11%
Africa
530 million

10.5%
Europe
490 million

8.5%
Latin America
400 million

5.5%
North America
258 million

0.5%
Oceania
25 million

now slowed in Western countries and in many nations in the Far East. *Family planning* means that men and women can choose if and when to have children; *contraception* provides a means of preventing unwanted pregnancies. Other medical methods of preventing births include abortion (See *Abortion, elective*) and *sterilization*. Political and social pressures are applied to couples in some countries by governments eager to reduce population growth.

Birth defects
Abnormalities obvious at birth or detectable early in infancy. Also called congenital defects, they encompass both minor abnormalities, such as *birthmarks*, and serious disorders such as *spina bifida* (a failure of the spinal column to close completely). About 2

percent of babies born in the US have a defect but only about half of them require treatment.

CAUSES
Birth defects may be due to one or more known causes, but unknown factors also play a part. Among the recognized causes are the following.

CHROMOSOME DEFECTS Some children are born with more or fewer than the normal 23 pairs of *chromosomes* (threadlike structures in cell nuclei that carry the information necessary for normal development)—or there are extra or missing bits of chromosomes, as in *Down's syndrome* (see *Chromosomal abnormalities*).

GENETIC OR HEREDITARY DEFECTS These types of defects may be inherited from one or both parents (see *Genes; Genetic disorders*).

Examples of genetic defects obvious at birth are *achondroplasia* and *albinism*.

DRUGS AND OTHER HARMFUL AGENTS Some drugs can damage the fetus if taken by the mother in early pregnancy, the most notorious being *thalidomide*, a sedative widely prescribed in the late 1950s and early 1960s.

Smoking by the mother can harm the fetus; the ingredients in tobacco smoke stunt the baby's growth. Alcohol can have the same effect and may also affect the development of the face and brain (see *Fetal alcohol syndrome*). Drugs and chemicals that can harm the fetus in this way are collectively called *teratogens*.

IRRADIATION Accidental irradiation of the embryo in early pregnancy—for example, if the mother is X-rayed or receives *radiation therapy* for cancer—can cause abnormalities. However, care is taken to avoid these procedures or to prevent radiation from reaching the embryo if the woman is known to be (or might be) pregnant.

Radiation damage to the unborn child from atomic radiation or radioactive fallout (following a nuclear explosion or leak from a nuclear reactor) is more than just a theoretical risk of modern living. Heavy doses of radiation (as occurred at Hiroshima in 1945, for example) can cause serious mental and physical handicaps at birth, such as *microcephaly*. Even very small doses of radiation increase the child's risk of developing leukemia later in life (see *Radiation hazards*).

MATERNAL INFECTIONS Certain illnesses during pregnancy can cause birth defects. If a woman who has not been immunized against *rubella* (German measles) contracts the disease during the first three months of pregnancy, there is a 50 percent chance that her child will suffer brain, eye, ear, or heart abnormalities. Other types of infection, such as *toxoplasmosis*, may cause inflammation of the eyes, spleen, liver, and other important organs in the fetus.

PHYSICAL FACTORS IN THE UTERUS If the developing baby has too little fluid around it, its limbs may become distorted. *Talipes* (clubfoot) is thought to occur in this way.

Apart from defects of known cause, many others occur, the causes of which are unknown. Among the more common are abnormalities of the brain and spinal cord. In the embryo these structures develop from a simple, fluid-filled tube of nerve tissue. Interference in development can lead to *spina bifida* and *hydrocephalus*.

BIRTH DEFECTS (for every 100,000 babies born live)

Defect	Number	Cause
Congenital heart disease	700	Multifactorial
Mental deficiency (without structural defect)	300	Multifactorial
Pyloric stenosis (structural stomach defect)	300	Multifactorial
Anencephaly (no brain)	200	Multifactorial
Spina bifida	150	Multifactorial
Down's syndrome	150	Chromosome abnormality
Cleft lip and palate	150	Multifactorial
Hypospadias	150	Multifactorial
Clubfoot	100	Multifactorial
Congenital hip dislocation	100	Multifactorial
Congenital deafness	70	Multifactorial
Cystic fibrosis	50	Recessive gene
Turner's syndrome	20	Chromosome abnormality
Hereditary spherocytosis	10	Dominant gene
Albinism	5	Recessive gene

The heart and blood vessels in a fetus develop from what in the embryo is a central muscular tube. If the development of this cardiovascular system is impaired, a congenital heart disorder may result—for example, patent ductus arteriosus, septal defect, transposition of the great vessels, or tetralogy of Fallot (see *Heart disease, congenital*).

Other common defects include *cleft lip and palate*, both of which result from a failure of the two halves of the fetal face and palate to join completely.

PREVENTION

Steps can be taken to minimize the risk of an abnormal child being born. For example, before starting a family, *genetic counseling* should be obtained if either parent has relatives who have genetic or hereditary abnormalities. All women should make sure they are immune to rubella.

A woman should not smoke during pregnancy and should drink alcohol in moderation only. Unless prescribed by a physician, drugs of any kind should be avoided during the first three months of pregnancy.

Various tests may be carried out when there is a possibility that a fetus may have some defect.

Tests include *amniocentesis* (taking a sample of amniotic fluid from the uterus), blood tests to detect the level of *alpha-fetoprotein* (AFP) in the mother, *chorionic villus sampling* (removing a sample of tissue from the placenta), and *ultrasound scanning*.

Birth injury

Damage sustained during birth. All babies suffer at least minor trauma, leading to bruising or swelling of the scalp, during a vaginal delivery. The swelling is sometimes marked (see *Cephalhematoma*) if delivery is by *vacuum extraction* or *forceps*.

More serious injury can occur during a complicated delivery, particularly if the baby is premature, is born by *breech delivery* (born bottom-first), or is too big to pass easily through the mother's pelvis. Birth injuries are less common today, partly because more babies are now being delivered by *cesarean section*.

In breech deliveries, nerves in the shoulder region are sometimes injured, causing temporary paralysis in the arm. The face, likewise, may be paralyzed temporarily if the facial nerve is traumatized by forceps. Broken bones such as the clavicle (collarbone), humerus (upper arm bone), and particularly the ribs, are another hazard of difficult deliveries. The bones usually heal easily.

Many cases of *cerebral palsy, mental retardation*, and *epilepsy* were attributed to birth injury, but it is now considered that these problems are more often due to prenatal factors. Poor nutrition, smoking, maternal alcohol intake, bleeding during pregnancy, and prematurity are among the various factors that can lead to brain damage in a baby. (See *Birth defects; Brain damage*.)

Birthmark

An area of discolored skin present from birth. The most common birthmarks are freckles and moles, also called melanocytic *nevi* (brown to blue-gray skin patches of various types), which are malformations of pigment cells. Strawberry marks (bright red, usually protuberant areas) and port-wine stains (purple-red, flat, often large areas) are *hemangiomas* (malformations of blood vessels). Strawberry marks often gradually disappear after the age of 6 months, but port-wine stains seldom fade. In rare cases (the *Sturge-Weber syndrome*), port-wine stains are associated with abnormalities in the blood vessels of the brain.

Unsightly moles can be removed from late childhood onward by *plastic surgery*. Port-wine stains can now be caused to fade by *laser treatment*; the most successful results have been in young people.

Very rarely, a mole may develop into a type of skin cancer called a malignant *melanoma*. A mole that is large or irregular or suddenly starts to change in appearance or bleed is a cause for suspicion.

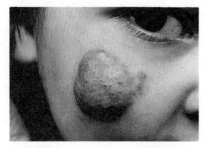

Birthmark
Strawberry marks—a common type of birthmark caused by malformation of blood vessels—are usually bright red, protuberant, and spongy.

Birth weight

The average full-term infant weighs 7.5 pounds at birth. Very few babies weigh less than 5.5 pounds (2,500 g) or more than 9.5 pounds (4,500 g).

A baby's birth weight depends on a number of factors, including the size and racial origin of the parents. Small parents tend to have small babies, and Asian infants tend to be smaller than white ones. Baby boys weigh, on the average, 8 ounces more than baby girls.

Babies who weigh less than 5.5 pounds at birth are classified as "low birth weight." About one half of these babies are small due to *prematurity*—that is, they were born before the 37th week of pregnancy. Others are small because they have been undernourished in the uterus, where the placenta was insufficient because the mother had *preeclampsia* or smoked heavily during pregnancy.

Oversized babies are often born to mothers who have *diabetes mellitus*.

During the first few weeks of life, babies lose up to 10 percent of their birth weight, but thereafter should steadily gain weight.

Bisexuality

Sexual interest in members of both sexes that may or may not involve sexual activity. Between what are regarded as being the two ends of the human sexuality spectrum—exclusive heterosexuality and exclusive homosexuality—there exists a continuous spectrum of bisexuality. Sexuality is determined by a person's sexual desires as well as his or her actual sexual behavior. Thus, the term bisexual includes those who suppress homosexual desires and behave exclusively as heterosexuals.

Sexual preference may vary during a person's lifetime. Alfred Kinsey, who conducted a broad study of human sexual habits in the US during the 1940s, developed a scale that allowed him to rate the relative amounts of heterosexual and homosexual activity and/or responses during different periods in an individual's life. He concluded that, at some stage in their adult life, half the population engaged in both heterosexual and homosexual activity, or reacted sexually to persons of both sexes.

Bismuth

A metal, the salts of which are used in various drug preparations including tablets and suppositories to treat *peptic ulcer*, *hemorrhoids* (piles), and inflammatory diseases of the intestine. Bismuth salts adhere to ulcers of the stomach and duodenum and form a protective coating, thus promoting healing. Preparations containing bismuth salts taken by mouth may color the feces black, simulating the presence of blood in the feces. Darkening of the tongue and nausea and vomiting may also occur. Certain bismuth salts enter the bloodstream and may be associated with abnormal behavior patterns.

Bite

See *Occlusion*.

Bites, animal

Any injury inflicted by the mouthparts of an animal—from the tiny puncture wounds of blood-sucking insects to the massive injuries caused by shark or crocodile attacks.

The bites of venomous snakes, other venomous animals, and insects cause special problems (see *Snake bites; Venomous bites; Insect bites*).

INCIDENCE

The greatest number of animal attacks worldwide come from dogs, mainly strays. In the US, more than 1 million people annually are bitten badly enough by a dog to seek hospital treatment. A small number of deaths each year result from dog bites, and also from the bites of other domestic animals, such as cattle, horses, pigs, and sheep.

Wild animals that have killed or caused serious injuries to humans include bears, buffalo, wolves, hyenas, wild pigs, lions, tigers, elephants, rhinoceroses, and hippopotamuses. Small mammals such as rodents cause less extensive injury, but they often have razor-sharp teeth and there is a high risk of infection.

About 100 shark attacks occur worldwide each year, of which half are fatal. In Africa, more than 1,000 people annually die from crocodile attacks. Other aquatic creatures capable of a serious bite include barracuda, groupers, and moray and conger eels.

THE MAIN HAZARDS

TISSUE DAMAGE The mouth's function is to obtain food and prepare it for digestion. Teeth, especially those of carnivores, are well adapted to tearing, crushing, and macerating tissues and bones, and can inflict severe and extensive mechanical injury.

BLOOD LOSS Severe injuries and lacerations to major blood vessels can sometimes lead to serious blood loss and physiological *shock*.

INFECTION An animal's mouth is heavily populated with bacteria and other microorganisms that thrive on food residue and debris. These organisms can produce serious secondary infection, especially in wounds where there is already extensive tissue damage. *Tetanus* is a particular hazard of animal bites.

RABIES In countries in which rabies occurs, any mammal may potentially harbor the virus and transmit it by its bite (see *Rabies*). Worldwide, dog bites are by far the most common source of human infection. In the US, however, there is relatively little rabies in dogs.

In 1983, for example, there were 132 cases in dogs compared with 168 cases in cats, from a total of 5,880 cases of animal rabies in the entire country. Skunks, raccoons, and bats accounted for most of the remainder (5,101).

TREATMENT

For anything more serious than a minor bite or scratch—or if there is any possibility of rabies—treatment should be sought. It usually includes wound cleaning and exploration (under anesthesia, if necessary). The wound will usually be left open and dressed, rather than stitched, as a closed wound tends to encourage the multiplication of bacteria transmitted by bites. Preventive antibiotic treatment, and an antitetanus injection, may also be given.

If possible, the animal that inflicted the bite should be held and checked for rabies. Sometimes, an antirabies vaccine or serum may have to be given. (See also *Bites, human*.)

Bites, human

Wounds caused by one person biting another. In general, wounds from human bites are more serious than those from animal bites due to higher complication and infection rates.

CAUSES

People bite each other more often than might be supposed—commonly in the course of fights or domestic arguments, or as part of a general pattern of *child abuse*. In New York in 1982, 10 percent of all bites were human. Occasionally, bite wounds occur unintentionally, such as in fistfights where a person is punched in the teeth, or as a result of sexual play.

HAZARDS

Human bites rarely cause serious tissue damage or blood loss. However, infection from any of the range of microorganisms (viruses and bacteria) in the mouth is as likely, or even more likely, than with animal bites, particularly if the bite is deep. There is a risk of *tetanus* infection.

The viruses responsible for *hepatitis B, herpes simplex, AIDS,* and *rabies* are present in the saliva of those affected by these illnesses. Transmission of hepatitis B and AIDS by a bite has never been documented but is a theoretical hazard. Human cases of rabies are extremely rare, and the risk of being bitten by a human victim would be generally confined to physicians and nurses.

TREATMENT

Treatment for any bite that penetrates the skin is as for an animal bite.

Black death

The medieval name for bubonic *plague*. One feature of the disease is bleeding beneath the skin with the formation of dark blue or black bruises. This, along with the fact that in medieval times the disease was fatal in over 50 percent of the cases, accounts for the name.

Black eye

The bruised appearance of the skin around the eye following an injury. Any direct blow damages the numerous small blood vessels beneath the skin, causing blood to leak and collect there.

Because the skin around the eyes is loose and transparent, bruising is darker in this area than on other parts of the body. A cold compress held over the eye will reduce inflammation and help relieve the discomfort.

Blackhead

A semisolid, black-capped plug of greasy material blocking the outlet of a sebaceous (oil-forming) gland in the skin. Blackheads occur most commonly on the face, chest, shoulders, and back, alone or in groups, and are associated with increased sebaceous gland activity, which is normal in adolescents. They are a characteristic feature of certain types of *acne*.

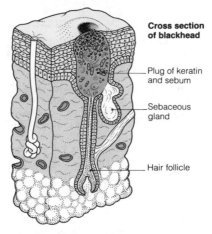

Cross section of blackhead

Plug of keratin and sebum

Sebaceous gland

Hair follicle

Blackout

A common term for loss of consciousness or syncope. (See *Fainting*.)

Black teeth

See *Discolored teeth*.

Blackwater fever

An occasional and life-threatening complication of falciparum *malaria* (the most dangerous form of the

disease). The condition is brought on by a sudden increased rate of destruction of red blood cells. The breakdown products of the cells find their way via the kidneys into the urine and cause it to darken, hence "blackwater." Other symptoms include loss of consciousness (cerebral malaria), fever, chills, and vomiting.

Bladder

The hollow, muscular organ that acts as a reservoir for urine. The adult bladder can hold a pint or more of urine. It lies behind the pubic bone, hidden within and protected by the pelvis.

The bladder walls consist of muscle and an inner lining called urinary epithelium. At the back are the two ureters, which carry urine to the bladder from the kidneys. At the lowest point within the bladder—the neck—is the opening into the urethra; this is normally kept tightly closed by a sphincter (circular muscle).

FUNCTION

The bladder's function is to collect and store urine until it can be expelled from the body at a suitable time.

Full control over bladder function takes some years to develop. In infants, bladder emptying is an entirely automatic or *reflex* reaction. When the bladder fills and stretches beyond a certain point, signals are sent to the spinal cord. Nerve centers in the spinal cord then cause the urethral sphincter to relax and the main bladder muscle to contract, thus expelling urine via the urethra.

As the child grows, he or she gradually develops the ability to delay emptying. Stretching of the bladder is registered consciously (as discomfort) in brain centers, which, if desired, can then send signals suppressing the emptying reflex. Eventually, the bladder becomes so stretched that the urge to pass urine is overwhelming.

Children vary in the age at which they achieve perfect bladder control and, in particular, night-time control. Most children are dry at night by the age of 5 years, but some take longer (see *Enuresis*).

Defective bladder function, leading to problems such as *incontinence* and *urine retention*, has various causes. (See *Bladder* disorders box.)

Bladder cancer

See *Bladder tumors*.

Bladder tumors

Growths originating in the urinary epithelium (inner lining) of the blad-

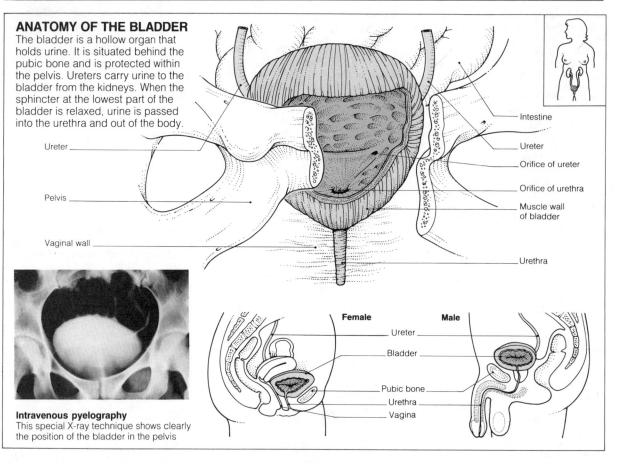

ANATOMY OF THE BLADDER

The bladder is a hollow organ that holds urine. It is situated behind the pubic bone and is protected within the pelvis. Ureters carry urine to the bladder from the kidneys. When the sphincter at the lowest part of the bladder is relaxed, urine is passed into the urethra and out of the body.

Ureter

Pelvis

Vaginal wall

Intestine

Ureter

Orifice of ureter

Orifice of urethra

Muscle wall of bladder

Urethra

Female   **Male**

Ureter

Bladder

Pubic bone

Urethra

Vagina

Intravenous pyelography
This special X-ray technique shows clearly the position of the bladder in the pelvis

---

der. Many bladder tumors are benign *papillomas* (small wartlike growths), but these tend to recur, and eventually one or more may become cancerous. Malignant growths tend to spread inward, into the bladder cavity, but may also spread through the bladder wall to nearby organs, such as the rectum, sigmoid colon, prostate gland, or uterus, and to the lymph glands and the bones of the pelvis.

INCIDENCE AND CAUSES

Bladder cancers account for about 4 percent of all cancers diagnosed in the US, with about 15 new cases (leading to about four deaths) per 100,000 population per year. If papillomas are included, the incidence is higher. Almost three times as many men as women are affected, and the average age at diagnosis is 65 years.

Certain groups are at increased risk, notably smokers and workers in the dye and rubber industries. Exposure to carcinogenic (cancer-inducing) substances used in these industries or in tobacco smoke is the presumed cause in these groups. The disease is

also common in areas of the tropics where the parasitic infection *schistosomiasis* is prevalent.

Avoiding smoking is the principal means of reducing the personal risk of bladder tumors. The incidence of occupational bladder cancer has been reduced by protective measures in the industries concerned and by regular screening of those who have been exposed in the past.

SYMPTOMS

Hematuria (blood in the urine) is the main symptom. Passing urine is usually painless, but a bladder infection may develop, and it then becomes painful and frequent. Sometimes, a tumor may obstruct the entry of a ureter into the bladder, causing back pressure and pain in the kidney region or may obstruct the urethral exit, causing difficulty in passing urine.

DIAGNOSIS AND TREATMENT

Bladder tumors are diagnosed primarily by *cystoscopy* (passage of a slim viewing tube up the urethra into the bladder) and by *biopsy*. If the tumor is still in its early stages, it is usually cut

out or treated by *diathermy* (heat destruction), via the cystoscope. Tumors recur in 80 percent of cases, so regular cystoscopy checkups are needed. Recurrences may be treated with surgery or *anticancer drugs*.

In the case of a more widely spread cancer, treatment is usually a combination of *radiation therapy* and more drastic surgery to remove the bladder (see *Cystectomy*).

OUTLOOK

This varies according to what stage the growth has reached when first diagnosed. If a tumor is diagnosed and treated early, the patient's long-term prospects are excellent (with regular follow-up checkups). If, however, it has spread beyond the bladder wall, the chances of survival for more than five years are not good.

Blastomycosis

A rare infection caused by breathing in a fungus, BLASTOMYCES DERMATITIDIS, found in wood and soil. The infection occurs mainly in the eastern part of the US and Canada.

DISORDERS OF THE BLADDER

The most important causes of bladder problems are infection, tumors, urinary tract *calculi* (stones), or impairment of the bladder's nerve supply.

INFECTION

Infection of the bladder, better known as *cystitis*, is particularly common in women, mainly because of the much shorter female urethra, which provides less of a barrier to bacteria. In men, infection is usually associated with obstruction to the flow of urine from the bladder by, for example, tumors of the bladder or prostate (the gland situated around the bladder neck in males). In some parts of the tropics, the parasitic worm infection *schistosomiasis* (bilharziasis) is a common cause.

TUMORS

Bladder tumors may be benign or malignant and are more common in men than in women. They are usually painless in the early stages and may cause *hematuria* (blood in the urine) or obstruction to the outflow of urine from the bladder. The latter may also be caused by a tumor of the prostate and result in partial or complete *urine retention* and stagnation in the bladder.

Tumors of the spinal cord may affect the nerves controlling the bladder, leading either to retention or *incontinence* (involuntary bladder emptying or leakage).

CALCULI

Calculi (stones) in the bladder, caused by the precipitation from solution of substances present in the urine, are an uncommon problem in the US. They mainly affect men and usually result from urinary retention and/or a long-standing urinary tract infection. In some other parts of the world, such as Southeast Asia, they are more common and are often associated with a low-protein diet.

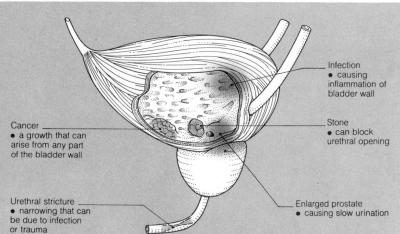

Cancer
• a growth that can arise from any part of the bladder wall

Urethral stricture
• narrowing that can be due to infection or trauma

Infection
• causing inflammation of bladder wall

Stone
• can block urethral opening

Enlarged prostate
• causing slow urination

INJURY

Injury to the bladder is uncommon. It may occur, however, if the pelvis is fractured when the bladder is full. Such injury typically occurs in traffic accidents. The bladder ruptures and urine leaks into the abdominal and pelvic cavities.

Damage to the nerves involved in bladder control may severely disrupt bladder filling and emptying, causing either incontinence or urinary retention, depending on the site of the injury. In the US, the most common cause of such damage is spinal cord injury due to motorcycle and automobile accidents or to bullet wounds. Nerves controlling the bladder may also be damaged by a prolapsed intervertebral disk.

OTHER DISORDERS

Disturbance of bladder control can also result from nerve degeneration found in conditions such as *diabetes mellitus* or *multiple sclerosis*.

An unstable or *irritable bladder* is a common condition in which the urge to empty the bladder occurs frequently. It is not fully understood but is sometimes associated with a *urinary tract infection* or prolapse of the uterus. Many other underlying conditions, most com- monly tension or anxiety, can cause frequent urination.

Failure to achieve bladder control by the age of 4 or 5 is termed *enuresis* (bed-wetting); this may be due to a treatable physical cause, such as urinary tract infection, or to emotional problems but more often results from delayed maturation of the nervous system.

INVESTIGATION

Many different methods are used to investigate bladder disorders. Urinary tract infection is diagnosed by culturing a urine sample. The bladder can be viewed directly by means of *cystoscopy*. X-ray studies include a voiding *cystourethrogram*, which shows only the bladder, and intravenous *pyelography*, which provides a picture of the whole urinary tract. *Cystometry* is a technique for measuring bladder capacity in relation to changing pressure.

The infection may cause acute pneumonia or a more chronic illness affecting the lungs, skin, and bones. It cannot be passed from one person to another. Treatment is with *antifungal drugs*, such as amphotericin B or ketoconazole.

Bleaching, dental

A cosmetic procedure for lightening endodontically treated or nonvital "dead" teeth that have become discolored (see *Discolored teeth*). The surface of the affected tooth is painted with oxidizing agents and may be exposed to special heat or light.

Bleb

A tiny *blister*. A common cause is the injection of a small amount of fluid under the outer layer of skin—for example, in the tuberculin skin test.

Bleeder

A term used to describe anyone who suffers from a *bleeding disorder*, which may be congenital or acquired.

Bleeding

Loss of blood from the *circulatory system* caused by damage to the blood vessels or by a *bleeding disorder*, which may be visible (external) or concealed (internal). Rapid loss of more than 10

B

percent of the blood volume can cause symptoms of shock with faintness, pallor, and sweating.

CAUSES

The most common cause of bleeding is an injury. The speed with which blood flows from a cut depends on the type of blood vessel damaged—it usually oozes from a capillary, flows from a vein, and spurts from an artery. If an injury does not break open the skin, blood collects around the damaged blood vessels close under the skin to form a *bruise*.

Damage to internal blood vessels may be the result of inflammation, infection, an ulcer, or a tumor. Any lost blood that mixes with other bodily fluids such as sputum or urine will be noticed quite readily; bleeding in the digestive tract may make vomit or feces appear darker than usual because the blood is partially digested. Internal bleeding, however, may not become visible but may gradually progress to where severe anemia is present.

Bleeding without injury usually requires investigation. The exceptions are an occasional *nosebleed* (epistaxis) and bleeding during *menstruation*. The amount of blood lost during menstruation varies and is only a problem if bleeding becomes very heavy or frequent, when it might lead to iron-deficiency *anemia*.

Bleeding disorders

Conditions that are associated with bleeding without injury or abnormally prolonged and excessive bleeding after injury.

Bleeding disorders are the result of one or more defects in the three mechanisms by which bleeding is normally stopped (see *Hemostasis* and *Blood clotting*). These mechanisms are blood coagulation, the plugging of damaged blood vessels by platelets, and the constriction of blood vessels.

Coagulation defects tend to cause deep bleeding into the gastrointestinal tract, the muscles, and the joint cavities, while defects of the platelets or blood vessels produce superficial bleeding into the skin, gums, or lining of the intestine or urinary tract. However, bleeding may occur anywhere with these defects.

COAGULATION DEFECTS

These defects usually result from too little of one or more of the enzymes (called coagulation factors) that take part in blood clotting, or from the enzymes being abnormal. The defect causes the blood to clot very slowly and produces clots that are weak and do not seal blood vessels securely. Coagulation defects may be congenital (present from birth) or acquired later in life.

CONGENITAL The main congenital coagulation defects are *hemophilia*, *Christmas disease*, and *von Willebrand's disease*. In each of these, one of the coagulation factors is either absent from the blood or is present in only small amounts.

Hemophilia and Christmas disease are similar disorders, resulting from deficiencies of two different coagulation factors, called factor VIII and factor IX, respectively. They are inherited as sex-linked disorders (see *Genetic disorders*), which means that normally only males are affected. In the US, about 10 people per 100,000 have hemophilia and about two people per 100,000 have Christmas disease.

Von Willebrand's disease is also a factor VIII defect but affects both sexes roughly equally. About five persons per 100,000 are affected.

Individuals with any of these disorders may bleed internally without warning and often have recurrent bleeding into joints such as the knee or elbow. The severity of the bleeding is variable.

ACQUIRED Deficiency of one or more coagulation factors may develop at any age as a result of severe liver disease, digestive system disorders that prevent the absorption from the diet of *vitamin K* (required to make some coagulation factors), or the use of *anticoagulant drugs*, such as warfarin, that prevent normal production of these enzymes. As with congenital bleeding disorders, a severe bleeding tendency may result.

One particularly complex coagulation disorder is disseminated intravascular coagulation (DIC); it may be triggered by a variety of circumstances. First there is aggregation of platelets and clotting within small blood vessels. Subsequently, coagulation factors are used and broken up in the blood faster than they can be replaced by the liver, and severe bleeding may result. Paradoxically, sometimes anticoagulants are given to interfere with the clotting activity, but this very serious condition generally does not improve until the underlying problem (for example, an infection or cancer) is brought under control.

Coagulation defects are investigated by *blood-clotting tests* such as the prothrombin time. Treatment of these disorders is based on giving the patient infusions of the missing coagulation factor or factors in fresh blood or fresh frozen plasma. Since these factors come from human blood, transmission of some viral infections (for example, hepatitis B or AIDS) is possible. Attempts are made to reduce the risk of contaminating viruses, such as the hepatitis B or AIDS virus, by checking for the presence of antibodies against the virus and, if they are present, discarding the blood or blood products.

PLATELET DEFECTS

Bleeding caused by a defect in the platelet system is usually due to too few of these cells in the blood—a condition called *thrombocytopenia*. The main features are surface bleeding into the skin and gums, which usually appears in the skin as multiple small bruises called *purpura*.

Occasionally, platelets are normal in number but function abnormally with resultant bleeding. Such defects may be inherited, may be associated with the use of many drugs (including aspirin), or may be a complication of certain bone marrow disorders such as myeloid *leukemia*.

Platelet defects are investigated by blood clotting tests such as bleeding and clotting times and various other tests of platelet aggregation (clumping). Whatever the cause, the main treatment of platelet disorders consists of transfusions of platelets from single donors or from "pools" (obtained from several normal blood transfusions). The transfusions need to be given daily until the underlying defect has been corrected and the body is producing its own healthy platelets again.

BLOOD VESSEL DEFECTS

Abnormal bleeding caused by blood vessel defects is rare today. In the past, *scurvy* (vitamin C deficiency) was a frequent and often fatal disorder of this type, affecting sailors, polar explorers, and anyone with a diet lacking fresh fruit and vegetables. Today, mild scurvy is occasionally seen in elderly people on a poor diet. Elderly people and patients on long-term *corticosteroid drugs* may also suffer mild abnormal bruising due to loss of skin support to the smallest blood vessels. These conditions are mild and treatment is rarely required.

Bleeding gums
See *Gingivitis*.

Bleeding, treatment of
The body's response to internal or external loss of blood is to contract the damaged blood vessels and to cause blood to clot at the site of injury. At the same time, blood flow may be reduced in the skin and muscles to make sure that the brain, kidneys, and other vital organs are adequately supplied. Loss of a large volume of blood quickly causes a dramatic fall in blood pressure accompanied by weakness, confusion, pallor, and sweating as the body tries to compensate; this state is known as *shock*.

First-aid measures have two objectives: to minimize blood loss and to help the body cope with the loss.

PROFESSIONAL TREATMENT
When bleeding is severe, infusions of saline solution and plasma preparations may be given to help replace fluids lost from the circulation. If a large amount of blood is lost, *blood transfusion* may also be required. Large wounds may need closing with *sutures* (stitches), which are effective in stopping bleeding from scalp injuries and also reduce the risk of scarring. If bleeding within the abdomen is suspected following an accident, *CT scanning* and/or exploratory surgery may be needed. If bleeding within the skull is compressing the brain, a hole will be drilled in the skull in order to relieve the pressure.

Severe bleeding may require treatment in the operating room. During operations, bleeding from small blood vessels is controlled by clamping them with forceps and then either tying them or sealing them with *diathermy*, the application of a high frequency electric current.

Blepharitis
Inflammation of the eyelids, with redness, irritation, and scaly skin at the lid margins. Older patients sometimes call marginal blepharitis "granulated eyelids." The patient may note burning and discomfort in the eyes and flakes or crusts on lashes. Occasionally, the surface of the eye may also be inflamed and red. In some cases the roots of the eyelashes become infected, and small ulcers form. Blepharitis is common, tends to recur, and is sometimes associated with dandruff or eczema of the scalp.

The problem can often be cleared up by removing the scales with cotton moistened with warm water. Mar-

ginal blepharitis frequently recurs, requiring more treatment. Ulcerated eyelids need the attention of your physician. Severe cases of blepharitis can lead to corneal problems.

Blepharoplasty
A cosmetic operation to remove wrinkled, drooping skin from the upper and/or lower eyelids. The operation is usually done using local anesthesia and takes about one and a half hours. Normally, the patient can go home the same day.

WHY IT IS DONE
As a person grows older, the skin loses some of its fat, and much of its elasticity, becoming droopy and creased. This process may be accelerated by grief, worry, or sudden loss of weight. As a result, the eyelids become baggy. Removing the excess skin can result in a greatly improved appearance.

FIRST AID: TREATING BLEEDING

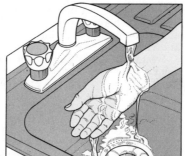

SIMPLE CUT

1 Wash your hands before dealing with the cut. Then, if the cut has dirt in it, rinse it lightly under lukewarm running water until it is clean, being careful not to touch the spout.

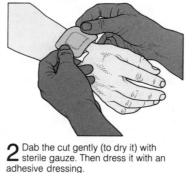

2 Dab the cut gently (to dry it) with sterile gauze. Then dress it with an adhesive dressing.

DEEP CUT

1 Raise the injured part and support it. Put a sterile dressing on the wound and apply firm pressure to control bleeding.

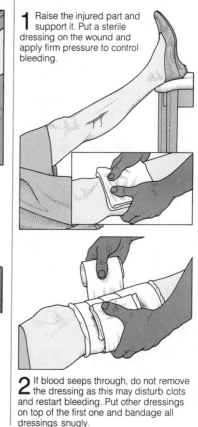

2 If blood seeps through, do not remove the dressing as this may disturb clots and restart bleeding. Put other dressings on top of the first one and bandage all dressings snugly.

HOW IT IS DONE
On the upper lids a horizontal fold of skin is removed from the center of each lid so that the resultant scar runs in a natural crease line. On the lower lids the incision is made just below the

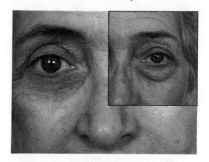

Appearance before (inset) and after blepharoplasty
The operation involves removal of a crescent-shaped section of skin and underlying fat from each eyelid.

eyelashes, so that the scar will be in the shadow of the lashes and extend into a smile wrinkle.

RECOVERY PERIOD

After the operation, ice packs and pads soaked with witch hazel solution are applied to both eyes, to reduce swelling and bruising. The patient is advised to repeat these applications at home. Swelling usually subsides within three days but bruising may last for two weeks.

Some of the stitches are removed three to five days after the operation, the rest seven to 10 days after. The scars usually fade to fine, unnoticeable marks within six to 12 months of the operation.

Blepharospasm

Involuntary prolonged contraction of one of the muscles that controls the eyelids, causing almost complete closure. It may be due to *photophobia* (sensitivity of the eyes to light), *blepharitis*, *anxiety*, or *hysteria*. Treatment is aimed at remedying the cause.

Blind loop syndrome

A condition leading to diarrhea with pale yellow, foul-smelling, bulky feces (called steatorrhea) that are difficult to flush away, along with general sickness, tiredness, and weight loss. The syndrome is caused by a redundant area or dead end in the small intestine, called a blind loop, which is usually the result of surgery but may be congenital (existing at birth).

Because there is not a constant flow of the bowel contents through the loop, its contents stagnate. Bacteria that are not the ordinary dominant inhabitants of the bowel multiply. They spread into other areas of the intestine where they interfere with absorption of nutrients, including fat and vitamin B_{12}.

Treatment with an antibiotic, usually a tetracycline, may be successful. If not, surgery to remove the blind loop usually cures the condition.

Blindness

Total or partial inability to see. Generally, blindness refers to a severe loss of vision that cannot be corrected with ordinary *glasses*. More commonly, vision is impaired to the extent that it markedly hinders everyday activities. Such partial loss—which may develop slowly or suddenly, according to the cause—can affect central vision, peripheral (side) vision, or both. The definition of blindness may vary by agency, but in the US it is usually defined as corrected *visual acuity* of 20/200 or less in the better eye, or a *visual field* of no more than 20 degrees in the better eye.

A person suffering from loss of central vision is usually aware of the fact, since it prevents reading and discernment of fine detail. However, loss of peripheral vision may pass unnoticed by the sufferer until it is well advanced, when it causes clumsiness of movement.

INCIDENCE

It is estimated that over 40 million people in the world are partially or totally blind. Vitamin A deficiency alone accounts for blindness in millions of children living in the poor countries of Africa, Asia, and South America.

In the US, about 214 persons per 100,000 are registered as legally blind, though the definition varies.

CAUSES

Blindness may result from injury, disease, or degeneration of the eyeball, of the optic nerve or nerve pathways connecting the eye to the brain, or of the brain itself.

EYEBALL Normal vision depends on the uninterrupted passage of light from the front of the eye to the light-sensitive retina at the back. Anything that obstructs the passage of light rays from the retina can cause blindness (see *Eye*; *Vision*).

Various disorders may impair the transparency of the cornea at the front of the eye. In *Sjögren's syndrome*, an inability to produce tears leads to *keratoconjunctivitis sicca*, which, if severe, causes the cornea to cloud over. Other causes of a cloudy cornea include *vitamin A* deficiency, accidental chemical damage, and injury. Ulcers on the cornea can also cause blindness since, when healed, they leave scars (see *Cornea* disorders box).

The common causes of such ulcers are severe attacks of certain infections, among them *ophthalmia* neonatorum

---

AIDS FOR THE BLIND

There are many ways in which life can be made easier for the blind person, and there are now a number of specially designed and adapted devices available. These include braille writers, mathematical apparatus, and home appliances, as well as aids for helping the blind person get around outside the home.

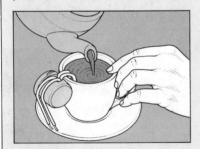

Liquid level indicator
This device measures liquid being poured into a cup or glass. Two sets of prongs are connected to a bleeper. A short set of prongs measures almost to the top, while the long set measures small amounts in the bottom. A bleep sounds when the liquid contacts the prongs.

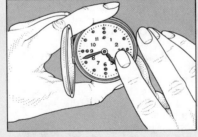

Pocket watch
Strengthened hands and raised dots make it easier for a blind person to "read" numerals: three dots are at 12, two are at 3, 6, and 9, and one is at each of the other hour positions.

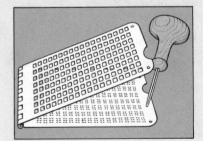

Pocket braille maker
This frame produces braille on one side of the paper. A special pointed stylus is used to make the braille indentations; a stencil keeps the stylus in the right place. The braille can be read without removing the paper from the frame.

(inflammation of the conjunctiva in newborn babies), *trachoma* (most common in hot, overcrowded regions), *herpes simplex*, and bacterial ulcers.

Inflammation of the iris, ciliary body, or choroid—a condition known as *uveitis*—can be caused by infections such as *tuberculosis*, *sarcoidosis*, *syphilis*, *toxocariasis*, or *toxoplasmosis*, but such inflammation frequently occurs for no known reason.

Cataract (cloudiness of the lens) is a common cause of blindness. It is usually the result of the lens deteriorating in old age, but is occasionally present from birth or develops during childhood.

Diabetes mellitus, *hypertension*, or injury can cause bleeding into the fluid that makes up the bulk of the eyeball. In *hyphema* blood enters the aqueous humor (watery substance) in front of the lens. *Vitreous hemorrhage* is bleeding into the jellylike vitreous humor behind the lens.

Disorders of the retina are a common cause of blindness. They include the age-related *macular degeneration* (degeneration of the central area of the retina, which occurs in old age), *retinopathy* due to diabetes or hypertension, *retinal artery occlusion* (blockage of the blood supply to the retina), *retinal vein occlusion*, *retinal detachment*, tumors such as *retinoblastoma* and malignant *melanoma* of the eye, and *retinal hemorrhage* (bleeding into the retina), caused by diabetes, hypertension, vascular disease, or injury.

In *glaucoma*, a common cause of blindness, pressure in the eyeball causes degeneration of the nerve fibers of the optic nerve disk. Many types of glaucoma exist; the more common types can cause loss of peripheral vision (side vision), which may be unnoticed until the disease is well advanced. *Amblyopia* ex anopsia (lazy eye from disuse in childhood) is subnormal vision that is associated with *strabismus* (misalignment of the eyes) or *anisometropia* (unequal focus between the eyes).

OPTIC NERVE AND NERVE PATHWAYS The light energy received by the retina is transformed into nerve impulses that travel along the optic nerve and nerve pathways into the brain. Conduction of these impulses may be impaired by pressure from a tumor in the orbit (the bony cavity that contains the eyeball) or in the brain; by interference with the blood supply to the optic nerve, which can be caused by diabetes mellitus, hypertension, tumors, in-

juries, or *temporal arteritis*; by *optic neuritis* (inflammation of the optic nerve that may occur in *multiple sclerosis*); or by toxic and nutritional deficiency amblyopia (optic neuropathy) caused by the poisonous effects of certain chemicals or by the lack of certain nutrients.

BRAIN Nerve impulses from the retina eventually arrive in a region of the *cerebrum* called the visual cortex. The nerve impulses are analyzed and interpreted to provide conscious images. Blindness can be caused if there is pressure on the visual cortex from a *brain tumor* or *brain hemorrhage* or if a *stroke* reduces blood supply to the visual cortex.

Finally, apparent blindness can be related to *hysteria*, a reaction to severe stress in which physical symptoms develop without there being any physical cause.

DIAGNOSIS AND TREATMENT

Anyone who suffers loss of vision, whether partial or complete, should consult a physician immediately. Various types of *vision tests* can be carried out.

Often, the cause can be ascertained by direct examination of the eye, including ophthalmoscopy, slit-lamp examination, tonometry, and perimetry. Electrical activity produced in the brain following visual stimulation can be measured by visual potentiometry (see *Evoked responses*). The age and medical history of the patient, the patient's account of the development of the sight loss, and other signs and symptoms, may provide important clues to the diagnosis. In a few cases, *ultrasound scanning*, *CT scanning*, or *MRI* may be performed to look for any abnormalities in the eyes, orbits, structures around the optic nerves, or brain. *Fluorescein angiography* (a technique for photographing the inside of the eye) may be used to study the retina and choroid.

Treatment depends on the underlying cause once discovered. If not correctable, and the loss of vision meets an agency's definition of blindness, certain services may be available. (See also *Color vision deficiency*; *Night blindness*; *Onchocerciasis*, also known as river blindness.)

Blind spot

The small, oval-shaped area on the retina of the eye where the optic nerve joins the eyeball. The area is not sensitive to light because there are no light receptors (nerve endings responsive to light) present there.

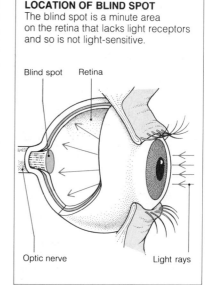

LOCATION OF BLIND SPOT
The blind spot is a minute area on the retina that lacks light receptors and so is not light-sensitive.

Blind spot   Retina

Optic nerve   Light rays

To demonstrate the presence of the blind spot, mark an X on a piece of paper and a dot 6 inches to the right. While holding the paper at arm's length, shut your left eye and look at the X with your right eye. Slowly move the paper toward you until the dot disappears. This is the point at which the dot has entered your right eye's blind spot.

Blister

A collection of fluid beneath the outer layer of the skin that forms a raised area, usually oval or circular in shape. Large blisters (more than a half inch in diameter) are sometimes called bullae; small blisters are called vesicles.

The fluid in a blister is serum that has leaked from blood vessels in underlying skin layers after minor damage. The fluid is usually sterile, and the blister provides valuable protection to the damaged tissue.

CAUSES

Common causes of blisters are *burns* (including *sunburn*) and friction—for example, from an ill-fitting shoe.

A number of skin diseases also can cause blisters. These include *eczema*, *impetigo*, and *erythema multiforme* (in which blistering is usually seen only in severe forms), and *pemphigoid*, *pemphigus*, and *dermatitis herpetiformis* (collectively called "bullous" disorders), in which blistering is the most important feature of the disease. Blisters also occur in the congenital disease *epidermolysis bullosa* and in some types of *porphyria*.

Small blisters develop at an early stage in the rashes of the viral infections *chickenpox*, *herpes zoster* (shingles), and *herpes simplex*; these blisters contain infectious virus particles that may spread the infection elsewhere or to another person.

TREATMENT

A blister is best left to heal on its own. It should not be burst, because the underlying damaged tissue could become infected. In the case of large, troublesome, or unexplained blisters, consult your physician. Bullous disorders are potentially serious and expert advice is needed.

Blocked nose

See *Nasal congestion*.

Blocking

Inability to express true feelings or thoughts, usually as a result of emotional or mental conflict. In Freudian-based psychotherapies, blocking is regarded as originating from the repression of painful emotions in early life. Successful treatment is thought to depend on putting patients in touch with these unconscious feelings.

A very specific form of thought blocking occurs in *schizophrenia*. In this disorder, trains of thought are persistently interrupted involuntarily, to be replaced by totally unconnected new ones. (See also *Psychotherapy*.)

Blood

The sticky red fluid that circulates in our veins and arteries. Its main function is to act as the body's transport system, but it also has a major role in the defense against infection.

Blood also contains ingenious mechanisms to halt its own loss from the body; it seals damaged blood vessels, protects the injury with a clot, and helps to repair the damage (see *Hemostasis; Blood clotting; Wounds*).

The average-sized adult has about 10 pints of blood. At rest, 10 pints a minute are pumped by the heart via the arteries to the lungs and all other tissues, then returned to the heart in veins, in a continuous circuit (see *Circulatory system*). During exercise the heart may pump blood at a rate of 40 pints or more a minute.

Almost half the volume of blood consists of cells, which include red blood cells (or erythrocytes), white blood cells (or leukocytes), and platelets or thrombocytes (see *Blood cells*). The remainder is a fluid called plasma, which contains dissolved proteins, sugars, fats, and minerals.

BLOOD CELLS

The main function of red blood cells is to act as containers for the pigment and protein *hemoglobin*. Hemoglobin carries oxygen from the lungs to the tissues, where it is exchanged for the waste product carbon dioxide (see *Respiration*). White blood cells play an important part in the defense against infection by viruses, bacteria, fungi, and parasites, and in inflammation of any cause (see *Immune system*). Platelets are essential to arrest bleeding and repair damaged blood vessels. They clump together to block small holes, and these clumps release chemicals that begin the process of blood clotting.

PLASMA

Blood plasma is a straw-colored fluid, consisting mainly of water (95 percent) with a salt content very similar to seawater. Levels of its many other dissolved constituents vary from time to time. Measurements of these constituents are useful to physicians in the diagnosis of disease states (see *Blood tests; Liver function tests*). Important constituents of plasma include the following.

NUTRIENTS These substances are transported to the tissues after absorption from the intestinal tract or following release from storage depots such as the liver. Nutrients include sugars (principally glucose), fats, amino acids required by cells to make proteins, and various vitamins and minerals. Immediately after a meal that is rich in fats, the plasma has a milky appearance as a consequence of its high fat content.

WASTE PRODUCTS The main product of tissue metabolism is urea, which is transported in the plasma to the kidneys; abnormally high blood urea levels occur in *renal failure*. The waste product from the destruction of hemoglobin is a yellow pigment called bilirubin. This is normally removed from the plasma by the liver and turned into bile. Bilirubin levels become abnormally high in liver disease, or in hemolytic *anemia*, where there is excessive destruction of red blood cells. Bilirubin causes the yellow color of the skin and eyes and the dark urine in patients with *jaundice*.

PROTEINS These include substances, such as fibrinogen, that are involved in the processes of coagulation and clotting, and others that act to inhibit coagulation (see *Blood clotting*). Plasma proteins, such as *immunoglobulins* (see also *Antibodies*), and complement (bacteria fighters) are part of the immune system. Another type of plasma protein is *albumin*. The large size of the protein molecules prevents them from escaping from the blood into the tissues; this helps to "hold in" the water content of blood (by osmotic pressure) and thus maintain blood volume.

HORMONES The hormones are chemical messengers transported in the blood from various glands to their target organs. (See *Endocrine system*.)

Blood cells

Cells present in blood for most or part of their life span. These include red blood cells, which make up about 40 percent by volume of normal blood, and white blood cells and platelets, which make up less than 5 percent of the total volume.

All types of blood cells are formed within the bone marrow by a series of divisions from a single type of cell called a stem cell.

RED BLOOD CELLS

 These are also called RBCs, red blood corpuscles, or erythrocytes. They carry oxygen from the lungs to the tissues, where oxygen is exchanged for carbon dioxide (see *Respiration*).

FORMATION RBC formation from stem cells in the bone marrow takes about five days. It requires an adequate supply of nutrients, including iron, amino acids, and the vitamins B_{12} and folic acid. The rate of RBC formation is influenced by a hormone called erythropoietin, which is produced by the kidneys.

Cells just released into the bloodstream from the marrow are called reticulocytes; over two to four days, these develop into mature RBCs. Reticulocytes are easily recognized in blood by means of special staining techniques, and a count of their numbers provides physicians with a helpful estimate of the rate at which RBCs are being formed (see *Blood count; Blood smear*).

STRUCTURE AND FUNCTION One cubic millimeter of blood contains about 5 million RBCs, each of which is doughnut-shaped, about 7.5 thousandths of a millimeter in diameter, and much thicker around the edge than at the center. This shape gives the cell a relatively large surface area, which assists it in absorbing and releasing oxygen molecules. The shape also allows the cell to distort and so helps it squeeze through narrow blood vessels.

CONSTITUENTS OF BLOOD

Blood is pumped around the body in veins and arteries, transporting oxygen from the lungs to the tissues, and carbon dioxide from the tissues to the lungs. Blood also carries nutrients such as sugars, fats, and proteins that have been absorbed from the intestine, and hormones produced by a variety of glands. Waste products that are released from cells are carried in the blood to be broken down in the liver or excreted from the kidneys.

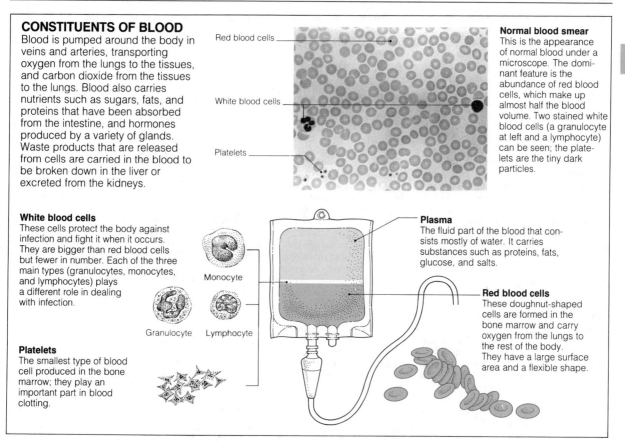

Red blood cells

White blood cells

Platelets

Normal blood smear
This is the appearance of normal blood under a microscope. The dominant feature is the abundance of red blood cells, which make up almost half the blood volume. Two stained white blood cells (a granulocyte at left and a lymphocyte) can be seen; the platelets are the tiny dark particles.

White blood cells
These cells protect the body against infection and fight it when it occurs. They are bigger than red blood cells but fewer in number. Each of the three main types (granulocytes, monocytes, and lymphocytes) plays a different role in dealing with infection.

Monocyte

Granulocyte Lymphocyte

Platelets
The smallest type of blood cell produced in the bone marrow; they play an important part in blood clotting.

Plasma
The fluid part of the blood that consists mostly of water. It carries substances such as proteins, fats, glucose, and salts.

Red blood cells
These doughnut-shaped cells are formed in the bone marrow and carry oxygen from the lungs to the rest of the body. They have a large surface area and a flexible shape.

Each cell is packed with large quantities of *hemoglobin*, a protein that contains iron. Hemoglobin is found in all animals—from insects and worms to birds, fish, and mammals—and is highly efficient at "binding" (combining chemically) with oxygen when the oxygen concentration is high (in the lungs), and releasing the oxygen again when the oxygen concentration is low (in the tissues). Oxyhemoglobin, formed when oxygen combines with hemoglobin, is responsible for the bright red coloration of oxygenated blood; the unbound (oxygen-free) hemoglobin in venous blood accounts for its darker color.

Each RBC also contains *enzymes*, minerals, and sugars, which give energy to maintain shape, structure, and elasticity (see *Cell; Metabolism*).

The surface structure of RBCs varies slightly among individuals, and this provides the basis for classifying blood into groups (see *Blood groups*).

AGING AND DESTRUCTION RBCs normally circulate in the blood for about 120 days, which is also their life span when removed for blood transfusion (within three to four weeks blood in blood banks contains a significant proportion of dead cells and must be discarded). As cells age, their internal chemical machinery wears out, they lose elasticity, and they become trapped in small blood vessels in the spleen and other organs; they are then destroyed by a type of white blood cell called a macrophage (see *Phagocyte*). Most components of the hemoglobin molecules are reutilized but some are broken down to a waste product called *bilirubin*.

DISORDERS Abnormalities can occur in the rate at which RBCs are formed or destroyed, in the number of RBCs in the blood, and in their shape, size, and hemoglobin content, causing various forms of *anemia* and *polycythemia* (see *Blood* disorders box).

WHITE BLOOD CELLS

These are also called WBCs, white blood corpuscles, or leukocytes; their principal role is to protect the body against infection and to fight infection when it occurs. The WBCs are bigger than RBCs (up to 15 thousandths of a millimeter in diameter) but much less numerous (about 7,500 per cubic millimeter of blood). They generally spend a much shorter part of their life span than RBCs in the blood itself. There are three main types of WBC, known as granulocytes, monocytes, and *lymphocytes*.

GRANULOCYTES WBCs of this type are also called polymorphonuclear leukocytes. Under the microscope, they are seen to contain granules and have an oddly shaped nucleus. Granulocytes are themselves of three types, called neutrophils, basophils, and eosinophils. Of these, the most important, making up 60 percent of all WBCs, which are responsible for isolating and killing invading bacteria (pus consists largely of neutrophils). The action of neutrophils in swallowing bacteria has led to their being called phagocytes (literally "engulfing cells"). Neutrophils remain in the blood for only about six to nine hours before moving through blood vessel walls into the tissues, where they survive for a few more days. Eosinophils play a part in allergic reactions and increase in numbers in certain parasitic infections.

MONOCYTES Also a type of phagocyte, these circulate in the bloodstream for about six to nine days and play an important part in the *immune system*.

LYMPHOCYTES Many of these are formed in the lymph glands rather than the bone marrow. They play a central role in the immune system, roving around the body between the bloodstream, lymph glands, and channels between the lymph glands.

T-type lymphocytes are responsible for the delayed hypersensitivity phenomena (see *Allergy*) and produce substances called lymphokines, which affect the function of many cells. T-type lymphocytes also moderate the activity of other lymphocytes called B-type cells. These lymphocytes form the antibodies that protect us against second attacks of diseases (e.g., measles). Individual lymphocytes survive for anywhere between three months and 10 years.

DISORDERS The *leukemias* are disorders in the numbers and maturity of WBCs. WBCs may also be too few in number (see *Blood disorders*). In *AIDS*, the T-lymphocytes are infected by a virus,

which results in dysfunction and increased risk of certain types of infection and cancers.

PLATELETS

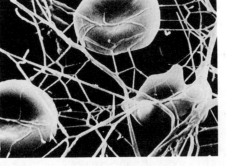

These are the smallest type of blood cell (two to three thousandths of a millimeter in diameter), more numerous than WBCs but less numerous than RBCs (about 250,000 per cubic millimeter of blood). Like other blood cells, they originate from stem cells in the bone marrow; they survive in blood for about nine days.

FUNCTION Platelets circulate in the blood in an inactive state, but under certain circumstances they begin to stick to blood vessel walls and adhere to each other. These activities are important in *hemostasis* (the arrest of bleeding) and in *blood clotting*. The same processes can also lead to the unwanted formation of thrombi (clots) in intact blood vessels (see *Thrombosis*), and to fatty deposits on blood vessel walls (see *Atheroma*). Because of their role in the formation of clots, platelets are sometimes also known as thrombocytes.

DISORDERS Abnormal platelets, or a lack of platelets, can lead to some types of *bleeding disorder*.

BLOOD CELLS IN DIAGNOSIS

Microscopic examination of blood preparations may reveal not only blood cell abnormalities characteristic of various diseases, but also healthy variations in the numbers of WBCs produced in response to infections. For example, the number of neutrophilic WBCs is raised in response to bacterial infections. The same is true of lymphocytes in some viral infections. The blood cell "picture" (numbers, shapes, and appearance of the various types) is thus of value to physicians in disease diagnosis (see *Blood count; Blood smear*).

Blood clotting

Solidification of blood. Blood begins to clot within seconds of the skin being cut. The clot helps seal the damaged blood vessels, which also contract to keep loss of blood to a minimum. Blood clotting is not always helpful, however. Thrombi (clots) formed inside major blood vessels are the cause of many heart attacks, strokes, and other disorders (see *Thrombosis*).

The blood clotting process has two parts (see illustration, below).

To prevent the formation of clots inside healthy blood vessels, the

---

HOW BLOOD CLOTS

Clotting describes the solidification of blood anywhere in the body. Clotting occurs almost immediately at the site of a cut and helps limit blood loss by sealing damaged blood vessels. However, if abnormal clotting occurs in major blood vessels, heart attacks, strokes, and other disorders may occur. The clotting process has two main parts—platelet activation and the formation of fibrin filaments.

Red blood cells enmeshed in fibrin filaments

Fibrin is formed by a chemical change from a soluble protein, fibrinogen, which is present in the blood. The fibrin molecules aggregate to form long filaments, which enmesh blood cells (see left) to form a solid clot. The conversion of fibrinogen to fibrin is the last step of the "coagulation cascade," a series of reactions in the blood triggered by tissue injury and platelet activation.

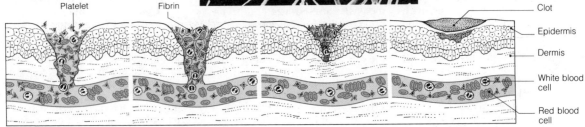

1 Platelets are activated by coming into contact with damaged blood vessel walls, where they become sticky and then clump at the site of injury and adhere to the damaged blood vessel wall.

2 Chemicals released by platelets and damaged tissues stimulate coagulation factors within the blood to form filaments of fibrin at the site of injury.

3 The fibrin filaments enmesh the platelets along with red and white blood cells.

4 Once the cut blood vessel is plugged by the mass of fibrin, platelets, and red and white blood cells, the fibrin filaments contract to form a solid clot.

Labels: Platelet, Fibrin, Clot, Epidermis, Dermis, White blood cell, Red blood cell blood also contains mechanisms that act to discourage clotting and dissolve clots. These balance the pro-clotting mechanisms; normally, the balance is tipped in favor of clot formation only when a blood vessel is damaged.

PLATELET AGGREGATION
Platelets have to be "activated" before they will clump together. This occurs when they come into contact with damaged blood vessel walls or artificial surfaces (such as glass), when blood flow is turbulent, or when platelets are acted on by certain chemicals secreted into the blood.

Once activated, platelets first become sticky, adhering to surfaces. They then change shape from disks into spiny spheres, enmeshing with each other. Finally, they release chemicals that activate other platelets, start the process of coagulation, and cause blood vessels to contract.

COAGULATION
Blood coagulation is triggered by chemicals released either by activated platelets or by tissues (following injury). Fibrin formation—the end product of coagulation—is the result of a complex series of reactions in the blood plasma called the "coagulation cascade." With each step in the cascade, a coagulation factor in the plasma is converted from an inactive to an active form.

The active form of the factor then activates several molecules of the next factor in the series—and so on until, in the final step, a factor called fibrinogen is converted into fibrin.

Provided all the participating factors are present, the activation of just one molecule of the first factor in the series can lead to the explosive production of up to 30,000 molecules of fibrin at the site of injury.

The factors involved in the coagulation cascade are numbered I, II, and V to XIII. Factor I is fibrinogen and factor II, its immediate precursor in the cascade, is called prothrombin. Most of the coagulation factors are made in the liver, which needs an adequate supply in the diet of *vitamin K*, found in green vegetables, for the manufacture of certain ones.

ANTICLOTTING MECHANISMS
Separate mechanisms act to prevent unwanted platelet activation and coagulation. Activation is inhibited mainly by a chemical known as prostacyclin (a type of *prostaglandin*), which is secreted by healthy blood vessel walls.

Coagulation is discouraged by various mechanisms. First, a number of inhibitory enzymes (types of protein) circulating in the blood neutralize activated coagulation factors. The most important of these is called antithrombin. Second, another series of enzymes is activated at the same time as the coagulation cascade. These enzymes form a substance called plasmin that breaks down fibrin (see *Fibrinolysis*). In addition, blood flow tends to discourage coagulation by washing away active coagulation factors from areas where they are being formed, and the liver deactivates any excess coagulation factors.

DEFECTS AND DISORDERS
Defects can occur for a wide variety of reasons in the clotting (or anticlotting) mechanisms, tipping the balance either in favor of a tendency to bleed or to form clots.

Some people carry a genetic defect that prevents them from producing sufficient amounts of one of the coagulation factors. In other cases, abnormally few platelets are made, insufficient vitamin K (required to make certain coagulation factors) is absorbed from the diet, or excessive amounts of the enzymes that inhibit coagulation of blood are produced. Abnormal bleeding may then result (see *Bleeding disorders*).

On the other hand, sometimes the balance is tipped abnormally in favor of coagulation and clotting. Possible causes include an increase in the levels of coagulation factors (as can occur in late pregnancy or when using some oral birth-control pills), a decrease in the level of enzymes that inhibit coagulation (as can occur in some forms of liver disease), or a sluggish blood flow through a particular area. The result may be abnormal clot formation (see *Thrombosis*).

Conditions in which there is a tendency for clot formation are often treated with *anticoagulants* such as heparin or warfarin. Heparin exerts its anticoagulant effect by increasing the level of antithrombin, which neutralizes activated coagulation factors; warfarin works by disrupting the production of coagulation factors. Because of the delicate balance between clotting and anticlotting mechanisms in blood, the use of these drugs has to be monitored frequently. Otherwise severe or persistent bleeding may develop.

Blood-clotting tests
Tests performed to screen for and diagnose *bleeding disorders*. These disorders usually result from deficiencies or abnormalities of the blood platelets or of blood coagulation factors (see *Blood clotting*).

Bleeding disorders caused by low numbers of platelets are detected by a *blood count* in conjunction with a test of the bleeding time.

Bleeding time may be measured by nicking the earlobe or puncturing the fingertip and timing the interval before bleeding stops. The normal range is three to eight minutes. Reduced platelet activity results in a prolonged bleeding time.

Various tests are used to assess the activity of blood coagulation factors—the most frequently performed being prothrombin time and partial thromboplastin time (named after two coagulation factors). The time taken for the patient's blood to clot is measured after addition of calcium and other factors that promote the coagulation process; the results are compared with the time taken for normal blood to clot under the same conditions. Abnormal results may indicate deficiency of a specific coagulation factor, as occurs in *hemophilia*, or of many coagulation factors, as in liver disease.

Anticoagulant therapy is designed to prolong the prothrombin time (clotting time) in order to reduce the risk of thrombosis (clotting) in susceptible subjects. People taking anticoagulants should have regular clotting tests to ensure that their therapy is adequate but not excessive, which could cause life-threatening bleeding.

Blood count
Also called complete blood count, this test measures hemoglobin concentration, and the numbers of red blood cells, white blood cells, and platelets in one cubic millimeter of blood. The proportion of various white blood cells is measured and the appearance of red and white cells is noted.

This is the most commonly performed blood test, important for diagnosing *anemia* and other conditions in which the number of blood cells is abnormally high (such as white blood cells in *leukemia* or red blood cells in *polycythemia*) or abnormally low (such as platelets in *thrombocytopenia*).

About 1 to 2 ml of blood are required for a blood count, which is usually performed in a laboratory by an automatic computerized analyzer, such as a Coulter counter.

Blood culture
See *Culture*.

DISORDERS OF THE BLOOD

Abnormalities can occur in any of the components of blood—the red blood cells (RBCs), white blood cells (WBCs), platelets, and numerous constituents of plasma.

Anemia (a deficiency of the red cell pigment *hemoglobin* and a consequent reduction in the blood's oxygen-carrying capacity) is by far the most common blood disorder. It has many different possible causes. In *polycythemia* there are too many red blood cells. In *leukemia* excessive numbers of immature white blood cells crowd out the normal cells from the bone marrow.

Defects in the platelets and in the clotting mechanisms may lead to any of various *bleeding disorders*. Unwanted clot formation (*thrombosis*) may result from circumstances that overactivate the clotting mechanisms.

Deficiencies of the proteins in blood plasma include hypoalbuminemia (*albumin* deficiency) and agammaglobulinemia (gamma globulin deficiency). Known causes of blood disorders include the following.

GENETIC DISORDERS

In these disorders there is an inherited abnormality in the production of some component of blood. People with *sickle cell anemia* and *thalassemia* produce an abnormal type of hemoglobin that makes their red blood cells more fragile; those with *hemophilia* fail to produce enough of one of the proteins involved in blood clotting. Disorders of this kind are present from birth and continue throughout life.

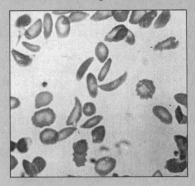

Sickle cell anemia
In this genetic (inherited) disorder, the red blood cells are abnormally fragile and have a characteristic sickle shape.

NUTRITIONAL DISORDERS

Loss of regular amounts of blood over an extended period may mean that iron (required to make hemoglobin) is lost faster than it can be replaced in the diet (see *Anemia, iron-deficiency*).

If insufficient amounts of the vitamins B_{12} or folic acid reach the bone marrow, it produces fewer red blood cells, which are abnormally large (see *Anemia, megaloblastic*). The vitamin deficiency may be due to a poor diet or, more often in developed countries, to a failure to absorb vitamin B_{12} correctly from the intestinal tract.

INFECTION

Multiplication of bacteria in the blood with the production of toxins is termed *bacteremia* and *septicemia*.

Many other microorganisms (i.e., viruses, fungi, protozoa, and other parasites) may infect the blood at some stage in their life cycle. Some organisms (notably those responsible for *malaria*) may actually attack and destroy red blood cells and so cause anemia (see *Anemia, hemolytic*).

TUMORS

All types of leukemia are the result of a type of cancer of the bone marrow, causing overgrowth of abnormal white blood cells and destruction of the healthy marrow. In *polycythemia* vera, a similar process occurs, except that mainly red cells are produced to excess. Another type of bone marrow cancer called *multiple myeloma* can cause an excess of certain proteins in the blood plasma.

POISONS

Carbon monoxide directly impairs the functioning of red blood cells by displacing oxygen bound to hemoglobin within the cells. Lead poisoning causes defective red blood cell production. Some snake and spider venoms destroy red cells and/or provoke clotting. *Septicemia* describes the presence of poisons produced in the blood by bacteria; toxemia describes the presence of metabolic poisons in the blood.

DRUGS

Certain drugs can cause blood abnormalities as a side effect. For example, co-trimoxazole, thiazide diuretics, and carbimazole may depress the production of white blood cells and/or platelets; chloramphenicol and sulfonamides may

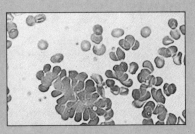

Cold agglutinin disorder
This is a rare blood disorder in which the body develops antibodies to its own red blood cells, causing them to clump together. This effect is especially marked in cold conditions when the clumps of cells reduce blood flow to the limbs.

depress all blood cell production; methotrexate and phenytoin may interfere with red cell production.

Too high a dose of *anticoagulant drugs* can cause a bleeding tendency through excessive disruption of clotting mechanisms.

RADIATION

High doses of radiation (received at the time of therapy or from nuclear explosions or radioactive leaks from nuclear reactors) can severely damage the bone marrow, causing depression of all blood cell production (see *Anemia, aplastic*).

OTHER DISORDERS

Albumin—an important protein in the blood plasma—may become deficient either as a result of liver disease (reduced production) or kidney disease (loss of albumin in the urine).

Liver disease may also cause *hyperbilirubinemia* (excess bilirubin in the blood), anemia, and deficiencies of some of the clotting factors. Kidney disease causes *uremia* (excess urea in the blood), sometimes anemia (possibly due to decreased production of the hormone erythropoietin), and also complex changes in blood chemistry.

INVESTIGATION

Blood disorders are investigated principally by various *blood tests*, such as the *blood count*, *blood smear*, and *blood clotting tests*.

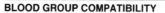

Blood donation

The process of giving blood so that it can be used in *blood transfusion*. Usually whole blood is taken from the donor and broken down later into components for storage. Recently, a new method called apheresis has been introduced, which involves extracting only a specific blood component from the donor. Whole blood donation takes about 45 minutes, including the medical check, while apheresis takes about two and a half hours.

Any healthy adult can potentially be a blood donor. Volunteer donors are first interviewed about their medical history. Anyone who has had anemia, cancer, heart disease, malaria, or hepatitis, or who has been exposed to the AIDS virus may be disqualified. Pregnant women are also disqualified. A blood sample taken from a finger or earlobe is then tested for anemia; body temperature, pulse, and blood pressure are also checked.

Most regular donors of whole blood give blood three or four times a year, but those with rare blood groups may be asked to give once every two months. Donors may safely give blood by apheresis as often as twice a week, provided a whole blood donation is not made between procedures.

HOW IT IS DONE

WHOLE BLOOD DONATION While the donor lies down and relaxes, a needle attached to a tube is inserted into the forearm. Up to a pint of blood (about one tenth of the total volume in the circulation) is slowly withdrawn into a plastic bag containing anticoagulant to prevent the blood from clotting. Most people feel fine after giving blood. A few may feel faint or sick and should rest or lie down for a few minutes. All donors should avoid strenuous exercise for about three hours after giving blood and should drink plenty of water and fruit juices.

The blood is taken to a local transfusion center, where it is tested for hepatitis B virus, syphilis, and antibody to HIV (the AIDS virus). The blood will not be used for transfusion if any of these is present. After being classified into blood groups, the blood is stored in a blood bank, either whole or separated into different components (see *Blood products*).

APHERESIS This technique allows only a blood component, such as plasma, platelets, or white cells, to be withdrawn from the circulation. About a pint of the donor's blood is taken from one arm, circulated through a closed, sterile separator system, and then returned to the other arm minus the component being collected. This withdrawal and return is repeated six to eight times, and collects the same amount of component normally requiring six to eight donors. Because only a single donor may be required to provide a patient with a sufficient quantity of a particular component, the risk of reaction or hepatitis transmission is reduced.

Blood gases

A test for determining the acidity-alkalinity (pH) and the concentrations of oxygen, carbon dioxide, and bicarbonate in the blood.

Blood oxygen and carbon dioxide values are useful in the diagnosing and monitoring of *respiratory failure*. Bicarbonate and acidity reflect the *acid-base balance* of the body. This may be disturbed in conditions such as diabetic ketoacidosis, aspirin poisoning, or repeated vomiting.

Modern apparatus can measure blood gases quickly using a few drops of blood, but full information requires samples to be taken from an artery as well as a vein and possibly from the interior of the heart.

Blood groups

Systems of classifying blood according to differences in the antigenic (able to provoke an immune reaction) make-up of red blood cells. Blood group typing is essential for a safe blood transfusion.

TYPES

ABO GROUPS Attempts in the nineteenth century and earlier at transfusing blood from one living person to another were sometimes successful but sometimes caused serious illness and even death. In 1900 the German pathologist Karl Landsteiner began mixing blood taken from different people and found that some mixtures were "compatible" while others were not. He discovered two types of marker proteins, or antigens, on the surface of the red blood cells—these he called A and B. According to whether a person's blood contains one or other antigen, both, or neither, it is classified as type A, B, AB, or O. Landsteiner found that the fluid part of the blood contained antibodies—anti-A and anti-B—that reacted with the protein markers.

The most common of the ABO blood groups is O, followed by A, then B, and finally AB. The precise frequency of each group differs among races.

BLOOD GROUP COMPATIBILITY

Recipient blood group	Donor blood group			
	A	B	AB	O
A	▲	●	●	▲
B	●	▲	●	▲
AB	▲	▲	▲	▲
O	●	●	●	▲

Key   ▲ Compatible   ● Incompatible

RHESUS FACTORS Another blood-group system, the Rhesus factors (Rh factors), was discovered in 1940 by Landsteiner during experiments on Rhesus monkeys. This system involves several antigens, the most important of which is factor D. This factor is found in the blood of 85 percent of people, who are called Rh positive, while 15 percent lack the factor and are Rh negative. Individuals are therefore classed as, for example, "O positive" or "AB negative" on the basis of their ABO and Rh blood groups. The main importance of this group is in pregnancy in Rh-negative women since, if the baby is Rh positive, the mother may form antibodies against the baby's blood (see *Hemolytic disease of the newborn*). Rh-negative women are given antibodies directed against factor D after delivery to prevent the development of anti-D antibodies in the mother, which would cause hemolytic disease of the newborn in Rh-positive infants. Transfusion of Rh-positive blood into an Rh-negative patient can also cause a serious reaction if the patient has had previous blood transfusions that contained the RH antigen.

OTHER GROUPS

Since the discovery of the ABO and Rh factors, about 400 other antigens have been identified, but, since these various antigens are widely scattered throughout the population, these rarely cause transfusion problems.

USES

TRANSFUSION AND CROSS MATCHING The ABO and Rh groups are used to categorize blood stored in blood banks so that if a patient who is, for example, A positive, needs a transfusion he or she can be given A-positive blood from the bank. In practice, however, each unit (about a pint) of blood to be given is first tested against a small sample of the patient's blood to exclude the small possibility that the two might be incompatible because of a reaction due to one of the other blood groups. This test is known as cross matching and takes a short time to perform. In an emergency, unmatched blood of the appropriate group may need to be given. (See *Blood transfusion*.)

ANTHROPOLOGY The ABO blood groups are found in all people, but the frequency of each group varies with race and geographical distribution. Study of blood groups can therefore aid anthropologists who are involved in investigating, for example, early population migrations.

PATERNITY CASES The blood group of an individual is determined by the genes inherited from his or her parents. Identification of blood group can be used in a paternity case to establish that a man could not have been the father of a particular child. It cannot

be shown positively that a man is the father by blood grouping, but, with modern techniques of gene analysis, paternity can now be proved with virtual certainty.

CRIMINAL INVESTIGATION Blood found at the scene of a crime can be grouped according to the various red blood cell antigens present. Although techniques are not yet sophisticated enough to allow positive identification of a specific individual, it is possible to exclude suspects if one of the red blood cell antigens does not match. Because ABO antigens are inherited, they occur in other tissue fluids, such as semen and saliva. Analysis of blood groups can also be useful in *forensic medicine* (the interrelation of medicine and the law).

INHERITED DISORDERS Some blood groups are associated with particular disorders. For example, blood group

A has been found to be more common in people suffering from cancer of the stomach. People who have blood group O are apparently more susceptible to peptic ulcer.

Blood loss
See *Bleeding, treatment of.*

Blood poisoning
A common name for *septicemia* or toxemia, a serious, often life-threatening illness caused by multiplication of bacteria and their formation of poisons or toxins in the bloodstream. Septicemia may be a complication of an infection (i.e., an infected wound or burn). It was formerly a feared and fatal complication of childbirth (see *Puerperal sepsis*). In some infective conditions, profound shock—called *septic shock*—may be caused by toxins released by bacteria. (See also *Bacteremia*.)

Blood pressure
The pressure of the blood in the main arteries, which rises and falls as the heart and muscles of the body cope with varying demands—exercise, stress, and sleep. Two types of pressure are measured. Systolic, the highest, is the pressure created by the contraction of the heart muscle and the elastic recoil of the aorta (great artery) as blood surges through it. Diastolic is when the ventricles relax between beats; it reflects the resistance of all the small arteries throughout the body and the load against which the heart must work. The pressure wave transmitted along the arteries with each heartbeat is easily felt as the *pulse*.

MEASURING BLOOD PRESSURE
A soft rubber cuff is inflated around the upper arm until it is tight enough to stop the flow of blood. The cuff is then gradually deflated until, by listening to the main artery through a stethoscope, the blood can first be heard as a beat forcing its way along the main artery in the arm. This is recorded as the systolic pressure. The cuff is then deflated further until the beat disappears and the blood flows steadily through the now open artery—giving the diastolic pressure.

Blood pressure may also be measured by miniature devices attached to an artery or by a continuous recording while an individual leads his or her daily life.

Blood pressure is recorded by giving the systolic pressure and diastolic pressure, expressed as millimeters of

mercury (mm Hg). This is because the earliest equipment used a glass column filled with mercury to measure the pressure directly. Today, some sphygmomanometers use a

spring gauge with a round dial. A healthy young adult has a blood pressure reading of about 110/75, which often normally rises with age to about 130/90 at age 60.

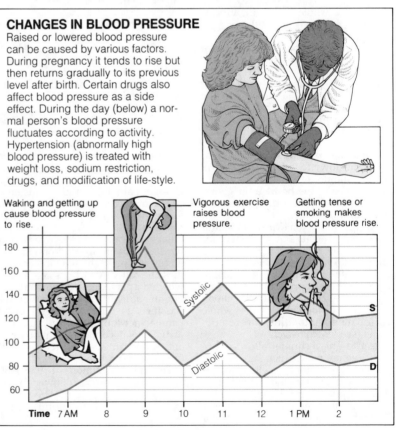

CHANGES IN BLOOD PRESSURE
Raised or lowered blood pressure can be caused by various factors. During pregnancy it tends to rise but then returns gradually to its previous level after birth. Certain drugs also affect blood pressure as a side effect. During the day (below) a normal person's blood pressure fluctuates according to activity. Hypertension (abnormally high blood pressure) is treated with weight loss, sodium restriction, drugs, and modification of life-style.

Waking and getting up cause blood pressure to rise.

Vigorous exercise raises blood pressure.

Getting tense or smoking makes blood pressure rise.

Systolic

Diastolic

S

D

Time 7 AM 8 9 10 11 12 1 PM 2

Blood products

After *blood donation*, blood is stored either whole or separated into its various components. Each product has a particular use in *blood transfusion*.

WHOLE BLOOD

Used to restore blood volume following sudden severe bleeding—for instance, after a traffic accident or during major surgery. Whole blood keeps three to four weeks after donation.

PACKED RED CELLS

Prepared by removing part of the liquid plasma. Concentrated red cells are used to treat patients with some forms of chronic anemia that have not responded to drug treatment. They provide the necessary hemoglobin without overloading the recipient with fluid, which can result in or aggravate heart failure. The cells can also be used to treat babies with *hemolytic disease of the newborn* ("Rhesus" babies).

WASHED RED CELLS

Blood that has had the white blood cells and/or plasma protein removed, thus reducing the chances of allergic reaction in patients, such as those with chronic anemia, who require transfusions over a long period.

FROZEN RED CELLS

Red cells can be preserved for long periods if stored at very low temperatures. This technique is used to preserve red cells belonging to rare blood groups.

PLATELETS

Extracted from whole blood and concentrated, they play an important part in normal blood clotting. Their low level in some blood disorders causes the patient to bruise easily and suffer internal bleeding. If necessary, platelets from several donors can be given during one transfusion.

WHITE BLOOD CELLS

Granulocytes, a type of white blood cell, can be separated from normal blood, or from the blood of patients with chronic granulocytic leukemia (who have an excess of these cells). Patients with life-threatening infections accompanied by abnormally low levels of granulocytes may be treated with granulocytes if they are not responding to antibiotics.

FROZEN FRESH PLASMA

Prepared by separating and freezing plasma as soon as possible after blood collection. Rich in clotting factors, fresh plasma is used to correct many types of bleeding disorders.

PLASMA PROTEIN SOLUTIONS

The liquid part of any whole blood not used within three weeks of collection that is converted into a concentrated solution of albumin (the main protein in plasma). The solution can be stored for long periods. Its chief use is in treating shock, resulting from severe blood loss, until whole blood compatible with the patient's blood group becomes available.

Purified albumin preparations are used to treat the nephrotic syndrome (a kidney disorder causing albumin loss in the urine) and chronic liver disease (in which production of albumin is deficient).

CLOTTING FACTORS

Concentrates of clotting factors VIII and IX can be prepared for the treatment of hemophilia and Christmas disease. Because blood from many donors is required to produce one small batch of clotting factor, it must be heat-treated to reduce the risk of hepatitis or AIDS transmission.

IMMUNOGLOBULINS

Antibodies (immunoglobulins) occur in the blood of patients recovering from certain viral diseases, such as rubella or hepatitis B, and in those who have recently been immunized—for example, against tetanus. These antibodies can be concentrated from plasma taken from such patients and used to protect people who are unable to produce their own antibodies or who have recently been exposed to a viral disease. This technique of inferring immunity is known as passive *immunization*.

A similar blood product, anti-D immunoglobulin, is obtained from the blood of patients sensitized to the Rh blood group factor. If given to an Rh-negative mother within 60 hours of her giving birth to an Rh-positive baby, it will prevent *hemolytic disease of the newborn* in her future babies.

Blood smear

A test that involves smearing a drop of blood onto a glass slide so that it can be examined under a microscope. The blood smear is stained with special dyes to make the blood cells show up more clearly.

The shape and appearance of blood cells are inspected for any abnormality, such as sickle-shaped red blood cells in sickle cell disease or abnormal lymphocytes in infectious mononucleosis. The relative proportions of the different types of white blood cells can also be counted. This examination, called a differential white cell count, may be helpful in diagnosing infection or leukemia. Blood smears are also used in diagnosing infections, such as malaria, in which the parasites can be seen inside the red blood cells.

Blood smears are usually done with a complete *blood count*.

Blood tests

Analysis of a sample of blood that gives information on its cells and proteins and any of the chemicals, antigens, antibodies, and gases that it carries. Since blood is the main transport system of the body, such tests can be used to check on the health of major organs, as well as on respiratory function, hormonal balance, the immune system, and metabolism.

TYPES

There are three types of blood test.

HEMATOLOGICAL TESTS These tests involve looking at the components of the blood itself, examining the numbers, shape, size, and appearance of cells, and testing the function of clotting factors. The most important hematological tests are *blood count*, *blood smear*, and *blood clotting tests*.

BIOCHEMICAL TESTS These look at chemicals in the blood, such as sodium, potassium, uric acid, and urea, and at vitamins, gases, digested foods, and drugs. (See *Acid-base balance*; *Kidney function tests*; *Liver function tests*.)

MICROBIOLOGICAL TESTS In these tests, the blood is examined for microorganisms, such as bacteria, viruses and viral particles, fungi, and parasites, and for antibodies that form against them. (See *Culture*.)

HOW THEY ARE DONE

The most convenient site for taking a blood sample is a vein at the bend in the elbow. A tourniquet is applied to the upper arm, and the blood is withdrawn through a needle into a syringe. The procedure causes only mild discomfort. Up to 20 ml of blood may be required, but, as the circulation contains 4 to 5 liters, loss of this small proportion has no harmful effect. If only a few drops are needed, they may be obtained by pricking a finger. Some tests require arterial blood, which is taken from the wrist or the groin. Obtaining such blood is a more difficult procedure that may cause some discomfort.

The sample may be allowed to clot, leaving its clear serum for examination, or an anticoagulant may be added to allow study of the cells and clotting factors. The sample is then sent to the laboratory, where one or more of the hundreds of available tests are performed. In some laboratories, modern computerized analyzers are

B

used to perform many different tests simultaneously on one small sample of blood. The printed results compare each value with the accepted normal range for that test. Each laboratory produces its own normal ranges that depend on the method and the ingredients of the test, and sometimes on the age and sex of the patient.

Blood transfusion

The infusion of large volumes of blood or blood components directly into the bloodstream, done mainly to remedy severe blood loss or to correct anemia.

Before the discovery of the major *blood groups* earlier this century, blood transfusion was a hazardous procedure, often causing severe reactions and even death. Growing knowledge of the complex properties of blood and its components has now made transfusion a safe procedure, although still not without possible complications.

WHY IT IS DONE

Blood transfusion may be needed by a patient who has bled severely after an accident or has lost a lot of blood during an operation. It may also be required after internal bleeding—for example, from a bleeding peptic ulcer. Chronic anemia that does not respond to medication may require treatment by blood transfusion (for example, in conditions such as thalassemia and leukemia).

In an exchange transfusion, nearly all of the recipient's blood is replaced by donor blood. It is most often needed in *hemolytic disease of the newborn* ("Rhesus babies") when abnormally high levels of bilirubin in the blood might cause brain damage.

HOW IT IS DONE

Before transfusion, blood must be cross matched to ensure compatibility. This procedure involves taking a sample of the recipient's blood, identifying the blood group, and matching it with suitable donor blood. This is done by mixing some of each blood sample on a microscope slide and examining it to make sure there are no antibodies in the recipient's plasma that would damage the donor blood cells. Blood can usually be cross matched in one hour or less. If the patient is losing blood very rapidly, it may not be possible to wait. In this case, O Rh-negative blood that has not been cross matched ("universal donor"), plasma protein solution, or an artificial plasma substitute may be given to the patient until tested blood becomes available.

Blood is transfused into an arm vein. Usually, each unit (about 1 pint) of blood is given over one to four hours; in an emergency 1 pint may be given in a couple of minutes. The amount of blood required depends on how much has been lost or on the severity of anemia. Usually, if transfusion is needed, more than one unit is given to justify the risks entailed in giving blood. During transfusion, the patient's pulse, blood pressure, and temperature are measured regularly, and, if there is any sign of a reaction, the transfusion is stopped.

COMPLICATIONS

If blood has not been cross matched reliably, antibodies in the recipient's blood may cause incompatible donor cells to hemolyze (burst). The most severe reactions can result in *shock* or kidney failure. Less severe reactions can produce fever, chills, a rash, or delayed anemia. Transfusion reactions can also occur as a result of allergy to transfused white cells, plasma proteins, or platelets.

Infections, such as hepatitis B, AIDS, syphilis, and malaria, can occur if donor blood has not been adequately screened. All blood for transfusion is now carefully tested and the risk of infection is very low.

In elderly or severely anemic patients transfusion can overload the circulation, leading to heart failure. *Diuretics*, which cause fluid loss, may need to be given simultaneously to avoid this. In patients with chronic anemia who require regular transfusion over many years, excess iron may accumulate (a condition called hemosiderosis) and cause damage to various organs, such as the heart, liver, and pancreas. Dangerous buildup of iron can be relieved by giving the drug deferoxamine.

Blood vessels

A general term for arteries, veins, and capillaries. (See *Circulatory system*.)

Blue baby

An infant with a cyanotic (blue-purple) complexion caused by a relative lack of oxygen in the blood. This is usually due to a structural defect of the heart or of the major arteries leaving the heart. The defect allows some of the deoxygenated blood returning to the right side of the heart to be pumped straight back into the general circulation instead of first going to the lungs to receive oxygen. Such defects can usually be corrected surgically. (See *Heart disease, congenital*.)

Blue bloater

A term physicians use to describe the appearance of some patients with the lung disease *emphysema*, with or without chronic *bronchitis*.

The person appears cyanotic (blue-purple) because of a deficiency in oxygen reaching the bloodstream from the lungs and appears bloated because of *edema* (swelling caused by fluid collection) in body tissues, mainly due to *heart failure* resulting from the lung damage.

Other patients with emphysema may have an alternative appearance known as *pink puffer*.

Blue Cross/Blue Shield

A private, not-for-profit health insurance association. The first local Blue Cross plan, covering hospital charges, began in 1929. Blue Shield's plans, to cover physicians' charges, were started a few years later by groups of physicians, in many cases by medical societies. The Blue Cross and Blue Shield associations merged in 1983. Blue Cross/Blue Shield plans in the US provide health insurance for more than 77 million people.

Blurred vision

A common term used to indicate a decrease or distortion of vision, or indistinct, fuzzy, or misty visual images. Blurred vision should not be confused with *double vision* (diplopia). Blurred vision can occur in one or both eyes, for episodes of varying lengths of time, and develop gradually or suddenly. Sometimes only part of the field of vision is affected. The need for proper glasses is probably the most common cause of blurred vision. Any change in vision should be brought to the attention of your physician.

CAUSES

Vision may be impaired, or blindness caused, by damage, disease, or abnormalities affecting the tear film, cornea, iris, lens, aqueous or vitreous humor, retina, or the nerve pathways behind the eye. These nerve pathways may be damaged by tumor, head injury, or *stroke*.

Many people notice gradual changes in near vision from the age of 40 onward—their vision for close work and for reading close-up becomes less sharp. They may also have problems with small print. Generally, distance vision does not worsen after age 40. After age 40 or 45, people generally need reading glasses or bifocals for close-up reading to correct the blur. This is due to *presbyopia* (decreased ability to focus close-up). If a person has been myopic (near-sighted), he or she may be able to take off the glasses to see close-up objects after age 40.

Blurred vision is most commonly due to refractive errors. They include *myopia* (nearsightedness), *hypermetropia* (farsightedness), and *astigmatism* (unequal curvature of the front of the eye). These defects can easily be rectified by glasses or contact lenses.

Blushing

Brief reddening of the face and sometimes the neck caused by the dilation of the blood vessels close to the surface of the skin. Blushing is usually an involuntary reaction to embarrassment. Some women blush during the *menopause* due to changes in hormonal activity (see *Hot flashes*). Flushing of the face occurs in association with the *carcinoid syndrome*.

Board certification

Formal recognition of a physician's qualifications in a medical specialty by one of the 23 organizations belonging to the American Board of Medical Specialties. To become board-certified in a medical specialty (i.e., dermatology, pediatrics, or surgery), a physician must usually complete an extended residency, demonstrate experience, complete special studies, and pass an exhaustive examination.

The 23 specialty boards, in addition to giving general certification, grant certification in 46 subspecialties (i.e., gastroenterology, hematology, or child psychiatry) after further study, experience, and examination.

The specialty boards consist of 15 to 25 physicians, representing the specialties and subspecialties in a given field, physicians in related fields and, often, physicians representing general medical organizations.

Body contour surgery

Operations performed to remove excess fat, skin, or both, from various parts of the body, especially the abdomen, thighs, and buttocks. Diet and exercise are the proper means of reducing the fat content of the body, and surgery is not a substitute. Operations may improve appearance where accumulations of fat or excess skin persist in certain areas after successful weight control.

ABDOMINAL WALL REDUCTION

In this contouring operation, often called abdominoplasty, excess skin and fat are removed from the abdomen. After the abdomen decreases in size, such as following weight loss or pregnancy, there remains an excess of skin in some people. These people may benefit from surgery.

The operation is carried out using general anesthesia and requires a hospital stay of from two to three days. The surgeon makes a horizontal "bikini" incision in the skin as low down on the abdomen as possible, then cuts upward between the fat and muscle layers. The flap of skin and fat is pulled down and the excess is removed. Sometimes, when the amount to be removed is particularly large, a vertical incision is required in addition to the horizontal one.

At the end of the operation the skin is stitched together. Drains are inserted into the wound and left in place for several days to prevent the risk of blood or serum collecting, which can lead to infection. The patient may sit on a chair soon after the operation, but should walk with the trunk slightly flexed for several weeks. Avoidance of tension on the wound will help minimize the size of the scar.

Despite care taken with movement after the operation, the final scar is often not as narrow as the patient and surgeon would like. In addition, the umbilicus (navel) usually must be moved to a higher position (with a resulting scar around it) because it has been pulled down with the flap during the operation.

REDUCTION OF THIGHS AND BUTTOCKS

In these operations, fat and skin are removed from the area of the crease separating these regions. The scar is planned to be in the "stocking-seam line," but the scars are often wide and unattractive and often end up in an undesired location. The wounds occasionally fail to heal properly, and the final appearance may not be symmetrical. Patients with generalized excess fat do not see improvement. Some people who ask for this operation may have a tilted pelvis because of prominent buttock muscles. Buttock and thigh reduction surgery yields a less satisfactory result than most other types of cosmetic plastic surgery operations.

SUCTION LIPECTOMY

To overcome the problem of noticeable scars, instruments have been developed to remove fat through "key-hole" incisions. A suction instrument is inserted through a small skin incision and moved back and forth under the skin to break up large areas of fat, which can then be suctioned through the instrument. However, because of the plentiful blood supply within the fat, there may be significant blood and fluid loss, which must be treated by the physician to prevent shock or anemia. In addition, the total amount of fat that can be removed at one time is limited. Suction lipectomy is useful in improving the appearance of people who have localized areas of excess fat, such as occurs on the hips, but cannot be used as a substitute for weight control. Minor irregularities and dimpling of the skin commonly occur after surgery.

Body odor

The smell caused by sweat on the skin surface. Sweat itself has no odor, but, if it remains on the skin for a few hours, bacterial decomposition may lead to body odor. The sweat may also smell strongly after garlic, curry, or other spicy foods are eaten. Bacterial decomposition of sweat occurs most noticeably in the armpits and around the genital area, because the *apocrine glands* in these areas contain proteins and fatty materials favorable to the growth of bacteria. Sweat from other areas of the body is mainly salt water, which does not encourage bacteria to form. Feet are an exception because they are subject to warm, airless conditions for hours on end—so making them a perfect environment for bacteria and fungi.

PREVENTING BODY ODOR

If body odor is a problem, the most effective treatment is to wash all over at least once daily. After washing, the use of a deodorant containing an antiperspirant will prevent sweat from reaching the surface of the skin.

Boil

An inflamed, pus-filled area of skin, usually an infected hair follicle (the tiny pit from which a hair grows). Common sites include the back of the neck, and moist areas such as the armpits and groin. A more severe and extensive form of a boil is a *carbuncle*.

The usual cause of boils is infection with the bacterium STAPHYLOCOCCUS AUREUS. Some people carry this organism in their nose or other sites; in many cases the source of an infection cannot be traced.

SYMPTOMS

A boil starts as a red, painful lump. As it swells it fills with pus and becomes rounded, with a yellowish tip (head). Recurrent boils may occur in people

B

with known or unrecognized *diabetes mellitus* or other conditions in which general body resistance to bacterial infection is impaired.

TREATMENT

Do not burst a boil, as this may spread the infection. A hot compress applied every two hours will relieve discomfort and hasten possible drainage and healing. Taking showers, instead of bathing, reduces the chances of spreading the infection.

If the boil is large and painful, consult your physician. He or she may prescribe an antibiotic, or may open the boil with a sterile needle to allow the pus to drain.

Occasionally, large boils have to be lanced using a surgical knife. This is usually done with a local anesthetic.

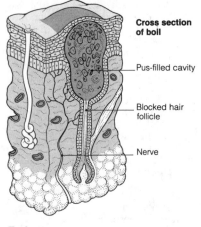

Cross section of boil

Pus-filled cavity

Blocked hair follicle

Nerve

Bolus

A soft mass of chewed food, ready to be swallowed, produced by the action of the tongue, teeth, and saliva. In this form, food is easily swallowed and passed through the esophagus.

A bolus also describes the rapid injection into a vein of a relatively large dose of a drug.

Bonding

The process by which a strong psychological tie is established between a parent and newborn child. Bonding is essential for a baby's healthy emotional development.

Ideas about bonding were first developed from studies of geese, monkeys, and other animals. Goslings were observed attaching themselves to and following the first moving object they saw after birth. Monkeys deprived of their mothers failed to develop normal maternal instincts. But most monkeys in the experiment developed normally when

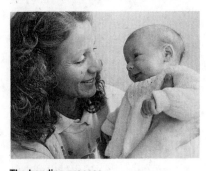

The bonding process
By maintaining eye-to-eye and frequent physical contact, bonding gradually becomes established.

given an inanimate mother substitute, especially a furry one that could be held and cuddled.

Bonding is a reciprocal process in which baby and parent respond to each other's gestures and expressions. A failure to bond may occur if a baby is sick or premature and has to be taken from his or her parent (by being placed in an incubator directly after birth), but most babies bond normally with special attention at a later stage. Bonding problems may occur if a new parent's own early family experiences failed to provide a good model of parent-infant interaction. However, such people can be taught successful ways to interact with their newborns.

Lack of bonding may increase the risk of neglect or child abuse and may lead to delayed mental development, depression, and inability to develop satisfactory relationships in adulthood. Most studies indicate that employed mothers can bond as successfully as nonemployed mothers and that children can fare well with more than one primary caregiver (of either sex) as long as all caregivers are loving and consistent.

Bonding, dental

The correction of tooth defects by using plastic materials, porcelain, or acrylic. The effects of bonding can be preventive (as with the use of sealants) or restorative.

WHY IT IS DONE

Bonding is used to treat teeth that are fractured, chipped, too widely spaced, malformed, or badly stained. Bonding is also used to close small gaps between front teeth, restore decayed back teeth, and, in some cases, substitute for a crown. Bonding has been used to protect exposed roots and is increasingly used to attach *orthodontic appliances*. Its use may also

make the teeth less sensitive to variations in temperature. One type of bonding, which incorporates sealants, is preventive in nature. Sealants, which are made of plastic, help prevent decay in the deep grooves of molars by keeping out bacteria.

HOW IT IS DONE

In many cases, bonding procedures require no anesthesia or drilling. Bonding techniques involve securing a plastic or porcelain material to the surface of the tooth. First, the dentist applies a weak acid solution to the tooth, creating a roughened surface to which the bonding material can adhere. This technique is sometimes called acid-etching. The liquid bonding material (resin) is then applied to the rough surface.

If a portion of a tooth needs to be rebuilt or a missing part replaced, a composite resin is shaped on the tooth and then hardened.

If work is being done on the front teeth or on badly stained teeth, a porcelain or acrylic laminate veneer may be bonded to the tooth's surface. For this procedure the enamel is acid-etched and an adhesive resin is attached. Finally, the preshaped laminate veneer is positioned on top of the resin.

EFFECTIVENESS

With bonding, the structure and appearance of teeth can be improved. Results of the bonding procedure last for about five years, so the procedure requires renewing. In addition, bonding is weaker than natural tooth enamel, so it chips more easily. Bonded areas may also become stained by certain foods and beverages. Because crowns are more durable than bonding materials, crowns may be more suitable for repairing badly damaged back teeth. Poorly aligned teeth may require orthodontic treatment.

Bone

The structural material of the body's framework, or *skeleton*. Bone contains calcium and phosphorus, which make it hard and rigid; the arrangement of bone's fibers makes it resilient.

STRUCTURE

The surface of bone is covered with periosteum, a thin membrane that contains a network of blood vessels and nerves. Beneath the periosteum is a hard, dense shell of compact, or ivory bone. Inside this shell the bone is cancellous or spongy. The central cavity of hollow bones and the meshes of spongy bone contain a fatty tissue,

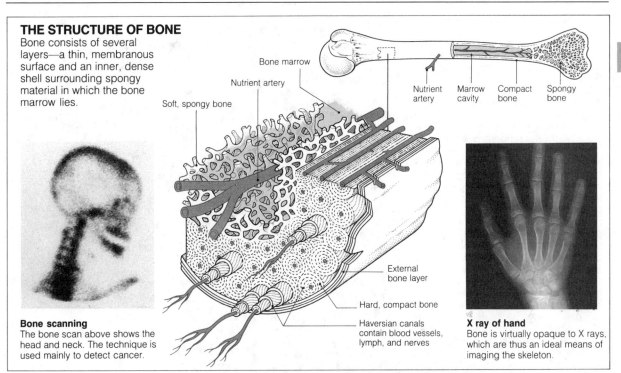

THE STRUCTURE OF BONE

Bone consists of several layers—a thin, membranous surface and an inner, dense shell surrounding spongy material in which the bone marrow lies.

Bone marrow

Nutrient artery

Soft, spongy bone

Nutrient artery

Marrow cavity

Compact bone

Spongy bone

External bone layer

Hard, compact bone

Haversian canals contain blood vessels, lymph, and nerves

Bone scanning
The bone scan above shows the head and neck. The technique is used mainly to detect cancer.

X ray of hand
Bone is virtually opaque to X rays, which are thus an ideal means of imaging the skeleton.

bone marrow, in which the red and most white blood cells and platelets are formed.

The hard structural part of bone underneath the periosteum is formed of columns of bone cells known as haversian canals. These are important for the nutrition, growth, and repair of the bone. The direction of the canals corresponds with the mechanical forces acting on the bone. Bone is insensitive; any sensation comes from the nerves in the periosteum.

FUNCTIONS

The long, short, flat, and irregular bones of the skeleton provide a rigid framework for the muscles; the muscles form surface coverings of the cavities that protect the body's organs (the heart and lungs in the bony thoracic cavity and the brain in the skull). Bones, with the joints and muscles, form the locomotor system.

GROWTH

The growth of bone is a balance between the activity of its two constituent cells, osteoblasts and osteoclasts. Osteoblasts encourage the deposit of the mineral calcium phosphate on the protein framework of the bone. Osteoclasts remove mineral from the bone. The actions of these cells are controlled by hormones: growth hormone secreted by the pituitary gland, the sex hormones estrogen and

testosterone, the adrenal hormones, parathyroid hormone, and the thyroid hormone thyrocalcitonin. These hormones also maintain the calcium level in the blood within close limits; any fall below the normal range affects the nerves and muscles.

Most bones begin to develop in the embryo during the fifth or sixth week of pregnancy, taking the form of cartilage. This cartilage begins to be replaced by hard bone, in a process known as *ossification*, at around the seventh or eighth week of pregnancy; the process is not complete until early adult life. At birth many bones consist mainly of cartilage, which will ossify later. The ends of the long bones are separate from the shaft, allowing the bones to grow. Some small bones of the hands and feet consist entirely of cartilage. Many of the bones of the skull do not begin life as bone. They are known as membranous bones.

Bone abscess

A localized collection of pus in a bone (see *Osteomyelitis*).

Bone cancer

Malignant growth in bone. Bone cancer may originate in the bone itself (primary bone cancer) or, more commonly, be a result of cancer that has spread from elsewhere in the body

(secondary bone cancer). The growth replaces bone, causing pain and sometimes swelling. It also makes the bone more likely to fracture without preceding injury. Bone cancer that affects the spine may cause collapse or crushing of vertebrae, damaging the spinal cord, and thus causing weakness or paralysis of the affected limbs.

PRIMARY BONE CANCER

The most common type of this rare form of cancer is *osteosarcoma*, which most frequently affects the leg bones of children and young adults. Symptoms of osteosarcoma are pain, tenderness, and swelling, typically just above or just below the knee. X rays, bone scans (see *Bone imaging*), and *biopsy* will confirm the diagnosis.

Other, even rarer, types of primary bone cancer include *chondrosarcoma* (originating from cartilage) and *fibrosarcoma* (from fibrous tissue). Cancer can also start in bone marrow (see *Ewing's tumor; Multiple myeloma*).

The treatment of osteosarcoma, chondrosarcoma, and fibrosarcoma depends on the extent to which the disease has spread. If it is confined to bone, amputation may be recommended. Alternatively, *radiation therapy* or *chemotherapy* may be used to control the tumor. With modern drugs, the outlook has improved and many patients have benefited.

SECONDARY BONE CANCER

Secondary, or metastatic, bone cancer, is more common than primary bone cancer; it usually occurs later in life. The cancers that spread readily to bone are those of the breast, lung, prostate, thyroid, and kidney. Bone metastases occur commonly in the vertebrae, pelvis, ribs, and skull.

In secondary bone cancer, pain is usually the main symptom and is often worse at night. Affected bones are abnormally fragile and may fracture, even without preceding injury. Such a fracture (a pathological fracture) may be the first indication that a person has cancer.

Imaging studies will confirm the presence of secondary bone cancer. If the original site of the cancer is not obvious, further tests may be needed to identify it.

Secondary bone cancers from the breast and prostate often respond to hormone therapy. Growth of prostate tumors may be inhibited with estrogen or hypothalamic hormones and in some breast tumors by *hormone antagonists*. Sometimes the most effective treatment is removal of the endocrine glands (ovaries, testes, or adrenals). Pathological fractures may require orthopedic surgery, with pins and plates inserted in the bone.

Bone cyst

A cavity in a bone, usually filled with fluid. It typically develops at one end of a long bone. The presence of a cyst is often discovered by chance after there has been a bone fracture at the site of the cyst. A minor operation that involves scraping the cyst and filling the cavity with bone chips usually cures the condition.

Bone graft

An operation in which a small piece of bone is taken from one part of the body to repair bone damage in another part. The bone graft is attached to the defective bone, and provides a bone growth stimulating protein. Although the bone graft eventually dies, it acts as a scaffold upon which new bone can grow.

WHY IT IS DONE

A bone graft has four main uses: to encourage a fracture to heal, to restore bone lost through injury, to replace bone removed surgically because of disease, and to provide a peg to join the bones of a diseased or unstable joint. A bone graft may also be used in cosmetic surgery to improve the shape of the face and skull.

DISORDERS OF THE BONE

Bone is affected by the same types of disorders as other body tissues, but its hard, rigid structure makes for extra complications. If a bone receives a direct blow or suffers from repeated stress it may *fracture*. If it becomes infected (for instance, due to *osteomyelitis* or a *bone abscess*), the resulting inflammation may interfere with the blood supply, leading to death of part of the bone.

GENETIC DISORDERS

Several genetic (inherited) conditions may affect bone growth; these include *achondroplasia* and *osteogenesis imperfecta*. People with these are usually of *short stature*.

NUTRITIONAL DISORDERS

Lack of calcium and vitamin D in the diet may result in *rickets* in children and *osteomalacia* in adults; in both conditions the bones become soft and lose their shape.

HORMONAL DISORDERS

If the pituitary gland produces excess growth hormone before puberty, there is an overgrowth of bones and other organs leading to *gigantism*. Excess parathyroid hormone causes *bone cysts*. *Osteoporosis* is also frequently due to other hormonal disturbances.

TUMORS

Several different types of benign and malignant growth can affect bones (see *Bone tumor*; *Bone cancer*).

DEGENERATION

Degenerative disorders of bone become more common in old age. In *osteoarthritis* there is wearing of the bone surface in a number of joints.

AUTOIMMUNE DISORDERS

Here the body's *immune system* attacks its own tissues. The main autoimmune disorder that may affect bones is *rheumatoid arthritis*.

OTHER DISORDERS

Paget's disease involves thickening of the outer layer of the bones while the inside becomes spongy.

INVESTIGATION

Bone disorders are investigated by techniques such as *X rays*, *CT scanning*, and *radionuclide scanning*, by *biopsy*, and by biochemical *blood tests* to look for any abnormalities in the levels of hormones or nutrients such as calcium and vitamin D.

HOW IT IS DONE

The bone from which the graft is to be taken is exposed and a portion removed. The most common sources are the iliac crests (upper part of the hip bones). These bones contain a large amount of cancellous bone, the inner, spongy part, which is especially useful for getting grafts to "take." Other sources are the ribs, which provide curved bone, and the ulna (in the forearm), which provides excellent bone pegs.

The bone that needs treatment is exposed and the graft fixed to it with screws or wires. After the area has been stitched, it is put into a plaster cast to keep the graft in place.

RECOVERY PERIOD

Bruising and pain at the site from which the graft was taken clear up within a week or two, and the only large scars left are those where bone has been taken from the iliac crests. X rays are taken to check the progress of healing, which usually is well under way after about six weeks.

Most bone graft operations succeed in permitting formation of new bone as strong and efficient as the old.

Bone imaging

Technique for providing pictures that show bone structure or function, used for the detection of disease or injury of the bone.

TYPES

Because *X rays* are more fully absorbed by bone than by other tissues, X-ray images show bone structure clearly. This makes them ideal for diagnosing fractures and injuries and also for revealing tumors and infections that cause changes in bone structure. A more detailed examination of small changes or abnormalities hidden by surrounding structures is provided by *tomography* (taking X-ray pictures at different depths of the structure being examined) or *CT scanning*. Magnetic resonance imaging (*MRI*), which is tomographic imaging using extremely high voltage magnets, shows tumors and infections and the effect of diseased bone on surrounding muscles, ligaments, and fat. Either CT scanning or MRI is useful in looking for *disk prolapse* in people with low back pain.

Radionuclide scanning is used to reveal bone function—the rate of blood flow to the bone and of cell activity within it. The technique is used mainly to determine whether cancer has spread to bone. It also can give useful information on bone injuries, infections, tumors, arthritis, and on metabolic bone diseases, such as rickets.

Bone marrow

The soft fatty tissue found in bone cavities; it may be red or yellow. Red bone marrow is a blood-producing tissue present in all bones at birth. During the teens, it is gradually replaced in some bones by less active yellow marrow. In the adult, red marrow is confined chiefly to the spine, sternum, ribs, clavicle (collarbone), scapulae (shoulder blades), hipbones, and skull bones.

Red bone marrow is the factory for most of the *blood cells*—all of the red cells and platelets and most of the white cells. Stem cells within the red marrow are stimulated to form blood cells by erythropoietin, a hormone originating in the kidney. The blood cells go through various stages of maturation in the red marrow before they are ready to be released into the circulation. Yellow marrow produces some white cells, but is composed mainly of connective tissue and fat.

Sometimes marrow fails to produce the normal amount of blood cells, as in aplastic *anemia* or when it has been displaced by tumor cells. It may overproduce only certain blood cells, as in *polycythemia* and *leukemia*.

Bone marrow biopsy

A procedure to obtain a sample of cells from the bone marrow (aspiration biopsy) or a small core of bone with marrow inside (trephine biopsy). Microscopic examination of the bone marrow gives information on the development of the various components of blood and on the presence of cells foreign to the marrow. It is useful in the diagnosis of many blood disorders, including anemia, leukemia, bone marrow failure, and certain infections. It can also show whether bone marrow has been invaded by lymphoma or cells from other tumors. Trephine biopsy requires a long, thick needle for removal of the bone core,

usually from the iliac crest. Trephine is used when tumor growth makes aspiration impossible, or when bone marrow structure needs to be examined. Bone marrow biopsy may be performed repeatedly to monitor the response of a disease to treatment.

Bone marrow transplant

The technique of using normal bone marrow to replace malignant or defective marrow in a patient. In allogeneic bone marrow transplantation (BMT), healthy bone marrow is taken from a donor who has a very similar tissue type to the recipient's—usually a brother or sister. In autologous BMT the patient's own bone marrow is used. Either type of BMT should be done only in centers specializing in this procedure.

WHY IT IS DONE

Because the procedure itself carries certain risks, BMT is used only in the treatment of potentially fatal blood and immune disorders, including severe aplastic anemia, leukemia, severe combined immunodeficiency and inborn errors of metabolism.

HOW IT IS DONE

ALLOGENEIC BMT (See box, overleaf.)
AUTOLOGOUS BMT Bone marrow is taken from the patient (usually someone with a malignant disease) while his or her disease is in remission (not active) and stored by *cryopreservation* (a tissue-freezing technique). Before freezing, the marrow may be treated in an attempt to eliminate any remaining malignant cells. This method remains investigational for most conditions. If the disease recurs, the stored bone marrow can be thawed and reinfused into the patient, after destroying all his or her bone marrow as in allogeneic BMT.

COMPLICATIONS

Infection can be a major problem during the recovery period, and isolation nursing procedures must continue for about four to six weeks until the new marrow is producing adequate numbers of white blood cells.

In allogeneic BMT, the other dangerous complication is the rejection process known as *graft-versus-host disease* (GVHD). GVHD occurs when lymphocytes in the donor bone marrow recognize their new host (recipient) environment as foreign. Symptoms include rash, jaundice, and diarrhea. *Immunosuppressant drugs*, such as *cyclosporine*, prevent and treat rejection.

Complications may continue to arise for long periods after BMT.

Bone tumor

A swelling of bone. Bone tumors may be *benign* or *malignant* (see *Bone cancer*). There are different types of benign bone tumors. The most common is *osteochondroma*, a mixed swelling of bone and cartilage that often begins in childhood. Other types are *osteoma*, a smooth, rounded bone swelling, and chondroma (see *Chondromatosis*), which is made up of cartilage cells and occurs mainly in the hands or feet. Osteoma and chondroma are painless and may affect any bone in the body. No treatment is necessary unless the tumor becomes very large or unsightly, or if pressure on other structures (such as arteries or nerves) causes symptoms. In such cases, the tumor can be removed surgically.

Another type of benign tumor of bone is the giant cell tumor, or osteoclastoma. This tumor occurs in young adults, usually in the arm or leg. The giant cell tumor is painful and tender and should be removed.

Booster

A follow-up dose of *vaccine* given to reinforce the effect of the first.

Borborygmi

Name for the audible bowel sounds that are a normal part of the digestive process. They are caused by movement of air and fluid through the intestine. In some people they may be accentuated during times of anxiety.

Borborygmi may be affected by some disorders of the *intestine*, and physicians listen to the bowel sounds as an aid to diagnosis.

Borderline personality disorder

A form of personality organization falling between neurotic and more primitive psychotic levels. Someone with a borderline personality disorder is usually incapable of maintaining stable relationships; mood changes are often rapid and inappropriate. Frequent, angry outbursts are common, as are impulsive, self-damaging acts such as gambling, shoplifting, or suicide attempts.

Boric acid

A weak *antiseptic* that may still be used in some antifungal skin lotions and ophthalmic ointments.

Bornholm disease

One of many names for epidemic *pleurodynia*, an infectious disease characterized by severe chest pains and fever.

PERFORMING A BONE MARROW TRANSPLANT

Normal bone marrow is used to replace malignant or defective marrow. In the allogeneic procedure, healthy marrow is taken from a donor. In the autologous procedure, the patient's own healthy marrow is used.

With one sibling there is a 25% chance of finding a compatible donor.

With three siblings there are three opportunities for a 25% chance of finding a donor.

Finding a donor

The more siblings one has, the greater the chance of finding a donor. With three or more siblings, the chances are good.

HOW IT IS DONE

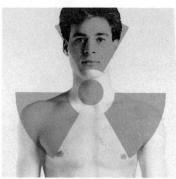

1 Before transplantation, all the recipient's marrow is destroyed by treatment with drugs or radiation. Destroying the marrow kills any cancer cells there.

3 After aspiration, the bone marrow is transfused intravenously into the patient. The bone marrow cells find their way through the circulation into the patient's marrow cavities, where they start to grow.

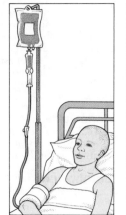

SITES OF BONE MARROW

Red or yellow in color, bone marrow is a soft, fatty tissue found in the cavities of bones. In newborn babies, red bone marrow is present in all bones; during the teen years, most is replaced by yellow marrow. The marrow used for transplants is red.

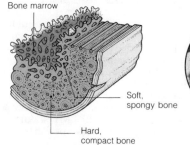

Bone marrow

Soft, spongy bone

Hard, compact bone

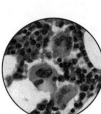

Bone marrow seen under the microscope

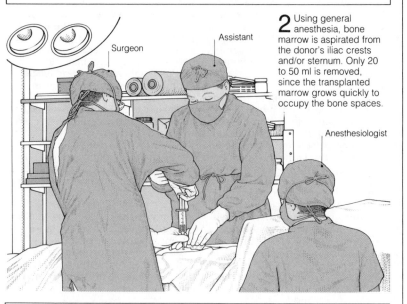

Surgeon

Assistant

2 Using general anesthesia, bone marrow is aspirated from the donor's iliac crests and/or sternum. Only 20 to 50 ml is removed, since the transplanted marrow grows quickly to occupy the bone spaces.

Anesthesiologist

ASPIRATION BIOPSY

A hollow aspiration needle is introduced into the bone (iliac crests or sternum). A stylet (a thin, sharp lance) is passed through the needle and advanced (using small, twisting movements) through the bone cortex. The stylet is removed. Bone marrow is sucked out from the cortex into a syringe connected to the needle.

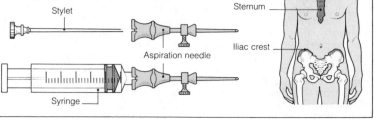

Stylet

Aspiration needle

Syringe

Sternum

Iliac crest

Bottle-feeding

A method of infant feeding using a formula usually based on modified cow's milk. Although *breast-feeding* is recommended where possible, many parents choose bottle-feeding for the convenience, certainty, and flexibility it offers. With bottle-feeding, there is no fluctuation in the quality or quantity of the milk, the baby's intake can be measured and regulated, and the mother's presence is not necessary.

PREPARING THE FEEDING

The formula must be measured accurately and made to the correct strength with water as instructed on the container. Some formulas may be purchased "ready-to-feed." No extra formula, sugar, or cereal should be added. Overconcentrated milk may injure a baby's kidneys and the extra calories may make him or her fat.

It is essential that strict hygienic rules be observed when preparing infant feedings because bacteria-causing infections thrive in warm milk. All equipment should be cleaned thoroughly and sterilized using one of two methods.

ASEPTIC STERILIZATION
This technique involves sterilizing all bottles, nipples, and caps before use by immersing them in boiling water. The feeding is then prepared using boiled water and can be used immediately after it cools to a lukewarm temperature.

TERMINAL STERILIZATION
This method involves sterilizing the prepared milk along with the bottles in a special steam sterilizing unit or saucepan. Up to six feedings—enough for one day—may be prepared at once and

BOTTLE-FEEDING

The parent's back should be supported firmly with feet flat on the floor. The baby should be cradled snugly with the head supported well above the level of the stomach. Eye contact should be maintained.

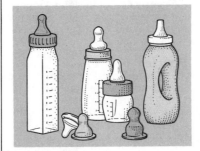

Types of bottle
Bottles, and their nipples, come in various shapes and sizes. Some come ready-filled with prepared formula.

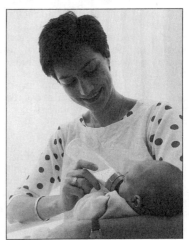

Technique
The bottle must be kept tilted and the flow of milk maintained at a good rate but not so fast as to cause choking.

stored in the refrigerator. The feeding may be warmed for use by standing the bottle in a pan of hot water, or by placing it in an electric warmer. Do not use a microwave oven; this method of warming may alter the nutritional value of the formula. Any unused milk must be discarded immediately.

PROBLEMS

If feedings are carefully prepared, equipment sterilized, and bottles given with warmth and cuddling, problems should be rare. However, parents should guard against overfeeding; the correct amount for an

infant is based on his or her birth weight and ideal growth rate.

A more serious long-term problem for some bottle-fed infants concerns the amino acids found in cow's milk. Early exposure to these amino acids (which are not present in breast milk) may sensitize the infant to cow's milk protein and result in allergic reactions in later life. If there is a history of allergy in the family, feeding an infant with a nonmilk formula may be recommended to prevent future allergic reaction. Consult your physician. (See also *Feeding, infant*.)

Botulism

A rare but serious form of poisoning caused by eating improperly canned or preserved food contaminated with a toxin, the most potent poison known to man, produced by the bacterium *CLOSTRIDIUM BOTULINUM*, which causes progressive muscular paralysis and other disturbances of the central and peripheral nervous system.

CAUSES

CLOSTRIDIUM BOTULINUM is found in soil and untreated water in most parts of the world and is harmlessly present in the intestinal tracts of many animals, including fish. It produces spores that resist boiling, salting, smoking, and some forms of pickling. These spores, which multiply only in the absence of air, cannot normally infect humans, but thrive in improperly preserved or canned food

where they produce the toxin. If such food is eaten, absorption of even minute amounts of toxin can lead to severe poisoning.

The foods most commonly responsible are home-preserved canned vegetables, cured pork and ham, and smoked or raw fish. Factory-canned foods are implicated occasionally, but are usually safe.

In infants, botulism can be contracted by another mechanism. The bacterium, which enters the intestinal tract in water or food (such as honey), colonizes the intestine, produces its toxin there, and causes a type of *hypotonia* (reduced muscle tone) known as the floppy infant syndrome. Botulism can also occur if the *CLOSTRIDIUM BOTULINUM* bacteria in the soil enter skin broken during an injury.

INCIDENCE

Botulism is more common in the US than anywhere else in the world (due to the popularity of preserving food at home). However, in an average year there are approximately 20 reported cases of food-borne botulism (causing fewer than 10 deaths), as many as 250 cases of infant botulism, and fewer than five cases of wound botulism in the entire country.

PREVENTION

Anyone who preserves food at home should make sure they sterilize it by pressure cooking at 250°F (120°C) for 30 minutes. Bulging cans or off-smelling preserved foods should not be taste-tested but should be discarded or investigated by health authorities.

SYMPTOMS AND TREATMENT

Symptoms of food-borne botulism usually first appear between eight and

B

36 hours after eating contaminated food. Symptoms include difficulty swallowing and speaking, nausea, vomiting, and double vision. Death occurs in about 70 percent of untreated cases and is usually due to suffocation caused by paralysis of the respiratory muscles. Prompt treatment with an antitoxin brings the risk of death down to less than 25 percent. (See also *Food poisoning*.)

Bougie
A soft flexible rod used to stretch narrowed passages in the body, particularly in the urethra and esophagus. The name is derived from the French word for candle, because bougies were often made from wax.

Bowel
A common name for the *intestine*.

Bowel movements, abnormal
See *Feces, abnormal*.

Bowel sounds
See *Borborygmi*.

Bowen's disease
A very rare skin disorder that sometimes becomes cancerous. The disorder consists of a flat, regular-shaped, patch of red, scaly skin, usually on the face or hands. Treatment consists of removing the diseased patch of skin surgically or destroying it by freezing or by *cauterization*. It is unlikely to recur. A person who has had Bowen's disease is much more likely than the average person to develop cancer of the lung, kidney, or large intestine later in life, therefore he or she should have periodic medical checkups to look for these.

Bow leg
An outward curving of bones in the legs. Bow legs are common in very young children and are a normal part of development. The curve usually straightens as the child grows, but, if the bowing is severe or persists beyond age 6, a physician should be consulted. A corrective operation may be needed.

Rarely, leg deformity is a result of bone disease, particularly *rickets* (a vitamin D deficiency) in children.

Brace, orthopedic
An appliance worn to support part of the body or hold it in a fixed position. One application is to correct or halt the development of a deformity. For example, a deformed spine is prevented from curving further by a rigid brace that fits closely to the back, chest, and pelvis.

A brace may also help the movement of a limb when movement would otherwise be impossible. For example, a person who has lost the ability to flex the foot upward, and, as a result, drags the toes on the ground with each step, can be fitted with a device (called a foot-drop splint) that keeps the foot permanently at right angles to the leg and thus allows walking. Some braces are used to relieve pain. The use of braces should be monitored because misuse can lead to weakness and joint stiffness.

Braces, dental
See *Orthodontic appliances*.

Brachialgia
Pain or stiffness in the arm. It is often accompanied by pain, tingling, or numbness of the hands or fingers, and weakness of hand grip. It may indicate an underlying disorder such as *frozen shoulder* or nerve compression from *cervical osteoarthritis*.

Brachial plexus
A collection of large nerve trunks that pass from the lower part of the cervical spine and upper part of the thoracic spine down the arm. These nerve trunks divide into the musculocutaneous and axillary, median, ulnar, and radial nerves that control muscles in and receive sensations from the arm and hand.

INJURIES
Injuries to the brachial plexus are an important and fairly common cause of partial or complete loss of movement and sensation in the arm. Damage to the brachial plexus sometimes occurs during birth, with an increased risk in breech delivery. In adults, a common cause of brachial plexus injury is a fall from a motorcycle.

Injury is usually a forcible separation of the neck and shoulder, due to a fall pushing the shoulder downward or to a blow to the side of the neck that stretches or tears upper nerve roots in the plexus. Damage to these roots causes paralysis in muscles of the shoulder and elbow.

Injury to lower nerve roots in the plexus, causing paralysis of muscles in the forearm and hand, can result from a forcible blow that lifts the arm and shoulder upward. In severe injuries, both upper and lower roots are damaged, producing complete paralysis of the arm.

TYPES OF BRACES
Braces are worn to support a part of the body or a limb or to keep a limb in a certain position. Braces also can help limb movement that would otherwise be difficult. A brace allows a person recovering from an injury or operation to exercise.

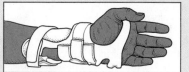

Wrist brace
Used to support a painful or weak wrist and as an alternative to surgery in the treatment of carpal tunnel syndrome. A wrist brace is usually made of plastic with foam padding.

Knee brace
Provides control of ligament instability while allowing the natural action of the knee. Knee braces are often used by athletes.

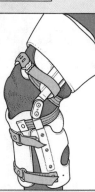

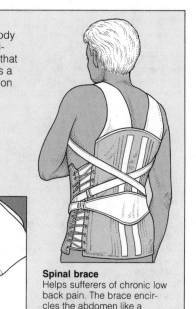

Spinal brace
Helps sufferers of chronic low back pain. The brace encircles the abdomen like a corset, preventing painful movement and decreasing the load on the lower spine. Braces are usually made of elastic material reinforced with metal or plastic.

Paralysis may be temporary if the stretching was not severe enough to actually tear nerve fibers.

TREATMENT The treatment of a brachial plexus injury depends on the extent of nerve damage, which is reflected in the amount of movement possible in the arm and shoulder. Electrical activity in the muscles, shown by *EMG* (electromyography) demonstrates those nerves that are still intact. *Myelography* (X-ray examination of the spinal cord after injection of a contrast medium) is used to assess nerve root damage. Sometimes, the exact situation will not be known until the neuroanatomy is inspected during the course of a repair operation.

Nerve roots that have been torn can be repaired by nerve grafting, a procedure done under a microscope, often with good results. If a nerve root has become separated from the spinal cord, attempts at repair will not restore function.

In the event of permanent paralysis of a particular group of muscles in the arm, function can be improved by doing a muscle or tendon transfer operation to provide an alternative structure to perform a particular movement. Physiotherapy, with exercises continued at home, will help restore function after a successful nerve graft operation and can reduce *contractures* in paralyzed muscles.

DISORDERS
Apart from injuries, the brachial plexus can be affected by the presence of a *cervical rib* (extra rib), infections, tumors, or *aneurysms*.

Bradycardia
An adult heart rate of below 60 beats per minute. Most people have a beat rate of between 60 and 100 beats, the average being 72 to 78. Many athletes and healthy people who exercise regularly and vigorously have bradycardia that is perfectly normal. In others, however, it may indicate an underlying disorder such as *myxedema* (an underactive thyroid gland) or *heart block*. Bradycardia may also be an effect of *beta-blockers*. Profound or sudden bradycardia may cause symptoms such as loss of energy, weakness, and fainting attacks.

Braille
A system of embossed dots that enables blind people to read and write. It was developed by the Frenchman Louis Braille and is now accepted for all written languages, music, mathematics, and science.

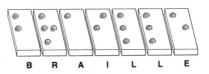

Example of Grade I braille
In this system, each letter is represented by its own pattern of dots.

The braille system is based on six raised dots, which can be arranged in different combinations to form 63 symbols. There are two types. In Grade I, each symbol represents an individual letter or punctuation mark. In Grade II, symbols represent common letter combinations or words. This second form is more widely used.

Brain
The major organ of the *nervous system*, located in the *skull*. The brain is the organ of thought, speech, and emotion, but its primary role is as the body's control center.

The brain and spinal cord constitute the *central nervous system* (CNS). The CNS controls basic functions such as rate of heartbeat, breathing, and body temperature. The brain receives, sorts, and interprets sensations from the nerves that extend from the CNS to every other part of the body; it initiates and coordinates the motor output involved in activities such as movement and speech.

The nerve pathways that control internal body functions, such as heart rate, temperature, sweating, and digestion, are called the *autonomic nervous system*.

The nerve pathways that carry sensations to the brain from the sense organs and messages from the brain to the muscles initiating movement are called the somatic nervous system.

Three main structures are easily recognized: the *brain stem, cerebellum,* and, above the brain stem, the large forebrain, much of which consists of the *cerebrum* (see illustration overleaf). Extending from the brain are 12 pairs of *cranial nerves*; some of these have a sensory function, some a motor function, and some have both.

BRAIN STEM AND CEREBELLUM
These parts of the brain are the oldest in evolutionary terms, and their structure and function differ little between humans and other mammals. The brain stem is concerned mainly with control of vital functions, such as breathing and blood pressure, and the cerebellum with muscular coordination, balance, and posture.

Both brain regions operate below the level of consciousness by *reflex* action, in which any particular stimulus or pattern of stimuli evokes a preprogrammed or automatic response. The brain stem and cerebellum receive sensory information (about temperature, pressure, position, or pain) from sensory receptors scattered throughout the body. The brain stem and cerebellum then transmit the appropriate response—for example, to muscles in the blood vessels to change blood pressure.

FOREBRAIN
The forebrain consists of a central group of structures and nerve nuclei (nerve cell groups) on the top of the brain stem and, enclosing these, the relatively huge cerebrum.

CENTRAL STRUCTURES These act mainly as links between parts of the cerebrum above and brain stem below. They include the two egg-shaped *thalami* which serve as relay stations for sensory information to the cerebrum. Beneath them, the *hypothalamus* is a tiny region involved in the regulation of body temperature, thirst, and appetite; it also influences sexual behavior, aggression, and sleep. The hypothalamus has close connections with the *pituitary gland*, which produces hormones that affect other glands and in this way controls growth, sexual development, metabolism, fluid balance, and many other physiological variables. Encircling the thalami, a further complex of nerve centers, the *limbic system*, is thought to be involved in the handling of emotions, some memory functions, and olfactory (smell) sensations.

CEREBRUM The two hemispheres that make up the cerebrum project upward and outward from the center of the forebrain to form an almost continuous egg-shaped mass. It constitutes nearly 70 percent of the weight of the entire nervous system.

The surfaces of the hemispheres are folded into deep clefts so that only one third of the total surface is visible. Certain of the sulci (fissures) separating gyri (folds) are particularly noticeable and divide the surface into distinct lobes—occipital, parietal, temporal, and frontal—named after the main bones of the skull that overlie them. The two halves of the cerebrum are connected by the corpus callosum.

The cerebral cortex (the outer surface of the cerebrum) consists of gray matter, with nerve cells arranged in six layers. This is the region of conscious thought, movement, and sen-

B

STRUCTURE OF THE BRAIN

The brain has three main parts—the brain stem (an extension of the spinal cord), the cerebellum, and the forebrain, much of which consists of the two large cerebral hemispheres. Each hemisphere consists of an outer layer, or cortex, which is rich in nerve cells and called gray matter, and inner areas rich in nerve fibers, called white matter. The surface of each hemisphere is thrown into folds called gyri separated by fissures called sulci. The two hemispheres are linked by a thick band of nerve fibers, the corpus callosum. Deep within the forebrain are various central structures, which include the thalamus, hypothalamus, basal ganglia, and pituitary gland.

The brain has a consistency like jelly and, in adults, weighs about 3 pounds. It is protected by membranous coverings, the meninges, within the skull.

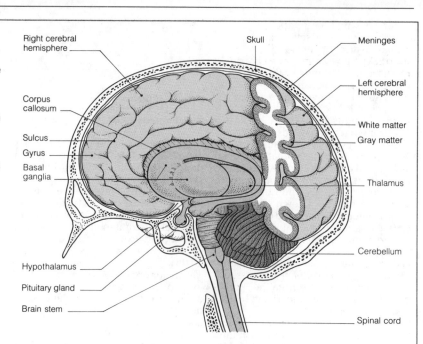

Lobes
These are broad surface regions of each hemisphere that are named after the overlying bones of the skull. The four main regions are the frontal, parietal, temporal, and occipital lobes.

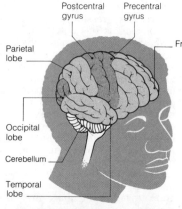

Special areas
Some brain areas are associated with specific functions—for example, the occipital lobe with vision, and the cerebellum with balance and coordination. Touch and pressure sensation is perceived within the postcentral gyrus. Muscle movements are controlled from the precentral gyrus; speech is controlled from an area in the frontal lobe of the dominant hemisphere.

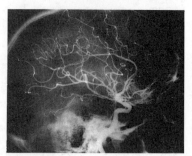

Angiography
This technique makes blood vessels clearly visible. The angiogram above shows the main blood supply to the brain—the carotid artery and its branches.

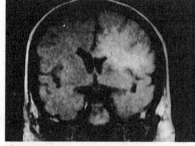

Magnetic resonance imaging
This technique is used mainly to reveal abnormalities that are otherwise undetectable. In the MRI scan above, the white mass to the upper right is a tumor.

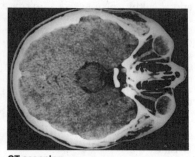

CT scanning
The CT scan above shows a "slice" through the head. The nose and eyeballs are visible at right; the small circular area in the center is the brain stem.

sation. It operates much like more primitive parts of the brain, except that incoming sensory information undergoes a much more detailed analysis. Various conscious factors, including perception, memory, thought, and decision-making, are interposed between the reception of sensory information and the output of a motor response. Actions initiated by output from the cortex—speech, movement, writing—can be highly complex in form.

Beneath the cortex, much of the cerebrum consists of tracts of nerve fibers forming "white matter"; these tracts connect various areas of the cortex to each other and to nerve centers in the center of the forebrain and brain stem. Deeper within the hemispheres are groups of cells named the *basal ganglia*; they are connected to the brain stem and cerebellum and are involved in relaying and modifying motor output from the cerebral cortex, signaling and coordinating movements to skeletal muscles.

Though the cerebrum is symmetrical in appearance, some higher activities such as speech and writing are controlled from one cerebral hemisphere, the dominant one. In right-handed people this is the left hemisphere; even in left-handed people the left side is usually dominant. The nondominant side is important in visual/spatial orientation and may be involved in artistic appreciation and creative thought.

PROTECTION AND NOURISHMENT

The whole of the brain and spinal cord is encased in three layers of membranes, called the *meninges*. The *cerebrospinal fluid* circulates between two of these layers and also within the four main brain cavities called *ventricles* (one in each cerebral hemisphere, a third in the center of the forebrain, and a fourth in the brain stem). This cerebrospinal fluid helps nourish the brain and also helps cushion it from trauma when the head is moved quickly or receives a blow.

The brain as a whole also has an extensive blood supply. Blood comes from a circle of arteries fed by the internal *carotid arteries* (which run up each side of the front of the neck to enter the base of the skull) and from two vertebral arteries that run parallel to the spinal cord. The brain receives about 20 percent of the cardiac output. (See *Brain* disorders box, overleaf; *Vision; Hearing; Smell; Pain; Consciousness; Thought; Memory; Speech; Intelligence; Perception; Psychology*.)

Brain abscess

A collection of pus, surrounded by inflamed tissues, in the brain or on its surface. Along with *brain tumors* and other space-occupying brain abnormalities, abscesses cause symptoms due to raised pressure and local damage to nerve tracts. The most common sites are the frontal and temporal lobes of the *cerebrum* in the forebrain.

CAUSES AND INCIDENCE

Brain abscesses, except with head injury, almost always result from the spread of infection from elsewhere in the body. About 40 percent of abscesses result from middle ear or sinus infections. Other causes include infection following a penetrating brain injury and blood-borne infection, most commonly in patients with acute bacterial *endocarditis* and certain *immunodeficiency disorders*. Abscesses that are due to blood-borne infection are often multiple.

SYMPTOMS

The most common symptoms are headache, drowsiness, and vomiting. There may also be visual disturbances, fever, epileptic seizures, and symptoms caused by local brain damage—for example, partial paralysis or speech disturbances.

DIAGNOSIS AND TREATMENT

The diagnosis is suggested by *CT scanning* or *MRI* (magnetic resonance imaging) of the brain. Treatment consists of a high dosage of antibiotics and usually surgery. A hole may need to be made in the skull (see *Craniotomy*) and the abscess is then either drained or removed; antibiotic drugs are also given.

OUTLOOK

Brain abscesses prove fatal in about 10 percent of cases, and the remaining patients often suffer some residual impairment of brain function. *Epilepsy* is common, so *anticonvulsant drugs* are often prescribed following removal or drainage of the abscess. (See also *Brain tumors; Brain hemorrhage; Brain syndrome, organic*.)

Brain damage

Degeneration or death of nerve cells and tracts within the brain. Damage may be localized to particular areas of the brain—causing specific defects of brain function, such as loss of coordination or difficulty with speech—or may be more diffuse, causing mental or severe physical handicap.

DIFFUSE DAMAGE

The most important cause of diffuse brain damage is prolonged cerebral *hypoxia* (not enough oxygen reaching the brain). This may occur during birth; a baby's brain cannot tolerate a lack of oxygen for more than about five minutes. At any age, hypoxia may occur as a result of *cardiac arrest* (stoppage of the heart) or *respiratory arrest* (cessation of breathing), and from causes such as poisoning, drowning, electric shock, or *status epilepticus* (prolonged convulsions).

Diffuse damage may also occur through the accumulation in the brain of substances poisonous to nerve cells—as in *phenylketonuria* (unless treated early) or *galactosemia*. Diffuse damage may also be a result of inhaling or ingesting environmental pollutants such as lead or mercury compounds (see *Minamata disease*).

Other possible causes include infections of the brain, such as *encephalitis* or, very rarely, vaccine damage following immunization.

LOCALIZED DAMAGE

Localized brain damage can occur as a result of *head injury*, especially penetrating injuries, at any age. It occurs later in life as a result of *stroke, brain tumor*, or *brain abscess*.

At birth, local damage to the *basal ganglia* (deep within the brain) caused by a raised blood level of *bilirubin* (formed from the destruction of blood cells in *hemolytic disease of the newborn*) leads to a condition called *kernicterus*, which is characterized by disorders of movement and sometimes mental deficiency. The basal ganglia may also be damaged by carbon monoxide.

SYMPTOMS AND TREATMENT

Brain damage that occurs before, during, or after birth may result in *cerebral palsy*, a condition characterized by paralysis and abnormal movements and often associated with mental retardation and sometimes deafness.

Victims of head injury, stroke, or other causes of localized or diffuse brain damage may also be left with any of a range of handicaps, including disturbances of movement, speech, or sensation, mental handicap, or epileptic seizures.

Nerve cells and tracts in the brain and spinal cord do not recover their function if they have been destroyed (nerves in the limbs or trunk regenerate slowly after being cut or crushed). Nevertheless, some improvement may be expected after brain damage as the victim learns to use other parts of the brain and other muscle groups in the body. Treatment often involves teamwork on the part of physicians and specialists in *physical therapy, speech therapy*, and *occupational therapy*.

B

DISORDERS OF THE BRAIN

Defects and disorders of the brain have much the same causes as disease in other body organs. One special feature of the brain, however, is that it is packed inside a rigid casing, the skull, so any space-occupying *brain abscess*, *brain tumor*, or *hematoma* (large blood clot) following a *head injury* or *brain hemorrhage* creates raised pressure that impairs the function of the whole brain. Another special feature is that brain cells destroyed through injury or disease cannot be replaced, so the loss in function can be more difficult to reverse.

Some diseases and defects in the brain are localized in a small region and may thus have a specific effect—for example, *aphasia* (speech loss). More often, damage is more diffuse and, because the brain has so many related functions, the symptoms can be varied and numerous.

CONGENITAL DEFECTS

Babies may be born with brain defects due to genetic or chromosomal disorders, as in *Down's syndrome*, *Tay-Sachs disease*, or *cri du chat syndrome* (all of which are associated with mental deficiency). Structural defects that arise during fetal development may be fundamental and untreatable, as in *microcephaly* (small head), or fatal, as in *anencephaly* (congenital absence of the brain). Others are potentially correctable, even while the fetus is still in the uterus, as in *hydrocephalus* (water on the brain).

IMPAIRED BLOOD AND OXYGEN SUPPLY

These are two of the most important causes of brain dysfunction because brain cells can survive only a few minutes without oxygen. *Hypoxia* (lack of oxygen) affecting the brain as a result of asphyxiation during the process of birth is one of the causes of *cerebral palsy*. Later in life, cerebral hypoxia can result from accidents such as choking or from arrest of breathing and heart beat following electrocution or drowning.

From middle age onward, the most important affliction of the brain is *cerebrovascular disease* impairing blood supply to one or several brain regions. If an artery within the brain becomes blocked or ruptures leading to hemorrhage, the result is a *stroke*.

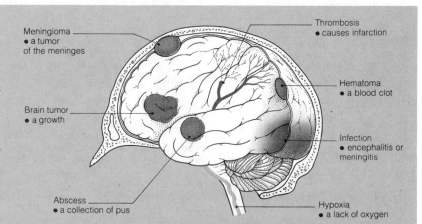

Meningioma
● a tumor of the meninges

Brain tumor
● a growth

Abscess
● a collection of pus

Thrombosis
● causes infarction

Hematoma
● a blood clot

Infection
● encephalitis or meningitis

Hypoxia
● a lack of oxygen

INJURY

Although protected by the skull, the brain may be damaged by heavy blows to the head or following skull fracture as a result of falls, high speed impacts, bullet wounds, or other physical violence (see *Head injury*).

INFECTION

Infection within the brain, called *encephalitis*, or of the membranes surrounding the brain, called *meningitis*, is uncommon today. Meningitis is usually caused by a bacterial infection. Encephalitis can be caused by any one of numerous viruses, of which the best known and most dangerous are the *rabies* and *herpes simplex* viruses.

An abscess (localized pocket of infection) in the brain may result from spread of infection from the ear, sinuses, or elsewhere in the body (see *Brain abscess*).

TUMORS

Tumors that affect the brain may be primary (arising from tissues inside the skull) as in *gliomas*, *meningiomas*, *acoustic neuromas*, and *pituitary tumors*, or secondary (arising from cancer cells that have spread through the bloodstream from tumors in the lungs, breasts, or elsewhere). See *Brain tumors*.

DEGENERATION

Multiple sclerosis, a progressive disease of unknown cause in which the nerve sheaths (composed of myelin) are destroyed, starts most commonly in early adulthood.

Degenerative brain diseases, such as *Alzheimer's disease* (a type of dementia) and *Parkinson's disease*, are particularly important causes of disability among the elderly.

OTHER DISORDERS

Disorders characterized by their symptoms rather than any obvious cause include *migraine*, *narcolepsy* (excessive episodic sleepiness), and idiopathic *epilepsy* (epilepsy of unknown cause), though epileptic seizures can also have specific causes, such as a tumor or infection.

Disorders of thought, emotion, or behavior are generally described as psychiatric or *mental illnesses*. Often, there is no obvious physical brain defect or disorder, although, with many important mental illnesses, such as *depression* and *schizophrenia*, there seems to be an underlying disturbance of brain chemistry. Some psychiatric illnesses, collectively called organic *brain syndromes*, by definition have a physical cause.

INVESTIGATION

Many different procedures may be used to investigate disorders of the brain. A full physical *examination* will include assessment of brain function by means of tests of mental abilities and state, sensation, movement, muscle tone, and reflexes. Electrical activity within the brain may be measured by means of an *EEG*. Physical abnormalities may be looked for using *brain imaging* techniques, such as *angiography*, *CT scanning*, or *MRI*. A *lumbar puncture* may be performed to look for evidence of bleeding or infection.

Brain death

The irreversible cessation of all functions of the entire brain, including the *brain stem*. The recognition of brain death, as defined above, has allowed physicians to certify death in situations where the lungs and heart continue to function (with machine assistance) but where death has occurred based on the absence of brain function. (See also *Death*.)

Brain failure

See *Brain syndrome, organic*.

Brain hemorrhage

Bleeding within or around the brain, caused either by trauma or spontaneous rupture of a blood vessel. There are four possible types: *subdural hemorrhage, extradural hemorrhage, subarachnoid hemorrhage,* and *intracerebral hemorrhage*.

Extradural and subdural hemorrhages usually result from a blow to the head (see *Head injury*); symptoms may include headache, drowsiness, confusion, and paralysis on one side of the body. These symptoms may develop within hours in extradural hemorrhage but possibly over months in subdural hemorrhage. Hospital treatment is urgently required.

Subarachnoid and intracerebral hemorrhage usually occur spontaneously (i.e., without any head injury) and are the result of rupture of *aneurysms* or small blood vessels in the brain. Middle-aged and elderly persons with untreated *hypertension* (high blood pressure) are at highest risk. Subarachnoid hemorrhage is characterized by a sudden violent headache and/or sudden loss of consciousness. Intracerebral hemorrhage is one of the three main types of *stroke*; symptoms may include sudden collapse, speech loss, and paralysis of the facial muscles or of an arm or leg. Both subarachnoid and intracerebral hemorrhages are emergencies.

Brain imaging

Obtaining pictures of the brain to detect injury or disease. The introduction of computerized scanning has revolutionized this field.

TYPES

CONVENTIONAL X-RAY TECHNIQUES The simplest and longest established method of obtaining images of the brain is to take *X-ray* films. X rays reveal distortion or erosion of the bony skull caused by a fracture, tumor, *aneurysm*, or abscess. Unless the brain substance itself is calcified in

SITES OF BRAIN HEMORRHAGE

Hemorrhages within the skull fall into four main categories—extradural, subdural, subarachnoid, and intracerebral hemorrhages— according to the site of the bleeding in relation to the brain and its protective coverings, the meninges. The causes and effects of the bleeding and the outlook of the patient vary among the categories.

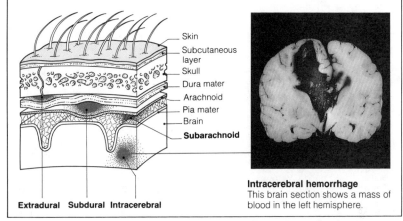

Skin
Subcutaneous layer
Skull
Dura mater
Arachnoid
Pia mater
Brain
Subarachnoid

Extradural Subdural Intracerebral

Intracerebral hemorrhage
This brain section shows a mass of blood in the left hemisphere.

a localized area due to disease, the plain X ray cannot detect disease of the brain matter.

Angiography involves injecting a dye into one of the arteries supplying the brain, and then taking X-ray pictures. This technique shows up the blood vessels in the brain, and is used to investigate subarachnoid hemorrhage, aneurysms, abnormalities of the blood vessels, and other disorders of the circulation.

SCANNING TECHNIQUES *CT scanning* was first conceived in 1971 specifically to study the brain. Unlike the conventional X-ray procedure, this method gives images of the brain substance itself. It gives especially clear pictures of the ventricles (the fluid-filled cavities of the brain) and can reveal tumors, blood clots, strokes, aneurysms, and abscesses. Contrast dye is often administered to help differentiate normal from abnormal brain tissue.

MRI produces better images of the brain than CT scanning. It is especially helpful in showing tumors of the posterior fossa (back of the skull). MRI does not involve radiation.

Radionuclide scanning uses radioactive isotopes to detect tumors, abnormalities of the blood vessels, and other lesions. It has been largely replaced by CT scanning and MRI.

Ultrasound scanning is used only in premature or very young babies because ultrasound waves cannot penetrate the bones of a mature skull.

Ultrasound scanning is particularly useful in detecting hydrocephalus and ventricular hemorrhage in premature babies and, because no radiation is involved, repeated scans can be performed safely.

PET scanning combines the use of radionuclides with CT scanning and gives information on activities in different parts of the brain.

Brain stem

The lowest section of the brain, which acts partly as a highway for messages traveling between other parts of the brain and the spinal cord, but also connects with ten of the 12 pairs of *cranial nerves* and controls basic functions such as breathing, vomiting, and eye reflexes. The activities of the brain stem are below the level of consciousness and operate largely on an automatic basis.

STRUCTURE

From the spinal cord upward, the brain stem consists of three main parts, called medulla, pons, and midbrain. Attached to the back of the brain stem is a separate brain organ, the *cerebellum*, concerned principally with balance and with coordinated movement. Running longitudinally through the middle of the brain stem is a canal, widening in the pons and medulla into a cavity, the fourth *ventricle* of the brain, which contains the circulating *cerebrospinal fluid*.

MEDULLA The medulla resembles a thick extension of the spinal cord. It

B

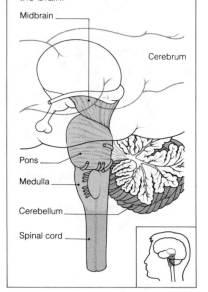

LOCATION OF THE BRAIN STEM
A 3-inch-long stalk of nerve cells and fibers joins the upper part of the spinal cord with the rest of the brain.

Midbrain

Cerebrum

Pons

Medulla

Cerebellum

Spinal cord

contains the *nuclei* of the ninth to twelfth cranial nerves and thus receives and relays taste sensations from the tongue and relays signals to muscles involved in speech and in tongue and neck movements. It also contains the vital centers—groups of nerve cells involved in the automatic regulation of heart beat, breathing, blood pressure, and digestion—and sends and receives information regarding these functions via the tenth cranial or *vagus nerve*.

Many of the tracts running through the medulla cross over in its lower portion so that the right side of the body links up with the left side of the brain and vice versa.

PONS This is considerably wider than the medulla and contains thick bundles of nerve fibers that connect with the cerebellum, which lies directly behind. The pons also contains the nuclei for the fifth to eighth cranial nerves and thus relays sensory information from the ear, face, and teeth, as well as the signals that move the jaw, adjust facial expressions, and produce some eye movements.

MIDBRAIN This is the smallest section of the brain stem, above the pons. It contains the nuclei of the third and fourth cranial nerves, which control eye movements and the size and reactions of the pupil. It also contains cell

groups such as the substantia nigra and red nuclei, which are involved in coordinating limb movements.

RETICULAR FORMATION Scattered throughout the brain stem are numerous nerve cell groups collectively known as the reticular formation. The reticular formation is believed to act as a watchdog on sensory information entering the brain, alerting the higher brain centers to new or important sensory stimuli that may require a conscious response. Our sleep/wake cycle is controlled by the reticular formation. Many *hypnotic drugs* (sleeping pills) and stimulants are believed to exert their actions by affecting this part of the brain.

DISORDERS
The brain stem is susceptible to the same disorders that afflict the rest of the central nervous system. Damage to the medulla's vital centers is rapidly fatal, while damage to the reticular formation may cause coma. Damage to specific cranial nerve nuclei can have specific effects—*facial palsy* in the case of the seventh cranial (facial) nerve and tongue-wasting with the twelfth cranial (hypoglossal) nerve. Degeneration of the substantia nigra in the midbrain is thought to be a cause of *Parkinson's disease*.

Brain syndrome, organic

Disturbance of consciousness, intellect, or mental functioning of organic (physical) as opposed to psychiatric origin. Possible causes include degenerative diseases (such as *Alzheimer's disease*), metabolic imbalances, infections, medication, toxins, vitamin deficiencies, or the effects of trauma, stroke, or tumor.

SYMPTOMS
In acute organic brain syndrome, symptoms range from slight confusion to stupor or coma, and may also include restlessness, disorientation, memory impairment, hallucinations, and delusions (see *Delirium*). The chronic form results in a progressive decline in intellect, memory, and behavior (see *Dementia*).

TREATMENT
Treatment relies on identifying and, if possible, dealing with the underlying cause. Treatment is more likely to be successful with the acute form. In chronic cases, irreversible *brain damage* may already have occurred.

Brain tumor

Abnormal growth in or on the brain. Although not always malignant, all brain tumors are serious because of

the buildup of pressure in the brain and compression of adjoining brain areas as the tumor expands.

TYPES
Brain tumors may be primary growths arising directly from tissues within the skull or metastases (secondary growths) spread via the bloodstream from tumors elsewhere in the body, most commonly the lungs or breasts.

The cause of primary brain tumors is not known. About 60 percent are *gliomas* (frequently malignant), which arise from the brain substance. Other primary tumors include *meningiomas*, arising from the meningeal membranes that cover the brain, *acoustic neuromas* arising from the acoustic nerve, and *pituitary tumors* arising from the pituitary gland, all of which are benign. Certain brain tumors mainly affect children and are often situated in the back of the brain. Included among these are two types of glioma called *medulloblastoma* and cerebellar *astrocytoma*.

Secondary growths, or metastases, are always malignant and may be found in more than one organ.

INCIDENCE
In the US, about six new cases of primary brain tumor, leading to about four deaths, are diagnosed per 100,000 population per year. They occur most commonly around the age of 50 years, although a significant number of children are also affected; about one child in 3,000 dies from a primary brain tumor before the age of 10 years.

In addition, about 30 persons per 100,000 annually die of cancer that includes metastases in the brain.

SYMPTOMS
Brain tumors cause symptoms by several mechanisms. Compression of brain tissue or nerve tracts within the vicinity of the tumor may cause muscle weakness, loss of vision, or other sensory disturbances, speech difficulties, and, in about one fifth of cases, epileptic seizures.

The presence of an expanding tumor can increase pressure within the skull, causing headache, vomiting, visual disturbances, and impaired mental functioning. If the circulation of cerebrospinal fluid is obstructed by the tumor, *hydrocephalus* (water on the brain) may result.

DIAGNOSIS
Many different techniques are used to locate the site of a brain tumor and to establish the extent of its spread. The most important are *CT scanning*, magnetic resonance imaging (*MRI*), special *X-ray* studies, and *angiography*.

TREATMENT
When possible, tumors are removed by surgery after opening the skull (see *Craniotomy*), but many malignant growths are inaccessible or too extensive for removal. The outlook in these cases is poor; fewer than 20 percent of patients survive for a year. In cases where a tumor cannot be completely removed, as much of it as possible will be cut away to relieve pressure in the brain. *Radiation therapy* or *anticancer drugs* may also be given. *Corticosteroid drugs* are often prescribed to reduce tissue swelling around a tumor, thus relieving symptoms.

Bran

The fibrous outer covering of grain. Eating bran regularly, either in breakfast cereals or added to food, raises *fiber* intake. This helps prevent constipation and thus lessen the risk of intestinal disease.

Branchial disorders
Branchial disorders include branchial cyst and branchial fistula.

A branchial cyst is a soft swelling that appears on the side of the neck in early adult life. The swelling contains a puslike or clear fluid that is rich in cholesterol. Diagnosis is made by identifying cholesterol crystals in a few drops of the fluid drawn from the cyst by means of a needle and syringe. Treatment is by surgical removal.

A branchial fistula is an abnormal passage between the back of the throat and the external surface of the neck, where it appears as a small hole usually noted at birth. Like a branchial cyst, the fistula results from an abnormality of fetal development. If the hole in the neck does not extend to the back of the throat, it is termed a branchial cleft sinus; it may be present at birth or may form if a branchial cyst becomes infected and ruptures. A branchial fistula or a branchial cleft sinus may discharge mucus or pus. If this is troublesome, the fistula or sinus can be excised (cut away).

Brash, water
Sudden filling of the mouth with tasteless saliva. It is not to be confused with *acid reflux* (the regurgitation of gastric juices), which has an unpleasant, sour taste. Water brash is usually accompanied by other symptoms such as abdominal pain before a meal. It usually indicates a disorder of the upper gastrointestinal tract, such as a *duodenal ulcer*.

Braxton Hicks' contractions
Short, relatively painless contractions of the uterus during pregnancy. These contractions allow the uterus to grow and also help circulate blood through the uterine vessels. In early pregnancy, they may be felt by a physician performing an internal examination. In late pregnancy, they may be felt by the woman and seen by looking at the abdomen. Sometimes they are mistaken for labor pains, although they occur as isolated contractions, have no effect on the cervix, and are not as uncomfortable as true labor.

Breakbone fever

A tropical, mosquito-spread, viral illness also known as *dengue*. One symptom is severe joint and muscle pain, hence the name "breakbone fever."

Breakthrough bleeding
Vaginal bleeding or staining ("spotting") between periods when taking an oral birth-control pill, especially the minipill. Breakthrough bleeding is most common during the first few months of taking the pill, when the body is adjusting to alterations in hormone levels. Loss of blood during pregnancy, or when an oral birth-control pill is not being taken, may be a symptom of an important underlying disorder (see *Vaginal bleeding*).

Breast
In addition to its primary function of nourishing a baby with milk, the female breast is a secondary sexual characteristic. It has always been regarded by society as a symbol of femininity, beauty, and eroticism. The size, shape, and appearance of breasts vary more than almost any other part of the body. Men's breasts are immature versions of women's breasts.

STRUCTURE
The female breast consists mainly of 15 to 20 lobes of milk-secreting glands embedded in fatty tissue. The ducts of these glands have their outlet in the

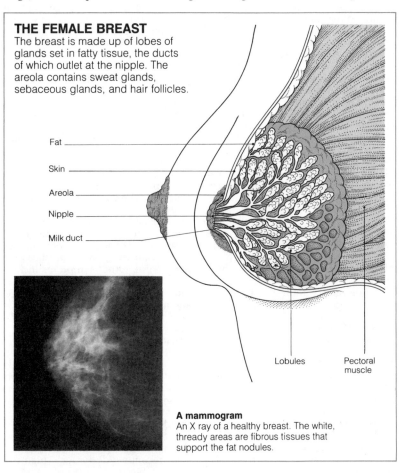

THE FEMALE BREAST
The breast is made up of lobes of glands set in fatty tissue, the ducts of which outlet at the nipple. The areola contains sweat glands, sebaceous glands, and hair follicles.

Fat
Skin
Areola
Nipple
Milk duct
Lobules
Pectoral muscle

A mammogram
An X ray of a healthy breast. The white, thready areas are fibrous tissues that support the fat nodules.

B

nipple, which is surrounded by the areola, the circular area of pigmented skin. The breast contains no muscle, but bands of fine ligaments that weave between the fat and lobules are attached to the skin and determine the breast's height and shape.

The skin over the breast is somewhat smoother, thinner, and more translucent than over much of the rest of the body. The areola skin is particularly thin, and contains sweat glands, sebaceous glands, and hair follicles. The nipple is very sensitive to the touch; contraction of its muscle fibers results in erection, a sign of sexual arousal or cold.

The size and shape of the breasts of mature women vary not only between individuals, but also vary at different times of a woman's life—during the menstrual cycle, during pregnancy and lactation, and after the menopause, for instance.

FUNCTION

During pregnancy estrogen and progesterone, secreted in the ovary and placenta, cause the milk-producing glands to develop and become active and the nipple to enlarge. Just before or after childbirth the glands in the breast produce a watery fluid called colostrum, which contains proteins and antibodies to protect the sucking baby against infection. Within about three days the colostrum is replaced with milk, whose production is stimulated by the hormone prolactin, released from the anterior pituitary gland (see also *Breast-feeding*).

BREAST DEVELOPMENT

The breasts, which are modified sweat glands, start to grow from mammary buds when the fetus is about 5 months old. At birth there is a nipple with rudimentary milk ducts. At *puberty*, a girl's breasts begin to develop—the areola swells and the nipple enlarges. This is followed by an increase in the production of glands and fat, which enlarges the breast. Ultimately the breast becomes rounded in shape and the areola gradually flattens.

Breastbone

A common name for the *sternum*.

Breast cancer

The most common cancer in women: one woman in every 14 develops breast cancer and one in every 20 dies from it. Fewer than one in every 100 breast cancers are in men.

Mortality from breast cancer (taking account of age) has hardly changed this century, but, in the early 1980s,

research studies in Sweden and the Netherlands suggested that deaths could be cut by about one third by mammographic screening of whole populations of women. Other studies indicate the great importance of breast examination by the physician and patient in diagnosing breast cancer in its early stages.

CAUSES AND INCIDENCE

Current theories of the cause of breast cancer are focused on hormonal influences. The incidence of breast cancer is known to be raised in women whose menstrual periods began when they were young and those whose menopause was late; in those who had no children or had their first child in their late 20s or 30s; and in those with mothers or sisters who had breast cancer. Diet also plays a part. The disease is rare in Japan, which has a low fat diet, but Japanese women living in the US and eating an American diet have the same rate of breast cancer as Americans. Tall, heavy women have more breast cancer than short, thin ones. Breast cancer may also be more common among women who have previously had nonmalignant cysts and tumors removed from their breasts.

There is no agreement on the part played by the oral birth-control pill in the cause of breast cancer. Some groups believe that women who take the pill in their teens have a slightly increased risk; others claim that it is protective. At present the evidence suggests that any increase in breast cancer from the pill, if at all, is small—and that it is outweighed by the effect of the pill in lowering the incidence of cancers of the ovary and uterus.

SYMPTOMS

The most common site of a malignant breast tumor is the upper, outer part of the breast. The lump is usually felt rather than seen, and in most cases is not painful. Other symptoms include a dark discharge from the nipple, retraction (indentation) of the nipple, and an area of dimpled, creased skin over the lump. In 90 percent of the cases only one breast is affected.

DIAGNOSIS

Monthly examination of the breasts (see *Breast self-examination*) should enable a woman to detect at an early stage any new or changed breast lump or any change in her nipples. The breast examination is important and should routinely be done by internists and gynecologists. In addition, X rays of the breasts, called mammograms, are recommended for high-risk

women (i.e., women with a family history of breast cancer) at age 40 and should be repeated every three to five years thereafter, or sooner, when advised. This procedure, called *mammography* is also of value for all women over 50 years old.

A woman who discovers a lump in her breast should report it to her physician immediately. A mammogram may be appropriate at this time. If the physician suspects that the lump is merely a *cyst* (a fluid-filled tissue sac), it can be aspirated (i.e., the fluid can be withdrawn) and may disappear completely. Where there is a possibility that the lump may be a malignant tumor, a *biopsy* will be carried out. This may be an outpatient procedure in which breast tissue is withdrawn with a hollow needle, causing little discomfort, or an operation to remove all or part of the lump; in either case the suspect tissue will be examined under the microscope.

If cancer is discovered, blood tests, X rays, and scanning will determine whether the disease has spread to other parts of the body.

TREATMENT

The high mortality from breast cancer is because the disease has spread beyond the breast when first detected. Surgical removal of the tumor achieves a cure in one third of women with early breast cancer. Studies have shown survival is not improved by extensive operations (such as radical *mastectomy*); many surgeons recommend *lumpectomy*, the simple removal of the tumor, combined with *radiation therapy* or *anticancer drug* therapy, or both. The extent of the primary treatment is influenced by the woman's age, the size of the tumor, whether or not there are signs of spread to the lymph nodes under the arm, and the sensitivity of the tumor cells to hormones as determined in the laboratory by a technique called estrogen receptor testing.

Tests carried out at the time of the initial diagnosis may show that the cancer is in the bones, liver, or other organs. Evidence of *metastasis* may develop years after apparently successful treatment. In either case, treatment with *anticancer drugs* and hormones usually relieves symptoms and prolongs life.

OUTLOOK

If cancer is treated at an early stage the outlook is optimistic; either a complete cure or many years of good health can be expected. Regular checkups are needed to detect any recurrence or

DISORDERS OF THE BREAST

Problems involving the breasts are usually minor and respond readily to treatment. The most important causes of problems are infection, tumors, and hormonal disturbance.

INFECTION

This is uncommon except during breast-feeding. Nursing mothers may suffer from *mastitis* (inflammation of the breast), usually due to a blocked milk duct. An *abscess* may follow if mastitis is not treated.

TUMORS

A *breast lump* may be a *cyst* (a fluid-filled sac), a *fibroadenoma* (a thickening of the milk-producing glandular tissue) or other benign tumor, or, rarely, *breast cancer*.

HORMONAL DISORDERS

It is common for women to notice that before *menstruation* their breasts become bigger and lumpy. Such lumps are swollen milk glands that shrink when menstruation is over. More common are breast pain and tenderness, which often occur just before menstruation or from taking hormones.

In men, *gynecomastia* (unusual breast development) may result from hormonal disturbance or treatment with certain drugs. Hormones may also cause the rare disorder *galactorrhea* (abnormal milk production).

INVESTIGATION

Disorders of the breast may be discovered during *breast self-examination* or by your physician during a physical examination. Special investigations for the breast are *biopsy* and *mammography*.

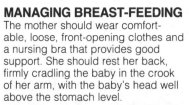

Fibroadenoma
• a common benign tumor

Cancer
• a malignant growth

Cyst
• a collection of fluid

Abscess
• a collection of pus

Nipple discharge

Galactorrhea
• abnormal production of milk

Mastitis
• inflammation of tissue

cancer in the other breast. Breast self-examination should be carried out monthly and mammograms should be performed periodically. If the cancer recurs, it can be controlled for many years by drugs, radiation therapy, and, in some cases, further surgery.

Breast enlargement

See *Mammoplasty*.

Breast-feeding

The natural method of infant feeding from birth to weaning. Human milk contains the ideal balance of nutrients for the human baby and provides valuable antibodies to protect the child against infections, such as *gastroenteritis*. Breast-feeding also provides the mother and child with a physical closeness that strengthens the bond between them.

HOW TO BREAST-FEED

Ideally, the baby should be put to the breast as soon after delivery as possible. Once sucking has begun, the mother should ensure that the whole of the areola (the dark area around the nipple) is in the baby's mouth. This helps to stimulate flow and can prevent soreness caused by the baby chewing on the nipple. In the first few days after birth, the baby should be encouraged to suck frequently, but for only a few minutes at a time. This provides him or her with valuable colostrum, and also stimulates the breasts so that a consistent and plentiful milk supply is established. During the first few weeks a baby should be fed on demand to make sure that the milk supply is maintained. Babies may want to nurse from once every hour or two to once every three or four hours.

PROBLEMS

Engorged (overfull) breasts are common in early lactation; they are uncomfortable and can prevent the baby from sucking properly. Expression of milk, either manually or with a *breast pump*, usually helps.

Sore or cracked nipples, often a problem in the early weeks, may be relieved by using a nipple shield. Alternatively, the milk may be expressed and given by bottle.

MANAGING BREAST-FEEDING

The mother should wear comfortable, loose, front-opening clothes and a nursing bra that provides good support. She should rest her back, firmly cradling the baby in the crook of her arm, with the baby's head well above the stomach level.

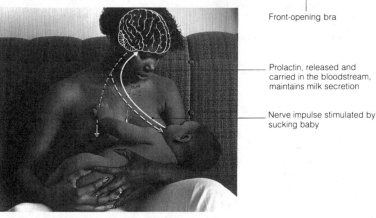

Front-opening bra

Prolactin, released and carried in the bloodstream, maintains milk secretion

Nerve impulse stimulated by sucking baby

A complication of breast-feeding is infection leading to an abscess, indicated by soreness and inflammation on the surface of the breast. Early antibiotic treatment may mean that breast-feeding can continue.

Sometimes breast-feeding problems have an emotional basis. A few women regard their breasts as having a primarily sexual function and find the whole feeding process distasteful. Others fear feeding may spoil the shape of their breasts and may resent the intensive commitment to the child that breast-feeding requires.

A woman whose baby always seems unsatisfied after feedings may doubt the quality or quantity of her milk. If she is in good health, eating a nutritious diet, and getting enough rest, then her milk supply should be adequate, and she may simply need reassurance and encouragement. Sometimes, despite continuing efforts by the mother, the baby remains hungry or the process of feeding is painful. A change to *bottle-feeding* is the likely answer, and should not be seen as failure or a reason for guilt. (See also *Feeding, infant*.)

Breast lump

Any mass, cyst, or swelling that can be felt in the breast tissue. At least 80 percent of lumps are benign; the remainder may be malignant. All breast lumps need assessment.

POSSIBLE CAUSES

The most common cause of a breast lump is fibrocystic disease, also known as chronic *mastitis* or fibroadenosis, in which one or more cysts (fluid-filled tissue sacs) and thickening of milk glands develop. Occurring mainly in women between the ages of 30 and 50, fibrocystic disease usually causes one or both breasts to become lumpy and tender in the week or so before a menstrual period starts.

Another common type is found most often in young women and usually results in a single lump called a *fibroadenoma*. This benign growth is usually round, firm, and rubbery, causes no pain, and can be moved around beneath the skin using the fingertips.

There are also several less common forms of breast lump: *breast cancer*, lipoma, intraductal papilloma, and cystosarcoma phylloides.

A lipoma is a benign, painless tumor, made up of fatty tissue, that sometimes changes the size and shape of the breast.

An intraductal papilloma is a wart-like growth within a duct of the milk-producing glands. The most common symptom is a discharge from the nipple, either clear or dark or bloody; there may be a pea-sized lump beneath the nipple. Intraductal papillomas are harmless but may become malignant.

A cystosarcoma phylloides is a tumor of connective tissue that can grow to an enormous size very quickly. Again, it is usually benign and only rarely becomes malignant.

SEEKING MEDICAL ADVICE

All women should examine their breasts each month (see *Breast self-examination*) to detect any significant changes. If a new lump or a change in a known lump is detected, or there is any discharge from a nipple, a physician should be seen.

DIAGNOSIS AND TREATMENT

Since a physical examination cannot reveal whether or not a growth is benign, tests (including *mammography*, needle aspiration *biopsy*, or tissue biopsy) will be arranged.

If fibrocystic lumps cause discomfort, they can be drained in a simple outpatient procedure if they are fluid-filled or be removed surgically if they are fibrous. Fibroadenomas, intraductal papillomas, and cystosarcoma phylloides are usually removed because it cannot be ascertained whether or not a lesion is benign and they continue to grow if they are left. All except very small lipomas are also usually removed. For the treatment of malignant tumors, see *Breast cancer*.

Breast pump

A simple device, consisting of a rubber bulb and a glass or plastic tube and reservoir, that is used to draw milk

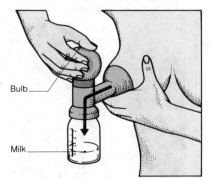

Bulb

Milk

Using a breast pump
Both parts of the pump must first be sterilized. The opening is placed firmly over the nipple to form a tight seal. The bulb is squeezed rhythmically until milk comes out.

from the breasts. The pump is used to relieve overfull breasts during early lactation and to express milk for future use. Most pumps are hand-operated but electric ones are available.

Breast reconstruction

See *Mammoplasty*.

Breast reduction

See *Mammoplasty*.

Breast self-examination

A visual and manual examination of the breasts carried out by a woman to detect lumps and other changes that might indicate the presence of early breast cancer. Although *mammography* (breast screening) has been shown to be more effective, it is not universally available. Self-examination is still important and should be carried out at about the same time monthly.

WHY IT IS DONE

Breast cancer is the leading cause of death among women aged 35 to 54 years. It is curable, however, if diagnosed at an early stage. Self-examination allows early changes and small lumps to be detected.

Breast tenderness

Soreness or tenderness of the breasts, often accompanied by a feeling of fullness in one or both breasts. Breast tenderness is relatively common just before menstruation (see *Premenstrual syndrome*), in early pregnancy, or during *breast-feeding*. Otherwise, it is comparatively rare and, in the absence of other symptoms, such as a *breast lump*, nipple discharge, or hot, inflamed skin over the breast, it is unlikely to be due to a serious underlying *breast disorder*. Malignant breast tumors are usually painless. Most cases of breast tenderness are thought to be due to hormonal changes (especially increased levels of *estrogen*) affecting the cells of the breast, causing them to retain excess fluid. This explains why the birth-control pill causes, or makes worse, breast tenderness in some women. Conversely, very low dose oral contraceptives may reduce breast tenderness in some women. Tenderness during breast-feeding may be due to engorgement with milk or to *mastitis* (inflammation of breast tissue as a result of infection).

Treatment of premenstrual breast tenderness may include dietary restriction of sodium and, when benefits justify the risk, *diuretics* (to reduce fluid retention) before each

EXAMINING YOUR BREASTS

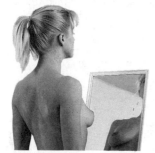 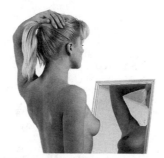

1 Once a month, after your period, examine your breasts. With arms by your side, look in a mirror and get to know their general appearance, shape, and size. Be alert to changes.

2 Raise each arm in turn above your head, looking for changes in appearance. Turn from side to side, looking at the outline of the breasts for any changes.

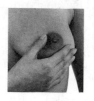

3 Gently squeeze the nipples to see whether there is any discharge.

4 Examine the skin surface for peculiarities. Orange-peel texture could indicate the presence of a lump.

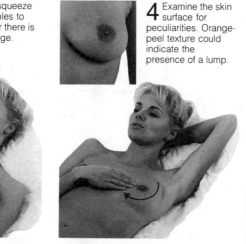

5 Lie on your back with a pillow under your shoulders and head, your arm by your side. Using the flat of your hand, work around the outer parts of the breast in a clockwise direction.

6 Raise your arm above your head and examine the inner parts of the breast. Stretching the tissue makes detection of lumps easier. Feel also along the top of the collarbone and into the armpit.

power over the environment. They may quickly learn that breath-holding attacks annoy or frighten parents, and use them as a means of manipulation.

MANAGEMENT
Breath-holding attacks should, as far as possible, be ignored. If the child is rewarded by gaining increased attention from parents, then he or she will continue to have attacks. As soon as the child realizes there is nothing to be gained, the attacks will stop. Firm, patient, and consistent handling will also help in avoiding attacks. The attacks will usually stop in any case by the age of 5 years, but, if they are causing parental anxiety, the physician should be consulted.

Breathing

The process by which air passes into and out of the lungs to allow the blood to take up oxygen and dispose of carbon dioxide (see *Respiration*). Breathing is controlled by the respiratory center in the brain stem; no conscious effort is needed to inhale and exhale air, but the depth and rate of breathing can be altered voluntarily. During exercise, when the heart and muscles need more oxygen, reflexes lead to a rapid increase in the breathing rate. This can vary in an adult from 13 to 17 breaths per minute at rest up to 80 breaths per minute during vigorous exercise. A newborn baby breathes at a rate of approximately 40 breaths per minute.

HOW AIR ENTERS THE LUNGS
When air is inhaled (inspiration), the diaphragm, which is dome shaped when relaxed, contracts and flattens. The muscles between the ribs contract and pull the rib cage upward and outward. This movement increases chest volume, causing the lungs to expand

period or the regular use of danazol (a drug that reduces changes in hormone levels) for a few months.

Breath-holding attacks

Periods during which a toddler holds his or her breath, usually as an expression of frustration or anger. Psychologists believe that children may unconsciously bring on these attacks to exert control over their parents. In some children, the attacks occur as a response to pain.

The child usually begins to cry, then holds his or her breath, becoming red or even blue in the face after a few seconds. The child may faint temporarily, but breathing quickly resumes as a natural reflex, ending the attack. Breath-holding sometimes results in twitching that resembles an epileptic seizure. However, a true epileptic seizure occurs with no obvious warning and is not preceded by breath-holding. Although breath-holding attacks may be alarming to parents, they are harmless.

CAUSES AND INCIDENCE
Breath-holding attacks occur in 1 to 2 percent of toddlers. They are most common between the ages of 1 and 2 years, particularly in children with determined personalities. Children at this age are just beginning to see themselves as individuals and are trying to determine the extent of their

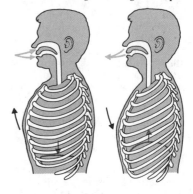

Inhaling and exhaling
When inhaling, the diaphragm flattens; the rib cage is pulled up and out. When exhaling, the diaphragm relaxes; the rib cage sinks.

B

and suck in air. When air is exhaled (expiration), the chest muscles and diaphragm relax, causing the rib cage to sink and the lungs to contract, squeezing out air.

The lungs do not fill completely during inhalation or empty completely during exhalation. In normal, quiet breathing only about one tenth of the air in the lungs passes out to be replaced by the same amount of fresh air. This new air (tidal volume), mixes with the stale air (residual volume) already held in the lungs.

A man's lungs hold about 1.5 gallons (6 liters) of air at one time, and a woman's lungs about 1 gallon (4.25 liters). At rest, about 0.1 gallon (0.4 liter) of air is taken into the lungs during normal inspiration; a deep breath can take in up to 0.8 gallon (3 to 4 liters) of air.

Breathing difficulty

Breathing difficulty is a change in the rate and depth of breathing. This happens when the effort required to breathe is increased, or when breathing movement is causing pain. Accompanying symptoms may include a feeling of tightness in the chest, coughing, wheezing, or chest pain.

Breathing difficulty may be due to any condition that affects the airflow into and out of the lungs, the transfer of oxygen from lungs to the blood, the circulation of blood through the lungs, or control of breathing by the brain stem. Breathing difficulty can occur at rest or when the body needs more oxygen during exercise or illness.

LACK OF FITNESS

The heart and lungs of an unfit person cannot respond adequately to the increased need for oxygen, so the increased effort needed to breathe causes discomfort. This problem can be overcome by fitness training.

OVERWEIGHT

Overweight people often experience difficulty breathing during exertion, partly because they are unfit and partly because of the increased effort needed to carry extra weight. In the very obese the brain-stem breathing center may not function efficiently and this may cause irregular breathing patterns (pickwickian syndrome).

ANXIETY

Severe anxiety during times of stress or tension can bring on attacks of *hyperventilation*. These attacks are associated with a feeling that one cannot get a good breath, itself leading to further overbreathing.

BRAIN-STEM DAMAGE

Damage to the breathing center in the brain stem due to a *transient ischemic attack* or a head injury can reduce or increase breathing activity. This may also happen as a side effect of certain drugs. In certain instances, a *ventilator* may be required.

ALTITUDE SICKNESS

This can cause breathlessness because there is less oxygen present in the surrounding air, so the lungs have to work harder to give the body sufficient oxygen. Swelling of the brain and fluid filling the lungs are serious stages of altitude sickness.

ANEMIA

When there is a shortage of red *blood cells* there is insufficient *hemoglobin* to carry oxygen around the body. If anemia is severe, the lungs need to work harder to supply the body with oxygen, resulting in breathlessness.

CIRCULATION DISORDERS

Breathing difficulty intensified upon exertion may be caused by a reduced circulation of blood through the lungs. This may be due to *heart failure*, where the heart pumps blood less efficiently, to blockage of blood vessels in the lungs by a blood clot (see *Pulmonary embolism*), or to increased pressure in the arteries within the lungs (see *Pulmonary hypertension*).

AIRWAYS BLOCKAGE

Breathing difficulty due to airflow obstruction may be caused by chronic *bronchitis* (in which mucus and thickened walls block the airways), by *asthma* or allergic reaction (where there is constriction of the lungs), or by *lung cancer* (in which a *tumor* blocks a large airway).

LUNG DAMAGE

Breathing difficulty may also be due to inefficient transfer of oxygen from the lungs into the bloodstream. This can be a result of damage to lung tissue, which may be temporary as in *pneumonia*, or a result of a *pneumothorax* (collapsed lung), pulmonary *edema* (fluid in the lung), or *pleural effusion* (fluid around the lung). Lung damage may also be permanent as in *emphysema*, where the walls of the *alveoli* are destroyed.

PAIN

Any pain in the chest that is made worse by chest or lung movement can make normal breathing difficult and painful. A fractured rib, for example, results in pain at the fracture site during breathing or movement of the torso. Pleurisy is associated with pain in the lower chest and often in the shoulder tip of the affected side.

Breathing exercises

Techniques for learning to control the rate and depth of breathing, used in therapy and to aid relaxation.

WHY THEY ARE DONE

PHYSICAL THERAPY Breathing exercises are often recommended for people with chronic chest diseases, such as bronchitis. They can also help people with anxiety disorders who breathe too deeply and rapidly and as a result disturb the chemical composition of their blood.

Breathing exercises are important after operations, when patients often breathe shallowly and are afraid to cough because of pain. In these circumstances, poor ventilation and the buildup of secretions can lead to collapse of segments of the lung or to collapse of a lobe of the lung, particularly in patients who are overweight or smokers. Deep breathing promotes coughing and keeps the lungs clear.

Many patients undergoing chest or upper abdominal surgery are given a device that, upon deep inhalation, causes three plastic balls to rise. This breathing exercise is called incentive spirometry and it promotes deep breathing and chest clearing.

RELAXATION In yoga, deep rhythmic breathing is used to achieve a state of relaxation. During labor and childbirth, breathing exercises relax the mother, help control contractions, and reduce pain.

HOW THEY ARE DONE

The person is taught to inhale through the nose, expanding the chest. He or she then exhales fully through the mouth, while contracting the abdominal muscles.

Hand lying on chest should hardly move

Hand lying on stomach should rise first

Practicing breathing
This exercise can be done unsupervised. A second person may apply gentle pressure to the chest or abdomen to help you become aware of the muscle groups used.

B

BREATHING DIFFICULTY Rapid breathing, or pain or tightness in the chest that makes you aware of your breathing.

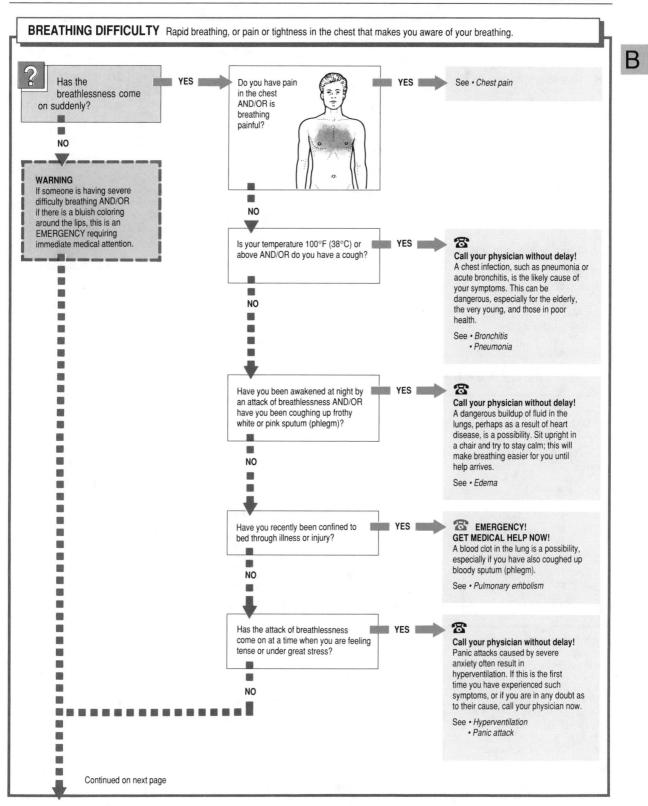

? Has the breathlessness come on suddenly?

YES → Do you have pain in the chest AND/OR is breathing painful?

YES → See • Chest pain

NO

WARNING
If someone is having severe difficulty breathing AND/OR if there is a bluish coloring around the lips, this is an EMERGENCY requiring immediate medical attention.

NO ↓

Is your temperature 100°F (38°C) or above AND/OR do you have a cough?

YES → ☎
Call your physician without delay!
A chest infection, such as pneumonia or acute bronchitis, is the likely cause of your symptoms. This can be dangerous, especially for the elderly, the very young, and those in poor health.

See • Bronchitis
    • Pneumonia

NO ↓

Have you been awakened at night by an attack of breathlessness AND/OR have you been coughing up frothy white or pink sputum (phlegm)?

YES → ☎
Call your physician without delay!
A dangerous buildup of fluid in the lungs, perhaps as a result of heart disease, is a possibility. Sit upright in a chair and try to stay calm; this will make breathing easier for you until help arrives.

See • Edema

NO ↓

Have you recently been confined to bed through illness or injury?

YES → ☎ **EMERGENCY!**
GET MEDICAL HELP NOW!
A blood clot in the lung is a possibility, especially if you have also coughed up bloody sputum (phlegm).

See • Pulmonary embolism

NO ↓

Has the attack of breathlessness come on at a time when you are feeling tense or under great stress?

YES → ☎
Call your physician without delay!
Panic attacks caused by severe anxiety often result in hyperventilation. If this is the first time you have experienced such symptoms, or if you are in any doubt as to their cause, call your physician now.

See • Hyperventilation
    • Panic attack

NO

Continued on next page

B

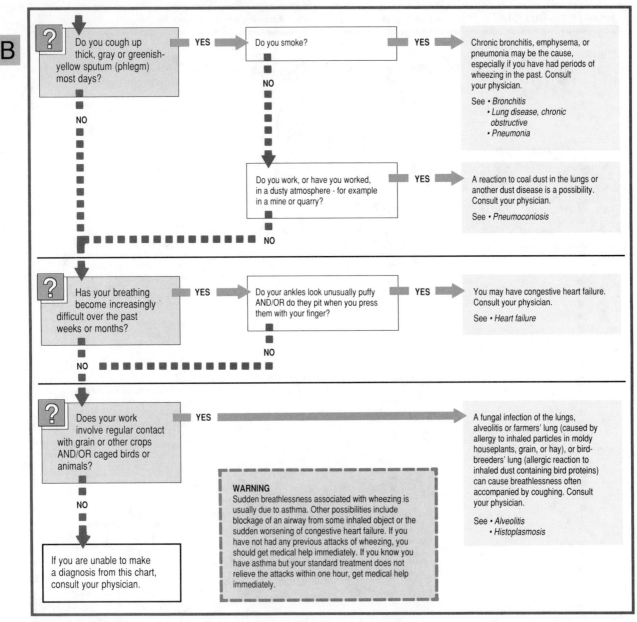

Do you cough up thick, gray or greenish-yellow sputum (phlegm) most days? — **YES** →

Do you smoke? — **YES** →

Chronic bronchitis, emphysema, or pneumonia may be the cause, especially if you have had periods of wheezing in the past. Consult your physician.

See • *Bronchitis*
• *Lung disease, chronic obstructive*
• *Pneumonia*

NO ↓ (from "Do you smoke?")

Do you work, or have you worked, in a dusty atmosphere - for example in a mine or quarry? — **YES** →

A reaction to coal dust in the lungs or another dust disease is a possibility. Consult your physician.

See • *Pneumoconiosis*

NO →

Has your breathing become increasingly difficult over the past weeks or months? — **YES** →

Do your ankles look unusually puffy AND/OR do they pit when you press them with your finger? — **YES** →

You may have congestive heart failure. Consult your physician.

See • *Heart failure*

NO

Does your work involve regular contact with grain or other crops AND/OR caged birds or animals? — **YES** →

A fungal infection of the lungs, alveolitis or farmers' lung (caused by allergy to inhaled particles in moldy houseplants, grain, or hay), or bird-breeders' lung (allergic reaction to inhaled dust containing bird proteins) can cause breathlessness often accompanied by coughing. Consult your physician.

See • *Alveolitis*
• *Histoplasmosis*

NO

If you are unable to make a diagnosis from this chart, consult your physician.

WARNING
Sudden breathlessness associated with wheezing is usually due to asthma. Other possibilities include blockage of an airway from some inhaled object or the sudden worsening of congestive heart failure. If you have not had any previous attacks of wheezing, you should get medical help immediately. If you know you have asthma but your standard treatment does not relieve the attacks within one hour, get medical help immediately.

Breathlessness
The need to breathe air in and out of the lungs very quickly. This is part of exercise or exertion in healthy people and not a cause for concern. The body requires more oxygen, so the lungs work harder. However, if breathlessness develops for any other reason it is a *breathing difficulty* that indicates some underlying disorder.

Breech delivery
Birth of a baby bottom-first instead of the usual head-first delivery.

By around the 32nd week of pregnancy, most babies have assumed a head-down position in the uterus, but about 3 to 4 percent take up breech presentation with the head at the top of the uterus. Often, one of two twins may present as a breech. At 34 weeks, some obstetricians try to turn a baby with a breech presentation into the head-down position.

If this attempt fails, the baby is left in the breech presentation until delivery. A breech delivery adds to the problems of mother and baby because

the baby's bottom does not mold a passage through the birth canal as efficiently as the head. Usually, an *episiotomy* will be performed to ease the baby's passage, and *forceps* are commonly used to ensure smooth emergence of the head.

If a baby with a breech presentation has a large head or the mother's pelvic girdle is small, delivery by *cesarean section* may be decided upon before she goes into labor. Some physicians recommend cesarean section for most breech babies, particularly if the baby is feet-first (footling presentation) or if a woman has not had a previous vaginal delivery, as there is an increased risk to the baby. In other instances, the decision is based on the results of *fetal heart monitoring*.

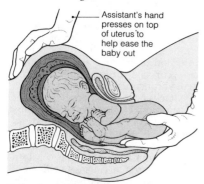

Assistant's hand presses on top of uterus to help ease the baby out

Delivering a breech baby
The buttocks are delivered first and then the legs. An episiotomy may be performed before the head is delivered.

Bridge, dental
False teeth (usually no more than four) attached to natural teeth on either side of a gap left by a missing tooth or teeth. Some bridges are removable. Unlike a *denture*, a bridge has no baseplate (artificial gum). Bridges are usually made of platinum or gold alloy faced with porcelain, but those at the back of the mouth may consist of only gold or gold-platinum alloy.

WHY IT IS FITTED
As with a denture, a bridge is fitted to fill any gap in the mouth to enable the person to bite properly, speak clearly, and avoid problems resulting from shifting or drifting of the remaining natural teeth. People who wear bridges usually do not have the option of wearing a denture.

Bright's disease
Another name for the kidney disease, *glomerulonephritis*, first described by the English physician Richard Bright (1789-1858).

Brittle bones
A term used to describe bones with an increased tendency to fracture. Brittle bones are a feature of the disorder *osteoporosis* (thinning of the bones), which is common in postmenopausal women and may occur in people confined to bed, on corticosteroid drugs, or with hormonal disorders. In *osteomalacia* (a vitamin D deficiency disease), the bones become soft, with an increased tendency both to deform and fracture.

A rare cause of brittle bones is the inherited connective tissue abnormality *osteogenesis imperfecta* (sometimes called brittle-bone disease). The disease is associated with blue sclerae (whites of the eyes) and with an increased susceptibility to many fractures throughout life.

Broken blood vessels
Any small, widened blood vessel visible beneath the skin surface, most commonly on the cheeks. Sometimes called a broken vein, it is the natural result of heavy alcohol consumption over many years, or of loss of supporting tissues in the skin due to overexposure to the sun. More rarely, a connective tissue disease, such as systemic *lupus erythematosus*, is the cause. Broken blood vessels may also be a feature of the facial redness seen in *rosacea*. Often, however, there is no obvious cause.

Broken blood vessels need not be any cause for concern. The only means of removal is *electrodesiccation*—electrical destruction of the upper layers of the skin—administered by a dermatologist. The procedure is successful only in some cases.

Broken tooth
See *Fracture, dental*.

Bromides
Substances formerly prescribed as sedatives in the treatment of *anxiety* or as anticonvulsants in the treatment of *epilepsy*. They are no longer prescribed due to their unpleasant side effects, which include loss of libido (sex drive), acne, tremor, and confusion.

Bromocriptine
By inhibiting the secretion of the hormone, prolactin, from the pituitary gland, bromocriptine is helpful in treating conditions associated with excessive prolactin production. Such conditions include *galactorrhea* (abnormal milk production by the breast), some types of female and male infertility, severe premenstrual breast discomfort, and benign pituitary tumors that cause *acromegaly* (abnormal tissue and bone growth). Bromocriptine is also used to suppress lactation in women who do not wish to breast-feed.

A few years after its development in the 1960s, bromocriptine was found to be effective for relieving the symptoms of *Parkinson's disease*. The reason is that it has almost the identical characteristics of dopamine, the chemical that is lacking in the brain of someone with Parkinson's disease. Bromocriptine is now widely used to treat those in the advanced stages of the disease when other drugs have failed or are unsuitable.

Serious adverse effects are uncommon when the drug is given in low doses. Nausea and vomiting, the most

---

FITTING A BRIDGE
The most common type of bridge consists of one or more false teeth attached to a crown on each side of a gap. The natural teeth are shaped to receive the crowns, which are then cemented into place.

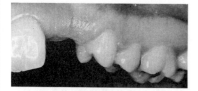

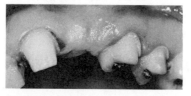

1 Two complete teeth are missing. A bridge of two false teeth and three crowns can be attached.

2 The three healthy teeth are shaped so that they can receive the crowns on either side of the gap.

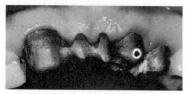

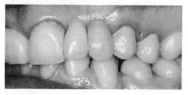

3 A cast-metal subframe made from an impression is tried out in the mouth and any necessary alterations are made.

4 The finished bridge is in position, showing the new porcelain teeth cemented to the metal base.

B

common problems, can be minimized by taking bromocriptine with meals. In rare cases, it may cause ulceration of the stomach. When taken in high doses, bromocriptine may cause drowsiness and confusion.

Bronchiectasis

A lung disorder in which one or more bronchi (the branching air passages that connect the windpipe to the lungs) are distorted and stretched, with a damaged lining. The abnormality usually occurs in childhood and results in chronic lung infections that may extend into later life.

CAUSES AND INCIDENCE

Bronchiectasis was formerly common and usually caused by childhood chest infections such as measles, whooping cough, tuberculosis, and severe bacterial pneumonias. As these infections have been controlled by immunization and antibiotics, so the incidence of bronchiectasis has plummeted. Bronchiectasis is now virtually extinct among children in the US and other developed countries.

When bronchiectasis occurs today, the cause is more often a congenital bronchial defect or blockage of a bronchus by a foreign body.

SYMPTOMS

The main symptom of chronic lung infection in bronchiectasis is a daily cough that produces large amounts of dark green sputum (phlegm) containing pus and occasionally flecked with blood. The sputum causes bad breath. If the disease is extensive it causes shortness of breath.

DIAGNOSIS AND TREATMENT

The diagnosis is usually made from the symptoms present. Occasionally a chest X ray or *bronchography* (X rays of the bronchi after they have been injected with a special dye) may be used to determine exactly how the bronchi have been affected.

Symptoms can usually be controlled by antibiotics and postural drainage; the patient is taught to lie in a position so that the pus and fluid drain from the affected segment or segments of lung and can then be coughed up.

If severe symptoms persist despite these measures, surgery may be recommended to remove the damaged lung areas.

Bronchiolitis

An acute viral infection of the lungs, mainly affecting babies and young children, in which the bronchioles (the smaller airways that branch off the bronchi) become inflamed.

CAUSES AND INCIDENCE

The most common cause of bronchiolitis is the respiratory syncytial virus (RSV), but various other viruses may also be responsible. Adult bronchiolitis may follow *bronchitis*, brought on by an influenza virus.

Winter epidemics of bronchiolitis tend to occur every two or three years, affecting thousands of children in the US. The viruses responsible can be transmitted from one person to another in airborne droplets, and a virus that may cause only a moderate head or chest infection in an adult can cause severe bronchiolitis in an infant. Hence, when suffering from a severe head or chest infection, contact with a baby is best kept to a minimum.

SYMPTOMS

The symptoms are a cough, shortness of breath, and, in severe cases, a cyanotic (blue-purple) complexion due to shortage of oxygen. The physician will also often hear crepitations (bubbling noises) in the lungs through a stethoscope.

TREATMENT

If a baby or young child has a cold and a cough that suddenly worsens, leading to rapid and labored breathing, a physician should be consulted. Sometimes no treatment is necessary, but, in more severe cases, the child may be admitted to the hospital, where oxygen and respiratory therapy (to clear the mucus from the bronchioles) is given.

Antibiotics and *corticosteroid drugs* (commonly used to treat bronchitis in adults) are ineffective against the viral infection, but antibiotics may nevertheless be prescribed to prevent any secondary bacterial infection. Occasionally, the child needs to be put on an artificial *ventilator* until normal breathing is restored.

With prompt treatment, even the most severely affected children usually recover completely within a few days.

Bronchitis

Inflammation of the bronchi, the airways that connect the trachea (windpipe) to the lungs, resulting in a persistent cough that produces considerable quantities of sputum (phlegm). Two forms of the disease are recognized—acute bronchitis (of sudden onset and short duration) and chronic bronchitis (persistent over a long period and recurring over several years). Both are more common in smokers and in areas with high atmospheric pollution.

ACUTE BRONCHITIS

This form comes on suddenly and usually clears up within a few days, except in those with a low resistance to infection, such as frail, elderly people and people with lung disease.

CAUSES AND INCIDENCE

Acute bronchitis is usually a complication of a viral infection such as a cold or influenza, but may also be caused by the effect of air pollutants. Bacterial infection may cause acute bronchitis or occur as a further complication of acute bronchitis with other causes.

Attacks occur most often in winter. In addition to smokers, those most susceptible are babies, the elderly, and people with lung disease.

SYMPTOMS

The inflammation of the mucosal lining of the bronchi causes swelling and congestion, and pus is formed. The main symptoms are wheezing, breathlessness, and a persistent cough that produces yellow or green sputum. There may also be discomfort behind the sternum (breastbone) and a raised temperature.

TREATMENT

Symptoms may be relieved by humidifying the lungs, either using a humidifier in the home, or by inhaling steam directly (be careful—inhaling steam that is too hot can cause serious burns). Drinking plenty of fluids is the best expectorant.

Most acute bronchitis clears up without further treatment and causes no further trouble. Complications such as *pneumonia* and *pleurisy* are exceptional. However, a physician should be consulted in any of the following cases: if there is severe breathlessness, if there is no improvement after three days, if blood is coughed up, if the temperature is above 101°F (38.3°C), or if the patient has underlying lung disease.

If your physician suspects there is a bacterial infection, antibiotics will be prescribed, but these are of no use if the infection is caused by a virus.

CHRONIC BRONCHITIS

Bronchitis is regarded as chronic when sputum is coughed up on most days during at least three consecutive months in at least two consecutive years. The disease commonly results in widespread narrowing and obstruction of the airways in the lungs. It often coexists with (and may contribute to the development of) another lung disease, *emphysema*, in which the alveoli (air sacs) in the lungs become distended. Chronic bronchitis and emphysema together are sometimes called chronic obstructive lung disease (COLD) or chronic obstructive pulmonary disease (COPD).

CAUSES AND INCIDENCE
Cigarette smoking is the main cause. It stimulates the production of mucus in the lining of the bronchi and thickens the bronchi's muscular walls and those of the bronchioles (smaller airways in the lungs), resulting in narrowing of these air passages. The passages then become more susceptible to infections, which cause further damage. Atmospheric pollution can have the same effect.

Approximately 3,000 persons per 100,000 in the US suffer from chronic bronchitis. Most are over 40 and male sufferers outnumber female sufferers two to one. The disease is most prevalent in industrial cities and in smokers, and is more common in manual and unskilled workers than among white collar workers (even after adjusting for differences in smoking habits). Chronic obstructive lung disease accounts for about 30 deaths per 100,000 in the US per year.

SYMPTOMS AND COMPLICATIONS
The symptoms are the same as in acute bronchitis—cough, breathlessness, and, rarely, chest pain—except that they are persistent instead of clearing up, and there is usually no fever. This persistence of symptoms also distinguishes the disease from chronic *asthma*, in which wheezing and breathlessness vary in severity from hour to hour and day to day.

As the disease progresses, often with the development of emphysema, the lungs become more resistant to the flow of blood, resulting in *pulmonary hypertension* (increased pressure in the arteries that supply blood to the lungs), and in strain on the right side of the heart due to its increased work in pumping blood through the lungs. The patient may become a *pink puffer*, with severe breathlessness. Sometimes, heart failure develops, further reducing the oxygen in the blood and causing a cyanotic (blue-purple) complexion. *Edema* (swelling caused by fluid collection) then develops in the legs and ankles due to the back pressure in blood vessels as a result of the heart failure. Patients with this condition are called *blue bloaters*.

Those with chronic bronchitis usually have two or more episodes of acute viral or bacterial infection of the lungs every winter. Occasionally, blood may be coughed up, requiring urgent medical investigation to exclude the possibility of *lung cancer*.

PREVENTION
A reduction in atmospheric pollution in some cities over the last few decades has helped reduce the incidence of chronic bronchitis, but the crucial advice is that smoking is by far the most common cause of chronic bronchitis. Most cases of chronic bronchitis could be prevented if people stopped smoking. Waiting until symptoms develop may be too late to halt the course of the disease.

DIAGNOSIS AND TREATMENT
Before starting treatment, the physician may decide the patient's condition requires investigation by chest *X rays*, *blood tests*, *sputum analysis*, and *pulmonary function tests*.

To relieve breathlessness, the physician may prescribe an inhaler containing a *bronchodilator* (a drug that relaxes and widens the bronchi). In certain specific cases, the patient may benefit from inhaling oxygen from oxygen cylinders or an oxygen concentrator kept at home. Efforts may be made to help the patient cough up sputum; to treat or prevent any bacterial lung infection, antibiotics may be given.

The disease often shows an inexorable progression with increasing shortness of breath leading to early retirement; eventually the sufferer may become housebound.

Bronchoconstrictor
A substance that causes narrowing of the airways in the lungs. Bronchoconstrictors such as *histamine* or dinoprost (a *prostaglandin*) are sometimes given by inhalation to provoke an attack of *asthma* in order to confirm the diagnosis or to test the effectiveness of a *bronchodilator drug*.

Bronchodilator drugs

COMMON DRUGS

Sympathomimetics
Albuterol Ephedrine Epinephrine Isoproterenol Metaproterenol Terbutaline

Anticholinergics
Ipratropium

Xanthines
Aminophylline Theophylline

WARNING
If your inhaler is not helping your symptoms, call your physician.

A group of drugs that widen the airways in the lungs.

Under certain conditions the bronchioles (narrow airways) become narrowed, either as a result of contraction of the muscle in their walls and/or as a result of mucus congestion within them. Narrowing of the bronchioles obstructs the flow of air into and out of the lung and causes breathing difficulty. Bronchodilator drugs are prescribed to widen the bronchioles, which increases the flow of air and improves breathing.

TYPES
There are three principal types: sympathomimetic drugs, anticholinergic drugs, and xanthine drugs. Sympathomimetics are primarily used for the rapid relief of breathing difficulty. Anticholinergics and xanthine drugs are more often used for the long-term prevention of attacks of breathing difficulty.

WHY THEY ARE USED
Bronchodilators may be prescribed for any condition in which there is a reduced flow of air into the lungs, as in chronic *bronchitis*, although they are of little benefit when damage to the bronchioles from repeated infections is severe. Most commonly, however, they are used in the treatment of asthma, both to relieve attacks that are in progress and to try to prevent such attacks from occurring. Some people find it helpful to take an extra dose of their bronchodilator immediately before an activity likely to provoke an attack of breathlessness. Drugs can be given by *inhaler* or in tablet form and one or a combination of drugs may be prescribed. In a severe attack of asthma that has not responded to an inhaler, bronchodilators can be given by *nebulizer* (a type of inhaler that uses air and/or oxygen under pressure to propel a watery suspension of the drug into the lungs) or by injection.

POSSIBLE ADVERSE EFFECTS
Bronchodilators can have a variety of minor side effects especially if taken in large doses or very frequently. Because sympathomimetic drugs stimulate the sympathetic branch of the autonomic nervous system which controls heart rate, they may sometimes cause palpitations and trembling. Anticholinergic drugs have the side effects typical of all drugs of this type, including dry mouth, blurred vision, and difficulty passing urine. Xanthine drugs may cause headaches and, like adrenergics, may cause palpitations. When bronchodilators are inhaled they are not absorbed by the body in large amounts and therefore do not commonly cause serious side effects. However, because of their possible effect on

B

HOW BRONCHODILATORS WORK

Bronchodilator drugs relax muscles surrounding bronchioles. Sympathomimetic and anticholinergic drugs interfere with nerve signals passed to the muscles through the autonomic nervous system. Xanthine drugs relax muscle in the bronchioles by a direct effect on the muscle fibers but their precise action is not known.

When bronchioles become narrow following contraction of the muscle layer and swelling of the mucous lining, the passage of air is impeded. Bronchodilators act on the nerve signals that govern muscle activity. Sympathomimetics enhance the action of neurotransmitters that encourage muscle relaxation. Anticholinergics block the neurotransmitters that trigger muscle contraction.

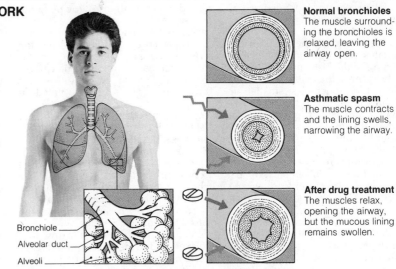

Bronchiole
Alveolar duct
Alveoli

Normal bronchioles
The muscle surrounding the bronchioles is relaxed, leaving the airway open.

Asthmatic spasm
The muscle contracts and the lining swells, narrowing the airway.

After drug treatment
The muscles relax, opening the airway, but the mucous lining remains swollen.

---

heart rate, sympathomimetic and xanthine drugs are prescribed cautiously for those with heart problems, high blood pressure, or an overactive thyroid gland. Anticholinergic drugs may not be suitable for men with enlarged prostate glands or for people who have a tendency to glaucoma.

Bronchography

An X-ray procedure for examining the bronchi, the main air passages of the lungs. Bronchography was formerly used to diagnose the disease *bronchiectasis*, but has now largely been replaced by other imaging techniques, such as *CT scanning* or lung *tomography*, and by using *bronchoscopy*.

HOW IT IS DONE

After the patient has been given mild sedation and/or a local anesthetic, contrast medium (an iodinated substance opaque to X rays) is introduced into the lung through a hollow flexible tube (either a cannula or a bronchoscope). X-ray pictures are then taken of the bronchi to detect any deformities in them. When the procedure is finished the contrast medium is partly coughed up and partly absorbed into the bloodstream.

Bronchopneumonia

The most common form of *pneumonia*, differing from pneumococcal or lobar pneumonia in that inflammation is spread throughout the lungs in small patches rather than confined to one lobe. It is often the cause of death in chronically ill patients.

Bronchoscopy

Examination or treatment of the bronchi, the main airways of the lungs, by means of a hollow tube or fiberoptic viewing tube with a light and lens attached.

WHY IT IS DONE

The two main uses of bronchoscopy are to aid in diagnosing and treating certain lung disorders. Apart from inspecting the bronchi for abnormalities, diagnostic procedures include collecting samples of mucus, obtaining cells from the outermost distant airways of the lungs, and taking biopsy specimens (small samples of tissue), all for analysis or microscopic examination. The bronchoscope is also sometimes used in a type of X-ray investigation called *bronchography*.

PERFORMING BRONCHOSCOPY

There are two kinds of bronchoscope. The rigid type is passed into the bronchi via the mouth and requires anesthesia. The flexible, fiberoptic bronchoscope (a narrower tube formed from light-transmitting fibers) can be inserted through either the mouth or nose. It is used after giving only a light sedative and/or local anesthetic and it reaches farther into the lungs. Both types of bronchoscope can be fitted with forceps, and the instrument also has attachments for performing laser therapy and cryosurgery. (See also *Endoscopy*.)

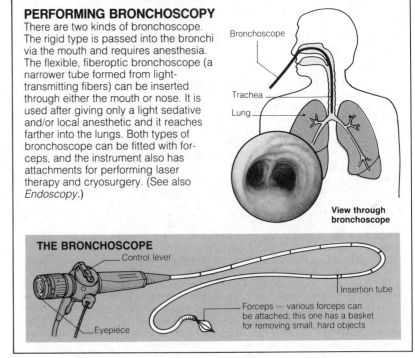

Bronchoscope
Trachea
Lung

View through bronchoscope

THE BRONCHOSCOPE

Control lever
Insertion tube
Forceps — various forceps can be attached; this one has a basket for removing small, hard objects
Eyepiece

Among the various forms of treatment possible are the removal of thick secretions of mucus or inhaled foreign bodies, destruction of growths, and the sealing off of damaged blood vessels. The last two are carried out by *laser treatment*, *diathermy*, or *cryosurgery* by means of attachments to the bronchoscope.

Bronchospasm

Temporary narrowing of the bronchi (airways into the lungs) caused by contraction of the muscles in the lung walls, by inflammation of the lung lining, or by a combination of both.

Contraction and relaxation of the airways is controlled by the autonomic nervous system. Contraction may also be caused by the release of substances during an allergic reaction.

When the airways are narrowed, flow of air out of the lungs causes wheezing or coughing. The most common cause of bronchospasm is *asthma*, though other causes include respiratory infection, chronic lung disease (including *emphysema* and chronic *bronchitis*), *anaphylactic shock*, or an allergic reaction to chemicals.

Bronchus

The air passage into the lungs. Each lung has one main bronchus, originating at the end of the trachea (windpipe), that is divided into smaller branches known as segmental bronchi. These then further divide into bronchioles.

Bronchus, cancer of

See *Lung cancer*.

Brown fat

A special type of fat, found in infants and some animals, but not in healthy adults. It is located between and around the scapulae on the back. Brown fat is a source of calories and so is useful in helping infants maintain a constant body temperature.

Brucellosis

A rare, bacterial infection caught from farm animals that causes fever.

CAUSES AND INCIDENCE

Three types of bacteria can cause the disease: BRUCELLA ABORTUS, B. MELITENSIS, and B. SUIS. These bacteria affect cattle, goats, and pigs, respectively. People who work with animals are at highest risk of infection. The bacteria enter the bloodstream through a cut or are breathed in. Up to 200 cases of brucellosis occur in the US each year.

In areas where milk pasteurization is not the rule—for example, Latin America and the Mediterranean—the disease can also be caught from drinking or eating unpasteurized dairy products from infected animals.

SYMPTOMS

The acute form of brucellosis consists of a single bout of high fever, shivering, widespread aching, and drenching sweats, which last for a few days. Other symptoms include headache, poor appetite, backache, weakness, and depression.

Sweating occurs by night as well as by day and can cause severe dehydration unless plenty of fluids are taken. The mental depression is sometimes severe; the patient may feel suicidal. In rare, untreated cases an acute attack is severe enough to cause sometimes fatal complications, such as *pneumonia* or *meningitis*.

In chronic brucellosis, bouts of the illness recur over months or years.

PREVENTION

The disease in livestock—and thus also human infection—is controlled by immunizing herds that have first been checked to guarantee that they are not infected. Infected animals are usually destroyed.

DIAGNOSIS AND TREATMENT

A definite diagnosis is made from blood tests. Treatment consists of tetracyclines, co-trimoxazole, or other *antibiotic drugs*, and the patient is advised to rest. After apparent recovery, the illness sometimes recurs a few months later, necessitating another course of treatment.

Bruise

A discolored area under the skin, caused by leakage of blood after injury. At first, the blood appears blue or black; then the breakdown of *hemoglobin* turns the bruise yellow.

To reduce the pain and swelling of a large bruise, place a cloth soaked in ice-cold water over it for 10 minutes. If a bruise does not fade after about one week, or if bruises appear for no apparent reason or are severe after only minor injury, a physician should be consulted as these may be signs of a *bleeding disorder*. (See also *Purpura*; *Black eye*.)

Bruits

The sounds made in the heart, arteries, or veins when blood circulation becomes turbulent or flows at an abnormal speed. This happens when blood vessels become narrowed by disease (as in *arteriosclerosis*), when

heart valves are narrowed or damaged (as in *endocarditis*), or if blood vessels dilate (as in an *aneurysm*). Bruits are usually heard through a *stethoscope*.

Bruxism

Rhythmic grinding or clenching of the teeth. This habit, which may develop at any age, usually occurs during sleep, but is sometimes done unconsciously when a person is awake. There are two underlying causes: unresolved stress and emotional tension, and some minor discomfort or unevenness when the teeth are brought together.

Continued bruxism may cause considerable wearing away and loosening of the teeth, and stiffness in the jaw. If the underlying problems cannot be resolved, a biteplate worn at night will minimize the damage.

Bubonic plague

The most common form of *plague*, characterized by the appearance of a bubo (swollen lymph node) in the groin or armpit early in the illness.

Buccal

An anatomical term, from the Latin word for cheek, relating to the cheek or mouth.

Buck teeth

Prominent upper incisors (front teeth), which protrude from the mouth and are often splayed out at an angle to each other. Buck teeth are easily damaged and may be susceptible to decay because they are not moistened by saliva.

CAUSES

The malpositioning of the teeth is probably an inherited trait rather than

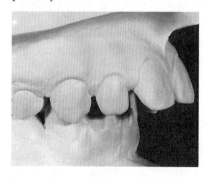

Buck teeth
Apart from the usually undesirable appearance protruding upper teeth produce, the upper and lower incisors do not meet satisfactorily. This produces stress on the jaw joint that can cause problems. A plaster cast of buck teeth is shown.

B

acquired—for example, by faulty eating habits. Often, the person's upper jaw is relatively large compared with the lower jaw, and the lips do not close over and exert a controlling influence on the position of the teeth. Rarely, the malpositioning may be the result of an abnormally large tongue gradually displacing the teeth forward. In many cases, there is an overall crowding of teeth within the upper jaw.

TREATMENT
Orthodontic treatment involves gradually coaxing the teeth back into position with a removable brace, or, in more extreme cases, with a fixed appliance (see *Orthodontic appliances*). To create room for the incisors, other crowded teeth may sometimes need to be extracted.

Budd-Chiari syndrome

A rare disorder in which the veins draining blood from the liver become blocked or narrowed. Blood then accumulates in the liver, which swells. The blockage leads to serious *liver failure*, and to *portal hypertension* (back pressure in the blood vessels due to slowed blood flow through the liver).

Treatment is aimed at removing the cause of the vein obstruction—which may be a blood clot, pressure on the veins from a liver tumor, or a congenital abnormality of the veins. In most cases, however, treatment has only a limited effect, and, unless a *liver transplant* can be performed, most patients die within two years.

Buerger's disease

A rare disorder, also called thromboangiitis obliterans, in which the arteries, nerves, and veins in the legs, and sometimes those in the arms, become severely inflamed. Narrowing of the arteries blocks off blood supply to the toes and fingers, eventually causing *gangrene*.

The disease occurs mainly in men under the age of 45 who smoke heavily. Most have a history of *phlebitis* (a type of vein inflammation). The main symptom is pain in the hands and feet; victims suffer cold sensitivity, with the hands turning white, then blue, then red (see *Raynaud's disease*) in cold conditions.

Sufferers must stop smoking to halt progress of the disease. *Vasodilators* (drugs that widen the blood vessels) may be prescribed, but are rarely, if ever, effective. If *gangrene* (tissue death) develops, the affected limb, toes, or fingers almost always have to be amputated.

Bulimia

An illness characterized by bouts of gross overeating usually followed by self-induced vomiting. These activities are often kept secret, so the exact prevalence of the illness is not known, but most sufferers are girls or women between the ages of 15 and 30.

CAUSES
Bulimia is often, though not always, a variant of another psychiatric disorder, *anorexia nervosa*, in which dieting is carried out to excess. In both illnesses there is a morbid fear of fatness. After months or years of eating sparsely, an anorectic may develop a constant craving for food and begin to binge—but the fear of becoming overweight remains and prompts the vomiting. Sometimes, large doses of *laxatives* are used as well as, or instead of, vomiting in an effort to expel food as quickly as possible.

Occasionally, a woman develops bulimia without a previous history of anorexia.

SYMPTOMS
Bulimics may be of normal weight or only slightly underweight, although some remain extremely thin. Bingeing and vomiting may occur once or several times a day. In severe cases, this can lead to dehydration and loss of potassium from the body, causing symptoms such as weakness and cramps. Gastric acid contained in vomit may damage the teeth. The sufferer is often highly distressed about her compulsive behavior and as a result may be depressed and sometimes suicidal.

TREATMENT AND OUTLOOK
Once the bulimic has been persuaded to accept it, treatment is similar to that given for anorexia nervosa. It consists of supervision and regulation of eating habits, *psychotherapy* aimed at improving emotional maturity, and, sometimes, the use of *antidepressant drugs*. To be successful, treatment usually must be given in a hospital over several weeks. In many patients there is a risk of relapse weeks or even months after their treatment has ended. (See also *Appetite*; *Obsessive-compulsive behavior*.)

Bulla

A large air- or fluid-filled bubble, usually in the lungs or skin.

In young adults lung bullae are usually congenital defects (abnormalities present from birth). In later life they develop in patients with the lung disease *emphysema* as the result of overdistention and coalescence of the alveoli (tiny air sacs) in the lungs.

A bulla in the skin is simply a large, fluid-filled *blister*.

Bundle-branch block

See *Heart block*.

Bunion

A firm, fluid-filled pad, or *bursa*, overlying the inside of the joint at the base of the big toe (which can become inflamed and very painful).

The underlying cause of the bunion is hallux valgus, an abnormal outward projection of the joint and inward turning of the toe.

HOW BUNIONS FORM

A bunion results from rubbing of a shoe against an abnormal outward projection of the joint at the base of the big toe (a hallux valgus), leading to irritation and inflammation. The joint abnormality is often itself due to the wearing of narrow, pointed shoes with high heels, although it can also result from an inherited weakness in the joint.

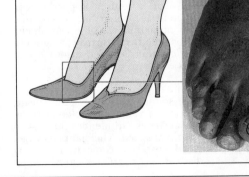

Valgus deformity of the joint between the first metatarsal bone and the adjoining phalanx.

TREATMENT
To remedy a small bunion, wear well-fitting shoes and a special toe pad or corrective sock that straightens the big toe and keeps it in position. Large bunions may require surgery to remove the swollen tissue; in some cases the big toe may have to be completely remodeled.

Unless treated, a bunion will get worse. People with recurring bunions should see a foot specialist.

Buphthalmos
Larger than normal eyeball due to *glaucoma*. In infants, increased pressure inside the eyeball due to glaucoma can result in abnormal eye development. Treatment usually involves surgery to reduce pressure.

Burkitt's lymphoma
A cancer of lymph tissues that is characterized by an enlarging tumor or tumors within the jaw and/or the abdomen.

INCIDENCE
Burkitt's lymphoma is confined almost exclusively to children living in low-lying, moist, tropical regions of Africa and New Guinea. A few cases have occurred among a wider age group in North America and Europe.

CAUSE
The growths are believed to be an abnormal response to a common virus, the Epstein-Barr virus. The distribution of the disease in Africa closely follows that of *malaria*; it is theorized that malaria in childhood alters the body's immune response to the Epstein-Barr virus, which triggers growth of the lymphoma.

TREATMENT
Injections of *anticancer drugs*, such as cyclophosphamide, or treatment by *radiation therapy* gives complete or partial cure in about 80 percent of cases. (See also *Lymphoma*.)

Burns
Each year in the US 2 million people are burned or scalded badly enough to need medical treatment, and about 70,000 require admission to a hospital. Burns are most common in children and older people; many are due to accidents in the home, which are usually preventable.

TYPES
The skin is a living tissue; even brief heating above 120°F damages its cells.
FIRST-DEGREE BURNS These burns cause reddening of the skin and affect only the epidermis, the top layer of the skin. Such burns heal quickly, but the

CARE OF BURN PATIENTS
Burn patients need specialized nursing care. Sterile linen should be used with sterile starch powder sprinkled on it. Drafts should be avoided and room humidity should be controlled. The revolving circular bed is useful in the treatment of burn patients since it can be moved into many different positions and stopped at any angle.

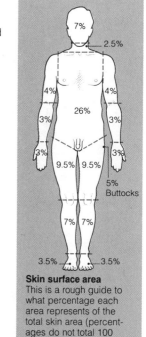

Skin surface area
This is a rough guide to what percentage each area represents of the total skin area (percentages do not total 100 due to rounding).

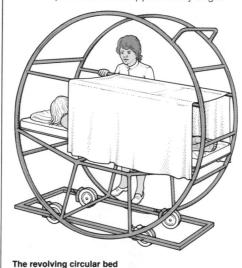

The revolving circular bed

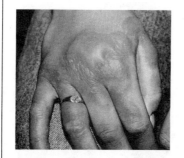

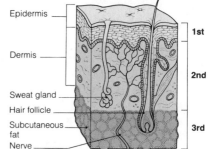

Degrees of burns
Burns are divided into three categories, depending on the depth of damage to the skin. First-degree burns affect the epidermis and skin may peel; second-degree burns cause the formation of blisters (above left); third-degree burns destroy the whole of the skin's thickness and require special treatment.

PRIMARY CAUSES OF FIRE AND BURN DEATHS, 1980

Cause	Number	% of total
House fire	4,509	75
Fire, other buildings	292	5
Ignition of clothing	364	6
Ignition of highly flammable material	105	2
Hot substances	194	4
Other causes	552	9
Total (percentages do not total 100 due to rounding)	**6,016**	101

B

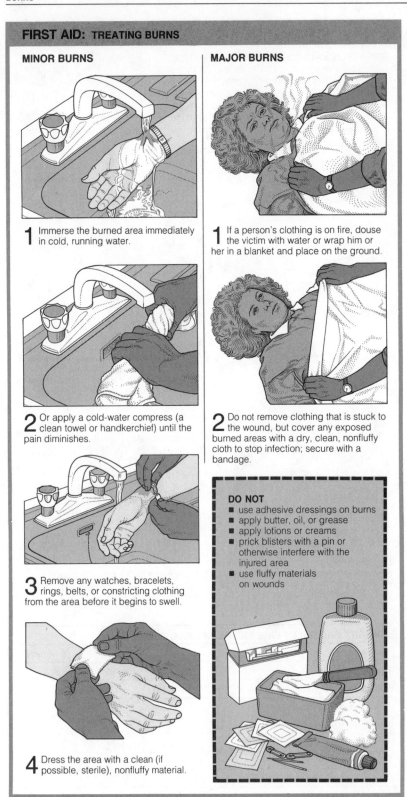

FIRST AID: TREATING BURNS

MINOR BURNS

1 Immerse the burned area immediately in cold, running water.

2 Or apply a cold-water compress (a clean towel or handkerchief) until the pain diminishes.

3 Remove any watches, bracelets, rings, belts, or constricting clothing from the area before it begins to swell.

4 Dress the area with a clean (if possible, sterile), nonfluffy material.

MAJOR BURNS

1 If a person's clothing is on fire, douse the victim with water or wrap him or her in a blanket and place on the ground.

2 Do not remove clothing that is stuck to the wound, but cover any exposed burned areas with a dry, clean, nonfluffy cloth to stop infection; secure with a bandage.

DO NOT
- use adhesive dressings on burns
- apply butter, oil, or grease
- apply lotions or creams
- prick blisters with a pin or otherwise interfere with the injured area
- use fluffy materials on wounds

damaged skin may peel away after a day or two. A *sunburn* is an example.

SECOND-DEGREE BURNS These damage the skin more deeply, causing blisters. However, some of the dermis (deep layer of the skin) is left to recover, and these burns usually heal without scarring, unless they are very extensive.

THIRD-DEGREE BURNS These burns destroy the full skin thickness. The affected area will look white or charred, and, if the burn is very deep, muscles and bones may be exposed. Even if very localized, these burns will need specialist treatment and skin grafts to prevent scarring.

ELECTRICAL BURNS These can cause extensive damage with minimal external skin damage. Since they can also cause heart damage, electrical burns require evaluation by a physician.

EFFECTS AND COMPLICATIONS
Extensive first-degree burns (such as sunburn) cause pain, restlessness, headache, and fever, but they are not life-threatening.

In second- or third-degree burns affecting more than 10 percent of the body surface, the victim will be in *shock* with a low blood pressure and rapid pulse. This is caused by the loss of large quantities of fluid (and its constituent proteins) from the burned area. It may be fatal if not treated by intravenous fluid replacement.

When skin is burned, it can no longer protect the body from contamination by airborne bacteria. The infection of extensive burns may cause fatal complications if effective antibiotic treatment is not given.

Victims who have inhaled smoke may develop swelling and inflammation of the lungs and may need specialist care for burns of the eyes. People who die in burning buildings usually suffocate long before their bodies are burned.

PROFESSIONAL TREATMENT
The burn will be either lightly dressed with an antibacterial dressing or left exposed to promote healing, with every effort made to keep the skin area scrupulously clean by reverse *isolation* nursing. If necessary, analgesic drugs (painkillers) will be given; antibiotics will be given if there is any sign of the wound being infected. Shock is treated by giving intravenous fluids through a drip inserted into a vein, usually in the arm.

For extensive second-degree burns, skin-grafting will be used early in the treatment to minimize scarring. Third-degree burns always require skin grafting if scarring is to be avoided.

Extensive burns may require repeated operations by a plastic surgeon.

Length of hospital stay can vary from a few days in some cases to many weeks in the case of severe and extensive burns. Extensive burns are usually treated at a burn center.

Burping

Another term for *belching*.

Burr hole

A hole made in the skull by a special drill with a rounded tip (burr). The hole permits access to the brain and the tissues surrounding it. The hole is made to relieve pressure on the brain, often resulting from the accumulation of blood between the inside of the skull and the brain after a head injury. The burr hole relieves the pressure, which can be fatal, by allowing the blood to drain. Burr holes also permit biopsy of the brain, injection of gas or drugs, drainage of abscesses or cysts, and placement of electrodes.

Bursa

A small, fluid-filled sac that acts as a cushion at a pressure point in the body—often near joints, where a tendon or muscle crosses either bone or other muscles. The most important bursae are around the knee, elbow, and shoulder.

A *bunion* is a bursa near the toe.

Bursitis

Inflammation of a *bursa*, causing it to swell and be painful.

Bursitis is usually the result of pressure, friction, or slight injury to the membrane surrounding the joint. Prepatellar bursitis ("housemaid's knee") is caused by prolonged kneeling on a hard surface, tibial tubercle bursitis ("clergyman's knee") from kneeling on a more upright surface, and olecranon bursitis ("student's elbow") from prolonged pressure of the elbow point against a desk or table. Another common form is subdeltoid (of the shoulder) bursitis, which, if left untreated, may result in "frozen shoulder."

The treatment is usually rest; often the bursitis will subside after a few days, with the fluid being reabsorbed into the bloodstream. Applying an ice-pack may help relieve pain.

Infection may be treated with antibiotics and drainage. The physician may apply a pressure bandage to stop the fluid from reforming. An injection of a *corticosteroid drug* may also be given.

In rare, recurrent cases, bursectomy (a minor operation to remove the bursa) may be performed. Using general anesthesia, a small incision is made in the skin over the bursa, and the lining of the bursal sac is completely removed to prevent it from regrowing.

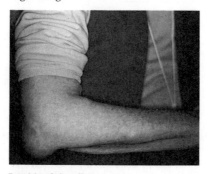

Bursitis of the elbow
This condition produces a fluid-filled swelling around the point of the elbow.

Bypass operations

Procedures to bypass the blockage or narrowing of an artery or vein or any part of the digestive system.

TYPES
Arteries can become blocked or narrowed by *atheroma*. Those most often affected are the carotid arteries (in the neck), the coronary arteries (in the heart), and the iliofemoral vessels

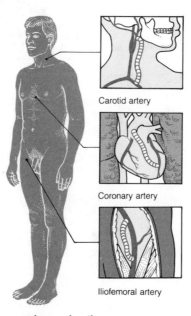

Carotid artery

Coronary artery

Iliofemoral artery

Common bypass locations
The carotid and coronary arteries and the iliofemoral vessels are the usual locations for bypasses.

(leading to the legs). These blocks can be bypassed using sections of artery or vein (taken from the patient) or using synthetic tubing.

Surgeons have attempted to bypass blocked arteries in the brain by joining points above the blockage to an artery in the neck. Known as extracranial-intracranial bypass, it has had little success, and is now rarely used.

Veins are bypassed most often in patients with diseases of the liver that cause portal hypertension (increased pressure in the veins draining the intestinal tract) and bleeding esophageal varices (enlarged veins in the lower esophagus). These bypasses are called *shunts*.

Intestinal bypasses are most commonly employed in patients with cancer. If tumor growth is too extensive for surgical removal, symptoms may be relieved by joining the sections of gut at either side of the blockage. Bypass for other conditions has been largely abandoned. An obstructed bile duct may be diverted into the intestine lower down the digestive tract. Intestinal bypass operations for treatment of obesity have largely been replaced by operations to reduce the capacity of the stomach. (See also *Coronary artery bypass*.)

Byssinosis

An industrial disease of the lungs caused by allergy to an unknown agent in the dust produced during the processing of flax, cotton, hemp, or sisal. It produces a feeling of tightness in the chest and shortness of breath that may become chronic. In the US, preventive measures in the textile industry have lowered the incidence of the disease, but it is common in India and other developing countries.

At first, symptoms are most pronounced at the start of the working week, but gradually they become troublesome on every working day. In chronic byssinosis (the risk of which is increased by smoking), the sufferer is short of breath even when away from work. *Respiratory failure* may eventually develop when lung damage has become extensive.

Drugs used to treat asthma, such as *bronchodilators*, can relieve symptoms, but the answer to the problem is prevention. This is achieved by treatment of raw textiles before processing, reduction of dust levels, and the wearing of face masks.

In the US, people who suffer from byssinosis have a statutory right to government compensation.

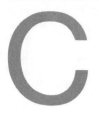

Cachexia

An appearance of profound illness and massive weight loss, usually due to either extreme starvation or a serious underlying disease such as cancer or tuberculosis.

Cadaver

A dead human body used as a source of transplant organs or preserved for anatomical study and dissection.

Cadmium poisoning

Poisoning by the fumes or dust of this tinlike metal, which is an industrial hazard. Cadmium varies in its effects according to the duration and severity of exposure. Exposure can lead to urinary tract *calculi* (stones), *renal failure* in severe cases, or inflammation in the lungs progressing to severe *emphysema*. In Japan, many cases of severe cadmium poisoning have occurred when people have eaten rice contaminated with industrial effluent. Cadmium poisoning can also be caused by eating vegetables grown in cadmium-rich soil, and by foods stored in cadmium-lined containers.

It is known that cadmium accumulates in the body (especially in the kidneys) throughout life. Cadmium has been implicated in causing high blood pressure, but this has not been proved in man. Minute amounts of cadmium may be essential for health.

Café au lait spots

Pale, coffee-colored patches, usually oval, and up to 3 inches across, that may develop anywhere on the skin. They usually have no significance, but the presence of several café au lait spots is sometimes a sign of *neurofibromatosis*, a hereditary disorder of the sheaths that surround nerve fibers. In such cases there are commonly (in addition to the café au lait spots) multiple small nodules in and on the skin.

Caffeine

A stimulant that occurs naturally in coffee beans, tea leaves, cocoa beans, and kola nuts. Several popular drinks contain caffeine, notably coffee. In medicine, caffeine is sometimes combined with certain analgesics.

CAFFEINE LEVELS (mg per cup)

Tea, weak	50
Tea, strong	80
Coffee, weak	80
Coffee, strong	200
Cocoa	10-17
Cola	43-75

The strength and method of preparation determine exact amounts of caffeine present (in mg per cup).

USES AND ABUSES

Few people consume so much caffeine that they experience unpleasant side effects, but some people are particularly sensitive and feel side effects from relatively small amounts.

People who regularly consume large amounts of caffeine (more than five cups of coffee a day) often find their system has adapted to this amount of caffeine so that their *tolerance* to the substance increases; the result is that they must increase their intake to continue any stimulant effect. Furthermore, if such people go without caffeine for some time—as little as a few hours in some cases—they may suffer withdrawal symptoms, such as tiredness, headaches, and

EFFECTS OF CAFFEINE ON THE BODY

Within a few minutes of consuming caffeine-containing drinks or tablets, there is a stimulant effect on all organs and tissues. Caffeine acts directly on individual cells by affecting the chemical reactions within them; it acts indirectly by increasing the release, from the adrenal glands into the circulation, of *epinephrine* (adrenaline) and norepinephrine (noradrenaline), hormones that stimulate cell activity.

Brain
Small amounts of caffeine stimulate the brain cells, helping to reduce drowsiness and fatigue. Concentration is improved and reactions are speeded up. Large amounts cause overstimulation, anxiety, irritability, and restlessness. This is why consuming caffeine before going to bed can cause insomnia and a hangover in the morning, with excessive fatigue and drowsiness on waking.

Skeletal muscles
Stimulation by caffeine may improve their performance during exercise, but excessive stimulation of the skeletal muscles can cause twitching.

Heart
With small amounts of caffeine, the heart muscle is stimulated, augmenting its pumping action. This causes the blood to circulate faster and blood pressure to increase for a short time. Too much caffeine results in overstimulation of the heart muscle and can result in palpitations.

Stomach
While small amounts of caffeine can actually help digestion by increasing production of stomach acid, too much can cause abdominal pain and nausea.

Kidneys
Caffeine action on the kidneys increases the production of urine.

irritability due to their physical and psychological dependence on the drug (see *Drug dependence*).

Because of increasing concern about the undesirable effects of caffeine, there has been a general decrease in its consumption in recent years. Moreover, because it can improve short-term athletic performance, caffeine has been included in the list of drugs banned in sports competitions (see *Sports, drugs and*).

The medical use of caffeine has also recently been reevaluated, in particular its inclusion in some combination analgesics. Caffeine was originally included in such preparations because it was thought to enhance their painkilling action, but studies indicate that it may not have this effect. Caffeine is combined with *ergotamine* in several drugs for the early preventive treatment of migraine.

Calamine

A pink substance consisting of zinc oxide and ferric oxide that is applied to the skin in the form of ointments, lotions, or dusting powders. It has a protective, cooling, and drying effect, and is used to relieve skin irritation and itching arising from *dermatitis*, *eczema*, *poison ivy*, *insect bites*, and *sunburn*. It is sometimes combined with topical local anesthetics, such as benzocaine (see *Anesthesia, local*), and with *corticosteroid drugs* or *antihistamine drugs*, which reduce any accompanying inflammation. Bandages impregnated with calamine are sometimes used to protect leg ulcers.

Calcaneus

The heel bone, which can be fractured as a result of falling from a height onto the heels. Minor fractures of this bone usually do not cause problems and are treated by putting the foot and leg in a cast. A more serious fracture, with compression of the bone, may cause permanent damage to the joints in the foot that are involved in turning the foot in and out. This usually leads to pain and stiffness in the foot that is aggravated by walking.

The *Achilles tendon* is fixed to the back of the heel bone and controls the up and down movement of the foot. The point at which the tendon joins the bone may be strained by excessive or prolonged stress from the pull of the tendon—for example, in some *running injuries*. In children this area of bone is still growing and occasionally becomes inflamed and painful (see *Osteochondrosis*).

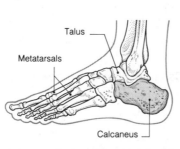

LOCATION OF THE CALCANEUS
This is the largest tarsal bone, projecting backward beyond the leg bones.

Talus

Metatarsals

Calcaneus

Tendons in the sole of the foot (see *Aponeurosis*) are fixed under the heel bone; the associated muscles are important in supporting the arches of the foot. Inflammation around these tendons (as in plantar *fasciitis*) causes pain and tenderness under the heel when standing or walking. A calcaneal spur (a bony protrusion from this part of the calcaneus) is sometimes seen on X rays of the foot in plantar fasciitis, but the spurs are also found on X rays of healthy feet.

Calciferol

An alternative name for vitamin D$_2$ (see *Vitamin D*); it is also known by the name ergocalciferol.

Calcification

The deposition of calcium salts in body tissues. Calcification is normal in bone and teeth formation and is necessary for the healing of fractures. Calcification can occur in an injured muscle and is common in arteries affected by *atherosclerosis*. It may also occur if the blood calcium level is raised as a result of a disorder of the parathyroid gland.

Calcification, dental

The deposition of calcium crystals in developing teeth. Calcium and phosphorous salts are brought to the teeth, where the crystals make up 96 percent of tooth enamel and 70 percent of dentin. Calcification of primary teeth begins in the fetus between three and six months; calcification of permanent teeth (other than wisdom teeth) begins between birth and 4 years.

Abnormal calcification occurs in amelogenesis imperfecta, an inherited disorder of the enamel (see *Hypoplasia, enamel*). The affected teeth have a thin, grooved covering due to incomplete

calcification. Another cause of abnormal calcification is the ingestion of high levels of fluoride (see *Fluorosis*).

Calcinosis

A condition in which there is abnormal deposition of calcium salts in various tissues (such as the skin) of the body, and in connective tissues including cartilage and tendons. Calcinosis tends to be associated with an underlying disorder of the connective tissue, such as *scleroderma* or *dermatomyositis*. The term "calcinosis" is usually combined with another word to signify which part of the body is affected—for example, calcinosis cutis affects the skin (and is apparent as nodules in the skin). (See also *Calcification; Calcium*.)

Calcitonin

PAGET'S DISEASE OSTEOPOROSIS									

Injection

Prescription needed

Not available as generic

A hormone produced by the thyroid gland. It controls the level of calcium in the blood by slowing the rate at which calcium is lost from bones.

WHY IT IS USED

A synthetic form of calcitonin is used to treat *Paget's disease*, in which the bones grow abnormally and become deformed, causing pain and an increased risk of fracture. Given by injection, calcitonin halts abnormal bone formation in about a week and can relieve pain within a few months.

Calcitonin is also used to treat *hypercalcemia* (abnormally high levels of calcium in the blood) caused by overactivity of the parathyroid glands or by cancer of the bone. Calcitonin helps relieve the nausea and vomiting that results from hypercalcemia by quickly reducing the level of calcium in the blood. It may be prescribed with a *corticosteroid drug* that decreases the calcium level in the blood.

POSSIBLE ADVERSE EFFECTS

Calcitonin does not generally cause any troublesome adverse effects. Gastrointestinal reactions, such as nausea, vomiting, and diarrhea, usually diminish with continued use.

Calcium

The most abundant mineral in the body— about 2 to 2.5 pounds (0.9 to 1.1 kg) in an average-

C

sized person—with several important functions. Calcium is essential for the functioning of cells, for muscle contraction, for the transmission of nerve impulses from nerve endings to muscle fibers, and for blood clotting. In the form of calcium phosphate it makes up the hard basic constituent of teeth and bones.

The main dietary sources of calcium are milk and dairy products, eggs, fish, green vegetables, and fruit.

CONTROL OF CALCIUM LEVELS

Vitamin D and certain hormones help control the overall amount of calcium in the body by regulating the amount of calcium absorbed from food, and the amount removed from the body by the kidneys (which filter excess calcium from the blood and excrete it in the urine).

Control of calcium levels is achieved by the actions of two hormones: parathyroid hormone (produced by the parathyroid glands) and calcitonin (produced by the thyroid gland). When the level of calcium in the blood is too low, the parathyroid glands release more parathyroid hormone, which raises the blood calcium level by helping to release calcium from the enormous reservoir of the mineral in the bones. When the blood calcium level is too high, the thyroid gland releases more calcitonin, which counteracts the effects of parathyroid hormone and lowers the calcium level.

DISORDERS OF CALCIUM METABOLISM

Some people have too little calcium in the blood, a condition known as hypocalcemia. The most common cause is vitamin D deficiency, due to a poor diet or, occasionally, lack of sunshine. Rarer causes include chronic kidney failure (which leads to a poor absorption of calcium from the diet), hypoparathyroidism (in which insufficient parathyroid hormone is produced), and unintentional removal of the parathyroid glands during thyroid surgery.

In mild cases hypocalcemia is symptomless. In severe cases it causes tetany (cramplike spasms in the hands, feet, and face) due to the effect of low blood calcium on muscle activity. Hypocalcemia may also lead to softening of the bones. In children this softening takes the form of rickets; in adults it takes the form of osteomalacia.

Too much calcium in the blood (hypercalcemia) is rarer. It is most commonly due to cancer (or the treatment of certain cancers) that has spread to the bones and caused excessive release of calcium into the blood.

Other causes include hyperparathyroidism (in which too much parathyroid hormone is produced), excessive vitamin D in the diet (as may occur by taking huge doses of vitamins), and certain inflammatory disorders (such as sarcoidosis). Hypercalcemia can result in depression and kidney stones. (See also Calcium channel blockers; Mineral supplements.)

Calcium channel blockers

COMMON DRUGS

Diltiazem Nifedipine Verapamil

A relatively new class of drug used in the treatment of angina pectoris (chest pain due to an inadequate blood supply to heart muscle), hypertension (high blood pressure), and certain types of cardiac arrhythmia (irregular heart beat).

HOW THEY WORK

In the treatment of angina pectoris and high blood pressure, calcium channel blockers work by interfering with muscle contraction. They prevent the movement of calcium across the membrane that lines muscle cells, which is an essential part of the mechanism of muscle contraction. As a result of this interference, the walls of the muscles relax and dilate. This action decreases the work of the heart's blood pumping, reduces the pressure of blood flow through the body, and improves the circulation of blood through heart muscle.

Calcium channel blockers also slow the passage of nerve impulses through heart muscle, which helps correct certain types of arrhythmia.

POSSIBLE ADVERSE EFFECTS

Adverse effects of calcium channel blockers are mainly related to their action of increasing blood flow through tissues. These effects include headaches, facial flushing, and dizziness (usually on standing). Such effects, however, generally disappear with continued treatment.

Calculus

A deposit on the teeth (see Calculus, dental) or a small, hard, crystalline mass formed from substances that have precipitated gradually from a fluid, such as bile or urine. The usual sites for such calculi are the gallbladder and bile ducts (see Gallstones), and the kidneys, ureters, or urinary bladder (see Calculus, urinary tract). Stones may be symptomless or may cause severe pain and require removal, dissolving, or shattering.

Calculus, dental

A hard, crustlike deposit found on the crowns and roots of teeth. Also known as tartar, calculus is formed when mineral salts from saliva are deposited in existing plaque. These minerals, mainly calcium and phosphorus, make up about 70 percent of the calculus; the rest is organic material and bacteria. Calculus commonly occurs on the inside surfaces of the lower incisors and on the outer surfaces of the upper molars—areas close to the duct openings of the salivary glands.

TYPES

Supragingival calculus, which forms above the gum margin on the crowns of teeth, is white or yellowish unless stained. Subgingival calculus, which forms below the gum margin, is more evenly distributed around all the teeth. Brown or black, possibly because of breakdown products of blood from the inflamed gums, it is visible if the gum is gently parted from the tooth and may show through the gum as a dark area. Both types of calculus are hard, and therefore difficult to remove; the subgingival variety may be more difficult to remove because of its location and degree of calcification.

EFFECTS AND TREATMENT

Being porous, calculus is impossible to keep clean and continually becomes covered by plaque. The irritant effect of toxins in plaque and calculus causes progressive inflammation and destruction of the gums and supporting structures of the teeth (see Periodontitis). Any calculus should be completely removed on a regular basis by professional scaling. Careful oral hygiene, professional cleaning, and elimination of stagnation areas, such as poorly finished fillings, should diminish or slow its recurrence.

Calculus, urinary tract

A stone that has formed or is present in the kidneys, ureters, or bladder, caused by precipitation from a solution of substances in urine.

INCIDENCE

Calculi differ in their incidence according to their site of origin. Kidney and ureteral stones are more common than bladder stones in developed countries and are three times more common in men than in women. In the US each year, about 100 persons per 100,000 are hospitalized with a ureteral calculus. Stones occur with different frequency in different sections of the country and the world.

Stones tend to be a recurrent problem; about 60 percent of patients treated for a stone develop another within seven years. The incidence is highest in the summer months, perhaps because we sweat more and pass a more concentrated urine.

COMPOSITION AND CAUSES

KIDNEY AND URETERAL STONES There are various types of kidney and ureteral stones; their composition is sometimes related to a specific cause. In the majority of cases, there is no identifiable underlying cause, although mild chronic dehydration (for example, due to inadequate water consumption in a hot climate) may play a part.

About 70 percent of kidney and ureteral stones consist mainly of calcium oxalate and/or phosphate. Oxalate is an end product of body *metabolism* and is present naturally in the urine. The salt it forms with calcium has a low solubility (dissolves poorly). An abnormally high level of oxalate in the urine encourages stone formation and may be related to a diet containing food or drinks with a high content of oxalic acid—for example, rhubarb, spinach, leafy vegetables, and coffee. Stones containing calcium are sometimes the first evidence of a disturbance of metabolism associated with *hyperparathyroidism*.

About 20 percent of calculi are termed infective stones and are linked with chronic infections of the urinary tract. These calculi consist of a combination of calcium, magnesium, and ammonium phosphate and are associated with a high ammonium content and alkalinity of the urine produced by the action of bacteria on urea (a substance in urine). In the kidney, an infective stone may fill the entire network of urine-collecting ducts and the top part of the ureter, forming a large, oddly shaped calculus.

Stones consisting mainly of uric acid comprise about 5 percent of the total and may occur in people with *gout*, people with some cancers, and people with chronic *dehydration*.

Other, uncommon types of stone occasionally occur. Those formed from the amino acid cysteine are most notable and affect people with a particular inherited metabolic disorder.

BLADDER STONES In poorer countries, bladder stones usually develop as a result of a diet low in phosphate and protein. In developed countries, such as the US, they result from obstruction to the flow of urine from the bladder and/or a long-standing urinary tract infection; they almost exclusively

URINARY TRACT CALCULI

Symptoms vary according to the site of the stone. Small stones in the kidney often cause no symptoms until they start to pass down the ureter, resulting in *renal colic*, a sudden pain in the flank that moves toward the groin. The pain is acute, sharp, and intermittent and may cause nausea and vomiting. There may also be hematuria (blood in the urine). Bladder stones, which affect men far more often than women, can cause difficulty in passing urine, a poor flow rate, and dribbling. Some stones may be associated with recurrent episodes of *urinary tract infection*. Any obstruction to urine flow may result in rapid kidney damage and acute severe infection termed *pyelonephritis*.

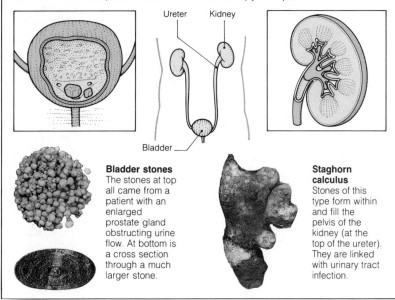

Ureter   Kidney

Bladder

Bladder stones
The stones at top all came from a patient with an enlarged prostate gland obstructing urine flow. At bottom is a cross section through a much larger stone.

Staghorn calculus
Stones of this type form within and fill the pelvis of the kidney (at the top of the ureter). They are linked with urinary tract infection.

affect men. The composition of bladder stones varies according to the acidity or alkalinity of the urine, but in the US the most common type consists of calcium oxalate.

DIAGNOSIS

Investigation of a suspected calculus usually starts with examination of the urine, which may reveal red blood cells and the presence of crystals. The degree of acidity or alkalinity of the urine may reflect the type of stone involved. About 90 percent of urinary tract calculi are visible on X rays, which will show the site of the stone; this can be confirmed by intravenous or retrograde *pyelography*. These techniques also indicate any obstruction of the urinary tract above the stone, which can be monitored by *ultrasound scanning*. If a metabolic disorder is a suspected cause of the stone, chemical analysis of the blood and urine may be performed to look for high levels of calcium, phosphate, or urate.

TREATMENT

Renal colic is treated with bed rest, pain relief using a narcotic analgesic (painkiller), and adequate fluid intake to encourage the passage of the stone through the ureter, bladder, and urethra. The majority of stones less than 0.2 inch (5 mm) in diameter are passed in the urine at home with relatively few problems.

With larger stones, or if an infection or obstruction to urinary flow is present, surgical treatment may be needed to prevent damage to the kidney. The traditional method of removing stones from the ureter and from the junction between the ureter and kidney is by surgery using general anesthesia. Stones in the bladder and lower ureter can be crushed and removed by *cystoscopy* (passage of a viewing tube and crushing device up the urethra into the bladder) or by ureterorenoscopy (passage of the same type of tube into the ureter).

In recent years new methods for removing kidney and ureteral stones have evolved and dramatically changed the way in which they are treated. Ultrasonic *lithotripsy* involves the use of an ultrasonic probe through

C

a telescopic tube to help break up stones that are too large to be removed whole. More advanced is the extracorporeal shock-wave lithotriptor, which is used to disintegrate kidney stones by focusing a shock wave on the stone from outside the body.

If a stone is thought to have developed because of some metabolic disorder, the patient may be prescribed a diet, and possibly drugs, to lower the content in the urine of the substance from which the stone is formed; it may also be necessary for the patient to maintain a high fluid intake. These methods may act to dissolve an existing stone and may help prevent recurrences.

Stones associated with hyperparathyroidism are treated by methods appropriate to their location; the parathyroid gland tumor that is usually responsible for the condition is removed.

Calendar method

A method of *contraception*, also called the rhythm method, that entails abstaining from sexual intercourse around the time of ovulation, which is predicted on the basis of the length of previous menstrual cycles.

The calendar method is unreliable because a woman's cycle may vary, and thus the time of ovulation can be estimated only approximately. There are now more scientific and effective contraceptive methods of this type. (See *Contraception, periodic abstinence*.)

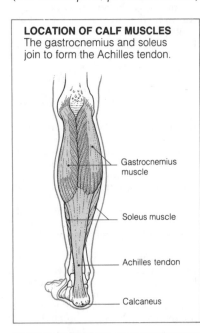

LOCATION OF CALF MUSCLES
The gastrocnemius and soleus join to form the Achilles tendon.

Gastrocnemius muscle

Soleus muscle

Achilles tendon

Calcaneus

Calf muscles

Muscles extending from the back of the knee to the heel. The gastrocnemius muscle starts behind the knee and forms the bulky part of the calf. Under it is the soleus muscle, which starts lower down from the back of the *tibia* (shin). These muscles join to form the *Achilles tendon*, which connects them to the heel.

Contraction of the calf muscles pulls the heel up to produce a springing movement through the toes. This movement is important in walking, running, jumping, and hopping.

Pain can occur because of *cramp*, *sciatica* (inflammation of one of the long nerves in the leg), or, more rarely, *claudication* (cramplike leg pain) or deep vein *thrombosis*.

Caliper splint

An orthopedic device used to exert control on a deformed leg or to support a leg weakened by a muscular disorder, making it possible for the person to stand and walk. A caliper splint consists of one or two vertical metal rods attached to leather or metal rings worn around the limb. A caliper splint extending only below the knee is sufficient to control the position of the ankle. Longer splints may be jointed to allow knee movement.

Callosity

See *Callus, skin*.

Callus, bony

A diffuse growth of new soft bone that forms around a *fracture* as it heals. The callus is eventually replaced by stronger bone with a more organized structure (see *Bone*).

A callus can be seen on an X ray and provides evidence that healing has started. A callus can sometimes be felt around a fracture site as a lumpy deformity. As healing continues, the original shape of the bone is restored.

Callus, skin

An area of thickened skin, caused by regular or prolonged pressure or friction. Manual laborers develop calluses on the palms of their hands, joggers on the soles of their feet, and guitarists on the tips of their fingers.

Calluses may also develop if body weight is borne unevenly—for example, if there is a *contracture* (persistent deformity) affecting one foot. A *corn* is a callus on a toe.

TREATMENT
If a callus on the foot becomes troublesome or painful, a podiatrist should be consulted. He or she can pare away the thickened skin in layers with a scalpel. Calluses caused by foot deformities almost always recur unless the underlying problem is corrected— either surgically or by using a molded insole in the shoe.

Caloric test

A method of discovering whether a person with *vertigo* (dizziness) and hearing loss has a diseased labyrinth (part of the inner ear). If so, *nystagmus* (reflex flickering of the eyes) stops sooner than normal or is absent.

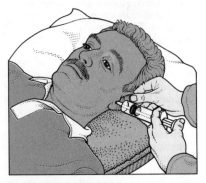

Checking for nystagmus
The outer-ear canal is flooded with water at varying temperatures, which induces convection currents within the lateral or horizontal semicircular canals. This stimulates them with resulting nystagmus, which is noted and its duration measured.

Calorie

A measure of energy. Strictly, it is the amount of energy needed to raise the temperature of 1 g of water by 1°C. In medicine and dietetics, the energy content of foods and the energy used to perform various activities is measured in units called kilocalories, which are equal to 1,000 calories. These two units are often confused because both are referred to as calories. However, the medical unit is abbreviated as Cal (with a capital "C") or kc, whereas the ordinary, "small" calorie is abbreviated as cal (with a small "c").

When the daily calorie intake is the same as the amount of energy expended, a person's weight remains constant. If intake exceeds expenditure, weight is gained; if expenditure exceeds intake, weight is lost. In general, fatty foods contain the most calories per unit weight while carbohydrate and protein have equal calories per unit weight, 56 percent less than fat. (See also *Calorimetry; Diet and disease*.)

Calorie requirements
See *Energy requirements*.

Calorimetry
A method of discovering the *calorie* (energy) value of foodstuffs by burning them in a container.

Direct calorimetry is the usual method of calculating the calorie value of small amounts of a particular foodstuff. This calorie value may then be converted to the number of calories in a typical serving. After being weighed and placed in a special sealed container, called a bomb calorimeter, the food is ignited; the calorimeter is then immersed in a known volume of water. The rise in the temperature of the water when the foodstuff is completely burned up gives the calorie value.

Cancer
Any of a group of diseases in which symptoms are due to the unrestrained growth of cells in one of the body organs or tissues. Most commonly, malignant tumors develop in major organs, such as the lungs, breasts, intestines, skin, stomach, or pancreas, but they may also develop in the nasal sinuses, the testes or ovaries, or the lips or tongue. Cancers may also develop in the blood cell-forming tissues of the bone marrow (the *leukemias*) and in the lymphatic system, muscles, or bones. Cancer is the second most common cause of death in the US, accounting for about one fifth of the total (the most common is heart disease).

Cancers are not the only type of abnormal growth, or *neoplasm*, that occur in the body. However, a cancer differs from a *benign* tumor, such as a *wart* or a *lipoma*, in two important ways. As it grows, it spreads and infiltrates the tissues around it and may block passageways, destroy nerves, and erode bone. Cells from the cancer may spread via the blood vessels and lymphatic channels to other parts of the body, where these *metastases* form new, satellite tumors that grow independently.

INCIDENCE
Cancer is a process that has affected humans since prehistoric times and is also common in domestic and farm animals, birds, and fish. Apart from childhood cancers, which may be associated with events during pregnancy, such as exposure to radiation, most cancers are a feature of aging.

CAUSES
The growth of a cancer begins when the *oncogenes* (genes controlling cell growth and multiplication) in a cell or cells are transformed by agents known as *carcinogens*.

Once a cell is transformed into a tumor-forming type (malignant transformation), the change in its oncogenes is passed on to all offspring cells. A small group of abnormal cells is thus established, and they divide more rapidly than the normal surrounding cells. Usually the abnormal cells show a lack of *differentiation*—that

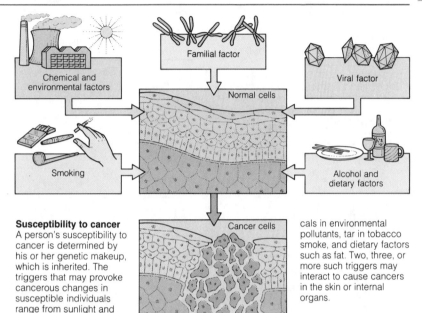

Susceptibility to cancer
A person's susceptibility to cancer is determined by his or her genetic makeup, which is inherited. The triggers that may provoke cancerous changes in susceptible individuals range from sunlight and viruses to alcohol, chemi-

cals in environmental pollutants, tar in tobacco smoke, and dietary factors such as fat. Two, three, or more such triggers may interact to cause cancers in the skin or internal organs.

is, they no longer perform the specialized task of the cells of their host tissue—and may escape the normal control of hormones and nerves. Thus, they are in effect parasites, contributing nothing to their host tissue but continuing to consume nutrients.

Years may pass before the growth of cells becomes large enough to cause symptoms, although the rate of growth varies according to the tissue of origin. Current estimates suggest that some cancers of the lung and breast have been present for more than five years before they cause symptoms. During this "occult" phase, metastases may be seeded in the liver, lungs, bones, or brain, and, in these circumstances, surgical cure is impossible because the cancer has already spread far beyond the primary site of origin.

CANCER-CAUSING AGENTS
The table gives a rough estimate of the contribution of various agents or behaviors to the causation of cancers. Smoking is particularly implicated in lung and bladder cancers, alcohol in cancers of the tongue, pharynx, and esophagus. Sexual and reproductive behavior affects the risk of cervical cancer (the more sexual partners a women has, the higher the risk) and of breast cancer (having children while relatively young protects against this cancer). Note the importance of dietary factors.

CANCER-CAUSING AGENTS

Agents	% of all cancers
Natural constituents of food (estimate)	35
Tobacco	30
Sexual and reproductive history	7
Occupational hazards	4
Alcohol	3
Food additives	1
Unknown	20

C

INCIDENCE OF CANCER
The likelihood of cancer developing varies with age. A 20 year old has a very low likelihood of it developing by the age of 30, but the risk roughly doubles between 30 and 40, and doubles again for each decade thereafter. Whatever the cause of death in someone aged 90, careful examination of the internal organs will often reveal a small cancer that may not have caused any symptoms. Localized cancer of the prostate is an almost universal finding in elderly men. Thus, while cancer seems to be much more common than in the past, this is mostly due to the increasing numbers of old people in the population.

CANCER WARNING SIGNS
Cancer may cause a variety of minor symptoms. Any that persist for several days should be checked by a physician. The earlier a cancer is diagnosed, the better the chance of there being a cure.

Rapid weight loss without apparent cause
A scab, sore, or ulcer that fails to heal within three weeks
A blemish or mole that enlarges, bleeds, or itches
Severe recurrent headaches
Difficulty swallowing
Persistent hoarseness
Coughing up bloody sputum (phlegm)

Persistent abdominal pain
Change in shape or size of testes
Blood in urine, with no pain on urination
Change in bowel habits
Lump or change in breast shape
Bleeding or discharge from nipple
Vaginal bleeding or spotting between periods or after menopause

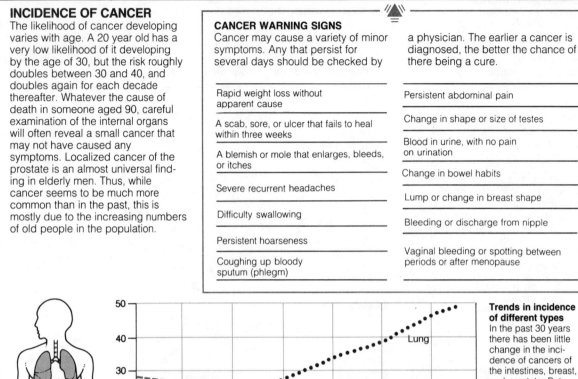

Trends in incidence of different types
In the past 30 years there has been little change in the incidence of cancers of the intestines, breast, and prostate. But stomach cancer has become less frequent because of improved diet, and lung cancer has become more common because of the dramatic increase in smoking.

WORLD INCIDENCE RATES FOR COMMON CANCERS

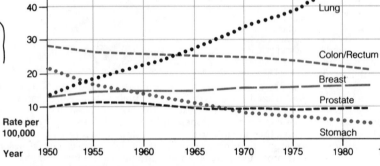

Site of origin of cancer	% affected in high-incidence area by age 75	Low incidence area
Skin	20 Queensland, Australia	Bombay, India
Esophagus	20 Northeast section of Iran	Nigeria
Lung and bronchus	11 England	Nigeria
Stomach	11 Japan	Uganda
Cervix	10 Colombia	Jewish Israel
Prostate	9 US (blacks only)	Japan
Liver	8 Mozambique	England
Breast	7 British Columbia, Canada	Non-Jewish Israel
Colon	3 Connecticut	Nigeria
Uterus	3 California	Japan
Mouth	2 Bombay, India	Denmark
Rectum	2 Denmark	Nigeria
Bladder	2 Connecticut	Japan
Ovary	2 Denmark	Japan
Nasopharynx	2 Chinese Singapore	England
Pancreas	2 Maori New Zealand	Bombay, India
Larynx	2 São Paulo, Brazil	Japan
Pharynx	2 Bombay, India	Denmark
Penis	1 Parts of Uganda	Jewish Israel

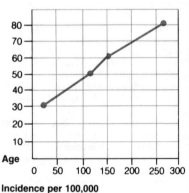

Incidence of breast cancer
Breast cancer most commonly affects women over the age of 30 and the incidence rises rapidly with age. At age 30, the rate is 20 per 100,000; at age 80, the rate is 260 per 100,000.

SYMPTOMS

The range of symptoms that may be produced by cancers is vast, depending on the site of the growth, the tissue of origin, and the extent of the growth. Symptoms may be a direct feature of the growth (e.g., lumps or skin changes) or derived from obstruction or bleeding into passageways, such as the lung airways, gastrointestinal tract, or urinary tract, or from disruption of the function of a vital organ. Tumors pressing on or disturbing nerve tracts can cause nervous system disorders and pain. Some tumors lead to the overproduction of hormones, with complications and effects far distant from the site of the growth. Unexplained weight loss is a feature of many types of cancer.

Some important warning signals that always warrant investigation by a physician are shown in the accompanying table.

DIAGNOSIS

Both the means of diagnosing cancer at an early stage (when the chances of cure are highest) and the range of treatments available have improved dramatically in the past decade.

Screening tests (for early breast cancer, cancer of the cervix, and intestinal cancer) have cut mortality from these tumors. For most tumors, however, diagnosis generally occurs after the appearance of symptoms, is based on the physician's examination of the patient, and is confirmed by microscopic examination of tissue cells obtained by *biopsy*; cancer cells look different from the normal cells of the host tissue. New scanning and imaging techniques give more information while causing less discomfort to the patient.

There are four main types of tests: cytology tests, imaging techniques, chemical tests, and direct inspection.

OUTLOOK

Almost half of all cancers are today cured completely, and cure and survival rates for various years after diagnosis continue to improve. For disease of certain organ systems, the diagnosis of a cancer may actually provide a better outlook than some of the alternative diagnoses. Cure and survival rates and the chances of recurrence do, however, vary markedly according to the organ or tissue affected.

For more information on cancers of individual organs—their incidence, causes, symptoms, treatment, and outlook—refer to the organ in question (e.g., *Breast cancer; Lung cancer; Stomach cancer*).

TREATMENT OF CANCER

The treatment of many cancers is still primarily surgical; excision of an early tumor will often give a complete cure. Because there may be small, undetectable metastases at the time of operation, surgery is commonly combined with *radiation therapy* and *anticancer drugs*. The aim of these treatments is to suppress, or arrest, the rate of cell division in any tumor cells left after surgery. Anticancer drugs often have unpleasant side effects because it is sometimes difficult to target specific drugs effectively, and normal cells and tissues may be disrupted along with the tumor cells.

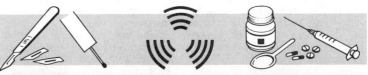

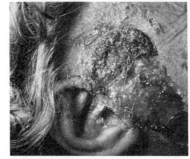

Before radiation therapy
The photograph shows a skin cancer in front of the ear before treatment.

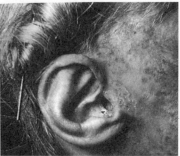

After radiation therapy
This was the appearance a few weeks later, after a course of radiation therapy.

TYPES OF CANCER TEST

Cytology tests	These tests reveal the shedding of abnormal cells. One example is the *cervical smear test* (Pap smear), an investigation in which cells are scraped from the cervix and examined microscopically to	detect potential or early cancer of the cervix. Another example is the urine cytology test, periodically carried out on those working in manufacturing industries where bladder cancer is a known risk.
Imaging techniques	These can sometimes reveal early cancerous changes in tissue. A notable example is the special low-dose X-ray technique used in *mammography* to detect early cancer of the breast. Research	with *ultrasound scanning*, which produces images of internal organs, suggests that it may provide a means of screening for cancer of the ovary.
Chemical tests	These tests can reveal the presence of substances indicative of cancer—for example, microscopic amounts of blood in	the feces and high levels of the enzyme acid phosphatase in the blood.
Direct inspection	Inspection of the interior of organs subject to cancer is usually carried out with an *endoscope* (a tube with a viewing lens), which is passed into the organ to be examined. Examples of this technique are	*colonoscopy, gastroscopy, cystoscopy,* and *laparoscopy*. These procedures are usually carried out only when clinical suspicion has been aroused.

Cancerphobia

An intense fear of developing cancer, out of proportion to the actual risk, so that the sufferer's behavior and lifestyle are significantly altered. Instead of paying sensible attention to diet and prevention (such as giving up smoking), the cancerphobe adopts extreme behavior (prolonged washing rituals, avoidance of social contact, bizarre eating habits) typical of *obsessive-compulsive behavior*. If the person experiences any symptoms (e.g., skin problems, constipation, or difficulty swallowing), he or she is convinced that they are signs of cancer. *Psychotherapy* may be of benefit. (See also *Phobia*.)

Cancer screening

Tests carried out on groups of people to detect cancer at an early stage. To warrant their use, screening tests must have a high rate of accuracy, must be safe, and must cause minimal discomfort. There must also be an effective treatment available. Screening tests are most effectively carried out among persons particularly susceptible to cancer.

In theory, regular annual checkups, including radiological and laboratory tests, might be expected to detect cancers at an early, treatable stage. In practice, several of the more common cancers—notably lung and stomach cancers—are rarely detected by screening tests before they cause symptoms. Nevertheless, in the past decade, screening tests have been developed for cancers of the cervix, breast, ovary, gastrointestinal tract, bladder, and prostate, and they are saving lives (see previous page).

Cancrum oris

A condition, also called *noma*, in which ulcers and tissue destruction occur within and around the mouth. It commonly affects malnourished children in poor tropical countries.

Candidiasis

Infection by the fungus CANDIDA ALBICANS, often within the vagina or, less commonly, on other areas of mucous membrane, such as inside the mouth or on moist skin. The infection is also known as thrush or moniliasis.

CAUSES AND INCIDENCE

The fungus that causes candidiasis grows in ecologic equilibrium in the vagina and mouth. Its growth is kept under control by the bacteria usually present in these organs. If a course of antibiotics destroys too many of the bacteria, or if the body's resistance to infection is lowered, as it is in *AIDS* and in patients being treated with *immunosuppressant drugs*, the fungus may multiply and overgrow. Certain disorders, notably *diabetes mellitus* and the hormonal changes that occur in pregnancy or when taking birth-control pills, may also encourage growth of the fungus.

Candidal infection of the penis is more common among uncircumcised than circumcised men, and may result from sexual intercourse with an infected partner. The condition can spread from the genitals or mouth to other moist areas of the body, such as the skin folds in the groin or under the breasts in women. In infants, candidiasis sometimes occurs in conjunction with *diaper rash*.

SYMPTOMS

Vaginal candidiasis may cause a thick, white, "cottage cheese" discharge from the vagina and/or itching and irritation in the area, which may cause discomfort when passing urine. Some women have no symptoms.

Infection of the penis usually results in *balanitis* (inflammation of the head of the penis). If the fungus spreads within the mouth, it produces sore, creamy-yellow, raised patches. Candidiasis in skin folds and as part of diaper rash takes the form of an itchy red rash with flaky white patches.

DIAGNOSIS AND TREATMENT

Candidiasis is diagnosed by examination of a sample of the white discharge or patches. If the cause proves to be CANDIDA ALBICANS, the physician will prescribe an *antifungal drug*, such as nystatin, clotrimazole, miconazole, or econazole nitrate. The drugs are usually prescribed in the form of a vaginal suppository or a cream for skin application.

OUTLOOK AND PREVENTION

Antifungal drugs usually clear up the trouble, but the infection may recur—sometimes as a result of reinfection by a sexual partner. Hence, treatment of both partners is preferable. People with a tendency to skin candidiasis should keep the skin as dry as possible, and women who take birth-control pills and suffer from candidiasis should consider changing to another method of birth control.

Canine tooth

See *Teeth*.

Canker sore

A small, painful ulcer that heals without help, occurring alone or in a group on the inside of the cheek or lip or underneath the tongue.

INCIDENCE

Minor canker sores affect about 20 percent of the population at any given time. They are most common between the ages of 10 and 40 and affect women more than men. The most severely affected people have continuously recurring ulcers; others have just one or two ulcers per year.

SYMPTOMS

Each ulcer is usually small and oval with a gray center and a surrounding red, inflamed halo. The ulcer usually lasts for one to two weeks.

CAUSES

The ulcer may be a hypersensitive reaction to hemolytic streptococcus bacteria. These organisms have been isolated repeatedly from canker sores. Other factors often associated with the occurrence of canker sores are trauma (such as an injection or a toothbrush abrasion), acute stress, and allergies (such as allergic *rhinitis*). In women, ulcers are most common during the premenstrual period. Ulcers may also be more likely to occur if other members of the family suffer from recurrent ulceration.

TREATMENT

The ulcers will heal by themselves if left alone. Topical painkillers may ease the pain and healing may be hastened by a corticosteroid ointment or a tetracycline mouthwash. The ulcer may also be covered with a waterproof ointment to protect it.

Cannabis

Any of the numerous psychoactive preparations derived from the hemp plant CANNABIS SATIVA (such as hashish and *marijuana*).

Cannula

A plastic or metal tube with a smooth, unsharpened tip for inserting into a blood vessel, lymphatic vessel, or body cavity to introduce or withdraw fluids. The physician first punctures the site with a long, thin needle, slides the cannula over it, and then withdraws the needle. Alternatively, he or she may insert a trocar (sharp-pointed rod) inside the cannula and remove it once the vessel has been entered. Cannulas are frequently used for *blood transfusions* and *intravenous infusions* and for draining *pleural effusions*. In certain circumstances, such as when blood is required for testing over a period of time, the cannula may be left in place for several days.

Cap, contraceptive

A barrier method of contraception in the form of a latex rubber device placed directly over the cervix to prevent sperm from entering. (See *Contraception, barrier methods*.)

Capgras' syndrome

The *delusion* (false belief) that a relative or close friend has been replaced by an impostor. Also known as the "illusion of doubles," Capgras' syndrome is seen most frequently in paranoid *schizophrenia*, but also occurs in organic disorders (see *Brain syndrome, organic*) and *affective disorders*.

Capillary

Any of the vessels that carry blood between the smallest arteries, or arterioles, and the smallest veins, or venules (see *Circulatory system*). Capillaries form a fine network throughout the body's organs and tissues. It is through the thin capillary walls that blood and cells exchange their constituents (see *Respiration*).

Capillaries have a diameter of approximately ten thousandths of a millimeter—not much wider than the red blood cells that flow through them. Their walls are permeable to substances such as oxygen, glucose, and water, which can thus move freely between the blood and the tissue fluid that surrounds all cells.

STRUCTURE OF CAPILLARIES
These minute blood vessels have permeable walls to allow transfer of oxygen, glucose, and water from blood to tissues.

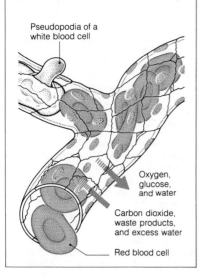

Pseudopodia of a white blood cell

Oxygen, glucose, and water

Carbon dioxide, waste products, and excess water

Red blood cell

The capillaries are not open to blood flow all the time; they open and close according to different organs' requirements for oxygen and nutrients. Thus, when running, most of the capillaries in the leg muscles are open, but at rest many are closed. The opening and closing of skin capillaries plays an important role in *temperature* regulation. Blood flow through each capillary is controlled by a tiny circle of muscle at its entrance.

DISORDERS
Because of their thin walls, capillaries are fragile. A direct blow to an area of the body can often rupture capillaries under the surface of the skin. Bleeding from them will cause swelling and bruising (around the eye this can cause a black eye).

Capillaries become more fragile in the elderly, in people taking high doses of steroids, and in victims of *scurvy* (vitamin C deficiency). These groups all have a tendency to *purpura* (small black and blue-purple areas of bleeding under the skin).

Capillary angiomas are benign tumors of the capillary wall that may be present at birth or may develop later in life. They may cause a red patch of variable size and shape on the skin and mucous membranes.

Capitation

A method of reimbursement based on constant dollar amounts per person rather than on variable fees reflecting services performed. For example, a group of physicians, contracting to provide medical services for the employees of a company, may charge the company so much per month per employee, collecting a capitation fee (so much "per head") rather than fees for the actual services rendered.

Capping, dental

See *Crown, dental*.

Capsule

A hard or soft shell, usually made of gelatin, that contains a dose of medication. Capsules are taken by mouth and have two main advantages over solid tablets. First, their elongated shape makes them easy to swallow. Second, they make it easier for patients to take solid or liquid medications that would have an unpleasant taste or smell if not administered in capsule form.

Some capsules have a special coating to prevent the release into the stomach of drugs that may have an irritant effect. Others are designed to release their contents into the small intestine at a slow steady rate so that a drug need be taken only once or twice a day.

Capsulitis

See *Bursitis*.

Captopril

The first member of a new class of drugs, the *ACE inhibitors*, used in the treatment of *hypertension* (high blood pressure) and *heart failure*.

Caput

Latin for head. The word caput is also used to refer to the face, skull, and all associated organs, to the origin of a muscle, or to any enlarged extremity, such as the caput femoris, the head of the femur (thighbone). However, the term most commonly refers to the caput succedaneum, a soft swelling in the scalp of newborn babies. It occurs as a result of pressure on the baby's head during labor and usually disappears after a few days.

Carbachol

A drug that mimics some of the actions of the *neurotransmitter* (chemical released from nerve endings) *acetylcholine*. It is used mainly as eye drops to treat *glaucoma* (raised pressure within the eyeball).

Carbamazepine

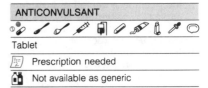

ANTICONVULSANT
Tablet
Prescription needed
Not available as generic

An *anticonvulsant drug*, introduced in 1960, chemically related to tricyclic *antidepressant drugs*.

WHY IT IS USED
Carbamazepine reduces the likelihood of seizures caused by abnormal nerve signals in the brain and is mainly used in the long-term treatment of *epilepsy*. It has less sedative effect than other anticonvulsants.

Carbamazepine is also prescribed to relieve *neuralgia* (the intermittent severe pain caused by damage to or irritation of a nerve). Carbamazepine is also occasionally prescribed to treat certain psychological or behavioral disorders, such as *mania*.

POSSIBLE ADVERSE EFFECTS
There may be some sedative effect, especially if alcohol is drunk while taking carbamazepine.

Carbohydrates

A group of substances that provides the body with one of its two main sources of energy (the other is *fat*) and is an essential ingredient of a healthy diet. Sugar and starch are probably the most familiar carbohydrates.

TYPES AND SOURCES

There are three main types of carbohydrate, differentiated by their chemical structure.

Monosaccharides	glucose, galactose, fructose
Disaccharides	sucrose, lactose, maltose
Polysaccharides	starch cellulose

Types of carbohydrates
Monosaccharides are the simplest, consisting of a single saccharide molecule. Disaccharides consist of two saccharide molecules linked together. Polysaccharides consist of a long chain of many saccharide molecules. The most important carbohydrate is starch.

Cereals and vegetables contain sugars, starch, and cellulose and are known as unrefined (complex) carbohydrate foods; they usually also contain vitamins and a little protein. Refined carbohydrate foods, such as white table sugar, are virtually pure energy sources; they usually contain neither cellulose nor other nutrients. Complex carbohydrates should constitute 50 to 60 percent of the diet.

CARBOHYDRATE METABOLISM

Before they can be used by the body, complex carbohydrates must be broken down to simple monosaccharide sugars—glucose, galactose, and fructose. This is accomplished by *enzymes* in saliva and other digestive juices. The enzymes break down polysaccharides into the monosaccharides glucose, galactose, and fructose. Cellulose is unaffected by digestive enzymes and passes out of the body largely unchanged.

The monosaccharides are then absorbed through the intestinal wall and into the bloodstream for distribution throughout the body. Certain cells, such as brain cells and red blood cells, must have glucose to survive. Some of the glucose is used immediately by these cells, which "burn" it in a series of biochemical reactions to generate energy and heat (see *Metabolism*). The rest of the glucose is conveyed to the liver, muscles, and fat cells where it is converted into *glycogen* (animal starch) and fat for storage. When more energy is needed, this glycogen is converted back to glucose, which reenters the bloodstream for distribution around the body. Fat cannot be converted to glucose but can be burned as fuel to save glucose. Unlike glucose, galactose and fructose cannot be used directly by cells and so must first be converted by the liver to glucose; thereafter, the fate of this glucose is the same as that of glucose absorbed directly into the bloodstream from the intestine.

When the blood sugar level is high, such as after a meal, carbohydrate metabolism is primarily controlled by *insulin* secreted by the *pancreas*. Insulin restores the glucose level to normal by stimulating the uptake of unneeded carbohydrate calories by the liver, muscles, and fat for storage as glycogen and fat. In the disorder *diabetes mellitus*, carbohydrate metabolism is disturbed by a deficiency of insulin, and carbohydrates cannot enter most cells for storage.

The action of insulin is balanced by that of glucagon, another pancreatic hormone. When the blood sugar level is low—after fasting overnight or after exercise—insulin secretion slows down and glucagon stimulates the conversion of glycogen to glucose for release into the bloodstream. Epinephrine and corticosteroids, adrenal hormones secreted at times of stress, have the same basic effect as glucagon (i.e., to increase the blood sugar level).

CARBOHYDRATE METABOLISM

Digestive enzymes act on carbohydrates

Carbohydrates
Starches, sugars, and cellulose

Carbohydrates are broken down into monosaccharides

Cellulose passes almost unaltered through the system

Glucose   **Galactose**   **Fructose**

Liver converts them to

Liver, muscle, and fat cells convert glucose to

Glucose, which is converted to

Glycogen, which is converted to

Fat, which may be burned as fuel

Glucose is absorbed into the bloodstream for distribution throughout the body or is used directly by body cells

Carbon

A nonmetallic element that is present in all organic molecules, the fundamental molecules of all living organisms. Pure carbon exists in nature as the major constituent of diamonds, coal, and graphite (pencil lead).

Carbon dioxide

A colorless, odorless gas (at normal temperatures) that is present in small amounts in the air and is also important as a by-product of normal metabolism in the body. Cooled and compressed carbon dioxide forms a white solid, *dry ice*, which is used in *cryosurgery*. Carbon dioxide consists of one carbon atom (symbol C) linked to two oxygen atoms (symbol O) and has the chemical formula CO_2.

Carbon dioxide is a waste product of the metabolic reactions that break down various substances, especially carbohydrates and fats, to generate energy. The carbon dioxide is carried by the blood to the lungs, where it is released and breathed out. One of the factors that controls the rate of breathing is the level of carbon dioxide in the bloodstream. When a person exercises strenuously, the amount of carbon dioxide produced increases rapidly, and the resultant high level in the bloodstream causes the person to breathe more rapidly to eliminate the carbon dioxide and take more oxygen into the body.

Carbon monoxide

A colorless, odorless, poisonous gas that is present in the exhaust fumes of oil- or gasoline-powered engines and is also produced by inefficient burning of coal, gas, oil, or propane in domestic heating appliances. It consists of one carbon atom (chemical symbol C) linked to one oxygen atom (symbol O) and has the chemical formula CO.

POISONING

Carbon monoxide is poisonous because it binds with *hemoglobin* (the oxygen-carrying molecule in red blood cells) and prevents it from carrying oxygen. As a result, the tissues are deprived of oxygen and asphyxiation occurs. If inhalation of the gas continues, it may lead to permanent brain damage or even death.

The initial symptoms of carbon monoxide poisoning—which may sometimes be mistaken for those of food poisoning—are dizziness, headache, nausea, and faintness. The most important step in first-aid treatment is to take the victim out into fresh air; continued exposure to the gas will lead to unconsciousness. If the victim has stopped breathing, get emergency medical aid, and give *artificial respiration*. Even if the victim seems to recover completely when taken into fresh air, it is advisable for him or her to consult a physician to make certain that there are no long-term effects.

Carbon tetrachloride

A colorless, poisonous, volatile liquid with a characteristic odor present in some home dry-cleaning fluids and also used as an industrial solvent. It consists of one carbon atom (symbol C) linked to four chlorine atoms (symbol Cl). Carbon tetrachloride has the chemical formula CCl_4.

Carbon tetrachloride is a dangerous chemical; it can cause liver and kidney damage if it is inhaled or drunk. Symptoms of poisoning include headache, nausea, pain in the abdomen, and convulsions.

Carbuncle

A cluster of interconnected *boils* (painful, pus-filled, inflamed hair roots). Carbuncles are usually caused by the bacterium *STAPHYLOCOCCUS AUREUS*; they generally begin as single boils, then spread. Common sites are the back of the neck and the buttocks.

Carbuncles are less common than single boils. They mainly affect people who have a lowered resistance to infection, in particular, diabetics.

TREATMENT

Anyone with a carbuncle should see a physician, who will usually prescribe an antibiotic and recommend the application of hot compresses (cotton soaked in hot salty water) or plasters. These may cause the pus-filled heads to burst, relieving pain. Subsequently, the carbuncle should be covered with a dressing until it has healed completely. Occasionally, incision and drainage (with removal of the core of the carbuncle) are necessary if drainage and healing do not occur on their own.

Carcinogen

Any agent capable of causing *cancer*, such as tobacco smoke, high-energy radiation, or asbestos fibers.

CHEMICAL CARCINOGENS

These form the largest group of carcinogens. Chief among them are the chemicals known as PAH (polycyclic aromatic hydrocarbons). They are found in, among other things, tobacco smoke, pitch, and tar fumes, all of which may cause lung cancer if inhaled over a long period; in solid pitch and tar, which may cause skin cancer in workers who handle them; and in soot, which was responsible for cancer of the scrotum among chimney sweeps in the eighteenth century.

Aromatic amines, which are used in the chemical and rubber industries, are other major chemical carcinogens, and prolonged exposure to them may cause urinary bladder cancer.

PHYSICAL CARCINOGENS

The best known physical carcinogen is high-energy radiation, such as nuclear radiation or X rays. In high doses, radiation usually first causes malignant change in cells, which divide quickly—for example, in the precursors of white blood cells in the bone marrow, causing leukemia. Everyone is exposed to some high-energy radiation from cosmic rays, radioactivity in rocks, and the like, but for many people the main source is X rays used in medical diagnosis.

Exposure over many years to ultraviolet radiation from sunlight can cause skin cancer, particularly in fair-skinned people.

Asbestos fibers are another known physical cause of cancer. White asbestos may cause lung cancer, particularly in workers who experience prolonged exposure to the fibers, who

already have the lung disease *asbestosis*, and who smoke. Blue asbestos and, to a lesser extent, brown asbestos can cause a tumor (mesothelioma) of the cells constituting the membranes that surround certain body cavities and organs. In the case of blue asbestos, this cancer can develop after very little exposure.

BIOLOGICAL CARCINOGENS

Very few biological agents cause cancer in humans. *SCHISTOSOMA HAEMATOBIUM*, one of the blood flukes that causes the tropical disease schistosomiasis, can cause cancer of the bladder, where it lays its eggs. *ASPERGILLUS FLAVUS*, a fungus that contaminates stored grain and peanuts, produces the poison aflatoxin, which is believed to cause liver cancer.

Certain viruses have been associated with cancer. The papilloma virus is believed to be responsible for cancer of the cervix, the hepatitis B virus has been implicated in liver cancer, and the Epstein-Barr virus is considered to be the cause of *Burkitt's lymphoma*, a malignant tumor of the jaw and abdomen that occurs mainly among children in Africa. *Kaposi's sarcoma* is probably caused by *HIV* (human immunodeficiency virus) or by one of the viruses associated with it.

SCREENING

Any substance that could possibly be carcinogenic, such as a food additive, cosmetic, or chemical for use in drugs, must be screened before it is allowed to be manufactured. One major preliminary test is to expose a certain strain of bacteria to the substance, and, if mutation (genetic change) occurs in the bacteria, the substance is regarded as a suspect carcinogen. It is then tested on laboratory animals, such as rats. If an increased incidence of tumors occurs, no license is usually granted to manufacture the substance for public sale.

AVOIDING CARCINOGENS

In industry, known carcinogens are either banned or allowed only if their use is considered essential, if exposure to them is strictly limited, and if regular medical screening is provided for workers using them, as, for example, in the nuclear fuel industry.

Outside of industry, the individual is exposed to very few known, unavoidable, high-risk carcinogens.

Carcinogenesis

The development of a *cancer* (a malignant tumor or blood disease) caused by the action of certain chemicals, viruses, constituents of the diet, radiation, and unknown factors on primarily normal cells.

Cancer-causing factors are called carcinogens. Carcinogens are believed to alter the *DNA* (genetic material) within cells, particularly the structure of certain genes called *oncogenes* that normally control the growth and division of cells. An altered cell divides abnormally rapidly and passes on the changes in its genetic material to all its offspring cells. Thus, a group of cells becomes established that is not affected by the body's normal restraints on growth.

Carcinoid syndrome

A rare condition characterized by bouts of facial flushing, diarrhea, and wheezing. It is caused by an intestinal or lung tumor, called a carcinoid, that secretes excess quantities of the hormone serotonin. Symptoms (profuse diarrhea and intermittent flushing of the skin) usually occur only if the tumor has spread to the liver or affects the lung.

DIAGNOSIS AND TREATMENT

Carcinoid syndrome is diagnosed by measuring the level of a breakdown product of serotonin in the urine. The condition is sometimes treated by removal of the tumor from the lung, intestine, and from the liver as well, if possible. In most cases, surgical treatment is thought unlikely to be helpful, and in these circumstances treatment with drugs that block the action of serotonin may be successful in relieving the symptoms.

Carcinoma

Any malignant tumor (*cancer*) arising from cells in the covering surface layer or lining membrane of a body organ. A carcinoma is thus distinguished from a *sarcoma*, which is a cancer arising in connective tissue, bone, or muscle. Carcinomas include all the most common cancers of the lungs, breast, stomach, skin, cervix, and the like. The terms cancer and carcinoma tend to be used interchangeably but are not strictly synonymous.

Carcinomatosis

The presence of one or more enlarging carcinomas in different sites of the body due to metastasis (spread of malignant cells) from an original malignant tumor. The sufferer experiences weight loss, lack of energy, and other symptoms depending on the site of the metastases (secondary or offspring tumors).

Metastases in the lungs may cause coughing or breathlessness; in the liver they may cause jaundice.

The clinical diagnosis of carcinomatosis may be confirmed by X rays or *radioisotope scanning* of the bones and lungs, by *liver function tests*, or during an operation or autopsy. An operation to remove the primary (original) tumor will not help someone with carcinomatosis unless the primary tumor is producing a hormone that is directly stimulating growth of the metastases. *Chemotherapy* or *radiation therapy* may be given to deal with the metastases, sometimes following removal of a primary carcinoma.

Metastases associated with some cancers (of the testis, prostate, and thyroid glands) may be treated with drugs or hormones, and a prolonged abatement of symptoms is now common. Metastases from lung and intestinal cancers are less amenable to treatment and, in such cases, the outlook is not good.

Cardiac arrest

A halt in the pumping action of the heart due to cessation of its rhythmic, muscular activity.

CAUSES

The most common cause is a *myocardial infarction* (heart attack), but other causes include *respiratory arrest*, *electrical injury*, *hypothermia*, loss of blood, drug overdose, and *anaphylactic shock*.

DIAGNOSIS AND TREATMENT

A person with cardiac arrest collapses suddenly, with loss of consciousness, absence of pulse, and no respiratory movements. A person who is breathing cannot have suffered a cardiac arrest. An absolutely certain diagnosis can be made only by measuring the electrical activity of the heart with an *ECG* machine, but emergency *cardiopulmonary resuscitation* should be started immediately to minimize the risk of irreversible brain damage.

As soon as adequate help arrives—in most hospitals there is a cardiac arrest team on standby to manage such emergencies—the diagnosis can be confirmed by ECG. This test distinguishes between two types of disturbance that can occur in the heart muscle. *Ventricular fibrillation* is the random contraction of individual heart muscle fibers. This abnormal activity may be corrected by *defibrillation* (application of electric shock to the heart).

Asystole is the complete absence of heart muscle activity and is more difficult to reverse. It may respond to

intravenous infusion of *epinephrine* and calcium or in extreme cases to direct injection of epinephrine into the heart. An electrical *pacemaker* may also stimulate the heart in asystole.

In all cases of cardiac arrest the balance of the chemical constituents of the blood is disturbed, making the blood more acidic; an intravenous infusion of sodium bicarbonate is usually given to correct it. Other drugs, such as lidocaine, also can be administered intravenously to stabilize the heart muscle.

OUTLOOK

Between one fifth and one third of patients whose heart beat is restored after cardiac arrest recover sufficiently to leave the hospital (however, a substantial number of these die within the following year). In the remainder, the damage to the heart or brain is too extensive for recovery to be possible.

Cardiac neurosis

Excessive anxiety or fear about the condition of the heart. Cardiac neurosis usually occurs after a *myocardial infarction* (heart attack) or heart surgery. However, it may occur in people who have had no previous heart trouble.

The sufferer experiences symptoms that mimic those typical of heart disease—chest pain, tightness in the chest, lethargy, palpitations, and breathlessness—and may be reluctant to exercise or return to work for fear of bringing on these symptoms. Examination and investigation of the heart by a physician will reveal no physical cause for the symptoms.

Psychotherapy may help the patient overcome fears and anxieties. If it does not, the patient may not be able to return to a normal, active life.

Cardiac output

The volume of blood pumped by the heart in a given time (usually per minute). It can be used as a measure of how efficiently the heart is working. At rest, a healthy adult heart pumps between 2.5 and 5 quarts (2.35 and 4.7 liters) of blood per minute; during exercise this figure may rise to 32 quarts (30 liters) per minute. A low figure during exercise is a sign that the heart muscle is damaged or that major blood loss has occurred.

Cardiac stress test

A type of *fitness* test carried out in people who have chest pain, breathlessness, or palpitations during exercise. The test is used to determine

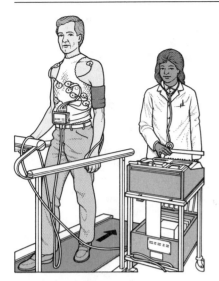

How the test is done
The patient is attached to an ECG machine, which records the pattern of the heart's electrical activity. He or she then performs an exercise, such as walking on a treadmill. A diagnosis of coronary artery disease is confirmed if there are specific changes in the wave pattern shown on the ECG recording as the intensity of the exercise is increased.

whether the cause of these symptoms is *angina pectoris* or another form of *coronary heart disease*.

The test is performed under close medical supervision, with resuscitation facilities immediately available. If at any time the patient has chest pains, becomes breathless, or feels sick, the test is stopped immediately. A cardiac stress test may also be performed with injection of a radioactive isotope, which outlines any damaged area of the heart.

Cardiologist
A specialist in diagnosing and treating problems related to the heart. Guided by symptoms such as shortness of breath, chest pain, or irregular heart rhythm, a cardiologist examines X rays, echocardiograms (see *Echocardiography*), and electrocardiograms (*ECGs*), or runs *cardiac stress tests* to determine the specific cause of a problem. Depending on the results of the tests, the cardiologist may recommend changes in diet or physical activity, prescribe medication, or refer the patient to a *cardiovascular surgeon*.

Cardiology
The study of the function of the *heart*; the investigation, diagnosis, and medical treatment of disorders of the heart and blood vessels, especially *atherosclerosis* and *hypertension*.

Anatomically and physiologically, the heart occupies a central position in the body. It has a single function—to pump blood first to the lungs and then to the rest of the body—but the sequence of events in each heart contraction is complex. Similarly, many heart disorders are variations of a single disorder. Reduced pumping efficiency can have various underlying causes, including *arrhythmias*, *coronary heart disease* (in which the blood supply to the heart muscle is impaired), *cardiomyopathy* (in which the muscle itself is abnormal), and *heart valve* disorders. Disease of the lungs and blood vessels can also have adverse effects on heart function. In addition, some babies are born with structural defects of the heart and/or major blood vessels that emerge from it (see *Heart disease, congenital*).

Heart disorders are now the leading cause of death in the US. The study of the heart in health and disease is thus a large part of the training of every physician; family physicians are familiar with the treatment of patients with common disorders, such as coronary heart disease and hypertension. For more expert investigation and treatment, a person with a heart problem may be referred to a cardiologist.

The past 10 years have seen rapid advances in the understanding of heart disease, its investigation, and its treatment.

Cardiomegaly
Enlargement of the heart. In some cases, it takes the form of hypertrophy (thickening) of the heart muscle; in others, one or more of the heart chambers increases in volume (dilatation).

CAUSES
Hypertrophy of the heart muscle occurs in any condition where the heart has to work harder than normal to pump blood around the body. Such conditions include *hypertension* (increased blood pressure associated with increased resistance against which the heart must pump), which causes the wall of the left ventricle to thicken; *pulmonary hypertension* (increased blood pressure in the lungs), in which the wall of the right ventricle thickens; and one type of *cardiomyopathy* (disease of the heart muscle), in which either or both ventricles may thicken.

Dilatation of a heart chamber may be due to heart valve incompetence (failure of a valve to close properly after a contraction). For example, in *aortic insufficiency*, failure of the aortic valve to close completely allows blood to flood back from the aorta into the left ventricle, eventually enlarging the chamber. Certain types of cardiomyopathy can also lead to swelling of a chamber.

SYMPTOMS
There are no symptoms of the enlargement until a critical point is reached in which added stress (e.g., hypertension, exercise, or infection) may reduce the efficiency of the heart as a pump. *Heart failure* will result, causing breathlessness and swelling of the legs and hands.

DIAGNOSIS AND TREATMENT
Cardiomegaly is diagnosed by a physician from a physical examination, chest X ray, and *ECG* (measurement of electrical impulses in the heart). Treatment is directed at the underlying disorder.

Cardiomyopathy
Any disease of the heart muscle that causes a reduction in the force of heart contractions and a resultant decrease in the efficiency of circulation of blood through the lungs and to the rest of the body. The disease may be infectious (viral), metabolic or nutritional, toxic, *autoimmune*, degenerative, or of unknown cause.

TYPES
Cardiomyopathies fall into the following three main groups: hypertrophic, dilated, and restrictive.

The hypertrophic type is usually a familial (inherited) disorder of unknown cause that leads to an abnormality of heart muscle fibers.

In dilated cardiomyopathy, muscle cell metabolism (chemical activity) is abnormal, and the walls of the heart tend to dilate (balloon out) under pressure. The cause of the abnormal cell metabolism is unknown.

Restrictive cardiomyopathy is caused by scarring of the endocardium (the inner lining of the heart) or by *amyloidosis* (infiltration of the muscle with a starchlike substance).

Heart muscle disorders may also be due to poisoning (e.g., by excessive consumption of alcohol) or to a vitamin or mineral deficiency (for example, lack of vitamin B_1).

INCIDENCE
Cardiomyopathies are less common than other types of heart disease. The specific incidence of the different types is unknown because in many cases there are few or no symptoms. Sometimes the damage to the heart

C

muscle is discovered only at an autopsy following death from an unrelated cause.

SYMPTOMS AND SIGNS

Symptoms usually include fatigue, chest pain, and palpitations due to an increased awareness of heart beat or to an abnormal heart rhythm such as *atrial fibrillation* (fast, irregular contractions of the upper heart chambers).

Heart failure (reduced efficiency of the heart's pumping action) can cause breathing difficulty and edema (swelling of the legs and hands).

DIAGNOSIS

A chest X ray usually shows enlargement of the heart outline. An *ECG* (measurement of electrical activity in the heart) often shows enlarged electrical impulses on the tracing due to heart muscle hypertrophy.

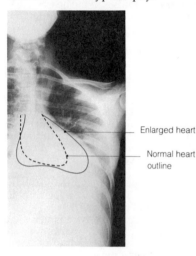

— Enlarged heart

— Normal heart outline

Chest X ray showing cardiomyopathy
The heart has become much enlarged, due to the heart muscle abnormality.

The diagnosis can be confirmed by examining a *biopsy* sample of heart muscle under the microscope to show muscle cell abnormalities.

TREATMENT

Since the causes remain unknown, there is no specific treatment. Treatment of symptoms may include the use of *diuretic drugs* to control heart failure and *antiarrhythmic drugs* to correct abnormal heart rhythm. For those with alcoholic cardiomyopathy, stopping all intake of alcohol is essential. Immunosuppresive drugs are occasionally helpful.

In many cases, heart muscle function steadily deteriorates, and the only option left, if available, is a *heart transplant*, which has successfully extended life in some individuals.

Cardiopulmonary resuscitation

The administration of the lifesaving measures of external cardiac compression massage and *mouth-to-mouth resuscitation* to someone collapsing with a *cardiac arrest* (cessation of effective heart beat).

It is vital to restore the circulation of oxygen-carrying blood to the brain as quickly as possible because permanent brain damage is likely if the brain is starved of oxygen for more than three to four minutes.

WHEN TO GIVE CARDIOPULMONARY RESUSCITATION

Before starting cardiopulmonary resuscitation it is important to establish that the victim has indeed suffered a cardiac arrest and has not simply fainted. The person will be unresponsive and have little or no breathing motion. Skin color will be pale, or blue-gray, especially around the lips. The person's heart will not seem to be beating. No pulse will be felt in the wrist or neck, and no heart beat will be heard when the chest is listened to. (If the person is breathing, no matter how slowly, then the heart will probably still be beating, even if no pulse can be felt.)

Cardiovascular

Of the heart and blood vessels.

Cardiovascular disorders

Disorders of the heart, blood vessels, and blood circulation. (See *Heart* disorders box; *Arteries, disorders of; Veins, disorders of.*)

Cardiovascular surgeon

A surgeon specializing in operations on the heart and the blood vessels to prevent or repair damage caused by, for example, birth defects, clogged arteries, or heart attacks. Procedures performed include *heart valve surgery, coronary artery bypass,* and *heart transplant.* Cardiovascular surgeons are generally seen by patients only on referral from other physicians.

Cardioversion

Another name for *defibrillation.*

Carditis

A general term for inflammation of any part of the heart or its linings. Carditis may be a *myocarditis,* inflammation of the heart muscle, usually caused by a viral infection; an *endocarditis,* inflammation of the internal lining of the heart chambers and heart valves, usually due to a bacterial infection; or a *pericarditis* (inflammation of the outer lining of the heart), possibly with *effusion.* The latter is usually due to a viral or bacterial infection, but may be associated with a *myocardial infarction* (heart attack) or occasionally may be caused by an *autoimmune disorder,* such as systemic *lupus erythematosus* (SLE).

Caries, dental

Tooth decay. The gradual erosion of enamel (the protective covering of the tooth) and dentin (the substance beneath the enamel).

CAUSES

Plaque is the main cause of tooth decay (see illustrated box).

The most common sites of initial decay are the grinding surfaces of the back teeth (which have minute grooves in them), the lateral surfaces of adjacent teeth, and near the gum line. Plaque easily becomes trapped in all these areas.

INCIDENCE

An encouraging sign in industrialized countries over the past 10 to 15 years has been the significant decline (of 35 to 50 percent) in dental caries among children. The evidence suggests that, of the various factors probably responsible, the most important is water fluoridation, which strengthens enamel. The addition of fluoride to toothpaste has also played a part in the reduction of dental caries.

SYMPTOMS AND TREATMENT

Early decay, the most easily treated, usually does not cause any symptoms. The chief symptom of advanced decay is toothache (brought on by eating sweet, hot, or cold food) that increases in severity as the decay progresses. Decay may also cause bad breath.

Treatment consists of drilling away the area of decay and filling the cavity with a dental restoration, usually made of amalgam (a metal alloy) or a cement (composite resin) that matches the color of the tooth (see *Filling, dental*). In cases of advanced decay it may be necessary to remove the infected pulp and replace it with a filling (see *Root canal treatment*) or to extract the tooth (see *Extraction, dental*).

PREVENTION

Our modern diet makes it unlikely that, even by taking the most scrupulous preventive measures at all times, we could avoid dental caries altogether. However, it is possible to reduce the risk of caries considerably by cutting down on the amount (and frequency) of sugar and other refined carbohydrates that is eaten and by practicing good *oral hygiene.*

FIRST AID: CARDIOPULMONARY RESUSCITATION

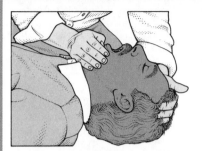

1 First make sure the airway is clear. Then look and listen for signs of breathing. Listen for air escaping and feel for air flow. Feel for the pulse.

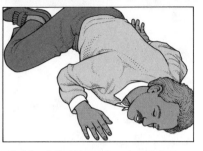

2 If the victim is breathing, place in the *recovery position*. If the victim is not breathing, place on a hard surface and start mouth-to-mouth resuscitation.

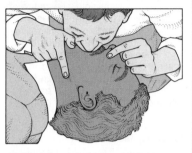

3 Pinch the victim's nose shut, take a breath, seal your lips around the mouth, and blow. Your breath contains enough oxygen for the victim's needs.

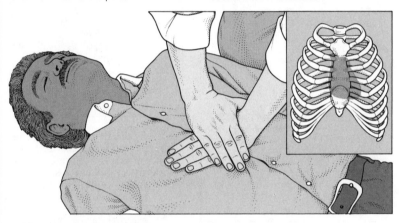

4 If breathing does not restart and you cannot detect a pulse or heart beat, start cardiac compression. Press with the heel of one hand placed on top of the other.

5 It is vital to apply pressure at the correct point—the lower part of the breastbone. Keep the pressure well clear of the victim's ribs.

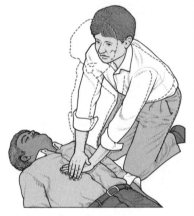

6 If you are on your own, the rate of compression should be 80 per minute, with two breaths given after every 15 compressions.

WARNING

Cardiopulmonary resuscitation is a life-support technique that is used in a medical emergency when the victim is not breathing and when it is possible that his or her heart has stopped beating.

Although opening the victim's airway and restoring breathing can be performed effectively at the time of the crisis by following the instructions here, restoring the victim's circulation if the heart has stopped beating (cardiac compression) cannot be learned effectively in a crisis situation.

Cardiac compression, and all phases of cardiopulmonary resuscitation, should be learned through formal instruction. Practicing the technique regularly and taking refresher courses are also recommended.

WITH TWO RESCUERS

If two rescuers are available, one should give mouth-to-mouth resuscitation (one breath every five compressions).

Sixty compressions should be given per minute, with a pause of 1 to 1.5 seconds allowed after every five compressions.

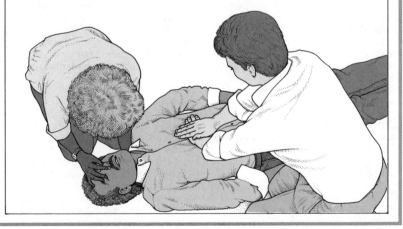

C

CAUSES OF TOOTH DECAY

The primary cause of tooth decay is dental *plaque*, a sticky substance that forms on the teeth. Plaque consists of food remains, mucus-saliva by-products, and the bacteria that live in the mouth. The bacteria feed mainly on the fermentable carbohydrates (simple sugars and starches) in food, and, in breaking them down, create an acid that gradually destroys enamel, forming a cavity. If the process is not checked, the dentin is eroded next, enlarging the cavity and enabling the bacteria to invade the exposed pulp at the center of the tooth.

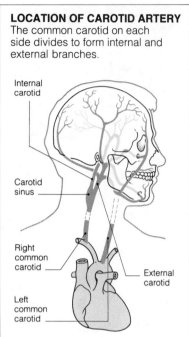

Severe dental caries
Example of caries affecting the necks of several upper and lower teeth.

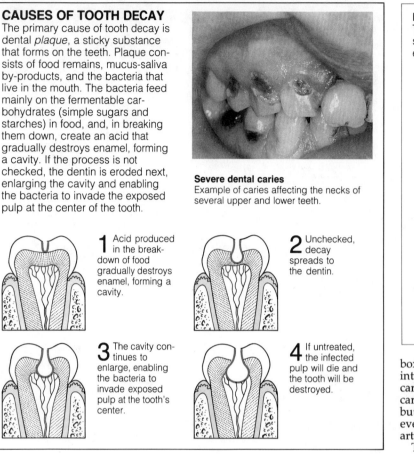

1 Acid produced in the breakdown of food gradually destroys enamel, forming a cavity.

2 Unchecked, decay spreads to the dentin.

3 The cavity continues to enlarge, enabling the bacteria to invade exposed pulp at the tooth's center.

4 If untreated, the infected pulp will die and the tooth will be destroyed.

LOCATION OF CAROTID ARTERY

The common carotid on each side divides to form internal and external branches.

Internal carotid

Carotid sinus

Right common carotid

Left common carotid

External carotid

Sweet food should be eaten only at mealtimes; snacks between meals should be limited. The harmful effects of simple carbohydrates (especially sugars) should be monitored from the beginning of a child's life. Babies should not be given a bottle of milk, fruit juice, or other sugar-containing liquid to comfort them or get them to sleep; this habit can cause extensive early tooth decay.

Teeth need brushing thoroughly each day with fluoride toothpaste. Dental floss should be used to clean between them. A dentist should be visited regularly for checkups. (See also *Oral hygiene*.)

Carisoprodol

A *muscle-relaxant drug* used mainly to treat muscle spasm caused by injury.

Carotene

An orange pigment found in carrots, tomatoes, and other colored plants, including leafy green vege-

tables. Carotene is converted in the liver to vitamin A, which is essential for normal vision and the health of the skin and other organs. Excessive intake of carotene-containing foods, especially carrots, results in carotenemia (high blood levels of carotene). This condition is harmless, but does cause yellowing of the skin, especially of the palms and soles. It can be differentiated from jaundice because the eyes remain white. The abnormal pigment rapidly disappears if carrots or other such plants are omitted from the diet.

Carotid artery

Any of the four principal arteries of the neck and head. There are two common carotid arteries (left and right), each of which divides into two main branches (internal and external).

The left common carotid artery arises from the *aorta*, just above the heart, and runs up the neck on the left side of the *trachea* (windpipe). Just above the level of the *larynx* (voice

box) it divides in two, forming the left internal carotid and the left external carotid arteries. The right common carotid artery follows a similar path, but on the right side of the neck. However, it arises from the subclavian artery, which branches off the aorta.

The external carotid arteries have multiple branches, which supply most of the tissues in the face, scalp, mouth, and jaws. The internal carotid arteries enter the skull to supply the brain (via cerebral branches) and eyes (via ophthalmic branches). At the base of the brain, branches of the two internal carotids and the basilar artery join to form a ring of blood vessels called the circle of Willis. Narrowing of these vessels may be associated with *transient ischemic attack* (TIA), while obstruction causes a stroke.

The carotid arteries have two specialized sensory regions in the neck, called the carotid sinus and the carotid body. The former monitors blood pressure; the latter monitors the oxygen content of the blood and helps regulate breathing.

Carpal tunnel syndrome

Numbness, tingling, and pain in the thumb, index, and middle fingers that often worsens at night. The condition may affect one or both hands and is sometimes accompanied by weakness in the thumb(s).

CAUSES AND INCIDENCE

The condition results from pressure on the median nerve where it passes into the hand via a gap (the "carpal tunnel") under a ligament at the front of the wrist. The median nerve carries sensory messages from the thumb and some fingers and also motor stimuli to the muscles in the hand; damage to the nerve causes sensory disturbances, particularly numbness or tingling, and weakness.

Carpal tunnel syndrome occurs most commonly among middle-aged women, usually for no obvious reason. It also occurs more commonly than average in women who are pregnant or have just started using birth-control pills, who suffer from *premenstrual syndrome*, and in people of either sex who suffer from *rheumatoid arthritis*, *myxedema*, or *acromegaly*.

TREATMENT

The condition often resolves itself without treatment. Resting the affected hand at night in a splint may alleviate symptoms. If symptoms persist, a small quantity of a *corticosteroid drug* may be injected under the ligament in the wrist. If this fails to help, surgical cutting of the ligament may be performed to relieve the pressure on the nerve.

Carrier

A person who is able to pass on a disease to others without actually suffering from it. Carriers may transmit infectious diseases to others, or may pass on inherited diseases to their offspring.

A carrier who harbors potentially harmful bacteria or viruses may unknowingly transmit an infectious disease such as typhoid or hepatitis B. The carrier may never have had symptoms of the disease, or may have had an infection in the past with apparently complete recovery.

Inherited disease may be transmitted if a parent who shows no signs of having a particular disease carries a gene for it. For example, a woman who carries the gene for hemophilia does not have the disease herself but may pass it on to her sons.

Cartilage

A type of connective tissue that, although not as hard as bone, forms an important structural component of many parts of the skeletal system, such as the joints. Much of the fetal skeleton is formed entirely of cartilage, which is then gradually converted to bone.

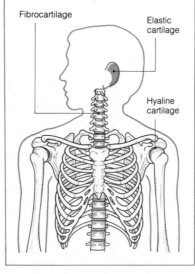

TYPES OF CARTILAGE
The three main types contain different proportions of collagen and vary in their toughness and elasticity.

Fibrocartilage

Elastic cartilage

Hyaline cartilage

Cartilage consists of specialized cells called chondrocytes embedded in a matrix, or ground substance, that comprises varying amounts of *collagen*, a gellike substance. There are three main types of cartilage: hyaline, fibrocartilage, and elastic, each with a different proportion of collagen and each with different functions.

TYPES

Hyaline cartilage is a tough, smooth tissue that lines the surfaces of joints, such as the knee, providing an almost frictionless layer over the bony parts of the joint. If the lining becomes worn (as occurs in *osteoarthritis*) or damaged, joint movement may be painful or severely restricted.

Fibrocartilage contains a large amount of collagen and is solid and very strong. It makes up the intervertebral disks between the bones of the spine and the shock-absorbing pads of tissue that are found in joints.

Elastic cartilage is soft and rubbery. It is found in various structures, notably the outer ear and the *epiglottis*.

Cast

A rigid casing applied to a limb or other part of the body to hold a broken bone or dislocated joint so that it will heal in the correct position. Most casts consist of bandages to which wet plaster of Paris has been applied; the plaster is positioned before it sets.

In some cases a half-plaster, known as a back slab, is applied. Held in place with straps, it covers only half the affected limb. It is used if swelling at the site of injury is likely, or as a temporary measure pending the insertion of a pin to secure a broken bone.

Modern fiberglass casts are stronger and lighter than plaster, but are more expensive and difficult to apply.

Castor oil

A colorless or yellow-tinged oil obtained from the leaves of the castor oil plant.

When given by mouth, castor oil irritates the lining of the small intestine and within two to six hours causes a powerful *laxative* action that completely empties the bowel. This effect helps in preparing patients for X rays of the intestine. Castor oil should not be used as a regular treatment of constipation because of its strong, rapid effect.

Zinc and castor oil ointment is an *emollient* used to soothe the skin and keep it moist in conditions such as diaper rash.

Castration

The removal of the testes (see *Orchiectomy*) or ovaries (see *Oophorectomy*). Castration is performed to remove a diseased organ or to reduce the amount of *testosterone* (male hormone produced in the testes) or *estrogen* (female hormone produced in the ovaries) in the body. Castration may be used in the treatment of breast and prostatic cancers since estrogen stimulates the growth of some breast cancers and testosterone stimulates the growth of prostatic cancer. In adults, the procedure has no immediate effect on libido (sexual desire), though in some cases libido may be affected in the long run.

Historically, castration was performed on some male singers during boyhood to preserve a high-pitched voice and on male slaves who guarded Muslim harems.

Catalepsy

A peculiar physical state in which the muscles of the face, body, and limbs are maintained in a semirigid position. Catalepsy may last for many hours, during which time neither the expression nor bodily position will alter no matter how uncomfortable (for example, an upraised arm or bowed trunk). Attempts to change the person's position will meet with resistance or the unyielding adoption of a new position. This state occurs mainly in those with schizophrenia, epilepsy, or hysteria, but may also be caused by some drugs or by various types of brain disease, such as a tumor.

C Cataplexy

A sudden loss of muscle tone, causing the victim to collapse, without any loss of consciousness. Cataplexy usually lasts for a few seconds and is triggered by emotions, particularly laughter. A rare cause of sudden involuntary falls, it occurs almost exclusively in those suffering from *narcolepsy* and other *sleep* disorders.

Cataract

Loss of transparency of the lens of the eye. The name arose many centuries ago from the fanciful idea that the whiteness behind the pupil was a kind of waterfall descending from the brain. In fact, the white appearance is due to changes in the delicate protein fibers within the lens, in a manner similar to that occurring in eggs when they are boiled.

Cataract never causes complete blindness, because even a densely opalescent lens will still transmit light. However, with increasing loss of transparency, the clarity and detail of the image is progressively lost. Even at a fairly advanced stage, a cataract may not be apparent to an external observer, and it is only when the front part of the crystalline lens becomes densely opaque that whiteness is visible in the pupil.

Cataract usually occurs in both eyes, but in most cases one eye is more severely affected than the other.

INCIDENCE

Almost everyone over the age of 65 has some degree of cataract, but usually the opacification is minor and often confined to the edge of the lens, where it does not interfere with vision. Opacification tends to progress with age, so that the majority of people over 75 have minor visual deterioration from cataract. Cataract in the elderly is so common that it is considered almost normal.

CAUSE

The majority of cataracts occur in old age; the cause in these cases is unknown. Progressive hardening of the center of the lens and increased permeability to water of the lens capsule (shell) occur in the natural aging process. Both lead to protein changes.

Congenital cataract (present at birth) may be due to maternal infection early in pregnancy, especially with the *rubella* virus, or to toxic effects from drugs taken by the mother. It may be due to *Down's syndrome* or to one of a variety of rare genetic conditions. *Galactosemia*, in which the sugar galactose accumulates in the body, almost always causes cataract unless a galactose-free diet is given.

Cataract may be caused by direct injury to the eye, either penetrating or concussive (caused by a hard blow to the head), and is almost inevitable if a foreign particle enters the crystalline lens. It may be associated with prolonged intake of corticosteroid drugs or caused by poisoning with substances such as naphthalene (found in mothballs) or ergot (formed in stored grain contaminated by a fungus). Severe *diabetes mellitus*, with high blood sugar levels, can be associated with cataract in young people. Finally, almost any form of radiation (other than light), including infrared, microwave, and X rays, can cause cataract to develop.

Cataracts with a known cause are rare compared to the large number of cases that occur in elderly people for no obvious reason.

SYMPTOMS

Cataract is entirely painless and causes only visual symptoms. The onset of these symptoms is almost imperceptible, and progress is nearly always very slow. The increased density in the lens often produces an increase in its light-refracting power so that the person concerned becomes nearsighted. This may temporarily permit a person who was previously hypermetropic (farsighted) to read without using his or her reading glasses. Color values are often disturbed, with dulling of blues and accentuation of reds, yellows, and oranges. The full perception of color is strikingly restored after surgery.

The main symptom, however, is progressive loss of visual acuity with increased blurring of vision. Often the opacities in the lenses cause scattering of light rays and, even at a fairly early stage, this may seriously affect night driving. Many patients, however, are barely aware of these effects and notice only that they cannot see as well as before.

TREATMENT

Once a lens has developed a cataract, there is no possible way of reversing the change and restoring transparency and vision by means of medications. If normal clear images are to be perceived, the lens must be removed and the refracting power of the eye restored either by means of a substitute (implant) lens or with a special type of contact lens. Cataract extraction is one of the less complex and most successful operations in all surgery and the expectation of an excellent result, provided the eye is otherwise healthy, is well over 90 percent. (See also *Cataract surgery*.)

Cataract surgery

Removal of an opacified lens, or *cataract*, from the eye, to restore sight.

WHY IT IS DONE

Cataract extraction is most often performed as soon as the lens opacification has developed to the point where the person feels it seriously affects his or her vision. It is no longer necessary to wait for a cataract to "ripen" (i.e., until its nucleus becomes hard). Ophthalmologists are usually relieved to find that a cataract, and not some other problem, is the cause of visual loss because the results of surgical treatment are now so good.

Together with the cornea at the front of the eye, the lens provides the eye with the light-refracting power needed to see the world in focus (see *Eye; Vision*). Once an opacified lens has been extracted, some method must be used to restore the lost focusing power. In the past, patients were forced to wear very strong, highly magnifying glasses, which were heavy and uncomfortable and caused much distortion at the edges of the narrowed field of vision. Such glasses are now seldom necessary; it has become usual during surgery to replace the removed lens with a tiny plastic implant, fixed permanently within the eye.

By taking preoperative measurements of the curvature of the cornea and (using an ultrasonic method) of the length of the eye, it is often possible to calculate the power of the implant lens needed to restore the patient to normal vision. Some patients, however, will need to wear glasses after the operation.

There are still, however, some cataract patients for whom intraocular lens implants are unsuitable. This group consists mainly of people with a history of other eye disease. Some surgeons also advise against intraocular lenses in young people because the life span of the implant has not been established. Contact lenses can offer these people excellent vision postoperatively, and many people now wear such lenses.

PROCEDURE FOR CATARACT SURGERY

In a normal, healthy lens there is no interference to the passage of light rays. Even with peripheral opacities, vision is not limited until the central zone is affected. Dense nuclear opacities, as that shown at right, result in deteriorating vision and cannot be restored to transparency, hence the need for surgical replacement.

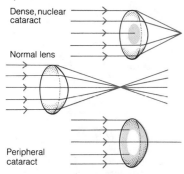

Dense, nuclear cataract

Normal lens

Peripheral cataract

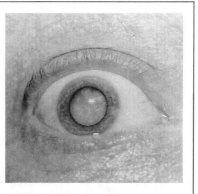

1 In preparation for surgery, measurements are taken of the cornea and of the length of the eye, in order to calculate the power of the lens implant needed to restore vision fully. The operation may be performed using general or local anesthesia; there is no pain in either case. Instruments of remarkable delicacy and precision are used to carry out the procedure, usually with the help of microscope magnification.

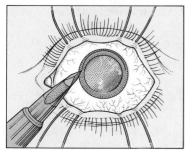

2 Before the operation, drops are used to widen the pupil so that most of the front surface of the lens is exposed. An incision is made around the upper edge of the cornea using an instrument with a diamond tip.

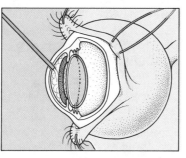

3 A small quantity of a clear gel (sodium hyaluronate) is injected to maintain a space between the back of the cornea and the lens.

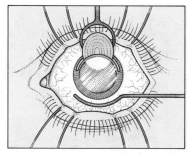

4 A large part of the center of the front capsule of the lens is then removed and the hard nucleus of the lens carefully squeezed out of the eye. The soft remaining parts of the lens are then cleared away, leaving the back of the capsule.

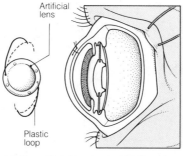

Artificial lens

Plastic loop

5 The artificial lens implant is slipped into the natural lens capsule; plastic loops hold it in place. The corneal incision is sewn up with fine nylon thread about half the diameter of a human hair.

HOW IT IS DONE

Surgeons use slightly different techniques, but a typical operation is described in the box at left.

Some surgeons remove the whole lens, in its capsule, by means of a probe that can be made to freeze to the lens. The lens may first be loosened by means of a digestive enzyme injected into the front chamber of the eye. In this case, the implant must be of a type that clips into the pupil or that is fitted in front of the iris. This method can also give excellent results.

Patients are no longer kept in bed after cataract surgery and, indeed, are encouraged to move about freely as soon as possible after the operation. The operation is commonly done today in an operating suite in the ophthalmologist's office. The corneal incision takes about a month to heal, but it is usually about ten weeks before the corneal curvature has ceased to alter. Glasses are not fitted until then.

OUTLOOK

The prospect of developing cataract need no longer cause concern. The results of treatment are usually excellent as long as no other cause of visual deterioration is present.

Catastrophic insurance

Insurance against a financially catastrophic illness. Though the term has not been specifically defined, it generally refers to the sort of health insurance that does not cover routine, moderately expensive procedures, but does protect a patient from the high costs of something such as a coronary artery bypass.

Catatonia

A state characterized by abnormalities of movement and posture. The sufferer's muscles usually become extremely rigid, but at other times he or she may be excessively active. Catatonia is a feature of a rare form of *schizophrenia*; it also occurs in people with certain brain diseases.

Catharsis

The process of expressing or acting out feelings and memories that were previously repressed. The term was originally used by Sigmund Freud, who believed that the revival of "forgotten" memories and the expression of the emotions associated with them could bring relief from anxiety, tension, and other symptoms.

The patient may be hypnotized or given drugs to bring on a suggestive state that allows the traumatic memory to be recalled and the emotions associated with the memory to be openly expressed. *Psychodrama*, which involves dramatic recreation of events, is another method used to help patients achieve emotional release. This cathartic method is claimed to be particularly successful in the treatment of battle fatigue and other forms of combat neurosis. (See also *Psychoanalytic theory*.)

Cathartic

A drug given by mouth or suppository that stimulates movement of the bowels, with production of liquid feces (see *Laxative drugs*).

Catheter

A flexible tube used either for draining fluid from or injecting fluid into the body. The most common type is the Foley catheter, which is used to drain urine from the bladder (see *Catheterization, urinary*). Other types of *balloon catheter* are used for unblocking or stretching open blood vessels, or for controlling bleeding.

A different variety of catheter is used to sample blood from the heart and to inject dye into the blood vessels during X-ray screening (see *Catheterization, cardiac*).

Catheterization, cardiac

A diagnostic test in which a fine tube called a *catheter* is introduced into the heart, via a blood vessel, to investigate its condition. The technique is used to diagnose and assess the extent of congenital heart disease (see *Heart disease, congenital*), *coronary heart disease*, and valvular defects (see *Heart valves*).

HOW IT IS DONE
The procedure, which causes little discomfort, is performed using local anesthesia. A small incision is made in a vein or artery and the catheter introduced through it. The tube is passed along the blood vessel and into the heart. Catheterization of the left side of the heart is carried out via an artery in the thigh or elbow. To investigate the right side of the heart, a vein in the groin or elbow is used.

Once in position, the catheter can measure blood pressure within the heart, withdraw blood to measure its oxygen content, or inject a dye that is opaque to X rays into the cavities of them so that X-ray photographs of them can be taken.

If an artery has been used, it is repaired with stitches after the catheter has been withdrawn; if a vein has been used, it is simply tied off.

COMPLICATIONS
Catheterization may disturb the heart rhythm, but, in a person in good physical condition, the rhythm is usually quickly restored to normal. For weaker patients the procedure does carry a slight risk of death from disturbed heart rhythm. However, since the disorders that it is used to investigate are life-threatening, the risk is regarded as acceptable.

Catheterization, urinary

Insertion of a sterile catheter into the bladder to drain urine.

WHY IT IS DONE
Catheterization is most often needed in a person who is unable to empty the bladder normally or who suffers from urinary *incontinence*. It may also be necessary during certain operations in which a bladder distended with urine might obstruct the surgeon's view of surrounding organs. Catheterization is performed in critically ill patients so that urine production can be carefully monitored; it is also used in tests of bladder function, such as *cystometry* and voiding *cystourethrogram*.

HOW IT IS DONE
The outlet of the urethra is cleaned before the catheter is inserted.

If it is not possible to pass a catheter up the urethra (because it is abnormally narrow, for example), a suprapubic catheter is inserted into the bladder through the abdominal wall. The skin of the lower part of the abdomen is cleaned with antiseptic solution, local anesthetic is injected under an area of skin overlying the bladder, and a small incision is made with a scalpel blade. The catheter surrounds a long needle that guides its insertion through this incision into the bladder. When urine flows back through the catheter, the guiding needle is withdrawn, leaving the catheter in place.

RISKS
Despite the use of sterile equipment, surgical gowns, gloves, and face masks, there is a risk of introducing infection into the bladder during catheterization.

Patients with incontinence associated with neurological disorders may have permanent catheters or may be

CATHETERIZATION OF THE BLADDER

The catheter is usually passed into the bladder through the urethra. Before this is done, the physician or nurse cleans the surrounding area with antiseptic solution to avoid introducing infection into the urinary tract. The procedure usually takes about ten minutes.

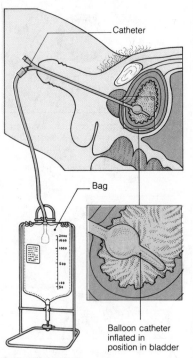

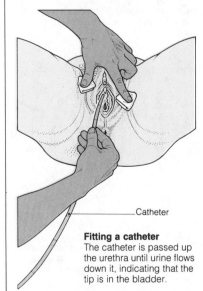

Fitting a catheter
The catheter is passed up the urethra until urine flows down it, indicating that the tip is in the bladder.

Self-retaining type
If the catheter is to remain in the bladder, a self-retaining type is used. This catheter has a balloon at its tip that can be inflated and filled with sterile water.

taught to carry out self-catheterization several times a day. Again, there is a substantial risk of infection, which can lead to urinary tract disorders, such as *cystitis* or *pyelonephritis*.

CAT scanning
Computerized axial tomographic scanning, more commonly known as *CT scanning*.

Cat-scratch fever
An uncommon disease that usually develops after a scratch or bite by a cat and is thought to be due to infection with a small bacterium transmitted by the cat. The cat itself is not ill. Three quarters of cases occur in children, and the disorder is more common in autumn and winter.

SYMPTOMS
Symptoms usually appear three to 10 days after a bite or scratch. In some cases there is no apparent break in the skin, although contact with a cat is sometimes reported. The main sign of illness is a swollen lymph node near the scratch. The node may become painful and tender and, in rare cases, it may discharge. A small, infected blister sometimes develops at the original site of skin injury. A fever, rash, and headache may also occur.

DIAGNOSIS AND TREATMENT
The diagnosis is made from a *biopsy* of a small sample of the swollen lymph node and from a skin test using a cat-scratch fever *antigen*. Analgesics (painkillers) may be needed to relieve fever and headache, and if a lymph node or blister is severely infected it may have to be drained. The prognosis is excellent. In most cases, the illness clears up within two months. The cat need not be destroyed.

Cats, diseases from
Cats carry various parasites and infectious organisms that can be spread to humans. Some are specific to cats, others affect dogs as well. A well-cared for cat poses no serious threat to human health, but cat owners should be aware of possible problems.

SPECIFIC DISEASES
Of the rare but serious problems, *rabies* can be contracted by the bite of an infected cat. Sudden unexplained aggression in a cat in any area where the disease is present, or in cats recently imported from such areas, should be treated with suspicion. Have a veterinarian see the animal as soon as possible and call your state health department to determine whether there have been any reported cases of rabies in your area.

Cat-scratch fever is an uncommon illness that usually follows the scratch or bite of a cat. The suspected cause of the illness is a small bacterium that has not yet been identified.

Cats commonly carry the protozoan (single-celled parasite) TOXOPLASMA GONDII, which is the cause of *toxoplasmosis*. A form of the parasite is present in the cat's feces. In most cases, the infection causes few or no symptoms, but, if a woman is infected during pregnancy, the parasites may gain access, via the placenta, to the fetus. Infections in early pregnancy can lead to spontaneous abortion or severe malformation; infections that occur later in pregnancy can cause nervous system disorders and sometimes blindness in early childhood. Pregnant women should not change cat litter boxes.

Cat feces may also carry eggs of the cat roundworm, a possible cause of *toxocariasis*. In very rare cases, a larva from an ingested egg may lodge in an eye, causing deterioration of vision or even blindness. This most commonly occurs in children who have been playing in soil or sand contaminated by infected dog or cat feces.

Of the more common problems, a substantial number of *tinea* (ringworm) fungal infections of the skin—particularly scalp ringworm—probably come from cats. Unlike dogs, cats are little affected by the fungus, but its presence can be demonstrated by examining the fur under ultraviolet light, which causes fluorescence of infected skin and hairs.

Bites from cat *fleas* are more common than is realized; many bites blamed on midges and mosquitoes are actually caused by fleas. The fleas may jump onto humans to feed, particularly in warm weather and if the cat is absent. Bites are most common around the ankles and can be very irritating. Look for these fleas in

places, such as beds or chairs, where the cat habitually rests.

Finally, some people develop allergic reactions to dander (tiny scales derived from animal skin and fur and present in the air) and consequently may suffer from *asthma* or *urticaria* when a cat is in the house.

PREVENTION
Serious diseases from cats are easily avoided by good hygiene—in particular, thorough washing of the hands if there is any chance they have been contaminated by cat feces. Young children should be discouraged from playing with cats and other animals, except under supervision, until they have become aware of the risks of poor hygiene. Animals that are obviously ill should be seen by a veterinarian, and routine health care should include regular worming and flea treatment.

HOW CATS TRANSMIT INFECTION
There are three main routes by which an infection or parasitic disease may be spread.

Direct contact
Mites or fungi from the animal's fur may be transferred.

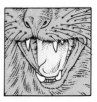

In feces
Worm eggs or parasites contained in feces may contaminate fingers or food.

Bites or scratches
Microorganisms contained in the cat's mouth or on its claws may be transmitted by a bite or scratch.

C

Cauda equina

A collection of nerve roots that descends from the lower part of the spinal cord and occupies the lower third of the spinal canal (the space in the backbone that contains the spinal cord). This "spray" of nerves resembles a horse's tail.

Caudal

Denoting a position toward the lower end of the spine. Caudal literally means "of the tail."

Caudal block

A type of *nerve block* in which local anesthetic is injected into the lower part of the spinal canal. Obstetric and gynecological procedures utilize this form of anesthesia.

Cauliflower ear

A painful, swollen, distorted ear resulting from blows or friction that have caused bleeding within the soft cartilage framework of the pinna (outer ear). The condition occurs most commonly among boxers. In other sports it is prevented by means of a protective helmet (as in football).

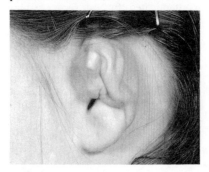

Example of cauliflower ear
Deformity of the shape of the ear, with loss of normal folds of skin.

TREATMENT

If the ear swells after injury in a game or fight, an ice pack should be used to reduce the swelling. In severe cases, a physician should be consulted. Blood can be drained from the ear using a needle and syringe, and a pressure bandage applied. Despite these measures, repeated injury will lead to a severely distorted ear, and plastic surgery is sometimes needed to improve the appearance.

Causalgia

A persistent, burning pain, usually in an arm or leg. The skin overlying the painful area may be red and tender or may be cold, blue, and clammy.

Causalgia is usually the result of injury to a nerve by a gunshot wound, a deep cut, or a limb fracture. The pain may be aggravated by emotional factors or by normal sensations, such as touch or a cold breeze.

Treatment is unsatisfactory, but, occasionally, a patient benefits from *sympathectomy*, an operation in which certain nerves are severed.

Caustic

Any substance with a burning or corrosive action on body tissues or that has a burning taste. An example is caustic soda, the common name for sodium hydroxide.

Caustic substances can destroy body tissues and so should not be used without adequate protection, such as rubber gloves. If a caustic chemical is spilled onto the skin or splashed into the eye, wash it off immediately with a gentle stream of running water, taking care not to wash the chemical onto other areas of skin or into the other eye.

Cauterization

The application of a heated instrument or a caustic chemical to tissues to destroy them, to stop them from bleeding, or to promote healing within them. In the past, heat was widely used to destroy hemorrhoids, to stop bleeding during operations, and to treat cervical erosion. It has now been largely replaced by *electrocoagulation* (the use of high-frequency electric current), which is more efficient and easier to use. Chemicals such as silver nitrate are still used to destroy warts.

Cavernous sinus thrombosis

Blockage by a thrombus (blood clot) of a venous sinus (collection of a group of veins) deep within the skull behind an eye socket. Usually it is a complication of a bacterial infection in an area drained by the veins entering the sinus. At first, only the veins behind one eye are affected but, within two or three days, the thrombosis may spread to the sinus behind the other eye. The condition has become rare since the advent of antibiotics to treat bacterial infections.

CAUSES

Among the infections that can lead to the thrombosis are *cellulitis* (a severe skin infection) occurring on the face; an infection of the mouth, eye, or middle ear; *sinusitis* (infection of the air spaces around the nose); and *septicemia* (infection in the bloodstream).

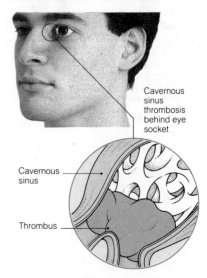

Thrombus in cavernous sinus
The cavernous sinus is found behind the eye socket, deep within the skull.

Picking at a small, infected pimple at the angle of the nose may also spread infection to the sinus.

Rarely, the thrombosis is caused by a tumor pressing on the veins or by *polycythemia* (an excessive concentration of red cells in the blood).

SYMPTOMS AND TREATMENT

The symptoms are severe headache, high fever, pain in and above the affected eye, loss of sensation in the cornea and on the forehead due to pressure on the fifth cranial nerve, and *exophthalmos* (protrusion of the eye) due to swelling around and behind the eye. Vision may become blurred and eye movements may be paralyzed due to pressure on the optic nerve and on other cranial nerves controlling the muscles that move the eyes.

The patient is usually critically ill. Treatment is with antibiotics to treat the infection and anticoagulants to help disperse the blood clot. Given promptly, treatment can save vision in the affected eye or eyes; if untreated, blindness will result, and the infection may prove fatal.

Cavity, dental

See *Caries, dental.*

CDC

See *Centers for Disease Control.*

Cecum

The chamber at the beginning of the large intestine and the large intestine's widest part. It takes its name from the

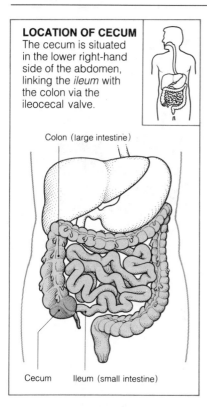

LOCATION OF CECUM
The cecum is situated in the lower right-hand side of the abdomen, linking the *ileum* with the colon via the ileocecal valve.

Colon (large intestine)

Cecum   Ileum (small intestine)

Latin word for blind, "caecum," because the large intestine terminates at this point. The *appendix* usually opens into the base of the cecum. (See also *Digestive system*.)

Cefaclor

A common cephalosporin-type antibiotic. (See *Cephalosporins*.)

Celiac sprue

An uncommon condition, known also as gluten enteropathy, in which the lining of the small intestine is damaged by gluten, a protein found in wheat, rye, and certain other cereals. The damage causes *malabsorption* (failure to absorb many important nutrients from the intestine), and the patient loses weight and also suffers from deficiencies of some vitamins and minerals. This can lead to anemia and skin problems. In addition, a large amount of fat and other nutrients remains in the stools, which are bulky and foul smelling.

CAUSE
Exactly how gluten damages the intestinal lining is not fully understood. However, it seems to be due to an abnormal immunological response. The *immune system* becomes sensitized to gluten and reacts in the same way as it would to an infection or foreign body. The abnormal reaction is limited to the intestinal lining, and the practical result is that the villi (frondlike projections) from the lining become flattened. Flattening of the villi seriously impairs their ability to absorb nutrients.

INCIDENCE
The proportion of people affected by the disease varies widely among different countries and populations. The severity of the disease varies, and many people who suffer some damage to the intestinal lining never develop symptoms.

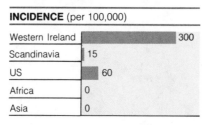

INCIDENCE (per 100,000)	
Western Ireland	300
Scandinavia	15
US	60
Africa	0
Asia	0

Celiac sprue tends to run in families—relatives of patients are much more likely than other people to have the disease themselves—which suggests that genetic factors may be involved (see *Genetic disorders*).

SYMPTOMS AND SIGNS
In babies, symptoms usually occur within six months of the introduction of gluten into the diet. The feces become bulky, greasy, pale, and offensive smelling, and the baby loses weight, becomes listless and irritable, and has a lot of gas, which makes the abdomen swell. Defective absorption of iron may lead to iron-deficiency *anemia* and defective absorption of folic acid (a vitamin) may lead to megaloblastic anemia. Vomiting may occur, and sometimes the baby develops acute diarrhea, becoming dehydrated and seriously ill.

In adults, symptoms, which usually develop gradually over months or even years, range from vague tiredness and breathlessness (due to anemia) to weight loss, diarrhea, vomiting, and abdominal pain and swelling of the legs.

In some patients, the damage to the intestinal lining is minimal, but a chronic, distinctive rash called *dermatitis herpetiformis* develops.

DIAGNOSIS
A firm diagnosis is made by means of jejunal *biopsy*, in which a small sample of tissue is taken from the lining of the upper small intestine. Three biopsies may be performed—one when the patient is eating foods containing gluten, another when he or she is on a gluten-free diet, and a third when gluten is again introduced into the diet. A change in the intestinal lining during the second and third stages indicates that gluten is causing the illness. Blood, urine, and feces tests show the level of malabsorption.

TREATMENT AND OUTLOOK
The only treatment required is a lifelong gluten-free diet; all foods containing wheat, rye, or barley must be avoided (many sufferers are also advised to avoid oats).

Specially manufactured substitute foods, including gluten-free bread, flour, and pasta, are available. There is no restriction on meat, fish, eggs and dairy products, vegetables, fruit, rice, and corn.

Within a few weeks of the start of a gluten-free diet, symptoms clear up and the sufferer starts to regain lost weight and to enjoy normal health.

Cell

The basic structural unit of the body. Each person consists of billions of cells, structurally and functionally integrated to perform the nearly infinite number of complex tasks necessary for life.

There is enormous variation among cells in the body. For example, mature red blood cells are only about 7 microns (about 0.0003 inch) across and are so highly specialized for their function of transporting oxygen that they lack some of the internal structures normally found within other cells, such as a nucleus. In contrast, nerve cells may be 3 ft (1 m) or more in length and are specialized to perform their function of transmitting electrochemical messages (nerve impulses).

Despite detailed differences, most human cells are basically similar in structure. Each cell is an invisibly small bag containing a fluid material called cytoplasm, surrounded by an outer skin called the cell membrane. Within the cytoplasm are the nucleus (except in red blood cells) and various other specialized structures, known collectively as organelles.

CELL MEMBRANE
Formed from a double layer of fatty material and proteins, the cell membrane holds the cell together. Its other main function is to regulate the passage of materials into and out of the cell, thereby enabling useful substances (such as nutrients and oxygen) to enter the cell, and waste materials

C

CELL TYPES

Despite their fundamental similarities, the cells of the body are differentiated to perform specific tasks, such as carrying oxygen (red blood cells), destroying invading microorganisms (white blood cells), manufacturing hormones (secretory cells in glands), and so on. Some cells (nerve cells, for instance) cannot be replaced once destroyed, while other cells (those that form fingernails, for instance) continue to function even after death. Cells can be grouped into four main types according to their underlying similarities.

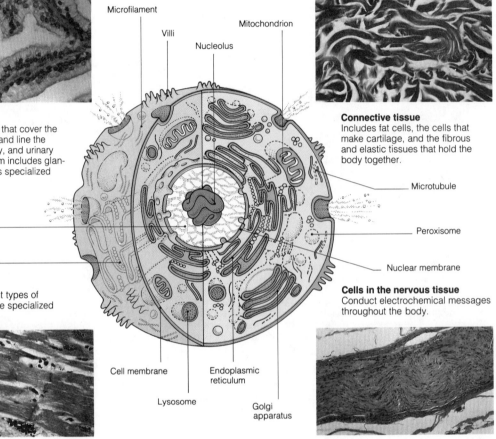

Epithelial cells
Make up the tissues that cover the outside of the body and line the digestive, respiratory, and urinary tracts. The epithelium includes glandular tissue, which is specialized for secretion.

Connective tissue
Includes fat cells, the cells that make cartilage, and the fibrous and elastic tissues that hold the body together.

Muscular tissue
Made up of different types of muscle cells that are specialized to contract.

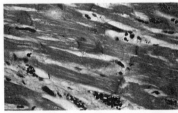

Cells in the nervous tissue
Conduct electrochemical messages throughout the body.

Diagram labels: Microfilament, Villi, Nucleolus, Mitochondrion, Nucleus, Ribosomes, Cell membrane, Lysosome, Endoplasmic reticulum, Golgi apparatus, Microtubule, Peroxisome, Nuclear membrane

(such as carbon dioxide) and substances for use elsewhere in the body (hormones, for example) to leave it. Small molecules pass freely through the membrane, but larger molecules require special molecular transport systems to cross the membrane.

NUCLEUS

The control center of the cell, the nucleus governs all major activities and functions. The nucleus exerts its influence by regulating the amount and types of *proteins* made in the cell. Proteins have two main functions. Large, structural proteins make up the tough building material of the body (such as muscle fibers). Smaller proteins called *enzymes* regulate all functions and activities of the cell.

The *chromosomes* (genetic material of the cell) in the form of DNA (see *Nucleic acids*) are situated in the nucleus. This DNA contains the instructions for *protein synthesis*, which are transmitted by a type of *RNA* to ribosomes (protein producers) in the cytoplasm. It is on the ribosomes that protein synthesis—the linking of various amino acids to form proteins—occurs.

OTHER ORGANELLES

In addition to the nucleus there are various other organelles within the cell, each with a specific role.

The endoplasmic reticulum is a single sheet of membrane twisted into complex folds. The sheet has rough and smooth areas. Rough endoplasmic reticulum is covered with small round "beads"; these are the ribosomes that produce proteins.

Once completed, the proteins are transferred to another membrane system, the Golgi apparatus, which resembles a series of stacked plates. Here protein structures are modified and packaged into vesicles budded from its surface.

Energy is generated (from the breakdown of sugars and fatty acids) by organelles called mitochondria. These are shaped like coffee beans and have a complex, folded inner surface. Cells that have high energy requirements, such as muscle or liver cells, have a large number of mitochondria. Many cell processes involve substances that would damage the cell if they came into contact with the cytoplasm, so they are contained within special vesicles called lysosomes and peroxisomes. Lysosomes are the cell's major digestive structures in which enzymes break down large particles, such as bacteria. Peroxisomes neutralize toxic substances.

CYTOPLASM

Modern cytological techniques have shown that the cytoplasm contains a network of fine tubes (microtubules) and filaments (microfilaments) known as the cytoskeleton. This network gives the cell a definite shape and allows it to move. In addition, microfilaments support microvilli (small projections from the surface of the cell), which help increase the surface area of the cell. Microfilaments also form micromuscles, which can produce contractions and movements of the cell.

Cell division

The processes by which cells multiply. There are two main types of cell division, *mitosis* and *meiosis*. The former gives rise to daughter cells that are identical to the parent cell. The latter gives rise to egg and sperm cells, which differ from their parent cells in that they have only half the normal number of *chromosomes*.

Cellulitis

A bacterial infection of the skin and the tissues beneath it. The most common form is caused by streptococci, which enter the skin via a wound.

SYMPTOMS

The face, neck, or legs are the usual sites. The affected area is hot, tender, and red, and the patient is often feverish and may have chills.

Untreated cellulitis complicating a wound may progress to *bacteremia* and *septicemia* or, occasionally, to *gangrene*. Before the advent of antibiotics the infection was an occasional cause of death. Facial infections may spread to the eye socket. Very rarely, cellulitis occurs after childbirth and may spread to the pelvic organs.

Any form of cellulitis is likely to be more severe in people with reduced resistance to infections, such as diabetics and those with any type of *immunodeficiency disorder*.

TREATMENT

The usual treatment is a penicillin antibiotic (or erythromycin in case of allergy). Drugs may need to be taken for up to two weeks to clear an infection. (See also *Erysipelas*.)

Celsius scale

A temperature scale in which the melting point of ice is zero degrees (0°C) and the boiling point of water is 100 degrees (100°C). On this scale, normal body temperature is 37°C (equivalent to 98.6°F). The scale is named for the Swedish astronomer Anders Celsius (1701-1744). Centigrade is an obsolete name for the same scale.

To convert Celsius to Fahrenheit, multiply by 1.8 (or nine fifths), then add 32. To convert Fahrenheit to Celsius, subtract 32 then multiply by 0.56 (or five ninths). (See also *Fahrenheit scale*.)

0°C	37°C	100°C
32°F	98.6°F	212°F

Cementum

The bonelike tissue that surrounds the root of a tooth (see *Teeth*).

Centers for Disease Control

A part of the US Department of Health and Human Services that is responsible for the analysis and timely reporting of significant variations in the normal patterns of morbidity (the occurrence of diseases) and mortality. In effect, the CDC is the nation's medical watchdog. The centers are located in Atlanta, Georgia.

Centigrade scale

The obsolete name for the *Celsius scale*.

Central nervous system

The anatomical term for the brain and spinal cord, often abbreviated as CNS. The central nervous system works in tandem with the *peripheral nervous system* (PNS), which consists of all the nerves that carry signals between the CNS and the rest of the body.

The overall role of the CNS is to receive sensory information from organs, such as the eyes, ears, and receptors within the body, analyze this information, and initiate an appropriate motor response (for example, moving a muscle).

The analytical stage may be very short and simple for information that goes no further than the spinal cord or lower areas of the brain (see *Reflex*), but may be complex and prolonged for information reaching higher, conscious brain centers.

In anatomical terms the CNS consists of nerve cells or neurons and supporting tissue; the PNS is made up of nerve fibers extending from cells in the CNS. In functional terms, injury or

disease to the CNS usually causes permanent disability; recovery is sometimes possible after damage to the PNS has been repaired surgically. (See also *Nervous system*.)

Centrifuge

A machine that separates the different components of a body fluid, such as blood or urine, so that they can be analyzed as an aid to diagnosis. The liquid is placed in a container that is spun at high speed around a central axis, and the centrifugal force (force moving away from the center) separates groups of particles of varying density. Blood, for example, can be separated into red cells, white cells, and its remaining constituents.

Cephalexin

A common cephalosporin-type antibiotic. (See *Cephalosporins*.)

Cephalhematoma

An extensive, soft swelling on the scalp of a newborn infant, caused by bleeding into the space between the cranium (skull) and its overlying fibrous covering, the periosteum. The swelling is due to pressure on the baby's head during delivery, causing rupture of some small blood vessels within the periosteum.

Although slightly alarming, a cephalhematoma is not serious and no treatment is necessary. The swelling should not be handled unnecessarily. It gradually subsides as the blood clot is reabsorbed, although this may take many weeks.

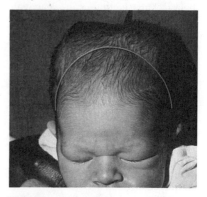

Bilateral cephalhematoma
This baby was born with a cephalhematoma on both sides of the scalp at the back of the head.

Cephalic

Relating to the head, as in cephalic presentation, the head-first appearance of a baby in the birth canal.

C

Cephalosporins

COMMON DRUGS

Cefaclor Cefadroxil Cefazolin Cefoperazone Cefoxitin Ceftriaxone Cephalexin Cephalothin Cephapirin Cephradine

A group of *antibiotic drugs* derived from the fungus *CEPHALOSPORIUM ACREMONIUM*. Cephalosporins were discovered in Sardinia in 1948. A large number of synthetic cephalosporins have since been produced, the most recent of which are effective against a wide range of infections.

WHY THEY ARE USED
Cephalosporins are widely used to treat ear, throat, and respiratory infections. They are also particularly useful in the treatment of urinary tract infections (which are often caused by bacteria resistant to penicillin-type antibiotics) and are used to treat *gonorrhea* that is resistant to other antibiotics. Cephalosporins are also sometimes used after surgery to reduce the incidence of wound infections.

The drugs in this group may be used in patients allergic to penicillin-type antibiotics. However, approximately 10 percent of those people allergic to penicillins are also found to be allergic to cephalosporins.

HOW THEY WORK
Cephalosporins interfere with the development of bacterial cell walls and inhibit the production of protein within the cells. As a result, the organisms die. However, some bacteria produce an enzyme (a protein that stimulates chemical reactions) called beta-lactamase that can inactivate some of the older cephalosporins. The newer drugs in the group are not affected by this enzyme.

POSSIBLE ADVERSE EFFECTS
Some people who take cephalosporins develop an allergic reaction. Reactions may include rash, itching, fever, and very rarely, *anaphylactic shock* (a severe allergic reaction causing collapse).

Cerebellum

A region of the brain concerned primarily with the maintenance of posture and balance and the coordination of movement.

STRUCTURE
The cerebellum is a rounded structure located behind the *brain stem*, to which it is linked by thick nerve tracts. The cerebellum accounts for about 11 percent of the whole brain weight and, with its convoluted surface, appears similar to the *cerebrum* (the main mass of the brain).

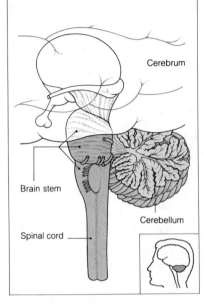

LOCATION OF CEREBELLUM
The cerebellum is found behind the brain stem and is connected to it by nerve tracts.

Cerebrum

Brain stem

Cerebellum

Spinal cord

Outwardly, the cerebellum consists of two hemispheres flanking a small protrusion from the brain stem, the vermis. The cortex (surface) of the hemispheres consists of numerous parallel ridges separated by deep fissures, so that only one sixth of the surface is visible. From the inner side of each hemisphere, three nerve fiber stalks, or peduncles, arise; these link up with different parts of the brain stem. All the signals between the cerebellum and the rest of the brain travel along these nerve tracts.

Microscopically, a cross section of the cerebellum shows the nerve fibers from these tracts fanning out toward the convoluted cortical surface. The cortex itself consists of gray matter (interconnected nerve cells) arranged in three main layers. Prominent among them are large cells in the middle layer, called Purkinje's cells, each of which may interconnect with up to 100,000 other cells.

FUNCTION
Via its connections to the brain stem, the cerebellum receives information from organs such as muscle tendons and the balance organ in the inner ear. Much of this information concerns the body's posture and the state of contraction or relaxation of its muscles. After receiving this information, the

cerebellum, working in concert with the *basal ganglia*, "fine-tunes" the orders sent to muscles from the motor cortex in the cerebrum, resulting in smoothly coordinated movements and balance.

DISORDERS
Disease or damage to the cerebellum can result in abnormalities of posture or movement. These include *ataxia* (jerky, staggering gait and other uncoordinated body movements); *dysarthria* (slurred speech); hand tremor and "overshoot" when an attempt is made to grasp or touch something; and *nystagmus* (jerky eye movements, with an inability to fix the gaze in one direction).

Alcohol intoxication impairs cerebellar function and thus may produce symptoms similar to those of cerebellar disease. *Stroke* may cause cerebellar damage, often associated with impairment of the function of one or more *cranial nerves*.

Cerebral hemorrhage

Bleeding within the brain caused by rupture of a blood vessel. (See *Intracerebral hemorrhage*.)

Cerebral palsy

A general term for nonprogressive disorders of movement and posture resulting from damage to the brain in the later months of pregnancy, during birth, in the newborn period, or in early childhood.

A child with cerebral palsy may suffer from *spastic paralysis* (abnormal stiffness and contraction of groups of muscles), *athetosis* (involuntary writhing movements), or *ataxia* (loss of coordination and balance). The degree of disability is highly variable, ranging from slight clumsiness of hand movement and gait to complete immobility. Other nervous system disorders, such as hearing defects or epileptic seizures, may be present. Many affected children are also mentally retarded, although a proportion are of normal or high intelligence.

In the US about two to six babies per 1,000 develop cerebral palsy. There has been only a slight reduction in cases in the past 20 years.

CAUSES
In over 90 percent of cases the damage occurs before or at birth. Probably the most common cause is cerebral *hypoxia* (poor oxygen supply to the brain).

A maternal infection spreading to the baby within the uterus is an occasional cause. A rare cause is *kernicterus*, which results from an excess of bilirubin (bile pigment) in babies with *hemolytic disease of the newborn*. The baby is severely jaundiced, and the bile pigment damages the *basal ganglia* (nerve cell clusters in the brain concerned with control of movement).

Following birth, possible causes include *encephalitis* or *meningitis* (infection of the brain or its protective coverings), or a head injury.

SYMPTOMS

Often cerebral palsy is not recognized until well into the baby's first year. Sometimes, but not always, some of the infant's muscles are initially hypotonic (floppy), and the parents may notice that the baby in some way does not "feel right" when held. There may also be feeding difficulties.

Once the disability is apparent, most affected children fall into one of two groups—a spastic group, in which the muscles of one or more limbs are permanently contracted and stiff, thus making normal movements very difficult, and a smaller, athetoid group, characterized by involuntary writhing movements.

The diplegic child (see below) has delayed development in many movement skills and has difficulty learning to walk. In hemiplegia the limbs on

---

TYPES OF CEREBRAL PALSY

There are three different categories of disability in the spastic group: diplegia, hemiplegia, and quadriplegia.

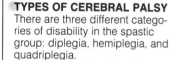

Diplegia
All four limbs are affected, the legs more severely than the arms.

Hemiplegia
The limbs on only one side of the body are affected, and the arm is usually worse than the leg.

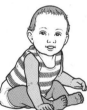

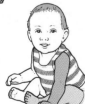

Quadriplegia
All four limbs are severely affected, not necessarily symmetrically.

---

the affected side grow slowly; there may be some sensory loss from the affected side of the body.

In quadriplegia, it may be difficult to know whether the child's arms or legs are the worst affected; mental retardation is usually severe. Often, the child never learns to walk.

The athetoid type of cerebral palsy results from damage to the basal ganglia, due either to birth asphyxia caused by hypoxia or to kernicterus.

Mental retardation, with an IQ below 70, occurs in about three quarters of all people with cerebral palsy, but the exceptions are important and occur particularly among athetoids; many athetoids and some diplegics are highly intelligent.

None of the various types of cerebral palsy is progressive (i.e., they do not worsen), but the features of the condition change as the child gets older, often for the better with patience and skilled treatment.

DIAGNOSIS

Parents of babies who are "at risk" from cerebral palsy—for example, babies born prematurely or during particularly difficult births—are generally encouraged to take the child more frequently for routine checkups by a physician, who will test with particular care for any abnormalities in the baby's muscle tone and reflexes, and for any delay in reaching various developmental milestones (see *Child development*). The diagnosis may rely on a combination of abnormalities.

TREATMENT

Although cerebral palsy is incurable, much can be done to help children affected by it. Abilities need to be recognized and developed to the full, as much stimulation as possible should be offered, and loving patience must always be shown.

Physical therapy is required to teach the child how to develop muscular control and maintain balance. This therapy is often given initially at a special school or clinic and then continued at home, possibly with the use of special equipment.

Inadequate speech can be helped greatly by *speech therapy*. For children who cannot speak at all, sophisticated techniques and devices have been developed to teach them how to communicate nonverbally.

Every attempt is made to place children with mild cerebral palsy in normal schools, but those who are severely affected need the special help available at schools for the physically and/or mentally handicapped.

OUTLOOK

Children with only moderate disability have a near-normal life expectancy and, with the help of social services, most of those who can move around and communicate effectively grow up to lead a relatively independent and normal life.

Cerebral thrombosis

The formation of a clot, or thrombus, in an artery in the brain. The clot may completely block the artery, cutting off the supply of blood and oxygen to a brain area, causing a *stroke*.

Cerebrospinal fluid

A clear, watery fluid that circulates between the ventricles (cavities) within the brain, the central canal in the spinal cord, and the space between the brain and spinal cord and their protective coverings, the meninges. Cerebrospinal fluid contains dissolved glucose, proteins, and salts, and some lymphocytes (roving cells—part of the immune system—that are also found in blood).

Examination of cerebrospinal fluid, usually obtained by *lumbar puncture*, is important in the diagnosis of many conditions affecting the brain and spinal cord, including *meningitis* and *subarachnoid hemorrhage*.

Accumulation of cerebrospinal fluid within the skull during fetal development or in infancy may cause the skull to become enlarged—a condition known as *hydrocephalus*.

Cerebrovascular accident

Sudden rupture or blockage of a blood vessel within the brain, causing serious bleeding and/or local obstruction to blood circulation.

Blockage may be due to *thrombosis* (clot formation) or *embolism* (obstruction by a plug of insoluble material formed and transported from elsewhere in the circulation). Rupture of different blood vessels may cause different patterns of bleeding, e.g., *intracerebral hemorrhage* (within the brain) or *subarachnoid hemorrhage* (around the brain).

Intracerebral hemorrhage, thrombosis, or embolism lead to neurologic features commonly called *stroke*.

Cerebrovascular disease

Any disease affecting an artery within and supplying blood to the brain—for example, *atherosclerosis* (narrowing of the arteries) or constitutional defects or weaknesses in arterial walls causing *aneurysm* (permanent swelling in an artery). The disease may eventually lead to a *cerebrovascular accident* (sudden blockage or rupture of a blood vessel), most commonly leading to the features of *stroke*. Extensive narrowing of blood vessels throughout the brain can be a cause of *dementia*.

Cerebrum

The largest and most developed part of the brain, and the site of most conscious and intelligent activities. The cerebrum consists of two large outgrowths from the upper part of the brain stem (an extension of the spinal cord) called the cerebral hemispheres. Together these growths form an almost continuous mass that envelops much of the rest of the brain.

For size relative to body weight, and also for sophistication, the human cerebrum is unmatched in the animal kingdom, except arguably by that of some marine mammals, such as dolphins. Its complexity dwarfs that of the most advanced man-made machines and, although its structure and function are understood in broad terms, much of its workings remain a complete mystery.

STRUCTURE

Like the rest of the brain, the cerebrum consists of billions of interconnected nerve cells, arranged in layers or in clusters called nuclei, together with nerve fibers, the long filamentous outgrowths from nerve cells along which electrical messages pass to other cells. These fibers are organized into bundles, or nerve tracts, like electrical cables. Both the nerve cells and their fibers lie in a matrix of supporting cells, called glia cells, which provide both physical support and some metabolic requirements (e.g., energy, nutrients, or structural components) for the nerve cells.

Each cerebral hemisphere contains a central cavity, called a ventricle, that is filled with cerebrospinal fluid. Much of the rest of each hemisphere falls into three main layers: an inner layer surrounding the ventricle and consisting of clusters of nerve cells called the basal ganglia, a middle layer of "white matter" consisting mainly of tracts of nerve fibers, and an outer surface layer, the cerebral cortex or "gray matter," which is about 0.3 inches (1 cm) deep and consists of several layers of interconnected nerve cells.

The surface of each hemisphere is thrown into a series of folds, called gyri, separated by fissures called sulci; much of the cortex is hidden within the folds. Broad surface regions, or

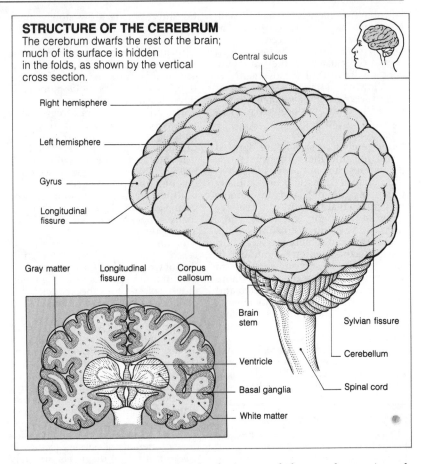

STRUCTURE OF THE CEREBRUM
The cerebrum dwarfs the rest of the brain; much of its surface is hidden in the folds, as shown by the vertical cross section.

Central sulcus
Right hemisphere
Left hemisphere
Gyrus
Longitudinal fissure

Gray matter — Longitudinal fissure — Corpus callosum
Brain stem
Sylvian fissure
Ventricle
Cerebellum
Basal ganglia
Spinal cord
White matter

lobes, of each hemisphere are named for overlying bones; the four main regions are the frontal, parietal, temporal, and occipital lobes.

The pattern of cortical folding is not precisely the same for everyone, but some of the gyri and sulci are constant and easily recognized on the surface of any brain. They have been given names by anatomists. The parietal and frontal lobes, for example, are separated by the central sulcus, and the temporal lobe from the frontal by the sylvian fissure. The longitudinal fissure is a deep cleft running front to back over the entire surface of the cerebrum, thus separating the two hemispheres. By reference to such landmarks, the location of any point on the surface of the cortex can be specified with some precision.

The nerve fibers forming much of the central white matter in each hemisphere are of three main types: association fibers link areas of cortex within a single hemisphere, projection fibers link areas of the cortex to central brain structures and to the

brain stem below, and commissural fibers, collected into a thick band called the corpus callosum, link the two hemispheres. A continuous stream of information, in the form of electrical impulses, flows along these fibers between groups of nerve cells.

FUNCTION

Much of the sensory information from organs such as the eyes and ears and from sensory receptors in the skin has its final destination in the cerebral cortex, where it is sorted, analyzed, and generally integrated until finally it is perceived as images, sound, touch sensations, and the like. Different levels of analysis are thought to correspond to the distinct layers of neurons in the cortex, with full conscious sensation probably occurring only in the top few layers.

Certain sensory modalities are specifically located within particular cortical regions—for example, visual perception is located within a part of the occipital lobe called the visual cortex. If this part of the brain is seriously damaged, vision is lost completely.

Touch and pressure sensations are consciously perceived along the postcentral gyrus, immediately behind the central sulcus that divides the frontal and parietal lobes. Other cortical regions, mainly in the temporal lobe, are associated with auditory (hearing), olfactory (smell), and gustatory (taste) sensations, although less specifically so. If these areas are destroyed, sensation is dulled considerably, but not lost altogether. It seems that some primitive sensations (e.g., smell and pain) may be perceived below the level of the cortex.

In addition to sensory areas, there are also specific "motor" areas concerned with the initiation of the signal for movement by the skeletal muscles. The main motor area of the cortex is in the frontal lobe, along the precentral gyrus, immediately in front of the central sulcus. Again, however, it seems that not all movements are initiated from the cortex. Some learned, semiautomatic programs of movement, such as those required for walking, are delegated to lower brain regions, leaving the cortex free to deal with newly formulated, skilled movements.

Linked to the more clearly defined sensory and motor areas are association areas of the cortex, which integrate information from various senses. The association areas also perform functions such as comprehension and recognition, memory storage and recall, arithmetic calculation, thought and decision-making, or are involved in the conscious experience of emotions. Whereas many of the sensory and motor areas are on both sides of the cerebrum (serving the opposite side of the body), some of these other cortical functions are localized to one hemisphere. The "dominant" hemisphere (the left in almost all right-handed and many left-handed people) tends to control logical functions such as word comprehension, language, speech, and numeration, whereas the nondominant hemisphere is concerned with spatial relationships and emotional responses such as color appreciation.

In general, the more complex the function, the less well localized it is. However, the areas responsible for the comprehension of words (heard and read) and for the formulation of speech are located within clearly defined areas of the dominant hemisphere. The comprehension region (Wernicke's area) is close to the part of the cortex concerned with sound perception; the speech region (Broca's area) is close to the motor region that controls the muscles used in speech.

Of all the regions of the cerebrum, the functions of the frontal lobe are the least understood, and for this reason it is sometimes termed a "silent area." Information on the activity of this and some other areas derives mainly from study of the symptoms of local damage or disease.

DISORDERS
Damage to the cerebrum may be the result of direct physical trauma, *intracerebral hemorrhage* or other forms of *stroke*, *brain tumors*, *encephalitis* (brain infection), some types of poisoning, nutritional deficiency, or degenerative processes.

Damage to particular regions may cause specific syndromes. Examples are mental apathy and self-neglect (or other personality change) resulting from frontal lobe damage, or the loss of sensory discrimination, tactile *agnosia* (loss of the ability to recognize objects by touch), and geographic disorientation (losing one's way even in a familiar neighborhood), which may occur with parietal lobe injury. Disease of the temporal lobe may cause *amnesia* (loss of memory), strange hallucinations of smell, sight, and sound, and *aphasia* (loss of verbal comprehension and/or speech) if in the dominant hemisphere. Specific visual defects result from damage to the occipital lobe.

Often, however, cerebral disease causes nonspecific symptoms such as epileptic convulsions or headaches.

Certificate-of-need
A measure aimed at holding down medical costs. In some areas of the US, a certificate-of-need satisfying governmental criteria is required before a health facility, such as a hospital, may be built, expanded, or acquire expensive medical equipment.

Certification
The process of completing the necessary legal documents during the procedure of *commitment* to a mental institution for compulsory detention and treatment. The term is also used to refer to death certification—the formal signing of a statement of cause of death issued by a medical practitioner. In addition, the term is used when a specialty board approves a physician candidate as a specialist. The candidate is then said to be "board certified" (see *Board certification*).

Certification, board
See *Board certification*.

Cerumen
The waxlike yellowish substance commonly found in the external ear canal (see *Earwax*).

Cervical
Relating to the neck or to the cervix (neck of the uterus).

Cervical cancer
See *Cervix, cancer of*.

Cervical erosion
A condition (also called cervical eversion) affecting the cervix (neck of the uterus) in which a layer of cells with a composition similar to that of its inner lining appears on its outside surface—as though the cervix had been turned slightly inside out. The layer of cells contains many that are column-shaped and of a glandular (mucus-forming) type. The term "erosion" is something of a misnomer as there is no loss of tissue or ulceration of the cervix. The cervix may, however, be more fragile and have a tendency to bleed and secrete more mucus.

CAUSES
Some women are born with cervical erosion and have no symptoms. Other causes include injury to the cervix during labor (which may cause glandular tissue to appear on the outer surface of the cervix during healing) and long-term use of oral contraceptives.

SYMPTOMS
Most women with an erosion have no or few symptoms. Those who do have symptoms usually complain of a vaginal discharge, especially in the week prior to a period, or bleeding between periods or after intercourse. Inspection of the cervix shows a reddened area on the surface that may bleed easily when touched. This appearance needs to be distinguished from cervical cancer by means of a *cervical smear test* (Pap smear) and *colposcopy*.

TREATMENT
Only women with symptoms need to be treated (after a cervical smear has been taken and inspected). Treatment by local destruction of glandular tissue includes *cauterization*, *cryosurgery* (freezing), *diathermy* (heat destruction), or *laser treatment*. The areas of destroyed glandular tissue are replaced in time by a layer of normal squamous (flat) cells.

Cervical eversion
See *Cervical erosion*.

C

Cervical incompetence

Abnormal weakness of the cervix (the neck of the uterus) that can result in recurrent *miscarriages* (spontaneous abortions). Normally, the cervix remains closed throughout pregnancy until labor begins. However, if the cervix is incompetent, it gradually widens from about the 12th week of pregnancy onward because of the weight of the fetus within the uterus.

CAUSES AND SYMPTOMS

Cervical incompetence may be suspected if a woman has had two or more miscarriages after the 14th week of pregnancy. About one fifth of women who have recurrent miscarriages have cervical incompetence.

The physician can detect the widening of the cervical opening by performing an internal pelvic examination. The condition can also be diagnosed by *ultrasound scanning*.

TREATMENT

When a woman with cervical incompetence becomes pregnant, a suture (stitch) is tied, like a purse string, around the cervix. This is performed during the fourth month of pregnancy with an epidural or spinal anesthetic. After the operation, the patient stays in the hospital for a few days, and should rest frequently in bed throughout the remainder of the pregnancy. The suture is left in position until the pregnancy is at or near full term. It is then cut so that the mother can deliver the baby normally.

Cervical mucus method

A form of contraception based on periodic abstinence from intercourse according to changes in the mucus secreted by a woman's cervix. (See *Contraception, periodic abstinence*.)

Cervical osteoarthritis

A degenerative disorder that affects the joints between the bones in the neck and causes neck pain, stiffness, and other symptoms. The affected joints are those between the cervical vertebrae (the neck segments of the spinal column).

Because the degenerative changes are associated with aging, middle-aged and elderly people are mainly affected. Occasionally, the degeneration may be started by an injury—for example, the repeated injury sustained by football players. Almost everyone over the age of 50 has some evidence of cervical osteoarthritis on X-ray imaging. However, in most cases it causes no symptoms or only minor ones.

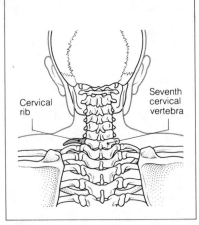

LOCATION OF CERVICAL RIB
The overdeveloped seventh cervical vertebra forms a rib parallel to a normal one.

Cervical rib

Seventh cervical vertebra

SYMPTOMS

In addition to pain and stiffness in the neck, there may be pain in the arms and shoulders, numbness and tingling in the hands, and a weak grip. These symptoms are caused by pressure on the nerves that run from the spinal cord into the arms as they pass between the affected vertebrae. The symptoms tend to flare up from time to time, with intervening periods of only mild discomfort.

Other symptoms can include dizziness, unsteadiness, double vision, and headache brought on by turning the head. These are caused by pressure on blood vessels running through the vertebrae up to the brain. Rarely, pressure on the spinal cord itself can cause weakness or even paralysis in the legs, and loss of bladder control.

DIAGNOSIS AND TREATMENT

People with persistent minor symptoms or symptoms that are becoming worse should consult their physicians. X rays will reveal the degenerative changes. If pressure on the spinal cord is suspected, other studies will be performed to decide whether decompression can be accomplished surgically.

Treatment of severe neck pain and stiffness may include resting at home with cervical traction, wet heat, supporting the neck in a collar, and the use of analgesics (painkillers). *Physical therapy* is useful when the pain has eased; it includes *diathermy*, ultrasound, massage, and exercises to improve neck posture and movement.

Cervical rib

A congenital disorder in which the lowest of the seven cervical vertebrae (neck section of the spine) has overdeveloped to form a rib. This rib lies parallel to the normal rib attached to the first thoracic vertebra (see *Spine*). The abnormality varies from a small bony swelling to a fully developed rib and may occur on one or both sides. The cause is unknown.

SYMPTOMS

Often, there are no symptoms and the rib is discovered only when an X ray of the chest or neck is taken for some unrelated reason. Symptoms may develop in early adult life, when the rib begins to press on the lower part of the brachial plexus (the group of nerves passing from the spinal cord into the arm), causing pain, numbness, and a *pins and needles sensation* in the forearm and hand. These symptoms can often be relieved by changing the position of the arm.

DIAGNOSIS AND TREATMENT

Pain and tingling in the hand and forearm have a variety of possible causes, and the presence of a cervical rib, which is easily detected on an X ray, does not necessarily mean that it is the cause. Other possible causes of the pain and tingling include *carpal tunnel syndrome* or a *disk prolapse* (herniated disk) in the neck.

If the cervical rib seems the most likely cause, the symptoms can sometimes be helped by exercises to strengthen the shoulder muscles and improve the posture. Severe or persistent symptoms may require surgery.

Cervical smear test

A test to detect abnormal changes in the cells of the cervix (the neck of the uterus) and thus prevent the development of cervical cancer. The procedure is also known as a Pap smear, for George Papanicolaou, the physician who devised it.

WHY IT IS DONE

The test offers a 95 percent chance of detecting dysplasia (abnormal cell changes) which, if not discovered and treated, could become cancerous.

Cervical smears are also used to detect viral infections of the cervix, such as *herpes simplex* and wart virus infection, and to assess the level of hormones in the body, particularly estrogen and progesterone.

WHEN IT IS DONE

A woman should have a cervical smear within six months of first having sexual intercourse. A second smear should be done six to 12 months

PROCEDURE FOR A CERVICAL (PAP) SMEAR

The procedure is risk-free and the smear test itself takes only a few seconds. It should be done as a matter of routine within six months of first having sexual intercourse, and then six to 12 months after. Thereafter, it should be performed at one- to three-year intervals.

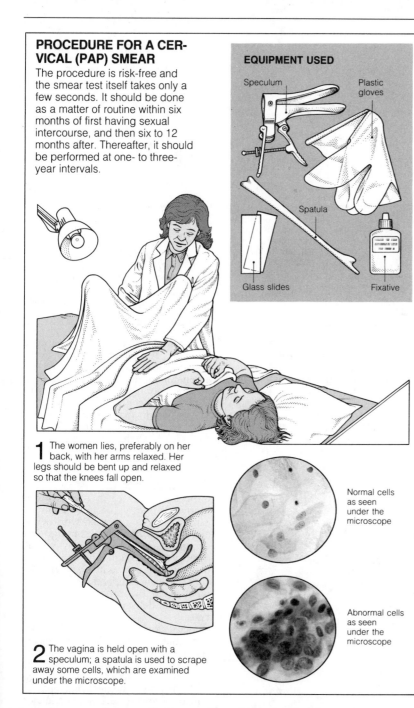

EQUIPMENT USED

Speculum

Plastic gloves

Spatula

Glass slides

Fixative

1 The women lies, preferably on her back, with her arms relaxed. Her legs should be bent up and relaxed so that the knees fall open.

2 The vagina is held open with a speculum; a spatula is used to scrape away some cells, which are examined under the microscope.

Normal cells as seen under the microscope

Abnormal cells as seen under the microscope

fication system: CIN1 (mild dysplasia), CIN2 (moderate dysplasia), or CIN3 (severe dysplasia/early cancer). All abnormal smears are followed by *colposcopy* (examination of the cervix through a system of lenses) and biopsy (removal of small samples of tissue for analysis) of any suspicious areas. There are two types of cervical biopsy: punch and cone. A punch biopsy is the less invasive and is used for diagnostic purposes only (see illustration, next page). Areas confirmed as abnormal by biopsy are treated by *electrocoagulation* or *laser* (both use heat to destroy tissue) or *cryosurgery* (which uses cold to destroy tissue). This treatment is sometimes carried out at the same time as colposcopy if the abnormal area is small and well defined. In pregnancy, treatment is usually delayed until after delivery.

If colposcopy is not available, or if the extent of the severe dysplasia cannot be identified, treatment is by *cone biopsy*, an operation to remove a core of cervical tissue.

Cervicitis

Inflammation of the cervix (the neck and outlet of the uterus). Cervicitis is usually due to a vaginal infection or a sexually transmitted disease, such as *gonorrhea*, a *chlamydial infection*, or genital *herpes*, but infection may also follow injury to the cervix during childbirth or an operation on the uterus. Both acute and chronic forms of the condition may occur.

SYMPTOMS

Acute cervicitis is often symptomless and may not be discovered until the cervix is examined for some other reason. The cervix is inflamed and there may be a discharge from it.

Chronic cervicitis may produce a vaginal discharge, bleeding from the vagina after sexual intercourse or between periods, and pain low in the abdomen, sometimes felt only during sexual intercourse.

COMPLICATIONS

Untreated cervicitis can spread to cause *endometritis* (infection of the lining of the uterus) or *salpingitis* (infection of the fallopian tubes). If a pregnant woman has cervicitis, her baby may be infected during delivery, resulting in neonatal *ophthalmia* (an eye infection leading to blindness), or, less commonly, pneumonia caused by chlamydial infection.

DIAGNOSIS AND TREATMENT

A woman with the symptoms described should see her physician, who will probably examine the cervix

later (because of the small chance of missing an abnormality on one smear) and, if no abnormality is found, subsequently at one- to three-year intervals for the rest of her life. More frequent tests may be needed in women who change sex partners often or whose partner changes sex partners frequently.

Most family planning clinics perform cervical smears; women may also be tested by their physicians.

RESULTS

If the cells appear normal, no further treatment is required. If the cells appear abnormal, the smear is graded according to the cervical intraepithelial neoplasia (CIN) classi-

BIOPSY OF THE CERVIX

If a woman has recurrent abnormal smears, colposcopy and biopsy of suspicious areas will be performed. If the abnormal area cannot be seen completely by colposcopy, a larger sample of tissue is removed by cone biopsy. This procedure is used for treatment as well as diagnosis.

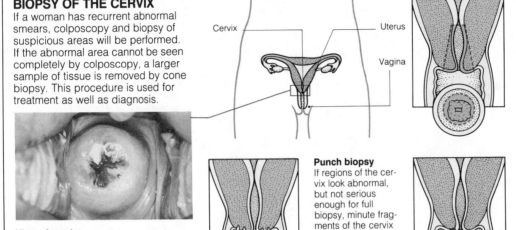

Cervix — **Uterus**

Vagina

Cone biopsy
Using general anesthesia, a cone-shaped piece of the cervix (containing an area with abnormal cells) is removed with a scalpel. The resulting crater is repaired by stitching flaps of tissue over the wound. Alternatively, the wound may be left open and diathermy or freezing used to stop any bleeding. Recently, lasers (left) have been used to destroy abnormal tissue.

Punch biopsy
If regions of the cervix look abnormal, but not serious enough for full biopsy, minute fragments of the cervix are removed for examination.

View of cervix
The photograph shows the end-on appearance of the cervix after a biopsy specimen has been taken from its tip.

and take swabs of any discharge so that the microorganism responsible for the discharge can be identified.

Treatment is with antibiotics, such as tetracyclines or penicillin, or antiviral agents, such as acyclovir, depending on the cause of the infection. If symptoms persist, the inflamed area of the cervix may be cauterized by *electrocoagulation*, *cryotherapy*, or *laser treatment* to destroy the infected tissue.

Cervix

A small, cylindrical organ, an inch or so in length and less than an inch in diameter, comprising the lower part and neck of the uterus. The cervix separates the body and cavity of the uterus from the vagina.

The bulk of the cervix consists of fibrous tissue with some smooth muscle. This tissue makes the cervix into a form of sphincter (circular muscle), allowing for the great adaptability in its size and shape required during pregnancy and childbirth.

FUNCTION

After puberty, mucus secreted from the glandular cells in the cervix aids the entry of sperm into the upper cervix, which acts as a sperm reservoir. In the middle of the menstrual month, this mucus becomes less viscous and more favorable for sperm transport. Within the cervix, the sperm are protected and provided with their energy requirements by the mucus.

During pregnancy, the internal muscular fibers increase in size, thus

ANATOMY OF THE CERVIX

The cervix contains a central canal for passage of sperm and menstrual blood, and for childbirth. Both the canal and outer surface of the cervix are lined with two types of cells: mucus-secreting glandular cells and protective squamous cells.

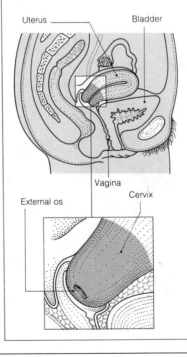

Uterus — Bladder

Vagina

External os — Cervix

lengthening the cervix, which acts as a barrier for retention of the fetus. Toward the end of pregnancy there is a general shortening of the cervix in readiness for labor and delivery. During labor the central canal widens up to 4 inches in diameter to allow the baby to pass from the uterus. Soon after childbirth the muscles in the cervix contract and the canal returns to its original size.

Cervix, cancer of

Cancer of the cervix (neck of the uterus) is one of the most common cancers affecting women worldwide, and in many areas is becoming more common. Untreated, it may spread directly and through the lymph nodes to most of the organs in the pelvis. The chances of cure depend very much on what stage the cancer has reached when first detected.

TYPES

Cervical cancer is one of the few cancers that has well-defined precancerous stages. Before any cancer appears, abnormal changes occur in cells on the surface of the cervix, referred to as various degrees of dysplasia, which are readily detected by a *cervical smear test* (Pap smear).

Mild dysplasia may later revert back to normal, but any woman who has an abnormal cervical smear should undergo further investigation and possible follow-up smears.

If more severe dysplasia or early cancer is detected, it can be treated and cured completely.

DISORDERS OF THE CERVIX

The cervix (neck of the uterus), with its central position in the female reproductive tract, is susceptible to injury, infections, and tumors.

INJURY

Minor injury to the cervix is common during childbirth, especially if labor has been prolonged or if forceps have been used to deliver the baby's head. These injuries usually take the form of a laceration (tear) in the side wall. Usually they can be repaired immediately after delivery, but rarely they may extend into the tissues surrounding the uterus and lead to internal bleeding, requiring major surgery.

Injury may also occur if the cervical canal is inexpertly dilated (widened) in the process of an abortion, especially if the woman has not had children. However, the risk of such injury is extremely small if the abortion is carried out in a well-equipped hospital or clinic by a qualified gynecologist.

When an injury does occur, there is a danger that the muscle fibers within the cervix will be damaged or weakened, leading to a condition called *cervical incompetence*. The ability of the cervix to retain a fetus in the uterus is impaired, with a risk of miscarriage unless the weakness is repaired.

INFECTION

Cervical infections are common and usually sexually transmitted, but may cause no or few symptoms. *Gonorrhea* and *chlamydial infections* are the two most frequent and are sexually transmitted. These infections may spread to the lining of the uterus or to the fallopian tubes with a risk of causing infertility (see *Cervicitis; Endometritis; Salpingitis*).

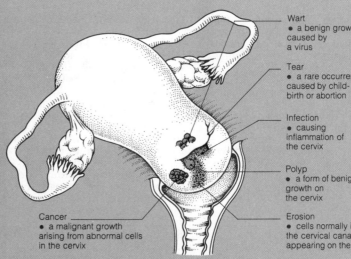

Wart
• a benign growth caused by a virus

Tear
• a rare occurrence caused by childbirth or abortion

Infection
• causing inflammation of the cervix

Polyp
• a form of benign growth on the cervix

Erosion
• cells normally in the cervical canal appearing on the cervix

Cancer
• a malignant growth arising from abnormal cells in the cervix

Trichomoniasis is another common infection affecting the vagina and cervix; it is also sexually transmitted and caused by a protozoan parasite.

Viral infections of the cervix are becoming more common, especially those due to the human papilloma or wart virus and the herpes simplex virus. These infections are sexually transmitted and are associated with warts or herpetic ulcers in other parts of the reproductive tract (see *Warts, genital; Herpes, genital*). Both have been incriminated in cancerous and precancerous conditions of the cervix.

TUMORS

Growths may be benign or malignant (cancerous). The former are usually present in the form of a polyp.

Malignant growths are always preceded by changes in the surface layer of cells, called cervical dysplasias. These changes can be detected by a *cervical smear test* (Pap smear) and alert the gynecologist to the need for

possible further investigation and treatment to prevent a cancer from developing (see *Cervix, cancer of*).

OTHER DISORDERS

Mucus-forming cells typical of those usually found in the cervical canal may appear as a layer on the outer surface of the cervix, causing a tendency to bleed. This relatively harmless condition is readily treated (see *Cervical erosion*).

INVESTIGATION

Investigation is by means of an internal examination (see *Pelvic examination*), a *cervical smear test*, and, in cases of suspected cancer or a precancerous condition, a *colposcopy*.

CAUSES AND INCIDENCE

Two main types of invasive (malignant) cervical cancer occur before or after the menopause.

SQUAMOUS TYPE This is by far the most common type of cervical cancer and is almost certainly the result of some process that occurs during sexual intercourse, probably transmission of an infectious organism to the cervix from the male partner. Recent evidence suggests that the culprit organism is a strain of the human papilloma, or wart, virus, which can

infect the penis (see *Warts, genital*). A woman in a sexual relationship with a man with genital warts has a high risk (about one in three) of developing a precancerous condition of the cervix. For this and other reasons, men with penile warts should seek treatment from their physicians.

There are 45 different strains of the human wart virus, but traces of one in particular, called HPV16, have been found in 90 percent of squamous-type cervical cancers and in 50 to 70 percent of precancerous conditions.

Other factors may predispose to the cancer. Female smokers are at higher risk than nonsmokers, possibly because smoking impairs the *immune system* (defenses against infection) in the vagina, allowing entry and proliferation of a causative virus.

The sexual behavior of a woman and her male partner(s) strongly influences the chances of her developing the disease. The earlier a woman and/or her partner(s) first started having sex, and the greater the number of sexual partners they have had, the higher the risk that she will develop a precancerous condition.

ADENOCARCINOMA The causes of this much rarer type of cervical cancer are unclear. Both sexually active women and those who have never had intercourse are susceptible.

The overall incidence of cervical cancer per 100,000 population in the US is about 17 new cases of cancer, leading to four to five deaths per year. Although the incidence of diagnosed cervical cancer and precancerous conditions has been increasing in the US for several years, the death rate has been decreasing for over 30 years, and should continue to do so due to more widespread, regular, and efficient cervical smear (Pap smear) testing.

SYMPTOMS
The precancerous stages cause no symptoms whatsoever. Symptoms of the malignant stage are also initially few. Eventually, a woman will notice vaginal bleeding or a bloodstained discharge at unexpected times—between periods, after intercourse, or after the menopause.

If left untreated, the cancer spreads from the cervical surface into the deeper parts of the cervix and then out into the pelvic tissues, causing pain. Eventually it enters the bladder, rectum, or surrounding pelvic tissue.

DIAGNOSIS
The precancerous stages are not visible to the naked eye and can be detected only by a cervical smear test or by *colposcopy* (inspection of the cervix under magnified illumination). All sexually active women are advised to have this test soon after their first experience of sexual intercourse, again six to 12 months later, and at regular intervals thereafter.

Diagnosis of more advanced stages may be made from a cervical smear, colposcopy, *cone biopsy*, or from a physician seeing areas of ulceration or cauliflowerlike growths on the cervix after symptoms are experienced.

TREATMENT
If a persistent area of abnormality or localized early cancer is diagnosed by colposcopy and biopsy and can be seen in its entirety, destruction is by *electrocoagulation, diathermy,* or *laser treatment* (all of which use heat to destroy tissue), or by *cryosurgery* (which uses cold). All methods except diathermy can usually be carried out painlessly using local anesthesia. Success rates for complete removal after one application of laser or diathermy are about 95 percent. In pregnancy, treatment of precancerous conditions

or early cancer is usually delayed until after delivery.

If an area of abnormality or cancer has spread into the canal, close inspection of a cone biopsy may show that this procedure has removed all the diseased tissue. In all other cases of spreading cancer, treatment will depend on the extent of the spread, the age of the patient, and the physician's recommendation for surgery or radiation therapy.

In more advanced cases, when the tumor has spread to the organs of the pelvis, radiation therapy is given. In specialized centers, radical surgical techniques may be employed for selected patients, in which bladder, vagina, cervix, uterus, and rectum may all be removed.

Survival rates (five or more years after treatment) are about 50 to 80 percent for early spreading cancer, whether treated by surgery or radiation therapy, dropping to 10 to 30 percent for later-stage disease. Among patients selected for radical surgery, the survival rate improves to about 30 to 50 percent.

Cesarean section

An operation to deliver a baby from the uterus through a vertical or horizontal incision in the abdomen. Cesarean section is performed when it is impossible or dangerous to deliver the baby vaginally. In the past 15 years the number of cesarean sections performed in the US has increased dramatically to around 25 percent of all births. This is partly because of the increased safety of the operation, but also because obstetricians fear litigation if a difficult birth leads to complications for the mother or baby.

The procedure is done under anesthetic (see illustrated box, opposite). For the first 24 hours, the bladder catheter remains in place and the patient is given analgesics (painkillers). Usually, the mother can drink 12 hours and eat 24 hours after the operation. The recovery period tends to be much quicker when an epidural rather than a general anesthetic has been used. Barring problems, hospital stay following the operation is a few days.

HISTORY
Cesarean section, which takes its name from the Latin "to cut," was first performed in ancient Rome when it was required by law in the event of maternal death. According to legend, Julius Caesar was born in this way. In the eighteenth century, desperate

women tried to perform the procedure on themselves, but most died in the attempt. Not until the present century has the procedure been considered safe for both mother and child.

Cestodes

 The scientific name for *tapeworms*—a group of long, flat, multisegmented parasites. Cestodes live in the intestine, where they may grow to more than 20 ft (6 m) long. Their larvae may infest other parts of the body, such as the brain (causing *cysticercosis*) or muscles. Tapeworms are acquired by eating raw or undercooked meat or fish. They may cause anemia.

Chagas' disease

An infectious parasitic disease found only in parts of South and Central America and spread by certain insects commonly called "cone-nosed" or "assassin" bugs. The disease is named after the Brazilian physician Carlos Chagas (1879-1934).

CAUSES AND INCIDENCE
The parasites responsible for Chagas' disease are single-celled organisms called trypanosomes, very similar to those that cause *sleeping sickness* in Africa. They live in the bloodstream and can also affect the heart, intestines, and nervous system.

Chalazion

A round, painless swelling on the upper or lower eyelid, sometimes known as a meibomian cyst. It results from obstruction (by its own secretion) of one of the meibomian glands that lubricate the edge of the eyelids. If the swelling is large, the pressure on the cornea at the front of the eye can cause blurring of vision.

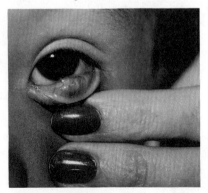

A chalazion on the lower lid
Many small chalazions disappear spontaneously. Larger ones may require surgery.

C

PROCEDURE FOR A CESAREAN SECTION

A cesarean section allows delivery of a baby through a horizontal or vertical cut in the abdominal and uterine walls. The mother is usually given epidural anesthesia, so that she remains conscious during the procedure, but general anesthesia is sometimes used.

HOW IT IS DONE

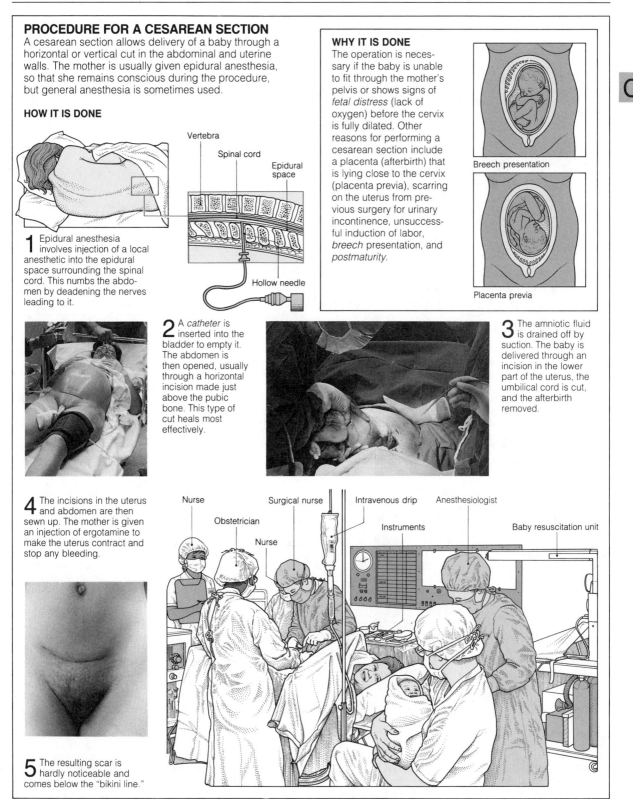

Vertebra

Spinal cord

Epidural space

1 Epidural anesthesia involves injection of a local anesthetic into the epidural space surrounding the spinal cord. This numbs the abdomen by deadening the nerves leading to it.

Hollow needle

WHY IT IS DONE

The operation is necessary if the baby is unable to fit through the mother's pelvis or shows signs of *fetal distress* (lack of oxygen) before the cervix is fully dilated. Other reasons for performing a cesarean section include a placenta (afterbirth) that is lying close to the cervix (placenta previa), scarring on the uterus from previous surgery for urinary incontinence, unsuccessful induction of labor, *breech* presentation, and *postmaturity*.

Breech presentation

Placenta previa

2 A *catheter* is inserted into the bladder to empty it. The abdomen is then opened, usually through a horizontal incision made just above the pubic bone. This type of cut heals most effectively.

3 The amniotic fluid is drained off by suction. The baby is delivered through an incision in the lower part of the uterus, the umbilical cord is cut, and the afterbirth removed.

4 The incisions in the uterus and abdomen are then sewn up. The mother is given an injection of ergotamine to make the uterus contract and stop any bleeding.

Nurse

Obstetrician

Nurse

Surgical nurse

Intravenous drip

Instruments

Anesthesiologist

Baby resuscitation unit

5 The resulting scar is hardly noticeable and comes below the "bikini line."

C

Chalazions can occur at any age and are particularly common in people suffering from the skin conditions *acne*, *rosacea*, or seborrheic *dermatitis*. If the cyst becomes infected the lid becomes more swollen, red, and painful. About one third disappear without any treatment, but large cysts usually need to be removed surgically using a local anesthetic.

Chancre, hard
An ulcer, usually on the genitals, that develops during the first stage of the sexually transmitted disease *syphilis*.

The chancre usually first appears as a dull red spot some 14 to 30 days after infection. It may occur on the penis, the anus, the vulva (the folds at the entrance of the vagina), or the inside of the vagina. The chancre can also occur on the lips or in the throat if oral sex has taken place. The spot gradually develops into a virtually painless ulcer, about one third of an inch in diameter, with a clearly defined edge and a thick rubbery base.

Diagnosis is made by microscopic examination of a smear of the chancre; blood test results may begin to be positive at this time.

TREATMENT
Any skin or mouth abnormality that might be a hard chancre should be reported to a physician immediately. A course of penicillin injections almost always prevents primary syphilis from developing into the later, more serious stages of the disease.

Chancroid
A sexually transmitted disease common in the tropics; it is characterized by painful ulcers on the genitals and enlarged lymph nodes in the groin. Also known as soft chancre and soft sore, the disorder is caused by the bacterium HEMOPHILUS DUCREYI.

The infection is relatively rare in the US and Europe; most cases that do occur involve sailors or travelers who have had contact with prostitutes in tropical countries.

TREATMENT
Prompt treatment with antibiotics usually clears up the problem. If the disease is left untreated, abscesses can form in the groin area and leave deep scars.

Chapped skin
Sore, cracked, rough skin on areas that have been repeatedly wet, inadequately dried, or exposed to the cold. The hands, face, and lips are most commonly affected.

Chapping occurs when the skin becomes excessively dry due to lack, or removal, of the natural oils that help keep it supple. This tends to happen in cold weather because the oil-secreting glands produce less oil. Repeated washing removes the oils.

Chapped skin can often be prevented by using protective gloves or barrier creams and by drying the skin carefully. Skin that has already become chapped usually responds well to applications of a rich, lanolin-based hand cream or face cream.

Character disorders
See *Personality disorders*.

Charcoal
A form of carbon. Charcoal's main medical use is as an emergency treatment for some types of poisoning and drug overdose.

Charcot-Marie-Tooth disease
An inherited muscle-wasting disease that mainly affects the legs. (See *Peroneal muscular atrophy*.)

Charcot's joint
A joint damaged by injuries that go unnoticed because of a neuropathy (loss of sensation) affecting the joint. Thus, the person cannot tell that certain activities are causing damage. (See *Neuropathic joint*.)

Checkup
See *Examination, physical*.

Cheilitis
Inflammation, cracking, and dryness of the lips. It can be caused by ill-fitting dentures, a local infection, allergy to cosmetics, too much sunbathing, or riboflavin (vitamin B_2) deficiency. In riboflavin deficiency, the corners of the mouth are chiefly affected. Until the underlying problem is remedied, a soothing skin cream will relieve the soreness.

Chelating agents
Chemicals used in the treatment of poisoning by metals such as lead, arsenic, and mercury. They act by combining with these metals to form less poisonous substances, which are usually excreted in the urine at a faster rate. Penicillamine is a commonly used chelating agent.

Chemonucleolysis
The injection of the enzyme chymopapin into a prolapsed intervertebral disk (see *Disk prolapse*) that is pressing on the spinal nerve root, causing *sciatica*. The enzyme dissolves the soft center of the disk, causing it to shrink, thus relieving the pressure on the nerve. Following initial enthusiasm, the frequency with which this procedure is performed seems to be declining. Chemonucleolysis is an alternative to surgical removal of the disk by *laminectomy* or to decompression of the spinal nerve root (see *Decompression, spinal canal*) in patients who have not been helped by conservative measures, such as bed rest or traction.

Chemotherapy
The treatment of infections or malignant diseases by drugs that act selectively on the cause of the disorder, but which may have substantial effects on normal tissue.

Infections are treated by *antibiotics*, which may be bactericidal (killing harmful bacteria) or bacteriostatic (stopping further bacterial growth and allowing the body's immune system to take over and destroy the bacteria). In the same way, *anticancer drugs* act either by destroying tumor cells or by stopping them from multiplying.

One problem with chemotherapy is that natural selection leads to the emergence of resistant bacteria or cells. This effect is minimized by the discriminatory use of antibiotics, and, in cancer chemotherapy, by giving several different types of drugs simultaneously. A further problem with cancer chemotherapy is that the drugs act on all rapidly dividing cells, not just tumor cells. Thus, they affect the bone marrow, the intestinal lining, the hair follicles (sometimes causing baldness), and the mouth, sometimes causing severe side effects. Antibiotics act more selectively because bacteria have a different structure from human cells, making side effects less of a problem for the patient.

Chenodiol
A chemical in *bile* that reduces the amount of cholesterol released by the liver into the bile.

Chenodiol is sometimes prescribed as a treatment for small *gallstones* if they contain mainly cholesterol and no calcium. Treatment takes several months, during which time progress is monitored by X rays or *ultrasound scanning* of the gallbladder. Chenodiol may cause diarrhea and, rarely, liver damage. It should not be taken during pregnancy because of possible adverse effects on the fetus.

Chest

The upper part of the body. Known technically as the *thorax*, the chest extends from the base of the neck to the *diaphragm*.

Chest pain

Chest pain usually does not have a serious cause, though occasionally it may be a symptom of a disorder that requires medical attention. The pain may occur in the chest wall (in the skin, underlying muscles, or ribs) or in an organ within the chest.

CAUSES

The most common causes of pain in the chest wall are a strained muscle (which is usually due to exercise) or an injury, such as bruising or a broken rib (due to a blow, fall, or other accident).

Pressure on a nerve root attached to the spinal cord may result in a sharp pain that travels to the front of the chest. This pain may be caused by *osteoarthritis* of, or injury to, the vertebrae, or, more rarely, a *disk prolapse*. Pain in the side of the chest may be due to *pleurodynia* (inflammation of the muscles between the ribs and the diaphragm associated with a viral infection). In rare cases, the viral infection *shingles* can cause pain in the chest wall. The pain, which is severe, runs along the course of a nerve and is followed by a rash of blisters in the *dermatome* (area of skin supplied by the same nerve). Inflammation of the junctions of the bony ribs and their cartilage or the junctions of the cartilage and the breastbone may cause chest pain that increases as the chest cage moves (*Tietze's syndrome*).

Within the chest, pain may be caused by *pleurisy* (inflammation of the pleurae, the membranes surrounding the lungs and covering the inner surface of the chest wall), which may be brought on by *bronchitis*, *pneumonia*, or, rarely, by *pulmonary embolism* (a blood clot lodged in an artery in the lungs). The pain of pleurisy is worse when the sufferer breathes in.

Malignant tumors of the lung (see *Lung cancer*; *Mesothelioma*) may cause pain as they grow and press on the pleura and ribs.

Acid reflux, a cause of heartburn, is a burning pain behind the breastbone produced by acid fluid from the stomach being regurgitated into the esophagus. It may occur as a symptom of *hiatal hernia*.

Various heart disorders can cause chest pain. The most common is *angina pectoris*, which is due to the

DIAGNOSING CHEST PAIN

To make an accurate diagnosis of the underlying cause, it is important for the patient to describe the location, quality (i.e., burning, pressing, or sharp), severity, and duration of the pain, any factors that relieve it or make it worse, and any other symptoms, such as breathing difficulty. In addition, the physician will perform a physical examination, including listening to chest sounds with a stethoscope and feeling for areas of tenderness in the chest wall. He or she may also arrange for other diagnostic procedures to be carried out.

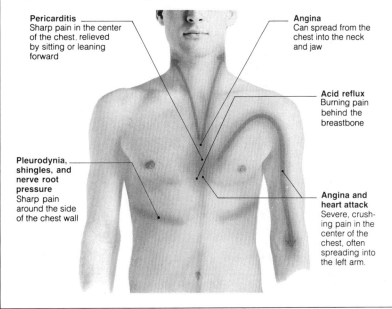

Pericarditis
Sharp pain in the center of the chest, relieved by sitting or leaning forward

Angina
Can spread from the chest into the neck and jaw

Acid reflux
Burning pain behind the breastbone

Pleurodynia, shingles, and nerve root pressure
Sharp pain around the side of the chest wall

Angina and heart attack
Severe, crushing pain in the center of the chest, often spreading into the left arm.

heart muscle receiving too little blood (and therefore oxygen), commonly as a result of *coronary heart disease*. The pain, which resembles that of severe indigestion or of a heavy weight pressing on the chest, is felt in the center of the chest and may spread outward to the throat, jaw, or arms (usually the left one). It usually is associated with effort or some acute stress that places an added work load upon the heart muscle. Stable angina pectoris may be present for many years. *Myocardial infarction* (damage to the heart muscle due to an inadequate blood supply) produces pain in the same areas as angina does but the pain is more severe. This is the crushing pain of a heart attack.

The pain of acute *pericarditis* (inflammation of the pericardium, the membrane that surrounds the heart) is also felt in the center of the chest. In some cases it is severe enough to resemble the pain of a heart attack. It can often be relieved by leaning forward. Acute pericarditis is rare and tends to occur in young adults after or with a viral infection.

Mitral valve prolapse has been associated with many symptoms, including chest pain. The chest pain may be sharp and left-sided. Chest pain may also be a result of anxiety and emotional stress. (See *Hyperventilation*; *Panic attack*.)

INVESTIGATION AND TREATMENT

Chest pain not associated with a trivial cause (such as bruising from a minor injury) should receive medical attention. Whether or not emergency treatment is necessary depends on the type and location of the pain and on the accompanying symptoms.

The treatment of chest pain depends on the underlying cause. For example, antibiotics may be prescribed for chest pain caused by pneumonia, and surgery may be necessary for the treatment of a malignant lung tumor or for some cases of coronary heart disease.

Chest X ray

One of the most frequently performed medical tests, usually carried out to examine the heart or lungs. The procedure is simple, quick, and painless,

C

CHEST PAIN Pain anywhere between the neck and the bottom of the rib cage that may be dull and persistent, stabbing, burning, or crushing.

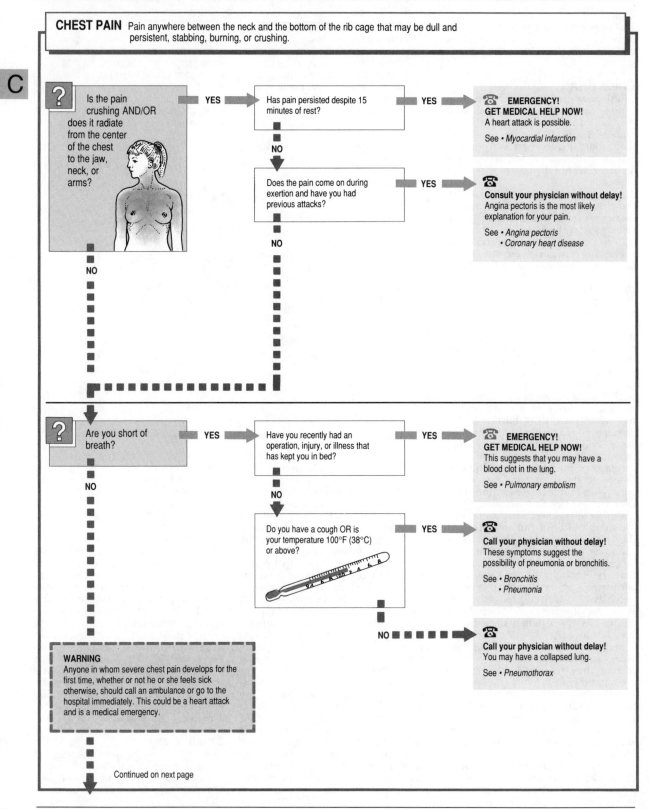

? Is the pain crushing AND/OR does it radiate from the center of the chest to the jaw, neck, or arms?

YES ▶ Has pain persisted despite 15 minutes of rest?

YES ▶ ☎ **EMERGENCY! GET MEDICAL HELP NOW!** A heart attack is possible.

See • *Myocardial infarction*

NO ↓

Does the pain come on during exertion and have you had previous attacks?

YES ▶ ☎ **Consult your physician without delay!** Angina pectoris is the most likely explanation for your pain.

See • *Angina pectoris*
• *Coronary heart disease*

NO ↓

NO ↓

? Are you short of breath?

YES ▶ Have you recently had an operation, injury, or illness that has kept you in bed?

YES ▶ ☎ **EMERGENCY! GET MEDICAL HELP NOW!** This suggests that you may have a blood clot in the lung.

See • *Pulmonary embolism*

NO ↓

Do you have a cough OR is your temperature 100°F (38°C) or above?

YES ▶ ☎ **Call your physician without delay!** These symptoms suggest the possibility of pneumonia or bronchitis.

See • *Bronchitis*
• *Pneumonia*

NO ▶ ☎ **Call your physician without delay!** You may have a collapsed lung.

See • *Pneumothorax*

NO ↓

WARNING
Anyone in whom severe chest pain develops for the first time, whether or not he or she feels sick otherwise, should call an ambulance or go to the hospital immediately. This could be a heart attack and is a medical emergency.

Continued on next page

C

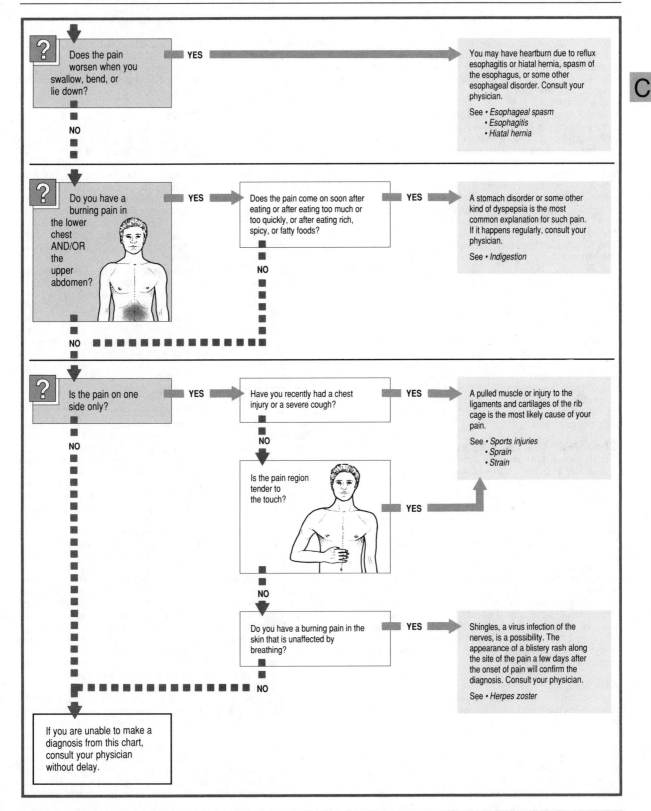

Does the pain worsen when you swallow, bend, or lie down?

YES → You may have heartburn due to reflux esophagitis or hiatal hernia, spasm of the esophagus, or some other esophageal disorder. Consult your physician.

See • *Esophageal spasm*
    • *Esophagitis*
    • *Hiatal hernia*

NO

Do you have a burning pain in the lower chest AND/OR the upper abdomen?

YES → Does the pain come on soon after eating or after eating too much or too quickly, or after eating rich, spicy, or fatty foods?

YES → A stomach disorder or some other kind of dyspepsia is the most common explanation for such pain. If it happens regularly, consult your physician.

See • *Indigestion*

NO

NO

Is the pain on one side only?

YES → Have you recently had a chest injury or a severe cough?

YES → A pulled muscle or injury to the ligaments and cartilages of the rib cage is the most likely cause of your pain.

See • *Sports injuries*
    • *Sprain*
    • *Strain*

NO

Is the pain region tender to the touch?

YES →

NO

Do you have a burning pain in the skin that is unaffected by breathing?

YES → Shingles, a virus infection of the nerves, is a possibility. The appearance of a blistery rash along the site of the pain a few days after the onset of pain will confirm the diagnosis. Consult your physician.

See • *Herpes zoster*

NO

NO

If you are unable to make a diagnosis from this chart, consult your physician without delay.

C

and is normally performed on an out-patient basis. Mobile equipment means that it can also be used (although somewhat less accurately) at the bedside of patients in the hospital, in the homes of immobilized people, and elsewhere.

WHY IT IS DONE
Chest X rays are usually used to confirm a diagnosis in patients suspected of having heart or lung disease, such as lung cancer, tuberculosis, or enlargement of a heart chamber.

HOW IT IS DONE
The X-ray machine contains a film in a large, flat cassette positioned at chest level. The patient stands facing the film cassette with the chest touching it and the chin projecting over the top. The hands are placed on the hips and the elbows swung forward, to move the shoulder blades to the side so that they do not obscure the lungs. A lead apron or screen protects the lower half of the body from radiation.

The patient takes (and holds) a deep breath and the radiographer then passes X rays through the upper trunk for a fraction of a second, from equipment behind the patient. The resultant X-ray picture provides an image not only of the heart and lungs but of major blood vessels, bones and joints, the esophagus, stomach, liver, and other organs and structures.

Cheyne-Stokes respiration
An abnormal pattern of breathing in which the rate and depth of respiration varies rhythmically. Deep, rapid breathing gradually becomes slower and shallower until breathing actually stops for some 10 to 20 seconds. Respiration then resumes, with deep, rapid breathing, and the cycle repeats itself. Each cycle lasts a few minutes.

Cheyne-Stokes respiration may be caused by disease or malfunctioning of the part of the brain that controls breathing (as occurs in some cases of *stroke*, head injury, metabolic dysfunction, or drug overdose). It may also occur as a result of *heart failure* and in some healthy people at high altitudes, especially during sleep.

Chickenpox
A common and mild infectious disease of childhood, characterized by a rash and slight fever. It is sometimes called varicella. Chickenpox is rare in adults; when it does occur it usually takes a more severe form.

INCIDENCE AND CAUSE
Throughout the world, most people have had chickenpox by the age of 10.

The disease is caused by the varicella-zoster virus. Although an attack confers lifelong immunity, the virus remains dormant within nerve tissues after the attack and may cause *herpes zoster* later in life.

The virus is spread from person to person in airborne droplets. Patients are highly infectious from about two days before the rash appears until about a week after.

All healthy children should be exposed to chickenpox so that they can catch the illness at an age when it is no more than an inconvenience. However, adults who have never had the disease should avoid it by staying away from children with chickenpox and also from anyone with shingles. Women in the final stage of pregnancy should be particularly careful since, if they catch the disease, the newborn child may develop a severe attack.

SYMPTOMS
One to three weeks after infection, a rash appears on the trunk, face, under the armpits, on the upper arms and legs, inside the mouth, and sometimes in the windpipe and bronchial tubes, causing a dry cough. The rash consists of a mass of small, red, itchy spots that become fluid-filled blisters within a few hours. After several days the blisters dry out and form scabs. Children usually have only a slightly raised temperature, but an adult may have severe pneumonia with breathing difficulties and fever. Those taking *immunosuppressant drugs* may also have a severe form of the disease.

Rarely, *encephalitis* (inflammation of the brain) occurs as a complication.

DIAGNOSIS AND TREATMENT
Diagnosis is usually obvious from a simple examination of the patient. In most cases rest is all that is needed for complete recovery, which usually takes place within 10 days in children, but over a longer period in adults. Acetaminophen can be taken to reduce fever, and calamine lotion relieves the itchiness of the rash. In severe cases the antiviral drug acyclovir may be prescribed. Children should be discouraged from scratching the blisters, which could lead to secondary bacterial infection (keeping the child's nails short is a good idea).

No vaccine against chickenpox is available or envisaged.

Chigger bite

An intensely irritating, itchy swelling, about half an inch in diameter, caused by the minute larva

of the harvest or red mite. Found on grass and weeds in summer, the mites attach themselves to the legs, particularly the ankles, of humans and feed on the blood. The swelling may become a blister, and sometimes the itching persists for weeks.

Chigoe

A painful, itchy, pea-sized swelling caused by a sand flea (also called the jigger or burrowing flea). When stepped on, the flea penetrates into the skin of the feet, under the toenails, or between the toes.

The chigoe flea lives in sandy soil only in Africa and tropical America. The burrowing fleas are pregnant females, which lay their eggs under the skin.

Avoidance involves wearing shoes or sandals outdoors in tropical countries (this also protects against *hookworms*). In the event of a suspected chigoe infestation, consult a physician. Chigoe fleas should be removed with a sterile needle and the wounds treated with an antiseptic.

Chilblain
See *Pernio*.

Child abuse
Any form of serious mistreatment of a child, whether physical or mental, including the use of a child for sexual gratification. Cases of child abuse today are coming to light with increasing frequency, probably not because such abuse is more widespread, but because there is a greater awareness of the problem.

Child abuse appears to be more common in lower socioeconomic groups, partly because of the greater stress on poor families with low living standards. However, the problem occurs at all levels of society, although it may be less easily recognized in higher socioeconomic classes.

The person injuring the child is usually a parent, but may be a step-parent, a parental friend or love interest, or someone to whom care of the child has been delegated.

CAUSES
Being ill-treated when young seems to predispose people to abuse their own children by repeating the pattern of their own experience. This is particularly likely if the abused people have become parents at an early age, when they are too immature and inexperienced to cope with the demands made on them by a young child.

Children under age 3 are at greatest risk of abuse (other than sexual) because at this time a child is most demanding and is not yet old enough to be reasoned with.

Alcoholism, drug addiction, or emotional disturbances are other causative factors, since they may lessen a parent's self-control.

PHYSICAL ABUSE

Physical injury is the most readily recognized and diagnosed type of abuse. The National Center for the Prevention of Child Abuse and Neglect estimates that approximately 1 to 2 million children in the US are maltreated each year. Of this number 200,000 are sexually exploited and 200,000 to 300,000 are psychologically abused. An estimated 4,000 children die annually from child abuse.

Inflicting injury on a child is in most cases an impulsive act, the result of a sudden loss of temper. Infants and toddlers may be picked up and shaken vigorously, which can damage the eyes and rupture blood vessels in the brain and eventually cause severe brain damage. Slapping or punching is usually delivered to the head, resulting in black eyes and other facial bruises, cuts on the inner lip, and, less commonly, bone fractures. Injuries of abuse present different characteristics than those that occur accidentally and may reveal to a physician or other examiner that, whatever the reason given for them by the parents, deliberate infliction is the real cause.

Premeditated, repeated physical assault is rare. When it does occur it is a sign that a parent is severely disturbed and that the risks to the child are grave. These types of assaults can lead to multiple fractures, damage to internal organs, and even to death. Such abuse is sometimes accompanied by deliberate neglect, with no attempt made to adequately feed or clothe the child.

A child with nonaccidental injuries is usually admitted to the hospital for full examination and tests. He or she may then be removed from the home while members of the health, social, and probation services, and often a police representative, assess the case and decide on the best course of action. The child's interests remain paramount, but the parents, who may be under considerable stress, should be treated sympathetically.

EMOTIONAL ABUSE OR NEGLECT

Neglect of physical and emotional needs, such as love, stimulation, and guidance, is another form of abuse

recognized only more recently by courts. Such abuse is usually unintentional, arising from the parents' lack of understanding of their child's needs. Intentional abuse indicates that the parents are emotionally disturbed and require psychiatric help.

Indications that a child is being emotionally abused include failure to thrive, slow development, and lack of normal emotional responses. The diagnosis usually is confirmed when the child begins to put on weight and become more responsive after he or she is taken into the hospital for observation. Management of the situation is the same as for physical abuse.

SEXUAL ABUSE

This form of abuse has been increasingly recognized in recent years. Most frequently sexual abuse occurs within the family; usually the victim is a girl, although there is some evidence that indicates adolescent boys may also be at risk. Sexual exploitation of both sexes occurs in pornography and prostitution.

Most cases of sexual abuse consist of a father, close relative, or family friend taking advantage of a girl's affection to obtain sexual gratification from her. This form of abuse is secretive, because of the man's awareness of the gravity of the offense, and morally coercive, because of the power he holds over the girl.

Sexual abuse may come to light because of an obvious complaint from the child, a relative, or friend, or the child may display disturbed behavior or have other symptoms, such as venereal infection. Police, psychiatrists, and social workers usually cooperate in management of the problem, the main aim being to prevent further sexual abuse and to rehabilitate the child through therapy. Although the offender may be convicted, every effort is made to keep the family unit together.

Childbed fever

See *Puerperal sepsis*.

Childbirth

The process by which an infant is moved from the uterus to the outside world. Childbirth normally occurs at between 38 and 42 weeks' gestation (pregnancy), timed from the mother's last normal menstrual period.

In previous centuries women of all social classes commonly died in childbirth; maternal mortality still remains high in developing countries. In Western countries, however,

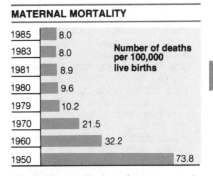

MATERNAL MORTALITY

Year	Deaths per 100,000 live births
1985	8.0
1983	8.0
1981	8.9
1980	9.6
1979	10.2
1970	21.5
1960	32.2
1950	73.8

Number of deaths per 100,000 live births

Mortality for complications of pregnancy and childbirth in selected years from 1950 to 1983 shows a dramatic decrease.

deaths and complications of childbirth have declined dramatically since the start of this century. Much of this decline is due to improvements in women's general health; the remainder has resulted from advances in the medical treatment of the complications of pregnancy and labor—most notably the availability of blood transfusion and antibacterial drugs.

Although the role of specialized equipment and drugs in improving safety during childbirth cannot be denied, women have become concerned about the increased mechanization of childbirth. Hence, the popularity of "natural childbirth," which advocates the avoidance of unnecessary medical intervention. Hospitals have begun to recognize the right of women to choose the type of birth they prefer (as long as it is compatible with safety). This choice may include the option of having people present during the birth and the type of pain relief, if any, the woman would like to have administered.

More flexibility is also being shown in allowing women to choose the position they prefer for giving birth. For many years, the supine position has been traditional in the US and many European countries. Historically, however, this position is a fairly recent innovation, not introduced until the eighteenth century.

Most hospitals still transfer the mother from the labor ward to a separate delivery room when she is ready to have the baby. Some hospitals now have alternative birthing rooms, where the mother can deliver in a homelike atmosphere with medical facilities at hand.

ONSET OF LABOR

It is often difficult to know when labor has started. During the last three months of pregnancy the uterus starts

C

STAGES OF BIRTH

The time it takes for a baby to be born depends on several factors, but primarily on whether it is a first or later baby. The first stage of labor can take 12 or more hours for a first baby, but only a few hours for a subsequent one. The mother is usually examined vaginally (or, on occasion, rectally) every two to four hours to assess the extent of dilation.

Fetal heart monitoring is performed throughout all stages of labor, and the frequency, strength, and duration of the mother's contractions are recorded.

Once delivered, the baby is usually placed on the mother's abdomen or warmed, dried, and quickly checked by a nurse or pediatrician.

ELECTRONIC FETAL MONITORING

This may be carried out if the fetus is at risk, or as a routine procedure. The detecting device is linked to a monitoring machine.

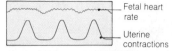

Printout

Fetal heart rate

Uterine contractions

Detecting devices

Here, the baby's heart beat is picked up by a metal plate strapped to the mother's abdomen (lower belt). A plate beneath the upper belt detects the mother's contractions.

An alternative method is to attach to the baby's head an electrode linked to the monitor by a wire led through the mother's vagina.

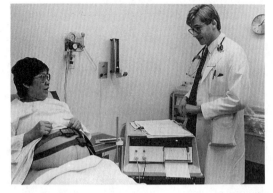

THE FIRST STAGE

With the first contractions, the normally thick, tough cervix becomes thinned and softened and is gradually pulled up until it becomes effaced (merged with the walls of the uterus). The cervix then begins to dilate (open) with each contraction. It is fully dilated when the opening is approximately 4 inches (10 cm) in diameter. This stage can take anywhere from a few hours to 12 hours or more for first babies.

Uterus

Cervix

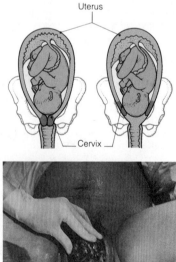

The head emerges
At this point, an episiotomy is sometimes performed to prevent tissues from tearing.

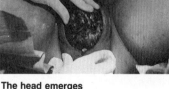

THE SECOND STAGE

As the baby's head descends, it reaches the pelvic floor muscles, which cause the head to rotate until eventually the baby's chin is pointing down to the woman's rectum. As the baby is pushed farther down, the anus and perineum (the area between the genitalia and anus) begin to bulge out, and soon the baby's head can be seen at the opening of the vagina. As the head emerges, the perineal tissues are stretched very thin; sometimes it is necessary to perform an *episiotomy* to prevent the tissues from tearing. As soon as the baby's head emerges, it turns so that it is once more in line with the rest of the baby's body; the physician usually helps this rotation.

With the next few contractions, first one shoulder and then the other is delivered; then the rest of the baby slides out. After delivery, the umbilical cord is clamped and cut.

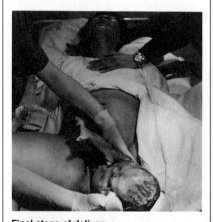

Final stage of delivery
Once both shoulders are out, the rest of the baby emerges easily.

THE THIRD STAGE

Within three to 10 minutes after the baby's birth, the placenta (afterbirth) is usually expelled. Drugs such as ergonovine or oxytocin may be used to aid in its expulsion, or the placenta may be manually removed by the physician. Any tears or incisions are cleaned and stitched. This may be done while the mother holds her baby.

Placenta

Umbilical cord

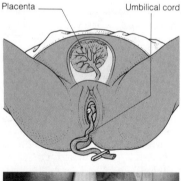

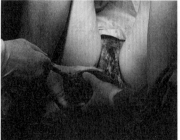

Placenta being delivered
The placenta is usually expelled within a few minutes of the baby's birth.

to contract in preparation for the birth, and these *Braxton Hicks' contractions* may be mistaken for the start of labor. However, when contractions become progressively more painful, regular, and at shorter intervals, then labor has probably started. Two other events may also happen. The mucous plug that has blocked the cervical canal during pregnancy may be expelled as a bloody discharge. This is called a "show" and means that the cervix is beginning to stretch. Rupture of the membranes surrounding the amniotic fluid in which the baby floats may occur at any time up to delivery. The leakage of amniotic fluid, called "breaking of the waters," varies from woman to woman. It may be a slow trickle of fluid from the vagina, or it may be a sudden gush.

STAGES OF LABOR

Labor is divided into several stages that are defined as though they are distinct, but which, in reality, can blend into one another. The latent phase (or prelabor) is a time of irregular contractions, when the cervix thins out and may dilate very gradually. This stage can last many hours. The first stage begins with rapid dilatation of the cervix and ends with full dilatation of the cervix.

After the cervix is fully dilated, the second stage begins; contractions become stronger and the women feels the urge to push (by contracting the voluntary muscles of the diaphragm and abdominal wall). She is advised to push only during a contraction.

The third stage of labor—expulsion of the placenta (afterbirth)—usually occurs within three to 10 minutes after delivery of the baby. Sometimes, medication such as ergonovine or oxytocin may be used to aid in the expulsion of the placenta, or the placenta may be removed manually by the physician reaching into the uterus. Any tears or incisions in the vagina are then cleaned and stitched.

Childbirth, complications of

Difficulties and complications occurring after the onset of labor. These complications may be associated with the mother or the baby, or both. Some are potentially life-threatening, especially to the baby, because they may impair its oxygen supply and cause brain damage (see *Fetal distress*).

MATERNAL PROBLEMS

If contractions begin, or if the membranes rupture, before 37 weeks' gestation, premature labor may occur, with the risk of delivery of a small, immature baby who may not be developed adequately to survive (see *Prematurity*). Drugs such as albuterol and ritodrine can sometimes stop premature labor. However, if the gestation period is more than 34 weeks and hospital conditions are suitable, the labor may be allowed to progress. Premature rupture of the membranes can also lead to infection in the uterus, which must be treated with delivery and antibiotics.

Slow progress early in a normal labor is most often the result of failure of the cervix to dilate, usually due to inadequate contractions of the uterine muscles. This is often treated by giving intravenous infusions of synthetic oxytocin to augment the naturally occurring oxytocin that causes the muscles of the uterus to contract during labor.

The mother may tire during a long labor so that she is unable to push strongly enough, or the muscular contractions of the uterus may be ineffective; in these cases *forceps delivery, vacuum extraction,* or even *cesarean section* may be required.

A major hazard in childbirth is blood loss. This may occur before the delivery (see *Antepartum hemorrhage*), either because the placenta separates from the wall of the uterus too early or, less commonly, because the placenta lies over the opening of the cervix instead of being attached to the wall of the uterus, a condition called *placenta previa*. Blood loss after the delivery (*postpartum hemorrhage*) is usually due either to failure of the uterus to contract normally after the child has been expelled or to retention of part of the placenta. With blood transfusions, complications from hemorrhage have decreased dramatically in the last 40 years.

In rare instances, women suffer from *eclampsia* (convulsions associated with raised blood pressure) during or just prior to the onset of labor. This is treated by giving anticonvulsant drugs and oxygen and inducing labor or performing a cesarean section.

FETAL PROBLEMS

If the baby is in a malposition (not lying in the normal headdown position in the uterus), vaginal delivery may be difficult or impossible. A baby in the breech position (bottom downward) can be delivered vaginally, although delivery by cesarean section may be preferable (see *Breech delivery*). A baby lying horizontally is always delivered by cesarean section because the arm and shoulder usually become jammed in the pelvis.

Multiple pregnancies (see *Pregnancy, multiple*) may be a problem during delivery because it is often difficult to predict the position of subsequent babies. It is also more likely that such babies will be born prematurely.

FETAL-MATERNAL PROBLEMS

Sometimes the mother's pelvis is too small in proportion to the baby's head (known as cephalopelvic disproportion), making vaginal delivery impossible or hazardous. In these cases, cesarean section is usually necessary.

PAIN RELIEF IN LABOR AND DELIVERY

Method	Why given	Possible effects on baby
Narcotic analgesics	Routine pain relief during labor	Less responsive at birth; respiratory problems, particularly in premature babies
Epidural	Routine pain relief during labor and childbirth, forceps delivery, and cesarean section	Brief drop in fetal heart rate; fetal monitoring is recommended during and after the procedure
Paracervical block	Pain relief during active labor (after the fetal head is engaged)	Drop in fetal heart rate; respiratory problems
Pudendal block	Forceps delivery	None
Local anesthetic into perineum	Forceps delivery, episiotomy, repair perineal tear	None
General anesthesia	Cesarean section	Reduced responsiveness at birth; respiratory problems, particularly in premature babies

C

FIRST AID: EMERGENCY CHILDBIRTH

PREPARING FOR THE BIRTH

1 Summon medical help and reassure the mother. Stay calm—most births are normal and natural.

2 Wash hands and scrub nails under running water. Do not dry them. Wash hands frequently during the birth. Make sure everything you use is clean: bedding, sheets, towels, and cloths.

3 Prepare a flat surface, using a clean sheet or towel, a plastic sheet, or fresh newspaper.

4 Prop the mother up with pillows. Her legs should be bent and apart, and the feet flat.

> **WARNING**
> DO NOT attempt to delay the birth by crossing the mother's legs or pushing in the baby's head. This is very harmful.

YOU WILL NEED

- Sterilized scissors (boil for 10 minutes and wrap in clean cloth).
- Clean pieces of string, boot laces, or strips of cloth about 9 inches (22 cm) long for tying the cord.
- Container in case the mother vomits.
- Container or plastic bag for the afterbirth (which must be taken to a physician for examination).
- Sanitary napkins or clean cloth to place over the mother's vagina after the birth.
- Cradle (or a box or drawer) and soft blanket for the baby.

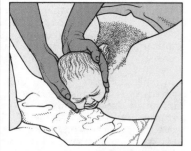

1 As the baby's head emerges, support it with cupped hands. If a membrane covers the face, tear it with your hands and remove quickly. If the cord is looped around the neck, ease it gently over the head. DO NOT touch the baby's head until it is out.

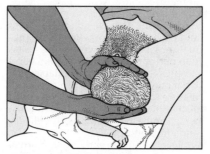

2 Support the shoulders as they emerge. One appears first, the second follows easily if you carefully raise the head. DO NOT pull on the baby's head.

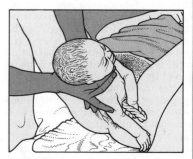

3 Support the body as it comes out. Using a clean cloth, wipe away any mucus or blood from the baby's mouth.

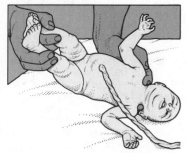

4 If the baby fails to breathe immediately, hold the head lower than the body to drain mucus away. DO NOT slap the baby on the back. Blow hard on the chest or tap the soles of the feet. If these methods fail, start *artificial respiration*.

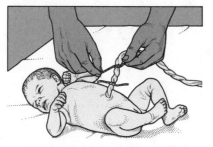

5 When the cord has stopped pulsating, tie it firmly once 6 to 8 inches (15 to 20 cm) away from the baby and again 2 to 4 inches (5 to 10 cm) away. Cut between the ties with sterilized scissors. Wrap the baby and place on the mother's abdomen.

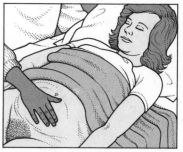

6 The afterbirth is delivered within 10 minutes. To help control blood flow, place a hand on the mother's abdomen and gently massage the uterus every few minutes until it feels firm. DO NOT pull on the cord to deliver the afterbirth.

Child development

Children acquire physical, mental, and social skills in well-recognized stages called developmental milestones. Although there is wide variation in the rate at which each child progresses, most children develop certain skills by a predictable age.

FACTORS AFFECTING DEVELOPMENT

A child becomes capable of developing certain skills only as his or her nervous system matures. The rate at which maturity occurs is determined genetically for each individual and modified by environmental factors in the uterus and after birth. For instance, girls often begin to walk and/or talk at an earlier age than boys. Premature children miss out on some growing time in the uterus; the time they take to progress should be calculated from the full-term pregnancy date, not the actual date of birth.

Sight and hearing are both crucial to a child's general developmental progress; any defect will affect the child's ability to watch, listen, learn, and imitate. Intelligence also affects a child's development, especially in the acquisition of speech and the ability to coordinate muscles for precise movements, such as holding a pencil.

The home environment plays an important part in developing the child's potential for certain skills. Speaking to and playing with children is essential for language development and for practicing new physical skills. Introducing children to other children at the age of 2 or 3 years provides them with plenty of stimulation.

HOW A CHILD DEVELOPS SKILLS

Reflex actions present at birth gradually disappear as the child learns to perform voluntary actions and develops sufficient muscle strength and control to perform them. Often, the child's actions progress from seemingly unconnected movements to the ability to control part of his or her body. In most children, development begins with control of the head and progresses down the body until control of the arms, trunk, and legs is attained. Walking is achieved in numerous stages, from lying with head raised, to sitting unsupported, to crawling, to toddling, to standing, and, finally, to walking unaided.

A baby begins to develop hand-eye coordination from birth. He or she watches objects, learns to focus and to judge distances, and develops the connection of seeing and doing by watching his or her hands. Both hand-eye and body-limb coordination can

be encouraged in an older child (by practicing ball games, for example).

At birth, a child communicates his or her needs by crying. After vision and hearing are sufficiently well developed, a child watches the parent's mouth intently to learn how to smile and listens to the parent speaking before attempting to imitate sounds. A child is able to concentrate on learning only one skill at a time, often forgetting a recently mastered skill that will appear again some time in the future.

DEVELOPMENTAL MILESTONES

When assessing the development of a child, specialists in child development look at abilities in four main areas: locomotion, hearing and speech, vision and fine movement, and social behavior and play. All children acquire skills in much the same order—for example, a child will not stand before learning to sit. The rate at which these skills are acquired varies enormously; a more detailed professional investigation is necessary (see *Developmental delay*) only if a child's progress is significantly out of line or if the parent is concerned for some other reason. (See next page.)

Child guidance

Multidisciplinary diagnosis and advice for a child who is suffering from emotional or *behavioral problems*. The problems may include poor school performance, disruptive behavior at school or at home, other behavioral problems, breaking the law, or using drugs.

SOURCES OF HELP

Trained professionals and lay workers from a number of fields offer help to such children and their families. A physician will arrange referral to the most appropriate team for assessment and, possibly, therapy.

Psychiatrists are medical doctors with a special interest and training in the field of mental problems. Their techniques may range from *psychotherapy* to treatment with drugs.

Clinical and educational *psychologists* are nonmedical specialists whose main role is diagnosis and assessment by means of intelligence and personality tests. They may also assess a child's progress during treatment. Many clinical psychologists also provide psychotherapy.

Psychiatric social workers are also nonmedical specialists. They are trained to deal with family problems and relationships within the family. In some instances they may be given

legal responsibility for children with severe personality or family problems.

These specialists often work closely together, either in hospital pediatric departments, schools, or special child-guidance clinics, using *counseling, group therapy,* or *family therapy.*

Chill

A shivering attack accompanied by chattering teeth, pale skin, goose bumps, and a cold feeling. It frequently precedes a fever, usually one caused by an infection. Treatment includes drinking plenty of fluids. A physician should be consulted if the condition persists.

Chinese medicine

Most of the various techniques of traditional Chinese medicine are based on the theory that there is a universal life force, called "chi," that manifests itself in the body as two complementary qualities known as "yin" and "yang." According to traditional beliefs, the vigorous yang and restraining yin must be balanced, and the chi must flow evenly for good health. An imbalance in the yin and yang and disruption of the flow of chi produce illness. Traditional Chinese treatments therefore aim to restore the yin-yang balance and normalize the flow of chi. To achieve this aim various techniques have evolved, notably *acupressure, acupuncture,* Chinese *herbal medicine,* and *t'ai chi.*

In general, these treatments are incompatible with orthodox Western medicine and most physicians do not recommend them. However, some techniques may help when standard treatment has not been effective.

Chinese restaurant syndrome

A short-lived illness that some people develop after eating food containing *monosodium glutamate* (MSG). Only about 5 percent of the population is susceptible to it.

SYMPTOMS AND PREVENTION

The most common symptoms, which usually occur within three hours of a meal, are pain in the neck and chest, a hot feeling, heart palpitations, and headache. Nausea, dizziness, and other symptoms have also been reported, and some people compare Chinese restaurant syndrome to the effects of migraine.

The symptoms pass and have no long-term effects. Affected people should avoid food containing MSG as an additive. Many "fast foods" may also contain the additive.

C

C

CHILD DEVELOPMENT

LOCOMOTION

By 6 months, babies lift up their heads and chests and roll from front to back and from back to front. They can sit up with support, bounce up and down, and bear weight on their legs if supported.

9-month-old children try to crawl, sit without support, pull themselves up to standing or sitting positions, and step purposefully on alternate feet if supported.

1-year-old children crawl on hands and knees, walk around furniture (holding on), and may walk alone or with one hand held.

At 18 months, children can walk well with feet closer together, can stoop to pick up objects, run with care, walk upstairs with one hand held, and crawl backward downstairs.

VISION AND FINE MOVEMENT

By 6 months, babies look intently at everything and everybody. They follow moving objects with their eyes and reach out for objects with one or both hands. Objects are transferred from hand to hand and brought to the mouth.

9 month olds are visually very alert. Grasp involves mostly the index and middle fingers. They can manipulate objects with both hands, but have difficulty voluntarily releasing grasped objects.

1-year-old children can grasp small objects well and release grasped objects easily. Both hands are used equally. They can hold a block in each hand and bang the blocks together.

At 18 months, children can build a tower of three blocks (when shown), enjoy turning pages of a book, can grip a crayon, scribble, and make dots. They may use one hand more than the other.

HEARING, UNDERSTANDING, AND SPEECH

By 6 months, babies turn their heads to locate sources of sound and have begun to understand the tone of their mothers' voices. They enjoy making vowel sounds and tuneful noises. They laugh, chuckle, and squeal.

9 month olds listen to sounds and understand "no" and other words. They babble in long strings (making sounds such as ba-ba, da-da, ma-ma) and start using sound to attract attention. (Deaf babies' utterances are monotonous and do not develop in complexity.)

1-year-old children turn when they hear their own names. They have some understanding of how other people feel, know what most household objects are used for, may babble meaningfully to themselves, and may say two or three words.

At 18 months, children comprehend short communications spoken directly to them, but do not understand the difference between statements, commands, and questions. Vocabulary may contain six to 20 words.

SOCIAL BEHAVIOR AND PLAY

6 month olds enjoy looking at their images in mirrors and playing peekaboo games. They can grasp objects and also shake, bang, and otherwise manipulate them. However, they will not look for objects that are shown and then hidden. They are shy with strangers.

9 month olds look for objects that are shown and then hidden, thus showing the beginnings of memory. They imitate hand clapping, wave bye-bye, and show great determination in getting objects. They continue to be shy with strangers.

1-year-old children spend less time putting objects in their mouths and more time releasing objects—throwing them, dropping them, putting them in boxes. They play pat-a-cake and like to be around a familiar adult to whom they demonstrate affection.

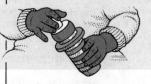

At 18 months, children actively explore their homes. They enjoy putting things in and taking things out of boxes and looking at picture books. They use spoons and cups and can take off their shoes and socks. They are also determined, impetuous, selfish, and cannot be reasoned with. They alternate between clinging to a familiar adult and struggling to break free.

C

LOCOMOTION

2 year olds climb furniture and walk up and down stairs (with two feet to each step).

3 year olds can climb with agility, throw and kick balls, ride tricycles, and run around corners.

4 year olds walk up and down stairs with one foot on each step, and can stand, walk, and run on tiptoe.

5 year olds can stand and hop on one foot, and are skillful in rolling, sliding, and swinging.

VISION AND FINE MOVEMENT

2 year olds can build towers of six or seven blocks, can unscrew a lid, and show a definite right- or left-handedness.

3 year olds hold crayons with an adult grasp and can undo buttons, but may need help buttoning them up. Their handedness is clearly established.

4 year olds hold a pencil with a mature grasp, can copy simple letters (i.e., O,T,H, or V), and can build a tower of more than 10 blocks.

5 year olds can match 10 or 12 colors, can copy many more letters, and can draw the full body of a person with a recognizable head and facial features.

HEARING, UNDERSTANDING, AND SPEECH

2 year olds begin to listen to general conversation. They obey simple instructions and can use 50 or more words meaningfully. They constantly talk to themselves and can put two or more words together to communicate.

3 year olds listen to general conversation and enjoy nursery stories. They understand the difference between statements, commands, and questions. They have large vocabularies and speak clearly in sentences, but there may be some errors.

4 year olds can repeat softly spoken words at a distance of three feet. They speak fluently and with correct grammar and can provide their full names, ages, and addresses. They tell long stories, confusing fact and fantasy.

5 year olds enjoy reciting rhymes, telling stories, and having books read to them.

SOCIAL BEHAVIOR AND PLAY

2 year olds ask the names of everything and enjoy participating in nursery rhymes and songs. They ask for food and drink and indicate toilet needs. They begin to play with toys more imaginatively, though they may not like to share them. They are constantly demanding and will throw tantrums if their desires are thwarted.

3 year olds constantly ask questions. They can dress and undress and eat with a fork and spoon. They are dry and clean during the day and sometimes at night. Three year olds can play with toys imaginatively and will share with others. They can be reasoned with and have fewer tantrums. They are also more affectionate to younger siblings.

4 year olds continue to ask questions constantly. They are more independent and skillful in dressing, undressing, eating, and washing. They need to play with other children and can share with others. They can understand past, present, and future.

5 year olds ask the meaning of abstract words. They like to build complex structures out of bricks or other objects. They continue in imaginative and dramatic play. They enjoy companionship and understand the need for rules and fair play. They have an understanding of time and are generally sensible, restrained, and independent.

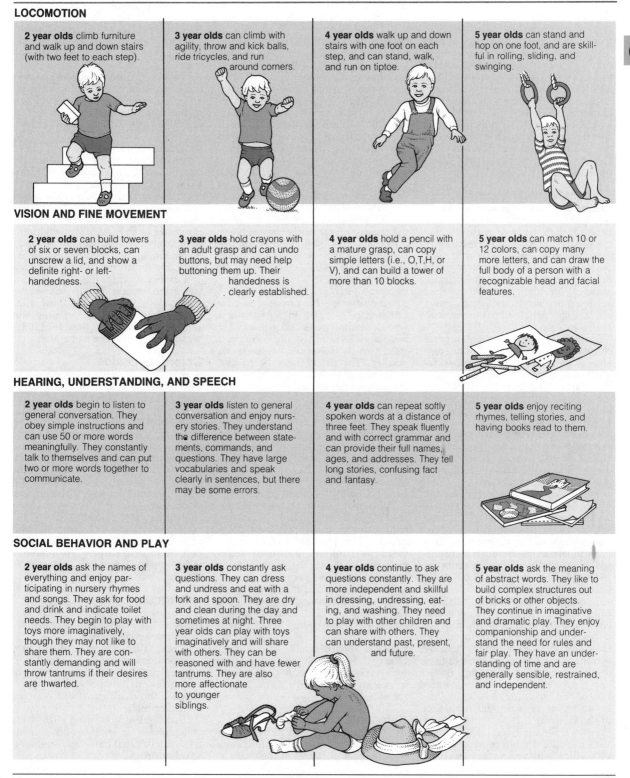

Chiropody
See *Podiatry*.

Chiropractic
A theory of healing based on the belief that disease results from a lack of normal nerve function. Chiropractic relies on physical manipulation and adjustment of the spine for therapy, rather than on drugs or surgery. Physicians believe that no scientific basis for chiropractic theory has ever been established and that it is ineffective in the treatment of such common ailments as hypertension, heart disease, stroke, cancer, diabetes, and infectious diseases.

Chlamydial infections
Chlamydiae are a group of microorganisms, intermediate in size between bacteria and viruses, that cause various infectious diseases in humans and animals (particularly birds). Like viruses, they can multiply only by first invading the cells of another life-form; otherwise, they behave more like bacteria than viruses and are susceptible to treatment with antibiotic drugs.

Two main species of chlamydiae cause disease in humans. Different strains of *CHLAMYDIA TRACHOMATIS* are responsible for various genital, eye, and lymph node infections. *CHLAMYDIA PSITTACI* mainly affects birds, but is occasionally spread to humans as a lung infection.

CHLAMYDIA TRACHOMATIS INFECTIONS
GENITAL INFECTIONS In the tropics, strains of *CHLAMYDIA TRACHOMATIS* cause the sexually transmitted disease *lymphogranuloma venereum*.

In developed countries, by far the most important impact of *CHLAMYDIA TRACHOMATIS* is its role as a cause of *nonspecific urethritis* (NSU), or nongonococcal genital infection. This is the most common sexually transmitted disease in the US, and in almost 50 percent of cases it is due to a chlamydial infection.

In men, nonspecific urethritis may cause a discharge from the penis and complications such as swelling of the testes, which, if untreated may lead to infertility. In women, NSU is usually symptomless, but may cause a vaginal discharge or pain on passing urine, and may lead to *cervicitis* (inflammation of the cervix) or cause complications such as *salpingitis* (inflammation of the fallopian tubes). In the US, an estimated 5 to 13 percent of all women have a chlamydial infection of the cervix (which is often symptomless).

Treatment is with antibiotics such as tetracycline or erythromycin and is usually rapidly successful. Treatment of sexual partners is advisable to prevent reinfection.

EYE INFECTIONS A child born to a woman with a chlamydial infection of the cervix may acquire an acute eye infection called neonatal *ophthalmia*.

In parts of Africa and Asia, usually where hygiene is lacking, certain strains of *CHLAMYDIA TRACHOMATIS* cause the serious eye disease *trachoma*. It is spread from eye to eye by flies and is the most important cause of blindness worldwide.

RESPIRATORY INFECTIONS *CHLAMYDIA TRACHOMATIS* is a major cause of pneumonia among infants in the US; up to three or four newborn babies per 1,000 are affected, and 50 percent of the children usually also have an eye infection. The main symptoms are breathing difficulty and a staccato cough, but no fever. Treatment is with antibiotic drugs.

CHLAMYDIA PSITTACI
The only disease that can be caused by *CHLAMYDIA PSITTACI* in humans is a type of pneumonia called *psittacosis*. It is a rare infection, usually contracted from parrots, parakeets, pigeons, or poultry. The disease can be treated with antibiotics, but it may be fatal in elderly and debilitated patients.

Chloasma
A condition, also called melasma, in which blotches of pale, green-brown skin pigmentation appear on the face. Chloasma may occur during pregnancy, around the time of the menopause, or in women who have been taking birth-control pills.

The blotches occur on the forehead, cheeks, and nose, and sometimes merge, forming the "mask of pregnancy." The pigmentation is aggravated by sunlight. It usually fades gradually, but may be permanent or recur in successive pregnancies.

There is no treatment, although avoiding direct sunlight and changing the brand of birth-control pill (if appropriate) may help.

Chloral hydrate
One of the oldest *sleeping drugs* in use today. It is mainly used as a short-term treatment for insomnia, especially in the elderly.

Chlorambucil
An *anticancer drug* used to treat some types of cancer, including Hodgkin's lymphoma and cancer of the ovary.

Chloramphenicol
An *antibiotic drug* widely prescribed as eye drops or an ointment to treat *conjunctivitis* caused by a bacterial infection. In tablet or injection form, chloramphenicol is used only in the hospital for the treatment of serious infections that are resistant to safer antibiotics. Chloramphenicol given in these ways carries a risk of causing aplastic *anemia* (a complete shutdown of the bone marrow's production of red cells, white cells, and platelets).

Chlorate poisoning
Chemicals present in some defoliant weed killers that, if swallowed, cause kidney and liver damage, corrosion of the intestine, and methemoglobinemia (a chemical change in the blood pigment hemoglobin). Even small doses can prove fatal, especially in children. Symptoms of poisoning include ulceration in the mouth, abdominal pain, and diarrhea.

If chlorate poisoning is known or suspected, medical help should be obtained immediately. If these substances have been spilled onto the skin or into the eyes, they should be washed off with plenty of water.

Chlordiazepoxide
A *benzodiazepine drug* used mainly to treat anxiety, but also in the management of alcohol withdrawal.

Chloroform
A colorless liquid producing a vapor that, if inhaled, acts as a general anesthetic (see *Anesthesia, general*). Formerly, it was used widely for operative procedures but it caused a high incidence of liver damage and heart problems and has now been replaced by safer drugs.

Chloroform is still occasionally used as an emergency anesthetic for major first aid or field surgery. Its main use today is as a flavoring and preservative for other medicines.

Chloroquine
A drug used in the prevention and treatment of *malaria* and occasionally as an *antirheumatic drug*.

When taken to prevent malaria, chloroquine is usually prescribed with other drugs to avoid problems of drug-resistant strains. Chloroquine remains the main treatment of acute attacks of malaria.

Chloroquine is used to treat *rheumatoid arthritis* and *lupus erythematosus* that have not responded to other drugs.

Possible side effects are nausea, headache, diarrhea, and abdominal cramps. Long-term treatment (as for rheumatoid arthritis) can damage the retina, causing blindness.

Chlorosis

A severe form of iron-deficiency *anemia* characterized by a yellow-green tinge to the skin. During the nineteenth century and before World War I, chlorosis was a common condition among underfed adolescent girls. This form of anemia has now virtually disappeared.

Chlorothiazide

One of the thiazide group of *diuretic drugs* often used as a treatment for *hypertension* (high blood pressure) and edema (fluid retention). It also reduces the amount of calcium excreted in the urine and is therefore sometimes used to prevent the recurrence of certain types of kidney stone.

Chlorpheniramine

An *antihistamine drug* used in the treatment of allergies such as allergic *rhinitis* (hay fever), allergic *conjunctivitis*, *urticaria* (hives), and *angioedema* (allergic facial swelling). It is also a common ingredient of over-the-counter *cold remedies*.

Chlorpromazine

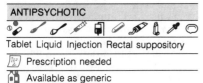

ANTIPSYCHOTIC			
Tablet	Liquid	Injection	Rectal suppository

Prescription needed	
Available as generic	

The first *antipsychotic drug* to be marketed. Introduced in the early 1950s, it remains one of the most widely used of this group of drugs. It suppresses abnormal behavior, reduces aggression, and has a tranquilizing effect.

WHY IT IS USED

Chlorpromazine is used in the treatment of schizophrenia, mania, dementia, and other disorders in which confused or abnormal behavior may occur. It does not cure the underlying disorder, but does relieve distressing symptoms.

Another use of chlorpromazine is in the treatment of nausea and vomiting, especially if caused by drug treatment, radiation therapy, or anesthetics.

POSSIBLE ADVERSE EFFECTS

Chlorpromazine sometimes produces serious side effects. These include uncontrollable movements of the face and limbs similar to those in *Parkinson's disease*, slowed reactions, and blurred vision; driving and operating machinery should be avoided. Alcohol should not be drunk when taking chlorpromazine because it increases the sedative effect.

Chlorpropamide

A drug used to treat *diabetes mellitus*. (See *Hypoglycemics, oral*.)

Chlorthalidone

One of the thiazide group of *diuretic drugs*, chlorthalidone is used to treat *hypertension* (high blood pressure) and *heart failure*. It reduces the amount of calcium in the urine and is sometimes used to prevent the recurrence of certain types of kidney stone.

Chlorzoxazone

A *muscle-relaxant drug* used mainly to treat painful muscle spasm caused by injury, strain, or misuse.

Choking

Partial or complete inability to breathe due to an obstruction of the airway, usually by food, drink, or an inhaled or swallowed foreign body. If the blockage is only partial, the choking person can usually inhale enough air to cough out the obstruction. If the airway is completely blocked, the person will be unable to breathe and, unless the blockage is cleared, he or she will die of suffocation.

CAUSES

Choking is caused by blockage of any part of the airway—the pharynx (throat), larynx (voice box), trachea

---

FIRST AID: CHOKING

CONSCIOUS VICTIM

1 A person clutching his or her throat is giving the universal distress signal for a foreign body blocking the air passage.

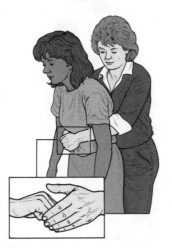

2 Clasp the victim, placing one fist just under the sternum and grasping the fist with the other hand. Then make a quick, hard, thrusting movement inward and upward.

UNCONSCIOUS VICTIM

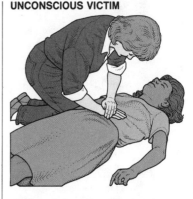

1 Place the heel of one hand against the middle of the victim's abdomen, slightly above the navel; place your other hand on top. Press in with a quick upward thrust.

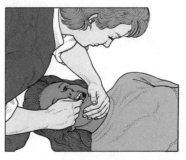

2 If this fails, try to remove the obstruction. If the victim is still unconscious, summon emergency help. If breathing has stopped, start *artificial respiration*.

C

FIRST AID: CHOKING

INFANT

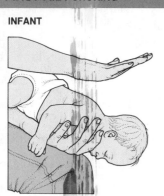

Straddle the baby over your arm with the head lower than the trunk, supporting the head by holding the baby's jaw. Deliver four back blows between the shoulder blades.

CHILD

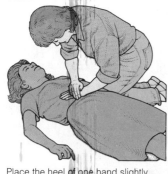

Place the heel of one hand slightly above the navel and well below the rib cage. Place the other hand on top and press down with a quick, upward thrust.

(windpipe), or bronchi (air passages from the trachea into the lungs). Most cases of choking occur when food or drink "goes down the wrong way," that is, when it enters the trachea (airway) and bronchi instead of passing from the pharynx into the esophagus. Although this can be an alarming experience, it is normally corrected by a bout of coughing.

Obstruction by something that partially blocks the airway is more serious. In adults the cause is usually a fishbone or a piece of meat. In children, who are more vulnerable to this type of choking because their airways are narrower, the obstruction is often a peanut or small plaything, such as a bead. Less commonly, choking may be due to aspiration (inhaling vomit) during a bout of coughing.

TREATMENT
Emergency medical help should be summoned if the obstruction cannot be cleared. The physician will probably try to clear the blockage manually; if this fails, an emergency *tracheostomy* (making an incision into the trachea and inserting a tube through it into the lungs), will be performed. With the airway restored, the physician can then use a laryngoscope, bronchoscope, or esophagoscope (viewing tubes through which instruments can be passed) to locate and clear the obstruction (see *Laryngoscopy*; *Bronchoscopy*; *Esophagoscopy*).

Cholangiocarcinoma
A malignant growth in one of the ducts that carries bile from the liver and gallbladder to the small intestine. The disease is rare, with less than one new case per 100,000 of the population each year in the US. The cause of the cancer is unknown. The main symptoms of cholangiocarcinoma are jaundice and weight loss.

Cholangiography
A procedure that enables the bile ducts to be seen on X-ray film after they have first been filled with a contrast medium (a substance that is opaque to X rays).

WHY IT IS DONE
Cholangiography is used when people who have had their gallbladders removed are suspected of having biliary stones. Biliary stones are similar to gallstones, but they form in the bile ducts instead of the gallbladder. Cholangiography is usually employed as a follow-up to *ultrasound scanning* if it has failed to establish the presence of stones. Cholangiography is also performed during an operation to remove the gallbladder to ensure that no stones have been left behind in the bile ducts. Cholangiography is also useful for diagnosing narrowing or tumors of the bile ducts.

HOW IT IS DONE
The contrast medium may be injected slowly into a vein, in which case the liver will excrete it several hours later in bile into the ducts (in this case, images are somewhat less satisfactory than those obtained by the following methods). Or the contrast medium may be injected directly into the ducts. This is done either through an endoscope (a flexible viewing instrument) passed into the ducts via the mouth, stomach, and duodenum (see *ERCP*), or by means of a long, fine needle inserted through the abdomen into

the liver. Once the ducts have filled, X-ray pictures are taken and any stones are apparent.

Cholangitis
Inflammation of the common bile duct (see *Biliary system*). There are two types: acute ascending cholangitis and sclerosing cholangitis.

ACUTE ASCENDING CHOLANGITIS
This type is usually due to bacterial infection of the duct and its content of bile. It generally occurs with a blockage of the duct—by a gallstone, tumor, following surgery, or, in some parts of the world, infestation of the duct by a worm or fluke (see *Bile duct obstruction*). The infection moves up the duct and may affect the liver.

The main symptoms are recurrent bouts of jaundice, abdominal pain, and chills and fever. Attacks may vary from mild episodes to a severe, life-threatening illness with *septicemia* (spread and multiplication of bacteria in the bloodstream) and *kidney failure* from toxins circulating in the blood.

The infection is usually diagnosed from the patient's symptoms, although investigations such as *liver function tests* and *ultrasound scanning* may also be carried out.

Mild cases are treated with antibiotics and a high intake of fluids. In severe cases, if there is no improvement within 24 hours, the infected material is drained from the bile duct by surgery or endoscopy.

Once the patient has recovered, the cause of the blockage must be determined and appropriate treatment of the cause of the obstruction provided (see *Bile duct obstruction*).

SCLEROSING CHOLANGITIS
In this rare condition, all the bile ducts, within and outside the liver, become narrowed; the liver is progressively damaged. No treatment is available other than the possibility of a *liver transplant*. The drug cholestyramine may relieve itching.

Chole-
A prefix relating to the bile or biliary system, as in cholelithiasis (the formation of stones in the biliary system).

Cholecalciferol
An alternative name for vitamin D_3 (see *Vitamin D*).

Cholecystectomy
Surgery to remove the gallbladder.
WHY IT IS DONE
Cholecystectomy is usually performed to deal with the presence in

PROCEDURE FOR CHOLECYSTECTOMY

If simple removal of the gallbladder is performed, it will take approximately an hour. However, more extensive exploration of the ducts may prolong the procedure.

With the patient under general anesthesia, an incision is made under the rib cage on the right-hand side; the cut may be vertical, horizontal, or oblique, according to the patient's build.

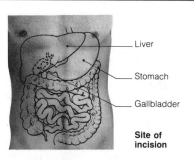

Liver

Stomach

Gallbladder

Site of incision

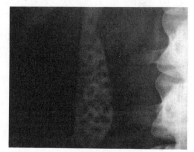

1 Gallstones, as shown by an ultrasound scan or by a cholecystogram (X-ray image of the gallbladder) such as the one above, increase in prevalence with age.

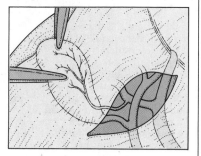

2 After an incision has been made, the liver is pulled up to expose the gallbladder. The thin membrane covering it is incised so that the cystic duct and artery can be identified.

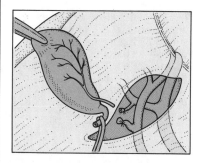

3 The artery to the gallbladder and the cystic duct leading from it are tied and cut, and the gallbladder is removed. If the person has jaundice, X rays are taken to ensure that there are no stones in the common bile duct. If the X ray reveals the presence of stones, they are removed.

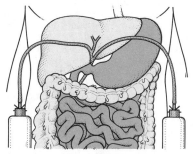

4 Drains are placed under the liver (and in the bile duct if it was opened) and the abdominal incision is closed. The two drains are removed, respectively, 48 hours and eight to 10 days later, after another X ray shows there are no more stones.

the gallbladder of troublesome *gallstones*, often because they are causing recurrent attacks of *biliary colic* (pain). Many surgeons advocate cholecystectomy at an early stage to treat acute *cholecystitis* (infection of the gallbladder). Emergency cholecystectomy is occasionally required for perforation (bursting) or *empyema* (pus formation) within the gallbladder.

Many gastroenterologists believe that gallbladders should not be removed if they contain stones that are not causing any symptoms.

HOW IT IS DONE

Simple cholecystectomy takes almost one hour, but duct exploration may add considerably to this time. Most patients are out of the hospital within five to seven days. (See box.)

RISKS AND OUTLOOK

The chief risk is inadvertent damage to the common bile duct. Severe inflammation sometimes obscures the anatomy and the surgeon may decide it is safer to perform a cholecystostomy (removal of gallstones by opening but not removing the gallbladder).

The outcome of cholecystectomy operations is generally good—symptoms are relieved completely in 90 percent of patients. About three weeks should be allowed for recovery from the operation.

Cholecystitis

Inflammation of the gallbladder, causing severe abdominal pain. There are two types: acute and chronic.

CAUSES

Acute cholecystitis is almost always caused by a *gallstone* obstructing the outlet (cystic duct) from the gallbladder. The trapped bile becomes concentrated by absorption of its water content and causes chemical irritation of the gallbladder walls; this is followed by bacterial infection of the stagnating bile.

Repeated mild attacks of acute cholecystitis can lead to chronic cholecystitis, in which the gallbladder walls thicken and the gallbladder shrinks and ceases to store bile. Whether chronic cholecystitis produces recognizable symptoms that justify surgery is controversial.

SYMPTOMS AND COMPLICATIONS

The main symptom of acute cholecystitis is severe constant pain in the right side of the abdomen, just under the ribs, which worsens on movement. The pain is accompanied by fever and, occasionally, jaundice.

In some people, complications develop. Complications may include *empyema* (in which the gallbladder fills with pus) and *peritonitis* (inflammation of the lining of the abdominal cavity) if the gallbladder bursts. In either event the patient is extremely sick and surgery is urgently needed.

The ill-defined gastrointestinal symptoms attributed to chronic cholecystitis are indigestion, vague pains in the upper abdomen, nausea, and belching. These symptoms may be aggravated by eating fatty food and are not invariably relieved by *cholecystectomy*.

DIAGNOSIS AND TREATMENT

A provisional diagnosis of acute cholecystitis is made by listening to a description of the symptoms and by performing a physical examination. The patient is usually admitted to the

C

hospital at once and given analgesics (painkillers), antibiotics, and an *intravenous infusion* to provide nutrients and fluid. *Ultrasound scanning* or *radionuclide scanning* may be used to make a firm diagnosis and exclude other possible causes of the pain, such as a perforated duodenal ulcer (see *Abdominal pain*).

Most cases subside without the need for urgent surgery, but, to prevent recurrences, the patient is usually advised to have a cholecystectomy (surgical removal of the gallbladder), which can be performed either during the initial attack or after an interval of several weeks. The same treatment is usually advised for chronic cholecystitis although the results are less certain. Loss of the gallbladder has little adverse effect on the digestive system.

Cholecystography

An X-ray procedure for examining the gallbladder and common bile duct after they have been filled with a contrast medium (a substance opaque to X rays). The main use of the technique is to detect gallstones, usually as a follow-up procedure to *ultrasound* if this test has failed to enable a definite diagnosis to be made. Cholecystography is not the procedure chosen first to study the gallbladder and is performed much less frequently than it once was.

HOW IT IS DONE
The patient swallows or is injected with contrast medium, which, after about 12 hours, is excreted by the liver into the bile. The opaque bile is stored by the gallbladder, which then shows up when X-ray pictures are taken. Gallstones, which do not absorb the contrast medium, appear on the film as "holes."

Cholera

An infection of the small intestine caused by the bacterium *VIBRIO CHOLERAE* (a vibrio is a comma-shaped bacterium). Cholera results in profuse watery diarrhea that in severe untreated cases can lead to rapid dehydration and death. Infection is always acquired by swallowing food or water that has been contaminated with the vibrio.

HISTORY, CAUSE, AND INCIDENCE
Cholera has been known for centuries in northeast India, where outbreaks of the disease occur regularly. In the nineteenth century, with the opening up of world trade routes and the increase in Muslim and Hindu

pilgrimages, cholera spread throughout the world, causing millions of deaths in a series of epidemics.

For the first half of the twentieth century the disease was confined to Asia, but since 1961 a new pandemic (worldwide epidemic) has spread from Indonesia to much of the rest of Asia, Africa, the Mediterranean, and the Gulf Coast of North America.

A handful of cases occurs in the US in most years, mainly among travelers who have returned from a visit to Asia or Africa. Occasionally, cases crop up in areas bordering the Gulf of Mexico and around the Mediterranean. Usually the victim has eaten shellfish, which appear capable of harboring the vibrio bacterium.

SYMPTOMS
Cholera starts suddenly, between one and five days after infection, with diarrhea, often accompanied by vomiting. Over a pint of fluid may be lost each hour in the diarrhea and, if not replaced, this loss of fluid causes death within a few hours. The fluid loss is brought about by the action of a toxin produced by a bacterium that greatly increases the passage of fluid from the bloodstream into the large and small intestines.

TREATMENT
Cholera is treated by replacing the lost fluid with drinks of water containing the correct proportions of various salts and sugar (see *Rehydration therapy*). If dehydration develops despite fluid replacement by mouth, the patient may be given extra fluid by means of intravenous infusion. Antibiotics, such as tetracycline hydrochloride, can shorten the period of diarrhea and infectiousness to others.

Given adequate rehydration, patients usually make a full recovery. In major epidemics following natural disasters, sufficient supplies of clean water may not be available—or so many people become ill simultaneously that there are few left to nurse the sick.

PREVENTION
Worldwide, cholera is controlled by improving sanitation—in particular by ensuring that sewage is not allowed to contaminate water supplies that will later be used for drinking. Travelers to cholera-infected areas should either restrict themselves to bottled drinks or boil all water before drinking.

A vaccine that provides some protection against the disease is advisable when traveling to Africa and to the Middle and Far East. The protection it

gives is short-lived (six months) and precautions still must be taken with drinking water. Usually, no country insists that travelers arriving directly from the US or Europe have a cholera vaccination certificate, but regulations change from time to time, and a certificate is sometimes required if travel has been via a cholera-infected area. International travelers should check vaccination requirements before departure. (See also *Dysentery; Gastroenteritis; Typhoid fever.*)

Cholestasis

Stagnation of bile in the small bile ducts within the liver, which leads to a characteristic type of jaundice and to liver disease. The obstruction to the flow of bile may be intrahepatic (within the liver) or extrahepatic (in the bile ducts outside the liver).

CAUSES
Intrahepatic cholestasis may be caused by viral *hepatitis* (inflammation of the liver) or may be a side effect of a number of drugs.

The bile ducts outside the liver can become blocked or constricted for a variety of reasons, including gallstones or tumors (see *Bile duct obstruction*); rarely, the ducts are absent from birth (see *Biliary atresia*).

TREATMENT
Extrahepatic bile duct obstruction and biliary atresia can often be treated surgically to guarantee a free passage of bile from the liver to the duodenum.

Drug-induced cholestasis usually disappears if the causative drug is stopped. In the case of viral hepatitis, there is no specific treatment; the flow of bile improves gradually as the liver inflammation resolves.

Cholesteatoma

A rare but serious condition in which skin cells proliferate and debris collects within the middle ear.

Cholesteatoma usually occurs as a result of a long-standing *otitis media* (middle-ear infection) that has caused the eardrum to burst (see *Eardrum, perforated*). In such cases, skin may grow inward from the ear canal into the middle ear. If the cholesteatoma continues untreated, it may grow and damage the small bones in the middle ear and surrounding bony structures.

Cholesteatoma requires surgical removal either through the eardrum or by mastoidectomy (excision of the mastoid bone behind the ear together with the cholesteatoma). If there is residual deafness, a hearing aid may be required.

Cholesterol

Chemically a *lipid*, cholesterol is an important constituent of body cells. It is also involved in the formation of *hormones* and bile salts and in the transport of fats in the bloodstream to tissues throughout the body. Most cholesterol in the blood is made by the liver from a wide variety of foods, but especially from saturated *fats*. However, some cholesterol is absorbed directly from cholesterol-rich foods, such as eggs and dairy products.

Both cholesterol and fats (triglycerides) are transported around the body in the form of lipoproteins. These are particles with a core, made up of cholesterol and triglycerides in varying proportions, and an outer wrapping of phospholipids and apoproteins ("carrier" proteins).

CHOLESTEROL-RELATED DISEASES

The level of cholesterol in the blood—which can be measured by analysis of a blood sample—is influenced by diet, heredity, and metabolic diseases such as *diabetes mellitus*. There is overwhelming evidence that a high blood cholesterol level increases the risk of developing *atherosclerosis* (accumulation of fatty tissue on the inner lining of arteries), and with it the risk of *coronary heart disease* or *stroke*. Recent research has shown that the risk of developing atherosclerosis can be assessed more accurately by measuring the proportions of different types of lipoproteins in the blood. In general, if most cholesterol in the blood is in the form of high density lipoproteins (abbreviated to HDLs), it seems to protect against arterial disease; conversely, if most cholesterol is in the form of low density lipoproteins (LDLs) or very low density lipoproteins (VLDLs), the risk of disease developing is increased.

A group of genetic metabolic disorders, the *hyperlipidemias*, cause abnormally high levels of LDLs in the blood; people with these disorders are susceptible to heart disease and stroke from an early age. Such people may need treatment with low fat diets and drugs to lower the level of LDLs in their blood. People with relatives who have had a heart attack or stroke before age 50 are at risk and should have their blood checked.

Cholestyramine

A *lipid-lowering drug* used to treat some types of *hyperlipidemia* (high levels of fat in the blood). Cholestyramine reduces the amount of bile and cholesterol absorbed into the blood from the small intestine. By reducing the level of bile in the circulation it increases the amount of cholesterol that can be converted into bile in the liver, thereby reducing high levels of cholesterol in the blood.

Cholestyramine is also used to treat diarrhea caused by abnormal digestion and absorption of fats in disorders such as *Crohn's disease*.

Chondritis

Inflammation of a cartilage, usually caused by mechanical pressure, stress, or injury. For example, in costal chondritis the cartilage between the ribs and the sternum (breastbone) becomes inflamed, usually after being stretched forcibly during a bout of coughing or heavy lifting. This causes tenderness over the sternum and pain if pressure is exerted on the ribs at the front of the chest.

The cartilage lining the hip and knee joints may also be affected, eventually leading to *osteoarthritis*.

Chondro-

A prefix that denotes a relationship to *cartilage*, as in chondroblast (or, alternatively, chondroplast), a cell that forms cartilage. The prefixes chondr-, chondri-, and chondrio- are also used to denote cartilage.

Chondromalacia patellae

A painful disorder of the knee, most commonly affecting adolescents, in which the cartilage directly behind the kneecap is damaged. When (rarely) it occurs in adults it is known as retropatellar arthritis.

CAUSE

The cause is uncertain. One theory is that actions such as bicycling or horseback riding, in which the knee is bent more than it is straight, or certain injuries to the knee, weaken the inner part of the main thigh muscle, the quadriceps. The result is that, when the knee is straightened, the kneecap is tilted; instead of sliding smoothly across the lower end of the thigh bone it rubs against it, roughening the smooth cartilage that covers both of the bones.

SYMPTOMS AND DIAGNOSIS

Pain is felt when the knee is straightened and is particularly bad when using stairs. After examination, the physician may use X rays to confirm the diagnosis.

TREATMENT AND OUTLOOK

Analgesics (painkillers) may be given to relieve tenderness in the knee. Treatment consists of strengthening the inner part of the quadriceps by exercises or electrical stimulation, which usually clears up the problem and the pain. If pain persists, it may indicate considerable damage to the cartilage; surgery may be necessary to alter the angle of the kneecap permanently, thus preventing further friction on the cartilage.

In rare, severe cases the kneecap must be removed—an operation that hinders mobility surprisingly little.

Chondromatosis

A condition in which multiple benign tumors, called chondromas, arise within bones. The tumors consist of cartilage cells and most commonly develop in bones of the hand. They occasionally develop in the pelvis.

Usually the tumors cause no symptoms, but occasionally they lead to thinning of the lining of the bone and a resultant fracture, which may occur on its own without injury.

Chondrosarcoma

A cancerous growth of cartilage that can develop within a bone or on its surface, occurring most commonly within large bones, such as the femur (thigh bone), tibia (shin), and humerus (long bone of the upper arm). Chondrosarcoma is one of the more common types of cancer arising in bone, but bone cancers in the overall population are rare.

Chondrosarcoma usually occurs in middle age and may develop from a benign tumor (see *Chondromatosis*; *Dyschondroplasia*) or from a previously normal area of bone. It causes pain, swelling, and, occasionally, tenderness. X rays will show an abnormal area of bone. The tumor grows slowly and does not spread elsewhere early in this stage, so that amputation of the bone above the tumor usually results in a permanent cure.

Chondrosarcoma is different from an *osteosarcoma* (cancer of bone cells), which has usually spread to other parts of the body (for example, the lungs) before it causes any symptoms.

Chordee

Abnormal bending or curvature of the penis. Chordee most often occurs in males with *hypospadias*, a congenital defect in which the urethral opening lies on the underside of the penis instead of at the tip. An operation to correct the condition is usually performed when the child is about 3 years old. Untreated chordee may make sexual intercourse very difficult.

C

C

Chorea

A condition characterized by irregular, rapid, jerky movements, or fidgets, usually affecting the face, limbs, and trunk. These movements are involuntary and, unlike *tics*, they are not predictable, but occur at random. Sometimes they resemble fragments of coordinated movements. They disappear in sleep.

TYPES AND CAUSES

Chorea arises from disease or disturbance of structures deep within the brain, in particular the paired nerve cell groups called the *basal ganglia*. Chorea is a feature of two specific diseases called *Huntington's chorea* and *Sydenham's chorea*. It may also occur in pregnancy, when it is called chorea gravidarum. Chorea may be a side effect of certain drugs, including birth-control pills, neuroleptics (for psychiatric disorders), and those used to treat Parkinson's disease; the choreic movements usually disappear when the drug is withdrawn.

In children with *cerebral palsy*, chorea may be combined with *athetosis*, a continuous writhing movement with the inability to maintain a posture. This combination is called choreoathetosis, and it may also occur as a drug side effect.

TREATMENT

If chorea has occurred as a drug side effect, a physician may withdraw the drug or prescribe a substitute. If there is an underlying disease, the physician may prescribe a drug that inhibits nervous system pathways concerned with movement.

Choreoathetosis

A condition that is characterized by uncontrollable movements of the limbs, face, and trunk, which combine the jerky, rapid fidgets characteristic of *chorea* and the slower writhing movements of *athetosis*.

Choriocarcinoma

A rare malignant tumor that develops from the placenta in the uterus. It is a type of *trophoblastic tumor* (a disorder of the tissues derived from the original placental attachment of the fertilized ovum to the wall of the uterus).

INCIDENCE AND CAUSES

Choriocarcinoma occurs in about one in 20,000 pregnancies, usually as a complication of a *hydatidiform mole* (a benign tumor of the trophoblast). Much less frequently, choriocarcinoma follows an abortion; very rarely, it develops after a normal pregnancy. Sometimes the tumor may develop months or even years after the pregnancy.

If untreated, the tumor invades and destroys the walls of the uterus and may spread to the vagina and vulva. Distant spread may occur to the liver, lungs, brain, and bones.

SYMPTOMS

The tumor may become apparent because of persistent bleeding from the vagina after an abortion or for more than eight weeks after childbirth. There may be no early symptoms, the disease being suspected and diagnosed only after the cancer has spread to the lungs and caused breathlessness and coughing up of blood, or to the brain, producing mental changes.

Any woman who has had a hydatidiform mole (an abnormal pregnancy resulting from an abnormal ovum) must have regular examinations for at least 12 months after it has been removed to check that she shows no signs of choriocarcinoma.

TREATMENT

Successful treatment depends upon diagnosing the disease at an early stage. Diagnostic tests include *ultrasound scanning* and measurement of blood and urine levels of human chorionic gonadotropin (HCG), a hormone normally produced by the placenta. Abnormally high levels of HCG may occur with choriocarcinoma.

Treatment is with *anticancer drugs*, especially methotrexate or dactinomycin. *Hysterectomy* (surgical removal of the uterus) may be necessary if persistent bleeding occurs despite drug treatment. The use of anticancer drugs has reduced the mortality from this formerly highly lethal cancer from 90 percent to 30 percent.

Chorionic villus sampling

A method of diagnosing abnormalities in the fetus during the first three months of pregnancy. A small sample of tissue is taken from the placenta and analyzed in the laboratory. The outpatient procedure provides earlier results than *amniocentesis*.

WHY IT IS DONE

The procedure is usually performed to determine whether a pregnant woman with a family history or an increased risk of a genetic disease, such as *Down's syndrome* or *thalassemia*, is carrying a child affected by the condition. Because the test can also identify the sex of the fetus, it can be used by a woman who is a known carrier of a sex-linked disease (such as *hemophilia*, which affects half the male

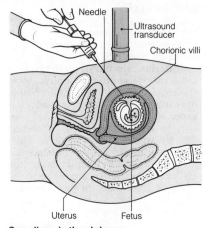

Sampling via the abdomen
A few chorionic villi are sucked through a hollow needle from the placenta.

but few female offspring) to predict the child's odds of having the disease.

HOW IT IS DONE

In some cases the woman is sedated before the sample is taken. The most common method of performing the test is to introduce a tube called a cannula, with a syringe attached, through the vagina and into the uterus. This procedure is controlled by the use of ultrasound or by an endoscope (a viewing tube with a light and lens attached). The syringe is used to suck a few chorionic villi (minute fingerlike projections) from the fetal side of the placenta. The chorionic villi are genetically identical to the fetus.

An alternative method is to insert a hollow needle through the abdominal wall and into the uterus, under ultrasound control, and withdraw some villi through the needle. Both procedures take about half an hour.

Chromosome analysis is done on the cultured villi; cell cultures may be set up if more cells are needed.

RESULTS

If the test reveals genetic abnormalities in the fetus, the parents may choose to terminate the pregnancy (see *Abortion, elective*).

RISKS

The procedure occasionally causes complications, such as perforation of the amniotic sac (the membrane that encloses the fetus), bleeding, and infection. The test itself seems to carry a 1 to 2 percent risk of pregnancy loss. (There is a 3 to 4 percent miscarriage rate in all pregnancies at this stage.) As the procedure becomes more routine, risks should decline.

The advantage lies in the woman's ability to secure an abortion in the first three months of pregnancy if this course is chosen rather than add to the risk to her life by having the abortion later (as is the case when amniocentesis is employed).

Choroid

A layer of blood vessels that lies at the back of the eye behind the retina. Pigment between the blood vessels gives color to the back of the eye that is visible through an *ophthalmoscope* (see *Eye, examination of*). The choroid supplies nutrients and oxygen to the light-sensitive cells in the retina and to surrounding tissues in the eye.

STRUCTURE OF CHOROID
The choroid thickens above and below the lens to form the ciliary body. Ciliary muscles found between it and the lens contract to control the lens' shape.

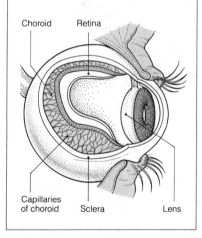

Choroid   Retina

Capillaries
of choroid   Sclera   Lens

Choroiditis

Inflammation of the choroid (network of blood vessels that line the back of the eye). It may occur on its own or as part of a generalized inflammation affecting the whole eye. It is commonly caused by infections such as *toxocariasis* or *toxoplasmosis*, more rarely by sarcoidosis, syphilis, and histoplasmosis, or may have no obvious cause.

Treatment may include *corticosteroid drugs* for the inflammation, and *antibiotic drugs* for the eradication of any causative infection.

Christian Science

A religious movement founded by Mary Baker Eddy. Following a near-fatal accident in 1862, she supposedly

was healed after reading one of the New Testament healing miracles. Eddy devoted the rest of her life to spreading the ideas of Christian Science. Strict Christian Scientists reject orthodox medicine and will, for example, refuse to allow themselves or members of their families to receive blood transfusions, opting to die rather than break the faith.

Christmas disease

A rare type of *bleeding disorder* caused by a defect in the mechanism of blood coagulation. Christmas disease has very similar features to another bleeding disorder, *hemophilia*, and is sometimes called hemophilia B. It is named for a man named Christmas, the first patient in whom the disease was shown to be distinct from hemophilia, and was first described in 1952.

Both Christmas disease and hemophilia are *genetic disorders* in which there is deficient production of one of the proteins in blood (see *Blood clotting*). In Christmas disease the deficiency is of a protein called factor IX, while in hemophilia the deficiency is of factor VIII.

Chromium

A metallic element that is essential for life because of its vital role in the activities of several *enzymes* (substances that promote biochemical reactions in the body). Chromium is required only in minute amounts (see *Trace elements*); chromium deficiency is unknown. In excess, chromium is toxic, although poisoning is rare. Chromium produces inflammation of the skin and, if inhaled, damages the nose. People exposed to chromium fumes also have a greater risk of developing lung cancer.

Chromosomal abnormalities

Variations from normal in the number or structure of chromosomes contained within a person's cells. In most cases, the chromosomal abnormality is present in all the cells; it may have anything from a lethal to virtually no effect, depending on the particular type of abnormality.

INCIDENCE AND CAUSES

About one in every 200 babies born alive has a chromosomal abnormality. Among spontaneously aborted fetuses, about one in three has such an abnormality; this suggests that most chromosome abnormalities are incompatible with life and that those seen in babies born alive are actually the less serious ones.

The cause in most cases is some fault in the process of chromosome division (see *Chromosomes*), either during the formation of the egg or sperm from which a person is derived, or during the first few divisions of the fertilized egg. Occasionally, one of the parents has an abnormal arrangement of his or her chromosomes.

TYPES

A complete extra set of chromosomes per cell is called polyploidy and is lethal. Other abnormalities can be classified according to whether they involve the 44 autosomes or the two sex chromosomes (see *Chromosomes*). Those affecting the autosomes are slightly less common than sex chromosome abnormalities, but tend to produce more serious and widespread effects.

AUTOSOMAL ABNORMALITIES

An extra autosome means that one of the 22 pairs of autosomes occurs in triplicate instead of as a pair—a phenomenon called *trisomy*. The most common trisomy, occurring in about one in 650 live births, is called *Down's syndrome*; it is due to the presence of three chromosomes labeled number 21. Other trisomies are rare and usually cause multiple physical defects and death soon after birth. All trisomies are more common with advancing maternal age.

Sometimes, a part of a chromosome is missing (for instance, in *cri du chat syndrome*) or an extra bit is present and joined to another chromosome.

All these autosomal abnormalities, as well as others causing physical defects of varying severity, tend to cause mental retardation as well.

Occasionally, a person has a normal chromosomal complement, but part of one autosome is not in its proper position; rather, it is joined to another chromosome—a phenomenon called *translocation*. The person is normal, but some of his or her children may suffer from an abnormality.

SEX CHROMOSOME ABNORMALITIES

About one girl in 2,500 is born with only one X chromosome in her cells instead of two—a condition known as *Turner's syndrome*. The annotation for this is 45 XO, meaning 45 instead of 46 chromosomes, with just a single X chromosome. The condition causes characteristic physical abnormalities, defective female sexual development, and infertility.

All other sex chromosome abnormalities involve extra chromosomes. A boy born with one or more extra X chromosomes has *Klinefelter's*

C

syndrome. The annotation for this is usually 47 XXY or 48 XXXY. Klinefelter's syndrome occurs in about one in 500 male births, although it is often not diagnosed until puberty. The condition causes defective male sexual development, infertility, and, in some cases, mental retardation.

Some women are born with an extra X chromosome (47 XXX) and men with an extra Y chromosome (47 XYY). These people are usually normal physically, but may have an increased risk of mental retardation and perhaps psychological problems. The presence of the extra chromosome is recognized only if a special attempt is made to discover it.

DIAGNOSIS AND TREATMENT

Abnormalities are diagnosed by *chromosome analysis*, which is now possible early in pregnancy using *chorionic villus sampling*. Because of the fundamental nature of these defects—affecting every one of a person's cells—no "cure" is possible. Most babies with autosomal chromosomal defects, apart from those with Down's syndrome, do not survive long. Children and adults with Down's syndrome, although handicapped, can usually integrate well into the community, living at home and even working at a modest job. Hormonal and/or surgical treatment can help correct some of the developmental defects characteristic of Klinefelter's and Turner's syndromes.

Anyone with a child or other member of the family with a chromosomal abnormality should obtain *genetic counseling* to establish the risk of his or her prospective children being affected and also to discuss other considerations of family planning.

Chromosome analysis

Study of the chromosomal material in an adult's, child's, or unborn baby's cells to learn whether a *chromosomal abnormality* is present or to establish its nature.

WHY IT IS DONE

Certain fetuses have a higher-than-average chance of being born with a chromosomal abnormality, in particular if the mother is over 35 years old, if she has previously given birth to a child with a chromosomal defect, or if either the mother or father is known to carry a defect or rearrangement of his or her chromosomes. In such cases, the parents are usually offered, at around the fifteenth week of pregnancy, chromosome analysis of cells that can be obtained from the fetus by a technique called *amniocentesis*. Some centers offer an alternative, *chorionic villus sampling*, which may have greater risks (regarding loss of the fetus), but which can be carried out as early as six to eight weeks into pregnancy.

If no abnormality is found, the test spares the parents any anxiety. If a serious abnormality is discovered, such as one that would lead to the infant having *Down's syndrome*, termination of the pregnancy may be considered, along with *genetic counseling* to assess the chances of a subsequent pregnancy being affected.

Chromosome analysis is also carried out when a baby is stillborn, or is born with physical abnormalities that suggest a chromosome defect. The analysis clarifies the nature and type of defect, which in turn affects the counseling given to the parents.

Finally, analysis of a person's sex chromosomes may be carried out to establish the chromosomal sex of a child with ambiguous genitals (see *Intersex*); to diagnose sex chromosome abnormalities such as *Turner's syndrome* and *Klinefelter's syndrome*; or to investigate *infertility*.

PROCEDURE FOR CHROMOSOME ANALYSIS

1 Fetal cells are obtained by amniocentesis or by chorionic villus sampling, or white blood cells are obtained from the blood of the baby, child, or adult being tested.

2 These cells are suspended in a medium containing substances that encourage the cells to divide. Chemicals are then added that stop the cells from dividing at a stage where their chromosome content is most easily visible.

3 The cells are then spread on a microscope slide, stained, and a selected few (in which the chromosomes are clearly visible and well separated) have their nuclei photographed or are closely examined through a high-power microscope.

4 The chromosomes are matched up or cut out from the photographic print and arranged into the 22 pairs of autosomes together with the sex chromosomes. Study of these reveals any abnormalities.

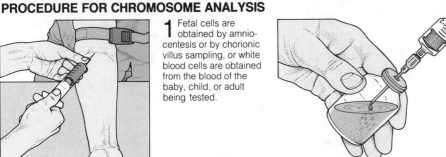

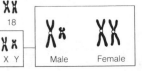

Male   Female

Chromosomes

Threadlike structures present within the nuclei of cells. Chromosomes carry the inherited, genetic information that directs the activities of cells and, thus, the growth and functioning of the entire body.

All the cells of any one person (with the exception of egg or sperm cells) carry precisely the same chromosomal material. This is because everyone is derived, by a process of cell division, from a single, fertilized egg cell and, with each cell division, the chromosomal material originally present in the fertilized egg is faithfully copied. A rare exception to this rule is seen in people with *mosaicism*, in which some cells contain one set of chromosomal material and other cells contain a slightly different set.

Although most chromosomal material is the same for everyone, certain parts differ from one person to another; these differences make each person (with the exception of identical twins) unique. Chromosomes determine physical characteristics, such as sex, hair texture and color, skin and eye color, nose shape, height, and (probably to a lesser extent) mental abilities and personality.

Each chromosome contains up to several thousand *genes* (hereditary units) arranged in single file along its length. A single gene is responsible for just one small aspect of body chemistry (e.g., enzyme synthesis).

STRUCTURE AND NUMBERS

Chemically, a chromosome consists of an extremely long chain of the hereditary substance deoxyribonucleic acid, or DNA, along with a coating of protein. This combination of DNA and protein is called chromatin. The sequence of chemical units, or bases, in the DNA provides the coded instructions for cellular activities. Each cell contains the chemical machinery for decoding these instructions (see *Genetic code; Nucleic acids*).

Although DNA chains are relatively enormous (compared, for example, with a molecule of water), their long, filamentous shape means that chromosomes cannot normally be seen in cell nuclei, even with the aid of a powerful microscope. But, shortly before any cell divides, its DNA molecules contract (probably by forming into tight coils) and, if cell division is chemically halted and the cell stained with a dye, the chromosomes can be seen with a microscope as dark rods in the nucleus, a few thousandths of a millimeter long.

EGG AND SPERM CELLS

These differ from other body cells in that they contain only 23 chromosomes—one from each of the 22 autosome pairs plus an X chromosome (in the case of an egg) and either an X or a Y (in the case of a sperm). Because they have only half the normal complement, they are said to be haploid, while other cells are called diploid.

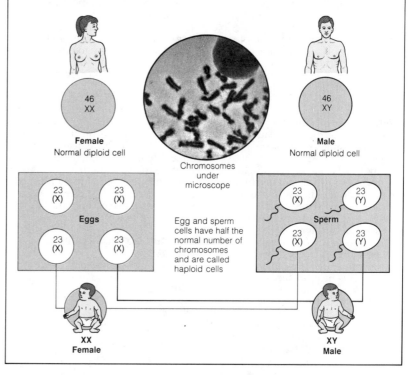

Female
Normal diploid cell

Male
Normal diploid cell

Chromosomes under microscope

Eggs

Sperm

Egg and sperm cells have half the normal number of chromosomes and are called haploid cells

XX
Female

XY
Male

This technique has shown that human cells (with the exception of egg and sperm cells) normally contain 46 chromosomes consisting of 23 pairs.

Most chromosomes have a constriction called a centromere that divides them into long and short "arms"

Appearance of chromosomes
This is the appearance just after a chromosome has copied itself. The two copies are joined at the centromere.

AUTOSOMAL AND SEX CHROMOSOMES

Of the 23 pairs of chromosomes, 22 are the same in both sexes and are called autosomal chromosomes. The two members of a pair cannot be told apart under the microscope—being alike in their length, the position of their centromeres, and in other aspects—but at the molecular level they differ slightly, in particular in the sequence of chemical bases in their DNA. One member of each pair is derived originally from a person's mother and the other from the father.

The other two chromosomes are called sex chromosomes. In women they form a pair and are called X chromosomes. Again, they look alike but differ slightly at the molecular level. In men, however, the two sex chromosomes are completely different. One is an X chromosome, but the other is a much shorter chromosome called the Y chromosome. The Y chromosome is believed to provide all the information for the development of male sexual characteristics. In its absence, the female pattern of development occurs.

As with the autosomal chromosomes, one of a person's sex chromosomes (an X) has come originally from the ovum of the mother and the other (an X in girls and a Y in boys) has come from the sperm of the father.

C

CHROMOSOME DIVISION

When a cell divides, its components are duplicated in the two offspring cells (see *Mitosis*); this applies also to the chromosomes. Shortly before division, the DNA in each chromosome is copied (see *Nucleic acids*). This means that, when the chromosomes are viewed just before division, they appear not as single but as double rods, conjoined in the region of their centromeres. This gives all 46 chromosomes (not just the sex chromosomes) an X-shaped appearance in the nuclei. As the normal cell division proceeds—a process known as mitosis—these duplicated chromosomes are pulled apart, dividing at the centromere, so that each daughter cell receives a single copy of each of the usual 46 chromosomes.

When egg or sperm cells are formed (a process known as meiosis) there are two important departures from the norm in the process of chromosome division. First, after the DNA has been copied, but before division takes place, some sections of chromosomal material are exchanged between the two members of all the paired chromosomes. This helps ensure that each of a person's eggs or sperm has a different combination of chromosomal material—and helps explain why all brothers and sisters (except identical twins) have a unique appearance.

The second difference is that, because eggs and sperm get only 23 chromosomes, their formation requires two consecutive divisions—a first one in which the 46 chromosomes in the parent cell are split into two groups of 23 (one group going to each daughter cell), followed by a second division in which the 23 chromosomes in each daughter cell (which at this point are still in duplicate form) are pulled apart. Thus, the original cell gives rise to four separate egg or sperm cells.

DISORDERS

Defective chromosome division during the formation of eggs and sperm—or more rarely during the first few divisions of a fertilized egg—can lead to various *chromosomal abnormalities*. The precise nature of the abnormality can be investigated by detailed *chromosome analysis*.

Chronic

Describing a disorder or set of symptoms that has persisted for a long time. In some disorders, such as chronic active *hepatitis*, the time is specified as six months or longer.

Chronic disorders are usually contrasted with acute ones. In addition to the duration difference between the two, the term acute suggests the presence of symptoms such as high fever, severe pain, or breathlessness, with a rapid change in the patient's condition from one day to the next. By contrast, a person with a chronic infection, such as some forms of hepatitis or a chronic form of *arthritis*, shows little change in symptoms from day to day and may be able, albeit with some difficulty, to carry out his or her regular daily activities.

A person with a chronic disease may experience an acute exacerbation (flare-up) of symptoms. Also, people who have had an acute illness such as a *stroke*, or who have been injured in an accident, may be left with permanent disabilities, but their condition is not chronic. A chronic disorder implies a continuing disease process with progressive deterioration (sometimes despite treatment).

Chronic obstructive lung disease

See *Lung disease, chronic obstructive*.

Cimetidine

ULCER HEALING

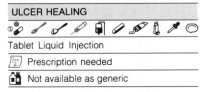

Tablet Liquid Injection

Prescription needed

Not available as generic

An *ulcer-healing drug* related to the *antihistamines*. Introduced in 1976, cimetidine reduces the secretion of hydrochloric acid in the stomach and, by doing so, promotes healing of gastric and duodenal ulcers and reduces esophagitis (inflammation of the esophagus).

Cimetidine generally relieves symptoms within one to two weeks and heals an ulcer in over 75 percent of cases after one to two months. Once the ulcer has healed, a maintenance dose of cimetidine is often prescribed; without such treatment the chance of an ulcer recurring is high.

There is a slight risk that cimetidine may temporarily mask the symptoms of stomach cancer by relieving symptoms in the early stages, thus delaying the diagnosis. It is therefore usually not prescribed for periods longer than two months unless investigations, such as *gastroscopy* and *barium X-ray examinations*, have ruled out the possibility of cancer.

Cimetidine interferes with the breaking down by the liver of certain drugs, such as *anticoagulants* and *anticonvulsants*.

Some people taking cimetidine suffer from confusion, headaches, and dizziness, which usually disappear when the drug is stopped.

Circadian rhythm

Any biological pattern based on a cycle approximately 24 hours long. (See also *Biorhythms*.)

Circulation, disorders of

Conditions affecting the flow of blood around the body. (See *Arteries, disorders of*; *Veins, disorders of*; *Capillary*.)

Circulatory system

The *heart* and blood vessels, which together are responsible for the continuous flow of blood throughout the body. Also called the cardiovascular system, the circulatory system provides all body tissues with a regular supply of oxygen and nutrients and carries away carbon dioxide and other waste products.

STRUCTURE AND FUNCTION

The circulatory system consists of two main parts: the systemic circulation (which comprises the blood supply to the entire body except the lungs) and the pulmonary circulation to the lungs (which is responsible for reoxygenating the blood).

The systemic circulation begins at the left side of the heart, where the left atrium receives oxygen-rich blood from the pulmonary circulation. The blood is ejected from the left atrium to the left ventricle, a powerful pump that sends the blood out through the *aorta*, the body's main artery. Other arteries branching off the aorta carry the blood all over the body, into the arterioles (small arteries) that supply the various organs. The arterioles branch further into a network of capillaries. These extremely fine blood vessels have thin walls to allow oxygen and other nutrients to pass easily from the blood into the tissues, and carbon dioxide and other wastes to pass in the opposite direction.

The capillaries deliver the deoxygenated blood into venules (small veins), which join to form veins. These carry the blood into the *venae cavae*, the body's two main veins, which then return the blood to the right atrium of the heart.

From the right atrium, the blood enters the pulmonary circulation. It passes to the right ventricle, which

CIRCULATORY SYSTEM

The heart and blood vessels create a continuous flow of blood around the body to provide tissues with oxygen and nutrients. The system also removes waste products. The systemic circulation deals with the supply of blood to all parts except the lungs; the pulmonary system reoxygenates the blood.

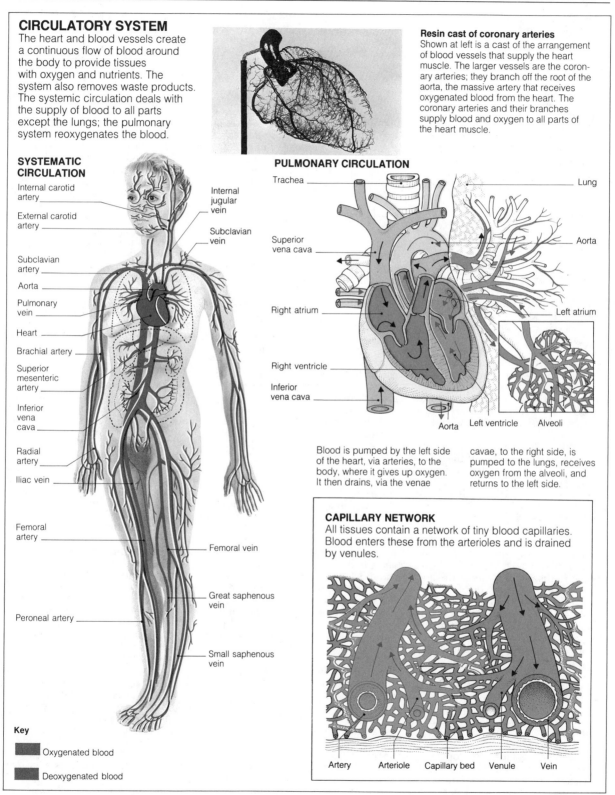

Resin cast of coronary arteries
Shown at left is a cast of the arrangement of blood vessels that supply the heart muscle. The larger vessels are the coronary arteries; they branch off the root of the aorta, the massive artery that receives oxygenated blood from the heart. The coronary arteries and their branches supply blood and oxygen to all parts of the heart muscle.

C

SYSTEMATIC CIRCULATION

Internal carotid artery
External carotid artery
Subclavian artery
Aorta
Pulmonary vein
Heart
Brachial artery
Superior mesenteric artery
Inferior vena cava
Radial artery
Iliac vein
Femoral artery
Peroneal artery

Internal jugular vein
Subclavian vein
Femoral vein
Great saphenous vein
Small saphenous vein

Key

Oxygenated blood

Deoxygenated blood

PULMONARY CIRCULATION

Trachea
Superior vena cava
Right atrium
Right ventricle
Inferior vena cava
Aorta

Lung
Aorta
Left atrium
Left ventricle   Alveoli

Blood is pumped by the left side of the heart, via arteries, to the body, where it gives up oxygen. It then drains, via the venae cavae, to the right side, is pumped to the lungs, receives oxygen from the alveoli, and returns to the left side.

CAPILLARY NETWORK

All tissues contain a network of tiny blood capillaries. Blood enters these from the arterioles and is drained by venules.

Artery   Arteriole   Capillary bed   Venule   Vein

C

pumps the blood through the pulmonary artery to the lungs. Here, carbon dioxide passes out of the blood, and oxygen enters. The reoxygenated blood then returns through the pulmonary veins to the left atrium of the heart, where it reenters the systemic circulation.

Within the systemic circulation there is a bypass to the liver called the portal circulation. Capillaries carrying nutrient-rich blood from the stomach, intestine, and other digestive organs join to form venules which, in turn, meet to form veins. These then merge to form the portal vein, which conveys the blood to veins, venules, and capillaries in the liver. Nutrients pass from the capillaries into the liver cells for processing and storage or reentry into the general circulation. Blood from the liver continues to rejoin the main systemic circulation via the inferior vena cava.

On its journey from the heart to the tissues, blood is forced along the arteries at high pressure. However, on the return journey through the veins and back to the heart, the blood is at low pressure. It is kept moving by the muscles in the arms and legs compressing the walls of the veins, and by valves in the veins preventing the blood from flowing backward. (See also *Lymphatic system; Respiration*.)

Circumcision

Removal of the foreskin of the penis. Circumcision is most often performed on newborn male babies, usually for religious reasons. It may also be carried out on adults.

WHY IT IS DONE
Circumcision is a religious ritual practiced for thousands of years by both Jews and Muslims. In some countries it is also routinely carried out for reasons of hygiene (because circumcision prevents the accumulation of secretions under the foreskin).

Medical reasons for performing circumcision include a tight foreskin that balloons on urination, or recurrent attacks of *balanitis* (infection under the foreskin due to retained secretions). In adults, the foreskin may be removed because it is tight and painful during intercourse, or because of attacks of paraphimosis (painful compression of the shaft of the penis by a retracted foreskin).

HOW IT IS DONE
In newborn babies, the operation takes only a few minutes. The foreskin is pulled forward over the tip of the penis and cut. The outer layer of the remaining foreskin retracts, leaving the glans covered by the thinner, inner layer. This is cut and pulled back. The two layers of the foreskin are then stitched and a waterproof dressing is applied.

In adolescents and adults, circumcision is usually performed using a general anesthetic. The foreskin is pulled back as far as it will go. It is slit along its upper surface and then all around so that it can be removed. The raw edges of the inner and outer layers are stitched, and a dressing is applied. The patient usually goes home the same day.

Circumcision, female

Removal of all or parts of the clitoris, labia majora, and labia minora, sometimes combined with narrowing of the entrance to the vagina. The operation is common in parts of Africa. In the early 1980s it was estimated that more than 84 million women in 30 countries had been circumcised.

There is absolutely no valid medical purpose for the procedure. Circumcision may cause retention of urine, injuries during coitus, and may also lead to frigidity and other psychological problems. Childbirth is likely to be made more hazardous.

There has been a strong move to end the practice, with little success. Legislation prohibiting circumcision in the Sudan was introduced in the 1940s, but has been ineffective.

Cirrhosis

A disease of the liver caused by chronic damage to its cells. Bands of *fibrosis* (internal scarring) break up the normal structure of the liver. The surviving cells multiply to form regeneration nodules (islands of living cells separated by scar tissue). Because these nodules are inadequately supplied with blood, liver function is gradually impaired—for example, the liver no longer effectively removes toxic substances from the blood (see *Liver failure*). The distortion and fibrosis of the liver leads to *portal hypertension* (high blood pressure in the veins from the intestines and spleen to the liver), which can cause serious complications.

INCIDENCE AND CAUSES
In the US, about one in 70 people dies as a direct result of chronic liver disease and cirrhosis—accounting for about 30,000 deaths each year.

Heavy alcohol consumption is the most common cause of cirrhosis both in Europe and the US; it is an increasing problem in most developed countries. The risk relates to the amount of alcohol consumed rather than the type, and women are more susceptible than men (see *Alcohol*).

Hepatitis (inflammation of the liver) can lead to cirrhosis. Chronic viral hepatitis (particularly that due to hepatitis B virus) is the most common cause of cirrhosis in the Middle and Far East and Africa (see *Hepatitis, viral*). A special pattern of liver inflammation called chronic active hepatitis is usually present before the cirrhosis develops (see *Hepatitis, chronic active*). Autoimmune chronic active hepatitis, with similar liver changes but with no obvious viral infection, is found in Europe and the US.

Rarer causes of cirrhosis include diseases and defects of the bile ducts, which can cause primary or secondary *biliary cirrhosis; hemochromatosis*, in which increased iron absorption occurs; *Wilson's disease*, in which there is an increase in copper absorption; *cystic fibrosis*, in which the bile ducts become obstructed by sticky mucus; and "cardiac cirrhosis," in which *heart failure* has led to long-standing congestion of blood in the liver.

SYMPTOMS AND SIGNS
There may be no symptoms of cirrhosis; the disease may be discovered initially during a routine medical examination or blood test because of some abnormality. The most common symptoms are mild *jaundice, edema* (fluid collection in the tissues), mental confusion, and *hematemesis* (vomiting of blood).

In men, enlargement of the breasts and loss of body hair are thought to be due to an abnormality in the sex hormone balance caused by liver failure associated with cirrhosis.

COMPLICATIONS
There are four main complications associated with cirrhosis and any may be the first sign of the condition. *Ascites* (collection of fluid in the abdominal cavity) can occur because of low protein levels in the blood (see *Albumin*) and high blood pressure in the veins leading to the liver. The high pressure in these veins also leads to *esophageal varices* (enlarged veins in the wall of the esophagus), which can rupture, causing vomiting of blood. *Confusion* and *coma* can result from the accumulation of toxic materials poisonous to the brain that would normally be processed and detoxified by a healthy liver. *Hepatoma* is a primary cancer of liver cells that complicates chronic hepatitis with cirrhosis.

DIAGNOSIS AND TREATMENT

Although the symptoms and signs of cirrhosis, or *liver function tests*, may suggest the diagnosis, the diagnosis is usually confirmed by *liver biopsy*, which may also show features that point to the underlying cause. Special blood tests and *cholangiography* (X rays of the bile ducts) may be performed to exclude the rarer causes.

The cirrhotic process itself can be treated by slowing the process causing liver cell damage. Abstinence from alcohol can lead to substantial improvement, and in some cases specific treatment for the underlying cause may be available. Ascites may be controlled by giving diuretics (drugs that increase the production of urine) and sometimes by reducing salt intake. Bleeding esophageal varices can be obliterated by injecting them with a sclerosant solution (a liquid that blocks off the affected veins) via a gastroscope (see *Gastroscopy*). The pressure in the veins can be reduced by using a *shunt* operation to divert the blood supply away from the engorged, dilated veins.

Confusion can be improved by measures that reduce the level of toxic waste products and other poisonous substances circulating in the blood. Such measures may include reducing the protein intake in the diet and giving special antibiotic treatment to reduce the number of bacteria in the intestines. In some cases a *liver transplant*, if available, may offer the only chance of a long-term cure.

Cisplatin

An *anticancer drug* used especially to treat cancers of the testis and ovary. It is used on its own or in combination with other anticancer drugs.

Cisplatin is being investigated to treat esophageal cancer.

Clap

A slang term used since the 16th century for the sexually transmitted infection *gonorrhea*.

Claudication

Lameness or limping. The term is associated with the Roman Emperor Claudius, who was notably lame. As a medical term it refers to a cramplike pain in one or both legs, which develops on walking and may eventually cause a limp.

The usual cause of claudication is blockage or narrowing of arteries in the legs due to *atherosclerosis* (see *Peripheral vascular disease*). Patients typically find that they have to stop walking after a set distance because of pain in the calves. After a short rest, they may be able to walk on. This is called intermittent claudication.

A rarer cause is spinal *stenosis* (narrowing of the canal carrying the spinal cord), causing pressure on nerve roots that pass into either leg.

Claustrophobia

Intense fear of being in enclosed spaces, such as elevators or small rooms, or of being in crowded areas. Claustrophobia may originate from a previous bad experience involving enclosed spaces (such as being locked inside a closet as punishment). *Psychotherapy* and/or *behavior therapy* is the usual treatment.

Clavicle

The collarbone. There are two of these bones, each slightly curved like an "f," that join the top of the sternum (breastbone) to the scapula (shoulder blade). The clavicles support the arms and transmit forces from the arms to the central skeleton.

The ligaments that link the clavicle to the sternum and scapula are very strong, which explains why the clavicle is rarely dislocated but frequently broken. Most fractures occur as a result of a fall onto the shoulder or an outstretched arm. When the clavicle is broken, the arm tends to sag and must be supported by a *sling* and a figure-of-eight bandage to keep the broken ends together until the fracture has healed, which may require six to 12 weeks of immobilization.

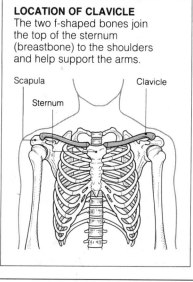

LOCATION OF CLAVICLE
The two f-shaped bones join the top of the sternum (breastbone) to the shoulders and help support the arms.

Scapula

Clavicle

Sternum

Clawfoot

A deformity of the foot that includes an exaggerated arch and turning under of the tips of the toes. The disorder may be present from birth or may result from disturbance or damage to the nerve or blood supply to the muscles of the foot.

Clawhand

A deformity of the hand in which the fingers are permanently curled. Clawhand is caused by an injury to the ulnar nerve, which controls some of the muscles involved in hand and finger movements.

Cleft lip and palate

Cleft lip is a vertical, usually off-center split in the upper lip that may be a small notch or may extend up to the nose. In some cases the upper gum is also cleft or notched, and the nose is crooked. Although cleft lip is also sometimes known as hare lip, this term properly refers only to a midline cleft lip, which is extremely rare. In some cases the lip or palate is cleft on both sides of the mouth.

Cleft palate is a gap in the roof of the mouth that runs along its midline, from behind the teeth to the nasal cavity. Many people with cleft palate are partially deaf and may have another *birth defect*.

Cleft lip and palate are present from birth, occurring either singly or together. About one in 600 babies is born with one or both deformities. Of every nine affected babies, two have only a cleft lip, three have only a cleft palate, and four have both. Inheritance is complicated but one third of those affected have relatives with one or both deformities.

DIAGNOSIS AND TREATMENT

All babies are routinely examined for both deformities immediately after birth. Babies with a cleft lip can breast-feed, but those with a cleft palate must be bottle-fed.

Surgery, usually at about 3 months, can restore a cleft lip so that it looks almost normal, and there are rarely any speech defects. A cleft palate is usually repaired at about 1 year; further operations and speech therapy are sometimes necessary.

Clergymans' knee

Inflammation of the bursa (fluid-filled sac) that acts as a cushion at the pressure point over the tibial tubercle (the bony prominence below the knee). The inflammation is caused by prolonged kneeling. (See *Bursitis*.)

C

Climacteric

The *menopause*, which indicates the end of menstruation (and thus fertility) in the female.

Clindamycin

An *antibiotic drug* used to treat serious infections that have not responded to other antibiotics. It is also used in the treatment of infections caused by bacteria (usually staphylococci or pneumococci) that are resistant to more commonly used antibiotics.

Clitoridectomy

An operation to remove the clitoris (see *Circumcision, female*).

Clitoris

Part of the female genitalia. The clitoris is richly supplied with nerves and blood vessels; during sexual stimulation, it swells and becomes even more sensitive.

LOCATION OF CLITORIS

The clitoris is a small, sensitive, erectile organ located just below the pubic bone, partly enclosed within the labia.

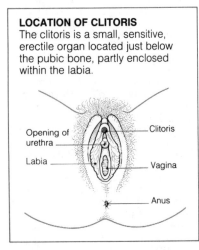

Opening of urethra — Clitoris

Labia — Vagina

Anus

Clofibrate

A drug that reduces high levels of triglyceride (a type of fat) in the blood; it is sometimes used in the treatment of certain types of *hyperlipidemia*. (See *Lipid-lowering drugs*.)

Clomiphene

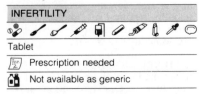

INFERTILITY
Tablet
Prescription needed
Not available as generic

A drug used to treat *infertility* caused by failure to ovulate in a woman and inadequate sperm production in a man. Multiple births may occur.

USE IN FEMALE INFERTILITY Normal ovulation (the release of a ripened egg from one of the ovaries) is stimulated by the action of two *gonadotropins* (follicle-stimulating hormone and luteinizing hormone) released from the pituitary gland. This secretion is stimulated by chemicals released by the hypothalamus (a part of the brain).

Failure to ovulate, one of the most common causes of infertility, is usually due to an abnormally low production of these gonadotropins. Clomiphene works by blocking the action of estrogens in the hypothalamus. Estrogens normally reduce the output of gonadotropins from the pituitary gland. As a result, the production of gonadotropins is increased and sometimes ovulation is stimulated. Occasionally, clomiphene must be given with gonadotropins before ovulation will occur.

USE IN MALE INFERTILITY Clomiphene is used to stimulate sperm production in some infertile men. Sperm counts are carried out regularly to check for increased sperm production and treatment is usually continued for six to twelve months or until his partner becomes pregnant.

POSSIBLE ADVERSE EFFECTS Minor side effects, some of which may occur in both men and women, include hot flashes, nausea, headache, breast tenderness, and, occasionally, blurred vision. All usually improve when the dose is reduced or if a gonadotropin is also taken. Between 5 and 15 percent of the women who take clomiphene develop ovarian cysts. These cysts shrink when the dose is reduced. Very rarely, alopecia (loss of hair) occurs in people taking the drug.

Clone

An exact copy. In medicine the term usually refers to one of three main types: clones of cells, clones of genes, and clones of organisms.

Clones of cells are all descended from one original cell. Many types of cancer are thought to be cellular clones derived from one abnormal cell. *Monoclonal antibodies* have been used to identify certain types of cancers and infections.

Clones of genes are duplicates of a single gene. Gene cloning is a valuable research tool because it enables numerous copies of a gene to be made so that they can be studied in detail.

Finally, clones of organisms can be produced by removing the nucleus from a cell of one individual and transplanting it into the egg cell of another individual. When this egg matures into a living plant or animal, it contains only the genes of the donor nucleus. To date, this process has been successful only in experiments with simple organisms.

Clonidine

An *antihypertensive drug* (used to treat high blood pressure). Clonidine is sometimes used with a diuretic, especially when the blood pressure is not being controlled by the diuretic alone. Clonidine works by reducing nerve impulses from the brain to the heart and circulatory system. Rarely, an unexpected rise in blood pressure develops when clonidine is given with a beta-blocker.

POSSIBLE ADVERSE EFFECTS

When given in high doses, sudden stopping of the drug may lead to a dangerous rise in blood pressure.

Other possible adverse effects, also usually occurring only in patients on high dosages, include drowsiness, dizziness, dry mouth, and constipation. Such effects often decrease with continued treatment or may require a reduction in dose.

Clonus

An abnormal response of a muscle to stretching. Normally when a muscle is stretched, it responds by contracting once and then relaxing (see *Reflex*). In clonus, stretching sets off a series of contractions of the muscle or muscles in quick succession.

Clonus is a sign of damage to nerve fibers that carry impulses from the motor cortex within the *cerebrum* of the brain to a particular muscle.

One typical example of clonus is called ankle clonus. A physician may demonstrate this type in the course of an examination by forcibly jerking the front of the foot upward, thus stretching the muscles of the calf, which are then triggered into a series of rhythmical contractions.

Clonuslike, or clonic, muscle contractions are also one feature of seizures in grand mal *epilepsy*.

Clorazepate

A drug used mainly in the treatment of anxiety. (See *Benzodiazepine drugs*.)

Closed panel

See *Health maintenance organization*.

Clotrimazole

A drug used to treat yeast and fungal infections, especially *candidiasis*. (See *Antifungal drugs*.)

Clove oil

A colorless or pale-yellow oil distilled from the dried flower buds of *EUGENIA CARYOPHYLLUS*. Clove oil is sometimes used to relieve flatulent colic, but its main use today is in flavoring pharmaceuticals. Applied externally, it is germicidal and mildly analgesic, and has been used as a domestic remedy for toothache. Repeated application, however, may damage the gums.

Cloxacillin

A penicillin-type antibiotic used to treat infections with staphylococcal bacteria. (See *Penicillin drugs*.)

Clubbing

Thickening and broadening of the tips of the fingers and toes, with increased curving of the fingernails and toenails.

Clubbing is associated with certain chronic lung diseases, including *bronchiectasis*, *lung cancer*, fibrosing *alveolitis*, and lung *abscess*; heart abnormalities that result in *cyanosis* (bluish complexion due to lack of oxygen in the blood); and occasionally with inflammatory bowel diseases such as *Crohn's disease* and *ulcerative colitis*. Rarely, clubbing may be inherited, in which case it is not a sign of any disease. (See also *Spatulate*.)

Clubfoot

A deformity of the foot, present from birth. (See *Talipes*.)

CNS

An abbreviation for *central nervous system* (the brain and spinal cord).

CNS stimulants

Drugs that increase mental alertness. (See *Stimulants*.)

Coagulation, blood

One of the main mechanisms by which blood clots (solidifies). Coagulation involves a complex series of reactions in the blood plasma (the fluid part of blood as distinct from the blood cells). The end result of this process is the formation of an insoluble substance called fibrin, which provides much of the framework for a clot. (See also *Blood clotting*.)

Coal tar

A thick, black, sticky substance, coal tar is a common ingredient of ointments and some medicinal shampoos. These preparations, which often also contain *antiseptics* and *corticosteroids*, are prescribed for skin and scalp conditions such as psoriasis, eczema, and certain forms of dermatitis.

Coarctation of the aorta

An abnormality, present from birth, in which there is a localized narrowing of the aorta (the large artery that supplies blood from the left side of the heart to the rest of the body).

The narrowing usually occurs just past the point where the left subclavian artery (which supplies blood to the neck, head, and the left arm) branches off the aorta. Thus, there is a reduced supply of blood to the lower part of the body, including the legs. In an attempt to compensate, the heart works harder, causing raised blood pressure in the upper part of the body, while the blood pressure in the legs is normal or low.

The cause is unknown. Coarctation of the aorta occurs in about 10 percent of babies born with heart defects (see *Heart disease, congenital*), affecting about one in 2,000 babies overall.

SYMPTOMS AND DIAGNOSIS

The symptoms often first appear in early childhood and depend on the severity of the hypertension. Symptoms may include headache, weakness after exercise, cold legs, and, rarely, breathing difficulty and leg swelling due to *heart failure*.

A physical examination of the child usually reveals the following abnormalities associated with the defect: a murmur (abnormal heart sound), weak or absent pulses in the groin, lack of synchronization between groin and wrist pulses, and higher blood pressure in the arms than in the legs. The diagnosis is confirmed by X rays of the chest that show bulging of the aorta on either side of the narrowed segment, among other abnormalities.

TREATMENT AND OUTLOOK

Surgery is necessary to prevent progressive hypertension, even when there are no symptoms. The narrowed segment of the aorta is removed and the two ends rejoined. The operation is usually performed between the ages of 4 and 8. Despite successful repair, high blood pressure may persist, requiring drug treatment.

Cobalamin

A cobalt-containing complex molecule that forms part of *vitamin B$_{12}$*.

Cobalt

A metallic element and a constituent of *vitamin B$_{12}$*. Radioactive cobalt is used in cancer treatment.

Cocaine

A drug obtained from the leaves of a South American plant.

WHY IT IS USED

Cocaine was once used as a local anesthetic (see *Anesthesia, local*), mainly for minor surgical procedures on the eye, ear, nose, or throat. It is sometimes sprayed onto the back of the throat before examination of the lungs or stomach with an *endoscope*. Because of its potential for abuse, cocaine has largely been replaced by other local anesthetics.

The onset of anesthesia is rapid and the effects last for about one hour. Cocaine also constricts blood vessels, helping to localize its effect. However, some cocaine is usually absorbed into the bloodstream; this may interfere with the action of chemical *neurotransmitters* in the brain, possibly producing feelings of euphoria and increased energy.

ABUSE

The effects of cocaine on the brain have led to its abuse. Regular inhaling of the drug can damage the lining of the nose. Continued use can lead to psychological dependence (see *Drug dependence*), and *psychosis* may develop if high doses are taken. Overdose can cause seizures and *cardiac arrest*. "Crack," a purified form of cocaine, produces a more rapid and intense reaction that also wears off very quickly; it has caused deaths due to adverse effects on the heart. (See also *Drug abuse*.)

Coccygodynia

A pain in the region of the coccyx. It usually starts after a fall in which the base of the spine strikes a hard surface, or through prolonged pressure on the coccyx (as can occur when slouching in a chair), or in women who have been in the *lithotomy* position (lying on the back with legs in the air) during childbirth. Occasionally there is no apparent cause.

Treatment may include the application of heat, injections of a local anesthetic, and manipulation, but these measures are not always successful. The pain usually eases in time with or without treatment. In very rare cases of persistent, incapacitating pain, surgical removal of the coccyx may be considered.

Coccyx

A small triangular bone at the base of the spine, positioned in front of the top of the cleft between the buttocks. The coccyx consists of four tiny bones

C

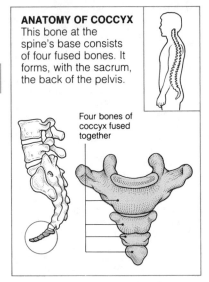

Four bones of coccyx fused together

fused together; it is all that remains of the tailbone structure of our evolutionary ancestors.

Along with a much larger bone called the sacrum, which lies above it, the coccyx forms the back section of the pelvis—a bowl-shaped, bony structure that provides protection to organs (such as the uterus and bladder) and supports the upper body.

The coccyx and sacrum can barely move relative to each other, although they do somewhat during childbirth. After middle age they fuse together.

Cochlear implant

A device for treating severe deafness that consists of one or more electrodes implanted by surgery inside or outside the cochlea (an organ in the inner ear that transforms sound vibrations into nerve impulses for transmission to the brain). Unlike a *hearing aid*, which amplifies sounds, the implant receives and passes on electrical signals. It cannot restore normal hearing, but, along with lipreading, allows a greater understanding of speech than is possible by lipreading alone.

WHY IT IS DONE

In rare cases, damage to structures in the cochlea (through disease, injury, or drug poisoning) is so great and the resultant deafness so profound that a hearing aid serves no useful purpose. If some nerve fibers have survived, it is sometimes possible to stimulate them electrically by an implant.

HOW IT IS DONE

An operation is carried out to implant one or more tiny electrodes either inside or outside the cochlea. At the same time, a miniature receiver is implanted under the skin, either behind the ear or in the lower part of the chest. A wire connecting the electrodes to the receiver is implanted at the same time.

Directly over the implanted receiver, the patient wears an external transmitter, which is connected to a sound processor and a microphone.

OUTLOOK

In general, an implant enables the user to hear the rhythms of speech, and sometimes also the intonation of the voice. Understanding obtained through lipreading is increased, and the deaf person is able to converse more effectively.

However, the usefulness of an implant for any particular person cannot be reliably predicted, and, in this respect, the technique is considered to be investigational. One quarter of patients make extremely good use of the implant and are able to repeat two thirds of simple words in unrehearsed sentences without lipreading. One

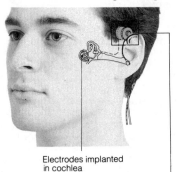

Electrodes implanted in cochlea

Subcutaneous fat

Receiver coil

Signals

Transmitter coil

Skin

Microphone (sometimes set into an ear mold)

Speech processor

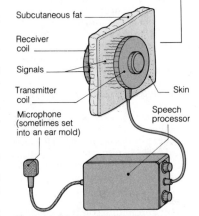

How a cochlear implant works
Sounds picked up by the microphone are converted into electronic signals by the processor and relayed to the external transmitter, which sends them through the skin to the receiver. The waves then travel along the wire to the electrodes in the cochlea.

quarter can repeat some words without lipreading and one quarter can repeat words only with lipreading. In the remainder, the signal is poor, an electrical fault occurs, or the patient develops an infection.

Codeine

 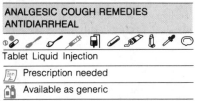
A narcotic *analgesic drug* (painkiller), derived from a poppy plant, in use since the early 1900s. It is not as strong as some other narcotic analgesics and is often combined with other drugs in tablets and mixtures.

WHY IT IS USED

Codeine is most useful in the relief of mild to moderate pain. It is also used as a *cough remedy*, because it suppresses the part of the brain that triggers coughing, and as an *antidiarrheal drug*, because it slows down muscle contractions in the intestinal wall.

POSSIBLE ADVERSE EFFECTS

Codeine may cause dizziness and drowsiness, especially if taken with alcohol. When taken over a long period, codeine may cause constipation and be habit-forming.

Cod-liver oil

A pale yellow oil obtained from the liver of fresh cod. It is a valuable source of *vitamin A* and *vitamin D* and is given to infants as a dietary supplement to ensure the healthy development of bones and skin. Cod-liver oil is available in capsule form and in a malt extract.

Cognitive-behavioral therapy

A method of treating mental disorders based on the idea that the way we think about the world and ourselves (our cognitions) affects our emotions and behavior.

A person suffering from depression may always think that undesirable events are due to his or her behavior and that desirable events are due to chance. The therapist shows the patient that these interpretations are false, suggests more positive ways of thinking, and encourages the patient to try out these new ideas during his or her everyday activities. Because cognitive-behavioral therapy is based on the manner in which each person relates to the environment, it allows treatment to be more specifically tailored to the individual's needs than do the more traditional forms of *behavior therapy*.

Coil
Any of the different types of intrauterine contraceptive devices (see *IUD*).

Coinsurance
A provision in a health insurance policy that requires the patient to pay a predetermined percentage of the various insured medical charges incurred during the life of the policy. (See also *Deductible*.)

Coitus
Sexual intercourse (from the Latin word for a coming together).

Coitus interruptus
The contraceptive technique in which the male partner withdraws his penis from the vagina before ejaculation occurs. This technique is not very reliable as a contraceptive method, because sperm may sometimes be released before orgasm occurs. In addition, coitus interruptus has been blamed for *psychosexual dysfunction* in both men and women. (See also *Contraception*.)

Colchicine
A drug extracted from the autumn crocus, colchicine has been in use since the nineteenth century as a treatment for *gout*. Although it has now been partly superseded by newer drugs, it continues to be used to treat acute and chronic gout and familial Mediterranean fever.

Cold, common
A viral infection that causes inflammation of the mucous membranes lining the nose and throat, resulting in a stuffy, runny nose and sometimes a sore throat and headache.

CAUSES
Almost 200 viruses, all broadly similar in their effects, are known to cause colds. The most common belong to one of two groups—the rhinoviruses and coronaviruses.

Most colds are contracted by breathing in virus-containing droplets that have been sneezed or coughed into the atmosphere or by rubbing the eyes or nose with fingers that have picked up a virus by hand-to-hand contact or by handling contaminated objects, such as playing cards.

INCIDENCE
Almost everyone occasionally gets a cold. The incidence is highest among schoolchildren (who may have as many as 10 colds a year) and declines with increasing age. On average, a young adult has two or three colds per year, an elderly person one or none at all. The reason for this is that children at school are exposed to a host of different viruses to which they have not yet had time to become immune and which they pass to one another. Adults gradually build up immunity against a wide variety of viruses responsible for colds.

Colds are most frequent in winter, probably because people tend to spend more time during these months crowded together indoors in places such as the movies and at parties, where there is a higher chance of viruses being spread.

SYMPTOMS
Most colds are what are popularly known as head colds—that is, infections confined to the nose and throat. The first symptoms are often a tickle in the throat, a watery discharge from the nose, and sneezing. Then the discharge may thicken and become yellow or green and other symptoms may develop—watering eyes, a low-grade fever, a sore throat, a cough, aching muscles and bones, a mild headache, listlessness, and chills.

In some cases, infection spreads to the larynx, windpipe, lungs, sinuses, or middle ear, leading to, respectively, *laryngitis*, *tracheitis*, acute *bronchitis*, *sinusitis*, or *otitis media*. At these sites a more serious secondary bacterial infection may then follow.

Colds can also aggravate existing respiratory disorders, such as asthma and chronic bronchitis, and chronic ear infections. They may also reactivate dormant *herpes simplex* virus, causing *cold sores*.

TREATMENT
Most colds clear up within a week or so. A physician should be consulted only if this fails to happen, if the infection has spread beyond the nose or throat, or if the cold has aggravated a chronic chest infection or ear disorder. If a secondary bacterial infection is suspected, antibiotics will be given.

PREVENTION
Many people believe there are ways of preventing colds—by avoiding exposure to cold drafts and dampness, for instance, or by taking large quantities of vitamin C—but there is no scientific evidence that any such measures work.

OUTLOOK
The search to find a cure for the common cold continues. The two most hopeful possibilities are the drug interferon and synthetic *antigens* (substances that stimulate the immune system to produce antibodies). In volunteer experiments, interferon has proved effective in preventing and reducing the severity of colds, but has caused local inflammation. Research is now centered on finding preparations of interferon that are less toxic.

Cold injury
Localized tissue damage caused by chilling—as distinct from *hypothermia*, which refers to generalized chilling; the two may occur together.

The most serious form of cold injury is *frostbite*, a hazard of very cold, dry conditions. The frostbitten area of skin and flesh is frozen, hard, and white; it is caused either by direct exposure to the air or restriction of the blood supply to the affected area.

Immersion foot is another type of cold injury, occurring when the legs and feet have been cold and damp for many hours or days, and blood supply to the feet has been restricted by tight-fitting footwear.

In established frostbite and immersion foot, the main risk is that blood flow will be slowed so much that the tissues will die, leading to gangrene. Treatment may take several months.

Less serious forms of cold injury include *pernios* (chilblains), caused by rapid skin rewarming after being out in cold weather, and *chapped skin* of the lips, nose, and hands from exposure to cold, windy conditions.

Cold remedies
Many preparations are available over-the-counter to treat different symptoms of the common cold. The main ingredient is usually a mild *analgesic drug* (painkiller), such as *acetaminophen* or *aspirin*, which helps to relieve aches and pains. Other ingredients include *antihistamines* and *decongestants*, which help to reduce nasal congestion, and *caffeine*, which acts as a mild stimulant and is thought to enhance the analgesic effects. *Vitamin C* is frequently included in cold relief products, but there is no evidence that it speeds recovery.

Cold sore
A small skin blister anywhere around the mouth caused by the *herpes simplex* virus. Usually, several such blisters occur together in a cluster.

C

CAUSE AND INCIDENCE

The strain of the virus usually responsible for cold sores is called HSV1 (herpes simplex virus 1). Most people—perhaps as many as 90 percent worldwide—are infected by HSV1 at some time in their lives. The first attack may pass unnoticed or may cause an illness resembling influenza and painful ulcers in the mouth and on the lips—a condition called gingivostomatitis.

Subsequently, the virus lies dormant in nerve cells, but in some people it is occasionally reactivated, causing cold sores. They tend to recur when the person is exposed to hot sunshine or a cold wind, has a cold or other infection, or is feeling run down; women seem more likely to develop cold sores around the time of their menstrual periods. Some people are afflicted regularly throughout the year. Prolonged attacks can occur in patients with an underlying disease that affects their immunity to infection, or in those taking immunosuppressive drugs (transplant or cancer patients, for example).

SYMPTOMS AND TREATMENT

An outbreak is often preceded by a telltale tingling in the lips. The blisters are small at first but soon enlarge, sometimes causing itching, irritation, and soreness. Within a few days they burst and become encrusted, but they usually disappear within a week.

If cold sores are particularly troublesome, a physician may prescribe idoxuridine paint or the antiviral drug acyclovir (by mouth or injection) to soothe them. No effective preventive treatment is available, although some people find that applying a lip salve before sun exposure does help prevent outbreaks.

Colectomy

The surgical removal of part or all of the colon (large intestine).

WHY IT IS DONE

A partial colectomy may be performed to relieve severe cases of *diverticular disease* or to remove either a malignant tumor in the colon or a narrowed part of the intestine that is obstructing the passage of feces. A total colectomy is carried out in cases of *ulcerative colitis* that cannot be controlled with drugs, in long-standing ulcerative colitis in which colonoscopic examination raises the question of a hidden malignancy, and in cases of familial *polyposis*, a rare condition in which potentially malignant growths stud the lining of the colon.

HOW IT IS DONE

In a partial colectomy, the damaged section of the colon is removed and the two ends of the severed colon are joined together; they fuse in a matter of weeks. A temporary *colostomy* (which allows the discharge of feces from the large intestine through an artificial opening in the abdominal wall) may also be required. The temporary colostomy is closed when the rejoined colon has healed.

In a total colectomy the whole of the large intestine is removed; the rectum may be removed or left in place. If the rectum is removed, an *ileostomy* (similar to a colostomy, but involving the small instead of the large intestine) is performed. If the rectum is left in place, the ileum (the lower part of the small intestine) may be joined directly to it—an ileorectal *anastomosis*.

RECOVERY PERIOD

The patient is in the hospital for eight to 12 days. After discharge, it may take up to two months or so at home to recover from the operation. A patient with an ileostomy or colostomy should receive training—before leaving the hospital and preferably from a specialist nurse—on caring for the opening in the abdomen.

OUTLOOK

The bowel usually functions normally after most partial colectomies. If a large section of the colon has been removed, or if the ileum has been joined directly to the rectum, the greatly reduced ability of the intestines to absorb water from the feces can cause diarrhea. Drugs such as codeine phosphate, loperamide, or diphenoxylate may be used to reduce the diarrhea.

Colic

Severe, spasmodic pain that occurs in waves of increasing intensity, reaches a peak, then abates for a short time before returning. The intermittent increase in the pain occurs when the affected part of the body contracts—for example, the bile duct (the tube between the gallbladder and small intestine) or the ureter (the tube from the kidney to the bladder).

Colic in the bile ducts or urinary tract is often the result of obstruction by a stone, but intestinal colic is usually due to an infection or to an obstruction. (See also *Colic, infantile*.)

Colic, infantile

Episodes during which an infant is irritable, cries or screams excessively, and draws up the legs. The baby may be red in the face and may pass gas. Episodes of colic tend to be worse in the evenings and do not respond to the usual means of comforting the infant, such as feeding, cuddling, or diaper changing.

CAUSES

Infantile colic is common, occurring in approximately one in ten babies. It often first appears around the third or fourth week of life. Usually it clears up on its own by the age of 12 weeks, hence its name, "three-month colic." Colic is thought to be due to spasm in the intestines, although there is no proof of this, and the cause of the presumed spasm is unknown.

Babies who have colic are otherwise well. The condition is harmless, although it can be highly distressing to a tired parent. If the baby seems sick between the bouts of colic or has diarrhea, constipation, or a fever, a pediatrician should be consulted as the baby may have a more serious underlying problem.

TREATMENT

Treatment essentially involves waiting for the baby to grow out of the condition. Attempts may be made to distract the baby by diaper changing, cuddling, or bathing. Treatment with *antispasmodic drugs* has been used in the past, but these drugs are now not usually recommended for babies under 6 months of age.

Don't overstimulate your child. Rapid changes coupled with parental anxiety will make the child even more irritable. A common mistake is to feed

TREATING COLIC

Take the baby for a ride in the car

Use white noise in the baby's room (e.g., radio static or an air conditioner)

Place a heating pad (set on a safe, comfortable setting) or a warmed washcloth under the baby's stomach

Place the baby facedown on your knees while stroking his or her back

Put the baby securely in a seat on top of a running washer or dryer (under diligent supervision)

Rock the baby in a rocking chair

Carry the baby in a front sling or pouch (this leaves your hands free)

Give the baby a pacifier

the child every time he or she cries. This causes a bloated stomach and more crying. Overall, rhythmic, soothing activities work best. It is most important that the parent avoid fatigue and exhaustion. A relative, spouse, friend, or sitter should provide some relief.

Colistin
One of the polymyxin group of *antibiotics*. It is used only to treat severe infections that are resistant to other antibiotics, due to a risk of damage to the kidneys and nerve tissue.

Colitis
Inflammation of the colon (the large intestine) causing diarrhea, usually with blood and mucus. Other symptoms may include abdominal pain and fever.
CAUSES
Colitis may be due to infection by a virus, an ameba, or a bacterium such as campylobacter that produces toxins that irritate the lining of the intestine. Other bacteria may directly infect the colon lining, causing colitis.

Antibiotics, especially if taken for a period of more than two weeks, may provoke a form of colitis. Antibiotics kill the bacteria that normally live in the intestine and may allow another type of bacterium, CLOSTRIDIUM DIFFICILE, to proliferate and produce an irritating toxin. Very commonly, prolonged use of antibiotics is associated with diarrhea that may be a direct irritative effect of the drug itself (antibiotic-associated diarrhea).

Ischemia, or impairment of the blood supply to the intestinal wall, which is usually due to *atherosclerosis* (narrowing of blood vessels), is a very rare cause in the elderly.

Ulcerative colitis and *Crohn's disease* are two serious intestinal disorders of unknown origin that usually start in young adulthood.

Other disorders that can cause symptoms similar to those of colitis include *proctitis* (inflammation of the rectum), which may be due to a form of ulcerative colitis or to *gonorrhea* or another sexually transmitted disease; inflammation of an area of colon affected by *diverticular disease*; or an intestinal cancer.
DIAGNOSIS
A physician will usually advise a patient with severe diarrhea to stop eating and to drink only clear fluids (e.g., water, tea, clear soups, and so on). If the diarrhea, with or without blood and mucus, persists for more

than five days despite these measures, the physician will usually send a sample of feces for investigation for parasites, and culture and smear staining for bacteria.

If digital examination of the rectum is normal and no infection is found, the rectum and colon will usually be examined with a sigmoidoscope (viewing tube for examining the rectum and colon, see *Sigmoidoscopy*) to see if there is any inflammation or ulceration of the lining. *Biopsy* samples of inflamed areas or ulcers may be taken and examined under a microscope to look for the changes of ulcerative colitis or Crohn's disease.

A barium enema of the colon may be performed (see *Barium X-ray examinations*) to look for any areas of narrowing or severe inflammation.
TREATMENT
Most infections that can cause a colitis resolve without treatment. Campylobacter infections are sometimes treated with the antibiotic drug erythromycin, amebic infections are treated with metronidazole, and clostridium infections are treated with metronidazole or vancomycin.

Colitis caused by ischemia is treated by surgical excision of the damaged section of colon. Crohn's disease and ulcerative colitis are treated with *corticosteroid drugs* (taken either by mouth or in an *enema* to settle an acute colitis), with different drugs (including sulfasalazine or newer forms of this drug that do not contain sulfa), or by a special diet and vitamin supplements. Surgery does not cure these diseases and is usually reserved for the treatment of complications.

Collagen
A tough, fibrous protein that is the single most common protein in the body. It is the body's major structural protein, forming an important part of tendons, bones, and connective tissues. Because of its tough, insoluble nature, collagen helps hold together the cells and tissues of the body.

Collagen diseases
Two groups of diseases are referred to as collagen diseases—true collagen diseases and connective tissue diseases. True collagen diseases are uncommon, usually inherited, and due to faulty formation of *collagen* fibers. Features of true collagen diseases include thin, slack skin and poor wound healing.

Connective tissue diseases are due to malfunctioning of the immune

system (see *Autoimmune disorders*). This malfunctioning often affects blood vessels and, as a result, produces secondary damage in connective tissues. For this reason, these diseases are sometimes called collagen vascular diseases. They are relatively common, and include *rheumatoid arthritis*, systemic *lupus erythematosus*, *periarteritis nodosa, scleroderma, dermatomyositis*, and other less clearly defined disorders.

Collarbone
The common name for the *clavicle*.

Collar, orthopedic
A device worn to treat neck pain or instability. A soft collar, usually made of foam, can relieve pain by limiting the movement of the neck, by transferring some of the weight of the head from the neck to the chest and by providing local warmth.

Stiff collars, commonly made of foam reinforced with plastic, are used when a fractured neck has almost healed but still needs support or when the vertebrae in the neck have otherwise become unstable.

Colles' fracture
A break just above the wrist in the radius (one of the two bones in the lower arm), usually resulting from a fall with the hand outstretched to break the fall. The fracture causes the wrist and hand to be displaced backward. Colles' fracture is the most common fracture in people over 40.

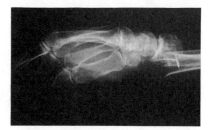

X ray of Colles' fracture
The wrist has been pushed back over the broken bone. This gives a classic "dinner fork" appearance when viewed from the side.
CAUSES AND INCIDENCE
The fracture usually occurs when someone stumbles when walking or slips on an icy sidewalk and puts out a hand to lessen the impact of the fall. Such a fall rarely produces a fracture in a young person, but it may be enough to break a bone weakened by *osteoporosis*, an invariable feature of aging. When a young person suffers a

C

Colles' fracture, it is usually the result of a more violent injury and often extends to the wrist joint itself.

SYMPTOMS

The wrist and hand are displaced and cannot be moved and there is severe pain and swelling in the area.

TREATMENT AND OUTLOOK

In most cases the two ends of the broken bone are manipulated back into position while the patient is under a local or general anesthetic, and a plaster cast is applied. Healing usually takes up to six weeks. When the cast is removed, the wrist may be stiff and exercise may be needed to restore its flexibility.

Minor deformity of the wrist may result from Colles' fracture, but movement of the hand and wrist is not usually impaired. In a young person, however, the more extensive damage may eventually lead to arthritis.

Colloid

A type of liquid similar to a suspension. A suspension—milk, for example—consists of insoluble particles of a substance suspended in a liquid. These particles are large and heavy enough to be separable from the liquid by centrifugation (spinning at high speed). A colloid is basically the same, except that its particles are significantly smaller and lighter than those of a suspension; they can be separated from the liquid part of the colloid only by ultracentrifugation (spinning at extremely high speed).

In medicine, colloid preparations containing *plasma proteins* (proteins in the fluid portion of blood) or certain complex carbohydrate molecules may be given to replace blood lost in cases of *shock* due to severe bleeding or burns. Such colloid preparations are called plasma expanders. Colloids containing gold or the metallic element technetium are used in some *radioisotope scanning* techniques.

The term colloid is also used to refer to the protein-containing material that fills the follicles of the *thyroid gland*.

Colon

The major part of the large intestine. A segmented tube about 2.5 inches (6.4 cm) wide and 4.5 feet (1.4 m) long, the colon forms a large loop, shaped somewhat like a distorted "M," in the abdomen. Its segments, or haustrations, give it an irregular outline.

The colon consists of four sections: the ascending, transverse, descending, and sigmoid colon. The first part, the ascending colon, starts at the

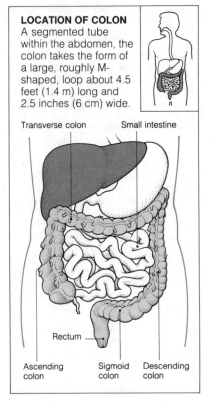

LOCATION OF COLON
A segmented tube within the abdomen, the colon takes the form of a large, roughly M-shaped, loop about 4.5 feet (1.4 m) long and 2.5 inches (6 cm) wide.

Transverse colon   Small intestine

Rectum

Ascending colon   Sigmoid colon   Descending colon

cecum, in the lower right-hand side of the abdomen, and extends up to a sharp bend just below the liver. This point, called the hepatic flexure, marks the beginning of the transverse colon, which loops across the abdomen, passing below the stomach to the spleen on the left-hand side of the abdomen. Here, there is a sharp downward bend (called the splenic flexure) that marks the start of the descending colon. From this point, the descending colon passes down the left side to approximately the brim of the pelvis, where it adopts an S-shaped course of variable length (the sigmoid colon) to connect with the *rectum* at the lower left-hand side of the abdomen.

STRUCTURE

The colon is a muscular tube with a lubricated inner lining. Its outermost layer, called the serous coat, is a tough, fibrous membrane with a smooth outer surface. This membrane protects the colon from damage when intestinal movements cause it to rub against the abdominal wall.

The muscular coat consists of three bands of longitudinal muscles and an inner layer of circular muscles. Rhythmic contractions and relaxations of these muscles (*peristalsis*)

squeeze the intestinal contents through the colon.

Inside the muscular coat is the third layer, the submucous coat. It consists of *connective tissue*, blood vessels, and lymphatic vessels.

The innermost layer is the mucous coat, which contains numerous tubular glands. These glands produce large amounts of mucus to lubricate the passage of digested material through the colon. Unlike the small intestine, the mucous coat of the colon (and the rest of the large intestine) is not folded into *villi* (tiny, fingerlike projections).

FUNCTION

The functions of the colon are, principally, to absorb water (and also a small amount of mineral salts) from the digested material passing through the colon and to concentrate indigestible waste for expulsion as feces.

When the intestinal contents enter the colon, digestion has been completed and the material is in the form of a liquid. As this liquid passes through the colon, the water and salts it contains are absorbed into the blood vessels in the submucous coat. By the time the intestinal contents pass out of the colon into the rectum, almost all the water has been absorbed and the contents are in the form of feces. (See also *Digestive system*; *Intestine* disorders box.)

Colon and rectal surgeon

A surgeon specializing in operations to correct disorders in or remove diseased tissue from the colon (large intestine) or the rectal area. Operations can range from the removal of *hemorrhoids* to the removal of part of the intestine. Patients are usually referred by another physician.

Colon, cancer of

See *Intestine, cancer of.*

Colon, disorders of

See *Intestine* disorders box.

Colon, irritable

See *Irritable bowel syndrome.*

Colonoscopy

Examination of the inside of the colon (the major part of the large intestine) by means of a long, flexible, fiberoptic viewing instrument called a colonoscope (see *Endoscopy*).

WHY IT IS DONE

Colonoscopy is used to investigate symptoms (such as bleeding from the bowel) and to look for disorders of the colon, such as colitis, polyps (small, benign, grapelike growths), and cancer. Attachments at the end of the instrument enable the physician to take biopsy specimens (remove small samples of tissue for analysis) or brushings for cytologic examination and to remove polyps.

HOW IT IS DONE
The patient takes laxatives for one or two days before the examination to empty the colon of feces. Because the procedure causes a little discomfort,

the patient is lightly sedated beforehand. The colonoscope is passed into the colon through the anus and guided along the length of the colon, which the operator examines through a viewing lens. A complete examination of the entire colon can take from 10 minutes to a couple of hours to perform.

Colon, spastic
See *Irritable bowel syndrome*.

Color blindness
See *Color vision deficiency*.

Color vision
The ability to discriminate among different parts of the color spectrum. It is an ability found in some, but not all, animals, and probably developed as an aid to finding or catching food.

THE COLOR SPECTRUM
Light perceived by the human eye consists of electromagnetic radiation

C

COLOR VISION

Light, consisting of radiation of various wavelengths, is focused on the retina, where light-sensitive rod and cone cells are stimulated to emit nerve impulses. Some initial processing of this "signaling" occurs in the ganglion cells of the retina, before impulses pass to the brain via the optic nerve.

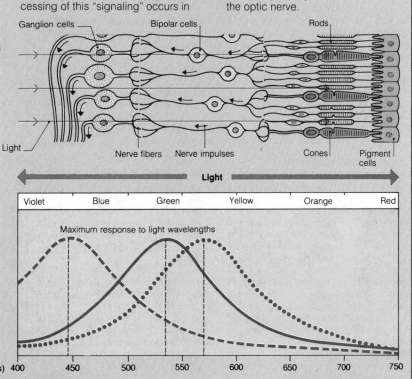

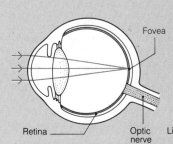

Location of color-sensitive cells
Light passes through the whole thickness of the retina before striking the rods and cones. Color vision depends mainly on the cones, concentrated in a region of the retina called the fovea.

Color response of cones
There are three classes of cone, and the graph shows how these vary in their response to the light spectrum. One class responds best to light of long wavelengths (red-sensitive cones), one to short wavelengths (blue-sensitive), and one to intermediate wavelengths (green-sensitive).

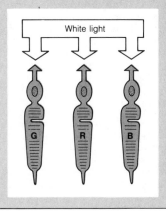

Response to white light
White light consists of a mixture of all wavelengths (colors), so it stimulates all three classes of cone to signal equally. This pattern of response produces the sensation of whiteness in the brain.

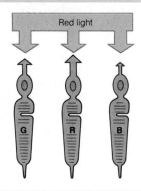

Response to red light
Light with a long wavelength (red light) produces a strong response from red-sensitive cones, a weak response from blue-sensitive cones, and an intermediate response from green-sensitive cones. This pattern of signaling is interpreted as the color red in the brain.

Key
G Green-sensitive
R Red-sensitive
B Blue-sensitive

C

(energy waves) with wavelengths between about 400 and 700 nanometers (a nanometer is 40 billionths of an inch). Going from the short to the long end of this spectrum, different wavelengths produce the sensations of violet, blue, green, yellow, orange, and red (colors of the spectrum, or rainbow) when they impinge upon the retina and stimulate nerve signals, which are processed in the rear portion of the brain (occipital lobe).

Light consisting of a single wavelength—pure spectral color—is rare in nature. The light reflected or emitted by most objects consists of a complex mixture of many different wavelengths, known as a spectral mixture. White light consists of a fairly uniform mixture of all wavelengths of the visible spectrum. The number of possible spectral mixtures is infinite, and a major task of the retina and brain is to sort and interpret the information available in order to produce a usefully large but finite number of perceivable colors (which is estimated at several million).

CONE FUNCTION

The light-sensitive cells in the retina are of two main types, rods and cones. Of these types, the rods vary little in their response to different light wavelengths, and thus play little, if any, part in color vision. The cone cells, of which there are roughly four million to seven million per eye, are more concentrated within a central area of the retina called the macula lutea; about 25,000 of the cones are in the central fovea in the center of this area. Consequently, color vision is most accurate for objects viewed directly and is poor at the periphery of vision. Color perception also requires a minimum level of total available light—below this level, only the rods respond, and everything is seen as shades of gray.

When light impinges upon a cone, it causes a structural change in pigment contained within the cone, which in turn causes the cone to emit an electrical impulse. Light of any wavelength and of sufficient intensity, in general, causes all cones to respond to some extent, but any single cone responds better (i.e., produces impulses more frequently) to certain wavelengths than others. Overall, it has been found that there are probably three classes of cone, responding maximally to light wavelengths of 445, 535, and 570 nanometers. Any particular light wavelength produces a unique overall pattern of response from all the cones together, and consequently any two wavelengths thus produce different patterns of response.

This offers some explanation of how the retina distinguishes light of different wavelengths, but gives few clues as to how information about complex mixtures of wavelengths is sorted, transmitted to the brain, and interpreted. The retina seems to contain other cells that receive, analyze, and compare the signals coming from several classes of cones. Further integration of the signals is accomplished as they are carried to the brain, where additional processing occurs, allowing for the perception of color. (See also *Eye; Perception; Vision*.)

Color vision deficiency

Any abnormality of the color vision system that causes a person to see colors differently from other people or causes difficulty distinguishing among certain colors. Such deficiencies are of various types and differ markedly in degree. Mild forms of deficiency are by far the most common; people with such mild defects generally have vision that is completely adequate for most purposes. True "color blindness" (monochromatism), in which the world is seen only in shades of black, white, and gray, is extremely rare.

CAUSES AND TYPES

Most cases of color vision deficiency are caused by an inherited defect of light-sensitive pigment in one or more classes of cone cell in the retina of the eye (see *Color vision*) and/or an abnormality or reduced number of the cone cells themselves. Acquired color vision deficiency may occur with certain retinal and optic nerve diseases and degenerations or trauma (injury).

The two common types of hereditary color vision deficiency are reduced discrimination of light wavelengths within the middle (green) and long (red) parts of the visible spectrum. The inherited defects are usually sex-linked (see *Genetic disorders*), which means that the majority of sufferers are male, although women may carry the defect and pass it on to some of their children.

A further very small group of people have a blue deficiency, called tritanopia, which may be inherited or due to the toxic effects of poisons or drugs on, or degenerative processes of, the retina or optic nerve.

INCIDENCE

Among whites of European origin, about 8 percent of males and less than 1 percent of females have either green or red deficiency. The prevalence is generally lower in people of Asian or American Indian origin and even lower among blacks. The prevalence of both blue deficiency and monochromatism may be as low as one affected person per 100,000.

SYMPTOMS

Most people with defective color vision have no reason to suspect there is anything abnormal about the way they see, because they have no ready access to how other people see the world and because most cases are mild and do not interfere with daily living. Most cases come to light only when a person is noticed making mistakes with color discrimination, such as confusing close shades of colors. Other cases are discovered when the person's color vision is tested.

DIAGNOSIS AND MEASUREMENT

Color vision is commonly tested, usually by means of special color plates under daylight conditions, during childhood or on entry to professions for which good color discrimination is needed.

More complicated testing, such as arranging sequences of colored chips or use of an anomaloscope, may also be used. The anomaloscope shines a variable mixture of green and red lights, and the person is asked to adjust the mixture until it appears the same as a fixed yellow light. If the adjusted mixture looks far too red or too green to the person with normal vision, the subject of the test is color defective. The severity of the defect is also measurable in this way.

OUTLOOK

People with the common, inherited, types of color deficiency retain the defect for life. It could be important for them to know about the abnormality, especially if considering an occupation that depends on color. The following occupations or careers may be unsuitable: train driver, airplane or marine pilot, electrician, jeweler, commercial artist, color photographer. In particular, the person who is severely color deficient can potentially be dangerous in some jobs (an electrician, for example, if color-coded wires cannot be properly identified). However, the more common mild color vision deficiencies do not interfere with most activities.

Colostomy

An operation in which part of the colon (large intestine) is brought through an incision in the abdominal wall and formed into an artificial opening to allow the discharge of feces into a lightweight bag attached to the skin. The colostomy may be temporary or permanent.

WHY IT IS DONE

In a severely ill patient, a temporary colostomy may be carried out as an emergency measure to deal with an obstruction or perforation in the large intestine that is preventing the patient from passing feces. The colostomy is made above the obstruction and, by allowing the feces to discharge, enables the patient to become well enough for a partial *colectomy* (an operation to remove part of the large intestine) to remove the obstruction. A temporary colostomy may also be performed at the same time as a colectomy to allow the repair to the colon to heal without feces passing through it. Temporary colostomies are closed when the rejoined colon has healed.

A permanent colostomy is needed when all or part of the rectum or anus, as well as part of the large intestine (for example, in cases of cancer of the rectum), require removal and normal defecation is no longer possible.

RECOVERY PERIOD

For two or three days after the operation the patient is fed intravenously. After that, the patient is given a light diet and begins to pass feces through the stoma (artificial opening) into a lightweight bag that is attached by adhesive seals to the skin around the stoma. After a bowel movement, the bag is exchanged for a new one.

During this period the patient should receive advice and training—preferably from a specialist nurse—on the care and management of the stoma and on how to apply and change the colostomy bag.

After leaving the hospital, the patient usually needs to convalesce for up to several weeks before returning to normal activities.

OUTLOOK

A person with a colostomy may eventually establish an almost normal bowel routine. The bowel usually discharges feces into the bag once or twice a day; the bag is then changed. The person with a temporary colostomy wears a bag over the stoma until the operation to close it is performed.

A person with a colostomy can expect to lead a normal life once fully recovered from the operation. The co-

PROCEDURE FOR COLOSTOMY

An incision is made in the abdominal wall and either a small loop of the colon or (if the rectum and anus have been removed) the severed end of the colon is pulled through. If a loop of the colon is used, an opening is made in it large enough for the feces to pass through. The edges of this opening or the edges of the severed end of the colon are stitched to the skin at the edge of the abdominal incision to create a stoma (artificial opening).

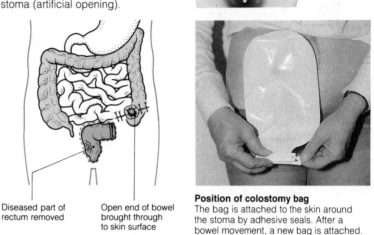

Large intestine

Possible sites of colostomy openings

Small intestine

Diseased part of rectum removed

Open end of bowel brought through to skin surface

Position of colostomy bag
The bag is attached to the skin around the stoma by adhesive seals. After a bowel movement, a new bag is attached.

lostomy usually causes no trouble, but occasionally a problem can occur. For example, the colostomy can prolapse (protrude too far from the abdomen) or become narrowed, blocking the passage of feces. In most cases these problems are overcome by surgery.

Colostrum

The thick, yellowish fluid produced by the breasts during late pregnancy and the first few days after childbirth. Colostrum is replaced by mature breast milk the week following birth. Compared with mature breast milk, colostrum contains less fat and sugar, and more minerals and protein. It has a high content of *lymphocytes* (a type of white blood cell) and *immunoglobulins* (antibodies), which help protect the baby from infection.

Colposcopy

Visual inspection of a woman's cervix (neck of the uterus) and vagina under illuminated magnification. A series of lenses is employed that can provide magnification of between five and 25 times.

WHY IT IS DONE

Colposcopy is performed to recognize or exclude the presence of any areas of precancerous conditions or early cancer in the tissues covering the cervix (see *Cervix, cancer of*). Usually, the gynecologist has been alerted by an abnormal *cervical smear test* (Pap smear), by smears that repeatedly show inflammation or infection, or by an abnormal appearance of the cervix during visual inspection at the time of a physical examination.

HOW IT IS DONE

Colposcopy is a painless procedure requiring no anesthetic. With the woman in the lithotomy position (lying on her back with legs apart and supported), the vagina and cervix are exposed using a speculum (an instrument that widens the opening and separates the collapsed walls of the vagina). The exposed tissues are first wiped with a dry sponge; the area is then washed with a solution of either dilute acetic acid or saline. The tissues are visually inspected under magnification to identify any suspicious-looking areas.

C

The applied solution causes any precancerous areas to show up either white (instead of their natural pink state) or with a characteristic surface pattern due to abnormal blood vessels. Once any such areas are seen, a *biopsy* sample of the tissue can be obtained. If, on examination by a pathologist, the tissue sample shows cells typical of severe dysplasia (abnormal growth) or an early cancer, and if the whole of the abnormal area can be seen, local destruction treatment (by *diathermy*, *cryosurgery*, or *laser treatment*) can be employed.

If any of the abnormal area is within the cervical canal, a *cone biopsy* (removal of a conical section of the cervix for inspection) is needed.

Coma
A state of unconsciousness and unresponsiveness distinguishable from *sleep* in that the person does not respond to external stimulation (e.g., shouting or pinching) or to his or her inner needs (e.g., a full bladder).

CAUSES
Coma results from disturbance or damage to areas of the brain involved in conscious activity or the maintenance of consciousness—in particular, parts of the *cerebrum* (the main mass of the brain), upper parts of the brain stem, and central regions of the brain, especially the *limbic system*.

The damage may be the result of a head injury, or of an abnormality such as a *brain tumor*, *brain abscess*, or *intracerebral hemorrhage*; all are shown by brain imaging techniques.

More often, there has been a buildup of poisonous substances that intoxicates brain tissues (due to a drug overdose, advanced liver or kidney disease, acute alcoholic intoxication, or in uncontrolled *diabetes mellitus*) or there has been impairment of blood flow to some brain areas, leading to cerebral *hypoxia* (lack of oxygen). *Encephalitis* and *meningitis* (respectively, inflammation of the brain and inflammation of the brain's protective coverings) can also cause coma.

SYMPTOMS
Varying depths of coma are recognized. In less severe forms, the person may respond to stimulation by uttering a few words or perhaps moving an arm. In severe cases, the person fails to respond in this way to repeated vigorous stimuli. However, even deeply comatose patients may show some automatic responses—they continue to breathe unaided, may cough, yawn, blink, and show roving eye movements, indicating that the lower brain stem, which controls these responses, is still functioning.

Measurement of variations in the depth of coma is important in assessment and treatment. Variations can be recorded by systems that classify the coma according to the person's verbal behavior, the movements he or she makes, and the state of the eyes (whether open, shut, or roving).

A person may remain in a state of deep coma for years, with little or no apparent activity in the cerebrum, but may be still alive because the brain stem is still functioning. By contrast, spread of the damage or disturbance to the lower brain stem may impair the vital functions of coughing, swallowing, and breathing. Artificial ventilation and maintenance of the circulation may be needed. Complete irreversible loss of brain-stem function leads to death (see *Brain death*).

Combination drug
One that contains more than a single, active, therapeutic substance. A common example is the antibiotic drug co-trimoxazole, which contains sulfamethoxazole and trimethoprim.

Comedo
Another name for a *blackhead*.

Commensal
A usually harmless bacterium or other organism that normally lives in or on the body. Occasionally, commensals may cause disease, especially in people with impaired immunity.

Commitment
The process by which an individual suffering from a severe mental disorder is legally deprived of his or her freedom. A person is committed if he or she is likely to harm him- or herself or other people. Physicians who have examined the person explain to the court, usually in writing, why they believe he or she should be placed in a mental institution.

Commode
A portable chair that contains a removable toilet bowl in its seat. Commodes are useful for patients who are not confined to bed but who are not mobile enough to use the bathroom.

Communicable disease
Any disease caused by a microorganism or parasite that can be transmitted from one person or animal to another. (See *Infectious disease*.)

Compartment syndrome
A painful cramp caused by compression of a group of muscles during exercise. Usually, the affected muscles are situated in a confined space, so that when they expand slightly during exercise they are thus compressed and the blood flow through them is obstructed. The muscles may have become slightly enlarged before exercise, through intensive training, or possibly through injury.

An example is tibial compartment syndrome, in which muscles on the outer side of the shin expand within their lining and cause a cramp in this area. Usually the pain subsides rapidly when exercise is stopped.

Compensation neurosis
Psychological reaction to injury affected by the prospect of financial compensation. Also called accident or "traumatic" neurosis, the symptoms vary with personality, but headache, dizzy spells, loss of concentration, anxiety, and mild depression are common, as are neurological symptoms, such as pain and tingling in the legs or numbness in the affected part.

Some specialists consider the neurosis to be a genuine and persistent psychiatric reaction; others insist it is an attempt, conscious or unconscious, to manipulate the situation for profit. Repeated medical assessments, legal wrangling, and contradictory experts make this one of the most difficult areas of psychiatric diagnosis. Backing the idea of a genuine organic disorder, recent studies have shown that some people's symptoms persisted over the period of observation even after a satisfactory settlement of their insurance claims.

Complex
A group of related ideas, beliefs, and memories that have great importance emotionally, but which are always unconscious. The term was first used by the early psychoanalysts Sigmund Freud and Carl Jung to sum up psychological states deriving from experiences and relationships in childhood. The *Oedipus complex* is an important example, affecting all levels of adult behavior and attitudes.

Compliance
The degree to which patients follow medical advice. One reason for poor compliance is that patients sometimes do not remember or understand the physician's advice. Good compliance

is more likely if the patient knows what to expect from taking the prescribed medicine. It is also important to know whether side effects are possible or likely, under what circumstances any medication should be stopped, and whether a prescribed drug has the potential to interact with other medicines the patient may be taking.

Complication
A disease or condition that results from, and is often more serious than, another condition. For example, in a case of *appendicitis*, the inflamed appendix may burst, spreading infection throughout the abdominal cavity and causing a serious complication called *peritonitis*. The childhood condition *mumps* occasionally has complications that may be serious, particularly *encephalitis* (inflammation of the brain) or *orchitis* (inflammation of the testes).

Sometimes a complication may be the result of treatment. Recovery from a surgical operation, for example, may be complicated by infection of the wound (caused by germs in the skin or in the operating room) or by cross infection from other patients.

Compos mentis
Latin for "of sound mind."

Compress
A pad of sheet lint or linen applied, under pressure, to an area of skin, and held in place by a bandage. The pad may be soaked in ice-cold water or wrapped around ice to provide a cold compress for reducing pain, swelling, and bleeding under the skin immediately after an injury (see *Ice pack*).

Compresses that have been soaked in hot water increase the circulation and are useful for bringing boils to a head. A dry compress may be used to stop bleeding from a wound (see *Bleeding* first-aid treatment box) or may be smeared with medication such as magnesium sulfate to draw pus from an infected area of skin.

Compression syndrome
A collection of symptoms caused by pressure on a nerve or nerves that supply the muscles and carry sensations from a particular area of the body. The symptoms may include numbness, tingling, discomfort, and muscle weakness. The best known is *carpal tunnel syndrome* (which affects the hand), caused by pressure on the median nerve as it passes under a ligament in the wrist.

Compulsive behavior
See *Obsessive-compulsive behavior*.

Computer-aided diagnosis
The physician makes a diagnosis by considering the patient's symptoms and medical history, examining the patient, and, when necessary, making use of imaging procedures, blood tests, and other diagnostic aids. Today, the computer has been added to the list of such aids.

PROBABILITY-BASED SYSTEMS
With probability-based systems the computer is used to store vast quantities of information involving cases of many different disorders. For example, it may be programmed with the details of thousands of cases of stomach pain—giving, for each patient, the exact type, location, and duration of the pain, accompanying symptoms, and relevant medical history, together with the eventual diagnosis. A physician confronted with a new case of stomach pain can enter the details into the computer, which, in a matter of seconds, will compare them with those already stored in its memory. It will then print out a list of the most likely diagnoses.

Although such computers are currently used in comparatively few hospitals, they are proving valuable in the treatment of people isolated from medical services, such as oil-rig crews or deep-sea divers. If someone becomes sick, the computer may be used to diagnose whether the case is an emergency requiring the sick person to be transported to a hospital.

PATTERN-RECOGNITION SYSTEMS
Computers can also be programmed to recognize and interpret visual data. One example is the examination of cells under a microscope. The computer has the ability to recognize abnormal cells. This could be of great future significance in certain types of *blood count* (for example, a differential white blood cell count) and also in *cervical smear tests* (Pap smears), in which cells taken from the cervix are microscopically examined for early signs of cancer. At present, each of the millions of smears taken annually needs examination by a laboratory technician, who can check only a comparatively small number at a time.

Computerized tomography
Another name for *CT scanning*.

Conception
Fertilization of a woman's *ovum* (egg) by a man's *sperm*, followed by implan-

tation of the resultant blastocyst in the lining of the *uterus*. (See also *Contraception*; *Pregnancy*.)

Concussion
Brief unconsciousness, usually lasting only a few seconds, that follows a violent blow to the head or neck. The loss of consciousness is due to disturbance of the electrical activity in the brain, and in most cases is not associated with any damage. Even so, concussion should always be treated seriously and reported to a physician.

Among the more common causes of concussion are traffic accidents, sports injuries, falls, industrial accidents, and blows received in fights.

SYMPTOMS AND TREATMENT
Common symptoms immediately following concussion include: confusion, inability to remember events immediately before the injury, dizziness, blurred vision, and vomiting. The more prolonged the period of unconsciousness, the more severe and persistent symptoms tend to be.

Repeated concussion—as happens, for example, to some boxers—can damage the brain and cause the "punchdrunk" syndrome: impaired concentration, slow thinking, and slurred speech.

Anyone who has been knocked out should see a physician, who will usually advise 24 hours of bed rest, either in a hospital or at home, under observation. The person should not drive a car or play any sport during this time. If new symptoms develop, such as drowsiness, difficulty breathing, repeated vomiting, or visual disturbances, they should be reported to the physician immediately since they could signify damage to a brain area or an *extradural hemorrhage* (bleeding between the skull and the outside of the brain).

The initial symptoms usually start to clear within a few days. If they fail to do so, medical opinion should be sought again, at which time the physician may wish to have the condition further investigated. (See also *Head injury*; *Drop attack*; *Syncope*.)

Conditioning
The formation of a specific type of response or behavior to a specific stimulus in the environment.
TYPES
Theories of conditioning are based largely on the work of the animal psychologists Pavlov and Skinner, whose names are identified with classical and operant conditioning.

C

In classical conditioning, if a stimulus that is known to consistently produce a response is paired consistently with a second "neutral" stimulus, eventually the second stimulus alone will produce the response. Pavlov demonstrated this occurrence in dogs. Each time food was presented to the dog, making it salivate, a bell was rung. Eventually the dog would salivate in response to the bell alone. Pavlov noted that the response would generalize to similar stimuli. Thus a dog conditioned to salivate when shown a round object would also salivate, although not as much, when shown an elliptical one. He also found that the conditioned response would eventually fade if not reinforced occasionally with the original neutral stimulus.

In operant conditioning, behavior is determined by rewards and punishments. Skinner placed a hungry rat in a box. It moved randomly about the cage, but occasionally accidentally pawed a lever, which released a pellet of food. Eventually the rat learned to press the lever whenever it wanted food; that is, it became conditioned.

EFFECTS

Behavioral psychologists believe that all behavior is learned in this way, and they regard psychiatric problems as learned behavior patterns. Many neurotic disorders are thought to arise because a previously neutral stimulus becomes associated with an anxiety-provoking stimulus. For example, someone who was punished as a child by being shut in a closet may develop claustrophobia (fear of enclosed spaces) because the enclosed space becomes associated with the fear of punishment. The anxiety may spread to fear of crowds or heights, for example, and does not diminish because it is continually reinforced by behavior; the claustrophobic person avoids using elevators or entering crowded shops.

Treatment for these disorders is based on the same principles of conditioning. A response that has been learned can also be unlearned, or a more appropriate form of behavior can be relearned (see *Behavior therapy*).

Condom

A barrier method of male contraception in the form of a thin latex rubber or plastic sheath placed over the penis before intercourse. Condoms provide both partners with some protection against sexual transmission of disease. (See *Contraception, barrier methods*.)

Conduct disorders

A group of behavioral disturbances, occurring in childhood or adolescence, in which the individual persistently and repetitively violates the rights and privileges of others. These violations may include vandalism, arson, assault, and robbery, as well as less aggressive forms of behavior such as truancy, substance abuse, and persistent lying (see *Behavioral problems in children; Adolescence*).

Condyloma acuminatum

See *Warts, genital*.

Condyloma latum

A small, moist, wartlike growth in the skin. In the second stage of the sexually transmitted disease *syphilis*, several develop at the side of the mouth, around the anus, and around the entrance to the vagina.

Cone biopsy

A surgical technique in which a section of the lower part of the cervix (neck of the uterus) is removed, either in the shape of a cone or a cylinder.

WHY IT IS DONE

A cone biopsy is performed if a woman has had an abnormal *cervical smear test* (Pap smear) or a series of abnormal smears, and if visual inspection of the cervix by *colposcopy* has failed to delineate the exact area of cancer or precancerous conditions (see *Cervix, cancer of*). Sometimes a cone biopsy is performed if a smear test suggests the presence of cancer, but colposcopy has failed to detect any abnormality on the outer surface of the cervix or at the entrance to the canal. In the latter cases there may be a precancerous area or cancer confined to the cervical canal.

Cone biopsy is now being accomplished using *laser* techniques or *cryosurgery*. (See also box on biopsy of the *cervix*.)

Confabulation

The use of a fictional story to make up for gaps in memory. Confabulation differs from lying in that it is motivated by the need to make sense of one's past rather than by a desire to deliberately deceive a listener. The phenomenon occurs most commonly in chronic alcoholics, when it is known as *Wernicke-Korsakoff syndrome*, and in people with head injuries.

Confidentiality

The ethical principle that a physician does not disclose to others information given in confidence by a patient. This concept was introduced by the ancient Greek physician Hippocrates and has been adopted by medical associations in all countries.

The physician's responsibility for maintaining confidential records has become more difficult with modern trends in medical practice. Clinics and health centers may have scores of medical and ancillary staff with access to records. In hospitals with computerized records, thousands of staff members may have such access. In theory everyone working in a medical setting is expected to understand and respect the code of confidentiality. In practice the code seems to be breached only rarely. More sophisticated computer systems make it possible to render the sensitive sections of medical records secure.

The patient's consent to disclosure is required before a physician may give confidential information to an employer, insurance company, or lawyer. When required by law to disclose confidential information, a physician does not have (as lawyers have) any "privilege" that allows refusal. A physician who persists in refusal is in contempt of court.

Physicians who treat children are expected to discuss their findings with the parents. As children mature, a point is reached at which their confidences merit the same respect as those of adult patients. In general, physicians believe that they should respect a child's request for confidentiality.

Most legal systems require physicians to override confidentiality in certain cases. For example, they are required to notify certain health authorities about specified infectious diseases; if patients with certain of these diseases refuse treatment, the health authorities may be informed so that treatment or isolation may be imposed by law. Physicians are generally required to notify the police if they treat gunshot wounds or know of other serious crimes.

Physicians who breach confidentiality without legal justification may be sued in the civil courts; damages may be awarded against them.

Confusion

A disorganized mental state in which the abilities to remember, think clearly, and reason are impaired.

TYPES AND CAUSES

Confusion can be acute or chronic. The acute condition can arise as a symptom of *delirium*, in which the activity of the brain is affected by fever, drugs, poisons, or injury. Elderly people are particularly prone to acute confusional states from these causes, especially from certain drugs (e.g., *barbiturates, tranquilizers,* or *alcohol*).

Chronic confusion is often associated with *alcohol dependence,* long-term use of tranquilizers, and certain organic mental disorders such as *schizophrenia.* Chronic confusion is a feature of *dementia,* a brain disorder commonly caused by the progressive degeneration and death of brain cells.

SYMPTOMS AND SIGNS

People who are acutely confused often suffer from terrifying hallucinations and may behave in a violent and abusive manner. However, acute confusion is usually only temporary, and few people remember the events after the attack has passed.

Chronic confusion is generally noticeable from features such as absentmindedness, poor short-term memory, and a tendency for the sufferer to repeat himself or herself. Chronically confused people may also become depressed and frustrated, but they are less likely to become aggressive or violent. Many of the conditions responsible for chronic confusion tend to be slowly progressive.

DIAGNOSIS AND TREATMENT

An accurate diagnosis is essential before confusion can be treated. A detailed description of the symptoms (often from a relative) and a general physical examination will suggest which studies should be performed.

If a treatable cause is found, the appropriate treatment can often produce a marked improvement. Undiagnosable acute confusion may be treated with sedatives. Medicine has little to offer the elderly, chronically confused patient apart from skilled, supervised care.

Congenital

A term that means "present at birth." Thus, a congenital abnormality is a defect that has been present since birth. It may have been inherited genetically from the parents, may have occurred as the result of damage or infection in the uterus, or may have occurred at the time of birth. Congenital abnormalities are often also called *birth defects.*

Note that "congenital" does not mean the same as "hereditary." Not all congenital abnormalities are inherited, and many hereditary diseases (such as *Huntington's chorea*) are not apparent at birth.

Diseases and disorders that are not congenital—for example, most infectious diseases, cancers, and degenerative disorders—are called "acquired."

Congestion

Usually a reference to the accumulation of an excessive amount of blood, *tissue fluid,* or *lymph* in part of the body. A major cause of congestion is an increased flow of blood in the area, as occurs in inflammation. Another possible cause is reduced drainage of blood from the area, as can occur in *heart failure,* venous disorders such as *varicose veins,* and *lymphatic* disorders. (See also *Congestion, nasal.*)

Congestion, nasal

Obstruction of the flow of air through the passages of the nose due to swelling of its lining. Congestion may be accompanied by the accumulation of thick nasal mucus, which further impedes breathing. These two factors produce the familiar feelings of a stuffy, "full" nose, and the frequent desire to blow the nose (which usually has little effect on the congestion).

Nasal congestion is a symptom of the common cold (see *Cold, common*) or hay fever (see *Rhinitis, allergic*). In these conditions, the swelling is due to inflammation of the nasal lining. This inflammation may become persistent in certain disorders such as *sinusitis* or nasal *polyps.*

Congestive heart failure

See *Heart failure.*

Conjunctiva

The transparent membrane covering the sclera (white of the eye) and lining the inside of the eyelids. Cells in the conjunctiva produce a fluid (similar to tears) that lubricates the lids and the cornea. Blood vessels within the conjunctiva are normally invisible to the naked eye, but become engorged in *conjunctivitis* (pinkeye) and other inflammatory conditions.

Conjunctivitis

Inflammation of the conjunctiva, causing redness, discomfort, and a discharge from the affected eye.

Conjunctivitis is very common. Each year, at least one person in 50 visits a physician because of this complaint. The common causes are infections (especially in children) and allergy (more common in adults).

INFECTIVE CONJUNCTIVITIS

Most conjunctival infections are caused by bacteria—for example,

LOCATION OF CONJUNCTIVA
This transparent membrane covers the white of the eye and lines the inside of the eyelids.

Sclera / Conjunctiva / Cornea / Iris / Lens

C

staphylococci—that are spread by hand-to-eye contact, or by viruses, associated with a cold, sore throat, or illness such as measles. Viral conjunctivitis can occur in epidemics, spreading rapidly (through schools and other group settings).

Newborn babies occasionally acquire a type of conjunctival infection called neonatal *ophthalmia,* caused by spread of infection from the mother's cervix during birth. This type of infection may be with common bacteria, with the microorganisms responsible for *gonorrhea* or genital *herpes,* or may be a *chlamydial infection* (any of which may be present on the mother's cervix without symptoms). The infection may spread to the whole of the baby's eye and can cause blindness.

Keratoconjunctivitis is an inflammation of both the conjunctiva and the cornea; it is often due to a viral infection. In some tropical countries, *trachoma* is a serious form of conjunctivitis caused by a type of chlamydial infection.

ALLERGIC CONJUNCTIVITIS

The following substances can provoke an allergic response of the conjunctiva: cosmetics (such as mascara), contact lens cleaning solutions, and pollen among allergic *rhinitis* (hay fever) sufferers. Prevention is by avoiding the causative substance.

SYMPTOMS AND DIAGNOSIS

All types of conjunctivitis cause redness, discomfort of an itchy, scratchy nature, a discharge, and occasionally photophobia (dislike of bright lights). In infective conjunctivitis the discharge is purulent (containing pus) and may occasionally stick the eyelids together in the morning. In allergic conjunctivitis the discharge is clear, and the eyelids are often swollen.

Diagnosis is made from the appearance of the eye. If an infection is suspected, swabs may be taken to find out the causative organism, especially in a newborn baby when an exact diagnosis may be needed.

TREATMENT

Warm water is used to wash away the discharge and remove any crusts on the eyelids. In babies the eye may be washed with sterile saline solution.

If an infection is suspected, antibiotic eye drops or ointment (with chloramphenicol, for instance) are instilled into the eye. These will not cure a viral conjunctivitis, which tends to resolve of its own accord.

Allergic conjunctivitis can be helped by the use of antihistamine drops. Occasionally, corticosteroid drops are used, but only when there is definitely no infection present (which could be made worse by corticosteroids).

Connective tissue

The material that holds together the various structures of the body. Some structures are made up of connective tissue, notably *tendons* and *cartilage*. Connective tissue also forms the matrix (ground substance) of *bone* and the nonmuscular structures of *arteries* and *veins*.

Connective tissue diseases

See *Collagen diseases*.

Conn's syndrome

A disorder caused by the secretion of excessive amounts of the hormone aldosterone by a benign tumor of one of the adrenal glands. This upsets the body's salt and water balance, causing *hypertension* (high blood pressure) and symptoms such as thirst, muscle weakness, and excessive passage of urine. (See also *Aldosteronism*.)

Consciousness

An awareness of self and surroundings, so that a person knows what he or she is doing and intends to do. The awareness is dependent on sensations (especially visual and auditory), memories, and experiences.

Such awareness requires intact brain function, particularly within the *cerebrum* (the main mass of the brain) and the reticular system in the *brain stem*. The content of consciousness relies heavily on the functions of the cerebrum—for example, on memory

and the interpretation of sensations—while wakefulness is linked with the reticular system.

Although a person may be conscious, much that goes on within the brain is still below the level of consciousness. In psychological terms this activity is referred to as subconscious activity.

Disturbance of consciousness leads to impaired attention, concentration, and understanding. The thinking becomes slowed and memory fails. There appears to be a lack of direction in thoughts and actions. Although patients can be stimulated to respond, their responses are faulty. As the level of arousal deteriorates, the person may eventually pass into a state of *stupor* and then *coma*.

Consent

The legal term describing a patient's agreement with a physician performing an operation, arranging drug treatment, or carrying out diagnostic tests. Consent is valid only if the patient has been fully informed about the purpose of the procedure, the likely outcome, and both common and rare complications and side effects that may arise.

AVAILABILITY OF INFORMATION

Even as recently as the 1960s many physicians in the US believed it necessary to conceal much of the information about an illness and its treatment from the patient and his or her family. At that time few physicians told patients they had cancer, even when the illness was at an advanced stage, and few told such patients that they would die. Similarly, few physicians discussed the risk of death or serious complications—small but unavoidable—in any surgical procedure requiring an anesthetic, or explained the full range of side effects possible from treatment with a particular drug.

This concealment was justified by the medical profession in the paternalistic belief that the physician knew best, and that patients were unable to understand technical terms or concepts. The consumer rights movements of the 1960s and 1970s swept away such ideas, and physicians now recognize that patients expect full and frank information about illness and its treatment. In the US, a physician has no defense if the patient suffers harm from a foreseeable hazard of treatment that was not disclosed at the time consent was given. In other countries (such as Britain), physicians are still allowed to conceal rare hazards if they

believe that such a policy is in the patient's best interests.

Nevertheless, even in the US the amount of detailed information offered to patients varies from physician to physician. Some distribute printed information sheets before asking patients to sign consent forms, while others discuss the issues at length. Many physicians tell patients that they will answer their questions honestly, but will not force unwanted information on them.

When the investigation or treatment is carried out solely for the patient's benefit the explanations may be fairly brief, but more detail is usually offered when patients are asked to take part in research studies that may be of no direct benefit to them as individuals. Under these circumstances the purpose of the study must be explained along with all its hazards. Consent to a research procedure is invalid if any pressure was placed on the patient (for example, by suggestions that participation in the study would ensure preferential treatment by a surgeon).

WITHHOLDING CONSENT

Consent cannot be given by children or by people with serious mental disorders. Consent may be given (or withheld) on their behalf by parents or relatives. On several occasions in recent years, however, the courts have intervened and overruled the consent of relatives to withhold treatment from newborn children with severe handicaps and from adults with permanent brain damage. This action by the courts is based on the doctrine that the law forbids euthanasia or assisted suicide, whether or not the patient consents or consent is given on his or her behalf. Consent may not be given on behalf of children or the mentally ill for research procedures that would be of no benefit to them as individuals.

Constipation

The infrequent or difficult passing of hard, dry feces. In most cases constipation is harmless, but occasionally it may be a symptom of an underlying disorder, especially if it is of recent onset in an adult over 40. Many people worry that they do not move their bowels often enough, but, in fact, regularity and comfort of bowel action are more important than frequency. However, any persistent change in the pattern of bowel movements should be investigated by a physician to rule out a serious disorder.

CONSTIPATION Infrequent or difficult passing of hard bowel movements.

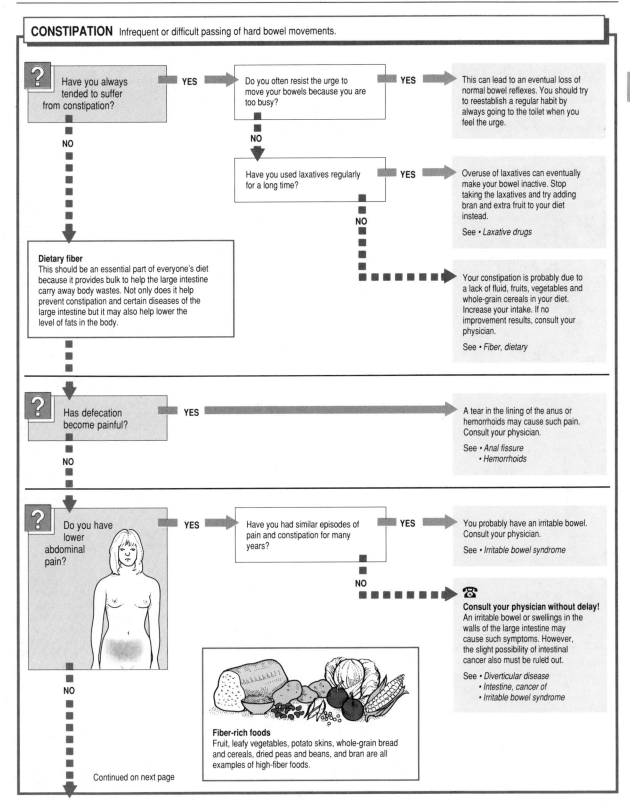

Have you always tended to suffer from constipation?

YES → **Do you often resist the urge to move your bowels because you are too busy?**

YES → This can lead to an eventual loss of normal bowel reflexes. You should try to reestablish a regular habit by always going to the toilet when you feel the urge.

NO ↓

Have you used laxatives regularly for a long time?

YES → Overuse of laxatives can eventually make your bowel inactive. Stop taking the laxatives and try adding bran and extra fruit to your diet instead.

See • *Laxative drugs*

NO →

Your constipation is probably due to a lack of fluid, fruits, vegetables and whole-grain cereals in your diet. Increase your intake. If no improvement results, consult your physician.

See • *Fiber, dietary*

NO ↓

Dietary fiber
This should be an essential part of everyone's diet because it provides bulk to help the large intestine carry away body wastes. Not only does it help prevent constipation and certain diseases of the large intestine but it may also help lower the level of fats in the body.

Has defecation become painful?

YES → A tear in the lining of the anus or hemorrhoids may cause such pain. Consult your physician.

See • *Anal fissure*
    • *Hemorrhoids*

NO ↓

Do you have lower abdominal pain?

YES → **Have you had similar episodes of pain and constipation for many years?**

YES → You probably have an irritable bowel. Consult your physician.

See • *Irritable bowel syndrome*

NO →

☎
Consult your physician without delay!
An irritable bowel or swellings in the walls of the large intestine may cause such symptoms. However, the slight possibility of intestinal cancer also must be ruled out.

See • *Diverticular disease*
    • *Intestine, cancer of*
    • *Irritable bowel syndrome*

Fiber-rich foods
Fruit, leafy vegetables, potato skins, whole-grain bread and cereals, dried peas and beans, and bran are all examples of high-fiber foods.

NO ↓

Continued on next page

C

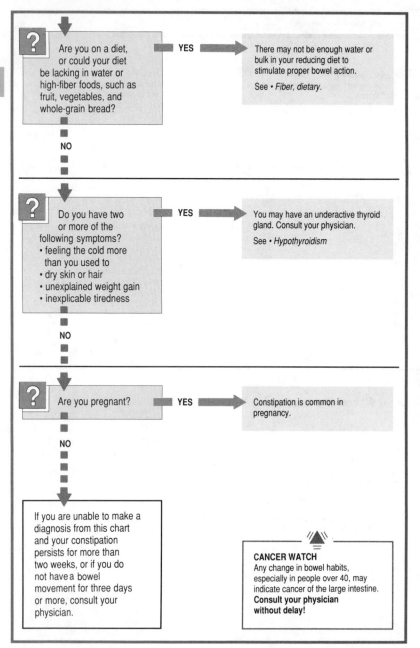

? Are you on a diet, or could your diet be lacking in water or high-fiber foods, such as fruit, vegetables, and whole-grain bread?

YES → There may not be enough water or bulk in your reducing diet to stimulate proper bowel action.

See • *Fiber, dietary.*

NO

? Do you have two or more of the following symptoms?
• feeling the cold more than you used to
• dry skin or hair
• unexplained weight gain
• inexplicable tiredness

YES → You may have an underactive thyroid gland. Consult your physician.

See • *Hypothyroidism*

NO

? Are you pregnant?

YES → Constipation is common in pregnancy.

NO

If you are unable to make a diagnosis from this chart and your constipation persists for more than two weeks, or if you do not have a bowel movement for three days or more, consult your physician.

CANCER WATCH
Any change in bowel habits, especially in people over 40, may indicate cancer of the large intestine. **Consult your physician without delay!**

CAUSES

The most common cause of constipation in Western countries is insufficient *fiber* in the diet. Fiber, which is found in foods such as whole-grain bread, fresh fruit, and vegetables, provides the bulk that the muscles of the colon (large intestine) need to stimulate propulsion of the fecal matter.

Lack of regular bowel-moving habits is another cause. This may be the result of inadequate toilet training in childhood or of repeatedly ignoring the urge to move the bowels. In the elderly the latter is sometimes due to immobility. Another cause of constipation in some elderly people is weakness of the muscles of the abdomen and pelvic floor, which prevents adequate pressure in the attempt to move the bowels.

In people suffering from *hemorrhoids* or an *anal fissure* (a crack, laceration, or

tear in the skin around the anus), the pain that results from passing feces can seriously inhibit efforts to initiate bowel movements.

In *irritable bowel syndrome*, the person may experience intermittent constipation, sometimes alternating with diarrhea. In *hypothyroidism*, colonic contractions are reduced, resulting in chronic constipation.

Finally, constipation may be caused by narrowing of part of the colon, due to *diverticular disease* or cancer (see *Intestine, cancer of*).

TREATMENT

In many cases constipation can be cured by following a few simple measures—establishing a regular routine for using the toilet (sometimes facilitated by the use of a glycerin suppository), acting on any urge to move the bowels, avoiding the use of laxatives and purgatives, increasing the amount of fiber in the diet, and drinking more fluids. If constipation continues despite these measures, medical advice should be obtained.

A physician should also be consulted if constipation occurs after years of normal bowel habits, or if it is accompanied by blood in the feces, pain on moving the bowels, loss of a sense of well-being, or weight loss.

A physician usually investigates the condition by obtaining a detailed case history, carrying out a physical examination, and sometimes arranging for tests.

Contact lenses

Very thin, shell-like disks fitted on the cornea (the transparent front part of the eye) to correct defective vision. Contact lenses alter the power of the cornea by replacing the existing outer surface with a plastic surface.

Leonardo da Vinci in 1508 was the first to describe the possibility of using contact lenses. The first lens was made by a German in 1887; it was made of glass and covered the entire front surface of the eye. The conventional small hard lens made of transparent plastic was first introduced in the 1940s and many millions have been used since.

WHY THEY ARE USED

Contact lenses can correct most of the defects in vision for which glasses are prescribed and can correct some conditions that glasses cannot.

Vanity and convenience account for most contact-lens wear. The lenses are almost undetectable when worn. Unlike glasses, these lenses generally do not fall off, do not get covered with rain, and normally do not mist up.

Some contact-lens wearers have a particular optical problem or medical condition. For people who are extremely nearsighted or those who have had cataracts removed, glasses can produce considerable distortion of vision, making contact lenses preferable. Contact lenses can also be useful for hiding scars on the surface of the cornea. Patients with irregular corneas (such as may follow corneal disease, corneal trauma, corneal ulceration, and corneal grafting) may be helped by contact lenses.

TYPES

HARD PLASTIC LENSES These give good optical vision, are long-lasting and durable (possibly five years or more of use), inexpensive, and easy to maintain. However, they sometimes are difficult to tolerate and occasionally fall out; severe pain can result if grit gets into the eye and under the lens. When the lenses are removed after prolonged wear, vision with glasses may be temporarily blurred.

HARD, GAS-PERMEABLE LENSES Introduced in the early 1980s, these have the same visual qualities as hard plastic lenses, but are more comfortable and easier to get used to because they allow oxygen to pass through the lens to the eye. However, they are less durable (possibly giving up to five years of wear) and more expensive.

SOFT LENSES Also called hydrophilic lenses (having a strong affinity for water), these are the most comfortable because of their high water content, which can range from 38 to 70 percent. They are usually easy to wear from the beginning, can be worn for long periods, and are ideal for occasional use since the eye generally tolerates them for short periods of time despite infrequent wearing. Classic soft lenses can correct nearsightedness and farsightedness, but not much astigmatism. Being flexible, they mold themselves to the shape of the eye, and thus cannot correct the irregularly shaped cornea that is the cause of astigmatism. However, special types of soft lenses are designed to correct some astigmatism. Other drawbacks include fragility, a shorter life (12 to 18 months), and more complicated maintenance than for hard lenses.

Extremely thin, specially designed soft lenses with a high water content can be worn for periods of up to one month. These extended-wear contact lenses may increase the risks and dangers of infection.

SPECIAL LENSES Rigid, scleral lenses, which cover the whole of the front of

CARE AND INSERTION OF CONTACT LENSES

Hard lenses may require several solutions, one for cleaning, one for wetting, and possibly one for storage. If used, the storage solution is washed off before lens insertion. The wetting solution is used before inserting a lens in the eye.

Care of soft lenses is more complicated. Because the lenses are permeable and absorb any chemi-cals they come in contact with, the solutions must be weaker. Disinfection with a chemical or heating system is required to prevent contamination and infection. Two or three solutions may be necessary, but intermittent cleaning with a third system, such as an enzyme tablet or an oxidizing agent, is also required to remove mucus and protein.

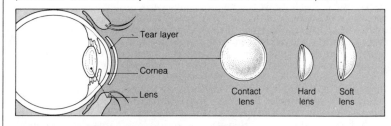

Tear layer
Cornea
Lens
Contact lens
Hard lens
Soft lens

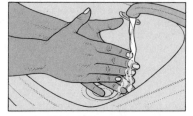

1 Wash your hands thoroughly under running water and carefully rinse off all traces of soap.

Inverted lens

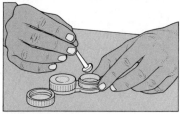

2 If you like, use a rubber sucker to remove a hard lens from its container. Rinse the lens thoroughly.

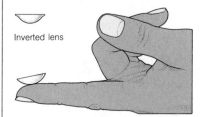

3 Place the lens on your index finger. If it is a soft lens, make sure that it has not turned inside out. If it has, you will see an out-turned rim.

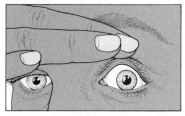

4 Keep both eyes open, hold the upper lid open, and look straight ahead or at the lens as you bring it up to your eye.

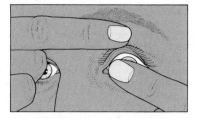

5 Place the lens on your eye. Look downward and then release the lid. If necessary, the lens may be centered by gently massaging the eyelid (the photograph on the right shows a hard lens correctly positioned).

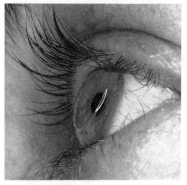

C

C

the eye, are used to hide disfigured eyes. Hard or soft bifocal contact lenses can be produced, but can be difficult to fit and vision may not be satisfactory. Toric contact lenses (thicker around the outside than in the middle) are used to correct high degrees of astigmatism and can be made in all materials.

PROBLEMS

Contact lens wearers can encounter problems with their lenses. A small group may be unable to wear contact lenses at all, because of hypersensitivity (for example, some hay-fever sufferers and very fair-skinned people), difficult optical requirements, or personal hygiene habits.

Lenses can irritate the eye because of dryness due to problems with tear production, which may be inadequate, especially in older people.

With hard plastic contact lenses, abrasion of the cornea can occur because of too rapid buildup of wearing time during the adaptation period, particularly with a tight-fitting lens. Wearing the contact lens too many hours per day can cause the same problem. Symptoms are pain and tearing. With patching and/or antibiotics applied to the eye, symptoms usually clear up within 24 hours.

A common problem that sometimes occurs with soft lenses is that people develop sensitivity of the eyes and lids, either to the maintenance solutions or to mucus forming on the lens surface itself. Symptoms include decreased lens tolerance, stinging, increased lens movement, increased mucus, and redness of the conjunctiva. The person generally must stop wearing contact lenses for several months and then start again with new lenses and a different type of maintenance solution.

Contact lens wear should be stopped if the eyes become red or infected, if vision is blurred, or if the lenses become uncomfortable.

Contact tracing

A service, provided by boards of health, that aims to control the spread of some infectious diseases.

WHY IT IS DONE

If a person is diagnosed as having a serious infectious disease, it may be possible to identify from whom it was caught and to whom it may have been passed on. If these contacts can be encouraged to have an examination and possible treatment, it can help reduce the spread of the disease. Many contacts do not, in fact, have the

infection; others are infected although they may have no obvious symptoms.

Contact tracing is undertaken for many types of sexually transmitted diseases (STDs), including *syphilis* and *gonorrhea*, and also for infections such as tuberculosis, meningitis, and sometimes some imported tropical diseases such as *Lassa fever*. Contact tracing is not carried out for less serious diseases or those for which the transmission mechanism is indirect or not clearly understood.

HOW IT IS DONE

At clinics involved in the treatment of sexually transmitted or other infections, trained nurses and health workers interview patients after their diagnosis to explain the nature of the disease, mode of transmission, and possible complications if left untreated. In strictest confidence, patients are asked for the names and, when relevant, addresses of contacts. These people may either be primary contacts (from whom they may have caught the disease) or secondary contacts (to whom they may have transmitted the disease).

Patients are not compelled to reveal the names of their contacts, nor are contacts compelled to consult a physician (although they are strongly encouraged to do so). If a patient is deemed to be a real danger to the community, the commissioner of health may legally quarantine the patient. This is rarely necessary.

It is important to remember that the principle of *confidentiality* is maintained throughout, and no patient or employer can be given the name or diagnosis of anyone else involved.

Contagious

A term describing a disease that can be transferred from one person to another by social contact, such as sharing the home or workplace.

Contraception

The control of fertility to prevent *pregnancy*. There are various contraceptive methods that work in differing ways, but their basic action is either to stop the sperm and the ovum from meeting in the fallopian tube (thus preventing conception or fertilization) or to prevent a fertilized ovum from implanting in the lining of the uterus.

METHODS

Contraception may be achieved in the following ways: by avoidance of intercourse; *coitus interruptus*; forms of periodic abstinence; various barrier methods; hormonal methods; postco-

ital methods; *IUDs*; and *sterilization*. Regarded today as highly unreliable, *breast-feeding* was once used as a method of contraception. If it is carried out frequently during both the day and the night, it causes changes in the hormone levels in the body that sometimes prevent ovulation until the baby is weaned.

MEASURING CONTRACEPTIVE EFFECTIVENESS

Contraceptives are measured not so much for their effectiveness as for their failure rate. The failure rate is the rate of pregnancies per 100 woman-years of use (i.e., the number of pregnancies among 100 women using the method for one year, or 50 using it for two years). The lower the failure rate, the more effective and useful the contraceptive. No account is taken of the fact that most failures occur in the first year of use, while the woman is getting used to the method.

There are two ways of defining contraceptive effectiveness: the theoretical, or method, effectiveness; and use effectiveness (i.e., the effectiveness in actual use).

THEORETICAL (METHOD) EFFECTIVENESS This is the effectiveness of a particular contraceptive method when used exactly as prescribed by the manufacturers, the physician, or the clinic. Theoretical failure rates are usually much lower than the failure rates of contraceptives in actual use.

USE EFFECTIVENESS Measures the effectiveness of the method under all circumstances. It takes into account pregnancies resulting from incorrect use (for example, forgetting to take the pill or not putting on a condom correctly). Use effectiveness is almost always markedly lower than theoretical effectiveness in "user-dependent" methods, such as barriers. With "nonuser-dependent" methods, such as IUDs and sterilization, there is less of a difference.

RISKS INVOLVED IN CONTRACEPTIVE METHODS

Risks vary a great deal depending on the method. Perhaps the greatest risk in all cases is failure of the method, which can lead to unwanted pregnancy and all that this entails (such as an elective *abortion*). Other risks include danger to the health or life of the mother or danger to the health of any other children.

Risks inherent in contraceptives themselves must also be weighed against the benefits. Hormonal contraceptives are linked with *cardiovascular* disease, particularly in women over 35 who smoke; IUDs may be associated with an increase in *pelvic*

C

METHODS OF CONTRACEPTION

There are various methods of contraception: the natural methods, barrier methods, hormonal methods, and postcoital methods. Sterilization interferes with part of the male or female reproductive system to render the individual infertile.

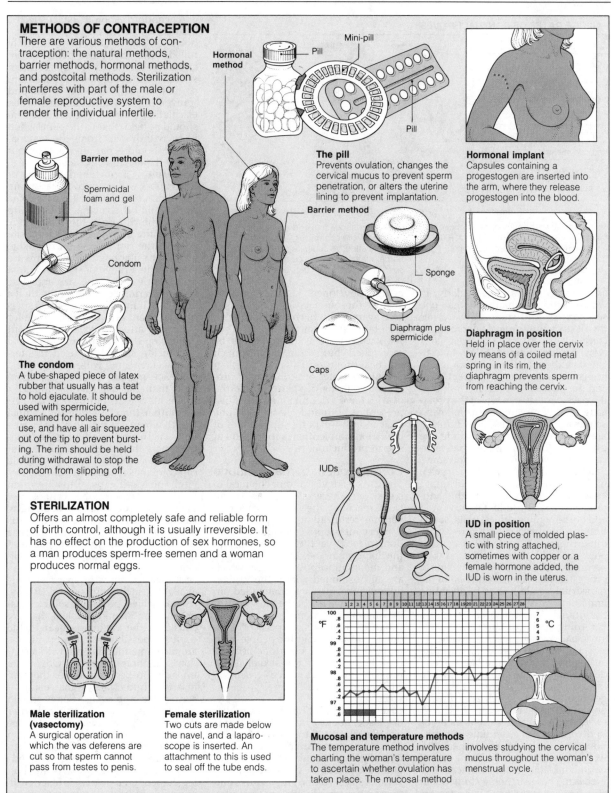

Barrier method

Spermicidal foam and gel

Condom

Hormonal method

Mini-pill

Pill

Pill

The pill
Prevents ovulation, changes the cervical mucus to prevent sperm penetration, or alters the uterine lining to prevent implantation.

Barrier method

Sponge

Diaphragm plus spermicide

Caps

IUDs

Hormonal implant
Capsules containing a progestogen are inserted into the arm, where they release progestogen into the blood.

Diaphragm in position
Held in place over the cervix by means of a coiled metal spring in its rim, the diaphragm prevents sperm from reaching the cervix.

IUD in position
A small piece of molded plastic with string attached, sometimes with copper or a female hormone added, the IUD is worn in the uterus.

The condom
A tube-shaped piece of latex rubber that usually has a teat to hold ejaculate. It should be used with spermicide, examined for holes before use, and have all air squeezed out of the tip to prevent bursting. The rim should be held during withdrawal to stop the condom from slipping off.

STERILIZATION

Offers an almost completely safe and reliable form of birth control, although it is usually irreversible. It has no effect on the production of sex hormones, so a man produces sperm-free semen and a woman produces normal eggs.

Male sterilization (vasectomy)
A surgical operation in which the vas deferens are cut so that sperm cannot pass from testes to penis.

Female sterilization
Two cuts are made below the navel, and a laparoscope is inserted. An attachment to this is used to seal off the tube ends.

Mucosal and temperature methods
The temperature method involves charting the woman's temperature to ascertain whether ovulation has taken place. The mucosal method involves studying the cervical mucus throughout the woman's menstrual cycle.

303

FAILURE RATES OF CONTRACEPTIVES

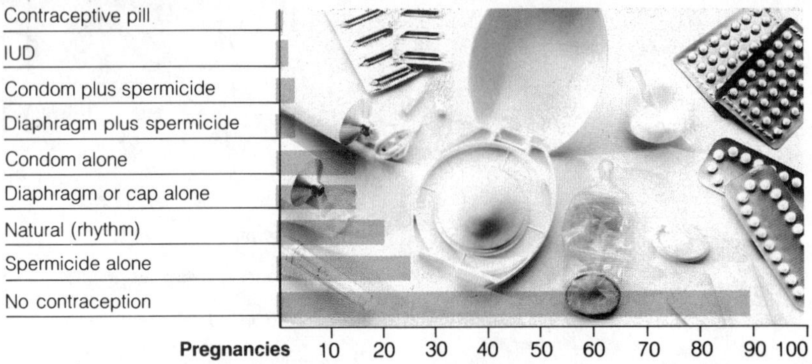

	Pregnancies	10	20	30	40	50	60	70	80	90	100
Contraceptive pill											
IUD											
Condom plus spermicide											
Diaphragm plus spermicide											
Condom alone											
Diaphragm or cap alone											
Natural (rhythm)											
Spermicide alone											
No contraception											

The chart shows the number of pregnancies that can be expected, on average, if 100 healthy young couples use a given contraceptive method (or none at all) for one year. Note that use of the pill or IUD, or barrier methods (condom or diaphragm) combined with spermicide, are all moderately to highly effective contraceptives. Using a barrier method without spermicide, or spermicide alone, is much less effective.

inflammatory disease, particularly in women who have had more than one sex partner; and sterilization carries the risks of any surgical operation.

CONTRACEPTIVE RESEARCH
New forms continue to be investigated although the constraints of licensing authorities, the great cost, and the paucity of funds have slowed the pace. However, a few of the promising lines of research are as follows.

HORMONAL CONTRACEPTION New forms of hormonal contraception include the use of *LH-RH* (a hormone that regulates the release of other hormones that control the ovulatory cycle), which may be given as a nasal spray.

RU-486 The development of this antiprogesterone is quite far advanced and is undergoing clinical trials, sometimes in conjunction with prostaglandins (hormonelike substances that play multiple roles in the body). It seems to act by stopping production of progesterone in the second half of the menstrual cycle, thus preventing implantation of a fertilized ovum in the uterus. It can also be used as a "morning-after" contraceptive.

STEROIDAL VAGINAL RINGS Made of silicone-rubber containing a progestogen, these are at a late stage of development. They are inserted into the vagina and release the progestogen locally, which acts directly on the reproductive organs.

PINPOINTING OVULATION Various methods to determine the exact time of ovulation continue to be researched; this would be of great help in the use of periodic abstinence for contraception.

VACCINES These are being studied, but still present problems. Vaccines are being developed against sperm, against the outer coat of the ovum, and against the hormone that helps maintain a pregnancy.

THE MALE PILL This continues to be researched, but so far without much practical progress. The main problem is that the testes are continually producing millions of sperm, while the ovaries have a definite number of ova present at birth and release only one each month—making suppression of ovulation simpler than suppression of sperm production.

Contraception, barrier methods

The use of a device and/or chemical to block or otherwise prevent sperm from reaching the ovum, thus preventing fertilization and pregnancy. Barrier contraceptives include the condom (placed over the erect penis), and the diaphragm, the contraceptive cap, and the contraceptive sponge, which are all positioned within the vagina. Spermicides are recommended in combination with barrier devices for maximum protection.

Barrier methods, especially condoms, are advisable for people with more than one sex partner because they help prevent the sexual transmission of diseases such as *gonorrhea*, *AIDS*, and *hepatitis B*.

TYPES

CONDOM A sheath of fine, latex rubber or plastic, about 7 inches long, that is usually lubricated for ease of application. A condom normally has a teat at its end to hold ejaculated sperm. Condoms are available over-the-counter in various sizes, colors, and textures and may be precoated with a spermicide.

A condom should be inspected before use to make certain there are no holes or tears, and then carefully rolled onto the erect penis before intercourse. The tip of the condom should be squeezed as it is rolled on, so that no air is trapped in the end (preventing it from bursting when ejaculation occurs). The condom rim should be held close to the penis when it is withdrawn from the vagina, which should occur after orgasm but before the erection subsides.

DIAPHRAGM A hemispherical dome of thin rubber with a coiled metal spring in the rim. It fits diagonally across the front wall of the vagina, with the top part of the rim up behind the cervix (neck of the uterus) and the opposite edge of the rim resting on the ledge above the pubic bone. Diaphragms are available in a range of sizes and must be properly fitted, the size and type being determined by an individual's anatomy. It must be used with a spermicidal agent and be left in place for six hours after intercourse. Without disturbing the diaphragm, additional spermicide should be used if intercourse is repeated within six hours.

CONTRACEPTIVE CAP Smaller and more rigid than the diaphragm, this latex rubber device fits tightly over the cervix (rather than covering the vaginal vault), where it is held in place by suction. There are three types: the cervical cap is thimble-shaped, the vault cap is bowl-shaped, and the vimule cap combines features of both the cervical and vault caps. Caps are often used by women who cannot use diaphragms because of anatomical changes, such as *prolapse* of the uterus or a *cystocele*. As with the diaphragm, a cap must be properly fitted and used with a spermicide. Caps became available in the US in 1988.

SPERMICIDE A range of spermicides is available, including aerosol foams, creams, jellies, pessaries, soluble plastic film, or foaming tablets that are placed in the vagina as near to the cervix as possible. Some preparations are recommended for use with a condom, diaphragm, or cap. Others are intended to be used alone; they are inserted into the vagina using a syringelike applicator. Some should not be used with rubber barrier devices. Spermicides should be applied shortly before intercourse; a fresh application is needed when intercourse is repeated or prolonged.

Pessaries are slightly waxy and bullet-shaped. One pessary is inserted 15 minutes before intercourse. Spermicides must be used in accordance with the manufacturer's instructions since the length of time for which they remain effective varies. They should not be washed away for six to eight hours after intercourse.

CONTRACEPTIVE SPONGE A disposable circular polyurethane foam sponge about 2 inches in diameter and 2 inches thick that is impregnated with spermicide. The sponge incorporates a loop for easy removal. Before being inserted high into the vagina, the sponge should be moistened with water to activate the spermicide. It should be left in position for at least six hours after intercourse.

EFFECTIVENESS

If used consistently and correctly, employing both mechanical and chemical barriers, these methods are highly effective in preventing conception. Failure rates in actual use vary between four and seven pregnancies per 100 woman-years of use for the condom, diaphragm, or contraceptive cap; nine to 16 pregnancies per 100 woman-years of use for the contraceptive sponge; and 30 to 40 pregnancies per 100 woman-years of use for spermicides used alone. (See *Contraception* for definition of woman-years.)

Contraception, hormonal methods

The use by women of synthetic progestogens, sometimes combined with synthetic estrogens, to prevent pregnancy. The best-known hormonal contraceptives are the various types of birth-control pill (see *Oral contraceptives*), but injectable contraceptives and implants are also available.

HOW THEY WORK

Most injectable contraceptives contain progestogens only. These contraceptives are administered every two or three months.

Contraceptive implants consist of six small silicone-rubber capsules containing a progestogen. These are inserted subcutaneously (under the skin) in the upper arm in a fanlike manner and are active for five years, releasing the progestogen steadily into the bloodstream.

Both methods suppress ovulation in most (although not all) menstrual cycles. All hormonal contraceptives act on the cervical mucus to make it thick and impenetrable to sperm. They also cause thinning of the endometrium (lining of the uterus).

Properly used, injectables and implants are extremely effective—the failure rate is about two pregnancies per 100 woman-years (see *Contraception* for definition of woman-years). The return of ovulation is sometimes delayed after stopping injectables, but a woman is fertile soon after implants are removed.

FOR WHOM ARE THEY RECOMMENDED?

Both methods are suitable for most women who want long-term protection against pregnancy and who cannot use estrogens or other hormonal contraceptives or IUDs. Injectable contraceptives are licensed and used in more than 80 countries; the Food and Drug Administration has not yet approved their use in the US.

Their main advantage is their excellent effectiveness and the relative lack of motivation necessary on the part of the user. Side effects include heavy bleeding in the first few months, irregular menstruation, or amenorrhea (cessation of periods). There is sometimes weight gain. Injections have the disadvantage of running their full two or three months of activity in the body after being administered. There is no way of neutralizing their action.

Contraception, periodic abstinence

Avoidance of sexual intercourse during part of the menstrual cycle in an attempt to avoid conception. Abstinence has been practiced with varying degrees of success in many parts of the world for many years. Often referred to as "natural" family planning, the term periodic abstinence describes more accurately what happens when couples abstain from sexual intercourse during those times when fertilization can take place.

TYPES

All forms of periodic abstinence attempt to pinpoint the time of ovulation. The oldest method (the calendar, or rhythm, method) attempted to predict ovulation on the basis of the lengths of previous menstrual cycles; it fell into disrepute because of its high failure rate. More up-to-date are the temperature and the cervical mucus (or Billings) methods. When these two are used together for greater accuracy, they are given the name symptothermal method.

TEMPERATURE METHOD Also known as the basal body temperature method, this involves the woman charting her daily temperature. This should be done at the same time each day—normally first thing in the morning while the body is in an inactive state—and using a special ovulation thermometer marked in fractions of degrees. Provided the woman is well (with no other cause for a rise in temperature), a sustained temperature rise for at least three days means that ovulation has taken place and that it is now considered safe to have sexual intercourse. However, to use this method properly, no intercourse should take place until after the sustained temperature rise has occurred; this can mean abstinence for more than half the cycle.

CERVICAL MUCUS METHOD This involves the observation and charting of the amount and appearance of the mucus secreted by the cervix (neck of uterus) throughout the menstrual cycle. Immediately after menstruation come the dry days when the mucus forms a thick plug that blocks the cervix. The mucus then becomes thick and viscid and appears at the vulva. About the time of ovulation it turns thin, watery, elastic, and slippery and flows more easily. A few days after ovulation it begins to become thick and viscid again, and this state lasts until the start of the next menstrual period. In this method, it is considered contraceptively safe to have sexual intercourse on alternate days during the dry days (alternate so that any semen remaining does not obscure the start of the thin mucus). As soon as any mucus appears, abstinence must begin. This should last until the fourth day after the peak day of the mucus (that is, the fourth day after the last appearance of fertile-type mucus). Intercourse can then continue until the next menstrual period.

SYMPTOTHERMAL METHOD This method combines the temperature and the cervical mucus methods and requires a closely supervised learning period of about six months. Intercourse can still take place during the dry days after the period, but must stop as soon as mucus is felt. It can be resumed only when both the sustained rise in temperature and the four days after peak mucus have been registered—thus giving a double sense of security.

EFFECTIVENESS

All these methods need great motivation on the part of the couple, with a strong commitment to abstain from intercourse when there could be a possibility of pregnancy. None of these methods is suitable for women who normally have irregular cycles, and they should not be used after a pregnancy until the cycle has regularized. Studies have shown the greatest use effectiveness with the

C

C

symptothermal method—6.24 pregnancies per 100 woman-years.

SIDE EFFECTS

Once the techniques have been mastered and a woman can observe and chart the necessary changes, there are no provable side effects, although there is a supposition that a higher incidence of miscarriages or congenital defects could occur because of fertilization by so-called "aged" sperm of "aged" ova. This supposition has neither been completely proved nor disproved.

Contraception, postcoital

The prevention of pregnancy after sexual intercourse has occurred, normally reserved for emergency situations. Rape of a woman who is not using contraception is a preeminent example; the bursting of a condom during intercourse is another.

Postcoital contraception must be provided very soon after intercourse, especially if the woman is ovulating. There are two main types, but neither of them is 100 percent effective; a woman should have a pregnancy test a month after treatment to ensure that she is not pregnant.

TYPES

HORMONAL CONTRACEPTIVE PROTECTION This must be started not later than 72 hours after unprotected intercourse. There are two methods: a five-day course of *estrogens* or a short, high-dose course of combined *oral contraceptives*. With the combined medication, often called the "morning-after" pill, two pills containing 250 micrograms of levonorgestrel (a progestogen) and 50 micrograms of ethinyl estradiol (an estrogen) are given at once and the dose is repeated 12 hours later. This sometimes causes nausea and vomiting, and an antiemetic treatment may be needed at the same time.

COPPER-BEARING IUD Insertion of a copper-bearing IUD within five days of unprotected sexual intercourse has been shown to be effective. However, it is not always advisable in women who have never been pregnant; its presence can also be one of the factors associated with an increase in *pelvic inflammatory disease*. Copper-bearing IUDs are not available in the US.

Contraceptive

Any agent that diminishes the likelihood of conception. Contraceptives can be hormonal (as in the oral birth-control pill), chemical (as in spermicides), or mechanical (as in condoms). (See *Contraception*.)

Contractions

The spasms of rhythmic, squeezing muscular activity that affect the walls of the *uterus* during *labor*. These true labor contractions should be distinguished from the *Braxton Hicks' contractions* that are often noticeable during the last few weeks of pregnancy. True contractions are characterized by their regularity and the discomfort they cause. Furthermore, they increase in strength and frequency from the start of the first stage of labor.

Contract practice

See *Corporate practice*.

Contracture

A deformity caused by shrinkage of scar tissue in the skin or connective tissues, or by irreversible shortening of muscles and tendons.

Skin contractures are common after extensive burns and may restrict movement. Other types of contracture may be caused by inflammation of the tendons and fascia (a sheet of fibrous tissue) that support muscle fibers, as in *Dupuytren's contracture*, which affects the hand. Sometimes there is damage to muscle fibers, usually due to ischemia (reduced blood supply). In *Volkmann's contracture*, this damage may be caused by a plaster cast being placed too tightly around a fractured bone in the arm, thus interfering with the circulation.

Contraindication

Any factor in a patient's condition that makes it unwise to pursue a certain line of treatment—such as drug therapy or surgery.

Controlled trial

A method of testing the value of a treatment—such as a new drug—or comparing the effectiveness of different treatments.

WHY IT IS DONE

The effectiveness of a treatment cannot accurately be assessed simply by administering it to a group of sick people and seeing if their conditions improve. With many illnesses, a large proportion of patients tend to get better even if the treatment they are given is useless and harmless. Reasons for this phenomenon include the healing properties of time, the psychological reassurance of a physician, and the fact that both patient and physician believe the treatment will work (the so-called *placebo* effect). A controlled trial is a scientific attempt to unravel

the true curative activity of a treatment from the psychological side benefits of "being treated."

HOW IT IS DONE

In a typical controlled drug trial, a randomly selected sample of patients with the illness that the drug is thought to cure is split into two carefully matched groups. One group is given a normal course of the drug—for example, a pill to be taken every day. The other patients—called the control group—are given an identical course of treatment, except that their pills are "dummy," or placebo, tablets, containing none of the drug being tested, but only an inert substance such as starch. Alternatively, the control group may be given a well-established drug treatment but with the drug disguised to appear identical to the test drug.

After a predetermined period, the two groups are medically assessed. If the improvement in the illness has been significantly greater in the patients given the drug over those given the dummy tablets, this suggests that the drug does have a real curative effect. Any benefits of treatment separate from the pharmacological effects of the drug have been accounted for (or "controlled") by comparing the two groups.

To be of any use, controlled trials must be conducted "blind"—that is, the patients do not know whether they are receiving the real or dummy treatment. In a further refinement—the *double-blind* controlled trial—neither the patients nor the physicians who assess them know who is receiving which treatment. The results of trials require detailed and careful statistical analysis before any conclusions can be drawn.

Contusion

Damage to the skin and underlying tissues from a blunt injury such as a fall; the skin may be grazed and the tissues bruised.

Convalescence

The recovery period following an illness or a surgical operation during which the patient regains strength before returning to normal activities. The convalescent period can vary from one or two days (following an infection such as influenza or tonsillitis) to several weeks (following a heart attack or a major operation). At one time special convalescent homes were popular, but today such places are generally reserved for the elderly.

Conversion disorder

A psychological illness in which painful emotions are repressed and unconsciously converted into physical symptoms. The repressed idea is expressed symbolically by the particular bodily symptom. For instance, a paralyzed right arm may represent guilt over an injury that the patient, using that arm, inflicted on another person; mutism (inability to speak) may represent sexual guilt, the mouth symbolizing the vagina.

This disorder serves mainly to relieve anxiety, but the sufferer may also "benefit" by gaining sympathy and avoiding responsibility.

Treatment requires *psychotherapy* involving exploration of the person's history and childhood experiences.

Convulsion

See *Seizure*.

Convulsion, febrile

See *Seizure, febrile*.

Cooley's anemia

One of the principal and most serious forms of *thalassemia*, an inherited blood disorder characterized by production of a defective *hemoglobin* (the protein that carries oxygen in red blood cells).

Copper

A metallic element that forms an essential part of several *enzymes* (substances that promote biochemical reactions in the body). Copper is needed in minute amounts (see *Trace elements*); deficiency is rare.

Copper poisoning is rare, occurring mainly in people who drink homemade alcohol distilled using copper tubing. Symptoms of poisoning include nausea, vomiting, and diarrhea. Copper excess may also result from *Wilson's disease*, an extremely rare inherited disorder of copper metabolism.

Cordotomy

An operation to divide bundles of nerve fibers within the spinal cord. Cordotomy is performed to relieve persistent pain that has not responded to treatment with strong analgesics (painkillers) or *TENS* (transcutaneous electrical nerve stimulation). In theory, cordotomy can treat pain anywhere in the body, depending on the part of the cord operated on. In practice, however, it is often difficult to locate precisely the nerves responsible for pain in the upper part

of the body, and the operation is most frequently performed for pain in the lower trunk and legs, usually on patients with cancer.

Corn

A small area of thickened skin on a toe, caused by the pressure of a tight-fitting shoe. People with high foot arches are affected most, because the arch increases the pressure on the tips of the toes when walking.

If a corn is painful, the obvious solution is to change to shoes that fit more comfortably; the corn should then gradually disappear. Until then, a spongy ring or corn pad—available at drug stores in various sizes—can be placed over the corn to ease pressure. If neither measure is successful, a podiatrist can remedy the problem by paring away the corn with a scalpel. (See also *Bunion; Callus, skin*.)

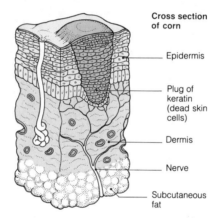

Cross section of corn

- Epidermis
- Plug of keratin (dead skin cells)
- Dermis
- Nerve
- Subcutaneous fat

Cornea

Front part of the tough outer shell of the eyeball. The cornea is transparent and is shaped like a thin-walled cap or dome. It is about 0.5 inches (12 mm) in diameter, less than 0.04 inches (1 mm) thick, and has a convex front surface like the front of a camera lens. At its circumference it joins the sclera (white of the eye), which is easily seen. The cornea itself, being transparent, is less obvious. The black pupil and the colored iris are visible beneath it.

The cornea performs two main functions; it helps focus light rays onto the retina at the back of the eye and it is a protective cover of the front of the eye. To warn of possible damage, the cornea's surface is extremely sensitive, and small scratches and foreign bodies are thus very painful.

The cornea must be kept moist (by tears), like the inside of the mouth, to remain healthy. This function is per-

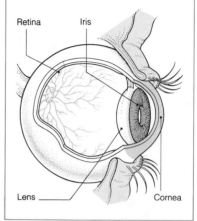

LOCATION OF CORNEA
The cornea is a transparent thin-walled dome forming the front of the eyeball. It consists of five layers of differing thickness.

Retina — Iris

Lens — Cornea

C

formed by the lacrimal gland and the mucus and fluid-secreting cells in the lids and conjunctiva (the thin lining of the rest of the surface of the eye and the inside of the eyelids). The endothelial cells (inner cell layer) in adults cannot reproduce themselves. If they are severely damaged there may be permanent corneal clouding, since they function to pump excess water out of the cornea to keep it clear and transparent.

Corneal abrasion

A scratch or defect in the epithelium (outer layer) of the cornea. The abrasion may be caused by a small, sharp particle in the eye (see *Eye, foreign body in*) or by an injury—for example, by a twig or hairbrush.

Usually, the scratch heals quickly, but may temporarily be very painful, causing intense photophobia (dislike of bright light) and increased production of tears.

Keeping the eye closed, such as with a patch, may help lessen the discomfort. Analgesics (painkillers) may be helpful to relieve the persistent pain, and a physician may prescribe eye drops containing a cycloplegic (a drug that relaxes muscles in the eye that may go into spasm with the abrasion), which makes the eye more comfortable. Antibiotic eye drops are usually also given to prevent any risk of bacterial infection, which could lead to a serious corneal ulceration, abscess, and blindness.

C

DISORDERS OF THE CORNEA
The cornea is a living structure, much like very specialized skin, and is prone to many disorders.

CONGENITAL DEFECTS
These are rare. Microcornea (smaller than normal) or megalocornea (bigger than normal) may occur in one or both eyes. In *buphthalmos,* or "ox-eye," the entire eyeball is enlarged and there is a strong tendency to *glaucoma.* This often leads to haziness of the cornea.

INJURY
Trauma to the cornea is common and is usually minor, a frequent occurrence being a *corneal abrasion* (scratch) caused by a particle in the eye or by overuse of contact lenses. An abrasion may become infected and progress to a *corneal ulcer.* Penetrating corneal injuries can cause scarring with loss of transparency, which may lead to a severe defect of vision.

Chemical injuries to the cornea can result from acid or alkali splashes, the latter being more serious. All contact with corrosive substances is dangerous, and immediate vigorous flushing with large volumes of water is essential if sight is to be saved. The term *keratopathy* can be applied to any corneal disorder, but is also used more specifically for certain types or causes of corneal damage.

Actinic keratopathy is damage to the outer layer of the cornea by ultraviolet light radiation. Exposure keratopathy is the damage done to a cornea deprived of the normal protection afforded by the tear film and the blink reflex.

INFLAMMATION
Keratitis means inflammation of the cornea. However, because the cornea contains no blood vessels, true inflammatory reactions are uncommon.

INFECTION
The cornea can be infected by viruses, bacteria, and fungi. Some of these cause ulceration, which may lead to penetration. *Herpes simplex* is especially dangerous.

NUTRITIONAL DISORDERS
Keratomalacia is the result of vitamin A deficiency and is common in severely undernourished children. The cornea becomes soft and often perforates. Keratomalacia is a major cause of blindness in some tropical countries.

DEGENERATION
Degenerative conditions of the cornea occur mainly in the elderly or may affect generally diseased eyes. The corneal changes include the deposition of calcium, thinning, and spontaneous ulceration.

OTHER DISORDERS
Keratoconjunctivitis sicca (dry eye) occurs when the tear film is inadequate. This is a feature of *Sjögren's syndrome,* the *Stevens-Johnson syndrome,* and various rheumatic disorders. Corneal dystrophies are inborn errors of corneal structure or function that may appear at various ages and may lead to opacification. One form of dystrophy is *keratoconus,* in which the cornea thins and bulges forward into a conical shape. Edema (fluid collection) in the cornea occurs when the endothelium (the inner layer) fails to prevent the internal fluid of the eye from entering the cornea. This may severely affect vision.

INVESTIGATION
Corneal disorders are examined under high magnification, using a slit-lamp microscope. In the majority of cases, the appearance of the various conditions is characteristic and diagnosis is straightforward. Corneal ulcers may require gentle scraping so that samples can be obtained for viral, bacterial, or fungal *culture* in the pathology laboratory.

Corneal abrasions usually heal completely within a few days, but (rarely) they may recur, probably because the new epithelium fails to stick properly to the underlying tissue. Patching the eye, application of bland ointments, and even prescription of a soft "bandage" contact lens may be tried.

Corneal graft
The surgical transplantation of corneal tissue. Most corneal transplants are homografts, meaning the tissue is taken from a human donor and put into the eye of a recipient with a corneal disorder. A much smaller number are autografts, in which a person's cornea is simply repositioned—for example, it may be rotated to a position in which the effect of a scar on the corneal surface is lessened. Donor corneal tissues can now be stored for days for future use. The term "eye bank" is used for the organization that handles the donor corneas.

WHY IT IS DONE
A corneal graft is carried out when a patient has an eye with possible good visual potential (most of the eye is healthy) but with substantially impaired vision caused by a cornea scarred or clouded by fluid collection in the tissues or for other reasons (see *Cornea disorders* box).

HOW IT IS DONE
With the patient under general or local anesthetic, the diseased area of the cornea is excised and replaced with a similarly shaped piece of donor tissue, which is fastened in place with stitches. Most corneal grafts are full-thickness, but, if the back part of the cornea is healthy, the cornea is sometimes split, with only the front, diseased part removed and replaced.

OUTLOOK
The success rate for corneal grafts is high, but depends on the type of corneal disorder (certain corneal problems have lower transplant success

rates than others). Generally, corneal grafts have a much better chance for success than other types of transplant. This is because the healthy cornea is free of blood vessels and there is therefore less access for the white blood cells, which bring about rejection of donor tissue. Matching certain features of the donor's and recipient's immune systems (see *Histocompatibility antigens*) has also improved the success rate of corneal grafts. Unlike other transplants, there is usually no need for the patient to receive immunosuppressant drugs to lessen the chances of rejection.

Corneal ulcer
A break, erosion, or open sore in the outer layer of the cornea, sometimes extending into the underlying stroma (middle layer).

CAUSES
The most common cause is a *corneal abrasion* or scratch, but an ulcer may

also be produced by chemical damage, by infection (particularly with the *herpes simplex* or *herpes zoster* viruses), or by various bacteria and fungi.

Certain eye conditions may make an ulcer more likely—for example, *keratoconjunctivitis sicca* (dry eye), eyelid deformities such as *entropion* or *ectropion*, or diminished sensation in the cornea, which more easily permits injury to occur.

SYMPTOMS, DIAGNOSIS, AND TREATMENT

Corneal ulcers are very painful, though chronic ones may become less so. They are easily recognized by a physician instilling some fluorescein dye into the eye and shining a blue light on it; the fluorescein fills the ulcer and reflects back green light.

Superficial, noninfectious ulcers caused by mechanical injury usually heal quickly. If an infection is suspected, swabs will be taken to identify the causative microorganism and the physician will then prescribe a suitable antimicrobial drug. Sometimes, a predisposing eye condition may need to be treated. Noninfectious ulcers that fail to heal quickly sometimes respond to a "bandage" contact lens or a tarsorrhaphy (a temporary joining of the eyelids).

Coronary

Strictly, a term used to describe any structure that encircles like a crown (from "corona," the Latin word for crown). In practice, the term usually refers to the coronary arteries that encircle and supply the heart. In popular usage, coronary often means a *coronary thrombosis* or a *myocardial infarction* (heart attack).

Coronary artery bypass

An operation to circumvent narrowed or blocked coronary arteries by grafting on additional blood vessels to receive blood flow.

Usually, symptoms of coronary heart disease can be controlled by drugs, weight loss (if appropriate), not smoking, and adopting a sensible diet and life-style. If this fails to relieve the symptoms, however, other treatment will be considered. When the disease is localized to one or two segments of artery it may be possible to relieve the blockage or blockages by using a technique called balloon *angioplasty*. In balloon angioplasty a small balloon is passed via catheter through the circulation into the coronary artery. The artery is then distended to stretch the narrowed segment. However, in most cases not re-

sponding to treatment with drugs, bypass surgery may be recommended rather than angioplasty.

HOW IT IS DONE

A decision to operate is based on identification of the sites of blockage using *angiography* (an X-ray technique). The operation itself is performed using general anesthesia. It usually requires two surgeons and lasts up to five hours. The heart is temporarily stopped and the circulation is maintained with a *heart-lung machine* that adds oxygen to the blood outside of the body. The procedure is illustrated on the following page.

RECOVERY PERIOD

After a coronary artery bypass, the patient spends two to four days in an intensive care unit, where his or her heart and other body functions are carefully monitored. Hospital stay is generally about ten to 12 days, and return to work is usually possible after about six weeks.

OUTLOOK

When candidates are appropriately selected, coronary artery bypass offers the patient another chance to feel well again and return to a normal life.

Coronary artery disease

Disease of the arteries that supply blood to the heart muscle, causing damage to or malfunction of the heart. (See *Coronary heart disease*.)

Coronary care unit

A small ward, specially staffed and equipped for the care of acutely ill patients who are suspected of being in the process of or who have suffered a *myocardial infarction* (heart attack involving damage to the heart muscle

from a blockage of one of the coronary arteries). In the unit, patients are kept under close surveillance and given immediate treatment if a complication such as *cardiac arrest* (cessation of heart beat), *arrhythmia* (irregular or very rapid or slow heart beat), or *heart failure* occurs.

A coronary care unit usually holds only five to 10 people, and the ratio of specially trained nurses to patients is high—one-to-one or one-to-two. The ward is equipped with monitoring equipment that provides a continuous record of each patient's heart rhythm, respiratory rate, blood pressure, and so on, and contains specialized equipment for providing treatment, such as *defibrillation* (to restore normal heart rhythm), and *ventilation*.

Coronary heart disease

Damage to or malfunction of the heart caused by narrowing or blockage of the coronary arteries, which supply blood to the heart muscle. Two of the manifestations of coronary heart disease (CHD) are *angina pectoris* (chest pain usually associated with effort or anxiety) and acute *myocardial infarction* (AMI, or heart attack).

INCIDENCE

CHD is an extremely common disorder in developed countries and is the cause of more deaths in the US than any other disorder. Many such deaths occur without warning in middle-aged men and women who are otherwise in good health, although most deaths from CHD are in people over 65.

In the past 20 years deaths and disability from CHD have declined. The mortality from CHD in men aged

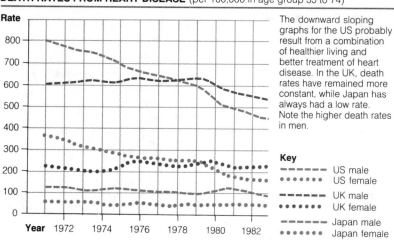

DEATH RATES FROM HEART DISEASE (per 100,000 in age group 35 to 74)

The downward sloping graphs for the US probably result from a combination of healthier living and better treatment of heart disease. In the UK, death rates have remained more constant, while Japan has always had a low rate. Note the higher death rates in men.

Key
- – – – – – US male
- • • • • • • US female
- – – – – – UK male
- • • • • • • UK female
- – – – – – Japan male
- • • • • • • Japan female

C

CORONARY ARTERY BYPASS

This is now the most common and successful major heart operation in the Western world. Each year some 500,000 Americans undergo the operation, which can relieve them from dependence on drug treatment for heart disease and restore them to active life.

HOW IT IS DONE

Coronary artery bypass is a major procedure, requiring two surgeons and lasting up to five hours.

1 The first surgeon makes an incision down the center of the patient's chest. The heart is then exposed by opening the pericardium.

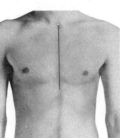

Site of incision

2 Simultaneously, several incisions are made in the leg, and a length of vein removed.

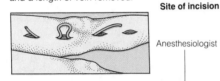

3 Before any incisions are made in the coronary arteries, the patient is connected to a heart-lung machine. This takes over the function of the heart and lungs while the surgeon repairs the heart.

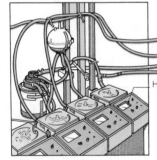

Heart-lung machine

4 A section of the vein taken from the leg is then sewn to the aorta and to a point below the blockage. If several arteries are blocked, they can be bypassed by using other sections from the same leg vein.

5 The heart-lung machine is disconnected, allowing blood to flow back into the coronary arteries.

WHY IT IS DONE

Narrowed coronary arteries are unable to supply the heart muscle with a sufficient amount of blood; as a result, it becomes starved of oxygen. This may cause angina (chest pain) or, if the narrowed artery becomes blocked, heart tissue damage. By attaching lengths of a vein taken from the leg to the aorta and to a point below the blockages, the narrowed or blocked sections can be bypassed.

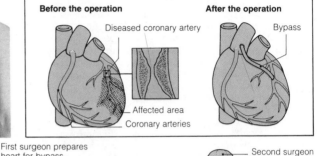

Before the operation

Diseased coronary artery

Affected area

Coronary arteries

After the operation

Bypass

First surgeon prepares heart for bypass

Anesthesiologist

Second surgeon removes vein from leg

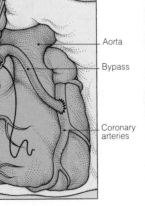

Oxygenated blood from heart-lung machine

Superior vena cava (tied off)

Deoxygenated blood to heart-lung machine

Inferior vena cava (tied off)

Pericardium

Aorta

Bypass

Coronary arteries

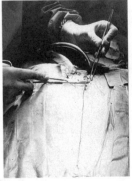

6 Finally, the breastbone is wired together, and pericardium and chest are sewn up.

35 to 64 declined by 35 percent between 1968 and 1982. Part of this decline is thought to be due to better medical treatment of elevated blood pressure, one of the causes of CHD, and part is due to improved surgical treatment of narrowed coronary arteries. Also, emergency treatment of heart attacks has improved.

CAUSES

CHD is caused by reduction in the blood flow to the heart muscle and to its electrical conducting system, which initiates and coordinates the contractions (beats) of the muscle (see *Heart*). The coronary arteries are first narrowed and may eventually be blocked by plaques (patches) of the cholesterol-rich fatty deposit called *atheroma*. Further narrowing or blockage may be caused by thrombi (blood clots) formed on the roughened surface of the plaques.

The causes of atheroma are numerous and interrelated (see *Atherosclerosis*). In addition to some genetic predisposition and diseases such as *diabetes mellitus* and *hypertension* (elevated blood pressure), the main causes are smoking, lack of exercise, being overweight, and elevated blood cholesterol (which itself is linked in part with a diet rich in dairy and animal fats).

The importance of personality traits, behavior, and stress as causes is still disputed. Some physicians believe that heart attacks are more frequent in people with "type A" personalities. Such individuals are always in a hurry, checking the time, impatient with delays, and interrupting colleagues in mid-sentence—but they are also doers and achievers. There is some evidence that heart attacks occur more frequently in people who are depressed after the death of a relative, loss of a job, or some other adverse life event. The medical consensus is that these psychological and behavioral factors are less important than physical factors—smoking, unhealthy diet, high blood pressure, and lack of exercise.

SYMPTOMS

In its early stages, atheroma of the coronary arteries causes no symptoms. The first symptom is usually either angina pectoris or heart attack.

Angina pectoris is discomfort or pain in the chest, typically brought on by exertion and relieved by rest. The pain is a dull ache in the middle of the chest or a feeling of pressure that may spread up to the neck or down the arms (on the left more often than the right). In some cases the pain occurs only in an arm or in the neck. The characteristic pain comes on predictably after a certain amount of exertion—after walking halfway up the stairs, for instance—and disappears after resting a minute or so.

Angina occurs when the heart muscle is working hard and getting too little blood for the amount of effort being expended. If the blood supply to part of the muscle is cut off completely by a blood clot or spasm in one of the coronary arteries, the result is an acute myocardial infarction (a coronary thrombosis or heart attack)—death of a portion of the heart muscle. The main symptom is intense chest pain of the same type as angina, but not relieved by rest and not necessarily brought on by effort; in addition the victim may become cold, sweat profusely, feel weak and nauseated, or even lose consciousness as the pumping action of the heart is weakened and shock ensues.

Angina and AMI may lead to disturbances in the electrical conduction system of the heart with resulting *arrhythmias* (abnormalities in heart beat) ranging from *ectopic beats* (occasional double beats) to *tachycardia* (rapid beats) and *ventricular fibrillation* (ineffective fluttering of the heart muscle). The latter causes rapid loss of consciousness and is fatal if not treated within a few minutes.

DIAGNOSIS AND INVESTIGATION

An AMI may produce such clear-cut symptoms that the diagnosis is in no doubt. Confirmatory tests may include electrocardiography and measurement of the level of serum creatine kinase enzymes released into the blood by damaged muscle. The conditions of patients who have intermittent attacks of angina are usually assessed by electrocardiography both at rest and during controlled exercise.

When the angina is persistent, severe, changing in quality, or of recent onset, the patient's condition is assessed by various *heart imaging* techniques. These imaging procedures, such as coronary *angiography* (injection of a radiopaque dye into the arteries followed by X ray), give the physician detailed, precise data on the extent of the narrowing of the coronary arteries and any damage to the heart muscle. The data aid in determining whether medical or surgical treatment is best.

TREATMENT

Angina may be relieved by a range of drugs that improves the blood flow through the coronary arteries and/or that reduces the work load on the heart during exercise. These drugs include glyceryl trinitrate and other *nitrates*, *beta-blockers*, *calcium channel blockers*, and peripheral *vasodilator drugs*. Arrhythmias are commonly treated with beta-blockers, calcium channel blockers, and specific *antiarrhythmic drugs*. If the heart's pumping action is weak, it may sometimes be improved by vasodilators or *digoxin*.

If drug treatment fails to relieve the symptoms, or if investigation shows extensive narrowing of the coronary arteries, blood flow may be improved by *coronary artery bypass* surgery (in which a vein graft is used to skip over the narrowed segment) or by transluminal *angioplasty* (in which the narrowed part of the artery is stretched apart when a balloon, passed to the site, is inflated).

An AMI is usually treated initially in a hospital coronary care unit. Treatment may be given with *thrombolytic drugs* in an attempt to dissolve the clot, the affected coronary artery may be widened by angioplasty or may be immediately bypassed by surgery, or treatment may simply be aimed at allowing the heart to recover by a natural process of healing.

OUTLOOK AND PREVENTION

CHD is a disease of middle to old age, but its foundations are laid in the teens and early adult life. The chances of developing the disease can be considerably reduced by an "anticoronary" life-style. The person who has never smoked, exercises regularly, has a normal weight and blood pressure, and eats a prudent diet is unlikely to develop symptoms of CHD until late in life.

Even when symptoms develop, treatment can do a great deal to halt their progression. Studies of patients treated by coronary bypass surgery for disease affecting all the major coronary arteries reveal that 80 to 90 percent are still alive five years after the operation. Survival is even better among those with less extensive disease; they can usually be treated with drugs. Survival is substantially improved in patients who quit cigarette smoking.

Coronary thrombosis

Narrowing or blockage of one of the coronary arteries (which supply blood to the heart muscle) by a thrombus (clot). This causes a section of the heart muscle to die because it has been deprived of oxygen.

C

Coronary thrombosis is one of the main processes involved in *coronary heart disease*, the major cause of death in the US. Sudden blockage of a coronary artery causes an acute *myocardial infarction* (death of a portion of heart muscle). The terms coronary thrombosis and myocardial infarction thus tend to be used interchangeably, but the latter is the more precise medical term for heart attack.

Coroner
A public officer appointed to look into any death in which the cause is unknown, or when it is suspected or known to result from unnatural causes. A coroner is most often called when the deceased was not attended by a physician during the final illness. Other circumstances vary from state to state. If there are any uncertainties about the cause of death, the coroner will order a postmortem examination before issuing a death certificate. If the death is thought to be due to unnatural causes, the coroner will hold an inquest.

Corporate practice
The employment of a physician by a lay-controlled corporation that sells the services of the physician for profit. Because the physician, as an employee, is presumed to owe greater loyalty to the corporation than to the patients, corporate practice has been opposed on ethical grounds. Physician employment by hospitals, health maintenance organizations, and similar providers is regarded as an independent contractor arrangement, the physician being free to make medical decisions independently of the corporation. Under these circumstances, no objections are raised.

Cor pulmonale
Enlargement and strain of the right side of the heart due to chronic lung disease. Damage to the lungs increases resistance to blood flow from the heart through the branches of the pulmonary artery and causes pulmonary hypertension (increased pressure in the pulmonary artery). The resultant "back pressure" strain on the heart may eventually cause right-sided heart failure with *edema* (fluid collection in the tissues). (See *Pulmonary hypertension*.)

Corpuscle
Any minute body or cell, particularly red and white *blood cells* or certain types of nerve endings.

Corset
A device worn on the trunk to treat back pain and spinal injuries or deformities. Soft corsets, usually made of cotton fabric stiffened with plastic or metal, have straps enabling them to be tightened. Most commonly prescribed for back pain, corsets work in the same way as weight-lifters' belts—by exerting increased pressure on the abdomen they take the weight of the trunk off the lower spine. They also restrict painful movements and help keep the back warm.

Rigid corsets are made of plaster or lightweight plastic and must be molded to the body. They immobilize and support the spinal column when it has become unstable as the result of injury or help to correct its faulty alignment, as in scoliosis (curvature of the spine).

Corticosteroid drugs

COMMON DRUGS

Beclomethasone Betamethasone Cortisone Dexamethasone Hydrocortisone Prednisolone Prednisone

---
WARNING

Sudden withdrawal of corticosteroid drugs may cause serious illness or death. Always inform a physician you are taking or have recently taken corticosteroids.

A group of drugs similar to the natural corticosteroid hormones produced by the cortex of the *adrenal glands*.

WHY THEY ARE USED
Corticosteroid drugs have a wide variety of uses. They are prescribed as hormone replacement therapy to patients with an inadequate level of natural corticosteroids caused by *Addison's disease* or following surgical removal of the adrenal glands.

Corticosteroid drugs are used in the treatment of inflammatory intestinal disorders, such as *Crohn's disease* and *ulcerative colitis*. *Temporal arteritis* needs urgent treatment with corticosteroids to reduce inflammation in the artery leading to the retina and so prevent blindness.

Other disorders that often improve with corticosteroid treatment include *asthma, rheumatoid arthritis, eczema, iritis* (inflammation of the iris), and allergic *rhinitis* (hay fever). The injection of corticosteroids around an inflamed tendon may relieve pain in disorders such as *tennis elbow*.

Corticosteroid drugs are also used to suppress the immune system to prevent rejection of a transplanted organ (see *Transplant surgery*) and in the treatment of some types of cancer, such as a *lymphoma* or *leukemia*.

POSSIBLE ADVERSE EFFECTS
The incidence and severity of any adverse effects depends on the dosage, the form in which the drug is given, and the length of treatment.

HOW CORTICOSTEROIDS WORK
When given as hormone replacement therapy, corticosteroids supplement or replace natural hormones. Large doses have an anti-inflammatory effect as they reduce the production of prostaglandins. They also suppress the immune system by reducing the release and activity of white blood cells.

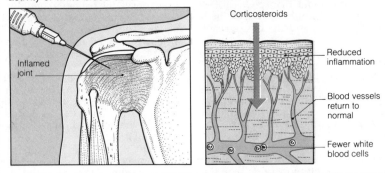

Inflamed joint

Inflamed skin

Dilated blood vessels

Increase in white blood cells

Corticosteroids

Reduced inflammation

Blood vessels return to normal

Fewer white blood cells

Adverse effects are uncommon when corticosteroids are given in the form of a cream or by inhaler because only small amounts are absorbed into the bloodstream.

Corticosteroid tablets taken in high doses for long periods may cause *edema* (tissue swelling), *hypertension* (high blood pressure), *diabetes mellitus*, *peptic ulcer*, *Cushing's syndrome*, *hirsutism* (excessive hairiness), inhibited growth in children, and, rarely, *cataract* or *psychosis*.

High doses of corticosteroid drugs also increase susceptibility to infection by impairing the body's *immune system* (natural defenses).

Long-term treatment with corticosteroid drugs suppresses the natural production of corticosteroid hormones by the *adrenal glands*. Sudden withdrawal of the drugs may lead to collapse, coma, and death (see *Adrenal failure*).

Corticosteroid hormones

A group of hormones produced by the *adrenal glands* that control the body's use of nutrients and the excretion of salts and water in the urine.

Corticotropin

An alternative name for *ACTH* (adrenocorticotropic hormone).

Cortisol

Another name for *hydrocortisone*, an important corticosteroid hormone produced by the *adrenal glands*.

Cortisone

A synthetic *corticosteroid drug* used to reduce inflammation in severe allergic, rheumatic, and connective tissue diseases. It is also used as a replacement hormone in *Addison's disease*, in which there is a corticosteroid hormone deficiency, and after adrenal gland removal.

Coryza

See *Cold, common*.

Cosmetic dentistry

Procedures to improve the appearance of the teeth. In many cases, these treatments are also necessary to restore or prevent further damage to the teeth and/or gums.

Teeth that are out of alignment can become decayed because the bite is incorrect and because the teeth are hard to keep clean. Such teeth can be moved into proper position by fitting a fixed *orthodontic appliance* (braces) that stays in place over a period of months. Correction is usually best carried out during childhood, when the teeth and jaws are still growing and developing, but can be done in adults as well.

The main use of a *crown* is to restore normal tooth structure and prevent further damage when a tooth is severely decayed or broken. However, crowns can also be important for appearance, particularly when a front tooth is damaged; in this case a porcelain crown is fitted because of its similarity in color to the natural teeth that surround it.

Bonding is a relatively new technique with a wide range of cosmetic uses. It can be used to treat chipped or malformed teeth, to close small gaps between front teeth, or to cover stained or discolored teeth. In some cases it can be used instead of a crown for front teeth.

Teeth that have become discolored because the pulp is dead or has been removed can be treated by *bleaching*.

Cosmetic surgery

An operation performed primarily to improve the appearance of an individual rather than to improve function or cure disease.

WHY IT IS DONE
Cosmetic surgery can improve appearance in a number of ways. Skin blemishes can be removed, and the appearance of an unsightly scar improved. The shape and size of the nose, chin, jaw, or breasts can be altered. Excess skin and fat, and any unsightly creases or marks that come with age or loss of weight, can be removed from the eyelids, face, breasts, or stomach.

An individual's expectations of the benefits of cosmetic surgery are often too great, however. Cosmetic surgery will not produce a dramatic change in personality or cure depression that a person attributes to his or her appearance. Nor can it reproduce an exact replica of someone else's features. Some procedures (such as face-lifts and hair transplants) may need to be repeated over the years; other procedures (such as *body contour surgery*) may result in uneven residual fat and unattractive scarring. Anyone contemplating cosmetic surgery should discuss the operation in detail with his or her physician.

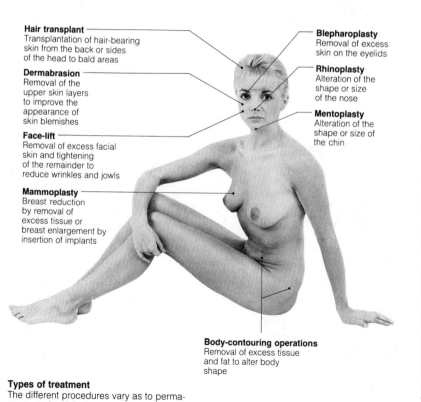

Hair transplant
Transplantation of hair-bearing skin from the back or sides of the head to bald areas

Dermabrasion
Removal of the upper skin layers to improve the appearance of skin blemishes

Face-lift
Removal of excess facial skin and tightening of the remainder to reduce wrinkles and jowls

Mammoplasty
Breast reduction by removal of excess tissue or breast enlargement by insertion of implants

Blepharoplasty
Removal of excess skin on the eyelids

Rhinoplasty
Alteration of the shape or size of the nose

Mentoplasty
Alteration of the shape or size of the chin

Body-contouring operations
Removal of excess tissue and fat to alter body shape

Types of treatment
The different procedures vary as to permanency and satisfactory results.

Costalgia

Pain around the chest due to damage to a rib or to one of the intercostal nerves (which run beneath the ribs). A broken rib produces pain and tenderness over the affected part of the rib cage. The pain is made worse by deep breathing and often persists for several weeks after the original injury.

Damage to one of the intercostal nerves is most commonly a result of an attack of the virus infection *herpes zoster* (shingles). The pain is difficult to treat successfully and tends to persist for several months or longer.

Cough

A reflex action to try to clear the airways of mucus, phlegm, a foreign body, or other irritants or blockages. Most coughs are due to irritation of the airways by dust, smoke, or mucus dripping from the back of the nose. However, in some cases a cough may be a symptom of an underlying disorder, most commonly a cold (see *Cold, common*), but sometimes a serious illness such as *lung cancer*.

A cough is said to be productive when it brings up mucus or phlegm, and unproductive, or dry, when it does not.

CAUSES

Among the more common causes of a cough are irritation of the upper respiratory tract—the pharynx (throat), larynx (voice box), and trachea (windpipe)—by inhaled particles, smoke, dust, or gases, or inflammation of these airways (see *Pharyngitis*; *Laryngitis*; *Tracheitis*), usually as a result of a viral infection.

In a child, inflammation of the upper respiratory tract can narrow the airways considerably (a condition called *croup*), causing a barking cough and breathing difficulty. Infection with the bacterium BORDETELLA PERTUSSIS produces a characteristic type of cough (see *Pertussis*).

Bronchitis (inflammation of the bronchi, the air passages into the lungs) produces thick mucus and phlegm and causes severe coughing. The disorder may be brought on by an infection, but is often the result of smoking (see *Cough, smokers'*). In *bronchiectasis* (distortion or dilatation of the bronchi), a large amount of infected phlegm collects in the bronchi, making the sufferer cough persistently in an attempt to bring up the phlegm, which may be associated with bleeding.

Bronchospasm (temporary narrowing of the bronchi) causes a dry cough that is usually worse at night. It is a feature of *asthma*, but also may be due to infection or allergic reaction.

The damage to lung tissues caused by *pneumonia* (inflammation of the lungs due to infection) results in painful coughing that brings up blood-flecked phlegm. Damage to the lungs brought about by pulmonary *edema* (accumulation of fluid in the lungs) produces a cough that is dry at first, but which later may bring up frothy, blood-stained phlegm. The cough associated with viral bronchitis and viral pneumonia is often dry and persistent, and may interrupt sleep.

Various chronic lung infections, notably *tuberculosis* and fungal infections (such as *histoplasmosis*), may cause a cough. Many *pneumoconioses* (dust diseases of the lungs) also cause a cough, which is usually accompanied by shortness of breath.

An inhaled foreign object, such as a peanut, that lodges in the larynx causes violent coughing to relieve *choking*. If the object travels further down and blocks a bronchus, inflammation and mucus will be produced at the site of obstruction, leading to a persistent cough.

Lung cancer and, less commonly, other tumors of the air passages usually first cause a mild cough, then a more severe one that may produce blood-stained phlegm.

Sometimes, especially in children, coughing develops as a nervous reaction to stress.

SELF-HELP

In some cases, a dry cough may be relieved by sucking on throat lozenges or by drinking warm, soothing drinks, such as honey and water. If ineffective, narcotic *cough remedies* afford symptomatic relief, particularly at bedtime to permit sleep.

Productive coughing is the body's way of unblocking airways obstructed by mucus or phlegm and, in such cases, cough suppressants should be avoided since they can do more harm than good. An expectorant cough medication or drinking lots of fluids can help loosen mucus or phlegm if there is difficulty coughing it up.

A physician should be consulted if any cough persists for more than two or three days, is severe, or is accompanied by symptoms such as chest pain, green phlegm, coughed-up blood, or breathing difficulty.

TREATMENT

Treatment depends on the underlying disorder. For example, antibiotics may be given for a bacterial infection, a *bronchodilator* and/or *corticosteroid drugs* for asthma, *breathing exercises* and *postural drainage* (lying in a position that allows mucus to drain from the bronchi) for bronchiectasis and chronic bronchitis, and surgery or *radiation therapy* for cancer.

Coughing up blood

Known medically as hemoptysis, coughing up blood is due to rupturing of a blood vessel in the airways, lungs, nose, or throat. The underlying cause can range from persistent coughing to a serious disorder, such as cancer. Coughed-up blood may be in the form of bright-red or rusty-brown streaks or clots in or on the phlegm, a pinkish froth, or, more rarely, pure blood. The form it takes depends as much on the size of the ruptured blood vessel as on the underlying cause. Because of the possibility of a serious underlying disorder, all cases of coughing up blood require medical assessment.

Coughing up blood should not be confused with blood in the mouth, which is usually due to a nosebleed or to bleeding gums.

CAUSES

The most common cause of coughing up blood is an infection—such as *pneumonia*, *bronchitis*, or *tuberculosis*—in which inflammation of the bronchi (airways into the lungs) and alveoli (air sacs) damages the wall of a blood vessel. Similarly, in *bronchiectasis* the bronchi become enlarged and distorted, which can lead to rupture of a blood vessel and coughing up blood.

Any disorder that causes persistent coughing, such as *tracheitis* (inflammation of the windpipe), can produce hemoptysis as a result of the coughing putting strain on the blood vessels in the airways.

Another cause of coughing up blood is congestion in, and subsequent rupture of, blood vessels within the lungs. Congestion can be due to *heart failure*, *mitral stenosis* (narrowing of the mitral valve in the heart), or *pulmonary embolism* (blood clot lodged in an artery in the lungs).

A malignant tumor can lead to coughing up blood by eroding the wall of a blood vessel in the larynx (voice box), bronchi, or alveoli.

Any *bleeding disorder* (such as *hemophilia*) can also cause hemoptysis.

INVESTIGATION AND TREATMENT

A *chest X ray* may be carried out. Anyone who smokes, who is older than 40, whose chest X rays are abnormal, or who has coughed up blood more than once may need *bronchos-*

COUGH A noisy expulsion of air from the lungs that may produce sputum (phlegm) or be "dry."

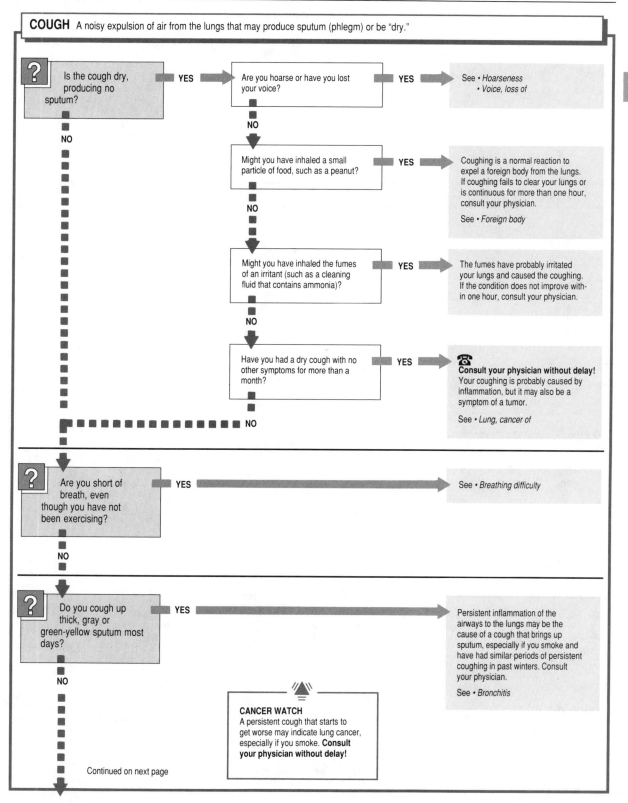

? Is the cough dry, producing no sputum?

YES → Are you hoarse or have you lost your voice?

YES → See • *Hoarseness*
• *Voice, loss of*

NO ↓

Might you have inhaled a small particle of food, such as a peanut?

YES → Coughing is a normal reaction to expel a foreign body from the lungs. If coughing fails to clear your lungs or is continuous for more than one hour, consult your physician.

See • *Foreign body*

NO ↓

Might you have inhaled the fumes of an irritant (such as a cleaning fluid that contains ammonia)?

YES → The fumes have probably irritated your lungs and caused the coughing. If the condition does not improve within one hour, consult your physician.

NO ↓

Have you had a dry cough with no other symptoms for more than a month?

YES → ☎ **Consult your physician without delay!** Your coughing is probably caused by inflammation, but it may also be a symptom of a tumor.

See • *Lung, cancer of*

NO →

? Are you short of breath, even though you have not been exercising?

YES → See • *Breathing difficulty*

NO ↓

? Do you cough up thick, gray or green-yellow sputum most days?

YES → Persistent inflammation of the airways to the lungs may be the cause of a cough that brings up sputum, especially if you smoke and have had similar periods of persistent coughing in past winters. Consult your physician.

See • *Bronchitis*

NO ↓

CANCER WATCH
A persistent cough that starts to get worse may indicate lung cancer, especially if you smoke. **Consult your physician without delay!**

Continued on next page

C

C

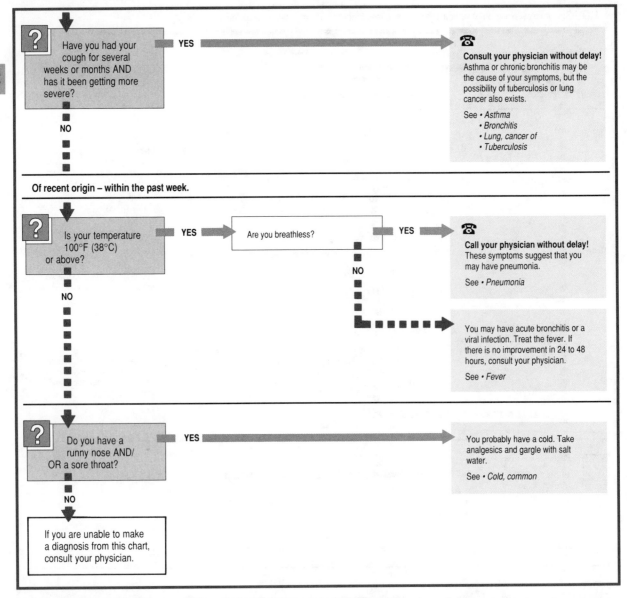

Have you had your cough for several weeks or months AND has it been getting more severe?

YES → ☎ **Consult your physician without delay!**
Asthma or chronic bronchitis may be the cause of your symptoms, but the possibility of tuberculosis or lung cancer also exists.

See • *Asthma*
• *Bronchitis*
• *Lung, cancer of*
• *Tuberculosis*

NO ↓

Of recent origin – within the past week.

Is your temperature 100°F (38°C) or above?

YES → Are you breathless?

YES → ☎ **Call your physician without delay!**
These symptoms suggest that you may have pneumonia.

See • *Pneumonia*

NO ↓

You may have acute bronchitis or a viral infection. Treat the fever. If there is no improvement in 24 to 48 hours, consult your physician.

See • *Fever*

NO ↓

Do you have a runny nose AND/OR a sore throat?

YES → You probably have a cold. Take analgesics and gargle with salt water.

See • *Cold, common*

NO ↓

If you are unable to make a diagnosis from this chart, consult your physician.

---

copy, a diagnostic procedure in which a flexible viewing tube is passed into the lungs. In about one third of cases, no underlying cause is found.

Treatment depends on the cause, but may include *antibiotic drugs, anticoagulant drugs,* and *diuretic drugs.*

Cough remedies

COMMON DRUGS

Expectorants
Ammonium chloride

Cough suppressants
Antihistamines Codeine Dextromethorphan

A bewildering variety of over-the-counter medications is available for treating a *cough.* Most cough remedies consist of a syrupy base to which various active ingredients and flavorings are added.

Two main groups of drugs are used: expectorants, intended for coughs that are producing sputum (phlegm), and cough suppressants, intended for dry coughs. It is important to select the correct type of medication—a cough suppressant taken for a sputum-producing cough may interfere with the coughing up of sputum and may delay recovery.

HOW THEY WORK
Expectorants "loosen" a cough by stimulating the production of watery secretions in the lungs. Some expectorants also have a mucolytic action (a direct effect on the sputum that makes it less sticky).

Cough suppressants act on the part of the brain that controls the coughing reflex. Drugs with this effect include some *antihistamine drugs* and the narcotic analgesic drug *codeine.*

POSSIBLE ADVERSE EFFECTS
All cough suppressants have a sedating effect and may cause drowsiness. Using cough remedies to alleviate the

symptoms of a persistent cough may delay diagnosis of a serious disorder.

Cough, smokers'

A recurrent cough that is very common among smokers, particularly heavy smokers and those who have smoked for a long time. In many instances, the sufferer becomes accustomed to his or her cough and regards it as normal.

Usually, coughing is triggered by the accumulation of large amounts of abnormally thick sputum (phlegm) in the airways (a feature of *bronchitis*), which is caused by inflammation of the airways due to smoking.

TREATMENT

Stopping smoking usually stops the persistent cough, though it does not happen immediately. The longer the person has been smoking, the longer the cough will persist after quitting.

Because of the health hazards of smoking, it is essential for the smoker to consult his or her physician about a cough, particularly if there is any change in its frequency or character. (See also *Tobacco smoking*.)

Counseling

Advice and psychological support given by a health professional and usually aimed at helping a person cope with a particular problem (for example, bereavement or cancer treatment). A more general exploration of a person's feelings and attitudes, not aimed at one particular problem, is sometimes included in the definition.

WHY IT IS DONE

Counseling can help people with problems at school, work, or within the family; provide advice on family planning, abortion, and sexual and marital problems; help people deal with drinking and drug problems; and provide support during life crises.

Counseling methods may be used by caseworkers as a means of history-taking and information gathering. Physicians, too, may use a counseling style when interviewing a patient whose medical problem is complicated by personal circumstances, or when the objectives of the consultation are not clear.

HOW IT IS DONE

Some counseling, especially for genetic disorders (see *Genetic counseling*) or the treatment of cancer, consists mainly of providing personalized information in a setting in which the patient, or client, is encouraged to ask questions and to express any doubts and uncertainties.

The techniques that are used in psychotherapeutic counseling are essentially similar. The counselor encourages the individual to make statements about his or her feelings, experiences, and problems. These statements can then be discussed and explored for inconsistencies as a means of helping the individual develop a greater and more realistic understanding of his or her problems.

Usually, counseling is a one-to-one activity. However, in some situations, such as *sex therapy*, representatives of a particular point of view or gender model may be incorporated (for example, one male and one female counselor). This is termed co-counseling. Counseling may also occur in small groups. (See also *Child guidance*; *Family therapy*; *Marital counseling*.)

Cowpox

An infection caused by the vaccinia virus, which usually affects cows.

An attack of cowpox used to confer immunity against *smallpox* (now presumed to be extinct) because the viruses responsible for the two diseases were very similar. This fact was the basis of smallpox vaccination. Vaccinia virus, which gave its name to "vaccination," continued to be used as smallpox vaccine until smallpox was considered to have been eradicated in the 1970s.

Coxa vara

A deformity of the hip in which the angle between the neck and head (ball) of the femur and the shaft of the femur (thigh bone) is reduced, causing shortening of the leg and a limp.

CAUSES AND INCIDENCE

The most common cause is injury—either a fracture of the neck of the thigh bone or, in adolescence, injury to the developing part of the head of the bone. The deformity can also occur if the bone tissue in the neck of the bone is soft instead of firm, so that it bends under the weight of the body. This softening may be congenital or the result of a bone disorder such as *rickets* or *Paget's disease*.

SYMPTOMS AND DIAGNOSIS

The symptoms are pain and stiffness in the hip and increased difficulty in walking. The disorder is diagnosed by X rays, which reveal the deformity.

TREATMENT AND OUTLOOK

When coxa vara is due to an underlying bone disorder, it can be treated to bring about hardening of the bone tissue; however, little can be done about bone that is soft from birth. To

relieve pain, stiffness, and limping, *osteotomy* is required. The neck of the bone is cut and the two ends are repositioned and secured at the correct angle. This usually eases the condition so that the patient can walk with only minor discomfort.

Crab lice

See *Pubic lice*.

Cradle cap

A condition common in babies in which thick, yellow scales occur in patches over the scalp. Cradle cap is harmless, although it tends to recur.

Cradle cap is a form of seborrheic *dermatitis*, which may also occur on the face, neck, behind the ears, and in the diaper area. The skin in these areas may look red and inflamed.

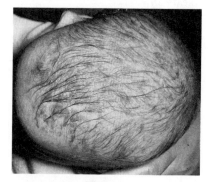

Appearance of cradle cap
Most prevalent between 3 and 9 months of age, it is not clear why cradle cap occurs, but it is not a result of poor hygiene.

TREATMENT

Rub warm olive or mineral oil into the baby's scalp and leave on overnight. This loosens and softens the scales, which can be gently washed off the next day with a mild, antidandruff shampoo. This procedure may need repeating for a few days until all scales have been loosened. The baby's hair should be brushed daily using a soft-bristled brush. This will also help loosen the scales so they can be removed with a fine-tooth comb. If the condition seems to be worsening or if the skin looks inflamed, a physician should be consulted. A mild corticosteroid cream may be prescribed until the condition improves.

Cramp

Painful spasm in a muscle caused by excessive and prolonged contraction of the muscle fibers. Cramps are a common occurrence and usually last only a few moments.

C

CAUSES

Cramps often occur during or immediately after exercise because of a buildup of lactic acid and other chemicals in the muscles (caused by increased muscular activity) and small areas of muscle fiber damage.

Cramps can also occur during any repetitive movement such as writing (see *Cramp, writers'*), or through sitting or lying in an awkward position. Any condition that causes profuse sweating, such as a fever, heat wave, or prolonged exercise, can lead to cramps in resting muscles; the loss of sodium salts in the sweat disrupts muscle cell activity.

Cramps at night may be due to poor circulation of blood into the legs (see *Peripheral vascular disease*), but often there is no known cause.

TREATMENT

The pain can be helped by massaging or stretching the muscles involved. If cramps occur regularly at night your physician may prescribe a drug containing calcium or quinine, which can help prevent painful recurrences. If cramps persist for longer than an hour they are likely to be due to a more serious medical condition and the attention of a physician should be sought immediately.

Cramp, writers'

Painful spasm in the muscles of the hand, making it impossible to write. In most cases the muscles in the hand are still able to perform other tasks, indicating that the problem may be psychological in origin. Contrary to this theory, however, writers' cramp fails to respond to psychotherapy. The use of muscle relaxants and other drugs has also met with little success in tackling the problem.

The condition sometimes improves if the hand is rested for months, but often it is permanent. Occasionally the other hand becomes affected.

Cranial nerves

Twelve pairs of nerves that emerge directly from the brain—as opposed to the *spinal nerves*, which connect with the spinal cord. All but two of the cranial nerve pairs connect with nuclei in the *brain stem* (the lowest section of the brain). The other two (the olfactory and optic nerves) link directly with parts of the *cerebrum* (the main mass of the brain). All the nerves emerge through various openings in the cranium (skull); many then soon divide into several major branches.

Craniopharyngioma

A tumor of the pituitary gland. The condition is very rare. There are about one or two cases per million population in the US each year.

Symptoms include headaches, vomiting, defective vision, stunted growth, and failure of sexual development. If untreated, the tumor may result in permanent brain damage.

FUNCTIONS OF CRANIAL NERVES

Some cranial nerves are principally concerned with delivering sensory information from organs, such as the ears, nose, and eyes, to the brain. Others carry messages that move the tongue, eyes, and facial (and other) muscles, or stimulate glands such as the salivary glands. A few have both sensory and motor functions. One of the nerves—the tenth cranial, or *vagus nerve*—is one of the most important components of the *parasympathetic nervous system*, concerned with maintaining the rhythmic automatic function of the internal body machinery. It has branches to all the main digestive organs, the heart, and the lungs.

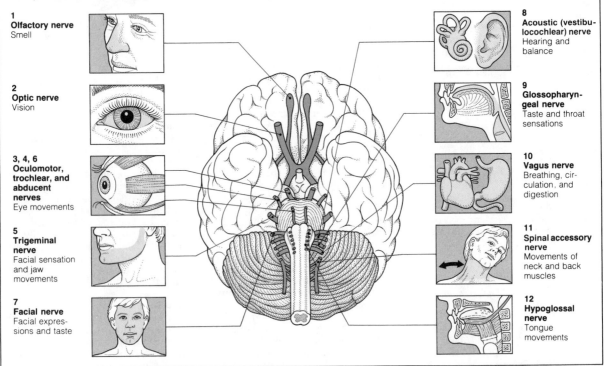

1 Olfactory nerve Smell

2 Optic nerve Vision

3, 4, 6 Oculomotor, trochlear, and abducent nerves Eye movements

5 Trigeminal nerve Facial sensation and jaw movements

7 Facial nerve Facial expressions and taste

8 Acoustic (vestibulocochlear) nerve Hearing and balance

9 Glossopharyngeal nerve Taste and throat sensations

10 Vagus nerve Breathing, circulation, and digestion

11 Spinal accessory nerve Movements of neck and back muscles

12 Hypoglossal nerve Tongue movements

Craniopharyngiomas are identified by imaging techniques for the brain (see *Brain imaging*) and are usually removed surgically.

Craniosynostosis
The early closure of one or more of the joints between the bones of the cranium (see *Skull*).

Craniosynostosis may occur in a baby affected by a bone disease, such as rickets, in a baby with multiple birth defects, or in an otherwise healthy baby. It may also occur if the baby's brain is abnormally small.

DIAGNOSIS AND TREATMENT
The physician's diagnosis is made from the outward appearance of the skull and by skull X ray. Treatment must be undertaken during the first few months of life to prevent brain damage. An operation is performed to separate the skull bones by cutting away the fused edges and separating the bony plates.

Craniotomy
Removal of part of the skull to carry out an operation on the brain, such as performance of a biopsy, removal of a tumor, or aspiration and drainage of an abscess or blood clot.

After the operation the bone is replaced and the membranes, muscle, and skin are sewn back into position.

Following successful surgery, the patient can usually leave the hospital within a week. He or she will generally experience mild headaches for a time, but little real pain.

Cranium
The part of the *skull* around the brain.

Cream
A thick, semisolid preparation used to apply medications to the skin for therapeutic or prophylactic (preventive) purposes. Creams are useful in the treatment of dry skin conditions because their high water content gives them a moisturizing effect.

Creatinine clearance
See *Kidney function tests*.

Cremation
Burning dead bodies to ash. Typically, the process takes between one and two hours and results in 5 to 7 pounds (2.3 to 3.2 kg) of ash. In some cases certain precautions must be taken before cremation can be performed. For example, if the deceased person was fitted with a pacemaker, it must be removed from the body because of

the risk of an explosion. Also, cremation involves additional formalities, principally to prevent destruction of a body before the possibility of a crime has been ruled out.

Crepitus
The grating sound heard, and the sensation felt, when two rough surfaces rub together. It may be experienced when the ends of a broken bone rub against each other or in *osteoarthritis*, when the cartilage that covers the bony surfaces of a joint has worn away and the roughened areas of the joint grind against each other. The sound is usually loud enough to be heard by the naked ear. Fainter sounds, audible through a stethoscope, are produced when lung *alveoli* rub together—as a result of inflammation due to pneumonia, for example.

Crepitus is also used to describe the sounds made when an area of subcutaneous *emphysema* (air under the skin) or gas *gangrene* (gas within infected tissues) is pressed.

Cretinism
A condition characterized by mental retardation, stunted growth, and coarse facial features. It results from decreased production of the hormone *thyroxine* by the thyroid gland. (See also *Hypothyroidism*.)

Creutzfeldt-Jakob syndrome
A very rare degenerative condition of the brain presumably caused by a slow virus (one that causes no signs of disease until many months or years after the original infection).

In most instances, no source of infection is discovered. However, rarely, infection has been linked with brain surgery when instruments contaminated by the virus have been used, transplantation of an infected cornea, and treatment with growth hormone extracted from pituitary glands after death (current growth hormone preparations are products of genetic engineering and carry no risk).

The condition causes progressive *dementia* and *myoclonus* (sudden

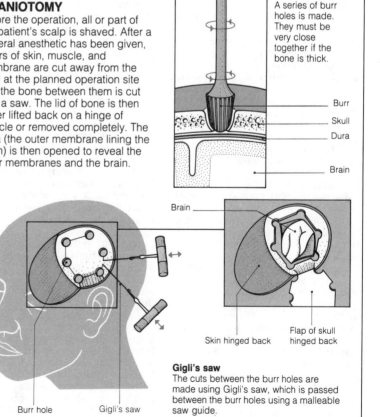

PROCEDURE FOR CRANIOTOMY
Before the operation, all or part of the patient's scalp is shaved. After a general anesthetic has been given, layers of skin, muscle, and membrane are cut away from the skull at the planned operation site and the bone between them is cut with a saw. The lid of bone is then either lifted back on a hinge of muscle or removed completely. The dura (the outer membrane lining the brain) is then opened to reveal the inner membranes and the brain.

Burr holes
A series of burr holes is made. They must be very close together if the bone is thick.

Burr
Skull
Dura
Brain

Brain

Skin hinged back

Flap of skull hinged back

Gigli's saw
The cuts between the burr holes are made using Gigli's saw, which is passed between the burr holes using a malleable saw guide.

Burr hole   Gigli's saw

muscular contractions). Muscular coordination diminishes, the intellect and personality deteriorate, and blindness may develop. As the disease progresses, the power of speech is lost and the body becomes rigid. There is no treatment and death usually occurs within three to 12 months of onset.

Crib death

See *Sudden infant death syndrome.*

Cri du chat syndrome

A congenital (present at birth) condition characterized by a catlike cry due to a small larynx. Mental handicap, unusual facial characteristics (such as a wide spacing between the eyes), a small head, and shortness of stature are other typical features.

Cri du chat syndrome is rare and the result of a *chromosomal abnormality*; a portion of one chromosome is missing in each of the affected individual's cells. No treatment is possible. The child needs special care and schooling if he or she survives infancy. (See also *Genetic counseling.*)

Crisis

A term that describes a turning point in the course of a disease (marking the onset of either recovery or deterioration), an emergency, or a distressing time of emotional difficulty (such as divorce or a death in the family). The term was in common use before the advent of antibiotics when patients with lobar *pneumonia* would be watched for the crisis.

Crisis intervention

The provision of immediate advice or help to people with acute personal or sociomedical problems.

Many voluntary organizations have been established to help people in crisis. Help may also be available at walk-in centers or social services departments. In addition to other crisis services, these centers may offer *counseling,* usually with the aim of helping clients cope with crises rather than of providing longer-term help.

Critical

A term used to mean seriously ill, or to describe a crucial state of illness from which it is uncertain whether or not the patient will recover.

Crohn's disease

A chronic inflammatory disease that can affect any part of the gastrointestinal tract from the mouth to the anus.

Crohn's disease may cause pain, fever, diarrhea, and loss of weight.

The most common site of inflammation is the terminal ileum (the end of the small intestine where it joins the large intestine). The intestinal wall becomes extremely thick due to continued chronic inflammation, and deep, penetrating ulcers may form. The disease tends to be patchy; areas of the intestine that lie between diseased areas may appear to be normal, but are usually mildly affected.

CAUSES AND INCIDENCE
The cause is unknown. It may represent an abnormal allergic reaction or may be an exaggerated response to an infectious agent, such as a bacterium or a virus. There is a slight genetic predisposition (inherited tendency to develop the disease).

The incidence of Crohn's disease varies between three and six new cases per year per 100,000 population in most developed countries, including the US; the incidence seems to have increased over the last 30 years. A person may be affected at any age, but the peak ages are in adolescence and early adulthood and after 60.

SYMPTOMS
In young people the ileum (small intestine) is usually involved, and the disease causes spasms of pain in the abdomen, diarrhea, and chronic sickness due to loss of appetite, anemia, and weight loss. The ability of the small intestine to absorb food is reduced. In the elderly, it is more common for the disease to affect the rectum and cause rectal bleeding. In both groups the disease may also affect the anus, causing chronic abscesses, deep fissures (cracks), and fistulas (passageways that create an abnormal link between organs of the body).

Crohn's disease can also affect the colon (large intestine), causing bloody diarrhea. It is rare in the mouth, esophagus, stomach, and duodenum (upper part of the small intestine).

Complications may affect the intestines or may develop elsewhere in the body. The thickening of the intestinal wall may narrow the inside diameter so much that an intestinal obstruction occurs.

About 30 percent of patients with Crohn's disease develop a fistula. Internal fistulas may form between loops of intestine. External fistulas to the skin of the abdomen or the skin surrounding the anus may follow a surgical operation (or rupture of an abscess) and may cause leakage of feces onto the skin.

Abscesses (pus-filled pockets of infection) form in about 20 percent of patients. Many of these abscesses occur around the anus, but some occur within the abdomen.

Complications in other parts of the body may include inflammation of various parts of the eye, severe arthritis affecting various joints of the body, *ankylosing spondylitis* (an inflammation of the spine), and skin disorders (including *eczema*).

DIAGNOSIS
If the symptoms suggest Crohn's disease, a physical examination may reveal tender abdominal swellings that indicate thickening of the intestinal walls. *Sigmoidoscopy* (examination of the rectum with a viewing tube) may confirm the disease's presence in the rectum. X rays using barium meals or barium enemas (see *Barium X-ray examinations*) will show thickened loops of bowel with deep fissures. It may be difficult to differentiate between Crohn's disease that affects the colon and *ulcerative colitis,* a form of inflammatory disease that is limited to the large intestine, but *colonoscopy* (examination of the colon using a flexible viewing tube) and *biopsy* (removal of a piece of tissue for microscopic examination) may help in doubtful cases. Blood tests may show evidence of protein deficiency or *anemia.*

TREATMENT
Sulfasalazine may be given by mouth to try to control the inflammatory process and *corticosteroid drugs* may be given by mouth or as enemas. Severe acute attacks may require admission to the hospital for blood transfusion, intravenous feeding, and treatment with corticosteroid drugs given intravenously. The severity of the disease fluctuates widely, and the patient is usually under long-term medical supervision.

Some patients find that particular foods exacerbate their symptoms. Others may benefit from a high-vitamin, low-fiber diet.

A surgical operation to remove damaged portions of the intestine may be needed to treat chronic obstruction or blood loss. If the small intestine is involved, the surgeon will remove as little of the intestine as possible, seeking only to remove the most affected parts since the surgery is not curative. If the large intestine is involved, surgery may involve removal of narrowed obstructing segments.

Emergency surgery may be required to deal with an abscess. Simple drainage of an abscess will produce an external fistula, but occasionally the patient is too ill for any further treatment. Surgery may also occasionally be required for obstruction, perforation, or severe bleeding.

OUTLOOK
The disease is chronic and the symptoms fluctuate over many years, "burning out" in time for some patients. Many patients eventually require surgical treatment to deal with the complications of the disease. The recurrence rate after surgery is high, although recurrences may be delayed for many years. Some patients with localized disease remain in normal health indefinitely after surgery and seem to be cured. There is no predisposition to intestinal cancer.

Cromolyn sodium

ALLERGY
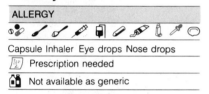
Capsule Inhaler Eye drops Nose drops
📋 Prescription needed
🔒 Not available as generic

A drug used in the treatment of some types of *asthma* and allergic conditions such as allergic *rhinitis* (hay fever), allergic *conjunctivitis*, and *food allergy*. Cromolyn sodium was introduced in the 1970s.

WHY IT IS USED
Cromolyn sodium is commonly given by inhaler to prevent attacks of mild to moderate asthma in children. It is also prescribed for allergic asthma in adults and for asthma induced by exercise or cold air. Cromolyn sodium has a slow onset of action, taking up to four to six weeks of regular dosing to produce its antiasthmatic effect. Its use sometimes permits a reduction in the dosage of other drugs taken to relieve attacks. It is not effective for the relief of an acute asthmatic attack in progress.

Taken as a nasal spray, cromolyn sodium is useful in treating allergic rhinitis. In the form of eye drops, it treats allergic conjunctivitis, and as capsules it can help in some types of food allergy.

HOW IT WORKS
Cromolyn sodium works by blocking the release of *histamine* (a chemical released into the body when an allergic reaction occurs).

POSSIBLE ADVERSE EFFECTS
Side effects are generally mild and rarely require the drug to be stopped. Coughing and wheezing on inhalation may be prevented by using a sym-

pathomimetic *bronchodilator drug* first. Hoarseness and throat irritation can be avoided by rinsing the mouth with water after inhalation.

Crossbite
A type of *malocclusion* in which the lower teeth overlap the upper teeth. In a normal bite, just the reverse is true.

Cross-eye
A type of *strabismus* (squint) in which one eye turns inward relative to the other eye.

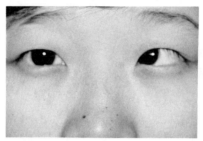

Appearance of cross-eye
Most types of cross-eye can, and should, be corrected to improve appearance and vision.

Cross matching
A procedure used to determine compatibility between the blood of someone requiring a *blood transfusion* and that of a blood donor.

Red blood cells from the donor are mixed with serum from the recipient, and red blood cells from the recipient are mixed with serum from the donor. After a short time, the mixtures are examined on a glass slide under a microscope. Clumping together of the red cells to form a small clot indicates the presence of antibodies in the serum, showing that the blood is not compatible. If no clotting occurs, the donor's blood may be safely transfused to the recipient.

Croup
Inflammation and narrowing of the air passages in young children, causing a barking cough, hoarseness, and stridor (a wheezing or grunting noise on breathing in). The condition is very common in children up to the age of about 4 years. In older children and adults, the air passages are too wide and the cartilage in the wall too stiff for any swelling or inflammation to cause the walls to collapse.

CAUSES
Croup is brought on by a viral infection, often a cold, affecting the larynx (voice box), trachea (windpipe), and bronchi (airways into the lung).

Several different types of virus can infect this part of the respiratory system, so one bout of croup does not confer immunity from subsequent attacks; some children are prone to recurrent bouts. Croup tends to occur in outbreaks in late fall and winter.

TREATMENT
Most cases are mild and pass quickly. A parent should remain calm and comfort the child; once soothed, the child will be able to breathe more easily. Providing cool mist for the child to inhale may also help (by utilizing a room humidifier or sitting in the bathroom with the shower running, for example). Cool night air has a beneficial effect as well.

If a child is struggling to breathe or turns blue, medical help should be obtained immediately. The child should be taken to the hospital and there given humidified oxygen in a tent. When breathing is seriously obstructed, treatment involves either passing a tube down the throat or an operation called a *tracheostomy* in which a tube is passed into the throat through the neck to bypass the obstruction. In either case, the tube can usually be removed within 24 hours. Complete recovery takes place within a few days.

Crowding, dental
A type of *malocclusion* that occurs when there is insufficient space along the jawbones to accommodate all the teeth in correct alignment.

Crown, dental
An artificial replacement for the crown of a tooth (the part above the gum) that has become decayed, discolored, or broken. A porcelain crown is usually used on front teeth because of its similarity in color to natural teeth, but back teeth require the greater strength of a crown made from gold or from porcelain fused to metal. (See illustration, next page.)

Cruciate ligaments
Two ligaments in the knee that pass over each other to form a cross (hence their name, from the Latin word "crux," meaning cross). The ligaments form connections between the femur (thigh bone) and tibia (shin) inside the knee joint.

The role of the cruciate ligaments is to prevent overbending and overstraightening at the knee joint. Consequently, if these ligaments are torn, the knee joint becomes unstable and may cause pain.

C

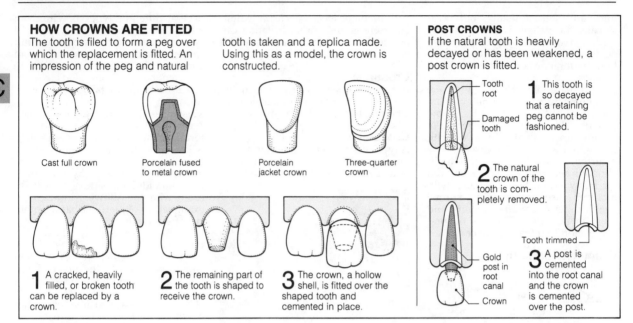

HOW CROWNS ARE FITTED

The tooth is filed to form a peg over which the replacement is fitted. An impression of the peg and natural tooth is taken and a replica made. Using this as a model, the crown is constructed.

Cast full crown

Porcelain fused to metal crown

Porcelain jacket crown

Three-quarter crown

1 A cracked, heavily filled, or broken tooth can be replaced by a crown.

2 The remaining part of the tooth is shaped to receive the crown.

3 The crown, a hollow shell, is fitted over the shaped tooth and cemented in place.

POST CROWNS

If the natural tooth is heavily decayed or has been weakened, a post crown is fitted.

Tooth root

Damaged tooth

1 This tooth is so decayed that a retaining peg cannot be fashioned.

2 The natural crown of the tooth is completely removed.

Tooth trimmed

Gold post in root canal

Crown

3 A post is cemented into the root canal and the crown is cemented over the post.

Crush syndrome

Damage to a large amount of body muscle—most commonly as a result of a serious auto accident—causing *renal failure*. Protein pigments released into the bloodstream from the damaged muscles temporarily impair the functioning of the kidney. As a result, some substances normally excreted in the urine build up to toxic levels in the blood. Without treatment the kidney failure may be fatal. Today, treatment by *dialysis* gives the kidneys a chance to recover their function.

Crutch palsy

Weakness or paralysis of muscles in the wrist, fingers, and thumb from a crutch pressed tightly under the arm, caused by pressure on the nerves that supply these muscles. The disorder occurs only after prolonged walking with a crutch that is too tall for the individual. A crutch should fit comfortably under the arm when standing upright, with the hand taking much of the weight.

Crutch palsy can also occur after falling asleep with one arm over the back of a chair with the top of the chair pressed into the armpit. Usually, the person has fallen asleep after a bout of drinking, giving the disorder its common name, Saturday night palsy.

Symptoms usually improve without treatment since the damage to the nerves is temporary. In rare cases, exercises are needed to strengthen the wrist and fingers.

Crying in infants

Occasional crying in a baby is normal behavior—it is the baby's only means of communicating a need. Only when crying is inconsolable or unusual in any way should it be regarded as signifying a problem.

CAUSES

Crying in infants is usually a response to needs or discomforts, such as hunger, thirst, a wet or soiled diaper, tiredness, interrupted sleep, a desire to be comforted, feeling hot or cold, boredom, or separation from parents. Most healthy babies stop crying when their needs are attended to.

Persistent crying, when it is not due to a continually ignored or unrecognized need, may be a baby's reaction to the overwrought state of a parent who is angry, resentful, or overtired. In a minority of cases, crying may be due to illness, commonly ear or throat infections, or to viral fevers. Persistent crying may indicate maltreatment (see *Child abuse*).

TREATMENT

A crying baby should always be attended to. The idea that attending to a crying infant is "giving in" is wrong. Persistent lack of attention is believed to have an adverse effect on emotional development in later life.

If a baby continues to cry after a feeding and a change of diaper, parents should make sure that their child is not too hot or cold, and should try to comfort the baby. A baby sling can be used to provide continuous physical contact. The baby may also prefer being propped up in a chair rather than lying flat, so that he or she can look around.

Parents should try to get as much sleep as possible, and mothers especially should put aside at least one period during the day for relaxation. If the baby cries at night, parents should take turns attending to him or her.

Medical advice is usually necessary only if a baby cries persistently despite all attempts to soothe him or her, if a normally quiet baby starts to cry a lot, if a baby also has diarrhea, vomiting, fever, or seems sick, or if a baby cries only weakly or not at all. Parents should not attribute persistent crying to teething or colic without consulting a physician.

Cryo-

A prefix meaning cold. It is often used to indicate that a procedure uses freezing or low temperatures.

Cryopreservation

The preservation of living cells by freezing. The technique is used chiefly to store human eggs, sperm, and blood for later use.

WHY IT IS DONE

In a woman who is infertile because of blocked fallopian tubes, eggs can be removed from her ovaries, frozen, and stored until they can be used for *in vitro fertilization*.

Treatment of cancer by radiation therapy or chemotherapy carries the slight risk of damaging sperm. If the man wants to retain the option of future fatherhood, a sample of his sperm is collected before treatment and frozen for possible later use in *artificial insemination*. Sperm from donors can also be frozen and used in this way to enable a woman whose husband is infertile to bear a child.

Plasma and blood from rare blood groups can be preserved by freezing and stored in a blood bank for long periods until needed.

HOW IT IS DONE

The cells to be preserved are first immersed in a fluid, usually glycerol. Glycerol enters and surrounds the cells so that they are protected from the normally destructive effect of freezing (see *Cryosurgery*). The temperature is lowered as the concentration of protecting fluid is increased until the final storage temperature of about -290°F (-180°C) is reached.

OUTLOOK

Apart from widespread cryopreservation of cells, there has also been some success with freezing and reusing small areas of tissue, such as the cornea and portions of skin. This has led to much experimental work on the possibility (as yet unfulfilled) of cryopreservation of major organs, such as the heart, liver, and kidneys, taken from people who have recently died, for the purposes of transplantation. This would enable transplants to be carried out on a normal surgical time scale rather than as a race against time, as at present.

Cryosurgery

The use of temperatures below freezing to destroy tissue. The term is also applied to the use of cold during surgery to produce adhesion between an instrument and body tissue. Cryosurgery has been in common use only for the past decade; in many cases it is proving to be a useful alternative to more traditional surgery or radiation therapy.

WHY IT IS DONE

Because cryosurgery causes only minimal scarring, it is particularly valuable for dealing with malignant tumors in the cervix and in major organs, such as the liver or bowel, in which heavy scarring can block vital openings or channels. For cosmetic reasons, it is also the best technique for removing skin cancers, such as basal cell carcinoma, and skin disfigurements, such as birthmarks. Hemorrhoids and other anal lesions can be treated rapidly and effectively.

Cryosurgery is also a good method for handling tiny structures in the eye; it has proved particularly useful in performing *cataract surgery* and for treating *retinal detachment*.

HOW IT IS DONE

Treatment of an internal tumor with cryosurgery is a major operation requiring a general anesthetic. The growth is destroyed in one of two ways—by applying a metal probe cooled to the temperature of liquid nitrogen, about -256°F (-160°C), or by spraying it with liquid nitrogen.

Skin cancers, disfigurements, and hemorrhoids are usually treated in the outpatient department, using a metal probe cooled to the same temperature as above. The procedure is virtually painless, since the extreme cold paralyzes the nerves in the skin as a local anesthetic does. After treatment, a blister develops, which may weep for a few days before healing. Although there is little scarring, the treated area may show up as a patch of paler skin.

Cryptococcosis

A rare infection caused by inhaling the fungus *CRYPTOCOCCUS NEOFORMANS*. It is found throughout the world, especially in soil contaminated with pigeon droppings. Infection with the fungus may cause *meningitis* (inflammation of the coverings of the brain) or granular growths in the lungs, skin, or elsewhere. Most but not all cases occur in people whose resistance to infection has been drastically lowered by diseases such as *AIDS* and *Hodgkin's disease* or by *immunosuppressant drugs*.

SYMPTOMS

Meningitis is the most usual, and serious, form that the illness takes. Symptoms include headache, stiffness in the neck, fever, drowsiness, blurred vision, and a staggering gait. If the infection is not treated, it may end in coma and death. When the disease attacks the lungs it causes chest pain and a cough, sometimes with sputum (phlegm); there may also be a skin rash of ulcerating spots.

DIAGNOSIS AND TREATMENT

Cryptococcal meningitis is diagnosed from a sample of fluid drawn from the spine. An X ray may be needed to detect any damage to the lungs, and laboratory examination of the sputum, lung *biopsy*, and *bronchoscopy* may be needed.

Most cases in which only the lungs have been infected need no treatment, clearing up of their own accord. When

the meninges have been affected, a combination of the antifungal drugs amphotericin B and flucytosine is usually given for about six weeks. Although these drugs are usually effective, relapses can occur.

Cryptorchidism

A developmental disorder of male infants in which the testes fail to descend normally into the scrotum. (See *Testis, undescended*.)

CT scanning

A diagnostic technique in which the combined use of a computer and *X rays* passed through the body at different angles produces clear cross-sectional images ("slices") of the tissue being examined. CT (computerized tomography) scanning—also known as CAT (computerized axial tomography) scanning or whole body scanning—provides clearer and more detailed information than X rays used by themselves. In addition, CT scanning tends to minimize the amount of radiation exposure.

WHY IT IS DONE

The first CT scanner, which came into operation in 1972, was developed to study the brain. Since then, CT brain scanning has marked a major advance in the diagnosis and treatment of tumors, abscesses, and hemorrhages in the brain, as well as strokes and head injuries. These once required tests, such as *angiography* and ventriculography (an outmoded technique for imaging the ventricles of the brain), that not only were difficult to perform, lengthy, and not always clear-cut in their findings, but also entailed some risk for the patient. CT scanning, on the other hand, is simple, quick, accurate, and carries a modest exposure to radiation.

As well as being essential for the study of the brain, CT scanning is invaluable in investigating disease of any part of the trunk. It is particularly useful for locating and imaging tumors, and for guiding the operator who is performing a needle *biopsy*.

RESULTS

Using the information produced by the scanner, a computer constructs cross-sectional images of the tissue under examination. These images, displayed on a TV screen, reveal soft tissues (including tumors) more clearly than normal X-ray pictures. The images are particularly valuable in brain scans due to their sharp definition of ventricles (fluid-filled spaces). The images can be manipulated

PERFORMING A CT SCAN

CT scanning combines the use of a computer and X rays passed through the body at different angles to produce clear cross-sectional images of areas of body tissue. Before the scan is carried out, a contrast medium may be injected to make blood vessels, organs, or abnormalities show up more clearly; a drink of contrast medium may be given to highlight loops of intestine.

1 The patient lies on a table that can be moved up or down to allow easy transfer and accurate positioning within the machine.

A central sliding cradle in the table moves the patient, at a controllable rate, into the machine

The machine can be tilted in either direction to allow precise areas to be X-rayed

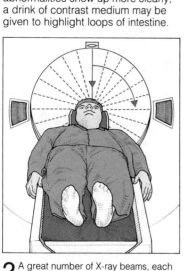

2 A great number of X-ray beams, each of low dosage and lasting only a fraction of a second, are passed through the body at different angles as the scanner rotates around the patient.

Right kidney
Spinal cord
Spine
Rib
Abnormal left kidney
Cysts
Gas in stomach
Liver
Cysts

3 The amount of X rays absorbed by different tissues is recorded by detectors in the scanner and transformed by a computer into an image, which is interpreted by a radiologist.

electronically to provide the best view of the area of interest, and adjacent two-dimensional "slices" can be reconstructed to produce three-dimensional representations as well as images in different planes.

Culture

A growth of bacteria or other microorganisms, cells, or tissues cultivated artificially in the laboratory.

WHY IT IS DONE

Microorganisms are collected and cultivated to enable the cause of an infection to be accurately diagnosed. Cultivation produces larger numbers of microorganisms in a form suitable for further tests.

Healthy cells are cultured to diagnose various disorders prenatally and for studying chromosomes. Human tissues, such as skin, may be cultured to produce larger amounts for use in grafting. Other tissues, notably human *amnion* (embryonic tissue) and monkey kidney, are cultivated to provide a medium in which viruses can be

grown and identified in the laboratory; viruses will multiply only within living cells.

HOW IT IS DONE

MICROORGANISMS The type of specimen collected from the patient depends on the suspected site of infection. For example, a throat swab is made if a streptococcal throat infection is suspected, a urine specimen is collected if urinary tract infection is thought likely, a sputum sample if respiratory infection is suspected, or a feces sample if gastrointestinal infection is suspected. Likewise, a blood sample is cultured (blood culture) if the bloodstream is thought to be infected. Bacteria, fungi, and, occasionally, viruses may be cultured directly from the blood.

The specimen is collected in a sterile container and is incubated at body temperature in a carefully chosen culture medium. Liquid or solid culture media, usually agar gel or meat-based broth, are used for culturing bacteria. These media contain various nutrients

chosen for the particular needs of the organism suspected of causing the infection; the media may also contain ingredients to discourage the growth of other organisms.

Any bacteria present will multiply to form visible colonies. The type of bacteria can be identified by noting the appearance of the colony, by chemical tests, and by examining the bacteria under the microscope. Bacterial cultures can be tested with various antibiotics to determine which antibiotic may be the most effective against a particular infection.

CELLS AND TISSUES For the diagnosis of prenatal abnormalities, cells are collected by *amniocentesis* or *chorionic villus sampling*. Cells for studying chromosomes (see *Chromosome analysis*) are cultured from white blood cells or cells gathered from the inside of the cheek. Cells and tissues to be used for analysis, for growing viruses, or to be used for grafting are cultured in a small amount of fluid containing nutrients essential for their growth.

Cupping

An ancient form of treatment used to draw blood to the surface of the skin. Cupping is still used in folk healing in some countries, particularly in China and Turkey.

A small vessel—commonly a glass jar, animal horn, ceramic vessel, or a closed-ended bamboo tube—is heated and applied to the skin. When it cools and the air inside contracts, a partial vacuum is created, causing the skin to be sucked into the vessel, producing a rounded area of inflammation. Believers in this form of treatment think the inflammatory response is therapeutic.

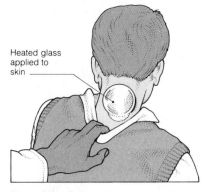

Heated glass applied to skin

Uses of cupping
Conditions treated by this technique include bronchitis, asthma, and musculo-skeletal pains.

Curare

An extract from the bark and juices of various trees that has been used for centuries by South American Indians as an arrow poison. The principal active ingredient is tubocurarine, a drug that inhibits muscle contractions by interfering with the action of *acetylcholine,* a *neurotransmitter* (chemical released from nerve endings).

Cure

To treat successfully; that is, to restore to normal health after an illness. The term usually means the complete disappearance of a disease rather than just a halt in its progress. Any medication or therapy used in the treatment of an illness may also be called a cure.

In general, infections may be cured, as may some tumors. By contrast, chronic conditions, such as *osteoarthritis,* or endocrine deficiency diseases, such as *hypothyroidism* (underactivity of the thyroid gland), are never cured but undergo remission or are controlled with long-term hormone treatment.

Curet

A spoon-shaped surgical instrument for scraping away material or tissue from an organ, cavity, or surface.

Curettage

The use of a sharp-edged, spoon-shaped surgical instrument called a curet to scrape abnormal tissue, or tissue for analysis, from the lining of a body cavity or from the skin. Curettage is commonly used to remove infected material from an abscess, to scrape tissue from the lining of the uterus as part of a *D and C* (dilatation and curettage) operation, and to remove small growths from the skin. (See also *Curettage, dental.*)

Curettage, dental

The scraping of the wall of a cavity with a dental *curet* (a narrow, spoon-shaped, scaling instrument). It is one method used in the treatment of simple periodontal pockets occurring in *periodontitis.* The curet is used to remove the lining and diseased tissue from the lateral walls of the root. This enables the healthy, underlying tissue to reattach itself to the root surface, which is cleared of calculus deposits before curettage.

Curling's ulcer

A type of *stress ulcer* (a disruption in the lining of the stomach or duodenum following any severe injury, infection, or shock) that occurs specifically in people who have suffered extensive skin burns. Ulcers develop about 24 hours after the burns and are usually small and multiple. Diagnosis and treatment are as for other types of stress ulcer.

Cushing's syndrome

A hormonal disorder caused by an abnormally high circulating level of corticosteroid hormones, produced naturally by the *adrenal glands.*
CAUSES AND INCIDENCE
Cushing's syndrome may be produced directly by an adrenal gland tumor, causing excessive secretion of corticosteroids, by prolonged administration of *corticosteroid drugs,* or by enlargement of both adrenal glands due to a pituitary tumor. Corticosteroid drugs are widely used for inflammatory conditions such as rheumatoid arthritis, inflammatory bowel disease, and asthma.

The pituitary gland controls the activity of the adrenal gland by producing a hormone known as *ACTH* (adrenocorticotropic hormone),

which stimulates the cortex (outer portion) of the adrenal gland to grow. Overactivity or a tumor of the pituitary can thus lead to overproduction of ACTH, overgrowth of the adrenal glands, and excess secretion of corticosteroids. Some lung cancers and various other tumors may also secrete ACTH, with similar results.

Cushing's syndrome can occur at any age, but is most common in middle age. Most cases today are caused by excessive, prolonged use of corticosteroid drugs, but these cases are usually mild. The patient is often described as having cushingoid features rather than full-blown Cushing's syndrome. Cases caused by pituitary overactivity (sometimes called Cushing's disease) are much more common in women, and those caused by lung tumors are more common in men.
SYMPTOMS
People with Cushing's syndrome have a characteristic appearance. The face appears round ("moon-faced") and red, the trunk tends to become obese with a humped upper back, and the limbs become wasted. Acne develops and purple stretch marks may appear on the abdomen, thighs, and breasts. The skin is thin and bruises easily. The bones become weakened and are at increased risk of fracturing (see *Osteoporosis*). Women may become increasingly hairy. Affected people are more susceptible to infection and may suffer from stomach or duodenal ulcers.

Mental changes often occur, including *depression, paranoia,* or sometimes *euphoria. Insomnia* may be a problem. Patients may develop *hypertension* (increased blood pressure) and *edema* (fluid collection in the tissues). About one fifth of patients develop *diabetes mellitus.* In children, Cushing's syndrome may suppress growth.
DIAGNOSIS
Anyone suspected of having Cushing's syndrome should be examined by an endocrinologist. Obese or depressed patients may have many of the clinical features of Cushing's syndrome, making diagnosis difficult. Diagnosis requires measurement of ACTH levels in the blood and corticosteroid levels in the blood and urine. *CT scanning* of the adrenal and pituitary glands is performed to look for abnormalities.
TREATMENT
If the cause is overtreatment with corticosteroid drugs, the condition is usually reversible with gradual withdrawal of drug treatment.

If the cause is shown to be a tumor or overgrowth of an adrenal gland, the gland is removed surgically. If the tumor lies in the pituitary gland, it is removed by surgery or shrunk by irradiation and medication. Patients subsequently need hormone replacement therapy; without it, they would be left completely deficient in adrenal or pituitary hormones.

Cusp, dental

One of the small, protruding areas occurring on the grinding surface of a tooth (see *Teeth*).

Cuspid

A name for a canine tooth (see *Teeth*).

Cutaneous

Pertaining to the skin. For example, a subcutaneous injection is an injection given beneath the skin.

Cutdown

The creation of a small incision in the skin over a vein to gain access to the vein. A cutdown may be necessary when it is essential to take blood or give intravenous fluid, and a vein cannot be identified through the skin.

CVS

See *Chorionic villus sampling*.

Cyanide

Any of a group of mostly highly toxic substances that contains the cyanogen chemical group. Chemicals in this group consist of a carbon atom linked to a nitrogen atom.

The poisonous effects of cyanides are due to their ability to block a specific *enzyme* (cytochrome oxidase) that plays an essential role in the uptake of oxygen by cells. This blocking action deprives cells of oxygen, which, in turn, produces a rapid progression of symptoms from breathlessness, through paralysis and unconsciousness, to death.

Because of their toxicity, cyanides have few applications. Hydrogen cyanide is used to kill rodents and fumigate buildings. It has also been used in gas chambers. Certain other cyanides are powerful eye irritants and are used in some tear gases.

Cyanocobalamin

A name for *vitamin B₁₂*.

Cyanosis

Bluish coloration of the skin and mucous membranes (such as the lining of the mouth) due to too much deoxygenated *hemoglobin* in the blood. Cyanosis is generally most obvious in the beds of the fingernails and toenails and on the lips and tongue.

Cyanosis occurs most frequently because of slow blood flow through the skin as a result of low temperatures (the familiar sign of turning blue with cold). In such cases, where no other symptoms are present, it does not indicate a serious underlying disease process.

In other cases, however, cyanosis may be a serious sign and requires medical investigation. Cyanosis may indicate poor peripheral blood circulation in which the fingers and toes turn blue even in relatively warm conditions. It may also be a sign of a heart or lung disorder, such as *heart failure*, lung damage, or pulmonary *edema* (fluid in the lungs). More rarely, cyanosis may be present at birth, when it may be a sign of a congenital heart disease in which some of the blood is not pumped to the lungs (where oxygen, and thereby a bright red color, is obtained). Instead, the blood goes directly to the rest of the body (see *Heart disease, congenital*).

Cyclacillin

A penicillin-type antibiotic commonly used to treat acute otitis media (acute infection of the middle ear), sinusitis, and cystitis. (See *Penicillins*.)

Cyclobenzaprine

A *muscle-relaxant drug* mainly used in the short-term treatment of painful muscle spasm caused by injury.

Cyclophosphamide

An *anticancer drug* used mainly in the treatment of Hodgkin's disease and leukemia, often in combination with other anticancer drugs. It is also useful as an *immunosuppressant drug*, helping prevent rejection of a transplanted organ by modifying the body's natural defense against abnormal or foreign cells. Cyclophosphamide has also been used to treat connective tissue diseases such as severe systemic *lupus erythematosus*.

Cycloplegia

Paralysis of the ciliary muscle, which controls the shape of the lens in the eye. With the ciliary muscle out of action, the process of *accommodation* is not able to work properly. Accommodation occurs when light rays from near objects are focused onto the retina (visual receptive layer) at the back of the eye.

Cyclosporine

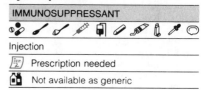

IMMUNOSUPPRESSANT
Injection
Prescription needed
Not available as generic

An *immunosuppressant drug* that suppresses the body's natural defense against abnormal cells; it was introduced in 1984.

WHY IT IS USED

Cyclosporine's immunosuppressant action is of particular use following *transplant surgery*, when the body may start to reject the transplanted organ unless the immune system is damped down. Cyclosporine is now widely used following many different types of transplant surgery, including heart, kidney, bone marrow, liver, and pancreas transplants. Its use has considerably reduced the risk of tissue rejection and also the need for large doses of *corticosteroid drugs*. Cyclosporine may need to be taken in oral form for an indefinite period following surgery.

POSSIBLE ADVERSE EFFECTS

Because cyclosporine reduces the effectiveness of the immune system, people being treated with this drug have an increased susceptibility to infection. Any flulike illness or localized infection requires immediate treatment by a physician.

Cyclosporine has also been found to cause kidney damage in some people. Regular monitoring of kidney function is therefore necessary for people being given this drug. If signs of kidney damage, such as protein in the urine, are detected, the dose of cyclosporine may need to be reduced or another drug substituted. Another adverse effect related to kidney damage is *hypertension*. A fairly common adverse effect of cyclosporine is swelling of the gums.

Cyclothymia

A type of personality characteristic that is associated with marked changes of mood. From being cheerful, energetic, and sociable people, these individuals may, for no apparent reason, quickly become withdrawn, gloomy, and listless. These swings of mood may be regular, may last for days or months, and may be separated by relatively "normal" periods of behavior. Sometimes an obvious *manic-depressive illness* results, or there may be a family history of such illness. There may be an associated pyknic (rounded and stout) body build. People with cyclothymia who are mainly "up" or "manic" often have very successful careers; others may resort episodically to heavy drinking or difficult behavior.

Cyst

An abnormal lump or swelling, filled with fluid or semisolid material, in any body organ or tissue.

The causes of cysts are numerous. They may result from blockage of the duct leading from a fluid-forming gland—*sebaceous cysts* in the skin, for example. Alternatively, there may be abnormal activity or growth of a fluid-forming tissue, with no means of the fluid escaping—in an *ovarian cyst*, for example. Finally, cysts may form

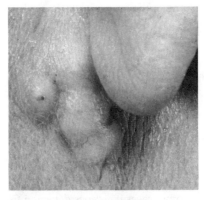

Sebaceous cysts under the ear
These cysts result from blockage of ducts leading from sebaceous glands in the skin. The cysts are benign; if they become unsightly, they can be surgically removed.

around parasites in organs such as the liver, brain, or intestinal wall in diseases such as *hydatid disease*, *cysticercosis*, and *amebiasis*.

Other types of cyst include *Baker's cyst* (behind the knee) and *dermoid cyst* (a type of skin cyst that may contain particles of hair follicles, sweat glands, nerves, and teeth).

Cysts are usually harmless in themselves, but they may disrupt the function of the organ or tissues in which they grow. Those in the skin are unsightly, but, if accessible, can be surgically removed.

Cyst-/cysto-

Prefixes that denote the bladder, as in *cystitis* (inflammation of the bladder) and *cystoscopy* (endoscopic examination of the bladder).

Cystectomy

Surgical removal of the bladder, after which urine is passed from the body via a specially constructed channel emerging in a *stoma* (mouthlike opening) on the lower abdomen.

WHY IT IS DONE

Cystectomy is performed either as a curative or palliative procedure for a widespread cancer of the bladder (see *Bladder tumors*). Once a cancer begins to invade the bladder muscle, treatment may be by surgery, radiation therapy, chemotherapy, or a combination of the treatments.

RISKS AND OUTLOOK

A cystectomy is likely to cause a major disturbance in life-style. In men, the operation in most cases causes impotence (due to damage to nerve tracts involved in penile erection) and in women it leads to infertility (although the majority of women who undergo the operation are past childbearing age). In addition, the patient needs to adapt to wearing an external pouch to collect urine and to learn about care of the stoma. Before undergoing surgery, cystectomy patients are thus advised to discuss their concerns about the operation and its consequences with the physician, surgeon, and enterostomy (stoma care) therapist. Many patients, however, are able to return to a fully active and healthy life. In recent years, the use of continent *urinary diversions*, with no external pouch, has been investigated. The newer pouches permit the patient to control the drainage of urine by emptying the pouch with a catheter. Results are encouraging, although they are still considered experimental.

HOW CYSTECTOMY IS DONE

The operation is a major procedure performed using general anesthesia. An incision is made in the abdomen, and the ureters are cut and tied. The bladder and other organs are removed (see below) and the stoma formed. After the operation, the patient is given intravenous infusions of fluids, salt, and glucose until the intestines function normally again.

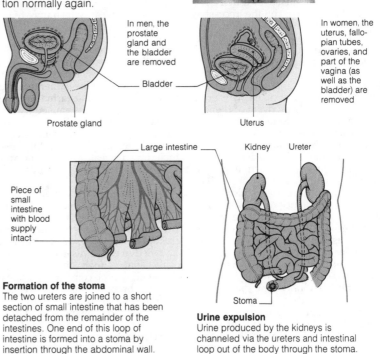

Ureters usually cut here

Line of incision

In men, the prostate gland and the bladder are removed

Bladder

In women, the uterus, fallopian tubes, ovaries, and part of the vagina (as well as the bladder) are removed

Prostate gland

Uterus

Large intestine

Kidney   Ureter

Piece of small intestine with blood supply intact

Formation of the stoma
The two ureters are joined to a short section of small intestine that has been detached from the remainder of the intestines. One end of this loop of intestine is formed into a stoma by insertion through the abdominal wall.

Stoma

Urine expulsion
Urine produced by the kidneys is channeled via the ureters and intestinal loop out of the body through the stoma.

C

Cysticercosis

An infection characterized by the presence, in tissues such as the muscle and brain, of cysts formed by the larval (immature) stage of the pork *tapeworm*.

Cysticercosis is an extremely rare disease in the US and most other developed countries, although cases occur in Latin America, Africa, parts of Asia, and Eastern Europe.

Cystic fibrosis

An inherited disease, present from birth, characterized by a tendency to chronic lung infections and an inability to absorb fats and other nutrients from food.

When cystic fibrosis (CF) was first identified in the 1930s, before effective antibiotics were available, almost all sufferers died in early childhood. More recently, however, and particularly since 1975, the outlook has changed dramatically. With more advanced methods of diagnosis and treatment, including the use of a wide range of antibiotics, over two thirds of CF sufferers now survive into adult life, although few of them are in perfect health. CF remains, however, a serious and potentially fatal disorder.

CAUSES AND INCIDENCE

CF (or mucoviscidosis, as it is sometimes called) is caused by a defective *gene*. The defect is of the recessive type, which means that a person must inherit it in a double dose (one gene from each parent) before any outward abnormality is apparent (see *Genetic disorders*). People who inherit the defective gene in a single dose (from one parent only) are called "carriers"; they are normally unaware of the fact and have no symptoms.

Among whites in the US and elsewhere, about one person in 22 is such a "carrier." The chance that any (random) procreating white couple are both carriers is roughly one in 500. In this event, each of their children has a one in four chance of inheriting the defective gene from both parents and of being born with CF. The incidence of the disease among whites is thus about one per 2,000 live births. In non-whites, however (for example, among black Africans), the disease is very rare (perhaps only one person in 90,000 is affected).

The mechanism by which the gene defect leads to the features of CF is unknown. It is known, however, that certain glands do not function properly. Most seriously, the glands in the

lining of the bronchial tubes produce excessive amounts of thick mucus, which predisposes the person to chronic lung infections. A further serious malfunction is failure of the pancreas to produce enzymes involved in the breakdown of fats and their absorption from the intestines; this deficiency causes malnutrition. Sweat glands are also affected.

SYMPTOMS AND SIGNS

The pattern of development of the disease, and the severity of its features, varies considerably among individuals. Hence, although the disease is sometimes obvious soon after birth, in other cases it escapes detection for months or years.

In a typical, or classical, case, the child passes feces that are pale, greasy-looking, and foul-smelling, and in some cases he or she may fail to thrive. The child also suffers from persistent chest infections, causing constant coughing and breathlessness. Pneumonia, bronchiectasis, and bronchitis commonly develop, and the lungs become damaged.

Sterility (not impotence) occurs in the majority of male sufferers but not in affected females; some otherwise healthy adult males have attended infertility clinics and been diagnosed subsequently as having CF. Other features of the disease include stunted growth in many cases, and also abnormally salty sweat, which may require salt replacement in hot climates, but is otherwise harmless.

DIAGNOSIS AND TREATMENT

Suspicious symptoms should be reported to a physician as soon as they are noticed, since the earlier treatment with antibiotics is started, the less lung damage will be caused by chest infections. Once the diagnosis is considered, it is easily confirmed or refuted by simple laboratory tests, including a sweat test. In some areas, screening of all newborn infants for CF is available.

Confirmation of the diagnosis and supervision of treatment is best carried out from a special center staffed by physicians, nurses, and physiotherapists who have a particular knowledge of the disease.

To enable food to be properly digested, replacement pancreatic enzyme preparations must be taken with meals. The diet needs to be rich in calories and proteins, and a vitamin supplement is often prescribed as an extra precaution. These measures bring about weight increase and more normal feces.

AFFECTED FAMILIES

The parents of a child with CF must assume that any subsequent child has a one in four chance of being born with the disease. Unaffected siblings of affected people have a two in three chance of being "carriers," creating problems if they plan to have children with someone who also has CF in the family. Advice can be obtained through *genetic counseling*.

Recent research has succeeded in establishing the location (on *chromosome* number 7 in a person's cells) of the gene involved in CF and has identified biochemical "markers" on the gene that are present when it is defective. It is now possible, therefore, to identify carriers of the defective gene, and also to detect CF before birth.

This service can sometimes be offered to parents who already have a CF child and are contemplating a second pregnancy. First, the presence of the markers for the defective gene is established in both parents. Between eight and 10 weeks into pregnancy, fetal cells obtained by *chorionic villus sampling* are analyzed to see if the markers of CF are present; alternatively, chemical tests on cells obtained by *amniocentesis* (at 17 or 18 weeks of pregnancy) can confirm whether or not the child will have CF. In either case, the parents may choose to terminate the pregnancy if the fetus is affected.

OUTLOOK

The highly specialized treatment given to CF sufferers today provides them with a much better quality of life than was formerly possible. Even so, most suffer permanent lung damage and have a considerably shortened life expectancy. Some people have been treated by heart and lung transplantation, while others have had a lung transplantation only; the results seem very encouraging.

Cystitis

Inflammation of the inner lining of the bladder, caused by an infection that is usually due to bacteria. Anything that obstructs the voiding of urine from the bladder, or leads to incomplete voiding of urine, tends to encourage infection; stagnant urine in the bladder or urethra (the tube leading from the bladder to the exterior) provides a good breeding ground for bacteria.

INCIDENCE AND CAUSES

In women, cystitis is common because the urethra is short, making it easier for infectious agents to pass from the mucous membrane around the urethral opening up into the bladder. The bacteria may come from the vagina or from the intestine via the anus. Most women have cystitis at some time. A *calculus* (stone) in the bladder, a *bladder tumor*, or a *urethral stricture* increases the risk of infection due to obstruction of urine flow.

In men, cystitis is rare (because of the longer urethra) and usually occurs only in the presence of an obstruction, which in most cases is due to an enlarged prostate gland compressing the urethra where it leaves the bladder. Rarely, the obstruction is due to a urethral stricture.

In children, cystitis is often due to a structural abnormality of the ureters (tubes that carry urine from the kidneys to the bladder) at the point at which they enter the bladder, allowing reflux (backward flow) of urine into the ureters when the bladder muscle contracts. This leads to incomplete voiding of urine and to subsequent infection.

Another possible source of infection is the introduction of a catheter (flexible tube) into the bladder—a procedure used to drain urine in a variety of circumstances (see *Catheterization, urinary*), including the treatment of incontinence and urinary retention. Diabetics are particularly susceptible to urinary tract infections.

SYMPTOMS
The main symptom of cystitis in both sexes is a frequent urge to pass urine, with only a small amount of urine passed each time. Passing urine is accompanied by pain, which is usually of a burning or stinging nature. Occasionally, the urine is foul smelling or contains blood. There may be a fever and occasionally chills and continuous discomfort in the lower abdomen. In children, there may be no urinary symptoms, only fever, or the child may cry when passing urine.

DIAGNOSIS
The diagnosis of a urinary infection can be confirmed by examining a sample of urine under the microscope, looking for pus cells, and in certain instances trying to grow the bacteria in a *culture*. When no infection is found in someone with symptoms of cystitis, the diagnosis may be *urethritis* (inflammation of the urethra), a bacterial prostatitis, or, in women only, the *urethral syndrome*, in which the cause is thought to be trauma to the urethra from sexual activity.

TREATMENT
Women with the symptoms of cystitis should drink large quantities of fluid,

---

AVOIDING CYSTITIS
A few simple measures can help women prone to cystitis reduce the chances of recurrence. In particular, women should drink a lot of fluid, especially cranberry juice, to encourage acidity of the urine.

Fluid consumption
Drink plenty of fluids—so that the urine is consistently pale—and ensure that the bladder is completely emptied at each visit to the toilet.

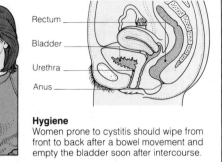

Rectum
Bladder
Urethra
Anus

Hygiene
Women prone to cystitis should wipe from front to back after a bowel movement and empty the bladder soon after intercourse.

---

including cranberry juice, which encourages acidity of the urine.

If an infection is present, antibiotics are prescribed to destroy the bacteria and prevent the infection from spreading to cause *pyelonephritis* (infection of the kidneys).

In many cases, the physician will have the patient start a course of antibiotics, especially when pus cells are in the urine, before waiting for the result of the urine culture. The physician will then check the results of the culture to confirm the presence of an infection. Cultures are more frequently performed when there have been recurrent urinary tract infections. Sensitivity of the bacteria to various antibiotics is ascertained from a culture.

In men, antibiotics are prescribed to treat the symptoms of cystitis, but more tests are arranged to look for any obstruction to urinary flow. In children, antibiotics are prescribed and usually more tests are performed to check for a disorder such as reflux of urine into the ureters.

OUTLOOK
Prompt treatment of cystitis with antibiotics usually settles the infection within 24 hours, with no complications. Occasionally, damage to the kidneys due to pyelonephritis occurs, usually because the infection has spread before significant symptoms have appeared.

More tests are performed when there are recurrent infections in women, any infection in men, and usually after one infection in children.

Cystocele
A swelling at the front and top of the vagina formed where the bladder

pushes against weakened tissues in the vaginal wall. Weakened tissues may be associated with descent of the uterus from its normal position down into the vagina (see *Uterus, prolapse of*). A cystocele may not cause symptoms, but occasionally the urethra (through which urine drains from the bladder) is pulled out of position. This may cause stress *incontinence* (leakage of urine on coughing, lifting, or sneezing) or the bladder may not empty completely when urine is passed. The urine remaining in the bladder may then become infected, causing frequent and very painful urination (see *Cystitis*).

Exercises to strengthen the pelvic floor muscles (which support the bladder, uterus, and other pelvic organs) may help relieve the symptoms (see *Pelvic floor exercises*). In severe cases, surgery is needed to lift and to tighten the tissues at the front of the vagina.

Cystometry
A procedure carried out to provide information about normal bladder function and about abnormalities either of the nerves supplying the bladder or of the bladder muscle itself. The procedure measures pressure changes in the bladder as it fills, and also the total bladder capacity and the presence of any residual urine after the bladder has fully contracted.

WHY IT IS DONE
Cystometry is used to investigate urinary *incontinence* or poor bladder emptying caused by damage to the bladder muscles (following childbirth or pelvic surgery, for example) or to disruption of the nerve control of these muscles (as in *Parkinson's disease* or *diabetes mellitus*).

C

HOW IT IS DONE

The examination, which takes about 20 minutes, is performed by a urologist or a trained urological technician. It is usually done on an outpatient basis and no anesthetic is required. A catheter (flexible tube) and pressure measuring probe are inserted into the bladder and sometimes the rectum. The bladder is gradually filled with water or carbon dioxide and a series of pressure readings is taken. They indicate the point at which reflex bladder emptying occurs.

Cystoscopy

The examination of the urethra and bladder cavity using a cystoscope (viewing tube inserted up the urethra). Modern cystoscopes have a metal sheath with interchangeable fiberoptic telescopes, allowing a viewing angle ranging from zero to 120 degrees. The zero-angle lens is best for examination of the urethra and prostate; the 70- and 120-degree angles are used to inspect the bladder wall.

WHY IT IS DONE

Cystoscopes have both diagnostic and therapeutic uses. Diagnostic uses include inspection of the bladder cavity for calculi (stones), *bladder tumors*, and sites of bleeding and infection, as well as the obtaining of urine samples from each kidney individually to look for infection or tumor cells. In addition, by means of radiopaque dye injected into the ureters via the cystoscope, X rays can be

taken to investigate the site of any obstruction to the flow of urine (see retrograde *pyelography*).

Many diseases of the urethra and bladder lend themselves to treatment via the cystoscope. Bladder tumors can be both biopsied and treated with diathermy or laser, calculi can be crushed or removed with basket forceps from the bladder or ureter, and stents (narrow tubes) can be inserted into the ureter to relieve any obstruction.

Cystostomy

The surgical creation of a hole in the bladder. A cystostomy is usually performed to drain urine when the introduction of a *catheter* (flexible tube) into the bladder via the urethra is inadvisable or impossible.

Cystourethrogram, voiding

An X-ray procedure for studying a person's bladder while he or she is urinating. The technique is most commonly used on young children who have had urinary infections to detect reflux of urine—that is, urine being forced back up the ureters (the tubes leading from the kidneys) as the bladder contracts. If severe, reflux leads to repeated infection, which can damage the kidneys.

-cyte

The suffix that denotes a cell. A *leukocyte* is a white blood cell; an *erythrocyte* is a red blood cell.

Cyto-

The prefix used to describe a relationship to a cell, as in cytomegalic, which means "giant cell."

Cytologist

A technician skilled in differentiating the appearance of normal from malignant cells.

Cytology

The study of individual cells, as distinct from *histology* (the study of groups of cells forming a tissue). The main application of cytology in medicine is to detect abnormal cells; it is thus used extensively to diagnose cancer. Cytology is becoming more important in *prenatal screening* for certain fetal abnormalities.

APPLICATIONS

The best known use of cytology is screening for cancer of the cervix, a procedure known as the *cervical smear test* (Pap test). A scraping of cells from the cervix and vagina is examined under a microscope; if they show precancerous changes, the woman's condition can be observed and she can be treated before cancer develops.

Cytology is also used to confirm (or exclude) the diagnosis of other cancers. Coughing up blood may be due to lung cancer, but a cytological examination of cells in a sample of sputum (phlegm) will help determine whether or not cancer actually is the cause. Similarly, cytology is valuable in detecting recurrent tumors in people who have already been treated for cancer. It is used particularly in cases of bladder cancer, in which tumors tend to recur after the original cancer has been successfully treated. Regular urinary cytology can detect any recurrent tumors at an early stage. Cytology may be helpful in determining the cause of conditions such as *pleural effusion* (fluid in the pleural cavity around the lungs) and *ascites* (fluid in the abdomen). Examination of cells in a sample of fluid usually indicates whether the condition is caused by cancer or an infection.

Fine needle aspiration *biopsy* of internal organs is growing as a method of diagnosis that utilizes cytology. A needle is guided to the organ (usually with the help of *ultrasound* or *CT scanning*) and a sample taken for examination. The procedure may eliminate the need for surgical biopsy or a major operation.

The other principal application of cytology is in various screening techniques for the early detection of fetal

---

PROCEDURE FOR CYSTOSCOPY

Cystoscopy allows inspection and treatment of the bladder using local anesthesia. There is no risk of damage to the genital organs or urinary tract, although the patient may feel some discomfort when passing urine for a few days afterward.

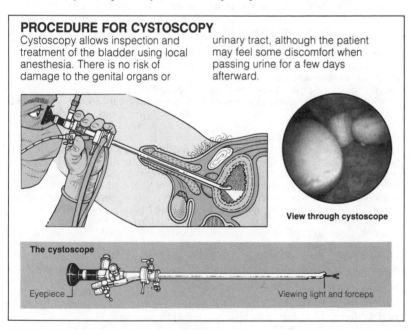

View through cystoscope

The cystoscope

Eyepiece   Viewing light and forceps

abnormalities such as Down's syndrome. The most widely used of these techniques is *amniocentesis*, in which a sample of the fluid that surrounds the fetus is removed and the cells in the fluid examined for abnormalities. *Chorionic villus sampling* is used earlier in the pregnancy. Usually, the cells must be cultured before a determination is made.

MODERN DEVELOPMENTS Various techniques are being developed to improve the ability to detect abnormal cells. Cells aspirated from various organs or tissues, as well as cells from cervical smears, can be studied further by the technique of *flow cytometry* (which uses a laser beam to scan cells and produce an image of the cells' DNA contents, thus differentiating between cells that are benign and those that are malignant).

The use of monoclonal antibodies—highly specific proteins that react with only one particular type of protein on the surface of a cell (see *Antibody, monoclonal*)—makes it easier to detect small numbers of abnormal cells in the midst of many normal ones, thereby improving the sensitivity of cytological tests for cancer. A refinement of this technique involves labeling the monoclonal antibodies with fluorescent stains, which makes them stand out against a dark background.

Other modern techniques have made it possible to detect abnormalities in *chromosomes* and even in individual *genes*. Such procedures have a potentially wide application for prenatal screening for congenital abnormalities, but many of them are still in the developmental stages and are not yet generally available.

Cytomegalovirus

One of the family of *herpes* viruses. It has the unique effect of causing the cells it infects to take on a characteristic enlarged appearance.

Infection with the cytomegalovirus (CMV) is extremely common. Approximately 80 percent of adults have *antibodies* to it in their blood (an indication of previous infection). In most cases, however, it produces no symptoms.

More serious CMV infections can occur in people with impaired immunity, such as the elderly and those with *AIDS*. A pregnant woman can transmit the virus to her unborn child; this could cause malformations and brain damage in the child.

Cytopathologist

A specialist in the microscopic appearances of cells in health and disease; also called a cellular pathologist. (See also *Cytology*.)

Cytotoxic drugs

A group of drugs that kills or damages cells; a type of *anticancer drug*. Cytotoxics primarily affect abnormal cells but they can damage or kill healthy cells, especially those that are multiplying rapidly. For example, they may affect noncancerous cells in bone marrow, causing anemia and increasing susceptibility to infection.

CYTOLOGY METHODS

Cells for cytological examination are obtained in several ways, depending on the part of the body being investigated. Recent improvements in imaging techniques have made it possible to collect cells from previously inaccessible sites. If the cytologist can make a definite diagnosis from a cell sample removed from a tumor using a very fine needle, the patient may be spared an exploratory operation.

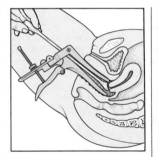

Cells from the cervix
These are scraped away with a spatula.

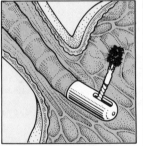

Cells from the respiratory tract, esophagus, or stomach
These are usually obtained by using an *endoscope* and small brush or suction tube.

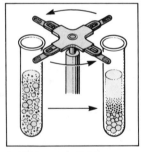

Cells from body fluids
These are obtained either by passing the fluid through a filter or by centrifugation.

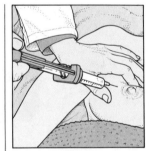

Aspiration biopsy
A very fine needle can be accurately passed into a suspected tumor and a biopsy sample of cells removed.

EXAMINATION UNDER THE MICROSCOPE

The cells are smeared on a microscope slide and stained with dyes. The cytologist then examines them, looking for abnormalities of size or shape in the cells or their nuclei. The smears are then graded—as normal, as displaying abnormalities, or as showing malignant cells.

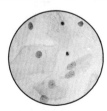

Normal cells in cervical smear

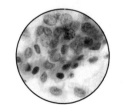

Smear showing abnormal cells

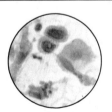

Smear showing malignant cells

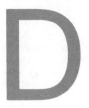

D

Dacryocystitis

Inflammation of the tear sac, which lies between the inside corner of the eyelids and the nose.

CAUSES

The inflammation usually results from blockage of the duct, which carries the tears from the tear sac to the nose. Inflammation may be followed by bacterial infection of fluid trapped in the tear sac. In infants, the tear duct may fail to develop an opening. In adults, the cause of the duct blockage is usually unknown. Rarely, it follows an injury; more often, it follows inflammation in the nasal region.

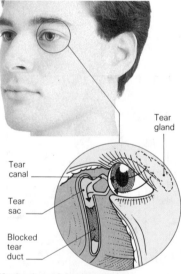

Mechanism of dacryocystitis
Inflammation of the tear sac occurs when the duct that carries tears from the tear sac becomes blocked.

SYMPTOMS

Usually only one eye is affected. There may be pain, redness, and swelling in the area between the inner corner of the eyelids and the nose. Occasionally, pus discharges from the inner canthus (corner). Prior to infection in the tear sac, the only symptom may be a watery eye and tearing due to obstruction of the duct.

TREATMENT

Irrigation can sometimes clear the obstruction. A *cannula* (fine tube) is introduced into one of the drainage openings into the tear duct and saline flushed through it. Antibiotic drops or ointment are prescribed to treat infection. In infants, massage of the tear sac can empty the sac and sometimes clear a blockage.

If irrigation and antibiotics fail to clear up the symptoms, a dacryocystorhinostomy (surgery to drain the tear sac into the nose) can be performed. In the infirm elderly, if recurrent infection is the main problem, the tear sac may be removed.

Danazol

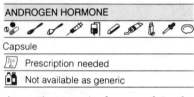

ANDROGEN HORMONE
Capsule
Prescription needed
Not available as generic

An antiestrogenic drug used in the treatment of *endometriosis* (a condition in which fragments of the lining of the uterus occur elsewhere in the pelvic cavity), fibrocystic breast disease (breast tenderness and lumpiness that worsen before menstruation), and *menorrhagia* (heavy periods).

HOW IT WORKS

Danazol suppresses the release of *gonadotropin hormones* (pituitary hormones that stimulate activity in the ovaries and testes). This reduces the production and release of estrogen from the ovaries. The change in hormone levels usually prevents ovulation, which results in irregularity or absence of menstruation.

Danazol is usually administered in courses lasting a few months. The disorder may recur once treatment has been discontinued.

POSSIBLE ADVERSE EFFECTS

Side effects may include nausea, dizziness, rash, back pain, weight gain, and flushing. Pregnancy should be avoided while taking (and shortly after taking) danazol because the drug can cause masculine characteristics in a female fetus.

D and C

A gynecological procedure in which the endometrium (lining of the uterus) laid down after each menstrual period is scraped away. Short for dilatation and curettage, D and C is commonly used in the diagnosis and treatment of *menorrhagia* (heavy menstrual bleed-

ing) and other disorders of the *uterus*. It is also used as a means of terminating a pregnancy (see *Abortion, elective*) and may sometimes be carried out following a *miscarriage*.

HOW IT IS DONE

D and C is usually carried out under general anesthesia. The cervix is dilated (stretched open) so that a *curet* (a spoon-shaped surgical instrument) can be inserted into the uterus to scrape away the endometrium. The scrapings may then be examined under the microscope to assess the condition of the uterus.

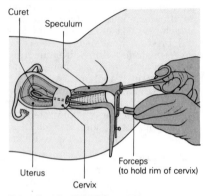

Procedure for D and C
The vagina is dilated with a speculum, the cervix is dilated, and a curet is inserted into the uterus to scrape away the endometrium.

RESULTS

Removal of the endometrium causes no side effects and it may be beneficial if the lining has thickened, causing heavy periods. The endometrium soon grows again normally as part of the menstrual cycle (see *Menstruation*).

Dander

Minute scales shed from an animal's skin, hair, or feathers. Both humans and pets produce such scales, which float in the air or settle on a surface, making up a large proportion of household dust. Human *dandruff* is a type of dander, except that the scales produced by the scalp are relatively large and easily visible.

Some people are allergic to animal dander and develop the symptoms of allergic *rhinitis* (hay fever) or *asthma* if they breathe in the scales.

Dandruff

A common, harmless, but irritating condition in which dead skin is shed from the scalp, often producing unsightly white flakes in the hair and on the collar and shoulders of clothes.

The usual cause of the condition is seborrheic *dermatitis*, an itchy, scaly rash on the scalp, which may also occur on the face, chest, and back.
TREATMENT
Shampoo frequently with an anti-dandruff shampoo. If this fails, a physician may prescribe a *corticosteroid* cream or lotion to apply to the scalp or an *antifungal* cream (even though dandruff is not a fungal infection), which sometimes helps. Whatever the treatment, dandruff usually requires constant control.

Dantrolene

MUSCLE RELAXANT

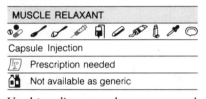

Capsule Injection
Prescription needed
Not available as generic

Used to relieve muscle spasm caused by *spinal injury*, *stroke*, or neurological disorders such as *cerebral palsy* or *multiple sclerosis*. It does not cure the underlying disorder, but often leads to a gradual improvement in mobility. Dantrolene is occasionally used to treat abnormal urine retention (see *Urine retention*).
POSSIBLE ADVERSE EFFECTS
Dantrolene acts predominantly on the muscles rather than the nervous system; consequently, it causes less sedation than many other muscle-relaxant drugs. Alcohol should be avoided during treatment, however, because it increases the sedative effect. Dantrolene may cause diarrhea, muscle weakness, and, rarely, kidney damage. In rare cases, dantrolene may also cause a skin rash on exposure to sunlight. Exposure to sun should therefore be avoided during treatment.

Dapsone
An antibiotic used in the treatment of *leprosy* and *dermatitis herpetiformis*, a rare skin condition.
POSSIBLE ADVERSE EFFECTS
Dapsone may cause nausea, vomiting, and, rarely, damage to the liver, red blood cells, and nerves. During long-term treatment, blood tests are carried out regularly to monitor liver function and the number of red cells in the blood.

Daydreaming
Conjuring up pleasant or exciting images or situations in one's mind during waking hours. Everyone daydreams to some extent, but it may be more common during unhappy or stressful periods in a person's life.

Children and teenagers may spend a considerable amount of time daydreaming. In general, this is not a cause for concern unless schoolwork and relationships suffer, at which time professional help may be needed.

DDT
The generally used abbreviation for the insecticide dichloro-diphenyl-trichloro-ethane. Developed in Switzerland in the early 1940s, DDT was much more effective than previous insecticides and it became an important weapon against insect-transmitted diseases, particularly in hot climates. A disadvantage of DDT is that some insects have adapted genetically to it so that their offspring become resistant to its toxic effects. (See also *Pesticides*.)

Deafness
Complete or partial inability to hear. Total deafness is rare and is usually congenital (present from birth). Partial deafness, ranging from mild to severe, is most commonly the result of an ear disease, injury, or degeneration of the hearing mechanism with age.

All deafness is either conductive or sensorineural. Conductive deafness is faulty transportation of sound from the outer to the inner ear, usually due to damage to the eardrum or the three connected bones in the middle ear—the malleus, incus, and stapes. In sensorineural deafness, sounds that reach the inner ear fail to be transmitted to the brain because of damage to the structures within the inner ear or to the acoustic nerve, which connects the inner ear to the brain.
CAUSES
CONDUCTIVE DEAFNESS In an adult, the most common cause of conductive deafness is *earwax* blocking the outer ear canal. Less commonly, *otosclerosis* (in which the stapes loses its normal mobility) may be responsible. In a child, *otitis media* (middle-ear infection) with effusion (a collection of fluid in the middle ear that is often sticky like glue) is by far the most common cause of this type of deafness.

Rarely, conductive deafness can be caused by *barotrauma* (damage to the eardrum or middle ear due to sudden pressure changes in an aircraft or under water) or by a perforated eardrum (see *Eardrum, perforated*) as the result of injury, a middle-ear infection, or surgery on the ear.

SENSORINEURAL DEAFNESS Defects of the inner ear are sometimes congenital, due to an inherited fault in a chromosome, to *birth injury*, or to damage to the developing fetus—for example, as the result of the mother having had *rubella* (German measles) during pregnancy. Damage to the inner ear may also occur soon after birth as the result of severe *jaundice*.

Sensorineural deafness that develops in later life can be caused by prolonged exposure to loud noise, by *Meniere's disease* (increased fluid pressure in the labyrinth), by certain drugs (such as streptomycin), or by some viral infections. All damage the cochlea and/or labyrinth. These structures also degenerate naturally with old age (*presbycusis*).

Damage to the acoustic nerve may be the result of an *acoustic neuroma* (a benign tumor on the nerve). As the acoustic neuroma enlarges, it causes increasing deafness.
INCIDENCE
Deafness at birth—which is sensorineural and incurable—is rare, occurring in only one in 1,000 babies. But deafness that develops in young children—usually conductive and curable—is common. As many as one fourth of the 5 year olds starting school have some degree of hearing loss as the result of previous middle-ear infections.

The hearing mechanism gradually degenerates with age, and about one fourth of the population over 65 need a hearing aid.
SYMPTOMS, SIGNS, AND DIAGNOSIS
A baby suffering from congenital deafness fails to respond to sounds, and, although crying is often normal, he or she does not babble or make the other baby noises that precede speech. This condition is usually first noticed by a parent, but the deafness is almost always diagnosed during one of the child's regular visits to a pediatrician.

Routine *hearing tests* are performed on children to detect any hearing loss, which is usually due to otitis media with effusion.

In an adult who has started to become deaf, sounds heard are not only quieter than before but are also distorted and less clear, high tones are less audible than low ones, the sounds "s," "f," and "z" are not heard, and speech may be difficult to understand if there is background noise. Deafness in one ear may be noticed only when that ear alone is used (for example, when the sufferer uses the affected ear when on the telephone).

D

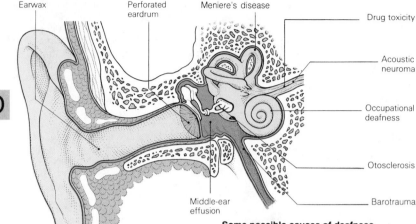

Earwax   Perforated eardrum   Meniere's disease

Drug toxicity

Acoustic neuroma

Occupational deafness

Otosclerosis

Barotrauma

Middle-ear effusion

Some possible causes of deafness
The affected part is shown in each case.
Some problems (e.g., earwax) cause conductive deafness; others (e.g., drug toxicity) cause sensorineural deafness.

Deafness may be accompanied by *tinnitus* (noises in the ear) and *vertigo* (dizziness and loss of balance). It sometimes causes confusion, *paranoia*, and auditory *hallucinations*, and can lead to withdrawal and depression.

Examination of the ear with an *otoscope* (a viewing instrument with a light attached) can show if the outer ear canal is obstructed by wax or if the eardrum is inflamed or there is fluid behind it. To determine whether deafness is conductive or sensorineural, hearing tests are used.

TREATMENT
Children born deaf need special instruction if they are to learn to speak. The process is a long and difficult one, but eventually many children can communicate effectively, often with sign language.

Conductive deafness in children due to otitis media with effusion is treated by an operation to drain the fluid from the middle ear through a hole in the eardrum (see *Myringotomy*). While awaiting surgery the child should sit at the front of the classroom to hear as much as possible.

When conductive deafness is caused by wax in the ear, the wax is removed by syringing the ear with warm water.

A perforated eardrum is usually allowed to heal of its own accord, but, if it has not done so after two or three months, a surgical repair, called *tympanoplasty*, is often carried out.

Conductive deafness due to otosclerosis is usually treated by *stapedectomy*, an operation in which the overgrown stapes is replaced with an artificial substitute.

Hearing aids are sometimes used to lessen deafness caused by otosclerosis, in which case the hearing aid takes the form of a bone-conducting device that transmits sound to the inner ear through a vibrating pad touching the bone behind the ear. The main use of hearing aids, however, is in treating sensorineural deafness, which cannot be cured because the structures of the inner ear are too delicate to allow surgery to be performed on them. These hearing aids increase the volume of sound reaching the inner ear by means of an amplifier and an earphone that fits into the outer ear.

A new development in the treatment of sensorineural deafness is the *cochlear implant*, in which electrodes that can receive sound signals are implanted in the inner ear. The single channel device has been replaced by one with multiple channels. Up to now, however, it has achieved only limited success.

Lipreading is an invaluable aid for all deaf people, whatever the type and severity of their deafness. People addressing a deaf person should remember to face him or her and not shout, which only distorts sounds.

Various household aids, such as an amplifier for the earpiece of a telephone, are available.

Death

Permanent cessation of all vital functions; the end of life. The classic indicators of death are the permanent cessation of the function of the heart and lungs; in most cases these remain the criteria by which a physician diagnoses and certifies death.

During the 1960s, however, medical technology advanced to allow the artificial (machine-assisted) maintenance of breathing and heart beat in cases where the lungs and heart would otherwise have stopped due to gross structural brain damage. This prompted a reexamination of the concepts of death and, in the late 1970s, state legislatures, at the urging of the medical profession, began recognizing an alternative criterion of death. This alternative is *brain death*, defined as the irreversible cessation of all func-

tions of the entire brain, including the brain stem.

An individual can thus now be certified legally dead if there is either irreversible cessation of circulatory and respiratory functions or if the criteria for brain death are satisfied.

DIAGNOSIS OF DEATH
The determination of death is considered a medical diagnosis. Physicians are expected to exercise their medical judgment within a defined legal framework.

The diagnosis of death under normal circumstances, when the individual is not on a *ventilator* (breathing machine), is based on absence of spontaneous breathing, absence of heart beat, and on the pupils being dilated and unresponsive to light.

The legal criteria for diagnosing brain death are based on the deter-

mination of the irreversible cessation of brain function. The guidelines state there must be clear evidence of irreversible damage to the brain; persistent deep coma; no attempts at breathing when the patient is taken off the ventilator; and absence of brain-stem function (such as the response of the pupils to light, grimacing in response to pain, and the involuntary blink when the surface of the eye is touched). The guidelines warn that this assessment might not be reliable if the patient is intoxicated, has an extremely low body temperature, or is in shock.

An *EEG* showing absence of electrical activity in the brain's cerebrum is not required, but sometimes provides useful confirmatory evidence of brain death diagnosed by the above criteria. (See also *Mortality*.)

SUDDEN DEATH

In infants (mainly up to 1 year of age), death that occurs without warning is called *sudden infant death syndrome* (SIDS) or crib death. The causes of SIDS are unknown, although there are several theories.

In adults, common causes of sudden death include injury, *myocardial infarction* (heart attack), *brain hemorrhage*, and *pneumonia*. Less common causes include *anaphylactic shock*, *asthma*, and *suicide*.

Cases of sudden death must be reported to the coroner or medical examiner, who decides if a postmortem examination (see *Autopsy*) should be performed.

Debility

Generalized weakness and lack of ambition and energy. Debility may be caused by a physical disorder (such as *anemia*) or a psychological disorder (such as *depression*).

Debridement

Surgical removal of foreign material and/or dead, damaged, or infected tissue from a wound or burn to expose healthy tissue. Such treatment promotes healthy healing of badly damaged skin, muscle, bone, and other tissue.

Decalcification, dental

The dissolving of minerals in a tooth. The first stage of decay, it is caused by the bacteria in *plaque* acting on refined carbohydrates (mainly sugar) in food to produce acid. After prolonged or numerous exposures, the acid causes changes on the surface of the tooth. The decalcified area can be seen as a chalky white patch when the plaque is brushed away. At this stage, the process is partly reversible if a mineralizing solution is applied.

If the decalcification penetrates the enamel, it spreads along the junction between the enamel and dentin, and then into the dentin. Lack of professional treatment at this point will permit bacteria to enter the pulp. Further destruction of dentin will then be caused by bacterial enzymes, and the pulp, once infected, may die. (See also *Caries, dental*.)

Decay, dental

See *Caries, dental*.

Decerebrate

The state of being without a functioning *cerebrum* (the cerebral hemispheres and associated structures), which is the main controlling part of the brain. This situation occurs when the *brain stem* (the upward extension of the spinal cord) is severed, which effectively isolates the cerebrum.

Deciduous teeth

See *Primary teeth*.

Decompression sickness

A hazard of scuba divers, also known as the "bends" and formerly known as caisson disease. Decompression sickness results from the formation of gas bubbles in the diver's tissues during ascent from depth.

CAUSES AND INCIDENCE

The amount of gas that can be held dissolved in a tissue (such as blood or body fat) increases with pressure (such as at great depth underwater) and decreases when the pressure is released. At depth, divers accumulate large quantities of inert gas in their tissues from the high-pressure gas mixture they breathe (see *Scuba-diving medicine*); if air is being breathed (as is usual for amateur divers), the main inert gas is nitrogen.

When the diver ascends, pressure falls and the gas can no longer be held within the tissues; if the pressure reduction is rapid, the gas may form bubbles—just as bubbles form in a bottle of beer when the cap is flipped off. The bubbles may block blood vessels, causing various symptoms.

Trained divers avoid problems by allowing the excess gas built up in their tissues to escape slowly via their blood into their lungs during controlled, very slow ascent.

SYMPTOMS

Symptoms may appear any time within 24 hours after a dive. Common symptoms include skin itching and mottling, and severe pains in and around the larger joints, particularly the shoulders and knees. Symptoms of nervous system impairment (such as leg weakness, visual disturbances, or problems with balance) are particularly serious, as is a painful, tight feeling across the chest, which may indicate the presence of bubbles in the vessels feeding the heart and in the circulation to the lungs.

TREATMENT

Any diver with the symptoms described should be transported immediately to a decompression chamber. Pressure within the chamber is raised by pumping in air; this causes the bubbles within the diver's tissues to redissolve, and symptoms to disappear. Subsequently, the

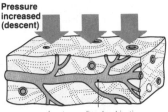

Pressure increased (descent)

Inert gas dissolved in tissue fluids and blood

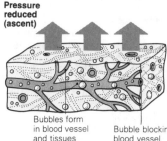

Pressure reduced (ascent)

Bubbles form in blood vessel and tissues

Bubble blocking blood vessel

How decompression occurs
On ascent, pressure is reduced rapidly and the gas may form bubbles that may, in turn, cause symptoms. Divers avoid this by ascending slowly.

pressure is slowly reduced, allowing the excess gas to escape safely via the blood and lungs.

OUTLOOK

If treated promptly by decompression, most divers with the bends make a full recovery. However, in serious, untreated cases, there may be long-term complications such as partial paralysis. Repeated episodes lead to degenerative disorders of the bones and joints.

Decompression, spinal canal

A surgical procedure to relieve pressure on the spinal cord or on a nerve root emerging from the cord.

WHY IT IS DONE

Pressure on the spinal cord may be due to a *disk prolapse*, to a tumor (in most cases benign) of the membranes surrounding the cord or of the cord itself, to a narrow spinal canal (spinal *stenosis*), which may be present from birth or caused by *osteoarthritis*, or to fracture of the vertebrae after an accident. Any of these conditions can cause weakness or paralysis of the limbs and also loss of bladder and bowel control.

HOW IT IS DONE

To treat major disk prolapses and tumors, a *laminectomy* (removal of the bony arches of one or more vertebrae) to expose the affected part of the cord or nerve roots must be performed.

D

Severely prolapsed disks are cut away and affected nerve roots are freed from surrounding tissues.

It is sometimes preferable to treat compressive conditions by using an anterior approach in which the spinal column is entered from the front.

When pressure is being caused by a tumor or abscess in a vertebra, the affected section of bone is removed. If a large portion of bone is removed, bone grafting is carried out at the end of the operation.

RECOVERY PERIOD
Confinement to bed in a flat position is necessary initially, with measures taken to prevent bedsores and physical therapy given to keep the leg muscles strong. Usually a patient can get up within a few days. Heavy lifting and carrying must be avoided for several weeks.

OUTLOOK
Recovery of movement, sensation, and bladder control, and achievement of pain relief after treatment, depend on the severity and duration of the pressure before the operation, the success of the surgery in relieving the pressure, and whether damage was sustained by the cord and nerves during the operation.

Decongestant drugs

COMMON DRUGS

Ephedrine Oxymetazoline
Phenylpropanolamine Pseudoephedrine
Xylometazoline

> **WARNING**
> Symptoms worsen when, after several days of treatment, decongestants are suddenly withdrawn. Use only in low doses for a short time.

Drugs used to relieve nasal congestion. Small amounts of these drugs are present in many over-the-counter cold remedies, which are available in tablet or nose-drop form. Decongestant drugs are commonly used in the treatment of upper *respiratory tract infections*, especially in patients susceptible to *otitis media* (middle-ear infection) or *sinusitis* (sinus infection).

POSSIBLE ADVERSE EFFECTS
Taken by mouth, decongestant drugs may cause tremor and palpitations; they are therefore not usually prescribed if a person has heart disease. In the form of nose drops, only small amounts are absorbed into the bloodstream and adverse effects are unlikely.

THE ACTION OF DECONGESTANTS

Decongestants work by narrowing blood vessels in the membranes that line the nose. This action reduces swelling, inflammation, and the amount of mucus produced by the nasal lining.

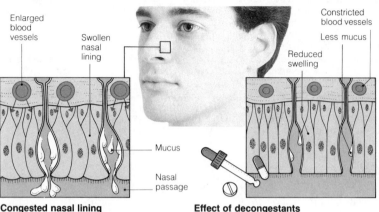

Congested nasal lining
When blood vessels enlarge in response to infection or irritation, increased amounts of fluid pass into the lining, which swells and produces more mucus.

Effect of decongestants
Chemicals stimulate constriction of the blood vessels in the nasal lining, which reduces swelling, mucus production, and nasal congestion.

If decongestant nose drops are taken for several days and then stopped, congestion frequently recurs ("rebounds") and may be worse than that for which the drug was taken. For this reason, decongestants should be taken for as short a time as possible.

Deductible
A provision in many health insurance policies that makes the patient responsible for a certain dollar amount of medical charges before the benefits of the insurance policy begin to apply. (See also *Coinsurance*.)

Defecation
The expulsion of feces from the body via the anus.

Defense mechanisms
Techniques used by the mind as a means of coping with unpleasant or unwelcome events, experiences, impulses, or emotions.

For example, death of a relative normally provokes grief and/or anger. One defense against these emotions may be repression—refusal to recognize these feelings and appearing to be unaffected by the event. Another reaction is denial—carrying on as though the relative is still alive.

A person who feels guilty about hating his or her father may transfer this hate to another person or turn the bad feelings toward himself or herself.

Disturbing impulses may take the opposite form in conscious thought. For instance, a person with strong sexual feelings may be excessively prudish or inhibited.

The body's defense mechanisms against infection are described under *immune system*.

Defensive medicine
The practice of ordering medical tests or procedures primarily to protect against any charge of malpractice.

Defibrillation
A technique in which a brief electric shock is administered to the heart, usually via two metal plates placed on the wall of the chest. Also called cardioversion, defibrillation is performed to treat some types of *arrhythmia* (irregular or rapid heart beat). The sudden burst of electricity through the heart converts *fibrillation* (rapid, uncoordinated heart beat) or *tachycardia* (rapid heart beat) back into a normal, regular heart beat. Occasionally a drug, such as lidocaine, is injected into a vein before the procedure to try to stabilize the heart rhythm.

Defibrillation can be carried out as an emergency procedure to treat *ventricular fibrillation*, which most commonly starts after a *myocardial infarction* (heart attack). It may also be used to treat an arrhythmia that has lasted several hours or days.

Defoliant poisoning

Defoliants are applied to plants to cause their leaves to drop off and the plants to die. Commonly used as weedkillers, defoliants are poisonous if swallowed. They should therefore always be kept in clearly labeled containers and stored out of the reach of children. The most widely used defoliant weedkillers are sodium chlorate, potassium chlorate (see *Chlorate poisoning*), and *paraquat*.

Another familiar defoliant is dioxin, which was used by US forces in Vietnam and has also occasionally been released into the atmosphere as a result of industrial accidents. Allegations have been made that this toxic substance caused nerve and other disorders in many Vietnam veterans and in others who have been exposed to it (as well as causing birth defects in their children). There is no convincing scientific evidence to support these allegations.

Deformity

Any malformation or distortion of part of the body. Deformities may be *congenital* (present at birth) or they may be acquired as a result of injury, disease, disorder, or disuse.

Most congenital deformities are relatively rare. Among the more common are clubfoot (*talipes*) and *cleft lip and palate*. The last two may occur separately or together.

Injuries that can cause deformity include burns, torn muscles, broken bones, and dislocated joints. Among the various diseases and disorders that may cause deformity are infections (such as *tuberculosis* and *leprosy*), damage to or disorders of nerves (such as paralysis of the facial nerves), some deficiency diseases (such as *rickets*), and a condition of unknown cause called *Paget's disease* of the bone. Disuse of a part of the body—as a result of being bedridden or confined to a wheelchair, for example—can lead to deformity through stiffening and *contracture* (shortening) of unused muscles or tendons.

Many deformities can be corrected by *reconstructive surgery*, various orthopedic techniques (including surgery), exercise, or by a combination of these methods. For example, cleft lip and cleft palate are now routinely treated during childhood by reconstructive surgery, with good results in most cases.

It is often possible to prevent the development of a deformity due to disuse by regular exercise.

Degeneration

Physical and/or chemical changes in cells, tissues, or organs that reduce their efficiency. Its true cause is unknown, but may be due to a disease process; degeneration is also a feature of aging. Other known causes include injury, reduced blood supply, poisoning (by alcohol, for example), or a diet deficient in a specific vitamin. (See also *Degenerative disorders*.)

Degenerative disorders

A blanket term covering a wide range of conditions in which there is progressive impairment of both the structure and function of part of the body. This definition excludes diseases caused by infection, inflammation, altered immune responses, chemical or physical damage, or malignant change. Many of the features of aging, such as wrinkling of the skin, are due to degenerative changes in body tissues, but, in degenerative disorders, the changes come on earlier in life, are more rapid, and typically affect some organs and not others.

Microscopic examination of an organ affected by degenerative disease often shows that the number of specialized cells or structures is reduced and that their place has been taken by connective or scar tissue.

Some diseases that were once thought to be degenerative disorders later proved to be due to slow viruses (such as *Creutzfeldt-Jakob syndrome*). Other degenerative disorders, such as *Parkinsonism*, may be traceable to poisoning—with carbon monoxide or with MPTP, an impurity formed during the illegal manufacture of one of the many *designer drugs*. Future research may identify specific infective or environmental causes for other degenerative disorders that are at present thought to be degenerative.

NERVOUS SYSTEM

Among degenerative disorders affecting the nervous system the most common is *Alzheimer's disease*, the main cause of presenile and senile dementia. In *Huntington's chorea*, dementia is combined with disorders of movement. Susceptibility to the degenerative changes in the brain is due to an abnormality in a single gene; the disease is transmitted from one generation to the next in a dominant pattern of inheritance (see *Genetic disorders*). In *Parkinson's disease* and in degenerative disorders that affect the *cerebellum*, abnormalities of movement are the main features. In *motor neuron diseases*, such as *Werdnig-Hoffmann*

disease and other diseases in their infantile forms, the prime symptom is muscular weakness.

EYES

Blindness in early adult life can be caused by a condition called Leber's *optic atrophy*, which is due to loss of nerve cells in the retina. *Retinitis pigmentosa*, another retinal degeneration, can cause blindness in childhood, but some vision may be preserved until late middle age. Both disorders have a genetic basis. By contrast, senile *macular degeneration* is not an inherited condition and rarely develops before the seventh decade.

JOINTS

The most familiar degenerative disorder is *osteoarthritis*, sometimes known as degenerative joint disease. Susceptibility to the condition seems to run in families; it also develops in sports enthusiasts and manual workers who have repeatedly damaged their joints. The prime features of osteoarthritis are thinning and destruction of the cartilage covering the surfaces of the joints and overgrowth and distortion of the bone around affected joints.

ARTERIES

Some hardening of the arteries seems to be a feature of aging. In some individuals, however, the degenerative changes in the muscle coat of these blood vessels are unusually severe and calcium deposits may be seen on X-ray films (as in Monckeberg's sclerosis, a type of *arteriosclerosis*).

MUSCLES

The *muscular dystrophies* are a group of genetic disorders that cause distinctive patterns of muscular weakness, sometimes associated with increased muscle bulk. *Myopathies*, by contrast, are muscle disorders for which an external cause, such as a chemical toxin, can usually be identified. Myopathies are not classed as degenerative disorders.

Deglutition

The medical term for *swallowing*.

Dehiscence

The splitting open of a partly healed wound, most commonly the splitting open of a surgical incision that has been closed with sutures or clips.

Dehydration

A condition in which a person's water content has fallen to a dangerously low level. Water accounts for about 60 percent of a man's weight and 50 percent of a woman's, and the total water

D

content must be kept within fairly narrow limits for healthy functioning of cells and tissues (see *Water*).

The concentration in the body's fluids of mineral salts and other dissolved substances also must be kept within a narrow range. In many cases of dehydration, salt will have been lost as well as water.

CAUSES

Normally, dehydration is prevented by the sensation of thirst, which encourages a person to drink when the body is short of water. This mechanism may fail because water is not available or because of high losses of water from the body.

Even in a temperate climate, a minimum of three pints of water continues to be lost every 24 hours through the skin via perspiration, from the lungs into the air, and in the urine to rid the body of waste products. Severe dehydration is likely to develop within a few days if no water is taken. Large amounts of water may be lost in vomit or diarrhea, particularly if the diarrhea is profuse and watery (as in *cholera*) or in the urine of anyone with uncontrolled *diabetes mellitus*, *diabetes insipidus*, and some types of *renal failure*. In all these cases, the thirst sensation may not encourage sufficient water intake to balance the losses.

SYMPTOMS AND SIGNS

Symptoms and signs of water depletion include severe thirst, dry lips and tongue, an increase in heart rate and breathing, dizziness, confusion, and eventual coma. The skin looks dry and loses its elasticity. Any urine passed is small in quantity and dark-colored. If there is salt depletion (usually as a result of heavy sweating, vomiting, or diarrhea), there may be lethargy, headaches, cramps, and pallor.

PREVENTION

When living in a hot climate, or when suffering from a fever, vomiting, or diarrhea, the simplest rule is to drink enough water to produce urine that is consistently pale. This often means drinking well beyond the point of thirst (possibly a pint of water every hour during the heat of the day).

Salt losses from heavy sweating need to be replaced either in the diet or by adding a quarter of a teaspoon of table salt to each pint of drinking water. Bottled mineral water can help maintain the intake of salts. For vomiting and diarrhea, special salt and glucose rehydration mixtures for adding to water may be purchased from drugstores.

TREATMENT

Once dehydration has developed, fluid and salt replacement may be required at a far faster rate than that required to simply prevent dehydration. Sometimes, fluids must be given intravenously and the water/salt balance requires careful monitoring with blood tests and adjustment.

Déjà vu

French for "already seen." A sense of having already experienced an event that is happening at the moment. Déjà vu is a common phenomenon that has never been properly explained. Some people believe that it is due to an unconscious emotional response caused by similarities between the current event and some past experience. Others believe that a neurological "short circuit" results in the experience registering in the memory before reaching consciousness. Frequent occurrence of déjà vu may sometimes be a symptom of temporal lobe *epilepsy*.

Delinquency

Behavior in a juvenile that in an adult would be considered a crime. The term is often extended to include noncriminal behavior, such as being truant, running away from home, drinking alcohol, or using drugs.

Juvenile delinquency is probably caused by a combination of factors—social, psychological, and biological—but relatively few offenders suffer from a definite mental disorder or mental retardation.

Child guidance or *family therapy* may be recommended for delinquents and their families. Persistent offenders are sometimes sent to special schools and may be taken into care or made wards of the court.

Delirium

A state of acute mental confusion, commonly brought on by physical illness. The symptoms are those of disordered brain function, and vary according to personality, environment, and the severity of illness. Failure to understand events or remember what has been happening, increased anxiety, physical restlessness, and sudden swings of mood occur as delirium worsens. At its most severe, the patient may hallucinate, suffer from *illusions* (for example, seeing nurses as threatening monsters), lapse into terrified panic, and resort to shouting and violence. Usually the symptoms are worse at

night, because of sleep disturbance and the fact that darkness and quiet make visual illusions more likely.

CAUSES

While any severe illness may underlie this state, high fever and disturbances of body chemistry are often present. Children and older people are most liable, particularly after major surgery or when there is a preexisting brain disturbance such as *dementia*. Drugs, various poisons, and alcohol are common precipitants.

TREATMENT

Treatment is of the underlying physical disorder, with appropriate nursing management to reduce anxiety. Suitable lighting, calm and clear communication, appropriate seclusion, and known, trusted attendants are all important. Particular attention must be paid to fluids and nutrition, but tranquilizers (e.g., chlorpromazine, haloperidol, or thioridazine) are often necessary for sedation of the physical restlessness. The control of infection by antibiotics has probably made this condition much rarer than it was 50 years ago.

Delirium tremens

A state of confusion accompanied by trembling and vivid *hallucinations*. It usually arises in chronic alcoholics after withdrawal or abstinence from alcohol, and often occurs following admission to the hospital with an injury or for a surgical operation.

SYMPTOMS, SIGNS, AND TREATMENT

In the early stages, symptoms include restlessness, agitation, trembling, and sleeplessness. Overactivity of sympathetic nerve pathways causes a rapid heart beat, fever, dilation (widening) of the pupils, and profuse sweating that may lead to dehydration. Confusion follows with visual and sometimes auditory hallucinations, and the patient appears terrified. Convulsions may also occur.

The symptoms usually subside within three days. Treatment consists of rest, rehydration, and sedation in a hospital. Sedative drugs used include chlorpromazine or chlordiazepoxide. Injections of vitamins, particularly thiamine (vitamin B), may be given, since some of the features of delirium tremens seem to be linked with thiamine deficiency (see *Wernicke-Korsakoff syndrome*).

Delivery

Expulsion or extraction of a baby from the mother's uterus. In most cases the baby lies lengthwise in the uterus with its head facing downward and is delivered head first through the vaginal opening by a combination of uterine contractions and maternal effort at the end of the second stage of labor (see *Childbirth*).

If the baby is lying in an abnormal position (see *Breech delivery; Malpresentation*), if uterine contractions are weak, or if there is disproportion between the size of the baby's head and the mother's pelvis, a *forceps delivery* or *vacuum extraction* may be required; these are called operative deliveries. In some cases, vaginal delivery is impossible or potentially dangerous to the mother or the baby, and *cesarean section* is necessary.

Deltoid

The triangular muscle of the shoulder region that forms the rounded flesh of the outer part of the upper arm, and passes up and over the shoulder joint. The wide end of the muscle is attached to the scapula (shoulder blade) and clavicle (collarbone). The muscle fibers converge to form the apex of the triangle, which is attached to the humerus (upper-arm bone) about halfway down its length.

The central, strongest part of the muscle raises the arm sideways. The front and back parts of the muscle twist the arm.

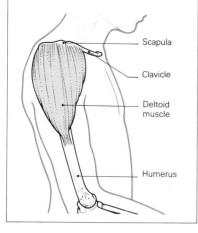

LOCATION OF THE DELTOID
Muscle of the shoulder region, forming the rounded, outer part of the upper arm, and attached to the scapula and clavicle.

Scapula

Clavicle

Deltoid muscle

Humerus

Delusion

A fixed, irrational idea not shared by others and not responding to reasoned argument. The central idea

in a paranoid delusion involves persecution or jealousy. For instance, a person may believe that he or she is being poisoned or that a partner is persistently unfaithful (see *Paranoia*). A person suffering from delusions of grandeur believes, for example, that he or she is related to royalty.

Persistent delusions are a sign of serious mental illness, notably *schizophrenia* and *dementia*. (See also *Hallucination; Illusion*.)

Dementia

A general decline in all areas of mental ability. Dementia is usually due to brain disease and is progressive, the most obvious feature being increasing intellectual impairment.

INCIDENCE

Dementia is the great health problem of modern developed societies, since long life is creating an increasing proportion of elderly citizens. Some 10 percent of those over 65 years and 20 percent of those over 75 years are affected to some degree by dementia.

CAUSES

Traditionally, dementing illnesses were divided into presenile (under 65 years of age at onset) and senile (over 65 years). This is now regarded as an artificial division, although treatable causes are more common in the younger age group. Causes include head injury, pernicious anemia, encephalitis, myxedema, syphilis, brain tumor, and alcoholism.

Such "reversible" illnesses account only for some 10 percent of dementias. The great majority of them result from *cerebrovascular disease* (including *strokes*) and from *Alzheimer's disease*. While the former can sometimes be helped by treatment of *hypertension* (high blood pressure) or heart disease, the recurrent loss of blood supply to the brain is often due to narrowed or blocked arteries within the brain, and a gradual deterioration occurs. Alzheimer's disease is at present completely irreversible, consisting as it does of gradual loss of brain cells and shrinkage of the brain substance.

SYMPTOMS

The person with dementia may not remember recent events, may become easily lost in a familiar neighborhood, may fail to grasp what is going on, and may become confused over days and dates. These symptoms tend to come on gradually and may not be noticed right away. People also tend to cover up their problems by *confabulation* (making up stories to fill the gaps in their memories). Sudden emotional

outbursts or embarrassing behavior (such as urinating in public) may be the first obvious signs of the illness.

Commonly the person's failures in judgment result in the magnification of his or her unpleasant personality traits; families may have to endure unreasonable demands, accusations, pilfering, and even physical assault. Paranoid and depressive illnesses (see *Paranoia; Depression*) with psychotic *delusions* may occur as dementia worsens. Irritability or anxiety, with the patient retaining some awareness of his or her emotional state, alters to a shallow indifference toward all feelings. Personal habits deteriorate, clothes and possessions become soiled and dirty, and speech becomes incoherent. Demented individuals lapse into "second childhood" and require total nursing care of their feeding, toilet, and physical activities.

TREATMENT

While appropriate treatment of certain illnesses is effective in arresting decline (such as surgery for a brain tumor or thyroid replacement for myxedema), management of the most common, Alzheimer-type illness is based mostly on the treatment of symptoms. The patient should be kept clean and well nourished in comfortable surroundings with good nursing care, and sedatives should be given for obvious restlessness or paranoid beliefs. These measures can help ease the distress for both patient and family. Timing of a transfer to suitable hospital or custodial care must be sensitively organized.

Research into medication to alleviate memory loss and intellectual decline has shown some promise, but no truly effective treatment is yet available commercially.

Dementia praecox

An outdated term for severe *schizophrenia*, especially that developing in adolescence or early adulthood. It means literally "prematurely out of one's mind."

De Morgan's spots

Harmless red or purple raised spots in the skin, about one tenth of an inch across, that usually affect middle-aged or elderly people. De Morgan's spots are also called cherry spots or cherry angiomas and consist of a cluster of minute blood vessels. With increasing age they become more numerous but do not increase in size.

The spots are of no significance but may bleed if injured.

D

Demyelination

Breakdown of the fatty sheaths that surround and electrically insulate nerve fibers. The sheaths provide nutrients to the nerve fibers and are vital to the passage of electrical impulses along them. Demyelination "short-circuits" the functioning of the nerve, causing loss of sensation, coordination, and power in specific areas of the body. The affected nerves may be within the central nervous system (CNS, comprising the brain and spinal cord) or may be part of the peripheral nervous system, which links the CNS to the body's sense receptors, muscles, glands, and organs.

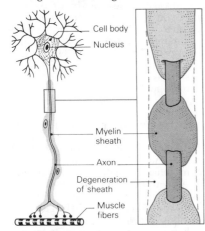

Mechanism of demyelination
The fatty myelin sheaths that surround and insulate nerve fibers break down, causing the affected nerves to "short-circuit."

Patches of demyelination are the prime feature of *multiple sclerosis*, a disease with symptoms that include blurred vision, muscle weakness, and loss of coordination. The cause of the demyelination is not known. In many cases, attacks of demyelination alternate with periods of partial or complete recovery of nerve function.

Encephalomyelitis is a rare disorder caused by inflammation of nerve cells within the CNS and sometimes areas of demyelination. It may be due to a viral infection or very rarely an allergiclike reaction following immunization. Symptoms vary from headache to brain damage.

Dendritic ulcer

A type of *corneal ulcer* characterized by threadlike extensions that branch out in various directions from the center. The ulcer is commonly caused by infection of the cornea by the virus that causes *herpes simplex*.

Dengue

A tropical disease caused by a virus spread by the mosquito *AEDES AEGYPTI*. It occurs in Southeast Asia, the Pacific region, parts of Africa, South and Central America, and the Caribbean. There have been occasional outbreaks in Mexico, Puerto Rico, and the US Virgin Islands in recent years, and a few cases have occurred along the Gulf coast.

Symptoms and signs appear five to eight days after a bite by an infected mosquito and include fever, rash, severe joint and muscle pains, and headache. These symptoms often subside after about three days, recur a few days later, and then subside again. Serious complications are uncommon. Full recovery may take several weeks. The symptoms of severe muscle and bone pain have led to dengue being called breakbone fever.

No specific treatment is available for dengue, though analgesics (painkillers) may relieve symptoms. No vaccine is available at present, so avoidance involves personal protection against mosquito bites in areas where the disease is prevalent (see *Insect bites*).

Densitometry

The measurement of bone density, as determined by the concentration of calcified material.

WHY IT IS DONE
Densitometry is used to confirm the presence of *osteoporosis* (wasting away of bone substance) or to diagnose *rickets* in young children. It is also useful in assessing the response of these conditions to treatment.

HOW IT IS DONE
The most accurate way to measure bone density is by analyzing the weight and content of a bone *biopsy* sample. However, this technique is time-consuming and requires an operation to remove the sample.

CT scanning provides more detailed pictures of the internal bone structure that enable smaller changes in bone density to be seen.

A relatively new and expensive technique is single or dual photon absorption, in which the pattern of absorption of a beam (or beams) of radiation as it passes through the bone is analyzed on an electronic counter. The dual photon method is used to evaluate the mineral content of the type of bone found in the vertebrae and most other bones where fractures from osteoporosis occur.

Density

The "heaviness" of a substance per unit volume. Density is a measure of how much a given volume of a substance weighs. For instance, a cubic inch of lead is considerably heavier than a cubic inch of wood; lead is therefore denser than wood.

In radiology, the term density relates to the amount of radiation absorbed by the structure being X rayed. Bone, which absorbs much radiation, appears white on X-ray film. By contrast, a lung, which contains mostly air, absorbs very little radiation and appears dark on film. The same holds true in *CT scanning*.

Dental assistant

A person who is trained to help a *dentist* at chairside and in the office.

The dental assistant is responsible for maintaining the cleanliness of the dentist's office and equipment, and for sterilizing and setting out instruments for each patient. During treatment of a patient, he or she passes instruments to the dentist and mixes any materials that are needed, such as cement for fillings. Other duties include record-keeping, processing X-ray films, and giving patients instructions on *oral hygiene*.

Dental emergencies

Injuries or disorders of the teeth and gums that require immediate treatment because of severe pain and/or because delay could lead to poor healing or complications.

A tooth that has become avulsed (completely dislodged from its socket) in an accident will be gently washed, reimplanted as rapidly as possible (see *Reimplantation*), and then immobilized with a splint. The success rate is about 90 percent if the tooth is out of its socket for 30 minutes or less, but falls to about 70 percent if the tooth is not reimplanted for 90 minutes. An extruded tooth (one that is partially dislodged from its socket) should be manipulated back into the socket within a few minutes of the injury.

A direct blow to a tooth may cause a fracture (see *Fracture, dental*). If the root is fractured so that the tooth is split in two, the halves will be brought closely together and splinted in position, usually for several months (see *Splinting, dental*). If the crown is fractured, but only the enamel and dentin are affected, a tooth-colored, composite filling will prevent pain from the exposed dentin, stop bacteria from entering the tooth, and restore appearance. If the fracture of the crown involves the pulp of a mature tooth, a root canal filling is needed (see *Root canal treatment*). In a young tooth, a dressing of calcium hydroxide placed over the pulp soon after the accident may allow a hard tissue barrier to form and prevent the pulp of the tooth from dying.

Sometimes a blow hard enough to fracture teeth may also fracture the jaw; the fractured parts may need to be wired together to allow them to heal (see *Wiring of the jaws*).

Toothache may be so severe that eating and sleeping are disturbed. Temporary pain relief can be gained by placing a sedative dressing in the tooth until the cause of the pain can be treated. The most severe dental pain is usually caused by an abscess (infection). This is treated either by antibiotics to reduce the swelling, or by draining the abscess (see *Abscess, dental*), followed by endodontic treatment. Swelling, pain, and inflammation also may occur around an impacted wisdom tooth, and the jaw may become stiff and difficult to open. This requires immediate treatment to prevent the infection from spreading (see *Impaction, dental*).

Acute necrotizing ulcerative *gingivitis* comes on suddenly and causes pain, inflammation, ulceration, and bleeding of the gums. It is a destructive condition, and professional treatment should be sought as quickly as possible.

Dental examination

Examination of the mouth, gums, and teeth by a dentist. A dental examination may be performed as a routine check at least once a year or as part of the assessment of the condition of a person complaining of a symptom.

WHY IT IS DONE

Routine examinations enable caries (cavities) and diseases of the gums and mouth to be detected and treated at an early stage before they cause serious damage. The examinations also allow the efficiency of *oral hygiene* to be checked.

It is particularly important for children to have their teeth examined by a dentist regularly so that the dentist can monitor replacement of the primary teeth by permanent teeth. If any problems occur, such as crowding, the dentist can refer the child for orthodontic treatment at the correct stage.

HOW IT IS DONE

Before the examination, the dentist or dental hygienist usually asks about

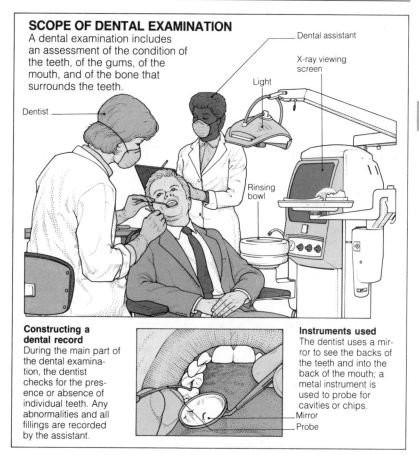

SCOPE OF DENTAL EXAMINATION
A dental examination includes an assessment of the condition of the teeth, of the gums, of the mouth, and of the bone that surrounds the teeth.

Dental assistant

X-ray viewing screen

Light

Dentist

Rinsing bowl

Constructing a dental record
During the main part of the dental examination, the dentist checks for the presence or absence of individual teeth. Any abnormalities and all fillings are recorded by the assistant.

Instruments used
The dentist uses a mirror to see the backs of the teeth and into the back of the mouth; a metal instrument is used to probe for cavities or chips.

Mirror
Probe

the patient's general health, especially if it is the person's first visit to a dentist or the first visit after a long time. Understanding the person's general health is important since it can affect the type of treatment that is recommended. A person with a heart valve disorder, for example, may be under increased risk of contracting bacterial *endocarditis* after extraction of a tooth or any other dental treatment. Particular care also is needed when treating diabetics and people who have had *hepatitis*. People with allergies may react dangerously to penicillin; people taking certain drugs can react badly to anesthesia. If the person feels pain, the dentist will ask him or her questions, such as when the pain was first noticed and whether it is continuous or intermittent.

The dentist begins by noting the general appearance of the patient and by examining the face and neck externally. The face is inspected for puffiness that might indicate a dental *abscess* and the neck is felt for swollen lymph glands, which may be caused

by an infection of the mouth or teeth. The dentist also feels the temporomandibular joint (jaw joint) for any abnormal movements (see *Temporomandibular joint syndrome*).

Next the dentist examines the patient's bite and the teeth as a whole, noting any tilted, rotated, overlapping, or missing teeth and observing points of contact between teeth, and the presence of any excessive movement in a tooth when the patient makes chewing movements.

Using a mirror to see the backs of the teeth and into the back of the mouth, the dentist then examines individual teeth, using a metal instrument to probe for cavities or chips. Fillings and crowns are inspected for fit, jagged edges, and signs of erosion or cracks. If teeth are missing, the alveolus (bone that surrounds and supports the teeth) is examined for signs of abnormality, especially if the patient is to be fitted with a prosthodontic appliance, such as a bridge. If the patient wears a denture, it is checked to ensure it still fits.

D

The gums and inside of the mouth are examined for signs of disease. Gums that are red, puffy, or receding or that bleed easily when touched with the probe may indicate *gingivitis* or *periodontitis*. White discoloration of the inside of the mouth may signify *candidiasis* or *leukoplakia*.

Finally, the dentist assesses the accumulation of plaque and calculus on the teeth; this indicates the efficiency of the patient's oral hygiene. Inspection of the teeth and gums is sometimes followed by *dental X rays*.

Dental hygienist

See *Hygienist, dental.*

Dental X ray

An image of the teeth and jaws that provides information essential for detecting, diagnosing, and treating conditions that can threaten oral and general health. The part to be imaged is placed between a tube emitting *X rays* and a photographic film. Because X rays are unable to pass easily through hard tissue, a shadow of the teeth and bone is seen on the film.

WHY IT IS DONE

X rays can reveal disorders of the teeth and surrounding tissues that a dentist would not see during a normal visual examination of the mouth. Small caries (cavities), abscesses, cysts, tumors, and other disorders can be detected and treated before obvious signs and symptoms have developed, avoiding serious long-term damage. Early identification of dental problems, such as impacted teeth, allows treatment to be carefully planned and carried out at an early stage.

RISKS

The amount of radiation received from dental X rays is extremely small, and the risk of any harmful effects is negligible. However, a woman who is, or suspects she may be, pregnant should tell her dentist, who may recommend the use of a leaded apron during the examination or postpone X rays until after the pregnancy.

Dentifrice

A paste, powder, or gel used with a toothbrush to clean the teeth. Although brushing without a dentifrice removes food debris and some plaque (see *Plaque, dental*), a slightly abrasive dentifrice is needed to remove the remaining plaque and the salivary pellicle (a thin protein film).

A dentifrice contains the following: an abrasive—usually an insoluble, organic salt, such as dicalcium phosphate, which ideally does not scratch the teeth; a synthetic detergent for foaming action; humectants to bind the ingredients together and keep them moist; thickening agents; flavorings; and colorings.

Fluoride has been added to dentifrices for many years, and the dramatic drop in caries has been partly attributed to its presence in the majority of preparations.

A variety of desensitizing dentifrices is available for teeth that are sensitive due to exposed dentin near the gum margin.

Dentin

Hard tissue surrounding the pulp of a tooth (see *Teeth*).

Dentist

The equivalent of the family practitioner for teeth. Dentists perform regular checkups, clean teeth, fill cavities, extract teeth (if absolutely necessary), correct problems with tooth alignment, and provide and fit bridges and/or dentures to replace missing teeth. They also check for cancer of the mouth, perform cosmetic procedures (such as bonding) and give general advice on how to care for the teeth and gums. Most dentists refer patients with complicated problems to dental specialists in different branches of *dentistry*.

Dentistry

The science or profession concerned with the teeth and associated structures of the mouth. Dentistry involves the prevention, diagnosis, and treatment of disease, injury, or malformation of the teeth, gums, and jaws. The majority of *dentists* work in

---

TYPES OF DENTAL X RAY

There are three different types of X ray. Each is useful for revealing particular problems.

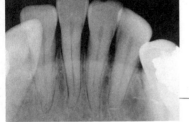

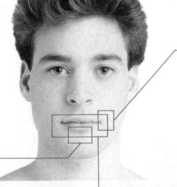

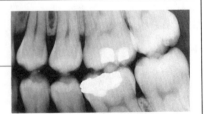

Bite-wing X rays
These X rays show the crowns of the teeth. They are useful for detecting areas of decay between teeth and changes in bone caused by periodontal (gum) disease. The film is in a holder with a central tab onto which the patient bites.

Periapical X rays
These X rays give detailed pictures of whole teeth and the surrounding gums and bone. They show unerupted or impacted teeth, root fractures, abscesses, cysts, tumors, and the characteristic bone patterns of some skeletal diseases. The film, in a protective casing, is placed in the patient's mouth and is held in position behind the teeth to be X rayed.

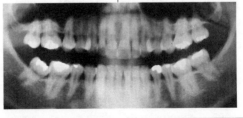

Panoramic X rays
These X rays show all the teeth and surrounding structures on one large film. They are invaluable for finding unerupted or impacted teeth, cysts, jaw fractures, or tumors. Pictures are recorded continuously onto film as the camera swings around from one side of the jaw to the other.

general dental practice (77 percent in the US). They are qualified to undertake all aspects of dental care, including cleaning teeth, filling cavities, extracting teeth, and fitting crowns, bridges, and dentures. Although they are qualified to diagnose and treat complicated problems, dentists may refer patients to a practitioner in one of the specialized branches of the dental profession.

Orthodontics concerns the moving of improperly aligned teeth to improve function and appearance. *Prosthodontics* concerns the provision of bridgework and dentures to replace missing teeth and the provision of substitutes for missing oral tissues.

Two branches specialize in the treatment of diseases: *endodontics* involves the treatment of diseases of the pulp, while *periodontics* involves the treatment of disorders that damage the supporting structures of the teeth, such as the gums.

Dentition

The characteristics of a person's *teeth*, including the number and arrangement in the jaw. The term is also used to describe the *eruption of teeth*.

Denture

An appliance that replaces missing natural teeth. A denture consists of an acrylic (tough plastic) and/or metal base mounted with acrylic or porcelain teeth. A natural appearance is achieved by choosing artificial teeth of the size, color, and shape that closely resemble the original teeth and that blend well with the contours of the person's face.

FITTING

The dentist takes impressions of the upper and lower gums. The impressions are removed from the mouth and allowed to harden. Models are then made by pouring plaster of Paris into the hardened impressions. Denture baseplates created from these models will fit the mouth accurately, but, to ensure that the bite will be correct when the artificial teeth are positioned, the dentist must also record the relationship of the upper and lower jaw. This is done by having the patient bite onto wax-rimmed plates (bite blocks) that can be trimmed to indicate the correct relative positions of the teeth.

Using the bite blocks as a guide, a temporary denture with the teeth waxed into position is then produced. The patient tries it on so the dentist can make adjustments to the position or choice of teeth. When the dentist and patient are satisfied with the bite and appearance, the wax is replaced by acrylic or metal, and the finished, polished dentures are fitted at the patient's next visit. Additional visits may be needed to modify any part of the base that is uncomfortable.

Dentures fitted immediately after tooth extraction usually require extra visits so that adjustments to the fit can be made as the tissues heal. Often a new acrylic lining is fused to the existing baseplate. Sometimes a soft lining (made of slow-setting impression material) is inserted temporarily to minimize pain.

Deodorant

A substance that removes bad smelling odors, especially body odors. Deodorants may contain *antiseptics* to destroy bacteria, perfume to mask odors, and *antiperspirants* (drugs that reduce the production of sweat).

Deodorant preparations are a useful aid against body odor caused by decomposition of sweat by bacteria on the skin. Deodorant liquids are also available to put into a *colostomy* or *ileostomy* bag. Deodorant drugs, such as bismuth, can be taken by mouth to reduce ostomy odor.

Deoxyribonucleic acid

See *DNA*; *Nucleic acids*.

Dependence

Psychological or physical reliance on persons or drugs. An infant is naturally dependent on parents, but, as he or she grows, dependency normally wanes. Some adults never become fully independent, continuing to demand excessive love, admiration, and help from others.

Alcohol and drugs (such as opiates, amphetamines, and tranquilizers) may induce a state of physical or emotional dependence in heavy, regular users. A person who is dependent may develop physical symptoms (sweating and abdominal pains) or emotional distress if deprived of the drug. The pattern of dependence varies with the drug and with the personality of the individual. (See also *Alcohol dependence*; *Drug dependence*.)

Depersonalization

A state of feeling unreal. The sufferer often describes feeling "like a robot" or "as though a glass screen came down." The sensation usually comes on suddenly, though it may be momentary or last for hours. It is often accompanied by *derealization* (experiencing the world as unreal).

An otherwise healthy person may experience depersonalization as an isolated event, especially if he or she is tired or worried. Although frightening, it is rarely serious. More often, people who have *anxiety disorders* experience depersonalization during *panic attacks*, especially if *hyperventilation* (rapid, shallow breathing) occurs. Other causes include drugs (e.g., LSD, antidepressants, or cannabis), migraine, and temporal lobe *epilepsy*.

TYPES OF DENTURES

Partial dentures	Partial dentures are used when only some teeth are missing. They fill unsightly gaps, make chewing easier, maintain clear speech, and keep the remaining teeth in position. Teeth on either side of a gap may tip (making cleaning more difficult) or drift (placing unnatural stress on the	tissues of the mouth). Partial dentures are held in place by metal clasps that grip adjacent teeth or by clasps combined with metal rests (extensions of the denture plate that rest on the tooth surface).
Full dentures	Full dentures are needed when there are no teeth left in the mouth. They stay in place by resting on the gum ridges and, in the case of upper dentures, by	suction. Fitting is usually delayed for several months after extraction of teeth to allow the gums to shrink and change shape as they heal.
Immediate dentures	Immediate dentures are fitted immediately after extraction of teeth. They protect the gum and control bleeding from extraction sites. Since a toothless period is avoided, they are particularly useful	for replacing front teeth. However, they can be expensive and require follow-up visits for refitting or relining so that they fit comfortably.

D

Depilatory

A chemical hair remover, such as barium sulfide, in the form of a cream or paste. Depilatories are used for cosmetic reasons and in the treatment of *hirsutism* (excessive hairiness).

HOW THEY WORK

Depilatories dissolve hair at the surface of the skin. They do not affect the hair root and therefore do not permanently remove the hair.

POSSIBLE ADVERSE EFFECTS

Depilatories may cause an allergic reaction, with inflammation and swelling. It is advisable to test them first on a small area of skin (they are not usually recommended for use on the face). Depilatories should not be used after a hot bath or shower. Heat increases blood flow to the skin and opens skin pores, thus increasing the amount of chemical that is absorbed into the body.

Depot injection

An intramuscular (into a muscle) injection of a drug specially formulated to give a slow, steady absorption of its active chemicals into the bloodstream.

Depot injections usually contain a much higher dose than that normally given by injection. Absorption of the drug is slowed by the inclusion of substances such as oil or wax. The release of the active drug can be made to last for hours, days, or weeks, depending on the formulation.

A depot injection is useful for patients who may not take their medication correctly. A depot injection also prevents the necessity of giving a series of injections over a short period. Examples of drugs given by depot injection include *corticosteroid drugs* and *antipsychotic drugs.*

Disadvantages of this type of injection include side effects caused by the uneven release of the drug into the bloodstream and prolonged adverse reactions caused by the long-acting nature of the treatment.

Patients who are receiving regular depot injections usually carry a warning card in case emergency treatment is required from another physician.

Depression

Feelings of sadness, hopelessness, pessimism, and a general loss of interest in life, combined with a sense of reduced emotional well-being. Most people experience these feelings occasionally, often as a normal response to a particular event. For example, it is natural to feel sad when a close relative dies. However, if the depression occurs without any apparent cause, deepens, and persists, it may be a symptom of a wide range of psychiatric illnesses. When a person's behavior and physical state are also affected, it then becomes part of a true depressive illness.

SYMPTOMS

Symptoms vary with the severity of the illness. In a person with mild depression, the main symptoms are anxiety and a variable mood. Sometimes he or she has fits of crying that occur for no apparent reason. A person with more serious depression may suffer from loss of appetite, difficulty sleeping, loss of interest and enjoyment in social activities, feelings of tiredness, and loss of concentration. Movement and thinking may become slowed; in some cases, the opposite occurs, and the person becomes extremely anxious and agitated. Severely depressed people may have thoughts of death and/or *suicide*, and feelings of guilt or worthlessness. In extreme cases, they may have *hallucinations* or *delusions* (believing, for example, that someone is poisoning them).

Intensity of symptoms often varies with the time of day. Most depressed people feel slightly better as the day progresses, but in some people the symptoms are worse at night. As a depressive illness progresses, the symptoms become more and more prominent. Finally, the person may become totally withdrawn and spend most of the time huddled in bed.

CAUSES

Usually, a true depressive illness has no single obvious cause. It may be triggered by certain physical illnesses (such as *stroke* or *hepatitis*), by hormonal disorders (such as *hypothyroidism*), or by the hormonal changes that occur after childbirth (see *Postpartum depression*). Some drugs, including the birth-control pill and sleeping pills, are contributing factors. If the depression is a part of a *manic-depressive illness*, inheritance may play a part, since this illness tends to run in families.

Aside from these biological causes, social and psychological factors may play a part. Lack of a satisfactory mother-child relationship may lead to depression in later life (see *Bonding*), especially when combined with difficult social circumstances. For example, a woman whose mother died early in her life may be particularly vulnerable if she has to cope with bringing up a child on her own.

Depression may also be related to the number of disturbing events or changes in a person's life.

INCIDENCE

Depression is the most common serious psychiatric illness. Some 10 to 15 percent of people suffer from it at some time in their lives, especially the milder forms. The more severe manic-depressive type affects only about 1 to 2 percent of depressed people, but the incidence of all forms of the illness increases with age. This may be due to social isolation, failing mental powers, and physical illness.

Depression appears to be more common in women, with about one in six seeking help for depression at some time in their lives (as opposed to only one in nine men). This may be a true difference or may result from the fact that women are more prepared to visit physicians for their depressive symptoms while men may be more likely to resort to alcohol, violence, or other expressions of discontent.

TREATMENT

There are three main forms of treatment for depression, depending on the type and severity of the illness.

Psychotherapy, whether individual or in a group, is most useful for those people whose personality and life experiences are the main causes of their illness. Many different types of therapy are available, ranging from an informal, purely practical approach to problem-solving, to the more structured approaches of *cognitive-behavioral therapy* and *psychoanalysis*.

Drug treatment is used for people who have predominantly physical symptoms. *Antidepressant drugs* are usually effective in over two thirds of these patients, provided the drugs are taken in a sufficient dosage over a long enough period of time.

Electroconvulsive therapy (*ECT*), which is given under a general anesthetic, is usually reserved for treating severely depressed people, especially if they are suffering from delusions or have failed to respond to treatment. ECT is effective and safe, and may be lifesaving; the only side effect may be a mild, temporary memory impairment. Trials have shown that ECT relieves severe depression faster than drugs.

OUTLOOK

Although depressive illness is a common cause of distress and social problems, the outlook is good for most sufferers, provided they are given appropriate treatment and advice. The main risk is suicide. In affluent societies the rate of suicide is about 20 per 100,000 population; at least 80 percent of these deaths are related to depression. The rate is highest in elderly men who are socially isolated and physically ill or in pain, but the rate is increasing in younger people.

Many people suffering from depression do not require hospitalization and make a good recovery. People with severe and prolonged depression (especially the elderly) may require continuous treatment and may be socially handicapped. However, spontaneous recovery is possible after many years of illness.

Derangement

An outdated term for severe mental disorder. It was first used in the nineteenth century to describe the idea of an orderly mind that had become "disarranged." Today it is usually applied to wild, disturbed behavior rather than a specific mental state.

The term derangement also applies to disorders of the ligaments in the knee joint (i.e., internal derangement of the knee).

Derealization

Feeling that the world has become unreal. It usually occurs with *depersonalization* and shares the sudden onset, symptoms, and causes of that condition. Sufferers commonly describe feeling that they are "looking at the world through a glass screen." Derealization may be caused by excessive tiredness, hallucinogenic drugs, or disordered brain function.

Dermabrasion

The removal of the surface layer of the skin by high-speed sanding to reduce the pitted scars of acne, to improve the appearance of unsightly raised scars, or to remove tattoos. The skin is numbed with a local anesthetic and the surface layer removed by a fast-revolving abrasive wheel. Healing takes about two weeks and the full effect of the treatment is apparent after two months.

Dermatitis

Inflammation of the skin, sometimes due to an allergy but in many cases occurring without any known cause. Many types of dermatitis are better known as *eczema* (for example, atopic, discoid, infantile, and hand eczema).

Apart from eczemas, the three main forms of skin inflammation are seborrheic dermatitis, contact dermatitis, and photodermatitis.

SEBORRHEIC DERMATITIS

This is a red, scaly, itchy rash that develops on the face (particularly the nose and eyebrows), scalp, chest, and back. On the scalp it is the most common cause of *dandruff*. The rash often develops during times of stress, but its exact cause is unknown. Generally, the treatment of dermatitis must be tailored to each case. Applying topical corticosteroids and/or antimicrobials is often helpful. Also, gentle handling of the involved skin is imperative (i.e., avoidance of scratching and irritating substances—like detergents).

CONTACT DERMATITIS

In this type, the rash is a reaction to some substance that comes in contact with the skin. The reaction may result from a direct toxic effect of the substance or may be an allergic response.

Among the more common causes of the reaction are detergents (including traces left in washed clothes), nickel (in watch straps, bracelets, necklaces, and the fastenings of underclothes), chemicals in rubber gloves and condoms, certain cosmetics, plants (such as poison ivy), and medications (among them the antibiotic neomycin in cream or droplet form).

The type of rash varies considerably according to the substance causing it, but it is often itchy, and may flake or blister; its distribution corresponds to the skin area in contact with the causative substance.

When it is not clear what substance is responsible, suspected chemicals are placed in contact with the skin of the back and are kept in place there with tapes for a few days to see whether any produces a patch of dermatitis. Once the offending substance is identified, it can then be avoided, if possible. A corticosteroid medication may be used for the treatment of an existing rash.

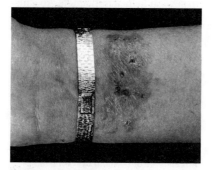

Contact dermatitis
Reaction to the nickel in a watch strap produced the itchy, blistering rash on the inside of the wrist shown above.

Dermatitis artefacta

Any self-induced skin condition. It may range from a mild scratch self-inflicted by someone under stress to severe and extensive mutilation by a psychologically disturbed patient.

The skin damage may take any form—ulcers, blisters, or scratches. The damage often has a symmetrical or bizarre pattern and, to the trained eye, does not resemble that seen in any skin disease.

Dermatitis herpetiformis

A chronic skin disease in which clusters of tiny, red, intensely itchy blisters occur in a symmetrical pattern on various parts of the body, most commonly the back, elbows, knees, buttocks, and scalp.

The disease usually develops in adult life and is believed to be related to *celiac sprue*, a condition in which the small intestine is allergic to gluten, a constituent of wheat and other cereals. One of the symptoms of celiac sprue is chronic diarrhea, which also occurs in some people with dermatitis herpetiformis. Both conditions often improve after treatment with a gluten-free diet.

Dermatographia

Sensitivity of the skin to mechanical irritation, to the extent that firm stroking leads to the appearance of itchy wheals (raised areas), which are slightly darker than the surrounding skin. The term dermatographia literally means "writing on the skin," and in fact it is sometimes possible with a few finger strokes actually to write visible words on the skin of a sufferer's back.

Dermatographia (also called dermographism) is a form of *urticaria* (hives) and is most common among fair-skinned people with a tendency to allergic conditions such as *eczema*.

Dermatologist

A physician who has been trained to treat problems relating to the skin, hair, and nails. Problems include everything from wrinkles, warts, and hair loss to acne, athlete's foot, and skin cancer. Treatment methods include medication (topical and/or oral), surgery, or the destruction of unwanted growths by freezing, burning, lasers, and radiation.

Dermatology

The study of *skin* diseases. Dermatology is involved with the study of the physiology and pathology of the skin and its appendages (e.g., hair, sweat glands, and oil glands). In the study of disease it includes investigation (such as examining skin scrapings under a microscope), diagnosis, and treatment, which principally consists of applying the appropriate creams, lotions, or ointments.

Dermatopathology is the study of the microscopic appearance of diseased skin tissue.

Skin diseases are relatively common, accounting for about 15 percent of all illnesses. In many instances no cause can be found or permanent cure provided. This is true for many cases of *psoriasis* and *eczema*, two of the most common skin conditions.

Dermatome

An area of skin supplied with nerves from one spinal root (see *Nervous system*). The entire surface of the body is an interlocking mosaic of dermatomes, the pattern of which is very similar from one person to another.

Loss of sensation in a dermatome signifies damage to a particular nerve root, the most usual cause of which is a *disk prolapse*.

Dermatome also refers to an instrument for cutting variable thicknesses of skin for use in skin grafting.

Dermatomyositis

A rare, sometimes fatal, disease in which the muscles and skin become inflamed, causing weakness of the muscles and a skin rash.

CAUSES AND INCIDENCE

The disorder belongs to a group of illnesses called the *autoimmune disorders*, in which, for reasons that are not fully understood, the body's defense system against disease starts attacking the body's own tissues. The condition is sometimes associated with underlying cancer of an internal organ. Two thirds of people suffering from dermatomyositis are middle-aged women.

SYMPTOMS

The first sign is often a red rash on the bridge of the nose and cheeks, followed by a purple discoloration on the eyelids and sometimes a red rash on the knees, knuckles, and elbows. Muscles then start to become weak, stiff, and painful, particularly those in the shoulders and pelvis where the limbs join the trunk. The skin over them feels thicker than normal. Sometimes the muscle pains precede the rash. The sufferer may also experience bouts of nausea, a loss of weight, and fever.

DIAGNOSIS AND TREATMENT

The diagnosis is confirmed by blood tests, electromyography (to detect the electrical activity of muscles; see *EMG*), and a *biopsy* (removal of a small piece of tissue for microscopic analysis) of skin or muscle.

Treatment is with *corticosteroid* and/or *immunosuppressant drugs* (to reduce the inflammation) and *physical therapy* (to prevent muscles from scarring and shrinking as they heal).

OUTLOOK

In about 50 percent of cases, full recovery occurs after a few years. In about 30 percent, the disease is persistent, causing muscle weakness. In the remaining 20 percent, it is progressive and affects the lungs and other organs and may be fatal.

Dermatophyte infections

A group of common fungal infections of the skin, hair, and nails, also called tineal infections (some are also called ringworm). Dermatophyte fungi can be spread from one person to another or from an animal such as a cat or dog to a person. The infections they cause usually have both a Latin name incorporating the term "tinea" and a common name—for example, tinea pedis (athlete's foot) and tinea capitis (ringworm of the scalp). (See *Tinea*.)

Dermoid cyst

A benign tumor with a cell structure similar to that of skin and containing hairs, sweat glands, and sebaceous glands. Fragments of cartilage, bone, and even teeth are also often found within such tumors.

About 10 percent of ovarian tumors are dermoid cysts. They are often readily diagnosed because the bony material within them is opaque to X rays. They very rarely become malignant (cancerous), but can enlarge up to several inches in diameter to cause discomfort and abdominal swelling. As with any enlarging ovarian tumor, surgery is recommended.

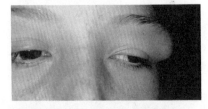

Appearance of dermoid cyst on head
The growth is firm, painless, and has an inner cavity that contains a fatty substance and sometimes hair, teeth, and bony material.

A dermoid cyst also sometimes develops in the skin of the head and neck, causing a small painless swelling, which may be removed for cosmetic reasons. This type of dermoid cyst is usually congenital and contains only skin structures.

Dermoid tumor

See *Dermoid cyst*.

DES

The abbreviation for the synthetic estrogen drug *diethylstilbestrol*.

Desensitization

A technique, used in *behavior therapy* for treating *phobias*, in which the patient is gradually exposed to the cause of the fear.

Desensitization, allergy

See *Immunotherapy*.

Designer drugs

> **WARNING**
> Designer drugs carry a high risk of *drug dependence*, with severe withdrawal reactions, and of *drug poisoning*, causing effects such as brain damage.

A group of illegally produced chemicals that mimics the effects of specific drugs of abuse. Made in illicit laboratories, these drugs are cheap to produce and thus undercut the street prices of drugs such as *LSD* and *amphetamine drugs*. Designer drugs are often made in such a way that their structures are subtly different from the drugs they imitate. As a result, these drugs escape the federal laws that control the manufacture and distribution of drugs listed under the Controlled Substance Act (CSA).

TYPES

Designer drugs can be divided into three major groups: those derived from narcotic *analgesics* (painkillers) such as meperidine and fentanyl; drugs that mimic amphetamine drugs (stimulants); and variants of phencyclidine (PCP), a drug originally used in animal anesthesia that causes hallucinations.

POSSIBLE ADVERSE EFFECTS

Designer drugs are highly potent. Some derivatives of fentanyl, for example, are between 20 to 2,000 times more powerful than *morphine*; this has led to a high incidence of death due to *drug poisoning*.

Amphetamine derivatives cause brain damage at doses only slightly higher than those required for a stimulant effect. Although they have been abused as aphrodisiacs, amphetamine derivatives commonly impair orgasm in both men and women and may prevent erection.

Many designer drugs contain impurities. For example, a substance known as MPTP, contained within an analogue (derivative) of meperidine, has caused permanent brain damage that has resulted in symptoms and signs of Parkinson's disease. Phencyclidine analogues often cause seizures and psychosis.

OUTLOOK

New laws are being introduced in many states to control the use of designer drugs. The Analogue Enforcement Act, if approved by Congress, will restrict the use of all such substances.

Desipramine

An *antidepressant drug*. It takes about 10 to 14 days before desipramine improves the condition of the person who is depressed. It has less of a sedative effect than some other antidepressants, and is therefore useful in treating patients for whom sedation is undesirable. Possible adverse effects include a dry mouth, and, rarely, constipation and blurred vision.

Desmoid tumor

A growth, usually in the abdominal wall. The tumor is hard, with a well-defined edge.

Desmoid tumors occur most frequently in women who have had children. Stretching or bruising of the abdominal muscle fibers during pregnancy may be a factor in their development. Desmoid tumors may also arise at the sites of old surgical incisions in the abdomen or elsewhere in the body, and they are often regarded as overgrowths of scar tissue.

Surgical excision is the usual treatment, although recurrence of the growth at the same site is common. *Radiation therapy* may arrest the growth of desmoid tumors.

Detergent poisoning

If swallowed, the cleaning agents in shampoos, laundry powders, and cleaning liquids cause vomiting, diarrhea, and a swollen abdomen. The treatment is to dilute the detergent by giving the victim plenty to drink. The same types of detergents can irritate the skin by removing its natural oils; people who constantly use them should protect their hands.

Developmental delay

A term used when a baby or young child has not achieved new abilities within the normal time range and has a pattern of behavior that is not appropriate for his or her age.

Development is an increase in the abilities—physical, intellectual, and social—and is a well-orchestrated process, with new abilities and new patterns of behavior appearing at given ages, while existing patterns of behavior change and sometimes disappear (see *Child development*).

Delays may be of varying severity and may affect any or all of the major areas of human achievement (i.e., development of the ability to walk upright, of fine hand-eye coordination, of listening, language, and speech, and of social interaction). Developmental delay is not a term used for slow increase in physical size (see *Growth; Short stature*) or for late appearance of sexual characteristics (see *Puberty*). The term developmental delay is not usually applied to children over the age of 5.

In general, the child who is slow in one or two aspects of development and of average or perhaps advanced ability in others needs to be distinguished from the child who is delayed in most aspects. When there is a significant delay in a few aspects, there may be a specific (although often not obvious) disability such as a visual or hearing impairment, which, if adequately treated, may allow the child to catch up. Children who are developmentally delayed in most aspects usually have a more generalized problem—for example, lack of adequate stimulation and teaching at home or a slowness to learn because of limited intellectual abilities.

CAUSES

Some important causes of generalized developmental delay are shown in the accompanying table. It is important to remember that a child born prematurely will reach most developmental milestones later than other children. Parents will want to recognize how old the baby would be if born at term rather than prematurely. Causes of delay in specific areas of development are outlined below.

WALKING AND MOVEMENT SKILLS There is an enormous time range within which most children learn to walk; children are not considered delayed unless they are not walking by themselves by 18 months.

In most late walkers, no serious cause is found. Late walking is an

inherited feature in some families and is probably due to delayed maturation of the nervous system. Such children learn to walk a few months later than other children, and from then on usually develop new skills at a normal rate. Other children develop slightly unusual patterns of locomotion—for example, creeping on their abdomens or shuffling on their bottoms. These traits also tend to run in families. Such children may miss out on the crawling stage. They eventually stand and walk and from then on follow the normal developmental sequence in all other developmental aspects.

A more specific reason for delayed walking and other skills is weakness of the leg muscles and other muscles. This can occur in boys with pseudohypertrophic *muscular dystrophy* and in children with *spina bifida*. *Cerebral palsy* is a disorder affecting all aspects of motor development; it may cause slowness and difficulty in gaining control of the head and neck muscles during the first months of life as well as delay in sitting and walking.

HAND-EYE COORDINATION Any defect of vision or of the nerves and muscles used to control fine finger movements may be a cause of delayed manipulative skills. However, the most common cause is not a specific abnormality but lack of experience—stimulation and encouragement are extremely important in the acquisition of these skills. If a child has only large toys to play with and is not encouraged to use the small finger muscles, skills involving the muscles will be delayed. Similarly, if a child is left lying down for most of the time instead of in a sitting position, the hands will not be in the correct position to acquire certain skills.

RESPONSE TO SOUND If a child is unresponsive to sound it may be due to deafness. However, children who are not talked to may show a lack of interest in the human voice, although they may respond normally to other sounds. Children exposed continually to a great deal of noise may show a general lack of interest in sound.

A rare cause of unresponsiveness to the human voice is the psychiatric condition of *autism*. An affected child can hear normally but shows little interest in human contact of any kind. Although unresponsive to human voices, autistic children often become obsessively interested in particular sound-producing toys.

SPEECH AND LANGUAGE The most important cause of delayed speech is deafness of any degree. Other common causes are lack of stimulation (when parents do not talk to the child sufficiently) and a familial pattern of delayed speech, which is more common in boys than girls. Twins are often late talkers, perhaps because they may receive less individual parental attention. Twins sometimes develop a private language that includes idiosyncratic words and nonverbal communication.

Children exposed to two or more languages may show signs of speech delay and may confuse the languages. However, many children become naturally bilingual or trilingual with no difficulties.

Any generalized difficulty with muscle control can affect speech production; muscle control can be a particular difficulty in children with cerebral palsy. Damage to, or structural defects of, the speech muscles,

larynx, or mouth may also cause speech difficulties, as may any disorder affecting the speech area of the brain (see *Dysarthria; Dysphonia; Aphasia; Speech disorders*).

BLADDER AND BOWEL CONTROL Children vary enormously in the age at which confident control of bowel and bladder function is acquired. Usually bowel function is acquired first. Delay in bladder control is much more common than delayed bowel control. There are many possible causes. (See *Incontinence, urinary; Enuresis; Incontinence, fecal; Encopresis*.)

ASSESSMENT AND TREATMENT
In many instances, the parents will be the first to notice that their child is not acquiring new skills at the same rate as his or her peers. A physician should be consulted. Problems are sometimes detected during one of the developmental checks that are carried out routinely in the US and other developed countries. These checks are performed by physicians or other health professionals at varying ages, but usually at birth, 6 weeks, 6 to 8 months, 12 to 15 months, 2 years, 3 years, and 5 years.

If a developmental delay is discovered, the first step is to establish the cause by undertaking a full assessment. This examination usually includes hearing and vision testing, a full physical examination, and thorough developmental assessment. Further investigation is arranged as necessary. It may include referral to a pediatrician, neurologist, psychologist, speech therapist, occupational therapist, or physical therapist.

Once the severity of the delay, and the probable cause, has been discovered, appropriate treatment can be arranged. In many cases, the parents can be reassured that there is no serious abnormality and that their child can be expected to develop normally without any specific treatment. Sometimes advice is given regarding suitable toys and other stimulation.

Specific treatment may include provision of glasses or a hearing aid; treatment may also include a lengthy course of speech therapy or psychiatric counseling for the whole family. In some cases it is felt that the child's best interests are served by admission to a special school for children with specific difficulties—for example, a language unit or a school for physically handicapped children. Whatever the cause, children can be helped to achieve their full potential by provision of appropriate therapy.

Professionals are usually involved in assessing the abilities of a child and deciding on the appropriate help. Parents are often of prime importance in providing this help.

Deviation, sexual

A form of sexual behavior in which intercourse between adults is not the final aim. Instead, the man (deviation is rare in women) achieves erection and orgasm in other ways, such as by being whipped or wearing women's clothes. Forms of sexual deviation include *exhibitionism, transvestism, fetishism, frottage, necrophilia, pedophilia, sadism,* and *masochism.*

Dexamethasone

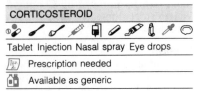

CORTICOSTEROID			
Tablet	Injection	Nasal spray	Eye drops

	Prescription needed
	Available as generic

Dexamethasone is a *corticosteroid drug* prescribed as a nasal spray to relieve nasal congestion caused by allergic *rhinitis* (hay fever) and as eye drops in the treatment of *iritis* (inflammation of the iris). It is given in tablet form to treat severe cases of *asthma* and to reduce inflammation of the brain due to *head injury, stroke,* or a *brain tumor.* Occasionally, dexamethasone is injected into an inflamed joint to ease pain and stiffness caused, for example, by osteoarthritis.

POSSIBLE ADVERSE EFFECTS
Taken as a nasal spray or in eye-drop form, minor local side effects, such as a nosebleed or eye irritation, may occur. When prescribed as a tablet, either for a prolonged period or in high doses, adverse effects common to other corticosteroids may occur.

Dextroamphetamine

A central nervous system stimulant (see *Stimulants*). Dextroamphetamine is prescribed for *narcolepsy* (a rare condition characterized by excessive sleepiness). Paradoxically, it is also used to treat children with *hyperactivity,* although the reason it helps in this condition is not known.

Dextroamphetamine is no longer recommended as an *appetite suppressant* for people who are attempting to lose weight.

ABUSE
Because of its stimulant properties, dextroamphetamine has become a drug of abuse. It is one of a group of

drugs commonly referred to as "uppers." If use is prolonged, the stimulant effects lessen and a higher dose must be taken to produce the desired effect. In an overdose, dextroamphetamine can cause seizures and hypertension.

Dextrocardia

A rare condition, present from birth, in which the heart is situated in, and points toward, the right-hand side of the chest instead of the left. The heart may also, but not necessarily, be malformed. Sometimes, the position of the abdominal organs is also reversed, so that the liver is on the left-hand side and the stomach on the right. When all organs are on the opposite side of the body from where they are customarily found, it is known as *situs inversus*.

The cause of dextrocardia is unknown. No treatment is necessary unless the heart is malformed, in which case surgery may be necessary (see *Heart disease, congenital*).

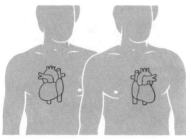

Abnormal position   Normal position

Heart positions
In dextrocardia, the heart is situated in, and points toward, the right-hand side of the chest instead of the left.

Dextrose

Another name for *glucose*, one of the monosaccharide sugars. Dextrose is absorbed from digested *carbohydrates* through the intestinal wall into the bloodstream. It is also available in the form of tablets, as an injection used in the emergency treatment of *hypoglycemia* (low blood sugar), and as a component of feedings given by infusion (see *Feeding, artificial*).

Diabetes, bronze

Another name for *hemochromatosis*, a rare disease in which excessive amounts of iron are deposited in tissues such as the liver, pancreas, and skin. Its name comes from the bronze skin coloration and *diabetes mellitus* that usually develop in people who suffer from this disorder.

Diabetes insipidus

A rare condition characterized by the passing of enormous quantities of dilute urine (polyuria) and excessive thirst (polydipsia). These symptoms also occur, in a milder form, early in *diabetes mellitus*, a much more common disease that in all other respects is different from diabetes insipidus.

CAUSES

Diabetes insipidus usually results from a failure of the *pituitary gland* to secrete antidiuretic hormone (*ADH*). Normally, this hormone diminishes the amount of water passed by the kidneys into the urine to maintain a constant dilution of the blood. Diseases of the pituitary, including damage from injury or a tumor, can cause failure of secretion.

In rare cases, the disease (called nephrogenic diabetes insipidus) is due to failure of the kidneys to respond to normal levels of ADH. This type is usually congenital (present from birth), but may result from a kidney disease called *pyelonephritis*.

SYMPTOMS, DIAGNOSIS, AND TREATMENT

A person with diabetes insipidus may pass between 10 and 40 pints of urine every 24 hours—provided this output is matched by a similar intake of water. If water is unobtainable or withheld, the signs and symptoms of *dehydration* will appear, leading to confusion, stupor, and coma.

Treatment is normally by administration of a synthetic variety of antidiuretic hormone. This, however, is ineffective in treating people with the nephrogenic variety of the disease. These people must be placed on a low-sodium diet and treated with a drug that slows the development of thirst symptoms.

Diabetes mellitus

A disorder in which the pancreas produces insufficient or no *insulin*, the hormone responsible for the absorption of glucose into cells for their energy needs and into the liver and fat cells for storage. As a result, the level of glucose in the blood becomes abnormally high, causing excessive urination and constant thirst and hunger. The body's inability to store or use glucose causes weight loss and fatigue. Diabetes mellitus also results in disordered *lipid* metabolism and accelerated degeneration of small blood vessels.

Apart from the symptoms of thirst and excessive urination, the disease has nothing in common with the much rarer disorder *diabetes insipidus*.

There are two main types of diabetes mellitus. Insulin-dependent (type I) diabetes, the more severe form, usually first appears in people under the age of 35 and most commonly in people between the ages of 10 and 16. It develops rapidly. The insulin-secreting cells in the pancreas are destroyed, probably as a result of an *immune response* after a virus infection, and insulin production ceases almost completely. Without regular injections of insulin, the sufferer lapses into a coma and dies.

The other main type, non-insulin-dependent (type II) diabetes, is usually of gradual onset and occurs mainly in people over 40. In many cases it is discovered only during a routine medical examination. Insulin is produced, but not enough to meet the body's needs, especially when the person is overweight. Often the body is resistant to the effects of insulin. In most cases, insulin-replacement injections are not required; the combination of dietary measures, weight reduction, and oral medication keeps the condition under control.

CAUSES AND INCIDENCE

Diabetes mellitus tends to run in families. However, of those who inherit the genes responsible for the insulin-dependent form, only a very small proportion eventually develop the disease. In these cases the disorder possibly occurs as the delayed result of a viral infection that had damaged the pancreas several years earlier.

In the case of non-insulin-dependent diabetes, the greater proportion of people predisposed to the disease by heredity (primarily those who are overweight) go on to acquire it.

Although obesity is the primary cause of unmasking latent diabetes, other causes that can unmask or aggravate diabetes are certain illnesses (among them *pancreatitis* and *thyrotoxicosis*), certain drugs (including some corticosteroids and some diuretics), infections, and pregnancy (see *Diabetic pregnancy*).

In the US about two persons per 1,000 have insulin-dependent diabetes by the age of 20; overall, the insulin-dependent form affects about 150 to 200 persons per 100,000. Non-insulin-dependent diabetes is more common, with as many as 2,000 persons per 100,000 affected.

DIAGNOSIS

A physician who suspects diabetes in a patient can often obtain confirmation from testing a sample of urine for its glucose level. Further confirmation

D

LIVING WITH DIABETES MELLITUS

As the level of glucose in the blood rises, the volume of urine required to carry it out of the body is increased, causing not only a continuous need to urinate but also constant thirst. The high levels of sugar in the blood and urine impair the body's ability to fight infection, leading to urinary tract infections (such as *cystitis* and *pyelonephritis*), vaginal yeast infections (*candidiasis*), and recurrent skin infections.

Because the body's cells are starved of glucose, the sufferer feels weak and fatigued. The cells are able to obtain some energy from the breakdown of stored fat, resulting in weight loss. However, the chemical processes involved in this breakdown of fat are defective (especially in insulin-dependent diabetics), leading to the production of acids and substances called ketones, which can cause coma and sometimes death.

Other possible symptoms of undiagnosed diabetes include blurred vision, boils, increased appetite, and tingling and numbness in the hands and feet.

Symptoms develop in all untreated insulin-dependent diabetics, but symptoms develop in only one third of those with the non-insulin-dependent type. There are many people suffering from a mild form of the disease who are unaware of it. The disease often is diagnosed only after complications of the diabetes have been detected.

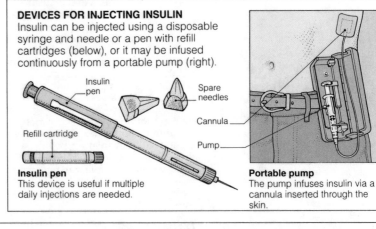

Fatigue
Blurred vision
Constant thirst
Muscle weakness
Pyelonephritis and continual need to urinate
Cystitis
Candidiasis
Tingling and numbness in hands and feet

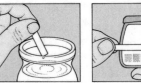

Testing urine for glucose
Urine can be tested for glucose by means of a chemically impregnated strip dipped into a sample of urine. The resulting color change in the strip is compared with a chart to indicate the glucose level.

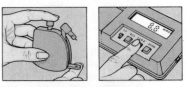

Direct testing of blood glucose
A pricking device is used to obtain blood, which is spread on a chemically coated strip. The strip is inserted into an instrument that reads the blood glucose.

DEVICES FOR INJECTING INSULIN

Insulin can be injected using a disposable syringe and needle or a pen with refill cartridges (below), or it may be infused continuously from a portable pump (right).

Insulin pen
Spare needles
Cannula
Pump
Refill cartridge

Insulin pen
This device is useful if multiple daily injections are needed.

Portable pump
The pump infuses insulin via a cannula inserted through the skin.

is secured when significantly high glucose levels are obtained from blood samples following an overnight fast or from samples taken two hours after a meal. Glucose-tolerance tests are not usually required.

TREATMENT

The aims of treatment are to prolong life, relieve symptoms, and prevent long-term complications. Success depends on keeping the level of blood glucose as near normal as possible through maintenance of normal weight, regular physical activity, and careful dietary management.

In people with insulin-dependent diabetes, treatment consists of regular self-injections, one to four times a day, with insulin (either obtained from animals or of a human type synthesized by *genetic engineering*). In addition, the person must follow a diet in which carbohydrate intake is regulated and spread out over the day according to a consistent timetable. In this way, marked fluctuations in the glucose levels in the blood can be avoided.

Disturbances in the careful balance between insulin and glucose intake can result in *hyperglycemia* (too much glucose in the blood), causing the symptoms of the untreated disease, or *hypoglycemia* (too little glucose), which can lead to weakness, confusion, dizziness, sweating, and even unconsciousness and seizures. To help prevent this, diabetics (of both types) are advised to regularly moni-

tor their blood and urine glucose levels with do-it-yourself testing kits.

For difficult-to-control diabetes, an insulin pump is an alternative treatment for those who are willing to monitor their blood glucose levels carefully. Insulin is continuously infused from a refillable pump through a needle implanted in the skin. Control is often no better than that for multiple daily injections.

As a precaution against an attack of hypoglycemia, insulin-dependent diabetics need to carry some sugar or glucose with them at all times. Because of the disabling effects of hypoglycemia, insulin-dependent diabetics who drive must declare their disorder to insurance companies and car-licensing authorities. Those with poorly controlled insulin-dependent diabetes are sometimes advised against doing jobs that involve working at a height or operating a public conveyance, and against engaging in activities like race-car driving or flying, where they may be a danger to themselves and others.

Because the pancreas does produce some insulin in non-insulin-dependent diabetics, the disorder can often be controlled by dietary means alone (regulating the carbohydrate intake with meals spaced out over the day). This not only lowers the blood glucose level, but also reduces weight. If diet fails to lower the glucose level sufficiently, *hypoglycemic* tablets (oral antidiabetic drugs that stimulate the pancreas to produce more insulin) may be prescribed, though these are ineffective unless dietary restrictions are observed.

All people with mild diabetes need regular advice from their physicians so that any complications can be detected and treated at an early stage. Diabetics should wear or carry information identifying them as diabetics in case of an emergency.

COMPLICATIONS
Complications eventually develop in a large number of diabetics. These complications tend to be more likely if the diabetes has not been well controlled, but they can occur even if there has been good control. Complications include *retinopathy* (damage to the retina, the light-sensitive area at the back of the eye, and the blood vessels serving it), peripheral *neuropathy* (damage to nerve fibers), and *nephropathy* (kidney damage). Ulcers on the feet, which in severe cases can develop into gangrene, are another risk, but with good foot care they can usually be prevented.

Diabetics also have a higher-than-average risk of *atherosclerosis* (narrowing of the arteries), *hypertension* (high blood pressure), other *cardiovascular disorders*, and *cataracts* (opacities of the lens of the eye).

There are, however, people who have lived full and active lives with diabetes mellitus for 50 years or more with few complications.

OUTLOOK
With modern treatment and sensible self-monitoring, almost all diabetics can look forward to a normal life. The life expectancy of people who have well-regulated, insulin-dependent diabetes is little different than that of nondiabetics. Those with the non-insulin-dependent illness have a slightly reduced life expectancy because of circulatory and heart disorders, which often are present when the diabetes is diagnosed.

Diabetic pregnancy
A small number of women acquire *diabetes mellitus* during pregnancy—a phenomenon called gestational diabetes. Diabetes mellitus may also have been present and under treatment before pregnancy. In both cases, special precautions are necessary.

PREEXISTING DIABETES
Nearly all women with established diabetes mellitus can have a normal pregnancy, provided the diabetes is well controlled throughout. It is important to plan the pregnancy and to make sure that the blood glucose level is under particularly good control before and at the time of conception; otherwise there is a slightly increased chance of the baby being malformed. If control is poor during the pregnancy, there may be an increase in the amount of glucose reaching the baby (which makes the baby grow faster than normal) and this may cause difficulties at birth. Also, the growth of infants of diabetic mothers may be stunted; these babies may have complications in the days immediately after birth.

GESTATIONAL DIABETES
Gestational diabetes is most often detected in the second half of pregnancy, when increased glucose appears in the urine or the baby is found to be bigger than expected when a physician examines the mother's abdomen (though these findings do not always mean the mother is diabetic). Apparently, not enough insulin is produced to keep the blood glucose levels normal during the pregnancy. Obstetricians now screen for diabetes at 26 weeks. Gestational diabetes usually disappears with the delivery of the baby, but can be a sign of future diabetes in up to three fourths of these mothers.

CARE
When feasible, diabetic pregnancies are treated at high-risk obstetrical centers (many of which offer prepregnancy clinics for those with established diabetes to help achieve good control before conception) and at antenatal clinics to supervise all aspects of the pregnancy.

The chances that the baby of a diabetic parent will become diabetic are about one in 100 and, if both parents are diabetic, about one in 20. If only the father is diabetic, no special precautions need to be taken at conception or during the pregnancy.

Diacetylmorphine
A synthetic drug similar to *morphine*, usually referred to by its popular name, *heroin*.

Diagnosis
The determination by a physician of the cause of a person's problem. Usually this entails identifying both the disease process—pneumonia or cirrhosis of the liver, for example—and the agent responsible, such as pneumonia due to legionnaires' disease, or cirrhosis due to alcohol. Diagnosis is part science and part art; an experienced physician relies not only on his or her scientific knowledge and experience, but also on intuition to recognize the pattern of an illness and establish a diagnosis.

THE MEDICAL HISTORY
The patient's own account of his or her illness is perhaps the most important part of the diagnostic procedure. This history provides vital clues, which can then be augmented by questions from the physician in an exchange that may last some 20 to 30 minutes in a complex case or if the physician has not previously seen the patient. What the physician is looking for is a pattern of symptoms that is strongly suggestive of a single disease. For example, the features of a migraine headache, duodenal ulcer, enlarged prostate gland, or angina pectoris are often unmistakable.

In some circumstances the physician may not attempt to reach a final diagnosis. If a patient has had only a sore throat for 48 hours, the physician may be content to treat the condition symptomatically, attempting to relieve the symptoms while awaiting the results of a throat culture or other laboratory tests.

However, when symptoms have been more prolonged, the physician will want to reach at least a provisional diagnosis before beginning treatment, partly because any treatment is likely to affect the symptoms and thus make diagnosis more difficult.

EXAMINATION AND TESTS
Tests may be ordered after a physical examination and the formation of a provisional diagnosis.

However, confirmation is obtained in a variety of ways, including tissue biopsy, culture of microorganisms, or finding the cause at surgery. If specific treatment (either with drugs or by

D

STEPS IN DIAGNOSING A CONDITION

A physician may go through several steps to ascertain the cause of a person's problem. The history, physical examination, and tests may provide vital clues. A physician usually makes at least a provisional diagnosis before beginning any treatment because treatment can mask symptoms, making the physician's job of establishing an exact diagnosis more difficult.

Taking the medical history

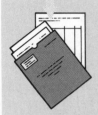

Perhaps the most important part of the diagnostic procedure is the patient's own account of his or her illness – the medical history. "Listen to the patients, they are telling you their diagnosis" is the traditional teaching given to medical students. Many physicians believe that the medical history provides the strongest basis for ascertaining a diagnosis. The added information derived from the physical examination is small, but at times, critical.

Conducting a physical examination

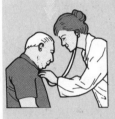

After the medical history has been obtained, the physician has in mind a short list of probable diagnoses. A physical examination helps shorten the list. The physician is then left with a differential diagnosis. A differential diagnosis is a group of possible diseases that could account for the patterns of symptoms and signs (i.e., physical findings, such as enlargements of lymph glands or tenderness in a specific region of the abdomen).

Ordering special tests

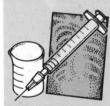

Next, based on his or her working diagnosis, the physician may order a series of laboratory tests on the blood (and sometimes the urine) and may also arrange for diagnostic imaging of suspect organs by techniques such as *ultrasound scanning, X rays,* *CT scanning, MRI,* or *radionuclide scanning.* The results of these tests either confirm the physician's working diagnosis or narrow the possibilities so the physician may be confident that he or she has found the correct diagnosis.

Using a computer

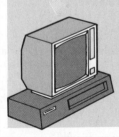

Physicians today also use computer systems and algorithms to help reach a diagnosis. Both approaches rely on analysis of large numbers of patient records to quantify probabilities and to devise an orderly series of questions – a decision tree. The main purpose of computer assistance is to remind the physician of the full range of possible diagnoses for a particular set of symptoms, thereby making it less likely that any possibility will be overlooked. It remains the task of the physician to integrate the facts and decide upon a diagnosis.

surgery) relieves the symptoms and cures the patient, the diagnosis is likely to have been correct—although it is also possible that the patient may have recovered spontaneously and the treatment may simply have coincided with the time of recovery. Alternatively, if the patient dies, a pathologist can usually, but not always, determine by postmortem examination (see *Autopsy*) what the disease process had been.

Diagnosis-related group

A system of payment for medical service to patients getting care from certain provider organizations and to *Medicare* patients. The system was established by amendments to the Social Security Act in 1983.

Under the diagnosis-related group (DRG) system, hospitalized patients are classified into one of 467 diagnosis-related groups; hospitals are then reimbursed at a set rate for each of the diagnosis categories. If the costs of a patient's care exceed the fixed rate, the hospital must absorb the cost. But, if the hospital's costs are less than the set rate, it may retain the difference. By determining costs prospectively, hospitals presumably have an incentive to manage patient care efficiently. Under the former system of retrospective payments, hospitals had little incentive to monitor costs.

Dialysis

A technique used to remove waste products from the blood and excess fluid from the body as a treatment for *renal failure* (kidney failure).

WHY IT IS DONE

The main function of the kidneys is the maintenance of *electrolyte* and water balance and the excretion of waste products. Fully one fifth of the blood pumped by the heart goes to the kidneys; the kidneys filter approximately 150 liters of blood daily. From this volume of blood, the kidney reabsorbs important elements, such as sodium, potassium, calcium, amino acids, glucose, and water. The kidneys excrete, as urine, the protein breakdown product nitrogen in the form of urea, as well as other excess minerals, toxins, and drugs.

In people whose kidneys have been damaged, this process may fail— either suddenly (in acute renal failure) or gradually (in the chronic form of the disease). Wastes start to accumulate in the blood, with harmful, sometimes life-threatening effects. In severe cases, the function of the kidneys must be taken over by the artificial means of dialysis. In cases of acute kidney failure, dialysis continues until the kidneys recover and start functioning normally again. However, in chronic kidney failure, patients may need to undergo dialysis for the rest of their lives or until they can be given a *kidney transplant.* Dialysis therapy may not always be chosen by the patient and physician when kidney failure is simply a part of an otherwise rapidly fatal disorder.

PROCEDURE FOR DIALYSIS

There are two methods of removing wastes from the blood and excess fluid from the body when the kidneys have failed. The first, hemodialysis, may also be used as emergency treatment in some cases of poisoning or drug overdose. It makes use of an artificial kidney (or "kidney machine") and can be carried out at home. Peritoneal dialysis, also done in the home, requires an abdominal incision (which is done in the hospital).

HOW HEMODIALYSIS IS DONE

1 Access to the bloodstream for rapid removal and return of blood is obtained by a shunt connecting an artery to a vein.

2 A needle connected to plastic tubing passes blood to the artificial kidney and back to the patient. The artificial kidney consists of many layers of special membrane.

Machine that prepares dialysate

Blood into dialyzer

Dialysate to and from dialyzer

4 The dialysate is discarded and the purified blood is returned to the patient. Each session lasts two to six hours.

WHY IT IS DONE

In people with damaged kidneys, the process of maintaining the balance of electrolytes and water, and of excreting waste products, may fail, causing harmful, if not life-threatening, effects. Dialysis can take over the function of the kidneys until they start working normally again. Or dialysis can function for the kidneys for the rest of a seriously affected person's life if a kidney transplant is not performed.

Diseased kidney
The kidney at right was removed from a person with adult polycystic kidney disease—one of many disorders that may damage kidney function to the extent that dialysis is needed.

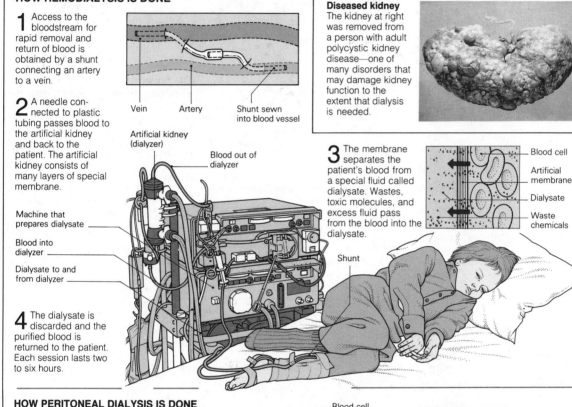

Vein   Artery   Shunt sewn into blood vessel

Artificial kidney (dialyzer)

Blood out of dialyzer

Blood cell

Artificial membrane

Dialysate

Waste chemicals

3 The membrane separates the patient's blood from a special fluid called dialysate. Wastes, toxic molecules, and excess fluid pass from the blood into the dialysate.

Shunt

HOW PERITONEAL DIALYSIS IS DONE

1 A small abdominal incision is made (using a local anesthetic); a catheter is inserted through it into the peritoneal cavity. Dialysate from a bag attached to the catheter passes into the cavity, where it is left for several hours.

Spinal column

Catheter

Fluid

Bag   Bladder

Blood cell

Fluid   Peritoneal membrane   Capillary wall

2 Waste products and excess water from the blood vessels lining the peritoneal cavity seep through the peritoneal membrane into the cavity and mix with the dialysate. The fluid is then allowed to drain out (by the release of a clamp) through the catheter and into the empty dialysate bag.

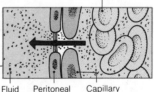

3 The bag is discarded and replaced with a bag containing fresh dialysate. The process, which takes about an hour, is repeated during the day or overnight.

D

HOW IT IS DONE

There are two methods of dialysis. Hemodialysis, which removes wastes by passing blood through an artificial kidney machine, was pioneered early in the 1940s. Peritoneal dialysis, which makes use of a natural filtering membrane within the body's abdomen, was developed in the early 1970s.

In most cases, hemodialysis is performed in outpatient dialysis centers by trained staff nurses, but, in the US, 5 percent of patients undergoing dialysis carry it out themselves with a kidney machine installed in the home.

Peritoneal dialysis may be performed in a hospital, but an increasing number of patients are now able, once the catheter has been inserted into the abdomen, to carry out the dialysis themselves at home, a procedure known as continuous ambulatory peritoneal dialysis.

For patients with chronic kidney failure, hemodialysis needs to be carried out several times a week. In the treatment of acute kidney failure, the process is carried out more intensively over a period of days or weeks until the kidneys are working normally again. Complications of hemodialysis may include weakening of the bones (see *Osteomalacia; Osteodystrophy*), anemia, infections, and pericarditis. Complications of peritoneal dialysis are the same as for hemodialysis along with peritonitis.

OUTLOOK

Long-term dialysis enables people who would once have died from chronic kidney failure to live relatively normal lives. Their diet and fluid intake must be restricted somewhat and they may not feel completely well. However, many do return to full or part-time employment. Since the patient's health is invariably affected in the long run, many physicians feel that dialysis should be replaced with a kidney transplant, which, if successful, can bring about a dramatic restoration of general health.

Diaper rash

A common condition affecting babies with otherwise healthy skin. Diaper rash results from skin irritation by substances contained in the feces or urine. Friction from rough diapers and prolonged wetting also play a part. Babies vary in their susceptibility to diaper rash. Occasionally, skin inflammation is severe. In some babies, diaper rash may be the first indication of sensitive skin and future skin problems, such as *eczema*.

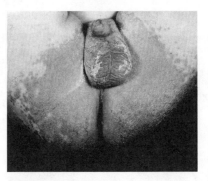

Symptoms of diaper rash
The skin over the buttocks, genitals, and inner thighs becomes red and sore at first, and may progress to blistering.

TREATMENT AND OUTLOOK

Prevention is better than cure. The aim is to keep the baby's skin dry for as long as possible. A newborn breast-fed baby passes urine about 20 times each day and has a bowel movement after each feeding, so this presents a major practical problem. Change diapers frequently and, after each change, apply a water-repellent emollient. Ideally, the diaper should be left off for an hour or so each day.

Cloth diapers should be well rinsed and kept soft. Sometimes an ointment containing a mild *corticosteroid drug* needs to be prescribed to suppress the inflammation. It is often prescribed in combination with an antifungal drug to kill any thrush organisms that are present (see *Candidiasis*).

Diaphragm, contraceptive

The most commonly used female barrier method of contraception, in the form of a hemispherical dome of thin rubber with a coiled metal spring in the rim. The diaphragm is individually fitted to each woman. (See *Contraception, barrier methods.*)

Diaphragm muscle

The dome-shaped sheet of muscle that separates the thorax (chest) from the abdomen. The diaphragm is attached to the spine, ribs, and sternum.

The diaphragm plays a vital role in breathing. For air to be drawn into the lungs, the muscle fibers of the diaphragm contract, thereby pulling the central tendon downward. This action enlarges the chest, and air passes into the lungs to fill the increased space. (See also *Breathing.*)

ANATOMY OF THE DIAPHRAGM

The diaphragm is attached to the spine, the lower pairs of ribs, and the lower end of the sternum (breastbone). The muscle fibers of the diaphragm converge on the central tendon, a thick, flat plate of dense fibers. There are openings in the diaphragm for the esophagus, phrenic nerve (which controls diaphragm movements and hence breathing), and the aorta and vena cava blood vessels.

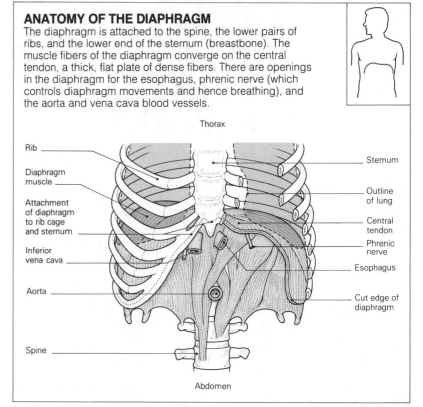

Thorax

Rib

Diaphragm muscle

Attachment of diaphragm to rib cage and sternum

Inferior vena cava

Aorta

Spine

Sternum

Outline of lung

Central tendon

Phrenic nerve

Esophagus

Cut edge of diaphragm

Abdomen

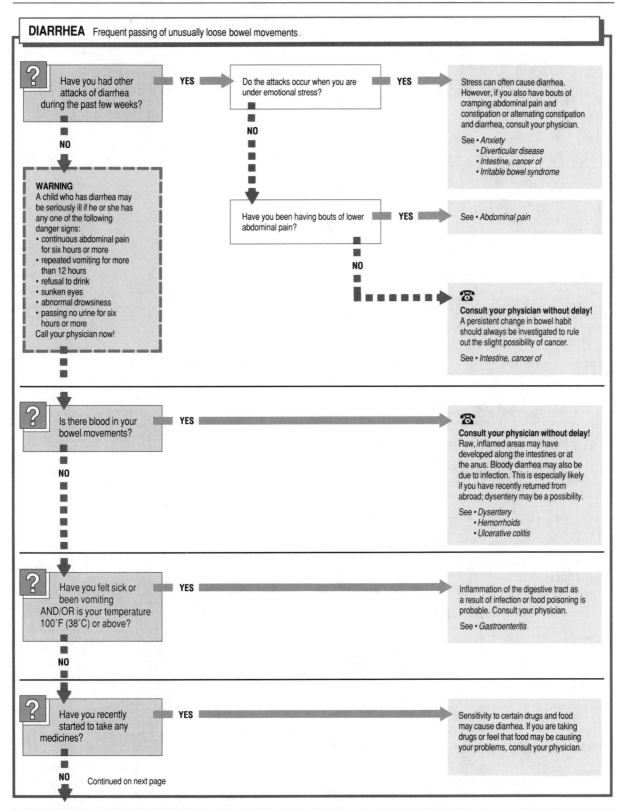

DIARRHEA Frequent passing of unusually loose bowel movements.

Have you had other attacks of diarrhea during the past few weeks?

YES → **Do the attacks occur when you are under emotional stress?**

YES → Stress can often cause diarrhea. However, if you also have bouts of cramping abdominal pain and constipation or alternating constipation and diarrhea, consult your physician.

See • *Anxiety*
• *Diverticular disease*
• *Intestine, cancer of*
• *Irritable bowel syndrome*

NO ↓

WARNING
A child who has diarrhea may be seriously ill if he or she has any one of the following danger signs:
• continuous abdominal pain for six hours or more
• repeated vomiting for more than 12 hours
• refusal to drink
• sunken eyes
• abnormal drowsiness
• passing no urine for six hours or more
Call your physician now!

Have you been having bouts of lower abdominal pain?

YES → See • *Abdominal pain*

NO ↓

☎ **Consult your physician without delay!**
A persistent change in bowel habit should always be investigated to rule out the slight possibility of cancer.

See • *Intestine, cancer of*

Is there blood in your bowel movements?

YES → ☎ **Consult your physician without delay!**
Raw, inflamed areas may have developed along the intestines or at the anus. Bloody diarrhea may also be due to infection. This is especially likely if you have recently returned from abroad; dysentery may be a possibility.

See • *Dysentery*
• *Hemorrhoids*
• *Ulcerative colitis*

NO ↓

Have you felt sick or been vomiting AND/OR is your temperature 100°F (38°C) or above?

YES → Inflammation of the digestive tract as a result of infection or food poisoning is probable. Consult your physician.

See • *Gastroenteritis*

NO ↓

Have you recently started to take any medicines?

YES → Sensitivity to certain drugs and food may cause diarrhea. If you are taking drugs or feel that food may be causing your problems, consult your physician.

NO ↓ Continued on next page

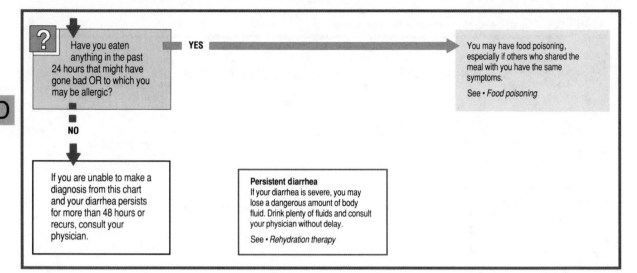

Have you eaten anything in the past 24 hours that might have gone bad OR to which you may be allergic?

YES → You may have food poisoning, especially if others who shared the meal with you have the same symptoms.

See • *Food poisoning*

NO ↓

If you are unable to make a diagnosis from this chart and your diarrhea persists for more than 48 hours or recurs, consult your physician.

Persistent diarrhea
If your diarrhea is severe, you may lose a dangerous amount of body fluid. Drink plenty of fluids and consult your physician without delay.

See • *Rehydration therapy*

Diarrhea

Increased fluidity, frequency, or volume of bowel movements, as compared to the usual pattern for a particular person. Diarrhea itself is not a disorder but is a symptom of an underlying problem.

Acute diarrhea affects almost everybody from time to time—usually as the result of eating contaminated food or drinking contaminated water. These attacks normally clear up within a day or two with or without treatment. Chronic diarrhea may be due to a serious intestinal disorder and requires investigation by a physician.

Diarrhea in infants is generally more serious than diarrhea in adults because it is more likely to cause severe, even potentially fatal, *dehydration*. However, elderly people also do not tolerate diarrhea well, and possible dehydration must be anticipated and treated immediately.

DIARRHEA IN ADULTS

In normal bowel activity the colon (large intestine) absorbs much of the water from the food residues (in liquid form) that pass through it, producing semisolid feces. If the intestinal contents pass through the colon too quickly, or if the small intestine is inflamed and secretes fluid into the fecal material, diarrhea may result.

CAUSES

Acute diarrhea starts abruptly and usually lasts from a few hours to two or three days. The most common cause is *food poisoning*. Diarrhea that starts within six hours of eating usually indicates that the food has been contaminated by toxins from *STAPHYLOCOCCUS* or *CLOSTRIDIUM* bacteria. If diarrhea develops 12 to 48 hours after eating, it is probably due to contamination by bacteria such as *SALMONELLA* or *CAMPYLOBACTER*, or by a virus such as the rotavirus or Norwalk virus. Infective *gastroenteritis* may also be acquired as a result of droplet infection, with adenoviruses or echoviruses, for example. Acute diarrhea may be caused by interference with the intestinal flora (harmless bacteria in the intestine) as a result of travel to a country where these bacteria are of a different type.

Other causes of acute diarrhea include anxiety and, less commonly, *shigellosis, typhoid* and *paratyphoid*, drug toxicity, *food allergy*, and *food intolerance*. In the case of shigellosis and *amebic dysentery*, there may be blood in the feces.

Chronic diarrhea generally takes the form of repeated attacks of acute diarrhea. Causes include *Crohn's disease, ulcerative colitis, diverticular disease*, cancer of the large intestine (see *Intestine, cancer of*), *thyrotoxicosis*, and *irritable bowel syndrome*. In all of these conditions, except thyrotoxicosis and irritable bowel syndrome, there may be blood in the bowel movements.

TREATMENT

The water and electrolytes (salts) lost during a severe attack of diarrhea need to be replaced to prevent dehydration. An effective means of doing this is to drink water to which salt and sugar have been added. To make up such an oral rehydration solution, dissolve one teaspoon of salt and four teaspoons of sugar (which helps the intestine absorb the water and salt) in one quart (0.95 liter) of water. It is important to be accurate with the measurements as too much salt may cause further dehydration. Alternatively, it is possible to buy ready-prepared electrolyte mixtures that also contain small amounts of potassium replacement that need only to be added to a specific amount of water. A pint of the oral rehydration liquid should be drunk every hour, and no solid food eaten, until the diarrhea subsides.

Antidiarrheal drugs should not be taken to treat attacks of diarrhea resulting from infection because they may prolong the illness.

Diarrhea that recurs, persists for more than a week, or is accompanied by blood in the bowel movements requires investigation to discover the underlying cause. In addition to taking the patient's case history, the physician will probably arrange for a stool *culture* to determine whether or not infection is the underlying cause. If it is not, other tests may be carried out, such as a barium enema or meal (see *Barium X-ray examinations*), *sigmoidoscopy*, and a *biopsy* of the rectum. These tests enable the physician to discover the underlying cause; treatment will be for that cause.

DIARRHEA IN INFANTS

Most cases of diarrhea in infants are of the acute form, which carries the risk of rapid dehydration (especially when accompanied by vomiting); it can be fatal unless countered quickly.

CAUSES

The most common cause is gastroenteritis resulting from a viral infection. Babies who are entirely breast-fed are less likely to contract the illness than those who have been bottle-fed. Viral gastroenteritis can damage the lining of the small intestine, thereby impairing its ability to absorb nutrients, and can cause a temporary deficiency of the enzyme lactase. The latter may lead to lactose intolerance (inability to absorb sugar from milk), which may produce secondary diarrhea that can last for several weeks.

TREATMENT

An infant who shows signs of dehydration (drowsiness, unresponsiveness, prolonged crying, loose skin, glazed eyes, a depressed fontanelle at the front of the head, and a dry, sticky mouth and tongue) needs urgent medical attention. In other cases, the baby should not be fed milk, and an electrolyte mixture (obtainable from a pharmacist) should be given to replace lost water and salts.

If the diarrhea persists for more than 48 hours, a physician should be consulted. However, if the diarrhea clears up within this period, milk can be gradually reintroduced over a 24-hour period. The first feeding should consist of one part milk to three parts water, the second of equal parts of milk and water, the third of three parts milk to one part water, and the fourth of undiluted milk.

Diastole

The resting period of the heart muscle; it alternates with the period of muscular contraction (*systole*).

Diathermy

The production of heat in a part of the body using high-frequency electric currents, microwaves, or ultrasound. The heat generated can be used to increase blood flow and to reduce deep-seated pain in rheumatic and arthritic conditions. By using large currents, enough heat can be produced to bloodlessly destroy tumors and diseased parts. A diathermy knife is used by surgeons to coagulate bleeding vessels or to separate tissues without causing them to bleed (see *Electrocoagulation*).

Diathesis

A condition of the body that makes the tissues react in a specific way to an outside stimulus. For example, a bleeding diathesis is present when a *bleeding disorder* (such as hemophilia) makes a person susceptible to prolonged bleeding after an injury. A diathesis may be inherited or acquired as a result of an illness.

Diazepam

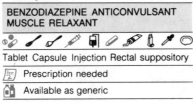

BENZODIAZEPINE ANTICONVULSANT MUSCLE RELAXANT

Tablet Capsule Injection Rectal suppository

Prescription needed

Available as generic

One of the best known and most widely used *benzodiazepine* drugs. Diazepam is used mainly to treat anxiety and insomnia. It is also prescribed as a *muscle-relaxant drug* (for example, to treat spasm of the back muscles), and as an *anticonvulsant drug* in the emergency treatment of epileptic seizures. Diazepam is also commonly used to treat the symptoms of alcohol withdrawal.

POSSIBLE ADVERSE EFFECTS

Diazepam may cause drowsiness, dizziness, and confusion; driving and hazardous work should therefore be avoided. Alcohol increases the sedative effect of diazepam and should therefore be avoided during treatment with this drug.

Like other drugs in this group, diazepam can be habit-forming if taken regularly, and its effect may diminish with prolonged use. Individuals who have taken diazepam regularly for more than two weeks should never stop their treatment suddenly. Instead, they should gradually decrease the dose under medical supervision to avoid withdrawal symptoms. Withdrawal symptoms include severe anxiety, sweating, and, in rare circumstances following large doses, seizures.

Dicumarol

An *anticoagulant drug* used to treat venous *thrombosis* and *pulmonary embolism* (blood clot in the lungs). It is also prescribed to prevent formation of an embolism in patients with a heart valve disorder or *arrhythmia* (irregular heart beat), or after heart surgery.

Dicumarol takes three to five days to have its full effect; a faster acting anticoagulant, such as *heparin*, is usually also given during the first few days of treatment. Frequent *blood-clotting tests* (prothrombin times) are usually given during treatment with dicumarol.

POSSIBLE ADVERSE EFFECTS

Adverse effects include flatulence, diarrhea, nausea, and, occasionally, bleeding in some part of the body, which may produce a nosebleed, bruising, or *hematuria*.

Dicyclomine

An *antispasmodic drug* used to relieve abdominal pain in *irritable bowel syndrome* and infantile *colic*. It is also used in the treatment of urinary incontinence caused by *irritable bladder*. Dicyclomine may cause dry mouth, blurred vision, and constipation.

Dideoxycytidine

Originally developed for use as an *anticancer drug*, dideoxycytidine (DDC) has been found to slow the multiplication of the *HIV* virus and is currently under investigation as a treatment for *AIDS*.

Dienestrol

An *estrogen drug* used as a cream to treat atrophic *vaginitis* (dryness of the vagina), which commonly occurs after the *menopause*.

Diet

See *Nutrition*.

Diet and disease

Until comparatively recently, medical concern about diet in Western countries was focused on dietary deficiencies in the poor. Today, however, deficiency diseases are very rare in developed countries (except in alcoholics, in people with malabsorptive intestinal disorders, and in people on extremely restricted diets) but are a major problem in many developing countries. In these countries, starvation or malnutrition may result in *marasmus* or *kwashiorkor*. Specific vitamin deficiencies in childhood may cause *rickets* or blindness due to *keratomalacia*; lack of certain vitamins in adult life may lead to *beriberi*, *pellagra*, or *scurvy*.

In the West, the pendulum has swung the other way, and many common disorders are due partly to overconsumption of certain types of food.

FATS

Virtually all people in developed countries have some degree of *atherosclerosis* (narrowing of arteries by deposits of fatty material), which can lead to cardiovascular diseases (such as *coronary heart disease, stroke*, and *peripheral vascular disease*). Most nutritionists believe that a major cause of atherosclerosis is a high level of the chemical *cholesterol* in the blood due to a high intake of saturated *fats*, which are found in meat, eggs, and dairy products. The disease is much less common in countries (such as Japan) in which fat in the diet is minimal and mostly polyunsaturated.

D

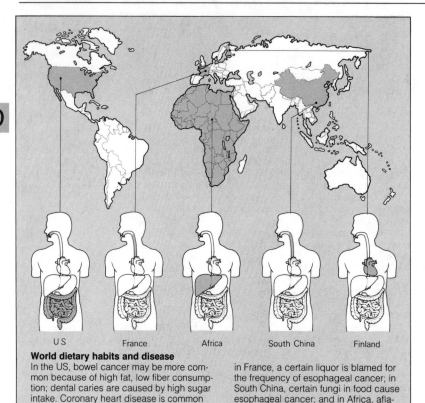

World dietary habits and disease
In the US, bowel cancer may be more common because of high fat, low fiber consumption; dental caries are caused by high sugar intake. Coronary heart disease is common among Finns because of their fatty diets; in France, a certain liquor is blamed for the frequency of esophageal cancer; in South China, certain fungi in food cause esophageal cancer; and in Africa, aflatoxins may cause liver cancer.

CALORIES
Obesity places a person at greater risk of acquiring serious disorders, such as *diabetes mellitus*, coronary heart disease, stroke, and *osteoarthritis*. Americans are among the most overweight of populations; the cause is simply an excess intake of *calories* (units of energy), mostly in the form of refined carbohydrates (such as are found in white bread, cakes, cookies, candy, and soft drinks), fatty meat and meat products, dairy products, and alcohol.

ALCOHOL
Apart from causing obesity, overconsumption of alcohol can lead to *cirrhosis* of the liver, brain damage (see *Wernicke-Korsakoff syndrome*), peripheral *neuritis*, and *cardiomyopathy*, and has been linked with *pancreatitis*, esophageal cancer (see *Esophagus, cancer of*), and many other disorders.

FIBER
The part played by diet in digestive disorders is less clear than the part played by diet in cardiovascular disease or obesity, but there is evidence suggesting that fiber may be an important factor in some illnesses. Fiber—found in foods such as wholegrain bread and vegetables—provides bulk to enable the large intestine to work effectively and also helps regulate the absorption of nutrients in the small intestine. Lack of dietary fiber has been implicated in intestinal disorders such as *diverticular disease*, chronic *constipation*, and *hemorrhoids*.

SALT
In Western countries, *hypertension* (high blood pressure) is far more prevalent than in primitive societies. Many nutritionists believe the main reason is the much higher intake of salt in the West. However, it is unlikely that some people would accept the large cut in salt from their diet that would be necessary to have any substantial effect on blood pressure.

DIET AND CANCER
Comparisons of the patterns of cancer in different countries suggest that diet may be as important a factor as tobacco in the cause of cancers. A high intake of fat (and possibly of meat) has been linked with cancer of the bowel (see *Intestines, cancer of*) and the breast (see *Breast cancer*). Moldy foods are known to cause cancer of the esophagus and liver (see *Liver cancer*), and research groups are examining many other associations.

FOOD ALLERGIES
It is fashionable to ascribe a great deal of illness to food allergy, but in fact the numbers of people in whom disease can definitely be traced to this factor are small. They include those who suffer from *celiac sprue*, as the result of an intolerance to gluten, a protein in cereals; some *migraine* sufferers, in whom foods such as chocolate, cheese, or red wine produce an attack; and people who develop a rash after eating shellfish or soft fruit (see *Urticaria*). In addition, some attacks of *asthma* and *eczema* may be due to an allergy to eggs and dairy products; and an allergy to food additives, such as artificial flavorings and colorings, may be a factor in eczema and *irritable bowel syndrome*. Some physicians believe that allergy to food additives is a major cause of behavioral disorders, such as *hyperactivity* in children, but research evidence suggests that this association is rare. Treatment for self-diagnosed food allergy should always be supervised by a physician.

A PRUDENT DIET
Although the connection between certain types of food and disease has not been proved in all cases, enough evidence exists to indicate that it is wise to make sure your diet is low in fats and refined carbohydrates, high in fiber, and free of artificial additives. (See also *Nutritional disorders*.)

GOOD DIETARY HABITS

Eat fresh rather than preserved, packaged, or convenience foods.

Eat plenty of vegetables and fruit. When raw or lightly cooked, they retain a higher nutritional value.

Eat whole-grain products including whole-grain bread.

Cut down consumption of red meat, instead, eat fish, poultry, and legumes.

Keep the fat content of your diet low and use polyunsaturated fats and vegetable oils rather than saturated fats.

Cut down on sugar in all foods.

When choosing filling foods, eat potatoes in their skins, pasta, or rice.

Dietetics

The study of *nutrition* and the application of nutritional science to people both sick and healthy. Dietetics involves not only a detailed knowledge of the composition of foods, the effects of cooking and processing, and dietary requirements, but also psychological aspects, such as eating habits.

Diethylstilbestrol

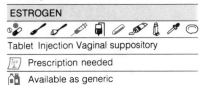

ESTROGEN

Tablet Injection Vaginal suppository

Prescription needed

Available as generic

A drug that mimics the natural estrogen hormone *estradiol*; it may be used to replace or supplement estrogen when natural hormone production is abnormal.

WHY IT IS USED

Diethylstilbestrol (DES) is used to treat the symptoms of *hypogonadism* (underdeveloped ovaries), symptoms of the *menopause* (such as hot flashes and sweating), and atrophic *vaginitis* (dryness of the vagina), which is common after the *menopause*.

DES is sometimes prescribed in high doses as a postcoital contraceptive (see *Contraception, postcoital*). It is also useful in the treatment of prostate cancer. It was formerly used as a treatment for threatened miscarriage, but this use has been abandoned as a result of evidence that vaginal cancer may develop many years later in daughters of women who took DES.

POSSIBLE ADVERSE EFFECTS

Side effects are as for other estrogen drugs. DES should not be taken during pregnancy.

Differentiation

The process by which the cells of the early *embryo*, which are almost identical and have not yet taken on any particular function, gradually diversify to form the distinct tissues and organs of the more developed embryo.

In cancer terminology, the word means the degree to which the microscopic appearance of the tissue resembles normal tissue.

Diffusion

The spread of a substance (by movement of its molecules) in a fluid from an area of high concentration to one of lower concentration, thus producing a uniform concentration throughout.

Diflunisal

A *nonsteroidal anti-inflammatory drug* (NSAID) used to relieve joint pain and stiffness in *osteoarthritis*, *rheumatoid arthritis*, and other types of arthritis. It is also prescribed to treat back pain, sprains, and strains. Occasionally, it is prescribed to ease pain after a minor operation or dental treatment. Diflunisal may cause nausea, indigestion, diarrhea, and a rash.

Digestive system

The group of organs that breaks down food into chemical components that the body can absorb and use for energy and for building and repairing cells and tissues.

The digestive system consists of the digestive tract (also known as the alimentary tract or alimentary canal) and various associated organs. The digestive tract is basically a tube through which food passes; it consists of the *mouth*, *pharynx* (throat), *esophagus*, *stomach*, *intestines* (the small intestine, comprising the *duodenum*, *jejunum*, and *ileum*, and large intestine, comprising the *cecum*, *colon*, and *rectum*), and the *anus*. The associated digestive organs—such as the *salivary glands*, *liver*, and *pancreas*—secrete digestive juices that break down food as it passes through the tract.

Food and digestion products are moved through the intestine, from the throat to the rectum, by *peristalsis* (waves of muscular contractions of the intestinal wall).

THE DIGESTIVE PROCESS

The human diet is made up of foods consisting of nutrients (*vitamins*, *minerals*, *carbohydrates*, *proteins*, and *fats*), residues (mainly vegetable *fiber*), and water. Most vitamins and minerals are absorbed into the bloodstream without change. However, before other nutrients can be absorbed, they must be broken down by digestive agents into simpler substances with smaller molecules.

Part of food breakdown is physical, performed by the teeth, which cut and chew food, and the stomach, which churns it. The rest of the process is chemical, performed by the action of *enzymes*, acids, and salts.

Carbohydrates, which are provided mainly by starchy and sugary foods, are the body's principal source of energy. The digestive process eventually converts all carbohydrates to three simple forms of sugar: glucose, fructose, and galactose.

Proteins, which are found in abundance in meat, fish, eggs, cheese, peas, beans, and lentils, are essential for the replacement and repair of cells. They are broken down into *polypeptides*, *peptides*, and *amino acids*.

Fats (also known as lipids), which are found not only in meat and dairy products, but also in oily plant foods such as peanuts, provide energy and some of the materials for cell building and maintenance. Fats also carry the fat-soluble vitamins A, D, E, and K. When fats are digested by lipases (enzymes that are secreted by the pancreas and intestine), they are broken down into *glycerol*, glycerides, and *fatty acids*.

The digestive process begins in the mouth, where the teeth chop food and the salivary glands secrete saliva, which lubricates the food and contains enzymes that begin to break down carbohydrates. The mouth also contains sensory nerves in the taste buds on the tongue. The tongue manipulates food in the mouth and forms it into small balls for easy swallowing.

From the mouth, food passes into the pharynx, which then pushes it into the esophagus. The esophagus does not contribute to the breakdown or absorption of food products; its sole function is to squeeze food down into the stomach. In the stomach, food is mixed with acids and digestive juices produced in the stomach lining; these help break down proteins. The stomach also breaks down food mechanically by its continual churning action. When the food has been converted to a semiliquid consistency, it passes into the duodenum.

The liver produces bile salts and acids, which are stored in the gallbladder and then released into the duodenum. These salts and acids help break down fats. The pancreas also releases digestive juices into the duodenum, and these juices contain enzymes that further break down carbohydrates, fats, and proteins. The final breakdown stages are completed in the small intestine, carried out by enzymes produced by glands in the lining of the intestine.

As the breakdown products of digestion pass through the small intestine, they are absorbed by its thin lining and pass into the bloodstream or the lymphatic system.

Finally food passes into the large intestine, where most of the water it contains is absorbed by the lining of the colon. Undigested matter and sloughed lining cells from the digestive tract are then expelled via the rectum and anus as feces.

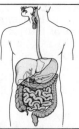

THE DIGESTIVE PROCESS

Digestion starts when food enters the mouth. It continues as the food is propelled through the digestive tract by waves of muscular contractions (peristalsis). The digestive process also involves other organs (the salivary glands, liver, gallbladder, and pancreas), which produce enzymes and acids that help break down the food.

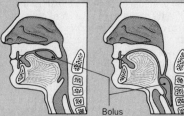

Bolus

Swallowing

In the mouth, food is cut and ground by the teeth and mixed with saliva, which softens food and breaks down certain carbohydrates. After swallowing, the food mass (bolus) enters the esophagus.

ACTION OF DIGESTIVE AGENTS

Agent or enzyme (where produced)	Digestive action
Amylase (mouth and pancreas)	Converts starch (a form of carbo-hydrate) to maltose
Sucrase, maltase, and lactase (pancreas and small intestine)	Break down vegetable and milk sugars into glucose, fructose, and galactose
Hydrochloric acid (stomach) Pepsin (stomach) Trypsin (pancreas) Peptidase (small intestine)	Assist in the breakdown of proteins into polypeptides, peptides, and amino acids
Lipase (pancreas) Bile salts and acids (liver—stored in the gallbladder)	Break down fats into glycerol, glycerides, and fatty acids

TIME SCALE

The approximate period food spends in each part of the digestive system is shown below.

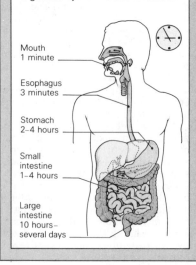

Mouth
1 minute

Esophagus
3 minutes

Stomach
2–4 hours

Small intestine
1–4 hours

Large intestine
10 hours–several days

Esophagus

Food is carried down the esophagus by peristaltic action and enters the stomach.

Stomach

Food is broken down further by churning and by the action of hydrochloric acid and digestive enzymes secreted by the stomach lining. Food remains in the stomach until it is reduced to a semiliquid consistency (chyme), when it passes into the duodenum.

Duodenum

As food travels along the duodenum, it is broken down further by digestive enzymes from the liver, gallbladder, and pancreas. The duodenum leads directly into the small intestine.

Small intestine

Additional enzymes secreted by glands in the lining of the small intestine complete the digestive process. Nutrients are absorbed through the intestinal lining into the network of blood vessels and lymph vessels supplying the intestine. Undigested matter passes into the large intestine (the colon).

Colon

Water in the undigested matter leaving the small intestine is absorbed through the lining of the colon. The residue passes into the rectum.

Rectum

Undigested matter enters this final part of the large intestine and is expelled.

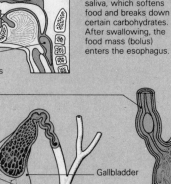

Gallbladder

Bile duct

Pancreas

Anus

D

DISORDERS

Digestive system disorders include a large number of conditions that disrupt the digestive process, either because they obstruct or prevent the passage of food along the digestive tract, or because they interfere with the breakdown or absorption of nutrients. Other conditions may have little effect on digestion but produce distressing symptoms such as difficulty swallowing, heartburn, flatulence, abdominal pain, diarrhea, constipation, or rectal bleeding.

The disease processes causing such disorders range from congenital abnormalities and inherited biochemical defects to inflammatory and autoimmune disorders, tumors, viral, bacterial, and parasitic infections, and chronic allergic conditions. (See also disorder boxes for *Mouth*, *Esophagus*, *Stomach*, *Liver*, *Gallbladder*, *Pancreas*, and *Intestines*.)

Digitalis drugs

A group of drugs extracted from the leaves of plants belonging to the foxglove family. They are used to treat various heart conditions. The most commonly used drugs in this group are *digoxin* and *digitoxin*.

Digital subtraction angiography

See *Angiography*.

Digitoxin

A *digitalis drug*, digitoxin is used to treat *heart failure* (reduced pumping efficiency) and certain types of *arrhythmia* (irregular heart beat). Digitoxin is usually prescribed as an alternative to *digoxin* for patients with kidney disease.

Digoxin

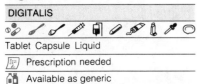

DIGITALIS

Tablet Capsule Liquid

Prescription needed

Available as generic

The most widely used of the *digitalis drugs*, digoxin is used in the treatment of *heart failure* (reduced pumping efficiency) and certain types of *arrhythmia* (irregular heart beat), such as *atrial fibrillation* (a rapid, irregular beating of the heart muscle).

HOW IT WORKS

Digoxin increases the force of heart muscle contractions, making the heart work more efficiently. It also slows

down abnormally rapid nerve impulses as they pass between the atria (upper chambers of the heart) to the ventricles (main chambers of the heart), which allows the ventricles time to fill up with blood and empty normally with each contraction.

POSSIBLE ADVERSE EFFECTS

If digoxin is to be effective, the dose must be just below that of a toxic dose. The patient must therefore be given regular blood tests to ascertain the digoxin level. An excessive dose may cause loss of appetite, nausea, vomiting, and headache. Digoxin occasionally interferes with the normal heart beat, causing *heart block* (an abnormally slow rate of contraction).

Adverse effects are more likely if the potassium level in the body is low. Patients who are also taking *diuretic drugs* (and therefore are more likely to become deficient in potassium) are given regular blood tests to monitor potassium levels.

Because digoxin is removed from the body mainly in the urine, patients with kidney disease are usually given *digitoxin* as an alternative drug because of the risk of a buildup of toxic levels of digoxin.

Dilatation

A condition in which a body cavity, tube, or opening is enlarged or stretched as a result of normal physiological processes (as in dilatation of the pupil), or because of disease (as in dilatation of the heart). Dilatation also refers to the process of achieving such enlargement, as in surgical procedures such as *D and C* (dilatation and curettage) of the cervix. Also called dilation.

Dilatation and curettage

See *D and C*.

Dilator

An instrument for stretching and enlarging a narrowed body cavity, tube, or opening.

Diltiazem

A *calcium channel blocker drug* used in the treatment of *hypertension* (high blood pressure) and *angina pectoris* (chest pain due to impaired blood supply to heart muscle). Taken regularly, diltiazem often reduces the frequency of angina attacks, but does not act quickly enough to relieve pain in an acute attack.

Diltiazem may cause headache, appetite loss, nausea, constipation, and ankle swelling.

Dimenhydrinate

An *antihistamine drug* used as an *antiemetic drug* to relieve nausea and vomiting caused by a number of disorders. Dimenhydrinate is especially effective when these symptoms occur with vertigo (dizziness with loss of balance)—for example, in *motion sickness*. It may also be used to relieve nausea and vomiting in early pregnancy. Like other antihistamine drugs, dimenhydrinate has a sedative effect that can be dangerous when operating machinery or driving.

Dioxin

A toxic defoliant chemical (see *Defoliant poisoning*).

Diphenhydramine

An *antihistamine drug* used to treat allergic disorders such as *urticaria* (hives) and allergic *rhinitis* (hay fever). It is given by injection to treat *anaphylactic shock* (a severe allergic reaction), which may occur, for example, as a result of an insect sting.

Diphenhydramine is also prescribed as an *antiemetic drug* to relieve nausea and vomiting in pregnancy and to prevent *motion sickness*. It is used as an ingredient in some *cough remedies* because of its cough suppressant effect. It has also been used to control abnormal movements in *Parkinson's disease*.

POSSIBLE ADVERSE EFFECTS

Diphenhydramine often causes drowsiness and, because of its sedative effect, has occasionally been used to treat insomnia. Driving and hazardous work should be avoided if the drug is causing sedation. Other possible side effects include dry mouth and blurred vision.

Diphenoxylate

An *antidiarrheal drug* (used to relieve diarrhea) chemically related to the narcotic *analgesics* (morphinelike painkillers). Diphenoxylate works by reducing the contractions of the muscles in the walls of the intestine, thus slowing down the frequency of bowel movements.

POSSIBLE ADVERSE EFFECTS

In normal doses, drowsiness and abdominal pain occur in rare instances. When taken in high doses, diphenoxylate produces euphoria due to its narcotic ingredient. Adding *atropine* to the preparation prevents abuse; a dose high enough to produce euphoria causes unpleasant side effects, such as dry mouth, flushing, blurred vision, and vomiting.

D

Diphtheria

An acute bacterial illness that causes a sore throat and a fever, and sometimes causes more serious or even fatal complications. Diphtheria was one of the most important causes of childhood death worldwide until the 1930s, but, since then, mass immunization has made it extremely rare in the US and other developed countries. However, diphtheria is still a hazard for people living in poor developing countries and is a particular risk for nonimmunized people who travel to such countries.

CAUSES AND INCIDENCE

Diphtheria is caused by the bacillus *CORYNEBACTERIUM DIPHTHERIAE.* It may live in the skin or in the nose of a person immune to the disease or, during an infection, may multiply in the throat or skin. Serious complications are caused by a toxin released by the bacterium into the bloodstream.

The few cases that occur in the US are invariably among immigrants from poor developing countries. In these countries, the disease is usually caught from a healthy "carrier" of diphtheria bacilli, who harbors the organisms in his or her nose or skin and spreads them through the air or by touch. These carriers have acquired immunity to the illness, having in the past recovered from a relatively mild infection.

SYMPTOMS

When a nonimmune person is infected by the bacterium spread from a carrier, the bacterium usually multiplies in the throat, giving rise to a membrane that appears over the tonsils and may spread over the palate or downward to the larynx (voice box) and trachea (windpipe). This may cause breathing difficulties and a husky voice. Other symptoms include enlarged lymph glands in the neck, an increased heart rate, and mild fever. Sometimes, an infection is confined to the skin, where it may cause no more than a few yellow spots or sores with an appearance similar to *impetigo.*

Life-threatening symptoms develop only in nonimmune people and are caused by the bacterial toxin. Occasionally, victims collapse and die within a day or so of getting the throat infection. More often they are recovering from this condition when heart failure or paralysis of the throat or limbs develops. These later complications can occur up to seven weeks after onset of infection in the throat. If victims survive the disease they make a complete recovery.

PREVENTION

In the US and other developed countries, the triple vaccine, also known as the *DPT vaccine* (against diphtheria, pertussis, and tetanus), is given routinely to children in the first year of life. The practice of immunizing against diphtheria must continue, despite the extreme rarity of the disease in these countries, because carriers can arrive from developing countries at any time; if large numbers of children were not immune, there could be a disastrous epidemic.

Those traveling to poor, developing countries who are in doubt as to whether they were immunized against diphtheria as children should have their immune status checked or simply be vaccinated.

Spread of effective immunization programs to all countries could eventually eradicate diphtheria (as smallpox has been eradicated), although this possibility is not envisaged at present.

TREATMENT

Penicillin kills diphtheria organisms in the throat, but is ineffective against the toxin in the blood. If the disease is suspected, an *antitoxin* (derived from the blood of immunized horses) must be given as soon as possible in addition to penicillin. If severe breathing difficulties develop in a patient, a *tracheostomy* (surgical introduction of a breathing tube into the windpipe) may be necessary.

Victims are kept in isolation until no diphtheria bacilli can be detected in the nose and throat (by swabs taken on six consecutive days).

Diplopia

The medical term for *double vision.*

Dipsomania

A form of *alcohol dependence* in which periods of excessive drinking and craving for drink alternate with periods of relative sobriety.

Dipyridamole

A drug that reduces the stickiness of platelets (cells in the blood that aid blood clotting) and, as a result, helps prevent the formation of abnormal blood clotting within the arteries. Possible adverse effects include headache, flushing, and dizziness.

Disability

Temporary loss or permanent impairment of a faculty, such as weakness of a limb or loss of sight. The distinction between disability and *handicap* is vague, and in practice the two terms are often used interchangeably. However, disability is sometimes defined as the physical disorder, and handicap as the extent to which a disorder impairs normal functioning. Thus two people with the same disability—blindness, for example—may suffer different degrees of handicap because one person manages to cope with everyday living better than the other. (See also illustrated box showing aids for the disabled; *Rehabilitation.*)

Discharge

Visible emission of fluid from a body cavity, such as the nose. Discharge may be part of the cavity's normal function, as in some types of *vaginal discharge*—during pregnancy, for instance. Alternatively, it may be due to infection or inflammation of the lining of the cavity, as in *rhinitis* (inflammation of the lining of the nose), *urethritis* (infection of the urethra, the tube that carries urine from the bladder to outside the body), *proctitis* (infection of the rectum), or *vaginitis* (infection of the vagina).

Disclosing agents

Dyes that make the plaque deposits on teeth more visible so that they can be seen and removed. As part of oral hygiene advice, the dentist or hygienist may apply a disclosing solution to the teeth to show the presence of harmful dental *plaque* and pellicle (a thin protein film), and to demonstrate an effective method of tooth cleaning.

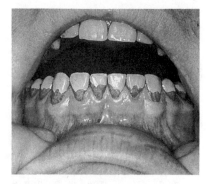

Plaque revealed by disclosing agent
The plaque appears here as the dark areas on the teeth near the gums. Plaque consists of bacteria, mucus, and food debris; it builds up quickly if the teeth are not brushed and flossed regularly.

AIDS FOR THE DISABLED

There are a variety of articles that are specially designed or adapted to assist disabled people in performing everyday activities. Aids include prostheses, supports, and mobility aids that enable people to function more efficiently, as well as equipment designed to help them perform specific tasks more easily.

Devices that help vision, hearing, and movement improve the ability of disabled people to cope with all aspects of everyday life. Such devices include walkers, glasses, hearing aids, artificial limbs, corsets, and wheelchairs. Ventilators, home dialysis, and enteral and parenteral feeding devices are life-sustaining aids.

There are various household aids available that can help people cook, feed and dress themselves, wash and use the toilet, and get in and out of beds and chairs. Specially designed furniture and devices can help disabled parents care for their children; sexual aids can facilitate an active sexual life.

D

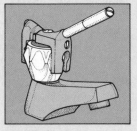

Faucet turner
Helps grip and turn faucet.

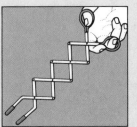

Tongs
Extending grippers to pick up dropped items. Closes up to fit in pocket or purse.

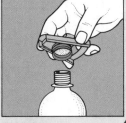

Bottle opener
A small hand-held device designed to grip and open small bottle tops.

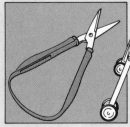

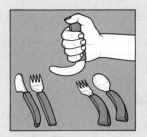

Cutlery
A range of knives, forks, and spoons with thick, molded handles for easy manipulating.

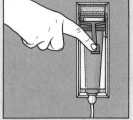

Toothpaste extruder
A wall-mounted device that dispenses toothpaste with minimal finger pressure.

Scissors
Self-opening scissors with easy-grip handles.

"A" frame
A lightweight walker that doubles as a seat and can be folded flat.

Discolored teeth

Teeth tend naturally to darken with age. The red pulp tissue in the center of the tooth, which makes young teeth look bright, gradually recedes while at the same time more dentin is laid down around it, resulting in the tooth's dull yellow color.

Both the tooth's surface and its internal structures are liable to be stained by a variety of substances brought to the mouth or carried by the blood supply. Extrinsic stains, those found on the tooth's surface, are common, but are easily removed by polishing and can be prevented by regular tooth-cleaning. Intrinsic stains, those within the tooth's substance, are permanent. Many stains, both extrinsic and intrinsic, can be covered or diminished with the newer cosmetic dental procedures that are available in the dentist's office.

EXTRINSIC STAINS
BROWNISH-BLACK DEPOSIT or TOBACCO STAIN
Usually found on the inside surfaces of the teeth, this staining is due to the accumulation of tars and resins.
BLACK STAIN A firmly attached, black or brown line, close to and following the contour of the gum, usually on the inside surfaces of the upper back teeth. More common in children, it is thought to be due to pigment-producing bacteria.
GREEN STAIN A heavy, "furry," grayish-green stain, firmly attached close to the gum, usually on the front surfaces of the upper front teeth. It is most commonly found in children and may be due to staining of remnants of developmental membrane by color-producing bacteria.
DULL YELLOW STAIN May be due to discoloration of *plaque* by dyes in foodstuffs; it is easily removed.

BROWN STAIN A thin, dark line near the gum, formed from little dots of pigmented plaque usually colored by iron salts taken internally or that come into contact with the mouth.
ORANGE-RED STAIN May be caused by pigment-producing bacteria; it is easily removed.
STAINED DENTIN With advancing age the full thickness of enamel may be worn away in parts and the dentin becomes stained by dyes in foods.
METALLIC STAINING May follow the use of medicines containing metallic salts. Iron-containing liquids stain the teeth brown. Inhalation of metallic dust by metal workers (prior to stringent safety measures) caused accumulation of metals in the plaque. Brass, copper, lead, bronze, and other copper alloys caused a bluish-green stain, iron produced brown staining, and mercury led to black staining.

D

INTRINSIC STAINS

BLACK TEETH Teeth may darken following the death of the pulp or the removal of the pulp during root canal treatment. This is caused by the decomposition of red blood cells that pass from damaged blood vessels in the pulp into the dentin.

TETRACYCLINE STAINING This antibiotic is absorbed by developing teeth and causes discoloration of primary or permanent teeth. Which teeth are affected depends on the stage of tooth development at the time it is absorbed, the amount taken, and the type of tetracycline prescribed. Tetracycline given to a pregnant woman often causes discoloration of her child's teeth. If mildly affected, the teeth will appear yellow but, if severely affected, they will be brown or blue-violet.

After the age of 7 years, discoloration is not such a problem, because all the cosmetically important teeth are already formed.

FLUOROSIS A mottling of the tooth enamel occurs if excessive amounts of fluoride are taken during development of the enamel (see *Fluorosis*).

Disinfectants

Substances that kill microorganisms and thus prevent infection. The term is usually applied to strong chemicals that are harmful to human tissue and so are used to decontaminate inanimate objects, such as pieces of equipment. Decontaminants that are safe for human tissue are called *antiseptics*.

Disk, intervertebral

A flat, circular, platelike structure containing *cartilage* that lines the surfaces of the ends of bones in the joints between adjacent vertebrae throughout the length of the spine.

Each of the intervertebral disks is composed of a hard, outer layer and a soft, jellylike core. The material acts as a shock absorber to cushion the vertebrae during movements of the spine, and to minimize jarring when jumping or running. With increasing age, intervertebral disks can wear out, becoming less supple and more susceptible to damage from injury. One of the most common forms of damage is a *disk prolapse*, in which part of the disk's soft center bulges out through a weak area in the hard, outer layer. This may compress a spinal nerve root and produce symptoms (such as interference with muscle strength and/or pain in the back and leg) along the course of the nerve.

Diskography

A diagnostic technique in which a dye visible on *X-ray* films is injected into an invertebral disk, one of the shock-absorbing structures between the vertebrae (bones of the spine).

WHY IT IS DONE

The technique is one of the methods used to diagnose *disk prolapse*. Ordinary X-ray films fail to reveal disks, which show on the film only as spaces between the vertebrae.

HOW IT IS DONE

After a local anesthetic has been given, a long thin needle is passed through the skin into the disk under X-ray control, dye is injected into the disk, and X-ray pictures are taken. Occasionally the site of the injection is sore afterward, but the pain usually clears up quickly.

RESULTS

The image obtained provides only a rough outline of the disk, but reveals clearly any leakage of dye, proving that the disk is ruptured. In some people the rupture may be due to small tears in the disk rather than a prolapse. However, if the procedure itself causes pain in the spine, and sciatica (pain down the back of a leg) or arm pain, it indicates a strong possibility of prolapse.

Because of its relative imprecision, diskography is of more limited use than *CT scanning* or *myelography*.

Disk prolapse

A common, painful disorder of the spine in which an intervertebral disk ruptures and part of its pulpy core protrudes. Disk prolapse causes a painful and at times disabling pressure on a nerve.

About 95 percent of disk prolapses occur in the lower back, but they can affect any part of the back or the neck.

CAUSES AND INCIDENCE

Although a prolapsed disk may sometimes be caused by a sudden strenuous action (such as lifting a heavy weight or twisting violently), it usually develops gradually as the result of disks degenerating with age.

People between the ages of 30 and 40 are the most likely to suffer from the disorder. Over the age of 30, disks start to dehydrate and become less resilient but, after 40, extra fibrous tissue forms around them, increasing their stability.

Disk prolapses are slightly more common in men than women, and their incidence is higher in people who spend long periods sitting without a break.

DIAGNOSIS

Many other disorders may cause back and leg pain or neck and arm pain, and various tests may be needed to arrive at a firm diagnosis. After the physician has examined the spine and tested movement and reflexes in the affected arm or leg, he or she may arrange for tests, including the following: *X rays*, *CT scanning*, *myelography* (the injection into the fluid around the spinal cord of a dye visible on X rays), *diskography* (the injection of the same dye into a disk), and electromyography (tests of electrical activity in muscles; see *EMG*).

If a certain nerve root is suspected of being compressed, a local anesthetic may be injected into its lining; if this relieves the pain, the location of the trouble is confirmed.

OUTLOOK

In most cases treatment without surgery clears the pain, but the pain tends to recur. An operation is performed when muscle function is impaired.

Dislocation, joint

Complete displacement of the two bones in a joint so that they are no longer in contact, usually as a result of injury. (Displacement that leaves the bones in partial contact is called *subluxation*.) Dislocation is usually accompanied by tearing of the joint ligaments and damage to the joint capsule (the membrane that encases the joint); it is the tearing that makes the injury so painful. Injury severe enough to cause dislocation often also causes fracture of one or both of the bones involved.

SYMPTOMS AND COMPLICATIONS

Dislocation restricts or prevents the movement of the joint and is usually accompanied by severe pain. The joint looks misshapen and soon swells. In some cases, dislocation is followed by complications. For example, dislocation of the spinal vertebrae resulting from a severe back injury can damage the spinal cord, sometimes causing paralysis below the point of injury. Dislocation of the shoulder or hip joint can damage major nerves in the arm or leg, again sometimes resulting in paralysis.

Rarely, the tissue around a dislocated joint, usually the shoulder, becomes so weakened that after the joint has mended only minimal pressure causes another dislocation.

TREATMENT

SELF-HELP A medically unqualified person should not attempt to manipulate the joint back into position because of

SYMPTOMS AND TREATMENT OF DISK PROLAPSE

A prolapsed disk in the lower back causes low back pain and, if the sciatic nerve root is compressed, *sciatica* (pain running down the back of the leg from the buttock to the ankle), sometimes accompanied by numbness and tingling. Low back pain and sciatica are usually aggravated by coughing, sneezing, bending, and sitting for long periods. Prolonged pressure on the sciatic nerve can lead to weakness in the muscles of the leg.

A prolapsed disk in the neck causes neck pain, stiffness, and, if the root of a nerve that is in the arm is compressed, tingling and weakness in that arm and hand.

In rare cases, pressure is exerted on the spinal cord itself, sometimes leading to paralysis of the legs and loss of bladder or bowel control.

Normal spinal nerve root

Disk

Lumbar vertebra

Normal position of disk

Pulpy interior protruding (prolapsed part of disk)

Compressed spinal nerve root

Cervical vertebrae

Thoracic vertebrae

Lumbar vertebrae (disks most commonly affected)

Sacrum

Coccyx

Cross section of a prolapsed disk
The fibrous outer layer is ruptured and some of its pulpy interior protrudes and presses on a spinal nerve root.

Before treatment
X ray showing the prolapsed disk protruding into the spinal cord, affecting the nerve from that point downward.

TREATMENT

Disk prolapse often responds to bed rest (lying flat on the back on a firm mattress for a few weeks) and analgesics; later, a supportive collar or corset and special exercises are helpful. If these measures fail and the nerve root compression is producing muscle weakness, an operation may relieve the pressure (see *Decompression, spinal canal*).

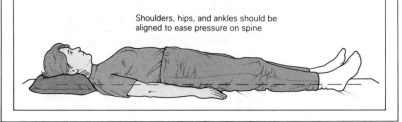
Shoulders, hips, and ankles should be aligned to ease pressure on spine

the risk of seriously damaging nerves around the joint or making an accompanying fracture worse. Movement of the joint should be prevented by means of a *splint* or, in the case of a dislocated shoulder, a *sling* on the arm. No food or drink should be taken, because a general anesthetic is usually required to reset the bones.

PROFESSIONAL The joint is usually X-rayed first to see whether a fracture is present. Then the bones are manipulated back into their proper position as quickly as possible, or, when manipulation is not feasible, an operation may be performed to reset them. After either procedure, the joint is usually immobilized by means of a splint or plaster cast to allow it to heal without disturbance. Recurrent dislocation is treated by surgery to shorten and tighten the ligaments of the joint, thus strengthening it.

Disopyramide

An *antiarrhythmic drug* used to treat abnormally rapid heart beats (for example, following *myocardial infarction*). Disopyramide reduces the force of heart muscle contraction and, as a result, may occasionally aggravate preexisting heart failure. This drug may also cause dry mouth, constipation, and blurred vision.

Disorientation

Confusion over time, place, or personal identity. The experience is similar to being awakened from a deep sleep. Disorientation is usually caused by head injury, intoxication, or a chronic brain disorder such as *dementia*.

The disoriented person's speech and behavior tend to be muddled, and he or she is often unable to answer simple questions about time, date, present whereabouts, or name and address. Although *hysteria* or inattention may cause such symptoms, if disorientation comes on suddenly, the cause is almost always an organic brain disease. (See also *Delirium*.)

Displacement activity

The transference of feelings from one object or person to another. This is usually a conscious act, performed to obtain emotional relief in a manner that will not cause harm to oneself or to another person. For example, a person who is angry may hit a wall or throw something rather than risk harming someone else.

Psychoanalysts regard displacement as an unconscious *defense mechanism*. Disturbing or unwelcome feelings are prevented from entering consciousness by being transferred onto another person or object. An understanding of this unconscious process is an important part of the interpretation of a patient's dreams during psychoanalysis.

Dissociative disorders

A group of psychological illnesses in which a particular mental function becomes cut off from the mind as a whole. While the process of dissociation is common in everyday life (for example, not hearing what is said because of intense concentration on another task), when taken to extremes it can lead to serious problems.

A common type of dissociative disorder is hysterical amnesia. The affected person is unable to remember his or her name or personal history, but can still speak, read, and learn new material (see *Hysteria*). Other forms of this disorder are *fugue*, *depersonalization*, and *multiple personality*. (See also *Conversion disorder*.)

Distal

Describing a part of the body that is farther away from a central point of reference, such as the trunk of the body. For example, the fingers are distal to the arm with the trunk as the point of reference. The opposite of distal is *proximal*.

Disulfiram

A drug that acts as a deterrent to drinking alcohol, disulfiram is prescribed for people who request help for an alcohol problem. Treatment with disulfiram is usually combined with a counseling program (see *Alcohol dependence*).

HOW IT WORKS

Alcohol is normally converted in the liver to acetaldehyde, which in turn is broken down to form acetic acid. Disulfiram reduces the breakdown of acetaldehyde, resulting in an increased level of this toxic substance and causing flushing, headache, nausea, dizziness, and palpitations.

These unpleasant symptoms generally start within an hour of drinking alcohol after taking disulfiram and can last for several hours.

POSSIBLE ADVERSE EFFECTS

Drowsiness and a metallic or garlic taste in the mouth frequently occur. These symptoms usually disappear within a few days as the body adapts to the drug.

Occasionally, large amounts of alcohol taken during treatment can cause unconsciousness, so a warning card indicating the person is taking disulfiram should be carried.

Diuretic drugs

COMMON DRUGS

Thiazide
Chlorothiazide Hydrochlorothiazide Metolazone

Loop
Bumetanide Furosemide

Potassium-sparing
Amiloride Spironolactone Triamterene

A group of drugs that helps remove excess water from the body by increasing the amount lost in the urine.

TYPES

The different types of diuretic drug vary markedly in their speed and mode of action.

THIAZIDE DIURETICS These diuretics cause moderate diuresis (increased urine production) and are suitable for prolonged use.

LOOP DIURETICS So called because they act on the region of the kidneys called Henle's loop, these are fast-acting, powerful drugs, especially when given by injection. Loop diuretics are particularly useful as an emergency treatment for heart failure.

POTASSIUM-SPARING DIURETICS These drugs are often used with thiazide and loop diuretics, both of which may cause potassium deficiency.

CARBONIC ANHYDRASE INHIBITORS Drugs that block the action of carbonic anhydrase (an enzyme that affects the amount of bicarbonate ions in the blood); these diuretics cause a moderate diuresis, but are effective only for short periods.

OSMOTIC DIURETICS These powerful diuretics are used to maintain urine production after serious injury or major surgery.

WHY THEY ARE USED

By increasing the production of urine, diuretic drugs reduce the amount of water in the circulation and thus reduce the *edema* (fluid retention) that causes breathlessness and ankle swelling in *heart failure*, *nephrotic syndrome* (a kidney disorder), *cirrhosis* of the liver, and bloating and breast tenderness before *menstruation*.

Diuretic drugs also lower the blood pressure and thus are used in the treatment of *hypertension* (high blood

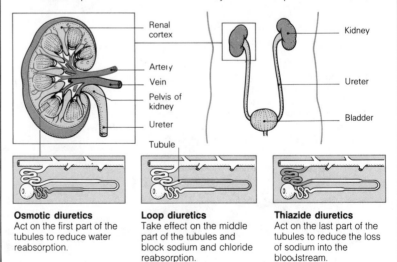

HOW DIURETICS WORK

The normal filtration process of the kidneys (which takes place in the tubules) removes water, salts (mainly potassium and sodium), and waste products from the bloodstream. Most of the salts and water are returned to the bloodstream, but certain amounts are expelled from the body along with the waste products in the urine.

Diuretic drugs interfere with this normal kidney action. Osmotic, loop, and thiazide diuretics reduce the amount of sodium and water taken back into the blood, thus increasing urine volume. Other diuretics increase blood flow through the kidneys and thus the amount of water they filter and expel in the urine.

Renal cortex
Artery
Vein
Pelvis of kidney
Ureter
Tubule
Kidney
Ureter
Bladder

Osmotic diuretics
Act on the first part of the tubules to reduce water reabsorption.

Loop diuretics
Take effect on the middle part of the tubules and block sodium and chloride reabsorption.

Thiazide diuretics
Act on the last part of the tubules to reduce the loss of sodium into the bloodstream.

pressure). Carbonic anhydrase inhibitors are sometimes used to treat *glaucoma* (increased fluid pressure in the eyeball).

POSSIBLE ADVERSE EFFECTS

Diuretic drugs may cause chemical imbalances in the blood, most commonly hypokalemia (low blood potassium). Symptoms of this condition include weakness, confusion, and palpitations. Treatment usually consists of a course of potassium supplements or a potassium-sparing diuretic drug. A diet rich in potassium (containing plenty of fruits and vegetables) may be helpful.

Some diuretic drugs may increase the level of uric acid in the blood, and thus the risk of *gout*. Certain types of diuretics increase the blood sugar level, an effect that can cause or aggravate *diabetes mellitus*.

Diverticular disease

The presence of diverticula (small sacs caused by the protrusions of the inner lining of the intestine or other hollow organs) and any symptoms or complications caused by their presence.

Diverticula may form in any part of the intestines but usually affect the lower part of the colon (the main section of the large intestine). The cause is not conclusively established, but diverticula are thought to arise when pressure forces the lining of the colon through areas of weakness in the intestinal wall. Diverticulosis merely signifies the presence of diverticula in the colon. Diverticulitis is a complication produced by inflammation due to obstruction and, occasionally, perforation (formation of a hole) in one or more diverticula.

DIVERTICULOSIS

Diverticulosis is rare in developing countries, but in Western Europe and the US it affects more than half the population by the age of 80. Its incidence increases progressively with age, being rare before the age of 20. Lack of adequate dietary fiber or roughage is believed to play an important role in its development.

SYMPTOMS

Symptoms occur in only 20 percent of patients with diverticulosis and usually result from spasm or cramp of the intestinal muscle near diverticula. Many patients have symptoms of *irritable bowel syndrome*, which may coexist with diverticulosis. In such patients, symptoms include a bloated sensation, episodes of pain in the lower abdomen, and changes in bowel habits, such as constipation, diarrhea,

or alternating attacks of both. Complications, which are uncommon, include hemorrhage (indicated by bleeding from the rectum), diverticulitis, and stricture formation (narrowing of the intestine). A physician should rule out the possibility of cancer in patients with symptoms of diverticulosis; tumors developing in areas affected by diverticulosis may be difficult to diagnose.

DIAGNOSIS

Diverticula are easily diagnosed by *barium X-ray examination* of the colon or by *colonoscopy* (visual examination via a flexible, fiberoptic instrument).

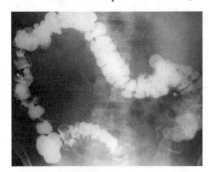

X ray showing diverticulosis
In this X ray taken after a barium meal, the bright, winding tube is the patient's colon. The knobs on its outer surface are diverticula.

TREATMENT

In patients with muscle spasms that cause cramps, a high-fiber diet, fiber supplements, and *antispasmodic drugs* may abolish symptoms. A high-fiber diet has also been shown to reduce the incidence of complications. Bleeding from diverticula usually subsides without treatment, but occasionally requires surgical treatment such as that for diverticulitis. Otherwise, surgery is rarely necessary.

DIVERTICULITIS

Inflammation and perforation of diverticula cause fever, pain, tenderness, and rigidity of the abdomen over the area of the intestine involved. Rarely, a large abscess can form in the tissues around the colon; it may be felt as a tender lump when a physician examines the abdomen. In exceptional circumstances, perforation may lead to *peritonitis* (inflammation of the lining of the abdomen). Complications of diverticulitis may also include the development of a stricture (narrowing of the intestine) at the site of the inflammation or of a fistula (narrow channel) connecting one part of the intestine to another.

TREATMENT

Diverticulitis usually subsides with bed rest and antibiotics. If the symptoms are severe, treatment may also include a liquid diet or intravenous fluids when oral feeding must be temporarily stopped. Surgical treatment may be needed if perforation causes a large abscess or peritonitis, if a tight stricture develops, or if hemorrhage cannot be controlled. In most cases requiring surgery, the diseased section of the intestine is removed and the remaining sections joined together. In some patients, a temporary *colostomy* (an operation to bring part of the large intestine to the body surface to form an artificial anus) is required.

Diving medicine

See *Scuba-diving medicine*.

Dizziness

A sensation of unsteadiness and lightheadedness. It may be a mild, brief symptom that occurs by itself, or it may be part of a more severe, prolonged attack of *vertigo* (characterized by a sensation of spinning, either of oneself or the surroundings) accompanied by nausea, vomiting, sweating, or fainting.

CAUSES

Most attacks of dizziness are harmless and are caused by a momentary fall in the pressure of blood to the brain, as can occur, for example, when getting up quickly from a sitting or lying position (a phenomenon called *postural hypotension*). Postural hypotension is more common in the elderly and in people taking drugs to treat *hypertension* (high blood pressure). Similar symptoms may result from a temporary, partial blockage in the arteries that supply the brain—a *transient ischemic attack*.

Other causes of dizziness include tiredness, stress, fever, *anemia*, *heart block* (impairment of the conduction of excitatory impulses through the heart muscle, causing slow, uncoordinated beating of the individual chambers), *hypoglycemia* (low blood sugar level), and *subdural hemorrhage* and *hematoma* (bleeding between the outer two membranes that cover the brain).

Dizziness as part of vertigo is usually due to a disorder of the inner ear, *acoustic nerve*, or *brain stem*.

The principal disorders of the inner ear that can cause dizziness and vertigo are *labyrinthitis* and *Meniere's disease*. In labyrinthitis, the labyrinth (the fluid-filled canals within the inner

D

DIZZINESS A sense of being dazed and unsteady sometimes accompanied by a sensation of spinning.

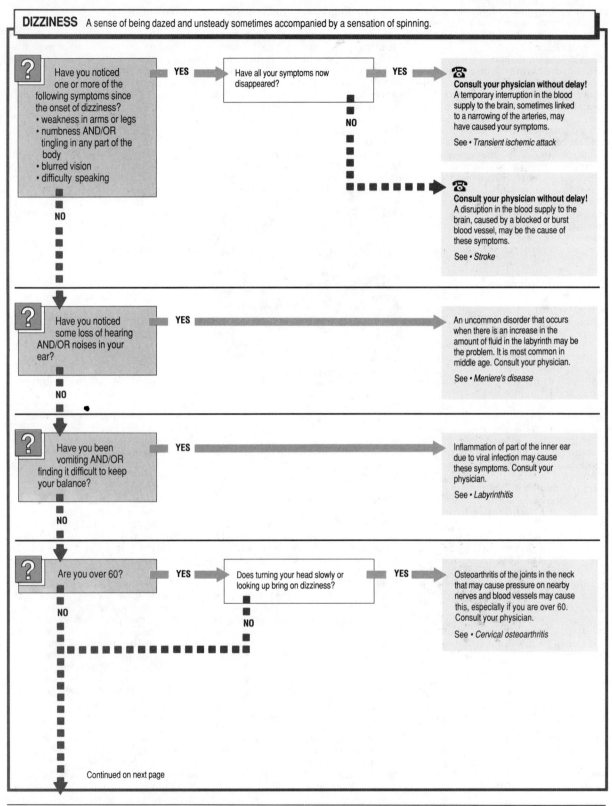

Have you noticed one or more of the following symptoms since the onset of dizziness?
• weakness in arms or legs
• numbness AND/OR tingling in any part of the body
• blurred vision
• difficulty speaking

YES ➡ Have all your symptoms now disappeared?

YES ➡ ☎
Consult your physician without delay!
A temporary interruption in the blood supply to the brain, sometimes linked to a narrowing of the arteries, may have caused your symptoms.

See • *Transient ischemic attack*

NO

☎
Consult your physician without delay!
A disruption in the blood supply to the brain, caused by a blocked or burst blood vessel, may be the cause of these symptoms.

See • *Stroke*

NO

Have you noticed some loss of hearing AND/OR noises in your ear?

YES ➡ An uncommon disorder that occurs when there is an increase in the amount of fluid in the labyrinth may be the problem. It is most common in middle age. Consult your physician.

See • *Meniere's disease*

NO

Have you been vomiting AND/OR finding it difficult to keep your balance?

YES ➡ Inflammation of part of the inner ear due to viral infection may cause these symptoms. Consult your physician.

See • *Labyrinthitis*

NO

Are you over 60?

YES ➡ Does turning your head slowly or looking up bring on dizziness?

YES ➡ Osteoarthritis of the joints in the neck that may cause pressure on nearby nerves and blood vessels may cause this, especially if you are over 60. Consult your physician.

See • *Cervical osteoarthritis*

NO

NO

Continued on next page

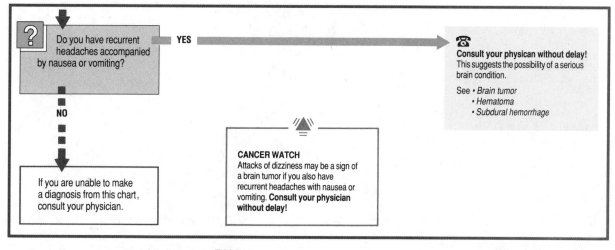

Do you have recurrent headaches accompanied by nausea or vomiting?

YES → ☎ **Consult your physican without delay!**
This suggests the possibility of a serious brain condition.

See • *Brain tumor*
• *Hematoma*
• *Subdural hemorrhage*

NO

If you are unable to make a diagnosis from this chart, consult your physician.

CANCER WATCH
Attacks of dizziness may be a sign of a brain tumor if you also have recurrent headaches with nausea or vomiting. **Consult your physician without delay!**

D

---

ear that play a vital role in balance) becomes inflamed, usually as a result of a viral infection. In severe cases, any movement of the head can cause vomiting and fainting. In Meniere's disease, a degenerative disease of the ear, the dizziness and vertigo are often associated with hearing loss and *tinnitus*.

Disorders of the acoustic nerve are relatively rare causes of dizziness and vertigo. They include *acoustic neuroma* and cases of *meningitis* in which the acoustic nerve is affected.

Disorders of the brain stem (specifically the part of the brain stem that connects with the acoustic nerve) that can cause dizziness and vertigo include narrowing of the blood vessels that supply this part of the brain stem (a condition called *vertebrobasilar insufficiency*); cases of migraine that involve blood vessels in the brain stem; and brain tumors that press on the brain stem. Vertebrobasilar insufficiency is itself often due to *cervical osteoarthritis* (arthritis of the neck region of the spine); it produces pain and dizziness on turning the head or moving the neck.

TREATMENT
Brief episodes of mild dizziness usually clear up after taking a few deep breaths, or, if this fails, after resting for a short time. Severe, prolonged, or recurrent dizziness should be investigated by a physician, who will try to determine the cause from a description of symptoms, examination of the ears, and, in some cases, further diagnostic tests.

In certain cases of dizziness and vertigo due to a disorder of the inner ear, the physician may prescribe *antiemetic* or *antihistamine drugs.*

DNA

The commonly used abbreviation for deoxyribonucleic acid, the principal carrier of genetic information in almost all organisms (the exceptions are certain viruses that use *RNA*, ribonucleic acid, to carry genetic information). DNA is found in the *chromosomes* of cells; its double-helix structure allows the chromosomes to be copied exactly during the process of cell division. (See also *Nucleic acids*.)

Dogs, diseases from

Infectious or parasitic diseases, acquired from contact with dogs, that may be caused by viruses, bacteria, fungi, protozoa, worms, insects, or mites living in or on the dog.

People and dogs have been sharing living quarters for more than three million years, so it is not surprising that they share some parasites. Many of these parasites show a marked preference for dogs, but may accidentally be transferred to humans who stroke a dog's fur or touch contaminated dog feces.

Overall, diseases contracted from dogs are uncommon—especially the more serious ones—and must be viewed in light of the tremendous psychological benefits and pleasure that owners derive from their pets.

Fleas and ticks
Ticks may transfer from a dog's fur; fleas inhabit the pet's resting places and can cause irritating bites.

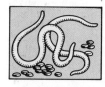

Worms and eggs
Worm eggs in dog feces are a more serious danger than adult worms.

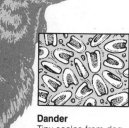

Dander
Tiny scales from dog fur (known as dander) may cause an allergy if they are inhaled.

Transmission of infection
Transmission from feces occurs when a person (often a child) directly handles a dog's feces or anus (or contaminates his or her fingers with fecal material from the soil or from the dog's fur) and transfers infective organisms to his or her mouth. Infection can also occur from eating food that has been contaminated with dog feces. Other means of transferring infection are through saliva and direct contact.

D

SPECIFIC DISEASES

The most serious disease that can be caught from a dog is *rabies*, usually transmitted by a bite. Any dog bite, particularly if the dog is a stray, should be treated with suspicion. Dog bites can also cause serious bleeding and shock and may become infected.

Two potentially serious, although rare, diseases caused by the ingestion of worm eggs from dogs are *toxocariasis* and *hydatid disease*. Toxocariasis is mainly an infection of children; the passage of worm larvae through the body can cause allergic symptoms such as asthma, and, rarely, a larva may lodge in an eye and cause blindness. Hydatid disease can lead to the development of cysts in the liver, lungs, brain, or elsewhere. Usually sheep, not people, pick up the infection and then reinfect dogs; the disease is most common in sheep-rearing areas.

In the tropics, walking barefoot on sand or soil previously contaminated with dog feces can lead to infection with dog *hookworms*.

Bites from dog *fleas* are an occasional nuisance. The fleas inhabit places in a house where the dog habitually rests and, if the dog is absent, may jump onto humans for a meal. *Ticks* and *mites* from dogs, including a canine version of the *scabies* mite, are other common problems. The fungi that cause *tinea* (ringworm) infections may come from dogs, although the disease is usually evident in the dog because it causes progressive hair loss.

Finally, some people become allergic to animal *dander* (tiny scales derived from fur or skin and present in household dust) and have such symptoms as *asthma* or *urticaria* when a dog is in the house. (See also *Cats, diseases from; Zoonoses*.)

Donor

A person who provides blood for transfusion, tissues or organs for transplantation, or semen for artificial insemination.

Many individuals carry donor cards to indicate that they have bequeathed all or parts of their bodies to be used, should they die unexpectedly, for the treatment of others. The bequest may also be made by the next-of-kin at the time of death.

Donors should be between the ages of 1 and 55 years, should be free of cancer (except primary brain cancer), should be free of serious infection (such as hepatitis B), and should not carry HIV (the AIDS virus).

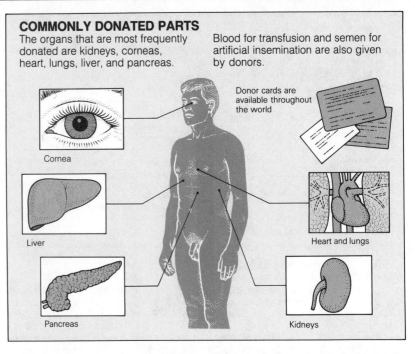

COMMONLY DONATED PARTS
The organs that are most frequently donated are kidneys, corneas, heart, lungs, liver, and pancreas.

Blood for transfusion and semen for artificial insemination are also given by donors.

Donor cards are available throughout the world

Cornea

Liver

Pancreas

Heart and lungs

Kidneys

In general, organs for transplantation must be removed within a few hours of *brain death*, and before or immediately after the heart beat has stopped. An organ is used only if it is completely healthy.

In about one third of kidney transplants, the kidney is provided by a living donor. The living volunteer is usually a sibling or parent whose body tissues match well on the basis of *tissue typing*. Tests are performed to make sure that both kidneys are healthy before one is removed for transplantation. A healthy donor's life is not shortened because the remaining kidney grows to compensate for the kidney that has been removed.

Suitable related donors whose tissue types match may also provide bone marrow for transplantation and sometimes skin for grafting. (See also *Artificial insemination; Blood donation; Bone marrow transplantation; Organ donation; Transplant surgery*.)

Do not resuscitate

The term used to request that hospital staff do not attempt heroic measures to save or restore life in patients with severe, progressive disease.

Doppler effect

A change in the frequency with which waves from a given source reach an observer when the source is in rapid motion with respect to the observer.

When a fast-moving train blows its whistle as it passes through a station, a person standing on the platform hears an apparent increase in pitch (frequency) as the train approaches and then a lowering of pitch once the train has passed and is moving away. In fact, the whistle gives off a constant pitch, but it seems to rise and then fall to the person on the platform because the train is moving. This change in the observed frequency of sound as a result of movement is called the Doppler effect or Doppler shift.

The Doppler effect is utilized in various medical *ultrasound scanning* techniques. In these techniques, an emitter sends out pulses of ultrasound (inaudible high-frequency sound) of a specific frequency. When these pulses bounce off a moving object—blood flowing through a blood vessel or the beating heart of a fetus in the uterus, for example—the frequency of the echoes is changed from that of the emitted sound (the Doppler effect in action). A special sensor detects the frequency change and, for the examples above, converts this data into information about how fast the blood is flowing or the rate at which the fetal heart is beating.

Doppler ultrasound techniques are used to measure blood pressure in superficial blood vessels and to detect air bubbles in *dialysis* and in *heart-lung machines*.

Dorsal

Relating to the back, located on or near the back, or describing the uppermost part of a body structure when a person is lying facedown. For example, dorsalgia is pain in the back, and the dorsal part of the tongue is the back of the tongue. In human anatomy, the term dorsal means the same as posterior. The opposite of dorsal is *ventral* (anterior or front).

Dose

A term used to refer to the amount of a drug taken at a particular time, or to the amount of radiation an individual is exposed to during one session of *radiation therapy*.

DRUG DOSE

The dose of a drug can be expressed in several ways: in terms of the weight of its active substance, usually in milligrams; in terms of the volume of liquid to be drunk, usually in milliliters; or in terms of its biological activity potential (its effects on body tissues as calculated in a laboratory). This last value is usually expressed in units or international units.

It is not possible to compare the effects of two different drugs from the same group on the body simply by comparing the size of the doses. Some are "stronger" (more potent) than others, just as different alcoholic drinks vary in their alcohol content.

RADIATION DOSE

The dose of radiation received during a session of radiation therapy is expressed in rads or grays (see box on *Radiation* units). These units are a measure of the amount of radiation absorbed by body tissues. Different types of body tissue are able to absorb different amounts of energy from the same beam of radiation.

Double-blind

A type of *controlled trial*—the aim of which is to test the effectiveness of a treatment or to compare the benefits of different treatments. Double-blind trials differ from other types of controlled trials in that neither the patients taking part nor the physicians who assess the treatments know which patients are receiving which treatment. This eliminates any conscious or unconscious expectations about which treatment will be most effective, thus affecting the results of the trial.

For example, a new drug and an older, standard treatment might be compared by placing the two drugs into identical capsules (by a person

who otherwise takes no part in the trial) and giving them to different groups of patients on a random selection (chance) basis. The patients are later examined by one or more physicians. Only after all assessments have been made is the identity of the drug that was given to each patient revealed—usually by the person who originally prepared the capsules.

Double vision

The seeing of two instead of one visual image of a single object, also known as diplopia. It should not be confused with *blurred vision*.

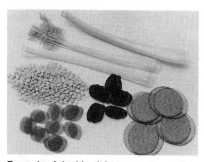

Example of double vision
Two images, rather than a single image, are seen. Prompt investigation by a physician is required.

CAUSES

Double vision is usually a symptom of *strabismus* (deviation or malalignment of the two eyes), although not all strabismus produces double vision. Paralytic strabismus is a type of strabismus that commonly causes double vision. In this condition movement of the eye in a particular direction is impaired due to paralysis of one or more of the muscles. Tilting or turning the head can sometimes overcome the double vision.

A growth in the eyelid pressing on the front of the eyeball can also cause temporary image separation by distorting the shape of the front of the eye and by causing a slight displacement in the path of light rays entering that eye (and thus variation in the points at which they are focused on the retina). Double vision may be caused by a tumor or blood clot behind the eye that prevents the normal motion of the eyeball.

In endocrine-related *exophthalmos*, protrusion of the eyeballs is the result of an underlying hormonal disorder and double vision results from swelling and scarring in the eye muscles, causing abnormal alignment and motion of the eyes.

Rarely, double vision arises because of an abnormality within the eye. For example, a dislocation of the *lens* in the eye may result in some light rays passing through the lens and others around it, so that separate images fall on the retina of one eye.

COMPLICATIONS AND TREATMENT

The brain of a young child with strabismus (congenital, accommodative, or paralytic) learns to suppress the second, unwanted image seen by the misaligned, strabismic eye so as not to see double. Continued misalignment of the child's eyes may eventually lead to poor vision in the affected eye. This poor vision is called *amblyopia*, or lazy eye. Patching of the better-seeing eye may improve the vision in the poorly seeing, deviated eye. The strabismus may need to be corrected early (by means of glasses and/or surgery) in children to prevent amblyopia from developing; otherwise, it may become permanent. A young child with strabismus should be seen by a physician to find the cause and to begin treatment.

The onset of double vision in adult life needs immediate investigation to exclude the possibility of a tumor, aneurysm, and/or neurologic abnormality. The double vision could be a symptom of a very serious underlying disorder that requires prompt attention and treatment.

Douche

Introduction of water and/or a cleansing agent into the vagina using equipment consisting of a bag and tubing with a nozzle attached. Intended to clean the vagina, a douche is unnecessary; the vagina is normally slightly acidic and cleans itself.

In the past, douches were widely used after sexual intercourse to cleanse the vagina and as a means of contraception. They were also used by women who were worried about having excessive or offensive vaginal discharge. Douches were sometimes recommended to treat vaginal infections and were also used after vaginal repair operations.

Today it is recognized that a douche carries the risk of introducing infection into the vagina, especially if the nozzle is not cleaned properly before use. A douche also may spread an existing vaginal infection into the uterus or fallopian tubes. A douche is completely ineffective as a contraceptive method. Today gynecologists rarely, if ever, recommend douches for any reason.

D

D

Down's syndrome

A *chromosomal abnormality* resulting in mental handicap and a characteristic physical appearance. Down's syndrome was originally named "mongolism" because it was thought that the facial features of affected children resembled those of Mongolians. The term is no longer used by the medical profession.

CAUSES

The cause of Down's syndrome remained a mystery until 1959, when researchers discovered that each of the body cells of people with Down's syndrome has one too many chromosomes—47 instead of the normal 46. Because in most cases the extra chromosome is number 21, the disorder is also called trisomy 21.

There are several possible reasons for the chromosomal abnormality. In most cases it is the result of a failure of the two chromosomes numbered 21 in a parent cell to go into separate daughter cells during the first stage of sperm or egg cell formation (see *Chromosomes*). Some eggs or sperm are therefore formed with an extra number 21 chromosome and, if one of these takes part in fertilization, the resulting baby will also have the extra chromosome. This type of abnormality is particularly likely if the mother is over 35, suggesting that defective egg formation, rather than sperm formation, is usually at fault.

A less common cause is a chromosomal abnormality in either parent, known as a *translocation*, in which part of one of the parent's own number 21 chromosomes has joined with another chromosome. The parent is not affected except for the risk of having a child with Down's syndrome.

INCIDENCE

About one in 650 babies born is affected by Down's syndrome. The incidence of affected fetuses rises steeply with increased maternal age to about one in 40 among mothers over 40. Pregnant women over 35, and

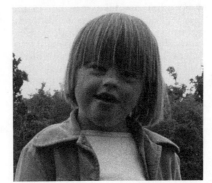

Typical features
The eyes slope upward at the outer corners and the inner corners are covered, the facial features are small, and the tongue is large and tends to stick out. The back of the head is usually flat.

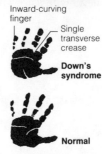

Inward-curving finger

Single transverse crease

Down's syndrome

Normal

those with a family history of Down's syndrome or other factors putting them at risk, are usually offered *chromosome analysis* of the fetus' cells after these have been obtained by *amniocentesis* or *chorionic villus sampling*. If the fetus is found to be affected, termination of the pregnancy may be one of the options.

SYMPTOMS

Most people with Down's syndrome have eyes that slope up at the outer corners and folds of skin on either side of the nose that cover the inner corners of the eye. The face and features are small, the tongue is large and tends to protrude, the head has a flattened back, and the hands are typically short and broad. The degree of mental handicap varies. A Down's syndrome child's IQ may be anywhere from 30 to 80. Virtually all affected children are capable of a limited amount of learning, including

in some cases the ability to read. Down's syndrome children are usually affectionate, friendly, and cheerful, and they get along well with other family members.

About one fourth of Down's syndrome children have a heart defect at birth (see *Heart disease, congenital*). They also have a higher-than-average incidence of intestinal *atresia* (narrowing at some point in the intestines), congenital *hearing* defects, and acute *leukemia*, and they are especially susceptible to repeated ear infections. For unknown reasons, *atherosclerosis* (narrowing of the arteries), which leads to an increased risk of heart disease, tends to develop in adults affected by Down's syndrome.

DIAGNOSIS

Because of the distinctive physical features, Down's syndrome is usually recognized soon after birth. The diagnosis is confirmed by a count of the chromosomes in white blood cells taken from a blood sample (see *Chromosome analysis*).

TREATMENT

There is no cure for the mental handicap, but Down's syndrome children can make the most of their capabilities through constant educational and environmental stimulation. Institutional care is sometimes necessary, but affected children are generally happiest in a sympathetic home environment. It is possible to alter the facial appearance by plastic surgery.

OUTLOOK

Until recently (less than a generation ago) most Down's syndrome children did not survive beyond their teens because of the high incidence of defects present from birth as well as their susceptibility to infection. Advances in medical and surgical techniques, together with improved long-term care facilities, have extended the life expectancy of Down's syndrome sufferers, but they still tend not to survive beyond early middle age.

Doxepin

An *antidepressant drug*, doxepin has a strong sedative effect and is useful in the treatment of depression accompanied by anxiety or insomnia.

Possible adverse effects include dry mouth, blurred vision, dizziness, drowsiness, and attacks of flushing, which may disappear if the dosage is reduced. This drug usually takes between two to six weeks to become fully effective.

Doxorubicin

An *anticancer drug* given by injection, usually in combination with other anticancer drugs of this group. Doxorubicin is used to treat a variety of cancers, including *leukemia, Hodgkin's disease*, and lung cancer.

Doxycycline

A *tetracycline* antibiotic drug. Doxycycline has been found to be more effective than most other tetracyclines

in the treatment of chronic *prostatitis* (prostate gland infection), *pelvic inflammatory disease*, and attacks of chest infection in chronic bronchitis.

Doxycycline is also used to treat severe attacks of traveler's diarrhea and is occasionally prescribed to prevent this condition before traveling to foreign countries.

Because its action lasts longer than that of some other tetracyclines, doxycycline must be taken only once or twice a day. It is also useful in treating people with kidney disease because it is broken down by the liver rather than excreted in the urine. Possible adverse effects, such as nausea and indigestion, can be reduced by taking doxycycline with food; absorption of doxycycline, unlike many other tetracyclines, is not impaired if the drug is taken with food.

DPT vaccination
A series of injections that provides immunity against *diphtheria*, *pertussis* (whooping cough), and *tetanus*.

HOW IT IS DONE
DPT vaccine is given initially as a course of three injections at the ages of 2, 4, and 6 months. More doses are given at 15 to 18 months and before school at the age of 4 to 6 years.

WHY IT IS DONE
DPT vaccination causes the body to produce antibodies to fend off diphtheria, pertussis, and tetanus infections. The vaccine does not provide complete immunity to diphtheria, but it does protect against the dangers of infection. Since DPT was not routinely administered in the US until the late 1940s, any adult exposed to diphtheria should be checked for immunity. If a blood sample shows no antibodies against the disease, diphtheria vaccine will then be administered.

The pertussis vaccine also does not provide absolute protection, but children who have been immunized get only a mild version of the disease and are unlikely to become seriously ill. The protection against pertussis gradually wanes, so adults can get the infection. In adults, the disease is mild, but adults can infect unimmunized children. The disease can be fatal in children.

Protection against tetanus is not permanent; it needs to be "boosted" with another shot every 10 years or at the time of any dirty, penetrating injury if vaccination has not been done within the last five years.

RISKS
In the cases of diphtheria and tetanus, the life-threatening feature of the infection is a toxin (poison) produced by the bacteria. The vaccine contains toxoids—modified versions of the diphtheria and tetanus toxins—that stimulate the formation of antibodies. Because the toxoids are chemicals and not organisms, physical reactions to them are rare.

Pertussis vaccine consists of killed bacteria, which stimulate antibodies (but are more likely to provoke a reac-

tion). The pertussis component commonly causes a slight fever and some irritability for a couple of days after the vaccination. More serious reactions, including signs of irritation of the brain and nervous system, including convulsions, occur in less than one in 100,000 vaccinations. Permanent damage from the vaccine is even more rare. Nevertheless, many babies are being given vaccine without the pertussis component. In England, when pertussis vaccinations were refused by many parents, an epidemic of pertussis occurred. It is estimated that, between 1977 and 1983, close to 500 children died as a result of pertussis infection; some cases of permanent brain damage or lung damage occurred as well. The benefits outweigh the minimal risk from the vaccine. Vaccine without pertussis is given to children who have reacted severely to DPT vaccine or who suffer from, or have a history of, brain abnormalities or seizures.

REASONS TO QUESTION THE ADMINISTRATION OF THE PERTUSSIS VACCINE TO YOUR CHILD
1. If your child is an infant with a neurologic disorder that is characterized by progressive developmental delay or seizures.
2. If your child's prior DPT immunization has caused any of the following:
■ Encephalopathy (severe alterations in consciousness and focal neurologic signs) within seven days (usually seen within three days) after receiving the vaccination.
■ Convulsions with or without fever within three days after receiving the vaccination.
■ Persistent, inconsolable screaming or crying (or an unusual, high-pitched cry) for three or more hours within 48 hours after receiving the vaccine.
■ Collapse or shocklike state within 48 hours after receiving the vaccine.
■ Temperature of 104.9°F (40.5°C) or more that is unexplained by any other cause within 48 hours after receiving the vaccine.
■ Allergic reaction to vaccine (such as anaphylaxis) after receiving the vaccine; this is extremely rare.

Drain, surgical
An appliance inserted by the physician into a body cavity or wound to release and permit drainage of fluid or air from it.

TYPES
The simplest drains are soft rubber tubes that pass from a body cavity into a dressing. More sophisticated drains are wide-bore tubes that connect to a

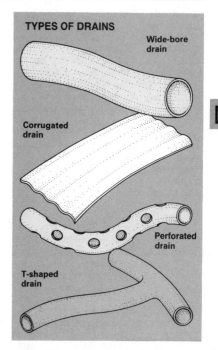

TYPES OF DRAINS
Wide-bore drain
Corrugated drain
Perforated drain
T-shaped drain

collection bag or bottle. A valve prevents fluid from refluxing back into the body. Another type, corrugated drains, have a series of curved ridges to help collect fluid from a wound. Suction drains consist of a thin tube with many small holes to help collect fluid, which is drawn into a vacuum bottle. Suction can also be applied to a drain by means of a vacuum pump.

A drain that removes bile from the biliary system (gallbladder and bile ducts) after surgery in that area is T-shaped to hold it in place.

Dream analysis
The interpretation of a person's dreams as part of *psychoanalysis* or *psychotherapy*. First developed by Sigmund Freud, the technique relies on the idea that a person's repressed feelings and thoughts are revealed in dreams, but in a disguised manner. The therapist unravels the significance of the dream by using a knowledge of the patient's character to interpret symbols, and by asking the patient for any associations suggested by the dream.

Dreaming
Mental activity that takes place during *sleep*. The evidence suggests strongly that dreaming occurs only during periods of REM (rapid eye movement) sleep, which last for about 20 minutes and occur four or five times a night.

D

PHYSIOLOGY

Although there are still arguments about the exact function of dreams, their physiological aspects are well understood. Using an electroencephalograph (a machine that records the electrical activity of the brain, see *EEG*), it is possible to describe various phases of sleep in terms of their different electrical patterns. Compared to other phases, the REM phase is active, as if the sleeper were awake but drowsy. At the same time, blood flow and brain temperature increase, and there are sudden changes in heart rate and blood pressure. All this may indicate that the brain is restoring itself for further activity.

Dreaming can be seen as a parallel process in which the mental impressions, feelings, and ideas that have been taken in during the day are sorted out. The content of dreams therefore closely represents the day's preoccupations—with the ideas and memories distorted by the lack of a conscious and awake mind.

People roused during periods of REM sleep report especially vivid dreams, but those who wake normally after normal dream activity has ended may not remember dreaming at all.

SIGNIFICANCE

As a proportion of total sleep, REM sleep is much greater in young babies and after head injury. This indicates that it may have an important role in promoting brain activity. Whether or not dreams have an important psychological role is more controversial. Depriving people of their dreams by constantly waking them during REM phases was once thought to cause severe psychological disorders, but this is now less generally accepted. Certain hypnotic drugs suppress REM sleep without causing any obvious psychological harm.

Dressings

Protective coverings for wounds. Dressings may be used to control bleeding, absorb secretions, or prevent contamination by bacteria. They are placed directly onto wounds and are large enough to cover them completely. They should be sterile so as not to introduce bacteria that could cause infection. A dressing should also be absorbent; if sweat cannot evaporate, the skin around the wound becomes moist and soft and the dressing sodden, thus encouraging the growth of bacteria and further infection. Unless a wound must be regularly cleaned, dressings should be

FIRST AID: DRESSINGS

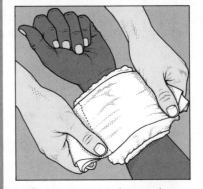

1 Remove outer protective wrapping, being careful not to touch the gauze. If possible, wash your hands before touching the unwrapped dressing. Then hold the dressing, gauze-side down, over the wound.

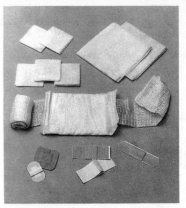

Assorted dressings
In addition to sterile dressings, plain gauze and a variety of adhesive-strip bandages can be used.

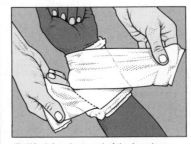

2 Wind the short end of the bandage once around the arm and dressing. Bandage firmly (not tightly) and cover pad.

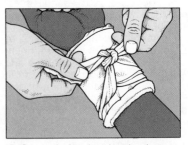

3 Secure the bandage by tying the two ends over the gauze pad using a square knot (left end over right end and under; right end over left end and under).

left undisturbed. A wound should be covered for the minimum length of time. (See also *Compress*.)

TYPES

ADHESIVE BANDAGES Available in a range of sizes, these consist of absorbent pads held in place by waterproof adhesive backings. They are commonly used to protect small wounds, such as cuts and abrasions, but may also be used to cover surgical wounds.

GAUZE Usually applied in layers, gauze is made of woven or nonwoven cotton or a synthetic material and is used to cover larger wounds. It is held in place by a bandage or a length of adhesive strapping. The gauze is usually applied dry, but ribbon gauze, soaked in a substance to promote granulation of the tissue, may be used to pack a deep wound. Sterile, unmedicated dressings consist of layers of fine gauze and a pad of absorbent cotton attached to a roller bandage.

NONSTICK DRESSINGS Of recent development, these dressings consist of a nonadherent contact layer of perforated polyethylene or viscose with an impregnated gauze pad backing. Such dressings do not adhere to wounds and can be removed without disturbing newly formed tissue.

IMPROVISED DRESSINGS In emergency first-aid treatment, any clean, dry, and absorbent material may be used to cover a wound (for example, a handkerchief or piece of sheeting) if a sterile dressing is not available. Absorbent cotton or woolly fibrous materials should not be used because the fibers may become embedded in the wound.

APPLYING A DRESSING
See illustrated box.

Dressler's syndrome

An uncommon condition, also called postinfarction syndrome, that may occur after a *myocardial infarction* (heart attack) or heart surgery. The condition is characterized by fever, chest pain, *pericarditis* (inflammation of the outer covering membrane of the heart), and *pleurisy* (inflammation of the outer lining of the lungs).

Dressler's syndrome is thought to be an *autoimmune disorder*. The body's immune system produces antibodies (proteins with a defensive role) that are directed against the damaged areas of heart muscle.

The features of the condition first appear any time between a few days and several weeks after a myocardial infarction or heart surgery. The diagnosis is confirmed by detecting specific antibodies in the blood. Treatment with aspirin usually clears the condition, although, in some more severe cases, treatment with *corticosteroid drugs* is needed.

DRG

The abbreviation for *diagnosis-related group*.

Dribbling

A term commonly used to denote involuntary leakage of urine (see *Incontinence, urinary*).

Drip

See *Intravenous infusion*.

Drooling

The involuntary leakage of saliva from the mouth—normal behavior in infants up to the age of about 12 months. Drooling in an adult may simply be due to poorly fitting dentures or may be the result of facial paralysis, *dementia*, or a serious underlying disorder, most commonly *Parkinson's disease*.

Drop attack

A brief disturbance affecting the nervous system, causing a person to fall suddenly to the ground without warning; the legs just seem to buckle. Unlike *fainting*, the person may not lose consciousness, but injuries can occur to the hands, face, or knees as a result of the fall.

CAUSES AND INCIDENCE
Although drop attacks can affect all age groups, elderly women are the most commonly affected. The causes are not fully understood, although in some cases there may be a fall in blood flow to nerve centers in the *brain stem*.

Occasionally, elderly men may experience a drop attack while passing urine or while standing. Lowered blood pressure or an abrupt alteration

in the heart's rhythm may be involved; it is advisable for these people to sit down while urinating.

Other rare causes of drop attacks include a block in the flow of cerebrospinal fluid around the brain—usually in patients with a type of *hydrocephalus*. One uncommon form of epileptic convulsion, an akinetic seizure, is sometimes also described as a drop attack. During this seizure, the sufferer falls suddenly to the ground and briefly loses consciousness, but does not convulse.

TREATMENT
Drop attacks in the elderly cannot be treated but usually disappear in time. Akinetic seizures respond to anticonvulsant drug treatment.

Dropsy

An outmoded term for generalized *edema* (fluid collection in body tissues). In the past, many people were certified as dead "due to dropsy."

Dropsy is not itself a disease, but merely a sign of malfunction in the body (especially congestive *heart failure* or kidney disease).

Drowning

Death caused by suffocation and *hypoxia* (lack of oxygen) associated with immersion in a fluid.

In about four fifths of cases the person has inhaled liquid into the lungs; in the other fifth, no liquid has entered the lungs—a condition called dry drowning (see *Drowning, dry*). People who are resuscitated after prolonged immersion are said to be victims of "near drowning."

INCIDENCE AND CAUSES
Drowning is the third most common cause of accidental death in the US (after motor vehicle accidents and falls). About one person in 280 in the US dies from drowning (or more than 7,000 people every year). Many more are victims of near drowning. Worldwide, possibly as many as 200,000 people drown annually.

Many victims are competent swimmers who have failed to take into account factors such as tidal currents (or undertow) and have tired and panicked. A relatively small number are nonswimmers. Other drowning circumstances include floods, sinkings, immersion in freezing cold water after falling through ice, and infant drownings, which can occur in as little as six inches of water.

Over one third of drowning victims have a significant amount of alcohol in their blood upon postmortem

examination. Alcohol intoxication impairs judgment and at the same time reduces physical coordination—an extremely dangerous combination before swimming.

Some methods of minimizing the risks of a drowning accident are shown in the table, next page.

MECHANISM OF DROWNING
When a person panics at the surface of the water, the thrashing movements are incapable of keeping the body afloat, and the person begins taking in small amounts of water. Initially, automatic contraction of a muscle at the entrance to the windpipe—a mechanism called the laryngeal reflex—prevents water from entering the lungs and instead it enters the esophagus and stomach. However, the laryngeal reflex impairs breathing, which can quickly lead to *hypoxia* and to loss of consciousness.

If the person is buoyant at this point and floats face-up, his or her chances of survival are reasonable because the laryngeal reflex begins to relax and normal breathing may recommence. On the other hand, the person may float face-down or may sink.

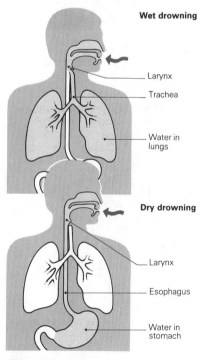

Wet drowning

Larynx

Trachea

Water in lungs

Dry drowning

Larynx

Esophagus

Water in stomach

Types of drowning
In four fifths of deaths due to drowning, the victim has inhaled liquid into his or her lungs. In the other fifth, no liquid is present in the lungs (dry drowning). In both cases, death is the result of suffocation.

FIRST AID AND TREATMENT

If a person is panicking at the surface of the water, he or she should be thrown any large item that will float. Ideally, the person should be approached in a boat and reached. If approached by swimming, an attempt should be made to calm the person before contact is made, otherwise he or she may struggle, possibly causing the rescuer to drown as well.

The victim should be supported with the head above water and towed to the nearest boat or shore. An ambulance should be called and the person's medical condition assessed. If breathing and/or the pulse (felt in the neck) is absent, resuscitative measures should be started (see *Cardiopulmonary resuscitation*). They should be continued until an ambulance or physician has arrived.

Often, a victim of near drowning will make an apparently remarkable recovery after being resuscitated. The person should nevertheless be sent to a hospital for investigation and observation. Water may have passed from the lungs into the blood, and the lining of the lungs may have been damaged. In either case, symptoms may develop some hours after rescue and may be life threatening.

Drowning, dry

A form of drowning in which no fluid enters the lungs.

About one fifth of fatal drowning cases are "dry"—illustrating the fact that death from drowning results mainly from lack of oxygen, whether or not water has entered the lungs (see *Drowning*). Victims of dry drowning have a particularly strong laryngeal reflex, which diverts water into the stomach instead of the lungs, but at the same time impairs breathing.

Drowsiness

A state of consciousness between full wakefulness and sleep or unconsciousness. It is medically significant if it is abnormal.

Abnormal drowsiness may be the result of a head injury, high fever, *meningitis* (inflammation of the membranes that surround the brain and spinal cord), a metabolic disorder such as *uremia* (excessive metabolic products in the blood), or liver failure. Alcohol or drugs may also produce this effect. In a diabetic, drowsiness may be due to *hypoglycemia* (low blood sugar), usually as a result of taking too much insulin, or to *hyperglycemia* (high blood sugar) due to inadequate control of the disorder.

If a person who is drowsy fails to awaken after being shaken, pinched, and shouted at—or wakes and then relapses into drowsiness—treat the situation as a medical emergency and call for professional help immediately. (See *Unconsciousness*.)

Drug

Any chemical substance that alters the function of one or more body organs or changes the process of a disease. Drugs include prescribed medicines, over-the-counter remedies, and the recreational, social, and illicit use of drugs, such as cocaine. Many foods and drinks contain small quantities of substances classed as drugs—tea, coffee, and cola drinks, for example, all contain *caffeine*, which is both a *stimulant* and a *diuretic drug*.

Each drug normally has three names: a detailed, descriptive chemical name; a shorter, generic name (see *Generic drug*) that has been officially approved; and a specific brand name chosen by the company that manufactures it. Drugs are either licensed for prescription by a physician only or are over-the-counter preparations available at a drugstore or supermarket.

SOURCES

Originally, all drugs were naturally occurring substances extracted from animals, plants, and minerals. Today, most drugs are produced artificially in the laboratory, ensuring a purer preparation with a predictable potency (strength) that is safer for medical use. Some drugs, such as *insulin* and *growth hormone*, are now sometimes synthesized using *genetic engineering* procedures.

New drugs are discovered in a number of ways: by screening a substance

---

DROWNING: RESCUE METHODS

Throwing the victim something to hold on to is useful if he or she is still conscious and has not panicked.

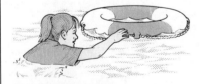

Otherwise, go to the person in a boat or, if no boat is available, reach him or her by swimming.

Throwing a buoy or line
If no life buoy is available, use any large object that floats. It should preferably have a rope attached to pull the person to safety (a rope alone may be sufficient).

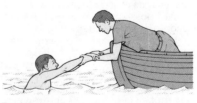

Rescuing from a boat
After grasping the person's arms, it may be necessary to "bounce" him or her in the water to gain momentum for a lift into the boat. With two rescuers, one can enter the water to assist.

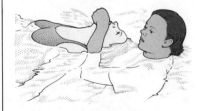

Towing
A panicky victim may need to be calmed before making contact; otherwise, he or she may struggle. During the tow ashore, it is important to keep the person's face above water.

MEASURES THAT MAY HELP PREVENT DROWNING ACCIDENTS

1 Never jump into deep water without ensuring that there is an easy and obvious method of exit.

2 Wear a life jacket or buoyancy device for all water sports (such as sailing and windsurfing).

3 Swim only in pools or from public beaches designated as safe and patrolled by lifeguards.

4 Do not drink alcohol before swimming or water sports of any kind.

5 Children should always be supervised when swimming and when they are taking baths.

6 Never walk on an iced-over pond or river unless the ice has first been tested by an adult.

for different types of activity against a disease; by making alterations to the structure of an established drug; or, occasionally, by finding a new application for a drug that is being used for another condition.

CLASSIFICATION

A drug is classified in one of the following ways: 1) according to its chemical make up (a *corticosteroid drug*, for example); 2) according to the disorder it treats (an *antihypertensive drug*, for example, is used to treat high blood pressure); or 3) according to its specific effect on the body (a diuretic drug, for example, increases the volume of urine).

EVALUATION

All new drugs are tested for their efficiency and safety. Tests usually go through three stages: laboratory trials on animals; laboratory trials on human volunteers; and, finally, clinical trials on patients.

The Food and Drug Administration (FDA) will issue a license if studies provide evidence of the drug's efficacy and safety according to strictly defined standards. The FDA also establishes standards of quality, purity of the preparation, and adequate labeling.

Evaluation continues even after a drug has become widely prescribed. A drug's license may be withdrawn if toxic effects are reported frequently or if even a few patients develop serious illness attributable to the drug.

WHY DRUGS ARE USED

Drugs can be used in the treatment, prevention, or diagnosis of a disease. They are prescribed to relieve physical or mental symptoms, to replace a deficient natural substance (such as a *hormone*), or to stop the excessive production of a hormone or other body chemical. Some drugs are given to destroy foreign organisms, such as bacteria or viruses. Others, known as *vaccines*, are given to stimulate the body's *immune system* (natural defenses) to form antibodies.

Antibiotic drugs, diuretics, *analgesics* (painkillers), and *tranquilizers* are among the most commonly prescribed drugs. The most frequently used over-the-counter remedies include analgesics, cough and cold remedies, vitamins, and tonics.

HOW DRUGS WORK

Drugs act on cells in the body or the infecting organism by stimulating or blocking chemical reactions. In many cases, this action occurs because the drug impersonates a chemical that occurs naturally in the body.

METHODS OF ADMINISTERING DRUGS

How taken	Action
By mouth 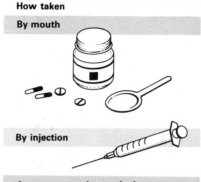	Drugs are digested and absorbed from the intestine in the same way as nutrients. How quickly the tablet or liquid works depends on how rapidly it is absorbed. This, in turn, depends on such factors as the drug's composition, how quickly the drug dissolves, and the effect of digestive juices on it.
By injection 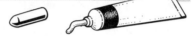	Drugs given by injection have a very rapid effect. Injection is also used if digestive juices would destroy a drug.
As a cream, anal or vaginal suppository, pessary, nasal spray, or by inhaler	These drugs have a local effect on the parts of the body that are exposed to them as well as a systemic (generalized) effect if some of the drug is absorbed into the bloodstream from the site of application.

Some drugs act by binding (becoming attached) to a drug receptor (a specific site on the cell's surface that matches the chemical structure of the drug). This triggers a change in chemical activity within the cell. Other drugs work by being absorbed into the cell, where they affect the chemical processes directly.

Drugs may also have a placebo effect, which occurs because of the individual's positive or negative expectations of the drug's action.

METHODS OF ADMINISTRATION

Drugs are given in different forms and in different ways (see table). These methods depend on many factors, including the severity of the illness, the part of the body being treated, the properties of the drug, and the speed and duration of action required.

ELIMINATION

Drugs taken by mouth that are not absorbed in the intestine are excreted in the stools. Drugs that have entered the bloodstream are eliminated through the kidneys in the urine. Some drugs are broken down into inactive forms in the liver by *enzymes* before elimination.

COMPLIANCE

If drug treatment is to be beneficial, the full course must be taken as instructed by a physician. It is estimated that as many as two out of every five people who are prescribed a drug do not take it properly, if at all. Reasons for noncompliance include failure to understand instructions for taking the drug, fear of possible reactions, or simply not bothering to take the drug.

DRUG INTERACTIONS

Taking drugs together or in combination with food or alcohol may produce effects on the body that differ from those occurring when a drug is taken on its own. Such drug interactions occur if chemicals in the different substances act on the same receptors or if one chemical alters the absorption, breakdown, or elimination of another chemical.

Physicians often make use of interactions to increase the effectiveness of a treatment; combinations of drugs are often prescribed to treat infection, cancer, or hypertension (high blood pressure). Many interactions, however, are unplanned; they may reduce the benefit from a drug or increase its level in the blood and cause adverse effects.

Patients undergoing long-term drug treatment may be advised to carry warning cards to avoid dangerous interactions from any treatment received during an emergency. Patients should tell their physicians about any other drugs they are taking to prevent interactions with drugs the physician may prescribe.

ADVERSE EFFECTS

Most drugs can produce adverse effects—harmful or unpleasant reactions that result from a normal dose of the drug. These adverse effects can be divided into predictable adverse reactions, which result from the effects of the chemical structure of the drug, and bizarre (unpredictable) reactions, which are unrelated to the drug's normal chemical effects on cells. Predictable adverse reactions are due to the difficulty experienced by the drug manufacturer in targeting the action of a drug to a single tissue or organ. For example, *anticholinergic drugs* prescribed to relieve spasm in the intestine also cause blurred vision and dryness of the mouth. Symptoms may wear off as the body adapts to the drug; otherwise, they usually are relieved by reducing the dose or increasing the interval between doses.

Any change in the absorption, breakdown, or elimination of a drug (caused, for example, by gastro-intestinal, liver, or kidney disease) that increases its concentration in the blood will increase the risk of predictable adverse effects.

Bizarre drug reactions may be due to a genetic disorder (for example, lack of a specific enzyme that usually inactivates the drug), an allergic reaction, or the formation of *antibodies* that damage tissue. Common side effects of this type include a rash, facial swelling, or jaundice. Occasionally, *anaphylactic shock* (a severe allergic reaction), characterized by breathing difficulty or collapse, may occur. All bizarre drug reactions usually necessitate withdrawal of the drug.

Many drugs cross the placenta and some adversely affect growth and development of the fetus. Most drugs pass into the breast milk of a nursing mother; some have adverse effects on the baby.

A drug is useful only if its overall benefit to the patient outweighs the risk and severity of any adverse effects. Research on new drugs partly aims to discover preparations that act selectively on target organs to avoid unwanted effects on other tissues.

Drug abuse

COMMON DRUGS
Stimulants *Amphetamines*
Depressants *Alcohol Barbiturates*
Psychedelics *LSD*
Narcotics *Cocaine Heroin*
Anabolic steroids

The use of a drug for a purpose other than that for which it is normally prescribed or recommended. The reasons for drug abuse include the desire to escape from reality or achieve a mystical experience, curiosity about its effects, and the search for self-awareness. Certain types of drugs (for example, anabolic steroids) are sometimes abused to improve performance in sports.

Problems resulting from drug abuse may arise from the adverse effects of the drug, from accidents during intoxication, and from the habit-forming potential of many drugs, which may lead to *drug dependence*.

Drug addiction
Physical or psychological dependence on a drug. (See *Drug dependence*.)

Drug dependence
The compulsion to continue taking a drug, either to produce the desired effects that result from taking it, or to prevent the ill effects that occur when it is not taken.

TYPES
Drug dependence takes two forms: psychological and physical. A person is psychologically dependent if he or she experiences craving or emotional distress when the drug is withdrawn. In physical dependence the body has adapted to the presence of the drug, causing the symptoms and signs of a withdrawal syndrome when the drug is withdrawn. Withdrawal is usually associated with severe physical and mental distress.

CAUSES AND INCIDENCE
Drug dependence develops as a result of regular and/or excessive use of a drug. Several million people in the US are dependent on nicotine, on the caffeine in coffee and tea, and on alcohol. Many thousands are dependent on tranquilizers.

Dependence occurs most frequently with drugs that alter the individual's mood or behavior. Narcotic *analgesics* used briefly to treat a disorder (for example, the use of *morphine* to treat a heart attack) hardly ever lead to dependence. Intravenous drug abuse carries a high risk of dependence; the rapidity with which the drug produces its effects reinforces the habit of injecting the drug.

Some people seem to be more susceptible to dependency than others. Factors that usually play a part include pressure from friends and associates, and environmental factors, such as poverty, unemployment, disrupted family life, and the availability of drugs.

SYMPTOMS AND SIGNS
A mild withdrawal reaction may cause yawning, sneezing, a runny nose, watering eyes, and sweating. More severe reactions include diarrhea, vomiting, trembling, cramps, confusion, and, rarely, seizures and coma. These symptoms are usually relieved if the drug is taken again.

Withdrawal symptoms probably occur because the body has become adapted to the continuous presence of the drug, which reduces the release of certain natural chemicals (for example, nicotine affects production of *epinephrine* and similar substances). When the drug is no longer taken or is withheld, the chemical deficiency is exposed.

COMPLICATIONS
Drug dependence may cause physical problems, such as lung and heart disease from tobacco smoking and liver disease from drinking excessive amounts of alcohol. Mental problems, such as anxiety and depression, are common during withdrawal. Dependence may also be associated with drug tolerance, in which an increasingly higher dose of the substance is needed to produce the desired effect.

Complications may occur as an indirect result of dependence. For example, people who inject a narcotic drug may get sick and die as a result of an infection, such as *hepatitis* or *AIDS*, introduced into the bloodstream on a dirty needle. In other cases, the abusers may suffer from an overdose because of confusion about the dosage or because they take a purer, more potent preparation than they are used to. In severe cases, social problems result from the disruption of family life and from criminal acts carried out to pay for drugs.

TREATMENT
Controlled withdrawal programs are available in special centers and larger hospitals. These programs usually offer supervised reductions in dose. Alternative, less harmful drugs may be given, as well as treatment for withdrawal symptoms. Social service agencies and support groups may provide follow-up care.

OUTLOOK
Successful treatment requires motivation on the part of the addict. Problems frequently recur when addicts return to the circumstances that originally gave rise to drug abuse and dependence.

Druggist
A *pharmacist*. A person who is licensed to dispense drugs and to make up prescriptions.

Drug overdose

The taking of an excessive amount of a drug, which may cause toxic effects. (See *Drug poisoning*.)

Drug poisoning

The harmful effects on various organs of the body as a result of taking an excessive dose of a drug.

CAUSES AND INCIDENCE

Drug poisoning may be accidental or deliberate. Accidental poisoning is most common in young children under the age of 5 years who swallow colored tablets thinking they are candies. Child-resistant drug packaging has helped reduce this risk. In adults, accidental poisoning usually occurs in the elderly because they are confused about their treatment and dosage requirements. Accidental poisoning may also occur during *drug abuse*.

Deliberate poisoning is usually unsuccessful and is done as a cry for help (see *Suicide*; *Suicide, attempted*). The drugs taken in overdose are usually *benzodiazepine drugs*, *antidepressant drugs*, *acetaminophen*, or *aspirin*. Homicide and suicide may involve administration of a drug by another person.

TREATMENT

In dealing with a drug overdose, first-aid measures depend on the condition of the patient. If the patient is unconscious, ensure that the *airway* is clear and that there is normal breathing and a pulse before rolling the patient into the *recovery position* and summoning emergency help. If the person is not breathing, *artificial respiration* should be started.

Any individual who has taken a drug overdose and any child who has swallowed tablets belonging to someone else should be seen by a physician. It is important to identify which drugs have been taken. Empty bottles may provide vital clues; save any you find. Contact the poison control center, hospital emergency room, or a physician for advice. If the victim is fully conscious, you may be advised to induce vomiting by sticking a finger down the throat or giving *ipecac* if this is available.

Some drugs taken in excess may cause *hypothermia*; if this occurs, keep the victim warm with blankets.

Treatment in the hospital may involve gastric *lavage* (emptying the stomach using several pints of water passed down a tube through the mouth and esophagus). This procedure usually is effective only if the drug has been taken within the previous four hours or a few hours longer for drugs (such as aspirin and antidepressants) that slow down normal stomach emptying.

Charcoal may be given in some cases to reduce the *absorption* of the drug from the intestine into the bloodstream. Diuresis (increased production of urine) may be induced using an *intravenous infusion* to speed up the elimination of the drug from the bloodstream.

Antidotes are available only for specific drugs. They include naloxone (given to reverse breathing difficulty caused by morphine), methionine (given to reduce the formation of toxic substances in the liver from acetaminophen), and *chelating agents* with deferoxamine (given to absorb and inactivate iron).

COMPLICATIONS

Drug poisoning may cause drowsiness and breathing difficulty (due to effects on the brain), irregular heart beat, and, rarely, cardiac arrest, seizures, and kidney and liver damage. *ECG* monitoring (electrical recording of the heart) is usually done for the first 24 to 48 hours after poisoning with a drug that is known to have effects on the heart. *Antiarrhythmic drugs* are prescribed to treat any heart beat irregularity as it develops. Seizures are treated with *anticonvulsant drugs*. In some serious cases, the patient requires artificial *ventilation* because of severe drug-induced breathing difficulty.

Blood tests to monitor liver function and careful monitoring of urine output are carried out if the drug is known to have any toxic effect on associated organs.

Dry eye

See *Keratoconjunctivitis sicca*.

Dry ice

Frozen *carbon dioxide*, also known as carbon dioxide snow. Unlike most substances, carbon dioxide changes directly from a gas to a solid when it is cooled, without first passing through a liquid phase. In practice, dry ice is produced by allowing carbon dioxide gas stored under pressure to escape through a small nozzle. This rapid expansion cools the carbon dioxide to about $-95°F$ ($-70°C$), and dry ice is formed as a powder. This powder is then compressed into cakes.

Dry ice is sometimes applied to the skin to destroy *warts* and *nevi*, which it does by virtue of its low temperature. (See also *Cryosurgery*.)

Dry socket

Infection at the site of a recent tooth extraction, causing pain, bad breath, and an unpleasant taste. A complication of about 2 percent of extractions, dry socket occurs most commonly when a blood clot fails to form in the tooth socket after a difficult extraction, such as removal of an impacted wisdom tooth. Infection may also develop following a normal extraction if the blood clot becomes dislodged (for instance, because of excessive rinsing of the mouth). In some cases, the clot itself may become infected, or infection may have been present before the extraction. The inflamed socket appears dry, and exposed bone, which may be dead and fragmented, is often visible.

TREATMENT

The socket is gently irrigated to remove debris, and then may be coated with a soothing, anti-inflammatory paste, such as zinc oxide or eugenol (oil of clove). Antibiotics may also be prescribed if drainage of the socket is incomplete. The infection usually begins to clear up within a few days.

DSM III

The third, and most recent, edition of the "Diagnostic and Statistical Manual of Mental Disorders," published by the American Psychiatric Association in 1980. DSM III provides criteria for classifying psychiatric illnesses for use by physicians when making diagnoses and by those compiling statistics and insurance forms.

Dual personality

See *Multiple personality*.

Duct

A tube or a tubelike passage leading from a gland to allow the flow of fluids—for example, tears through the tear ducts.

Dumbness

See *Mutism*.

Dumping syndrome

Symptoms including sweating, faintness, and palpitations resulting from the rapid passage of food from the stomach into the upper intestine. It mainly affects people who have had a partial or total *gastrectomy* (surgical removal of the stomach). Symptoms may occur within 30 minutes of eating (early dumping, usually associated with a lowered blood volume) or after 90 to 120 minutes (late dumping,

D

usually due to low blood sugar and potassium). Some tense people may have symptoms of dumping with an intact stomach.

CAUSES

Gastric surgery interferes with the normal mechanism by which food is emptied from the stomach. If a meal that is rich in carbohydrates is "dumped" too quickly from the stomach, it may cause the upper intestine to swell. In addition, certain hormones are released in excess into the bloodstream. These hormones, with the intestinal swelling, cause the symptoms of early dumping.

As sugars are absorbed from the intestine, they rapidly increase the blood glucose level, causing an excess amount of *insulin* to be released, which in turn may later lower the blood sugar level below normal, causing the symptoms of late dumping. A person who has had a gastrectomy can avoid symptoms by eating frequent, small, dry meals that do not contain refined carbohydrates such as white sugar. Symptoms may also be prevented by lying down after a large meal. Drug treatment is not often successful, but adding guar gum to food to slow the emptying of the stomach and the absorption of sugars is sometimes effective.

Duodenal ulcer

A raw area in the wall of the duodenum, caused by erosion of its inner surface lining. Duodenal and gastric ulcers (similar raw areas in the lining of the stomach) are also called *peptic ulcers* and have similar causes, symptoms, and treatment.

Duodenitis

Inflammation of the duodenum of uncertain cause, vague symptoms, and no physical signs. Treatment (which has never conclusively proved to be effective) is similar to treatment for a duodenal ulcer (see *Peptic ulcer*).

The diagnosis of duodenitis is made by *gastroscopy* (examination of the walls of the duodenum with a gastroscope, a fiberoptic viewing tube passed through the esophagus, stomach, and pylorus). Instead of an ulcer there is a diffuse area of inflammation, with redness and swelling of cells in the duodenal lining and bleeding after contact with the tip of the gastroscope. A direct correlation between the gastroscope findings and any symptoms that could be considered duodenitis has yet to be made from clinical studies.

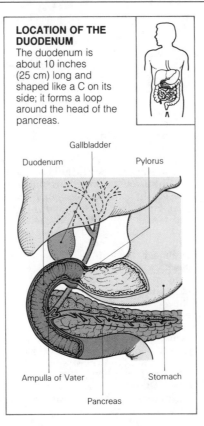

LOCATION OF THE DUODENUM
The duodenum is about 10 inches (25 cm) long and shaped like a C on its side; it forms a loop around the head of the pancreas.

Gallbladder

Duodenum

Pylorus

Ampulla of Vater

Stomach

Pancreas

Duodenum

The first part of the small intestine, extending from the pylorus (the muscular valve at the lower end of the stomach) to the ligament of Treitz, which marks the boundary between the duodenum and the jejunum (the second part of the small intestine).

Ducts from the pancreas, liver, and gallbladder feed into the duodenum through a small opening called the ampulla of Vater, which is surrounded by the sphincter of Oddi. Digestive enzymes (proteins that break down food) contained in bile and the pancreatic secretions are released into the duodenum through this opening.

Dupuytren's contracture

A disorder of the hand in which the ring and little fingers become fixed in a bent position and can be straightened only by an operation. In about half the cases, both hands are affected. The disorder is named after the French surgeon who first described it, Baron Guillaume Dupuytren (1777-1835).

CAUSES AND INCIDENCE

The cause of the disorder is unclear. In most cases there is no apparent or known cause, although the condition is slightly more common in certain groups—for example, in people whose work involves gripping tools, especially those that vibrate. The condition is a common feature in people with alcoholic liver *cirrhosis*. There is a slight tendency for the condition to run in families, though this does not necessarily mean it is inherited genetically. Men over 40 are the most commonly affected.

SYMPTOMS AND SIGNS

The tissues under the skin in the palm of the hand become thickened and shortened, with tethering of the tendons that run into the fingers. A small, hard nodule forms on the palm of the hand and it spreads to form a band of hard tissue under the skin, with puckering of the skin itself. The affected fingers start to bend more and more over a period of months or years and cannot be pulled back straight.

TREATMENT

The only treatment is surgical and is performed when the deformity has become unsightly or has started to impede hand function. During surgery the bands of thickened tissue under the skin are cut and separated to free the tendons.

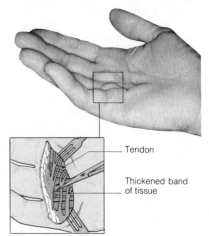

Tendon

Thickened band of tissue

Surgery for Dupuytren's contracture
Bands of tissue under the skin that have become thickened are cut and separated so that the tendons are freed.

Dust diseases

A group of lung disorders caused by inhalation, usually over several years at work, of dust particles that are absorbed into the lung tissues. There they cause *fibrosis* (formation of scar tissue) and progressive lung damage with crippling symptoms.

The main symptoms are a cough (with dark sputum) and breathing difficulty. It usually takes at least 10 years of exposure to dusts containing coal, silica, talc, or aluminum before serious lung damage develops (see *Pneumoconiosis*). Inhalation of asbestos dust can cause damage in much less time (see *Asbestosis*).

Workers in relevant industries show considerable variation in their susceptibility to dust disease. These people should have regular medical checkups to ensure that any signs of disease are detected early and serious damage is thus prevented.

Dwarfism

See *Short stature*.

Dying, care of the

People who are near death should be provided with physical and psychological care so that their final period of life is as free from pain, discomfort, and emotional distress as possible. Today, with good quality medical care, many deaths, even those from cancer, are pain-free and are associated with little physical discomfort. Emotional distress can be minimized by perception, understanding, and sensitive communication on the part of all those caring for the dying person. Usually, these people include physicians and other medical professionals, counselors, social workers, clergy, family, and friends. Family and friends should realize that they may undergo great emotional strain and may sometimes experience guilt for not being able to do more for the dying person. They, too, may benefit from counseling.

WHEN AND WHAT TO TELL THE DYING PERSON

Over the last 20 years it has become more common for physicians to tell dying people, particularly cancer patients, the facts related to their diagnoses. Generally, if a person can discuss the likely outcome of his or her illness and can prepare for death, then dying itself is eased. However, there are people who prefer not to know or block out the knowledge. The wishes of the patient should be paramount; these wishes may not always be clear and those caring for the patient need considerable perception and understanding. Careful probing should be attempted before any blunt statements are made.

Sometimes, even though the dying person has made it clear that he or she would prefer to talk about death, family members feel unable to do so, and this can cause the patient much isolation and suffering. Sometimes, the dying person may find it easier to talk to someone who is not a relative. In both cases, specially trained people, counselers, and members of the clergy may be able to help promote communication between the patient and the family.

PHYSICAL CARE

For most dying people, pain is often the most feared problem. Today, however, virtually all pain can be relieved by the use of analgesics (painkillers). Regular, low doses of the drugs are given so that pain never builds up and the patient remains alert. Powerful analgesics, such as morphine and other opiates, are commonly given to relieve severe pain.

When analgesic drugs are not adequate, other methods may be needed. These include nerve blocks (in which a nerve carrying pain from the body to the brain is interrupted by an injection or surgery), cordotomy (also called rhizotomy, or severing of nerve fibers in the spinal cord), or *TENS* (nerve stimulation with small electric currents), which is less likely to be effective once narcotic analgesics have been used.

Physical symptoms other than pain may also cause great distress. Nausea and vomiting may be a problem when the kidney and liver have ceased to function adequately. A combination of two or three drugs may occasionally control the symptom. An obstruction in the esophagus can cause vomiting or difficulty swallowing and may need to be relieved by an operation or by laser treatments through an esophagoscope. Another common problem is breathlessness, which usually responds to morphine.

The patient may develop aches or become stiff from being in bed. Comfort can be improved by keeping the patient as active as possible.

Toward the end, the dying person may become restless and breathing may become difficult, either because the lungs become waterlogged as the heart fails or because of a constant trickle of saliva into the windpipe. These symptoms can be relieved by medication and by placing the patient in a more comfortable position.

PSYCHOLOGICAL CARE

Emotional care is every bit as important (if not more so) as the relief of pain. Many people feel anger or depression at the thought of dying; feelings of guilt or regret over the past are also common. Ultimately, however, given loving, caring support from family, friends, and others, most terminally ill people come to terms with the thought of death. Sometimes antidepressant drugs are prescribed to relieve severe depression.

A great cause of anxiety and worry may be fear of a painful end. Patients should be reassured that adequate pain relief will be maintained at all times and that even when death is very close they need not fear suffering. Most people sink into unconsciousness just before the end and die "in their sleep." Fear of dependency and loss of dignity may also cause worry. The dying person should be allowed to participate as much as possible in family discussions and decisions regarding the future.

Preparing for death may include practical matters, such as writing a will, or other less tangible things such as saying "I'm sorry," "thank you," or "goodbye." Confession and reassurance from a priest or spiritual counselor are also important for some people. Perhaps the most pressing need for the terminally ill person is communication. Relatives, friends, and caregivers must be willing to share the dying person's concerns.

HOME OR HOSPITAL?

The treatment of most types of cancer requires hospital facilities at one time or another. However, once an illness has a foreseeable end, many people prefer and many families choose to care for a dying relative at home. Few terminally ill patients require complicated nursing for a prolonged period, and the sort of loving understanding and emotional care needed may be best provided at home. At home, too, the dying person can maintain some dignity and independence, avoid isolation, and participate in family life. By contrast, a hospital is better equipped to deal with acute illness.

HOSPICES

Hospices are small units, sometimes linked to a general hospital, that have been established specifically to care for the dying and their families. Their numbers have grown considerably during the last few years. Hospital routine is generally absent; instead, the efforts of the hospice staff, which includes nurses specially trained in terminal care, are directed toward the relief of physical and emotional pain. Basic to the hospice philosophy is the idea that dying people and their families need help, care, and understanding. It has been argued that a dying person might find the sight of other people dying depressing, but it has been found that most people who die in a hospice are reassured because death occurs peacefully.

Dys-

A prefix meaning abnormal, difficult, painful, or faulty, as in dysuria (pain on passing urine).

Dysarthria

A speech disability caused by disease or damage to the physical apparatus of speech, or to nerve pathways controlling this apparatus.

Dysarthria differs from *aphasia* (another type of speech disorder) in that dysarthric patients have nothing wrong with the speech center in the brain. They are able to formulate, select, and write out words and sentences grammatically; it is only vocal expression that causes problems. *Dysphonia* is a speech disability with a more restricted meaning than dysarthria, referring only to defects of sound production caused by some disease or damage to the larynx.

CAUSES

Dysarthria is a common feature of many degenerative conditions affecting the nervous system, such as *multiple sclerosis*, *Parkinson's disease*, and *Huntington's chorea*. It also affects some children who have *cerebral palsy*. Dysarthria may result from a *stroke*, *brain tumor*, or an isolated defect or damage to a particular nerve (such as the hypoglossal nerve that controls tongue movements). Structural defects of the mouth, as occur in *cleft lip and palate*, or even ill-fitting false teeth may also affect speech.

TREATMENT

There is no specific treatment for dysarthria. In some cases, drug or surgical treatment of the underlying disease or structural defect may restore the ability to speak clearly. In other instances, patients may benefit from *speech therapy*. (See also *Speech*.)

Dyschondroplasia

A rare disorder, present from birth, characterized by the presence of multiple tumors of cartilaginous tissue within bones. Dyschondroplasia is caused by a failure of normal bone development from cartilage. Usually only the bones in one limb are affected; the bones and limb are shortened, with resultant deformity.

Dysentery

A severe infection of the intestines, causing diarrhea (often mixed with

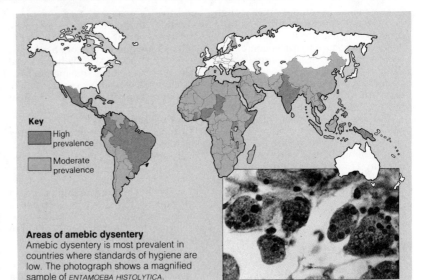

Key
High prevalence
Moderate prevalence

Areas of amebic dysentery
Amebic dysentery is most prevalent in countries where standards of hygiene are low. The photograph shows a magnified sample of ENTAMOEBA HISTOLYTICA.

blood, pus, and mucus) and abdominal pain. The person may spend hours straining on the toilet, producing little but blood-stained watery mucus.

There are two distinct forms of dysentery. *Shigellosis*, also called bacillary dysentery, is caused by infection with any of a group of bacteria called shigella. The diarrhea starts suddenly and is watery; sometimes toxemia (the presence of bacterial toxins in the blood) develops.

Amebic dysentery is caused by the protozoan (single-celled) parasite ENTAMOEBA HISTOLYTICA. It starts more gradually and often runs a chronic course.

The main risk with acute dysentery is *dehydration* from loss of fluid in the diarrhea. (See also *Colitis*.)

Dyskinesia

Abnormal muscular movements caused by a brain disorder. Uncontrollable twitching, jerking, or writhing movements occur that cannot be suppressed and may impair the performance of voluntary (willed) movements. The disorder may involve the whole body or may be restricted to a group of muscles, such as those around the eye.

Different types of dyskinesia include *chorea* (mainly jerking movements), *athetosis* (writhing movements), *choreoathetosis* (a combined form), *tics* (repetitive fidgets), *tremors*, and *myoclonus* (muscle spasms).

Dyskinesias may result from brain damage at birth or it may be a side effect of certain drugs, particularly some drugs used to treat psychiatric illnesses and the antiemetic drug metoclopramide. The affected brain region is a group of linked nerve centers called the *extrapyramidal system*, which includes the *basal ganglia*.

Dyskinesias due to drugs often resolve when drug use is stopped. Otherwise they are difficult to treat. Drugs such as tetrabenazine may help reduce choreic movements, but often the physician must prescribe several drugs in turn before one (if any) is effective. (See also *Parkinsonism*).

Dyslexia

A specific reading disability characterized by difficulty in coping with written symbols. The term is not used to describe other types of reading difficulty, such as problems arising from brain damage or mental handicap, or from speech or visual defects. In addition, dyslexia does not include reading problems caused by educational or social neglect.

CAUSES AND INCIDENCE

Emotional disturbance, minor visual defects, and failure to "train" the brain have all been suggested as possible causes of dyslexia, but there is now good evidence that a specific, sometimes inherited, neurological disorder underlies true dyslexia. Some 90 percent of dyslexics are male.

SYMPTOMS

The key feature of dyslexia is that in other respects the child has entirely normal intelligence. Thus, his or her attainment of reading skills lags far behind other scholastic abilities and overall IQ. Usually, the child can read numbers or musical notes much more easily than words.

Furthermore, while many first- and second-grade children tend to reverse letters and words (for example, writing or reading p for q, b for d, was for saw, no for on), the majority soon correct such errors. Dyslexic children continue to confuse these symbols. Letters are transposed (as in pest for step) and spelling errors are common. These children may even be unable to read words they can spell correctly. Writing from dictation may be difficult even though most dyslexics can copy sentences.

TREATMENT

It is important to recognize the problem early to avoid any added frustrations. Specific remedial teaching can help the child develop "tricks" to overcome the deficit, and avoidance of pressure from parents combined with praise for what the child can do is equally important. Given the right support and training, sufferers can usually overcome their difficulties. Many dyslexics have developed notable careers while still retaining some features of dyslexia.

Dysmenorrhea

Pain or discomfort during or just before a menstrual period. Most teenage girls and young women suffer to some degree from what is called primary dysmenorrhea. It usually starts two or three years after the first period, once ovulation is established; often it diminishes after the age of about 25, and it is rare after childbirth.

Dysmenorrhea is known to be associated with the hormonal changes that occur during a period, but the exact mechanism of the link between them remains uncertain. One possibility is that dysmenorrhea is due to excessive production of, or undue sensitivity to, prostaglandin, the hormone that stimulates muscular spasm of the uterus.

Secondary dysmenorrhea is, by definition, due to an underlying disorder (such as *endometriosis* or *pelvic inflammatory disease*).

Either type of dysmenorrhea may or may not be accompanied by *premenstrual syndrome*, a bloated feeling and irritability, depression, and other changes that commonly occur in the days preceding *menstruation*.

SYMPTOMS

Dysmenorrhea is typically felt as cramplike pain or discomfort in the lower abdomen, which may come and go in waves. There may also be dull lower backache and, in some women, nausea and vomiting. In primary dysmenorrhea the pain starts shortly before a period and usually lasts for less than 12 hours. About 10 percent of women have symptoms severe enough to interfere with their work or leisure activities. In secondary dysmenorrhea the pain begins several days before a period and lasts throughout it.

Mild primary dysmenorrhea is often relieved by analgesics (such as aspirin) or prostaglandin inhibitors (drugs that block the action of prostaglandin) such as naproxen. Rest in bed with a heating pad or hot-water bottle is a traditional and sometimes effective remedy. If symptoms are severe, they can usually be relieved by suppressing ovulation, either with the birth-control pill or with non-contraceptive hormones.

Treatment of secondary dysmenorrhea depends on the cause.

Dyspareunia

The medical term for painful sexual intercourse. (See *Intercourse, painful.*)

Dyspepsia

The medical term for *indigestion*.

Dysphagia

The medical term for *swallowing difficulty*.

Dysphasia

A term sometimes used to describe a disturbance in the ability to select the words with which we speak and write (and/or to comprehend and read) caused by damage to regions of the brain concerned with speech and comprehension. (See *Aphasia*.)

Dysphonia

Defective production of vocal sounds in speech, caused by disease or damage to the larynx (the voice box at the top of the windpipe) or to the nerve supply to the laryngeal muscles. Dysphonia should be distinguished from *dysarthria*, in which speech is defective because of damage or disease involving the controlling nerve pathways or muscles of other speech apparatus (e.g., respiratory muscles, throat, tongue, or lips); it is also to be distinguished from expressive *aphasia*, in which the ability to speak may be profoundly disturbed by damage to the speech center in the brain. (See also *Larynx* disorders box; *Speech*; *Speech disorders*.)

Dysplasia

Any abnormality of growth. The term applies to misshapen structures such as the skull (cranial dysplasia) and to abnormalities of single cells (cellular dysplasia). Abnormal cell features include the size, shape, and rate of multiplication of cells.

Dyspnea

The term for difficult or labored breathing. (See *Breathing difficulty*.)

Dysrhythmia, cardiac

The medical term, sometimes used as an alternative to *arrhythmia*, meaning disturbance of heart rhythm.

Dystonia

Abnormal muscle rigidity, causing painful muscle spasms, unusually fixed postures, or strange movement patterns. Dystonia may affect a localized area of the body, or it may be more generalized.

The most common types of localized dystonia are *torticollis* (painful neck spasm) and *scoliosis* (abnormal curvature of the spine) caused by an injury to the back that produces muscle spasm.

More generalized dystonia occurs as a result of various neurological disorders, including *Parkinson's disease* and *stroke*, and may also be a feature of *schizophrenia*. Dystonia may be a side effect of *antipsychotic drugs*.

Dystrophy

Any disorder in which the structure and normal activity of cells within a tissue have been disrupted by inadequate nutrition. The usual cause is poor circulation of blood through the tissue, but dystrophy can also be due to damage to nerves or to lack of catalytic protein (a specific enzyme) in that tissue.

In *muscular dystrophies*, muscle cells fail to develop normally, causing weakness and paralysis. In the leukodystrophies, there is *demyelination* (loss of the sheath surrounding nerves) within the brain, causing a variety of disturbances of sensation, movement, and intellect.

Corneal dystrophies are a rare, usually inherited, cause of blindness. In this condition, cells lining the cornea are damaged and the eye's surface becomes opaque.

Dysuria

The medical term for pain, discomfort, or difficulty in passing urine. (See *Urination, painful*.)

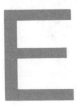

Ear

The organ of hearing and balance. The ear consists of three parts: the outer ear, the middle ear, and the inner ear. The outer and middle ear are concerned primarily with the collection and transmission of sound. The inner ear is responsible for analyzing sound waves; it also contains the mechanism by which the body keeps its balance.

OUTER EAR

The outer ear consists of the pinna (also called the auricle), which is the visible part of the ear, composed of folds of skin and cartilage. The pinna leads into the ear canal (also called the meatus), which is 1 inch (2.5 cm) long in adults and closed at its inner end by the tympanic membrane (eardrum). The part of the canal nearest the outside is made of cartilage. The cartilage is covered with skin that produces wax, which, along with hair, traps dust and small foreign bodies.

The eardrum separates the outer ear from the middle ear. The eardrum is a thin, fibrous, circular membrane covered with a thin layer of skin. It vibrates in response to the changes in air pressure that constitute sound and works in conjunction with the other components of the middle ear.

MIDDLE EAR

The middle ear is a small cavity between the eardrum and the inner ear. It conducts sound to the inner ear by means of a chain of three tiny, linked, movable bones called ossicles. They link the eardrum to an oval window in the bony wall on the opposite inner side of the middle-ear cavity. The bones are named because of their shapes. The malleus (hammer) is joined to the inside of the eardrum. The incus (anvil) has one broad joint with the malleus (which lies almost parallel to it) and a delicate joint to the third bone, the stapes (stirrup). The base of the stapes fills the oval window, which leads to the inner ear.

The middle ear is cut off from the outside by the eardrum, but it is not completely airtight; a ventilation passage, called the eustachian tube,

ANATOMY OF THE EAR

The outer ear comprises the pinna and ear canal; the middle ear—the eardrum, hammer, anvil, stirrup, and eustachian tube; and the inner ear— the vestibule, semicircular canals, and cochlea. Sensory impulses from the inner ear pass to the brain via the vestibulocochlear nerve.

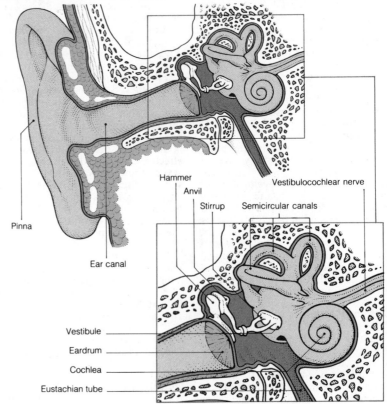

runs forward and down into the back of the nose. The eustachian tube is normally closed, but it opens by muscular contraction with yawning and swallowing.

The middle ear acts as a transformer, passing the vibrations of sound from the air outside (which is a thin medium) to the fluid in the inner ear (which is a thicker medium).

INNER EAR

The inner ear is an extremely intricate series of structures contained deep within the bones of the skull. It consists of a maze of winding passages, collectively known as the labyrinth. The front part, the cochlea, is a tube resembling a snail's shell and is concerned with hearing. (For a detailed discussion of how this system works, see *Hearing*.) The rear part (three semicircular canals and two other organs) is concerned with balance. The semicircular canals are set at right angles to each other and are connected to a cavity known as the vestibule. The canals contain hair cells bathed in fluid. Some of these cells are sensitive to gravity and acceleration; others respond to positions and movements of the head (i.e., side to side, up and down, or tilted). The information concerning posture or direction is registered by the relevant cells and conveyed by nerve fibers to the brain. (See also *Ear* disorders box.)

Earache

The most common cause of earache is acute *otitis media* (infection of the middle ear), most commonly occurring in young children. The pain is likely to be severe and stabbing; there may also be loss of hearing and a raised temperature. If the eardrum bursts, there is a discharge of fluid and immediate relief from the pressure and therefore the accompanying pain.

DISORDERS OF THE EAR

The ear is susceptible to a large variety of disorders, some of which can lead to *deafness*. *Vertigo* (dizziness associated with a disturbance of balance) as a result of ear disease is not common, but it occurs in some disorders of the inner ear.

CONGENITAL DEFECTS

Very rarely, a baby is born with an absent or extremely narrowed external ear canal, and sometimes the small bones of the middle ear are deformed or absent.

Occasionally, the pinna (external ear) is missing or distorted. *Rubella* (German measles) affecting a woman during the first three months of pregnancy can cause severe damage to the baby's hearing apparatus, leading to deafness.

INFECTION

Infection is the most common cause of ear disorders. Infection may occur in the ear canal, leading to *otitis externa*, or may affect the middle ear, causing *otitis media*, which often leads to perforation of the eardrum (see *Eardrum, perforated*). Persistent *middle-ear effusion* (buildup of fluid within the middle ear), often due to infection, is the most common cause of hearing difficulties in children.

Middle-ear infection can spread to cause *mastoiditis* (infection of the mastoid process, the bone behind the ear) or brain abscess, but these complications have become extremely rare since the introduction of antibiotics.

Virus infection of the inner ear may cause *labyrinthitis* with severe vertigo and/or sudden hearing loss.

INJURY

Cauliflower ear is the result of repeated injury to the pinna. Injury to the external ear canal and perforation of the eardrum can result from poking objects into the ear or, rarely, from careless syringing. A sudden blow, especially a slap, to the ear or a very loud noise may also perforate the eardrum. Prolonged exposure to loud noise or close proximity to a loud explosion can cause *tinnitus* (noises within the ear) and/or deafness. Pressure changes associated with flying or scuba diving can also cause minor damage and pain (see *Barotrauma*).

TUMORS

Tumors in the ear are rare, but occasionally a *basal cell carcinoma* (rodent ulcer) or a *squamous cell carcinoma* affects the pinna. The latter may also involve the ear canal. Cancers of the middle and inner ears are extremely rare. *Acoustic neuroma* is a benign (nonmalignant), slow-growing tumor of the acoustic nerve that may press on structures within the ear to cause deafness, tinnitus, and imbalance. *Cholesteatoma*, a growing collection of skin cells and debris, is not a tumor, but may be equally dangerous.

OBSTRUCTION

Ear canal obstruction is most often caused by dried *earwax*, but may also result from otitis externa. In children, a frequent cause is putting a foreign body into the ear (see *Ear, foreign body in*).

DEGENERATION

Deafness in many elderly people is due to *presbycusis*, deterioration of the hair cells in the cochlea.

POISONING/DRUGS

The inner ear is especially sensitive to damage by certain classes of drugs. The most important—the aminoglycoside *antibiotic drugs*—include such drugs as streptomycin and gentamicin. These drugs can cause damage to the cochlear hair cells, especially if used in high concentration and particularly in the presence of kidney disease, which can delay the excretion of the drugs from the body.

There are other drugs that can damage ear function, including quinine, aspirin, and the *diuretic drugs* furosemide, ethacrynic acid, and bumetanide.

OTHER DISORDERS

In *otosclerosis*, a hereditary condition, the base of one of the small bones in the middle ear becomes fixed, causing deafness. *Meniere's disease* is an uncommon disorder in which deafness, vertigo, and tinnitus result from the accumulation of fluid within the labyrinth in the inner ear.

INVESTIGATION

The function of hearing is investigated by various tuning-fork and audiometric *hearing tests*, which reveal different types and levels of hearing loss. The external ear canal and the eardrum may be examined with an *otoscope* and mirror; an otoscopic microscope may also be used.

The function of the balancing mechanism of the inner ear is investigated by observing *nystagmus* (jerky eye movements) when the head is placed in different positions or the whole body rotated, and when the ear is gently syringed with hot or cold water (*caloric tests*). These tests may be refined and recorded by *electronystagmography*.

Another common cause of earache is *otitis externa* (inflammation of the outer ear canal), which is often caused by infection. Infection may be localized or affect the whole canal, sometimes taking the form of a boil or abscess. The earache may be accompanied by irritation or itching in the ear, a discharge, and mild deafness.

A much rarer cause of earache is *herpes zoster* infection, which causes blisters in the ear canal. The earache may persist for weeks or months after the infection has cleared.

Intermittent earache may also occur in people with dental problems, tonsillitis, throat cancer, pain in the lower jaw or neck muscles, and other disorders affecting areas near the ear. Earache in this case is caused because the ear and many nearby areas are supplied by the same nerves; in these cases the pain is said to be "referred" to the ear.

INVESTIGATION

The physician inspects the outer ear manually and then examines the ear canal and drum with an *otoscope* and, if necessary, a binocular microscope; he or she may arrange for X rays and other tests to be carried out (see *Ear, examination of*). The mouth, throat, and teeth are also examined.

TREATMENT

Analgesics (painkillers) may be given and the underlying cause of the earache treated. Antibiotic drugs are prescribed for an infection. Pus in the outer ear may need to be aspirated (sucked out), usually as an office procedure. Pus in the middle ear may require draining through a hole made in the eardrum; this operation is known as *myringotomy*.

Ear, cauliflower

See *Cauliflower ear*.

Ear, discharge from

Fluid emitted from the ear, usually as the result of an infection of the outer ear (see *Otitis externa*) or middle ear (see *Otitis media*).

INVESTIGATION AND TREATMENT

Any discharge from the ear should be reported to your physician. Tests may include performing *hearing tests* and taking a swab of the discharge to produce a *culture* for laboratory analysis. It may be necessary to clean and carefully inspect the ear using a special microscope and/or take special X rays to rule out *cholesteatoma* (a benign condition associated with chronic drainage from the ear).

Eardrum, perforated

Rupture or erosion of the eardrum, usually as the result of acute *otitis media* (infection of the middle ear).

CAUSES

In acute otitis media, pus builds up in the middle-ear cavity and, unless the infection is treated, the pressure may burst the eardrum. A hole may also be eroded in the eardrum as the result of chronic otitis media. Less common causes of rupture are inserting a sharp object into the ear to relieve irritation, a blow on the ear (usually a hard slap), a nearby explosion, fracture of the base of the skull, *barotrauma* (caused by air pressure change during flying or diving), or, very rarely, a tumor of the middle ear. The physician may puncture the eardrum to drain the middle ear and prevent rupture in a more critical area.

TREATMENT AND OUTLOOK

Anyone who suspects a perforated eardrum should first cover the ear with a clean, dry pad to prevent infection from entering the middle ear; next, consult a physician. An analgesic (painkiller) may be taken.

The physician will prescribe *antibiotic drugs* to treat any infection. Except in chronic otitis media that has damaged the sound-transmitting

bones in the middle ear, no other treatment is usually required, since the eardrum generally heals on its own. Normal hearing is restored within a month.

If a perforation fails to heal or close sufficiently within six months, a *myringoplasty* (an operation in which the eardrum is repaired with a tissue graft from elsewhere in the body) may be performed. Many perforations can be healed with an office treatment that "freshens" the edges of the perforation so that it has another chance to heal on its own.

Ear, examination of

The ear requires examination any time the following symptoms develop: earache, discharge from the ear, loss of hearing, a feeling of fullness in the ear, disturbance of balance, tinnitus (noises in the ear), or swollen or tender lymph nodes below or in front of the ear.

The physician can inspect only the pinna (the visible outer ear), the ear canal, and the eardrum. To investigate the middle and inner ears, more specialized tests are required.

HOW IT IS DONE

The physician inspects the pinna manually for any evidence of swelling, tenderness, ulceration, or deformity and examines the skin above and behind the ear for signs of previous surgery. To inspect the ear canal and eardrum, the physician usually uses an *otoscope* (a viewing instrument for examining the ear). If necessary, a more magnified, three-dimensional image can be obtained by using a binocular microscope.

To obtain images of the middle and inner ears, the physician may arrange for plain X rays, *tomography*, *CT scanning*, or *MRI* to be carried out. Hearing and balance may require assessment by means of *hearing tests*, *caloric tests*, and *electronystagmography*.

Ear, foreign body in

The external ear canal is a common location for foreign bodies. Children often insert small objects, such as beads, peas, or stones, into their ears. It is also possible for insects to fly or crawl into the ear.

TREATMENT

SMALL OBJECTS These must always be removed by a physician. Under no circumstances should removal be attempted by poking with cotton swabs, hair pins, or similar objects; these efforts usually drive the object farther into the ear canal.

FIRST AID: FOREIGN BODY IN EAR

DO NOT
- attempt to dislodge the object by probing. Small objects must be removed by a physician
- pour liquid into the ear unless you are certain the object is an insect

TO REMOVE AN INSECT

Tilt the victim's head so that the affected ear is facing upward. Pour lukewarm water into the ear and the insect may float to the surface. If this fails, call your physician.

The physican will remove the object either by syringing or by grasping it with a pair of fine-toothed forceps. A brief general anesthetic may be required if the object is impacted, as often occurs with organic foreign bodies, such as beans, which swell when moistened by ear secretions.

INSECTS An insect can sometimes be removed from the ear by having the person tilt his or her head so that the affected side is uppermost and then pouring oil or lukewarm water into the ear. If this is not successful, a physician will need to syringe the ear after killing the insect with chloroform or drowning it with oil. It is impossible for insects to penetrate the brain from the ear.

Ear piercing

Making a hole in the earlobe or, occasionally, another part of the external ear, to accommodate an earring. Ear piercing was once performed with a needle, but the risk of transmitting diseases through the use of unsterile needles caused this method to be replaced by a special ear-piercing gun.

HOW IT IS DONE

A local anesthetic is not necessary, since the procedure causes only minor discomfort. The ear lobe is pierced by a post or stud (sometimes called a sleeper), fired into it by the gun, which does not come into contact with the ear. The posts are of gold or gold-plate (cheaper metals can cause contact *dermatitis*), are kept sealed in a sterile pack before use, and are not handled during the procedure.

For six weeks after insertion, the posts must be cleaned regularly with hydrogen peroxide or rubbing alcohol to prevent infection; the posts are kept in the ears and turned twice daily to prevent the hole from closing.

Ears, pinning back of

See *Otoplasty*.

Ear tube

A small tube that can be inserted through the eardrum at *myringotomy* (a surgical incision made in the eardrum) to treat persistent *middle-ear effusion* in children. The tube equalizes the pressure on both sides of the eardrum, permitting drainage. Tubes are usually allowed to fall out on their own, which generally occurs between six and 12 months after insertion. Children should not swim unless they wear special earplugs.

Earwax

A deep yellow or brown secretion, medically known as cerumen, produced by glands in the outer-ear canal. In most people, wax is produced in only small amounts, falls out on its own, and causes no trouble; in other people, so much wax forms that it regularly obstructs the canal, sometimes as often as every few months.

Excess earwax may produce a sensation of fullness in the ear and, if the canal is blocked completely, partial deafness. These symptoms are made worse if water enters the ear and makes the wax swell. Prolonged blockage may also inflame the skin of the canal, causing irritation.

Wax completely blocking the ear should always be removed. A firm plug of wax can be removed by a physician with a ring probe, right-angle hook, or *forceps*. If the wax is too soft for this, it can be softened further with oil and then flushed out with an ear syringe containing warm water. If there is a possibility that the eardrum is damaged, the physician uses suction instead of syringing.

A person can remove his or her own earwax with mineral oil drops (for hard wax) or hydrogen peroxide drops (for soft wax) or with commercially available preparations. Cotton swabs should not be used. They can push wax deep into the canal, making the problem worse.

Ecchymosis

The medical term for a *bruise*.

ECG

Also sometimes called EKG, the abbreviation for electrocardiogram, a record of the electrical impulses that

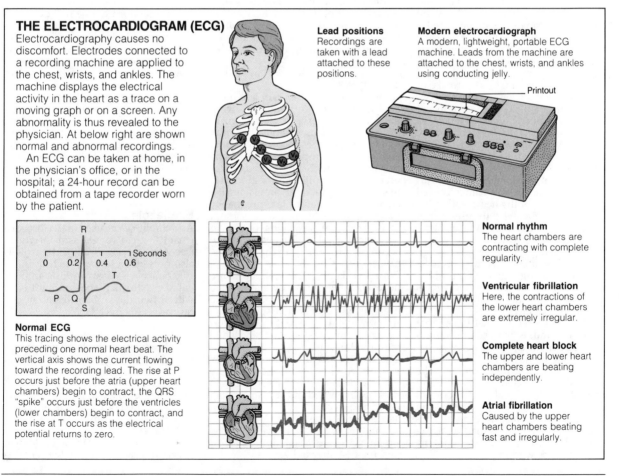

THE ELECTROCARDIOGRAM (ECG)

Electrocardiography causes no discomfort. Electrodes connected to a recording machine are applied to the chest, wrists, and ankles. The machine displays the electrical activity in the heart as a trace on a moving graph or on a screen. Any abnormality is thus revealed to the physician. At below right are shown normal and abnormal recordings.

An ECG can be taken at home, in the physician's office, or in the hospital; a 24-hour record can be obtained from a tape recorder worn by the patient.

Lead positions
Recordings are taken with a lead attached to these positions.

Modern electrocardiograph
A modern, lightweight, portable ECG machine. Leads from the machine are attached to the chest, wrists, and ankles using conducting jelly.

Printout

Normal ECG
This tracing shows the electrical activity preceding one normal heart beat. The vertical axis shows the current flowing toward the recording lead. The rise at P occurs just before the atria (upper heart chambers) begin to contract, the QRS "spike" occurs just before the ventricles (lower chambers) begin to contract, and the rise at T occurs as the electrical potential returns to zero.

Normal rhythm
The heart chambers are contracting with complete regularity.

Ventricular fibrillation
Here, the contractions of the lower heart chambers are extremely irregular.

Complete heart block
The upper and lower heart chambers are beating independently.

Atrial fibrillation
Caused by the upper heart chambers beating fast and irregularly.

E

immediately precede contraction of the heart muscle. The waves produced are known as the P,Q,R,S, and T waves. An ECG is a useful means of diagnosing disorders of the heart, many of which produce deviations from normal electrical patterns. Among these disorders are *coronary heart disease*, *coronary thrombosis*, *pericarditis* (inflammation of the membrane surrounding the heart), *cardiomyopathy* (heart muscle disorders), *myocarditis* (inflammation of the heart muscle), and arrhythmia (see *Arrhythmia, cardiac*).

Echocardiography

A method of obtaining an image of the structure of the heart using *ultrasound* (inaudible, high-frequency, sound waves). The sound is reflected differently by each part of the heart and a complex series of echoes results.

WHY IT IS DONE

Echocardiography is a major diagnostic technique used to detect structural, and some functional, abnormalities of the heart wall, the heart valves, and the heart's large blood vessels. Blood flow across valves is also measured.

The procedure is especially valuable for studying disorders of the heart valves. Abnormal opening and closing of the valves can be detected because they deviate from normal patterns of valve movement. Other diagnostic uses include detection of congenital heart disease (such as ventricular *septal defect*, a hole in the wall between the two lower chambers of the heart), various abnormalities of the large blood vessels, *cardiomyopathy* (enlargement or damage of the heart muscle), *aneurysms* (swellings caused by weakening of the heart wall or the walls of blood vessels), the presence of a blood clot within the chambers of the heart, and *pericarditis*.

HOW IT IS DONE

Echocardiography is harmless and the patient feels nothing; it has the added advantage of producing recordings without having to place an instrument inside the patient's body.

The transducer (the instrument that sends out and receives sound signals) is placed on the chest in a position that allows its sound waves to reach the structures under investigation. The echoes are detected, amplified, and then displayed visually as a series of lines on an oscilloscope screen or a paper tape. This information is interpreted by cardiologists as a picture of the heart and its valves and the way they are working.

Echocardiography has become more sophisticated and methods have been developed that incorporate a moving transducer, or a set of transducers, attached to a computer. This allows a series of different views of the heart to be obtained, and a two-dimensional scan can thus be produced. When recorded on videotape, an easily recognizable picture of the activity of the interior of the heart can be seen. Another recently developed feature is Doppler echocardiography. This technique can indirectly measure the flow velocity of blood as it passes through the heart. It can be useful in assessing malfunctioning valves (e.g., in *aortic stenosis* or *mitral insufficiency*) and in assessing patients with congenital heart disease.

Echolalia

The compulsive repetition of what is spoken by another person. The tone and accent of the speaker are copied as well as the actual words. It is an unusual symptom of catatonic *schizophrenia* and sometimes also occurs in people suffering from *autism* and some forms of *mental retardation*. Echolalia may be accompanied by echopraxia (imitating the behavior of another person).

Eclampsia

A rare, serious condition of late pregnancy, labor, and the period following delivery. Eclampsia is characterized by seizures (convulsions) in the woman, sometimes followed by coma and death; eclampsia also threatens the life of the baby. The disorder occurs as a complication of moderate or severe (but not mild) *preeclampsia*, a common condition of late pregnancy that is marked by *hypertension* (high blood pressure), *proteinuria* (protein in the urine), and *edema* (an excessive accumulation of fluid in the tissues).

CAUSES

Both preeclampsia and eclampsia are believed to be caused by a substance or toxin produced by the placenta, the organ in the uterus that sustains the unborn child. To date, however, extensive investigations have failed to identify the cause.

Eclampsia occurs more commonly in women who have had little or no *prenatal care*. Preeclampsia develops in these women without it being recognized and treated.

INCIDENCE

About half of all cases develop in late pregnancy, one third during labor, and the rest after delivery.

SYMPTOMS AND SIGNS

In eclampsia the symptoms that characterize severe preeclampsia are present. In addition, before the onset of seizures, the woman may suffer from headache, confusion, blurred vision, and abdominal pain. The seizures consist of violent, rhythmic, jerking movements of the limbs caused by involuntary contraction of the muscles; there may also be breathing difficulty caused by constriction of the muscles of the larynx. The seizures may sometimes be followed by coma.

TREATMENT

The seizures are treated by ensuring that the woman can breathe properly (sometimes by inserting an endotracheal tube down her throat) and by giving *anticonvulsant drugs*, which prevent further seizures.

The baby's condition is monitored throughout. Rapid delivery (often by emergency *cesarean section*) is usually performed, since the condition often clears once the baby is born.

OUTLOOK

About one third to one half of babies fail to survive eclampsia, usually because of lack of oxygen in the uterus. Of these deaths, half occur before delivery, the others soon after.

After delivery, the mother's blood pressure usually returns to normal within a week and proteinuria clears within six weeks. In about 5 to 10 percent of cases, however, serious complications develop in the woman before, during, or after delivery. These may include failure of the heart and lungs, kidney, or liver, *intracerebral hemorrhage*, *pneumonia*, or pulmonary *edema*.

Econazole

An *antifungal drug* used in the form of a cream to treat fungal skin infections (see *Athlete's foot*; *Tinea*). Econazole is also prescribed to treat *candidiasis*.

Econazole is a fast-working antifungal drug (usually beginning to act within two days). Skin irritation is a rare adverse effect.

ECT

The abbreviation for electroconvulsive therapy, which uses an electric shock to induce a *seizure* as a form of psychiatric treatment. Muscle-relaxant drugs are used to minimize movements of the body and the effects of ECT are limited primarily to the brain.

WHY IT IS USED

ECT is used almost exclusively to treat severe depressive illness that is causing symptoms such as weight loss or apathy. It is used less widely to treat *postpartum depression,* catatonic *schizophrenia,* and some cases of *mania* that have not responded to other treatments. ECT is not used to treat people with severe physical illness or those who have had a recent myocardial infarction (heart attack).

HOW IT IS DONE

The patient is given an anesthetic and a muscle relaxant before two padded electrodes are applied to the temples, one on each side or both on the same side. A controlled electric pulse is delivered to the electrodes from a small machine until the patient experiences a brain seizure. The seizure is indicated by brief muscular rigidity, followed by twitching of the limbs and eyelids. Afterward, patients experience only a mild discomfort similar to the discomfort felt after a minor dental operation.

Treatment usually consists of six to 12 seizures (two or three per week).

OUTLOOK

If a true brain seizure has been induced at each session, the patient's condition usually begins to improve

by the third treatment, often dramatically. Temporary *amnesia* is a possible side effect.

Ectasia

A medical term for widening or distention, usually used to refer to a disorder affecting a duct that carries secretions from a gland or organ. For example, mammary duct ectasia—a rare disorder that affects mainly menopausal women—is widening of the ducts that carry secretions from the tissues of the breast to the nipple (see *Breast*).

-ectomy

A suffix denoting surgical removal. Tonsillectomy is surgical removal of the tonsils.

Ectoparasite

A parasite that lives in or on its host's skin and derives nourishment from the skin or by sucking the host's blood. Various *lice,* ticks, mites, and some types of *fungi* are occasional ectoparasites of humans. By contrast, endoparasites live inside the body.

Ectopic

A medical term used to describe a structure that occurs in an abnormal location or position or an activity that occurs at an abnormal time.

Ectopic heart beat

A contraction of the heart muscle that is out of the normal timed sequence. An ectopic heart beat occurs shortly after a normal beat and is followed by a longer than usual interval.

Ectopic beats can occur in a heart that is otherwise functioning normally and may cause no symptoms. Multiple ectopic beats can sometimes cause *palpitations.*

After a *myocardial infarction* (heart attack), the occurrence of multiple ectopic beats is a sign of damage to the conduction system of the heart muscle. Multiple ectopic beats may lead to ventricular *fibrillation,* a rapid uncoordinated heart beat that can cause collapse and death.

Multiple ectopic beats that are causing palpitations, or that occur after a myocardial infarction, are often treated with an *antiarrhythmic drug.* (See also *Arrhythmia, cardiac.*)

E

Ectopic pregnancy

A pregnancy that develops outside the uterus, most commonly in the fallopian tube, but sometimes in the ovary or, rarely, in the abdominal cavity or cervix. It is a cause of acute abdomen (see *Abdomen, acute*).

INCIDENCE AND CAUSE

About one in every 100 pregnancies is ectopic. The fertilized ovum (egg) may become "stuck" in the fallopian tube if the tube is damaged or abnormal in any way. Ectopic pregnancies are more common if there is some congenital abnormality of the fallopian tubes, if the tubes have been previously operated on or infected, or if the woman has an *IUD.* They are also more likely if the woman has been taking the progesterone-only birth-control pill, has ingested postcoital hormonal contraception, or has undergone a (failed) sterilization, especially if the fallopian tubes have been cauterized.

SYMPTOMS AND SIGNS

Most ectopic pregnancies are discovered in the first two months, often before the woman realizes she is pregnant. In most cases a menstrual period is missed, but, in about 20 percent of the women, menstruation occurs. Symptoms of ectopic pregnancy usually include severe abdomi-

nal pain and vaginal spotting. After rupture or internal hemorrhage, the symptoms of internal bleeding appear—pallor, sweating, weakness, and faintness.

COMPLICATIONS

An ectopic pregnancy may cause the woman to go into *shock* due to severe loss of blood when the developing fetus damages the surrounding struc-

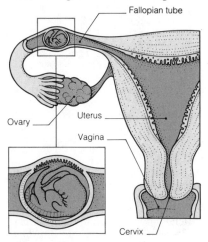

Location of an ectopic pregnancy
The pregnancy usually develops in the fallopian tube; occasionally it develops in the ovary, abdominal cavity, or cervix.

tures. Ectopic pregnancies are life-threatening and are responsible for about 10 percent of maternal deaths (deaths as a result of pregnancy or its complications). In the US approximately 50 women die each year as a result of ectopic pregnancy.

DIAGNOSIS

The physician usually performs a *pregnancy test* on any sexually active woman of childbearing age who has persistent, unexplained lower abdominal pain. *Ultrasound scanning* and a *laparoscopy* (examination of the abdominal cavity with a viewing instrument) may also be performed.

TREATMENT

Once an ectopic pregnancy is confirmed, an operation is performed to remove the developing fetus, the placenta, and any damaged tissue at the site of the pregnancy. Any torn blood vessels are repaired and, if the fallopian tube cannot be repaired, it is removed. If blood loss has been severe, transfusions are needed.

OUTLOOK

It is still possible to have a normal pregnancy even if one fallopian tube has been removed, although the chances of conception are slightly reduced. Women with two damaged tubes may require *in vitro fertilization* to achieve an intrauterine pregnancy.

Ectropion

A turning outward of the eyelid so that the inner surface is exposed.

INCIDENCE AND CAUSE

Ectropion most commonly occurs in elderly people because of weakness of the muscle surrounding the eye; it usually affects the lower lid. It may also be caused by the contraction of scar tissue (from wounds, burns, or surgical treatment) in the skin near the lids. In these cases, the upper lid may be affected. Ectropion often follows *facial palsy*, in which the muscles surrounding the eye (and other facial muscles on that side) are paralyzed.

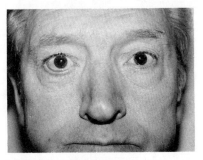

The appearance of ectropion
An example of ectropion affecting the lower eyelid of one eye. The lid is turned outward to reveal the lining of its inner surface.

SYMPTOMS AND SIGNS

Even slight ectropion interferes with normal drainage of tears by distorting the opening of the tear duct. Chronic *conjunctivitis* may result, with redness, discomfort, and overflow of tears so that the skin becomes damp and inflamed. Constant wiping tends to pull the lid farther from the eye.

TREATMENT

Lid-tightening surgery (the removal of a wedge of tissue from the lid) is simple and effective in the early stages of ectropion. Even plastic surgery with skin grafting is liable to fail if the condition is long-standing.

Eczema

An inflammation of the skin, usually causing itching and sometimes accompanied by scaling or blisters. Some forms of eczema are better known as *dermatitis* (such as seborrheic dermatitis, contact dermatitis, and photodermatitis). Eczema is sometimes caused by an *allergy*, but often occurs for no known reason.

TYPES

ATOPIC ECZEMA This chronic, superficial inflammation occurs in people who have an inherited tendency toward allergy. They, or members of their family, may also have other allergies, such as *asthma* or allergic *rhinitis*.

Atopic eczema is common in babies and often appears between the ages of 2 and 18 months. A mild but intensely itchy rash occurs, usually on the face, in the inner creases of the elbows, and behind the knees. The skin often scales in these areas, and small red pimples may appear. As the baby scratches, the pimples begin to "weep" (leak) and join to form large weeping areas. Infection may occur, particularly in the diaper area.

For mild cases, treatment consists of applying emollients, such as petroleum jelly, which help keep the skin in the infected area soft. In severe cases, corticosteroid ointments may be prescribed, and *antibiotic drugs* may be given for infection. *Antihistamine drugs* may be prescribed to reduce itching, particularly if it keeps the baby awake at night. It is important to prevent the baby from becoming too hot (e.g., by wearing too many clothes), which aggravates the condition. Only cotton clothing, which is nonirritating and absorbent, should be in direct contact with the skin.

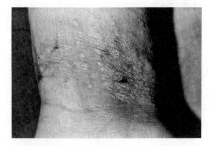

Atopic eczema
An example of atopic eczema on the creases of the inner wrist, showing the characteristic pimples and raw, scaling skin. Because the rash is intensely itchy, scratching is usually inevitable and aggravates the condition.

Atopic eczema often clears of its own accord as the child grows older, although it may come and go for several years before disappearing finally. Most children outgrow the condition by the time they reach puberty.

NUMMULAR ECZEMA This type usually occurs in adults. The cause is unknown. Nummular eczema takes the form of circular, itchy, scaling patches anywhere on the skin, similar to those of the fungal infection *tinea* (ringworm), from which the eczema needs to be distinguished. Corticosteroid ointments may be applied to the affected skin to help reduce inflammation, although the disorder is persistent and often resistant to treatment.

HAND ECZEMA This type is usually a result of irritation by substances such as detergents, household cleansers, and dishwashing liquid, but may occur for no ascertainable reason. Itchy blisters, up to about 1 inch (2.5 cm) across, develop, usually on the palms, and the hand may be covered with scales and cracks. Tests are performed to check for allergy.

Hand eczema usually improves if rubber gloves are worn over white cotton gloves when in contact with any irritants. The hands should be thoroughly patted dry after washing. An unscented hand cream should be applied several times a day. If severe, corticosteroids may be prescribed for the inflammation and antibiotics may be given for infection.

STASIS DERMATITIS In people with varicose veins, the skin on the legs may become irritated, inflamed, and discolored. The most important factor is swelling of the legs, which may be controlled with compression bandages or special stockings. Mild corticosteroid ointments may give temporary relief.

GENERAL TREATMENT

To reduce irritation and the likelihood of scratching, a soothing ointment should be applied to the affected areas, which should then be covered by a dressing to prevent scratching. Absorbent, nonirritating materials such as cotton should be worn next to the skin; irritating fabrics such as wool, silk, and rough synthetics should be avoided.

Edema

An abnormal accumulation of serum-like fluid in the body tissues. It may or may not be visible (as a swelling) and can be either local (as following an injury) or general (as in *heart failure*). Generalized edema (also called anasarca) was once popularly known as dropsy.

WATER BALANCE IN THE BODY

Water accounts for roughly three fifths of body weight and it is constantly exchanged between blood and tissues. Water is forced out of the capillaries and into the tissues by the pressure of blood being pumped around the body. By a reverse process, which depends on the water-drawing power of the proteins in the blood (see *Osmosis*), it is reabsorbed into the capillaries from the tissues. These two mechanisms normally are in balance, keeping the levels of water in the blood and the tissues more or less constant.

Another factor involved in maintaining this balance is the action of the kidneys, which pass excess salt from the blood into the urine to be excreted from the body.

CAUSES OF EDEMA

Various disorders can interfere with these processes. Heart failure leads to blood congestion in the veins, creating backward pressure in the capillaries. This backward pressure overcomes osmotic pressure in the capillaries and thus causes more fluid than normal to be forced into the tissues at various places throughout the body. Backward pressure can also be created by a tumor pressing on veins. The edema produced is confined to the area drained by the obstructed vein.

In the *nephrotic syndrome*, there is an abnormal loss of protein from the blood, which reduces its osmotic pressure and prevents enough fluid from being drawn from the tissues into the blood. *Renal failure* prevents salt from being excreted from the body, allowing it to accumulate in the tissues and attract water to it.

Other disorders that can cause edema include *cirrhosis* of the liver, which leads to blood congestion in the veins of the liver, lowers blood protein (and therefore osmotic pressure), and causes salt retention. A deficiency of protein in the diet, as may occur in alcoholics, can also reduce osmotic pressure; edema in alcoholics may also be due to deficiency of thiamine (vitamin B_1), leading to *beriberi*.

Injury may cause edema by damaging capillaries and thus allowing fluid to leak out of them. *Lymphedema* may result from blocked lymphatics.

Finally, certain drugs may cause edema. These include *corticosteroid* and *androgen drugs*, and high-estrogen *oral contraceptives*, which act on the kidneys, causing a certain amount of salt retention. Antidiuretic hormone (see *ADH*) increases water retention by the kidneys.

SYMPTOMS AND SIGNS

Until the excess fluid in the body increases by more than about 15 percent, edema may show itself only as an increase in weight. After that it is evident as a swelling, often in the lower part of the body, commonly in the lower back and around the ankles.

In severe cases, fluid accumulates in one or more of the large body cavities. For example, in *ascites*, fluid collects in the peritoneal cavity of the abdomen,

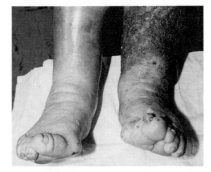

Chronic edema
An example of chronic edema, showing the characteristic swelling and stretched, shiny skin. In this patient, the skin of the left leg is also ulcerated.

causing abdominal swelling. In *pleural effusion*, fluid fills the pleural cavity of the lungs, resulting in compression of the lungs and breathing difficulty. In pulmonary edema, the air sacs of the lungs become waterlogged, again causing breathing difficulty.

If a finger is pressed into skin swollen by edema, it makes an indentation that slowly flattens out as the fluid seeps back.

TREATMENT

The aim is always to remedy the underlying cause of the edema. In many cases, however, the underlying cause is not remediable and the only treatment is to make the body excrete the excess fluid by increasing the output of urine by the kidneys. This is done by restricting dietary sodium and taking *diuretic drugs*, which the patient may need indefinitely.

Edentulous

Without teeth, either because they have not yet grown or because they have fallen out or been removed.

EEG

The abbreviation for electroencephalogram. An EEG records the minute electrical impulses produced by the activity of the brain. The technique of electroencephalography was first

E

HOW ELECTROENCEPHALOGRAPHY IS DONE

A number of small electrodes are attached to the scalp. Shaving of the scalp is unnecessary. The electrodes are connected to an instrument that measures the brain's impulses in microvolts and amplifies them for recording purposes. The technique is painless, produces no side effects, and takes about 45 minutes. Recordings are taken with the subject at rest, with eyes open and then shut, during and after *hyperventilation,* and while looking at a flashing light. It is also helpful, especially when epilepsy is suspected, to record activity as the patient goes to sleep.

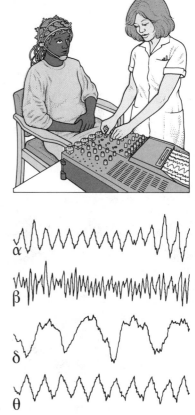

EEG wave patterns

Alpha waves
The prominent pattern of an awake, relaxed adult whose eyes are closed.

Beta waves
The lower, faster oscillation of a person who is concentrating on an external stimulus.

Delta waves
The typical pattern of sleep, but also found in young infants; rarely, they are caused by a brain tumor.

Theta waves
The dominant waves of children aged 2 to 5; also produced by frustration and found occasionally in psychopaths.

E

used in medicine in 1928, although it was known since the nineteenth century that electrical impulses could be recorded from animal brains.

WHY IT IS DONE

An EEG indicates, by the frequency of the recorded activity, the mental state of the subject—that is, whether he or she is alert, awake, or asleep. Also, by revealing characteristic wave patterns, the EEG can help in diagnosing certain conditions, especially *epilepsy* and certain types of *encephalitis*, *dementia*, and tumors.

Electroencephalography can also be used to monitor the conditions of patients during surgery and to assess the depth of anesthesia on the brain and spinal cord. It is also used as a test for *brain death*, but it is not required to make the determination.

Effusion

The escape of fluid through the walls of a blood vessel into a tissue or body cavity, often as a result of a vessel being inflamed or congested. For example, *pleural effusion*, a symptom of *heart failure*, occurs when raised blood pressure in the veins leads to fluid being forced out of the blood and through the walls of capillaries into the pleural cavity that surrounds the lungs.

Effusion, joint

Accumulation of fluid within a joint space, causing swelling and sometimes pain and tenderness. A joint is enclosed by a capsule lined with a membrane called the synovium. This membrane normally secretes small amounts of fluid to lubricate the joint, but if it is damaged or inflamed (by arthritis, for example) it produces excessive amounts of fluid.

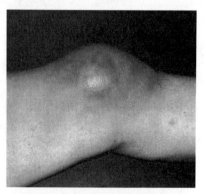

Location of knee joint effusion
Excessive production and accumulation of fluid within a knee joint may be caused by injury or inflammation.

TREATMENT

Analgesics (painkillers), anti-inflammatory drugs, and corticosteroid injections help relieve pain and inflammation. The swelling can be reduced by rest, firm wrapping with a bandage, ice packs, and, when possible, keeping the affected joint raised. In some cases, the fluid may need to be aspirated (drawn out) with a hypodermic needle and syringe. Antibiotics may also be given if the cause is infective arthritis (also called septic arthritis). *Physical therapy* may be necessary later to restore full movement to the joint.

Egg

See *Ovum*.

Ego

The conscious sense of oneself, equivalent to "I." In Freudian *psychoanalytic theory*, this part of the personality maintains a balance between the primitive, unconscious instincts of the id, the controls of the superego (or conscience), and the demands of the outside world.

Egomania

An unhealthy overconcern with oneself. People described as egomaniacs talk constantly about themselves or their own activities, to the exclusion of everything else. Egomania is not regarded as a mental disorder, but such extreme self-conceit is sometimes said to indicate underlying mental instability.

Ehlers-Danlos syndrome

An inherited disorder of collagen, the most important structural protein in the body. Affected individuals have abnormally stretchy, thin skin that bruises very easily. Wounds are slow to heal and leave paper-thin scars. Sufferers tend to bleed easily from the gums and gastrointestinal tract. The joints are exceptionally loose and are prone to recurrent dislocation.

Ehlers-Danlos syndrome is usually (although not always) inherited in an autosomal dominant pattern (see *Genetic disorders*). This means that many affected individuals have an affected parent; each of an affected person's children has a 50 percent chance of being affected.

There is no known specific treatment for Ehlers-Danlos syndrome, although unnecessary accidental injury, as may occur in contact sports, should be avoided. The outlook for a normal life expectancy is good.

Eisenmenger complex

A complication of ventricular *septal defect* (a hole in the heart between the two pumping chambers). Normally, the ventricles are separate and no blood flows between them. The pressure of blood flow from the left ventricle is normally much higher than from the right; when a ventricular septal defect exists, the shunt of blood from the left to the right ventricle raises the pressure of blood flow to the lungs, and there is a gradual rise in blood pressure in the pulmonary (lung) arteries.

If the defect is not corrected surgically within the first few years of life, the prolonged pulmonary hypertension damages small blood vessels in the lung tissue and increases the resistance to blood flow, making it harder and harder to pump the blood through the lungs. As the pressure increases, it reverses the flow of blood through the septal defect so that blood then flows from the right ventricle to the left. At first this reversal is intermittent, often associated with exercise. Deoxygenated blood (blood that is on its way to receive oxygen) instead of going to the lungs to get oxygen, gets passed directly into the body.

SYMPTOMS AND SIGNS

Eisenmenger complex causes breathing difficulty, fainting during exercise, and *cyanosis* (blue skin) due to *hypoxia* (lack of oxygen in the blood). The diagnosis is confirmed by cardiac *catheterization* (the insertion of a thin tube into the heart via a blood vessel under X-ray control).

TREATMENT AND OUTLOOK

Once permanent changes have developed, surgical correction of the ventricular septal defect does not help because the lung damage has already occurred. Most affected people die in their 30s or 40s. The only treatment in a severely disabled individual is a *heart-lung transplant*. (See also *Heart disease, congenital*.)

Ejaculation

The emission of semen from the penis at *orgasm*. Ejaculation is a reflex action that depends on regular and rhythmic pressure on the penis, usually during intercourse or masturbation. This stimulation acts on spinal nerves and triggers ejaculation.

Shortly before ejaculation the muscles around the epididymides (ducts where sperm are stored), the *prostate gland*, and the seminal vesicles contract rhythmically, forcing the

EJACULATORY DISORDERS

Premature ejaculation	Premature ejaculation is the most common sexual problem in men and is especially common in adolescents. Most adult men occasionally experience premature ejaculation, often because of overstimulation or	anxiety about sexual performance. If premature ejaculation occurs frequently, the cause may be psychological. Sexual counseling and techniques for delaying ejaculation may help (see *Sex therapy*).
Inhibited ejaculation	Inhibited ejaculation is a rare condition in which erection is normal, or even prolonged, but ejaculation does not occur. It may be psychological in origin, in which case sexual counseling may help, or it may be a	complication of other disorders, such as *diabetes mellitus*. Inhibited ejaculation may also occur during treatment with certain drugs, such as some antihypertensives.
Retrograde ejaculation	In this disorder, the valve at the base of the bladder fails to close during ejaculation. This forces the ejaculate backward into the bladder. Retrograde ejaculation can occur as a result of a neurological disease, after	surgery on the neck of the bladder, after prostatectomy, or after extensive pelvic surgery. There is no treatment, but intercourse with a full bladder can sometimes lead to normal ejaculation.

sperm from the epididymides to move forward and mix with the secretions from the seminal vesicles and prostate. At ejaculation, this fluid is propelled through the *urethra* and out of the body.

Because both semen and urine leave the body by the same route, a valve at the base of the bladder closes during ejaculation. This not only prevents ejaculate from going into the bladder but also stops urine from contaminating the semen.

Ejaculation, disorders of

Conditions in which ejaculation occurs before or very soon after penetration, ejaculation does not occur at all, or in which the ejaculate is forced backward into the bladder (see box, above).

EKG

See *ECG*.

Elbow

The joint between the lower end of the humerus (upper arm bone) and the upper ends of the radius and ulna (forearm bones). The joint is stabilized by ligaments at the front, back, and sides. The elbow enables the arm to be bent and straightened, and the forearm to be rotated through almost 180 degrees around its long axis without movement of the upper arm.

DISORDERS

Disorders include arthritis and injuries to the joint and its surrounding muscles, tendons, and ligaments.

ANATOMY OF THE ELBOW

The elbow is a hinge joint between the lower end of the humerus and the upper ends of the radius and ulna. The biceps muscle bends and rotates the arm at the elbow.

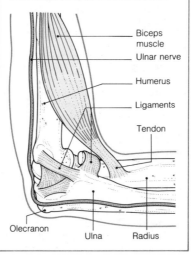

- Biceps muscle
- Ulnar nerve
- Humerus
- Ligaments
- Tendon
- Olecranon
- Ulna
- Radius

SOFT TISSUE INJURY AND INFLAMMATION
Repetitive strain on the tendons of the forearm muscles at the points at which they attach to the elbow (at the bony outgrowths called epicondyles) can lead to an inflammation at these points called *epicondylitis*. The two main types of epicondylitis are *tennis elbow* and *golfers' elbow*. Alternatively, a *sprain* of the joint ligaments can occur, especially in children.

Olecranon *bursitis* occurs over the tip of the elbow in response to local irritation. Repeated overstraightening of the joint can cause *baseball elbow*. Strain on the joint produces an *effusion* or traumatic *synovitis*.

A sharp blow on the olecranon process (the bony tip of the elbow, also called the "funny bone") may impinge on the ulnar nerve as it passes in a groove in this area, causing temporary discomfort—a pins and needles sensation and lancing pains that shoot down the forearm into the fourth and fifth fingers.

FRACTURES A fall onto an outstretched hand or onto the tip of the elbow can lead to any of various types of fracture around or at the lower end of the humerus. Children may alternatively sustain an injury to the epiphyses (growing areas) at the ends of the humerus, radius, or ulna. Dislocation of the elbow can occur at any age as a result of falling onto an outstretched hand; dislocations and fractures of the elbow frequently occur together.

ARTHRITIS *Osteoarthritis*, *rheumatoid arthritis*, and infective arthritis can affect the elbow joint.

Elderly, care of the

As people age they become prone to an increasing number of physical disorders and are more likely to suffer from loneliness and isolation. Efforts to stress personal pride and independence (along with appropriate medical care) can minimize physical and mental deterioration. Sensitive attention to psychological needs can help the elderly enjoy old age and can encourage them to feel that they are useful members of society rather than a burden.

PHYSICAL CARE

Elderly people often ignore symptoms of illness, either because they do not want to be a nuisance to those caring for them or because they are afraid of being "put away" in a home. Some conditions, such as *hypothyroidism* (underactive thyroid gland) and *anemia* (often due to a poor diet) cause a very gradual deterioration, which may incorrectly be assumed to be a natural effect of old age; as a result, these conditions tend not to be diagnosed and treated.

Failing vision and hearing are frequently regarded as inevitable features of old age, but in many cases surgical removal of a cataract or provision of a hearing aid can enable the individual to lead a more independent and active life.

E

E

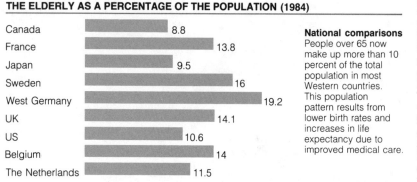

Country	Percentage
Canada	8.8
France	13.8
Japan	9.5
Sweden	16
West Germany	19.2
UK	14.1
US	10.6
Belgium	14
The Netherlands	11.5

National comparisons
People over 65 now make up more than 10 percent of the total population in most Western countries. This population pattern results from lower birth rates and increases in life expectancy due to improved medical care.

To ensure that medical problems are detected early and treated, it is important that caregivers remain alert to the symptoms and signs of illness. In addition, all people over age 65 should have regular checkups by a physician.

PSYCHOLOGICAL CARE
Common causes of depression in the elderly are isolation, inactivity, and a feeling of not being wanted. Elderly people can be helped by making them part of family activities. Attending a day-care center or senior citizen club can provide contact with other people and the opportunity to develop new interests. *Dementia* (loss of normal brain function) becomes more common as a person ages; it increases the level of supervision required.

DAY-TO-DAY CARE
Many elderly people prefer to live with their families, ideally in a separate section of the house, where they can have some degree of independence. If this is not possible, they may be able to live near relatives so that help can be provided with daily activities, such as shopping, cooking, and laundry. Assistance with personal care, such as bathing or getting in and out of bed, may also be required.

While this type of arrangement may be ideal for the elderly person, the responsibility can be a great strain on other members of the family. Voluntary agencies can sometimes help by providing a daily meal or occasional domestic help.

The elderly person's home, or that part of the house set aside for his or her use, should be well-heated in winter and cooled in summer to prevent *hypothermia* or *hyperthermia*; a high level of artificial illumination should be provided to make activities such as reading and sewing easier. The risk of falls can be reduced by ensuring that there are no loose rugs or slippery surfaces (see *Falls in the elderly*) and the

person living alone can be provided with an alarm that enables him or her to summon help in an emergency.

Sheltered housing is becoming a popular choice for many elderly people. It allows independence while providing discreet supervision and assistance when needed.

Elective
A term used to describe the degree of urgency and thus the timing of any procedure that a patient may be advised to undergo. When there is no need for urgency, the patient—in consultation with his or her physician—can select the most convenient time. A second surgical opinion is recommended for elective procedures that may be unnecessary.

Elective surgery
Surgery of a nonemergency nature. It includes correction of conditions such as hemorrhoids or a hernia as well as some cosmetic procedures.

Electrical injury
Damage caused by the passage of an electric current through the body and by its associated heat release.

INCIDENCE AND CAUSES
More than 1,000 people die from electrical accidents in the US each year and many others are injured, some seriously. Most fatal cases occur in the electrical generating and construction industries as the result of workers coming into contact with high voltages, but hundreds of people also die at home each year through handling frayed electric cords or by using electrical appliances near water. In addition, lightning causes about 300 deaths in the US annually.

The internal tissues of the body, being moist and salty, are good conductors of electricity; the main limitation to current flow is the electrical

resistance of the skin. Dry skin provides a high resistance (several tens of thousands of ohms), but moist skin has a resistance of only a few thousand ohms and thus allows a substantial current to flow. In these circumstances, voltage levels in the home are high enough to prove fatal. This is particularly so if the person is "well-grounded"—that is, if he or she is sitting or standing on a good conductor of electricity. Thus, a person in a bathtub of water is likely to suffer a fatal shock, whereas someone in a dry environment, and especially someone wearing shoes soled with rubber (which is a poor conductor of electricity), is less likely to be harmed by exposure to the same hazard.

EFFECTS
All except the mildest electric shocks are liable to cause unconsciousness. The extent of tissue damage depends on the size and type of the current flowing through the body. Alternating current (AC) is more dangerous than direct current (DC), because it causes sustained muscle contractions, which, by preventing hand movement, may prevent the victim from releasing his or her grip on the source of the current.

A current as small as one tenth of an amp passing through the heart can bring about a fatal *arrhythmia* (disturbance of the heart beat). This quantity is about the size of current passing through the filament of a very low-power bulb. The same current passing

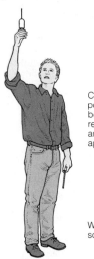

Check that the power is off before attempting repairs on any electrical appliance.

Wear rubber-soled shoes.

Electrical injury in the home
A small electric current may cause death through heart damage. Shoes with rubber soles reduce the effect of an electric shock.

FIRST AID: ELECTRICAL INJURY

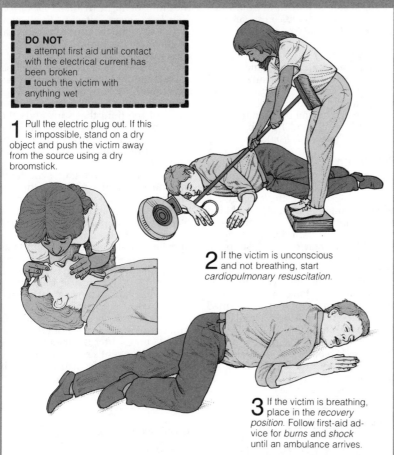

DO NOT
- attempt first aid until contact with the electrical current has been broken
- touch the victim with anything wet

1 Pull the electric plug out. If this is impossible, stand on a dry object and push the victim away from the source using a dry broomstick.

2 If the victim is unconscious and not breathing, start *cardiopulmonary resuscitation*.

3 If the victim is breathing, place in the *recovery position*. Follow first-aid advice for *burns* and *shock* until an ambulance arrives.

through the brain stem may cause the heart to stop beating and breathing to cease. Larger currents, generated by high voltages, may also char tissues, especially at points where resistance is highest, usually where the current enters and exits the body.

Electric shock treatment
See *ECT* (electroconvulsive therapy).

Electrocardiography
See *ECG*.

Electrocautery
See *Electrocoagulation*.

Electrocoagulation
The use of high-frequency electric current to seal blood vessels by heat and thus stop bleeding. Electrocoagulation may be used during all forms of surgery to close freshly cut blood vessels. It is also used to destroy

spider nevi and other kinds of abnormal blood vessel formations and to stop nosebleeds. The current is applied through a fine needle or, in surgery, may be delivered through a knife, enabling the surgeon to make bloodless incisions.

Electroconvulsive therapy
See *ECT*.

Electrodesiccation
The use of high-frequency electric current to destroy tissue by heat. Electrodesiccation is used to treat small *skin cancers*, *cervical erosion*, early *cervical cancer*, *warts*, and precancerous changes in the soft, moist tissue in the mouth. It is also used to destroy small tumors spread from other areas.

The procedure, which may be performed using a local anesthetic, consists of applying an electric probe to the tissue for one or two seconds.

Electroencephalography
See *EEG*.

Electrolysis
Permanent removal of unwanted hair by means of short-wave electric current, which destroys the hairs' roots.

WHY IT IS DONE
Hair on the face and body can be removed temporarily by shaving or plucking, or by the use of depilatory creams, abrasives, or wax preparations. Electrolysis is the only means of permanent removal.

Unskilled electrologists abound. Before embarking on treatment a person should first ensure that the operator is fully trained; damage from incompetent treatment can cause permanent disfigurement.

AREAS THAT CAN BE TREATED
With a few exceptions, electrolysis can be safely used on any part of the body where excessive hair is regarded as unsightly. Its use should be avoided on the lower margins of the eyebrows, where the skin above the eyelids is delicate and easily damaged, and it is questionable whether it should be used on the armpits because of a risk of bacterial infection. Electrolysis has no harmful effect on the breasts (where hair sometimes grows around the areola, the dark area surrounding the nipple) or on the ability of mother or infant to breast-feed.

The legs are not well suited for electrolysis; treatment of large areas requires so many sessions that it is too time-consuming and expensive for most people.

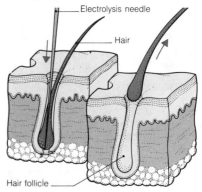

Electrolysis needle

Hair

Hair follicle

How electrolysis is done
To remove each hair, a fine needle is inserted into the follicle and a small electric current is passed through it. The current destroys the root of the hair, which is then pulled out. The procedure may cause some pain, but, in skilled hands, it is harmless. If the treatment is successful, there should be no more hair growth from that follicle.

Electrolyte

A substance whose molecules dissociate (split) into its constituent *ions* (electrically charged particles) when dissolved or melted. For example, sodium chloride (table salt) dissociates into positive sodium ions and negative chloride ions when dissolved in water. Ions that play an important role in regulating body processes include sodium, potassium, hydrogen, magnesium, calcium, bicarbonate, phosphate, and chloride.

Electromyography

See *EMG*.

Electronystagmography

A method of recording the various types of *nystagmus* (uncontrollable eye movements) to investigate their cause. Electrical changes caused by eye movement are picked up by electrodes placed near the eyes and recorded on a graph for analysis.

Electrophoresis

The movement of electrically charged particles suspended in a *colloid* solution under the influence of an electric current. The direction, distance, and rate of movement vary according to factors such as the size, shape, and electrical charge of the particle. Because of this, electrophoresis can be used to analyze mixtures of substances, particularly to identify different proteins in a mixture. For example, it can be used to identify and quantify the various proteins in blood; furthermore, by comparing the results from a particular blood sample with normal values, it is possible to diagnose disorders such as *myeloma*, a tumor of the bone marrow that produces abnormally high levels of a specific *immunoglobulin* in the blood.

Elephantiasis

 A disease encountered in the tropics, characterized by massive swellings of the legs, arms, and scrotum, with thickening and darkening of the overlying skin so that it resembles the skin of an elephant. Most elephantiasis is due to chronic lymphatic obstruction occurring as a feature of *filariasis* (a worm infestation).

ELISA test

A laboratory blood test commonly used in the diagnosis of infectious diseases. ELISA stands for enzyme-linked immunosorbent assay. (See also *Immunoassay*.)

Elixir

A clear, sweetened liquid, often containing alcohol, that forms the basis for many liquid medicines, such as cough medicines.

Embolectomy

Surgical removal of an embolus, a fragment of material—usually a blood clot—that has been swept into an artery after formation elsewhere in the bloodstream; an embolus can threaten life if it blocks blood flow through a vital artery (see *Embolism*).

Embolism

Blockage of an artery by a clump of material traveling in the bloodstream. The particle causing the blockage is called an embolus and may be a blood clot, a bubble of air or other gas, a piece of tissue or tumor, a clump of bacteria, bone marrow, cholesterol, or fat, or any of various other substances.

TYPES

Blood clots are the most common type of embolus; they have usually broken off from a larger clot that has formed elsewhere in the blood circulation. Pulmonary embolism is usually the result of a fragment from a deep vein *thrombosis* (a blood clot formed deep in a vein, usually in a leg) breaking off and being carried via the heart to block an artery supplying the lungs; this is a common cause of sudden, unexpected death. Similar blood clots may form in the lining of the heart after a *myocardial infarction* (heart attack); they may travel as emboli toward the vital arteries of the brain and cause a cerebral embolism, leading to a *stroke*.

Fat embolism is a blockage of blood vessels caused by fat globules, particularly after fractures of the arm or leg. Amniotic fluid embolism is when some of the fluid that surrounds the baby in the uterus is forced into the mother's circulation toward the end of a normal pregnancy.

SYMPTOMS

Factors that determine symptoms include the extent of blockage, the size and type of embolus, and the size, nature, and location of the affected blood vessel. In pulmonary embolism the sufferer feels faint and breathless, and has chest pains. If the embolus causes a stroke, the symptoms depend on which part of the brain is affected; it may, for example, cause inability to speak, inability to move a part of the body, loss of consciousness, or a disturbance of vision. In the small number of serious cases of fat embolism, 48 hours after the major fracture occurs the patient's heart rate and rate of breathing rise dramatically; this is accompanied by restlessness, confusion, drowsiness, and *cyanosis*.

TYPES OF EMBOLISM

Embolisms are named after the part of the circulation affected or the embolus involved (e.g., a fat embolism is caused by fat globules released from a bone fracture). When an embolus is released, it is carried through branches of an artery until it becomes lodged. Blood is prevented from reaching parts of the body beyond the blockage.

Cerebral embolism
A blockage of one of the arteries that supplies blood to the brain; it is one of the most common causes of a stroke.

Pulmonary embolism
A blockage of one of the arteries that supplies blood to the lungs. This may cause chest pain, breathlessness, and sudden death.

Amniotic fluid embolism
The escape of some of the fluid that surrounds the baby in the uterus into the mother's circulation. This may cause blockage of an artery in one of her lungs.

Leg embolism
An embolism that blocks one of the arteries that supplies blood to the leg. Gangrene may occur below the blockage.

Arm embolism
This X ray of the upper arm was taken after the injection of a radiopaque dye into the blood vessel. It shows, near the top, an embolus obstructing the normal flow of blood through one of the main arteries.

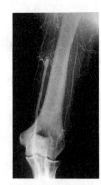

TREATMENT

If a pulmonary or other severe type of embolism causes the person to collapse, emergency lifesaving procedures are carried out to keep breathing and circulation going. If the person survives, *embolectomy* (surgery to remove the blockage) may be possible. Under general anesthesia, an incision is made in the artery and the embolus is aspirated (sucked out). The incision is closed with stitches. If surgery is not possible, *thrombolytic drugs* (to dissolve blood clots) and *anticoagulant drugs* (to prevent clot formation) may be given.

OUTLOOK

In all severe types of embolism, survival depends on the success of resuscitation attempts, the importance of the vessel obstructed, and the speed with which blood flow is reestablished. If the source of the embolus is treated, the long-term prospects for the patient are good.

Embolism, therapeutic

Also called embolization, the deliberate obstruction of a blood vessel to stop internal bleeding or cut off blood flow to a tumor.

WHY IT IS DONE

Therapeutic embolism is increasingly being performed to stop otherwise uncontrollable bleeding, particularly when the patient is too sick to undergo surgery. Among its uses are the control of bleeding from small vessels in the lining of the intestines, often due to a malformation of blood vessels (similar to a birthmark in the skin).

Using the technique to deprive a tumor of its blood supply has several effects. It can relieve the pain caused by the growth; it can cause the tumor to shrivel, making it easier to remove surgically; or it may stop the tumor from spreading. Therapeutic embolism may be used to treat tumors that would be difficult to remove surgically, such as tumors in the liver. It is also used to treat certain vascular tumors on the face, such as *hemangiomas*, in preference to surgery that might leave unsightly scars.

HOW IT IS DONE

The procedure is usually carried out by a radiologist with the patient under a general anesthetic. The first step is to obtain an image of the blood vessel to be blocked and those leading to it. This image is obtained by means of *angiography*, an X-ray procedure in which an opaque dye is introduced into the blood vessels through a *catheter* (a flexible tube).

The catheter is then guided, by means of television monitoring, as close as possible to the vessel to be blocked, and the embolus that will block the blood vessel is released. Emboli are made of many materials, such as blood-clotting agents (such as fibrin), metal coils, silicone balloons, wool, and medicinal glue.

RISKS

There is always a risk that an embolus may lodge in the wrong place; an embolus that blocks a vessel in the brain may cause a *stroke*. The procedure is still being refined.

Embolus

A clump of material that is present (usually as a result of an accident or a disease of the heart and blood vessels) in the blood circulation, where it travels eventually to cause an arterial obstruction. (See *Embolism*.)

Embryo

The unborn child during the first eight weeks of its development following conception; for the rest of the pregnancy it is known as a *fetus*.

Development of the embryo is governed internally by genes inherited from the parents, and externally by factors such as the woman's diet and any medication taken during pregnancy. (See box, overleaf.)

THE FIRST TWO WEEKS

The embryo develops from an egg, fertilized by a sperm (see *Fertilization*). It starts as a single cell—just large enough to be seen by the naked eye. As the fertilized egg travels along the tube to the uterus, the cell divides in two. These cells divide further, eventually forming a spherical mass of cells; a hollow depression develops in the center of the sphere. The cells form into two groups: one makes up the wall lining the sphere; the other expands to form the embryo itself.

On about the sixth day the sphere of cells becomes attached and then embedded in the lining of the uterus. At the site of attachment the outer layer of cells obtains nourishment from the woman's blood; the outer layer later will become the placenta.

Two bubbles form side by side within the cell mass. Between the bubbles a flat disk forms, consisting of layers of cells from which all the baby's tissues and organs will form. The amniotic sac develops around the growing embryo.

THE THIRD WEEK

Early in the third week the disk of cells becomes pear-shaped. The head of the embryo forms at the rounded end and the lower spine at the pointed end. A group of cells develops along the back of the embryo to form the notochord, a rod of cells that constitutes the basis for the spine. From this time on, the embryo has two recognizable halves that develop more or less symmetrically. The notochord then furrows and the edges grow toward each other. They fuse to form the neural tube, which later will develop into the brain and spinal cord.

THE FOURTH WEEK

During the fourth week the embryo becomes recognizable as a mammal. The back grows more rapidly than the front, giving the embryo a C-shape, and a tail becomes visible. Within the embryo, buds of tissue form that will later develop into the lungs, pancreas, liver, and gallbladder.

The neural tube extends toward the head of the embryo, where a broad fold becomes visible that eventually will grow into the brain. The developing ears first appear as pits. Rudimentary eyes develop in the form of stalks. The outer layers begin to form the limb buds and the branchial arches (folds of tissue) that will become the jaws and other structures in the neck.

Paired bulges appear on the sides of the neural tube that will become the cartilage, bone, and muscle of the back. On the front of the embryo, just beneath the head, a rudimentary heart develops in the form of a straight tube. As the branchial arches develop, the heart is pushed down into the chest. It is during this period that the embryo is at the greatest risk of birth defects caused by abnormal genetic or external factors (see *Birth defects*).

THE FIFTH WEEK

The external ears become visible, pits mark the position of the developing nose, the upper and lower jaws form, and the limb buds extend, becoming flattened at the end where the hands and feet will develop.

The two folds of tissue meet at the front of the embryo and fuse to form the front wall of the chest and abdomen. The umbilical cord develops.

THE SIXTH TO EIGHTH WEEKS

The face becomes recognizably human, the neck forms, the trunk becomes less curved and the head more erect, the tail between the buttocks disappears, the limbs become jointed, and fingers and toes appear.

After eight weeks the embryo is 1 inch (2.5 cm) long. Most of the internal organs have formed and all the external features are present.

E

THE DEVELOPING EMBRYO

From the time of conception until the eighth week, the developing baby is known as an embryo. At conception, the fertilized egg consists of a single cell, the zygote, which contains genetic material from the sperm and the egg. The zygote divides several times to form a ball of cells, which then implants into the lining of the uterus. At the point of attachment, the outer layer of cells forms the placenta, while a group of cells within one area of the cell ball develops into the embryo. A sac filled with amniotic fluid forms around the embryo to protect it. As the embryo grows, it begins to form features and, by the fifth week, it has developed a recognizable head and limb buds.

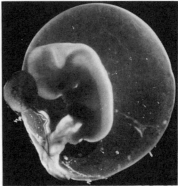

Embryo at about six weeks
The embryo is floating in the amniotic sac. The smaller sac at left (the yolk sac) provides nourishment for the early embryo.

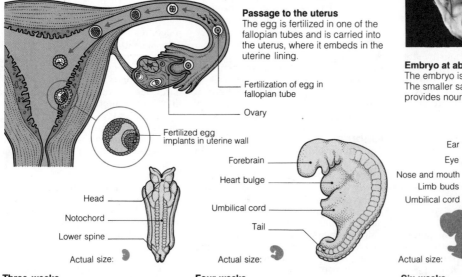

Passage to the uterus
The egg is fertilized in one of the fallopian tubes and is carried into the uterus, where it embeds in the uterine lining.

Fertilization of egg in fallopian tube

Ovary

Fertilized egg implants in uterine wall

Head

Notochord

Lower spine

Actual size:

Three weeks
The embryo becomes pear-shaped, with a rounded head, pointed lower spine, and notochord running along its back.

Forebrain

Heart bulge

Umbilical cord

Tail

Actual size:

Four weeks
The embryo becomes C-shaped and a tail is visible. The umbilical cord forms and the forebrain enlarges.

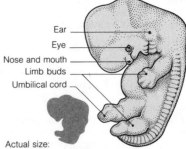

Ear

Eye

Nose and mouth

Limb buds

Umbilical cord

Actual size:

Six weeks
Eyes are visible and the mouth, nose, and ears are forming. The limbs grow rapidly from initial tiny buds.

INTERNAL ORGANS AT FIVE WEEKS

All the internal organs (such as the liver, pancreas, stomach, heart, lungs, kidneys, and sex organs) have begun to form by the fifth week. During this critical stage of development, the embryo is highly vulnerable to harmful substances consumed by the mother (such as alcohol and medication), which may cause birth defects.

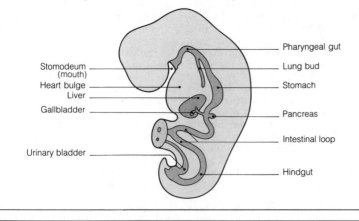

Stomodeum (mouth)

Heart bulge

Liver

Gallbladder

Urinary bladder

Pharyngeal gut

Lung bud

Stomach

Pancreas

Intestinal loop

Hindgut

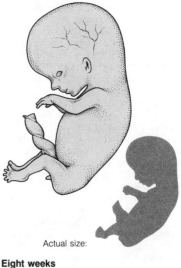

Actual size:

Eight weeks
The face is more "human," the head is more upright, and the tail has gone. Limbs become jointed and digits appear.

Embryology

 The study of the development and growth of the *embryo* and then the *fetus* from conception until birth.

Embryology is an essential part of the medical student's training, since it leads to a greater understanding of adult anatomy and of the ways structural defects in the body arise. For example, the occurrence of congenital heart defects (such as "holes in the heart" and transposition of the main blood vessels) is easier to understand when the stages of fetal heart development have been explained.

Until recently, embryology was based on the study of animal embryos and dead human embryos at different stages of development. More details about the nature of physical and chemical processes involved in embryo development have been established by examination of live embryos grown in the laboratory (see *Embryo, research on*).

Embryo, research on

Human embryos are regularly grown in laboratories as part of the treatment of infertility (see *In vitro fertilization*). Physicians usually fertilize more eggs than they need, since they do not know how many will "take" (begin the process of cell division and growth); the unwanted embryos may then be frozen for use in later attempts at achieving a pregnancy. Surplus embryos are being used for research aimed at improving the results of in vitro fertilization, at finding better methods of contraception, and at detecting genetic disorders at an early stage in pregnancy.

In several countries, such research has been prohibited or the physicians concerned have agreed not to perform it for ethical reasons. As yet there is no consensus on the circumstances under which research on embryos is ethically acceptable.

Emergency

Any condition that requires urgent medical treatment, such as cardiac arrest, or any procedure that must be performed immediately, such as *cardiopulmonary resuscitation*.

Emergency physician

A physician who has been specially trained to deal with a broad range of life-threatening conditions, ranging from acute asthma attacks to bullet wounds. The first concern of the emergency-care physician is to save the life of the patient and then to stabilize the condition as much as possible before transferring the patient to an appropriate hospital unit for further care.

Emesis

The medical term for *vomiting*.

Emetic

A substance that causes vomiting, used to treat some types of poisoning and drug overdose. Emetics work by stimulating the part of the brain that controls vomiting and/or by irritating the lining of the stomach.

The most widely used emetic is *ipecac*. Emetics should not be given to a person who is drowsy because he or she may inhale the vomit.

EMG

The abbreviation for electromyogram, a test in which the electrical activity in muscle is analyzed after being amplified, displayed, and recorded.
WHY IT IS DONE
An EMG can reveal the presence of muscle disorders, such as *muscular dystrophy*, or disorders in which the nerve supply to muscle is impaired, such as *neuropathy* or *radiculopathy*. In cases of nerve injury, the actual site of nerve damage can often be located.
HOW IT IS DONE
The technique for obtaining an EMG (called electromyography) is harmless and takes 30 to 60 minutes to perform, depending on the number of muscles to be tested. There are no side effects. Impulses are recorded by attaching small disk electrodes to the skin surface over the muscle or by inserting needle electrodes into the muscle. The electrical activity is evaluated during muscle contraction and at rest. Impulses are seen on an oscilloscope screen or heard over a loudspeaker. Changes in the electrical wave forms and sounds associated with them allow the electromyographer to determine whether nerve or muscle disorders are present.

Emollient

A substance such as olive oil, lanolin, or petroleum jelly that has a soothing, softening effect when applied to the skin, eyes, or mucous membranes (for example, the lining of the nose and mouth). By forming an oily film, emollients prevent the loss of water from these surfaces and therefore have a moisturizing effect. Emollients are used in creams, ointments, nasal sprays, and suppositories.

Emotional deprivation

Lack of sufficient loving attention and warm, trusting relationships during a child's early years, leading to difficulty in normal emotional development. Emotional deprivation may result if *bonding* does not occur in the early months of life, if a child is frequently separated from his or her parents for long periods during the first five years, or if parents cannot meet the child's emotional needs.

Emotionally deprived children are often impulsive, crave attention, cannot cope with frustration, and may even be mildly mentally retarded.

Emotional problems

A common term for a wide range of psychological difficulties. The problems may be due to upbringing, relationships, or psychiatric illness, but external feelings of *anxiety* and *depression* generally predominate. Age, sex, and social and cultural factors influence the most suitable methods of coping with emotional problems.

Empathy

The ability to partake in and understand the thoughts and feelings of others. It is possible to share an emotion with another person by comparing it with our own experiences.

In *psychoanalysis* the therapist relies on empathy to establish a relationship with a patient. Empathy can also help in making a diagnosis.

Emphysema

A disease in which the alveoli (tiny air sacs) in the lungs become damaged. The disorder causes shortness of breath and in severe cases can lead to respiratory and/or heart failure.
CAUSES
In almost all cases, emphysema is caused by cigarette smoking. Atmospheric pollution is sometimes a predisposing factor. Rarely, a predisposition to emphysema is inherited due to a deficiency of a chemical called alpha$_1$-antitrypsin in the lungs; the disease appears early in life, but its development is hastened and intensified by smoking.

The alveoli, of which there are many millions in each lung, are groups of air sacs at the end of bronchioles (tiny air passages). Through their thin walls, inhaled oxygen is passed into the bloodstream and carbon dioxide is removed from the capillaries to be breathed out. Tobacco smoke and other air pollutants are believed to cause emphysema by provoking the release of chemicals within the alveoli that damage the alveolar walls. Alpha$_1$-antitrypsin is thought to protect against this chemical damage; hence, people with a deficiency of this substance are particularly badly affected. The damage is slight at first, but in heavy smokers it becomes progressively worse, with the alveoli bursting and blending to form fewer, larger sacs with less surface area, and with consequent impairment of oxygen and carbon dioxide exchange. Over the years the lungs become less and less elastic, which further reduces their efficiency.

Eventually—sometimes after many years—the level of oxygen in the blood starts to fall, with one of two effects. In some cases *pulmonary hypertension* (raised blood pressure in the pulmonary artery) develops, leading to *cor pulmonale* (enlargement and strain on the right side of the heart) and, subsequently, *edema* (accumulation of fluid in the tissues), particularly in the lower legs. Other sufferers are able to compensate for oxygen deficiency to some extent by breathing faster. Why individuals react in these different ways is not known.

Emphysema is often accompanied by chronic *bronchitis*, also brought on by air pollutants and smoking. Emphysema and chronic bronchitis together are sometimes called chronic obstructive lung (or airways) disease.

INCIDENCE

Several hundred people per 100,000 in the US suffer from some degree of emphysema. About 30 people per 100,000 in the US each year die from chronic obstructive lung disease; of these, about six deaths are ascribed to emphysema alone.

SYMPTOMS AND SIGNS

Initially, and for a considerable time in mild cases, there may be no symptoms, but as the disease progresses it results in increasing shortness of breath. At first this may be noticed only when climbing stairs or steep inclines, but gradually it becomes more severe until eventually it occurs after only mild exercise or is present even at rest.

A sign of emphysema is a barrel-shaped chest associated with air being trapped in the outer part of the lungs. There may also be a chronic cough (caused by accompanying bronchitis) and a slight wheeze.

As the disease progresses, sufferers in whom cor pulmonale develops start to turn purple-blue due to oxygen deficiency in the blood and their legs

swell because of edema; these people are known as blue bloaters. Those who breathe rapidly and retain normal coloring are called pink puffers. Many people, however, show signs somewhere in between these two extremes. As respiratory and/or heart failure develops, sufferers find it increasingly difficult to breathe.

DIAGNOSIS

The diagnosis is made from the patient's symptoms and signs, from a chest examination, and from various tests. Tests include taking a blood sample from an artery to measure the concentration of the blood gases (e.g., oxygen and carbon dioxide) and sometimes a sample from a vein (to determine whether the disease is due to alpha$_1$-antitrypsin deficiency). Chest X rays are taken to exclude the possibility of another lung disease being responsible for the symptoms and to determine how great an area of the lungs has been affected. *Pulmonary function tests* are carried out to assess breathing capacity and the efficiency of the alveoli in exchanging gases.

TREATMENT

Because emphysema is incurable—lung tissue that has been damaged cannot be replaced—treatment can only control the disease. This means preventing more damage to the lungs by a total and lifelong ban on smoking, and improving the efficiency of remaining lung tissue, which is done in various ways. *Bronchodilator drugs* are given to widen the bronchi (the airways linking the windpipe to the lungs) and the bronchioles. These drugs can be taken by means of a hand-held aerosol inhaler or an electrically operated *nebulizer* that produces a fine spray. Occasionally, *corticosteroid drugs*, taken by inhaler to reduce inflammation in the lungs, are also beneficial.

To treat edema, a sodium-restricted diet and *diuretic drugs* may be given to reduce the volume of fluid within the body by promoting output through increased urine production.

If the oxygen level of the blood falls considerably, oxygen may need to be given by mask or *cannula*. The patient may be given oxygen equipment to use at home.

OUTLOOK

The course of the disease depends on how far it has progressed before the patient gives up smoking. If extensive areas of lung have been damaged or if cor pulmonale has developed, death occurs sooner or later from respiratory and/or heart failure.

Emphysema, surgical

The abnormal presence of air in tissues underlying the skin. It most often occurs as a complication of *pneumothorax* (the abnormal presence of air in the pleural cavity between the lung and chest wall). This can itself result from injury, chest surgery, or as a result of a diving accident.

Empirical treatment

Treatment undertaken when a precise diagnosis cannot be made. In the case of a fever of undetermined origin, for example, a physician might prescribe antibiotics on the basis of experience with similar cases.

Empyema

An accumulation of pus in a body cavity or in certain organs.

Pleural empyema occurs as a rare complication of a lung infection such as pneumonia or pleurisy; it may also develop after a severe injury to the chest that penetrates the pleural space. The main symptoms are chest pain, breathlessness, and fever.

The diagnosis is confirmed by taking X rays of the chest and aspirating some of the pus for smear and culture. Treatment is an operation to open the infected cavity and drain the pus; antibiotic therapy is also used.

Empyema of the gallbladder may occur as a complication of *cholecystitis*, when it usually causes abdominal pain, fever, and sometimes jaundice. It is treated by *cholecystectomy* (surgical removal of the gallbladder).

Enalapril

An *ACE inhibitor drug* used in the treatment of *hypertension* (high blood pressure) and *heart failure* (reduced pumping efficiency). It may be given in conjunction with a *diuretic drug*. Enalapril was introduced in 1986.

Enamel, dental

The hard outer layer of a tooth that covers and protects the inner structures (see *Teeth*).

Encephalitis

Inflammation of the brain, usually caused by a viral infection. In many cases the *meninges* (the membranes that cover and enclose the brain) are also affected. An attack may be so mild that it is barely noticeable, but in most cases it is a serious condition.

CAUSES AND INCIDENCE

The virus most commonly responsible for encephalitis is the *herpes simplex* virus type 1, which also causes cold sores. In the US, another cause is a virus transmitted to humans by mosquito bites, which causes an illness known as St. Louis encephalitis. In addition, an increasing number of cases are caused by infection with HIV (human immunodeficiency virus), the organism responsible for *AIDS*. Rarely, the condition may be a complication of certain other viral infections, including measles and mumps.

SYMPTOMS AND SIGNS

Encephalitis has variable effects but often starts with headache, fever, and prostration, and progresses to hallucinations, confusion, paralysis of one side of the body, and disturbed behavior, speech, memory, and eye movement. There is a gradual loss of consciousness and sometimes coma. Epileptic seizures may also occur.

If the meninges as well as the brain are inflamed, the neck usually becomes stiff and the eyes become abnormally sensitive to light.

DIAGNOSIS

Diagnosis is based on symptoms, signs, and the results of *CT scanning* of the brain, an *EEG* (which records the electrical activity of the brain), and a *lumbar puncture* (taking a sample of cerebrospinal fluid from the spinal canal for analysis). Blood tests and, rarely, a brain *biopsy* (removal of a small sample of tissue for analysis) may also be required to confirm the diagnosis, which permits lifesaving treatment of some patients.

TREATMENT AND OUTLOOK

The antiviral drug acyclovir, administered by an intravenous drip, has proved an effective treatment for encephalitis caused by the herpes simplex virus. When the disease results from other viral infections, there is no known effective treatment. Depending on the infecting agent, some patients die and some of those who recover are left with brain damage, resulting in mental impairment, behavioral disturbances, and persistent epilepsy.

Encephalitis lethargica

An epidemic form of encephalitis (inflammation of the brain). There have been no major outbreaks since the 1920s, although rare sporadic cases still occur.

The symptoms are as for encephalitis, with additional lethargy and drowsiness—hence the illness's popular name of "sleeping sickness."

About 40 percent of sufferers died during the major epidemics; of those who survived, many later developed postencephalitic *parkinsonism*, a movement disorder marked by symptoms such as tremor, rigidity, immobility, and disturbed eye movements.

A small number of survivors from the post-World War I epidemics were still alive in the 1970s, when administration of a new antiparkinsonian drug, levodopa, brought a remarkable improvement in their conditions. However, after half a century of almost complete immobility, most sufferers were seemingly unable to cope with this "awakening," and lapsed back into their torpid state.

Encephalomyelitis

Inflammation of the brain and spinal cord, resulting in damage to the nervous system. The condition occurs as a complication of about one in 1,000 cases of measles, developing a few days after the rash appears. Rarely, it may occur after other viral infections, such as chickenpox, rubella (German measles), or infectious mononucleosis (glandular fever), or it may follow vaccination against rabies.

SYMPTOMS

Symptoms include fever, headache, drowsiness, confusion, epileptic seizures, partial paralysis or loss of sensation, and sometimes coma.

DIAGNOSIS AND TREATMENT

Diagnosis is as for *encephalitis*. Critically ill patients require careful nursing in a hospital. There is no cure for the disease, but *corticosteroid drugs* are given to reduce inflammation and *anticonvulsant drugs* are given to control epileptic seizures.

OUTLOOK

About 10 to 20 percent of patients die; those that recover may suffer permanent damage to the nervous system, causing mental retardation, epilepsy, paralysis, pituitary insufficiency, loss of sensation, or incontinence.

Encephalopathy

Any disease or disorder affecting the brain, especially chronic degenerative conditions (see *Brain* disorders box).

Wernicke's encephalopathy is a degenerative condition of the brain caused by a deficiency of thiamine (vitamin B_1) and is most common in alcoholics. Hepatic encephalopathy is caused by the effect on the brain of toxic substances having accumulated in the blood as a result of liver disease and liver failure, and is characterized by symptoms such as impaired consciousness, memory loss, personality change, tremors, seizures, stupor, and coma.

Encopresis

A type of *soiling* in which children pass normal feces in unacceptable places after the age at which bowel control is normally achieved (usually 2 to 3 years). These children have no specific physical problem, but often refuse to use a potty or toilet; they defecate in their clothes or in other, secretive, places, such as behind furniture, usually during the day. The problem almost invariably improves with time and is rare after the age of 10.

E

Endarterectomy

An operation to remove the lining of an artery narrowed by *atherosclerosis*, the buildup of fatty tissue. Removing the diseased lining restores normal blood flow to the part of the body supplied by the artery.

WHY IT IS DONE

Endarterectomy is performed to treat *cerebrovascular disease* (in which there is a serious reduction of blood supply to the brain) or to treat *peripheral vascular disease* (in which blood supply to the legs is impaired).

HOW IT IS DONE

Before surgery, the site of narrowing is located by means of an X-ray procedure called *angiography*, which requires a local anesthetic. For the operation itself the patient is given a general anesthetic.

Endarterectomy is a delicate procedure that may take several hours to perform. The artery is exposed, clamps are applied, an incision is made, and the diseased lining is removed along with any thrombus (blood clot) that has formed. The incision is closed with stitches.

RESULTS

New lining grows in the artery within a few weeks of surgery. The operation often brings about a considerable improvement in symptoms (for example, it can greatly reduce pain in the legs in peripheral vascular disease), but its long-term effect is more limited, since narrowing of an artery is rarely confined to one site. When narrowing is widespread, *arterial reconstructive surgery* may have to be carried out.

Endemic

A medical term applied to a disease or disorder that is constantly present in a particular region or specific group of people, in contrast to an *epidemic*, which is not generally present but occasionally affects a large number of people. *AIDS*, for example, has become endemic in central Africa and

E

has also spread to many other parts of the world. The lung disease *pneumoconiosis* was formerly endemic in coal miners before safety regulations enforced controls over coal dust, the causative agent.

Endocarditis

Inflammation of the endocardium (internal lining of the heart), particularly the heart valves, usually due to infection. It may occur alone or as a complication of another disease. The various types of endocarditis include acute bacterial, subacute bacterial, fungal, and nonbacterial.

CAUSES AND INCIDENCE

In both types of bacterial endocarditis, causative microorganisms enter the bloodstream and infect the lining of the heart and valves, eventually causing damage. This process is encouraged if the endocardium is already damaged (by congenital *heart disease* or *rheumatic fever*, for example) because clots form on the injured surface and then trap the microorganisms, which multiply rapidly at the site of damage.

Bacteria may be introduced into the bloodstream during cardiac surgery, particularly in places where foreign bodies such as stitches, monitoring tubes, or an artificial heart valve are inserted. Large numbers of microorganisms pass into the bloodstream when people undergo major dental treatment, especially tooth extraction. Surgical and investigative procedures of the gastrointestinal and genitourinary systems—for example, *cystoscopy* (passing a viewing tube through the urethra to inspect the bladder)—carry the same risks.

Drug addicts are susceptible to endocarditis (even if their hearts are healthy) because of the possibility of introducing bacteria and fungi from a dirty syringe and because of the risk of transmitting infection from unclean skin at the site of injection.

Fungal endocarditis may occur in people with previously damaged tissue and in people who have low resistance to infection, especially those on *immunosuppressant drugs*.

Endocarditis that is nonbacterial is a rare feature of some cancers as well as *autoimmune disorders* such as systemic *lupus erythematosus*.

SYMPTOMS

In the subacute form, the disease smolders undetected, sometimes for many months, during which time it causes serious damage to a heart valve. Symptoms are general and nonspecific; the sufferer may complain of fatigue and weakness, feverishness, night sweats, and vague aches and pains. On examination the only evident abnormality may be a heart murmur that changes from time to time.

Acute bacterial endocarditis, which occurs less frequently, comes on suddenly. The patient suffers from severe chills, high fever, shortness of breath, and rapid or irregular heart beat. The infection progresses quickly and may destroy the heart valves, leading to rapidly progressive heart failure (reduced pumping efficiency).

Apart from the inflammation and its effects on the heart, the clots attached to the valves tend to break up and fragments of infected tissue are carried in the blood. This may cause an *embolism* (blockage of an artery) and may carry the infection to other parts of the body.

DIAGNOSIS AND TREATMENT

Any patient suspected of having endocarditis is given a thorough physical examination. Blood samples are examined for bacteria or fungi and, if possible, the organisms are grown in culture so that their sensitivity to antibiotics can be determined. Tests on the heart may include the *ECG*, *echocardiography*, and *angiography*.

Once the diagnosis is confirmed by blood tests, patients are treated with high doses of *antibiotic drugs*. The drugs are usually given intravenously; treatment is started in the hospital, may be continued at home, and may last for as long as 6 weeks.

If a valve has been extensively damaged by erosion due to infection it may have to be replaced surgically with an artificial one. Artificial valves often become infected, in which case they must be replaced. Heart valve replacement may need to be done as an emergency procedure.

PREVENTION AND OUTLOOK

People who are known to have heart valve defects are prescribed antibiotics before undergoing any procedure that runs a significant risk of introducing bacteria into the bloodstream. People with heart valve defects should also be aware of the warning signs of endocarditis and call the physician should they appear.

Before the introduction of antibiotics, endocarditis was practically incurable and the bloodstream infection and valve damage resulted in death in 95 percent of patients; today, 65 to 80 percent recover. The disease is usually fatal if not treated.

Endocrine gland

A gland that secretes chemicals directly (that is, not through a duct) into the bloodstream. Examples include the thyroid gland, ovaries, and adrenals, which release thyroxine, estrogens, and hydrocortisone, respectively. The endocrine glands in the body make up the *endocrine system*. (See also *Exocrine gland*.)

Endocrine system

A collection of glands that produces hormones (chemical substances necessary for normal body functioning) that regulate the body's rate of metabolism, growth, and sexual development and functioning. Unlike *exocrine glands*, the secretions of which pass through ducts to local areas, endocrine glands are ductless and release their hormones directly into the bloodstream to be transported to organs and tissues throughout the body. (See also box, opposite.)

Endocrinologist

An internist who specializes in diseases and disorders of the *endocrine system*. Patients include people with *thyroid* disorders or *diabetes mellitus*.

Endocrinology

The study of the endocrine glands and the hormones they secrete, including the investigation and treatment of their disorders.

The hormones produced by the endocrine glands are responsible for numerous body processes, including growth, metabolism, sexual activity, temperature regulation, and response to stress. Any increase or decrease in the production of a specific hormone interferes with the process it controls.

One example of overproduction is *Graves' disease*, in which the thyroid gland produces too much thyroxine.

The symptoms and signs of an endocrine disorder may lead a family physician to suspect such a disease, but confirmation usually requires referral to an endocrinologist for specialized tests, including measurement of the amounts of various hormones in the blood and urine.

Endodontics

The specialized branch of dentistry concerned with the causes, prevention, diagnosis, and treatment of disease and injury affecting the nerves and pulp in teeth and the periapical (surrounding) tissues in the gum. Endodontics includes *pulpotomy* and *root-canal treatment*.

ENDOCRINE SYSTEM

The system consists of a collection of hormone-producing glands, many regulated by trophic (stimulating) hormones secreted by the pituitary. The pituitary is itself influenced by hormones secreted by the hypothalamus in the brain. Shown are the principal glands, with a note on the hormones they produce.

Pancreas
Secretes insulin and glucagon, which control the body's utilization of glucose.

Adrenal cortex
When stimulated by ACTH, produces hydrocortisone, which has widespread effects on metabolism; also produces androgen hormones and aldosterone, which maintains blood pressure and the body's salt balance.

Ovaries
Produce the hormones estrogen and progesterone, which influence multiple aspects of female physiology. These processes are controlled by gonadotropic hormones secreted by the pituitary.

Pituitary gland
Secretes hormones that stimulate the adrenals, thyroid, pigmentation-producing skin cells, and gonads; also secretes growth hormone, antidiuretic hormone, prolactin, and oxytocin.

Thyroid gland
Produces the hormones thyroxine, triiodothyronine, and calcitonin, which stimulate metabolism, body heat production, and bone growth. Thyroid activity is controlled by TSH, secreted by the pituitary.

Parathyroid glands
Secrete parathyroid hormone, which maintains the calcium level in the blood.

Testes
Produce testosterone in response to gonadotropins secreted by the pituitary. A combination of gonadotropins and testosterone stimulates sperm production and the development of other male characteristics.

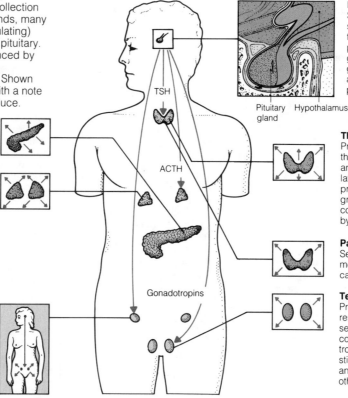

Pituitary gland   Hypothalamus

E

CONTROL OF HORMONE PRODUCTION

Production of too much or too little hormone by a gland is prevented by feedback mechanisms. Variations in the blood level of the hormone are detected by the part of the brain known as the hypothalamus, which prompts the pituitary to modify its production of trophic (gland-stimulating) hormone accordingly.

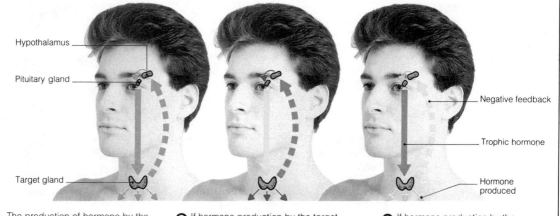

1 The production of hormone by the target gland (in this illustration, the thyroid gland) and of trophic hormone by the pituitary gland is normal.

2 If hormone production by the target gland rises too high, the feedback effect causes less trophic hormone to be produced, which tends to return the situation to normal.

3 If hormone production by the target gland drops too low, the feedback lessens and more trophic hormone is produced, which tends to return the situation to normal.

ENDOCRINE DISORDERS

In all endocrine disorders, there is either deficient or excess production of a hormone by a gland. Common causes of abnormal hormone production include a tumor or an autoimmune disease affecting a gland, or a disorder of the pituitary or the hypothalamus, which control many other glands. Abnormal hormone production often has a feedback effect on the secretion of trophic (stimulating) hormones by the pituitary and the hypothalamus – as in two of the examples shown. The blood levels of different hormones may need to be measured to pinpoint the cause of a disorder.

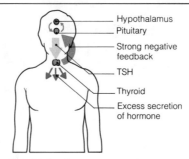

Thyrotoxicosis
This disorder is usually due to an autoimmune disease of the thyroid. Excess hormones cause the symptoms; the output of TSH and its hypothalamic releasing hormone is reduced, but the thyroid continues to overproduce.

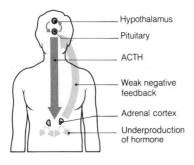

Addison's disease
Symptoms are caused by reduced hormone production by the defective adrenal cortices. Feedback is weak, so the pituitary pours out adrenocorticotropic hormone (ACTH), but it fails to stimulate the adrenals.

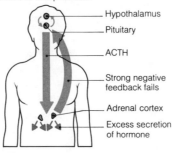

Cushing's syndrome
This disorder is caused by excess ACTH secretion by a pituitary tumor. This stimulates the adrenal cortices to make excess hydrocortisone, leading to the symptoms of the syndrome. Feedback fails to suppress ACTH secretion.

Endodontist

A dentist who is specially trained to treat the nerves and pulp in teeth and the periapical (surrounding) tissues in the gum. *Root-canal treatment* is a common endodontic procedure.

Endogenous

Arising from causes within the body. For example, an endogenous infection may occur if bacteria from around the anus invade the urinary tract.

The term endogenous depression was formerly used to describe depression with no discoverable external cause that was thought to be due to a chemical imbalance in the brain.

Most disorders, however, are exogenous (caused by external infections, poisoning, or injury).

Endometrial cancer

See *Uterus, cancer of.*

Endometriosis

A condition in which fragments of the *endometrium* (lining of the uterus) are found in other parts of (or on organs within) the pelvic cavity.

INCIDENCE AND CAUSE
Endometriosis is most prevalent between 25 and 40 and is a common cause of *infertility*. About 10 to 15 percent of infertility patients have endometriosis and about 30 to 40 percent of women suffering from endometriosis are infertile.

The exact cause of endometriosis is uncertain, but in some cases it is thought to occur because fragments of

SITES OF ENDOMETRIOSIS

Fragments of the *endometrium* may travel from the uterus into the pelvic cavity via the fallopian tubes. They then implant on parts of the pelvic organs (such as the uterus, ovaries, vagina, cervix, bladder, and rectum). The patches of endometrium continue to respond to the menstrual cycle and bleed every month, causing the formation of painful cysts, which can be very small or as large as a grapefruit.

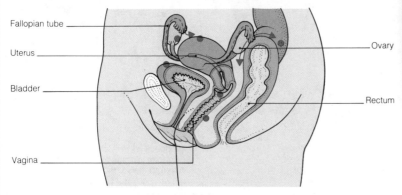

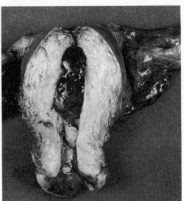

Severe endometriosis
The uterus, fallopian tubes, and ovaries shown above had large cysts growing around them due to endometriosis. As the patient was nearing the menopause, the affected organs were surgically removed.

the endometrium that are shed during *menstruation* do not leave the body with the menstrual flow. Instead, they travel up the fallopian tubes and into the pelvic cavity. There, they may adhere to and grow on any of the pelvic organs.

These displaced patches of endometrium continue to respond to the menstrual cycle as if they were still inside the uterus, so each month they bleed. This blood cannot escape, however, and causes the formation of slowly growing cysts from the size of a pinhead to the size of a grapefruit. The growth and swelling of the cysts are responsible for much of the pain associated with endometriosis.

SYMPTOMS AND SIGNS
The symptoms of endometriosis vary widely, with abnormal or heavy menstrual bleeding being most common. There may be severe abdominal and/or lower back pain during menstruation, which is often most severe toward the end of a period. Other possible symptoms include dyspareunia (see *Intercourse, painful*) and digestive tract symptoms such as diarrhea, constipation, or painful defecation. Rectal bleeding that happens only at the time of the menses may occur. In some cases, however, endometriosis causes no symptoms.

DIAGNOSIS AND TREATMENT
Laparoscopy (examination of the abdominal cavity with a viewing instrument) confirms the diagnosis.

Treatment depends on many factors, including the age and health of the patient, the severity of the condition, and the desire of the woman to have children. Some cases are mild and require no treatment. Drugs to prevent menstruation (including danazol, progesterone, or the combined birth-control pill) may be given. In some cases, pregnancy can suppress endometriosis.

In severe cases, surgical removal of the cysts may be necessary in addition to drug therapy. This may relieve symptoms and aid fertility. If the woman is planning to have no children or she is nearing the menopause, a *hysterectomy* may be considered.

Endometritis
Inflammation of the *endometrium* (uterine lining) due to infection.

Endometritis is a feature of *pelvic inflammatory disease* (PID). It may also occur as a complication of abortion or childbirth, after the insertion of an *IUD*, or as the result of a sexually transmitted infection.

Symptoms include fever, vaginal discharge, and lower abdominal pain. Treatment includes removing any foreign body (such as an IUD or retained placental tissue) and the administration of antibiotics.

Endometrium
The membrane that lines the inside of the *uterus*. It increases in thickness during the menstrual cycle until ovulation occurs. The surface layers are shed during *menstruation* if conception does not take place.

Endorphins
A group of substances formed within the body that relieves pain. Endorphins have a similar chemical structure to *morphine* (it is because of this similarity that morphine has an analgesic effect).

In 1973 morphine was found to act at specific sites (called opiate receptors) in the brain, spinal cord, and at other nerve endings. This discovery led to the identification of small protein molecules produced by cells in the body that also act at opiate receptors; these morphinelike proteins were named endorphins (short for endogenous morphines).

Two other small proteins produced within the brain were originally considered to be examples of endorphins, but they have now been reclassified as *enkephalins* because they are released from different nerve endings.

FUNCTIONS
Since their discovery, endorphins have been found at several sites in the body apart from the nervous system, including the pancreas and testes. Research is being performed to elucidate their full range of functions.

In addition to their analgesic effect, endorphins are thought to be involved in controlling the body's response to stress, regulating contractions of the intestinal wall, and determining mood. They may also regulate the release of hormones from the pituitary gland, notably growth hormone and the *gonadotropin hormones* (which act on the ovaries or testes).

Addiction and *tolerance* to narcotic analgesics, such as morphine, are thought to be due to suppression of the body's production of endorphins; the withdrawal symptoms that occur when the effects of morphine wear off may be due to a lack of these natural analgesics. Conversely, acupuncture is thought to produce analgesia partly by stimulating the release of endorphins and enkephalins.

Endoscope
A lighted viewing instrument that is inserted into a body cavity for the purpose of investigating and treating disorders. (See also box, overleaf.)

Endoscopy
Examination of a body cavity by means of an *endoscope*, a tubelike instrument with lenses and a light source attached. The procedure is safe and in only some cases is a general anesthetic required. Endoscopes may be used with a camera or video recorder, which enable permanent records of the appearance of the internal organs of the body to be obtained and used for reference.

HISTORY
Attempts to view the interior of the body through a rigid, lighted, telescopelike tube were made in the early 1900s, but endoscopy really began in the 1930s with the invention of a semiflexible gastroscope for viewing the stomach. In the late 1950s, a second revolution came with the introduction of *fiberoptics* (flexible bundles of glass or plastic fibers along which light is transmitted). This enabled more versatile instruments to be developed and led to the acceptance of endoscopy as a routine part of hospital medicine.

USES
There are two main uses of endoscopy—diagnostic and therapeutic. For patients suspected of having a tumor or other disorder in the stomach, bladder, lungs, or other organs, endoscopy enables the physician to study the relevant organ and to take a *biopsy* sample (small piece of suspicious tissue for testing), procedures that once required a major operation. Since endoscopy is safe and can be repeated at frequent intervals, it is also useful in assessing how well an ulcer of the stomach or duodenum is healing.

Endoscopy is valuable in the treatment of acute emergencies such as bleeding from the stomach. It allows the cause and site of the bleeding to be identified and, in some cases, to be treated with electrocautery or a *laser*.

Many minor disorders of the knee joint that formerly required a major operation can now be treated quickly and easily. Other uses include removal of polyps (small growths) and swallowed foreign bodies, local application of drugs, and sterilization operations for women. (See also *Arthroscopy; Bronchoscopy; Colonoscopy; Cystoscopy; ERCP; Gastroscopy; Laparoscopy; Laryngoscopy*.)

E

E

ENDOSCOPES

A typical flexible fiberoptic endoscope consists of a bundle of light-transmitting fibers (see *Fiberoptics*). At one end is the head (featuring a viewing lens and steering device) and a power source. The tip has a light, a lens, and an outlet for air or water. Side channels enable attachments to be passed through to the tip of the endoscope.

A rigid endoscope is a straight, narrow viewing tube that is not flexible. Attached to it is a light source, which is usually fiberoptic.

COMMON TYPES OF ENDOSCOPES

Instruments	Region	Nature
Cystoscope	Bladder	Rigid
Bronchoscope	Bronchi (main airways of the lungs)	Flexible or rigid
Gastroscope	Esophagus, stomach, and duodenum	Flexible
Colonoscope	Colon (large intestine)	Flexible
Laparoscope	Abdominal cavity	Rigid
Arthroscope	Knee joint	Rigid

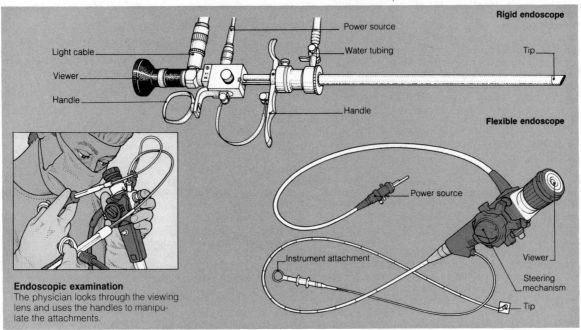

Rigid endoscope

Light cable
Viewer
Handle
Power source
Water tubing
Tip
Handle

Flexible endoscope

Power source
Instrument attachment
Viewer
Steering mechanism
Tip

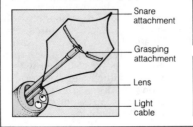

Endoscopic examination
The physician looks through the viewing lens and uses the handles to manipulate the attachments.

ATTACHMENTS

Various specialized attachments are available for use with the endoscope. They enable the physician to perform diagnostic and therapeutic procedures such as taking a biopsy specimen (a small piece of tissue for analysis).

Snare attachment
Grasping attachment
Lens
Light cable

Grasping forceps
Sharp-toothed forceps that allow foreign bodies to be grasped firmly and removed.

Biopsy forceps
Used for taking small samples of tissue for microscopic analysis.

Scissors
Tiny surgical scissors are used for cutting through tissue and removing small growths.

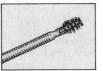

Brushes
Small brush attachments are used to obtain cells for cytologic examination.

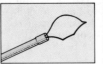

Snare
A thin wire loop, used to remove polyps, through which an electric current is passed.

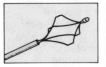

Basket
A wire basket is sometimes used to trap and remove stones from the bile duct.

Endothelium

The layer of cells that lines the heart, blood vessels, and lymphatic ducts. The cells are squamous (thin and flat), providing a smooth surface that aids the flow of blood and lymph and helps prevent the formation of thrombi (blood clots). See also *Epithelium*.

Endotoxin

 A poison produced by certain bacteria but not released until after the death of the bacteria; until then the toxin remains in the cell wall of the bacteria. Released endotoxins produce two major effects. First, they cause a fever by acting on the temperature-regulating center in the brain. Second, they make the walls of blood capillaries more permeable. This causes fluid to leak into the surrounding tissue, sometimes resulting in a serious drop in blood pressure, a condition called endotoxic shock. (See also *Enterotoxin*; *Exotoxin*.)

Endotracheal tube

A narrow plastic tube passed through the mouth or nose into the trachea (windpipe) by an anesthesiologist. The tube is held in place by an inflatable cuff at its lower end, giving an airtight fit. Endotracheal intubation is performed to deliver oxygen to the lungs if a patient is not breathing adequately and needs mechanical *ventilation*. It may be necessary in a comatose or anesthetized patient, or in a person with respiratory disease.

Enema

A procedure in which fluid is passed into the rectum through a tube inserted into the anus, either as treatment or for diagnostic reasons.

WHY IT IS DONE

An enema is performed for one of three reasons. It can be used to clear the intestine of feces to relieve constipation or to make the tract suitably clean for surgery of the abdominal cavity. Traditionally, this enema was performed by passing soap and water into the rectum. The soap irritated the wall of the intestine, causing contractions and thus stimulating defecation. Soap and water has now largely been replaced by prepacked, small volume enemas containing medication that has the same effect.

Another use of the enema is to administer medicine, such as corticosteroids dissolved in small volumes of fluids to relieve bleeding and inflammation in ulcerative colitis, or, less commonly, electrolyte solutions to treat severe dehydration.

A third use is in *barium X-ray examinations* to investigate the large intestine for the presence of disease. Barium sulfate, a metallic chemical impervious to X rays, is introduced by enema and outlines the intestine on X-ray pictures.

HOW IT IS DONE

No anesthetic is needed, although the procedure may cause slight discomfort as the fluid distends the intestine. The patient lies on his or her side with hips raised on a pillow. A catheter (flexible tube) with a soft, well-lubricated tip, is gently inserted into the rectum and the fluid for the enema, warmed to prevent sudden contraction of the intestine, is slowly introduced through it.

Energy

The capacity to do work or effect a physical change; nutritionists now also refer to the fuel content of a food as its energy content.

There are many different forms of energy—including light, sound, heat, chemical, electrical, and kinetic (the energy possessed by an object by virtue of its motion)—and most of them play a role in the body. For instance, the retina converts light energy to electrical nerve impulses, thereby making vision possible. Muscles use chemical energy—obtained from food—to produce kinetic energy (movement) and heat.

Energy is measured in units called calories (symbol c), which are becoming obsolete, or joules (symbol J). One calorie is defined as the amount of energy needed to raise the temperature of 1 gram (about 0.033 ounce) of water by 1°C (about 0.6°F); 1 calorie is equivalent to about 4.2 joules (therefore, 1 joule equals approximately 0.24 calories). However, these units are too small for many practical purposes. In medicine, especially in nutrition, the most commonly used units of energy are the kilocalorie (1,000 calories, often called simply a Calorie and represented by a capital C) and the kilojoule (1,000 joules, or 1 kJ).

METABOLIC ENERGY

The most important forms of energy in the body are chemical and heat. The body's *metabolism* comprises thousands of different chemical reactions, some of which liberate energy and some of which use it. Overall, there is a balance between the amount liberated and the amount consumed (see *Energy requirements*).

In general, the energy liberated from the breakdown of nutrients such as glucose and fats (protein is broken down for energy only in extreme situations) is stored as chemical energy in the form of ATP (adenosine triphosphate) molecules. The energy in the molecules is then available to power processes that consume energy, such as muscle contraction or the building up of complex substances needed for repair and maintenance of body structures. Some body processes (muscle contraction, for instance) produce energy in the form of heat. A certain amount of this energy is needed to maintain body temperature, but any excess cannot be used and must leave the body by mechanisms such as radiation of heat from the skin or sweating.

Energy requirements

The amount of *energy* needed by a person for cell metabolism, muscular activity, and growth. This energy is provided by nutrients in the diet, primarily carbohydrate, fat, and protein, and from stored nutrients in the liver and muscles.

ENERGY EXPENDITURE

Energy is needed to keep the heart beating and the lungs functioning and to maintain body temperature. The rate at which these processes use energy is known as the basal metabolic rate (BMR). The BMR accounts for three quarters of the total daily expenditure of energy of the average sedentary person. Any form of movement increases energy expenditure above the BMR. The greater the muscular effort required, the more energy is expended.

Additional energy is needed during growth to provide for extra body tissue. During pregnancy and lactation the mother's energy requirement increases because she must meet the needs of the baby as well as her own. (See also *Nutrition*; *Obesity*.)

Engagement

The arrival of the head of the fetus into the mother's pelvis. In a woman's first pregnancy, engagement usually occurs by the 37th week but, in subsequent pregnancies, it may not occur until labor begins. Rarely, engagement may fail to occur—if, for example, the baby's position in the uterus is abnormal, the baby's head is too big for the mother's pelvis, or if there is *placenta previa* (abnormal position of the placenta across the opening of the uterus).

Enkephalins

A group of small protein molecules that are produced in the brain and by nerve endings elsewhere in the body (in the digestive system and adrenal glands, for example) that have an analgesic effect. In addition, they are thought to produce sedation, to affect mood, and to stimulate motivation.

Enkephalins were initially considered to be *endorphins* (endogenous morphines), but it has since been discovered that they are released by different nerve endings and that they differ slightly chemically.

Enophthalmos

A sinking inward of the eyeball. The most common cause is fracture of the floor of the orbit (bony cavity making up the eye socket).

Enteric-coated tablet

A form of drug preparation whose surface is covered with a substance that is resistant to the action of stomach juices. Enteric-coated tablets pass undissolved through the stomach into the small intestine, where the covering dissolves and the contents are absorbed.

Such tablets are used either when the drug might harm the stomach lining (as may occur with certain corticosteroids, such as prednisone) or when the stomach juices may destroy the efficacy of the drug, as can happen with sulfasalazine.

The drawback of some enteric-coated tablets is that they may pass through the gastrointestinal tract without dissolving.

Enteric fever

An alternative name for either *typhoid fever* or *paratyphoid fever*.

Enteritis

Inflammation of the small intestine. Enteritis may result from infection, particularly *giardiasis* and *tuberculosis*, or from *Crohn's disease*, which is sometimes called regional enteritis. Enteritis usually causes diarrhea. (See also *Gastroenteritis; Colitis*.)

Enteritis, regional

Another name for *Crohn's disease*.

Enterobiasis

An infestation of the intestines by a small roundworm, ENTEROBIUS VERMICULARIS. (See *Pinworm infestation*.)

Enterostomy

An operation in which a portion of small or large intestine is joined to another part of the gastrointestinal tract or to the abdominal wall. When part of the colon (large intestine) is brought through an incision in the abdominal wall to allow the discharge of feces into a bag attached to the skin, the operation is called a *colostomy*. When the ileum (last section of the small intestine) is used for the opening, it is called an *ileostomy*.

Enterotoxin

A type of *toxin* (poison released by certain bacteria) that inflames the lining of the intestine, causing vomiting and diarrhea. Staphylococcal *food poisoning* is due to eating food contaminated with an enterotoxin that is produced by staphylococci bacteria; the toxin is resistant to heat and thus is not destroyed by cooking. The severe intestinal purging that occurs in *cholera* is also caused by an enterotoxin, but by one that is actually produced in the intestine by the cholera bacteria. (See also *Endotoxin*.)

Entropion

A turning in of the margins of the eyelids so that the lashes rub against the cornea and the conjunctiva.

CAUSES

Entropion is sometimes congenital, especially in fat babies. It is common in the elderly, when weakness of the muscles surrounding the lower part of the eye allows the lower lid plate to turn inward. Entropion of the upper or lower lid may be caused by scarring on the inner surface of the lid—for example, due to *trachoma* (a bacterial eye infection).

SYMPTOMS AND SIGNS

Entropion is easily recognized by the sufferer or his or her family. The lid margin is rolled inward so that the lashes are concealed, which sometimes irritates the conjunctiva. When gentle pressure is applied with the fingertip over the lid, the margin pops out, revealing the lashes again.

COMPLICATIONS

In babies, entropion rarely causes any complications because the lashes are very soft and unlikely to damage the cornea. In later life, entropion can cause irritation, conjunctivitis, or corneal ulceration. Persistent entropion may permanently damage the cornea and cause problems with vision and, in some people, blindness.

TREATMENT

Entropion that affects babies usually disappears spontaneously within a few months and seldom requires treatment. In the elderly or in sufferers from trachoma, surgery to correct the entropion prevents damage to the cornea.

ENT surgeon

See *Otolaryngologist, head and neck surgeon*.

Enuresis

The medical term for bed-wetting. Enuresis is a common phenomenon; about 10 percent of children still wet the bed at the age of 5 years, and many of these continue to do so until the age of 8 or 9. A slightly higher number of boys than girls are bed-wetters, and the problem tends to run in families.

CAUSES

In most cases, bed-wetting is due to slow maturation of nervous system functions concerned with control of the bladder. Occasionally it results from psychological stress. In a small number of bed-wetters, there is a specific physical cause—for example, a structural abnormality of the urinary tract present from birth, *diabetes mellitus*, infection of the urinary tract, or a nervous system defect, such as *spina bifida* or spinal cord damage. In each of these cases, the child also has difficulty with daytime bladder control (see *Incontinence, urinary*).

INVESTIGATION

The physician tries to discover, by a full physical examination, urine testing, and other procedures, whether the problem is due to psychological stress or to a nervous system or other physical disorder. If these diagnoses are excluded, tests may be needed to assess bladder function (see *Cystometry*). However, these tests are usually performed only on older children. They involve inserting a catheter into the bladder, which is difficult for a young child to tolerate.

TREATMENT

In the absence of an ascertainable cause, or until the problem can be more fully investigated, treatment starts with training the child to pass urine regularly during the day. This helps the child recognize when the bladder is full, even during sleep. Systems such as rewarding the child with a star on a chart for each dry night are often successful.

If such simple measures fail to work, a nighttime alarm system may be recommended by the physician. The system consists of a pad, placed in the child's bed between the lower sheet and the mattress, that is sensitive to moisture and that triggers a loud alarm when urine is passed. This awakens the child, who can then use the toilet. Eventually, the child wakes whenever urine is about to be passed. Alarms are said to help over two thirds of bed-wetting children over 7 years old.

Other measures that can help include encouraging the child not to drink for two or three hours before sleep, getting him or her to go to the toilet each night immediately before bed, and waking the child to use the toilet two or three hours after going to bed. Antidepressant drugs have also been used successfully in the treatment of bed-wetting.

Parents should not punish a child for bed-wetting or focus undue attention on it, as this may only make the child more anxious and make the problem worse. The vast majority of bed-wetting children eventually become dry at night.

Environmental medicine

The study of the effects on health inherent in different naturally occurring phenomena, such as climate, altitude, sunlight, and the presence of various minerals. The effects of working environments, such as in coal mining, is a separate study (see *Occupational medicine*).

CLIMATE

Certain regions, such as the south of France and the Canary Islands, have long been considered generally beneficial to health; more recently, these sites have been joined by Florida and California.

There is also convincing evidence that particular types of illness respond well to certain climates. For example, sufferers from chest disorders, such as chronic bronchitis and asthma, usually obtain some relief from their symptoms in warm, dry climates. In the US and Europe, where most respiratory complaints are more common in winter, sufferers benefit from spending their winters in a warm environment. Until the introduction of chemotherapy in the 1940s, the prime treatment for pulmonary tuberculosis was to move the patient to a mountain sanatorium to enjoy cool, clean, dry air.

ALTITUDE

Although mountainous regions have much less atmospheric pollution, they are not necessarily beneficial to health because air becomes thinner as altitude increases. Anyone with a chest disease who ascends quickly from sea level to 5,000 feet (about 1,500 meters)—the altitude of Denver, Colorado—may find that his or her breathing difficulty becomes worse. Above 10,000 feet (about 3,000 meters), breathing becomes difficult even for healthy people. Rapid ascent from sea level to 12,000 feet (3,600 meters) or higher carries the risk of altitude sickness, which can produce symptoms ranging from nausea and sleeplessness to coma or death. Only a few communities in the high Andes of South America live permanently above that level.

Sustained living seems to be impossible above 20,000 feet (about 6,000 meters) since at that level the blood cells increase to compensate for lack of oxygen. This strains the heart and causes a predisposition to thrombosis (blood clotting).

SUNLIGHT

White people who live in sunny climates may more easily suffer ill effects from repeated exposure to sunlight, including wrinkling of the skin and an increased risk of skin cancers, such as *basal cell carcinoma* and malignant *melanoma*, and the precancerous condition actinic *keratosis*.

MINERALS

Variations in the distribution of certain *minerals* in the environment are known to have an effect on health. For example, it has recently been discovered that, in areas where the radioactive gas radon is emitted (from rocks of the granite type), there is a higher-than-average incidence of cancers. In contrast, communities that are located in regions where the water has a high fluoride content have a lower-than-average incidence of dental caries.

E

THE GROWING IMPORTANCE OF ENVIRONMENTAL MEDICINE

Large areas of the world are naturally hostile to humans and were, in the past, avoided. Today, exploitation of natural resources has lured people into these regions and has highlighted the importance of environmental medicine.

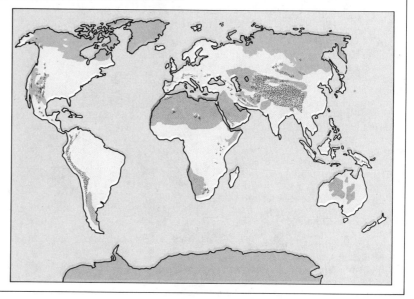

Key

Desert regions

Cold regions with average winter temperature below −10°F (−23°C)

Mountain regions above 10,000 feet (3,000 m)

Enzyme

A protein that regulates the rate of a chemical reaction in the body. There are thousands of enzymes, each with a different chemical structure. It is this structure that determines the specific reaction regulated by an enzyme. To function properly, many enzymes need an additional component called a coenzyme, which is often derived from a vitamin or mineral.

Every cell in the body produces various enzymes; different sets of enzymes occur in different tissues, reflecting their specialized functions. For example, the pancreas produces the digestive enzymes lipase, protease, and amylase; among the numerous enzymes produced by the liver are some that metabolize drugs.

INDUCTION AND INHIBITION

Enzyme activity is influenced by many factors. Liver enzyme activity is increased by certain drugs, such as barbiturates, which affect the rate at which other drugs are metabolized by the liver. This effect, known as enzyme induction, is responsible for many important *drug* interactions.

Conversely, many drugs inhibit or block enzyme action. Some antibiotics destroy bacteria by blocking bacterial enzymes while leaving human ones unaffected. Similarly, some anticancer drugs work by blocking enzymes in tumor cells, affecting normal body cells to a lesser degree.

ENZYMES AND DISEASE

Measuring enzyme levels in the blood can be useful for diagnosing disorders of certain organs or tissues. For example, the level of heart enzymes is raised after a *myocardial infarction* (heart attack) because the damaged heart muscle cells release enzymes into the bloodstream; muscle enzyme levels are raised in *muscular dystrophy*; and liver enzymes—measured in *liver function tests*—may be raised as a result of certain liver disorders.

Many inherited metabolic disorders, such as *phenylketonuria, galactosemia,* and *G6PD deficiency,* are caused by defects in, or deficiencies of, specific enzymes.

ENZYMES AND TREATMENT

Enzymes can play a valuable role in treating certain diseases and disorders. Pancreatic enzymes may be given as digestive aids to patients with *malabsorption* related to pancreatic disease; enzymes that loosen phlegm in the airways may be given to people with chronic lung disease who find it difficult to cough up the phlegm; enzymes such as streptokinase from bacteria and activated tissue plasminogen are used to treat acute *thrombosis* (especially in the coronary arteries) and arterial *embolism* (especially pulmonary embolism). Papain from the papaw fruit can be used in the dressing of wounds and ulcers because it dissolves dead tissue and coagulated blood and may also reduce bruising and swelling.

HOW ENZYMES WORK

An enzyme is a type of protein that acts as a catalyst for a chemical change in the body – that is, it greatly speeds up the rate at which the change occurs. The change may be a small modification to the structure of a substrate (chemical) in a body tissue, the splitting of a substrate, or the joining of two substrates.

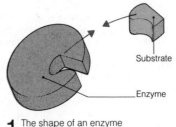

1 The shape of an enzyme determines its activity. It will combine only with a specific substrate that has molecules of a complementary shape.

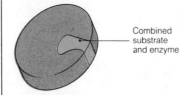

2 When enzyme and substrate combine, their interaction causes a chemical change within the substrate – in this case, splitting it into two products.

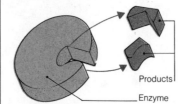

3 After the reaction, the enzyme molecule is unchanged and can move on to combine with another substrate molecule and repeat the process.

Ependymoma

A type of *brain tumor* that occurs commonly in children. It is a *glioma,* a tumor arising from the glial (supporting) cells within the nervous system.

Although ependymomas are one of the more common types of tumor in childhood, in overall terms they are rare. In the US, there are about two to three cases annually per million people. The cause is unknown.

Symptoms, diagnosis, and treatment of ependymomas are as for other types of brain tumor.

Ephedrine

A drug that stimulates the release of *norepinephrine* (a chemical *neurotransmitter* released from nerve endings).

Ephedrine is used in eye drops to narrow dilated blood vessels and to relieve redness of the eyes caused by minor irritation, such as smoke.

Other uses occasionally include the relief of motion sickness, bed-wetting in children, and delayed ejaculation. Ephedrine is prescribed as a *decongestant drug* and as a *bronchodilator drug.*

Epicanthic fold

A vertical fold of skin extending from the upper eyelid to the side of the nose. It is a normal feature in Orientals. In other races, it is rare except in babies; the folds usually disappear as the nose develops.

Epicondylitis

A painful inflammation of an epicondyle, one of the bony prominences of the elbow at the lower end of the humerus (upper arm bone). Various forearm muscles that bend or straighten the wrist or fingers are attached by tendons to the epicondyles. Overuse of these muscles can lead to epicondylitis due to repeated tugging of the tendons at their point of attachment to the bone.

Epicondylitis affecting the prominence on the outer side of the elbow, caused by overuse of the muscles that straighten the fingers and wrist, is called *tennis elbow.* When the prominence on the inner side of the elbow is affected, caused by overuse of muscles that bend the fingers and wrist, it is called *golfers' elbow.*

Epidemic

A medical term applied to a disease that for most of the time is rare in a community, but which suddenly spreads rapidly to affect a large number of people. Epidemics of new strains of influenza are probably the most common, occurring periodically when the influenza virus changes to a form to which the population has no resistance. (See also *Endemic*.)

Epidemiology

The study of disease as it affects groups of people, as opposed to individuals. Originally, as its name suggests, epidemiology dealt mainly with epidemics of infectious diseases (such as cholera, plague, and influenza) and outbreaks of infections (such as gastroenteritis) associated with food poisoning. More recently, it has been applied to widespread noninfectious diseases, such as cancer and heart disease.

Members of a population (or, in comparative studies, populations) under study are carefully counted and defined in terms of each person's race, sex, age, occupation, social class, marital status, and the like. Then the incidence of the disorder (the number of new cases per week, month, or year) and its prevalence (the number of people with the disorder at any given time) are determined. These observations may be repeated at regular intervals to detect changes occurring over time. The result is an exact statistical record that often yields many valuable findings.

Groups that spend all their lives in one defined area often provide more useful information than highly mobile populations whose environments change considerably over the course of their lives. For example, a high incidence of cancer of the esophagus has been studied among the inhabitants of one region of China and among other inhabitants of Iran. This incidence has been compared to similar groups in other regions of the countries; certain foods have been implicated.

COMPARATIVE EPIDEMIOLOGY

In the attempt to conquer cancer, heart disease, and other widespread diseases that afflict people in the West today, comparative epidemiology is proving to be one of the most potent weapons. Two or more groups are chosen—one having, the other not having, a characteristic that may affect the frequency of a disease. For example, in a study of the link between smoking and lung cancer, one group may consist of smokers and the other of nonsmokers; the proportion with cancer in each group is then calculated. In such cases, the epidemiologist is careful to make the two groups as nearly identical as possible in other respects, carefully

matching such factors as age, sex, weight, and socioeconomic status.

Another approach is to compare a group of people that has a certain disease, such as hypertension, with a control group (people without the condition but similar in other respects); the aim is to isolate identifying factors, such as obesity, that differ between the two groups.

The links discovered by comparative epidemiology—such as the correlation of a high level of fish oils in the diet and low prevalence of heart disease—do not demonstrate cause and effect. For example, epidemiologists have discovered that the prevalence of heart disease is high in countries in which most people have an automobile. This association obviously does not mean that owning an automobile causes heart disease, but, since such ownership suggests a more sedentary life-style, the link does reinforce the belief that lack of exercise increases the risk of heart disease. The study thus justifies more research on the subject.

Epidermolysis bullosa

A rare, inherited condition in which blisters appear on the skin after minor damage. The disorder mainly affects young children and has a wide range of severity, from the type in which blisters form on the feet in hot weather, to a form with widespread blistering and scarring.

CAUSES AND OUTLOOK

The condition is caused by a genetic defect that may show either an autosomal dominant or autosomal recessive pattern of inheritance (see *Genetic disorders*). It is diagnosed by skin *biopsy* (removal of a small amount of skin for microscopic analysis).

No special treatment for the condition is available, although injury to the skin should be avoided and simple protective measures should be taken to prevent rubbing of affected areas when blisters appear.

The outlook varies from a gradual improvement in mild cases of epidermolysis bullosa to progressive serious disease in the most severe cases.

Parents of affected children should obtain *genetic counseling* so that the risks of any future children being affected can be calculated.

Epidymal cyst

A harmless swelling, usually painless, that may develop in the upper rear part of a testicle. Small cysts are very

common in men over the age of 40 and need no treatment. Rarely, they may become tender or may enlarge and become uncomfortable, in which case it may be necessary to remove the cysts surgically.

Epididymis

A long, coiled tube connecting the vasa efferentia (small tubes leading from the testicle) to the vas deferens (the sperm duct leading to the urethra). Sperm cells produced in the testicle pass slowly along the epididymis, maturing there until they are capable of fertilizing an egg. They are then stored in the seminal vesicles until *ejaculation*.

Disorders affecting the epididymis include *epididymo-orchitis* (inflammation of the epididymis and testicle) and *epididymal cysts* (fluid-filled swellings). Infection or injury can block the epididymis; if this occurs in both testicles, it can cause infertility.

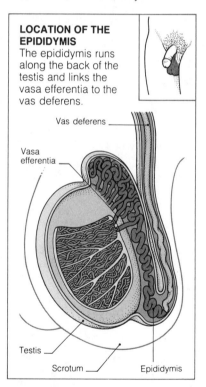

LOCATION OF THE EPIDIDYMIS
The epididymis runs along the back of the testis and links the vasa efferentia to the vas deferens.

Vas deferens

Vasa efferentia

Testis

Scrotum

Epididymis

Epididymitis

See *Epididymo-orchitis*.

Epididymo-orchitis

Acute inflammation of a testicle and its associated epididymis (the coiled tube that carries sperm away from it) characterized by severe pain and swelling at the back of the testicle and accompanied by swelling and redness of the scrotum in severe cases.

The inflammation is caused by infection. Often there is no obvious source of infection, but sometimes the cause is a bacterial infection spread from the urinary tract via the vas deferens (sperm duct). Rarely, epididymo-orchitis occurs through spread of a tuberculosis infection.

DIAGNOSIS AND TREATMENT
The symptoms of severe pain and swelling are similar to those of torsion of the testicle, in which the testicle cord becomes twisted and blocks its own blood supply (see *Testis, torsion of*). An exploratory operation may be necessary to make a firm diagnosis and save the testicle. In some cases testicular scans may be helpful.

Treatment is with antibiotics and rest. If there is an underlying urinary tract infection, its cause is investigated. The tuberculous form of the disease usually responds to treatment given for tuberculosis elsewhere in the body. In all cases it may take several months for the testicle to return to its normal size. Sometimes normal size is never attained. (See also *Orchitis*.)

Epidural anesthesia
A method of pain relief for surgery in which local anesthetic is injected into the epidural space in the middle and lower back to numb the nerves leading to the chest and the lower half of the body. Epidural anesthesia may be combined with a light general anesthesia. Usually a catheter (a flexible, fine tube) is introduced into the

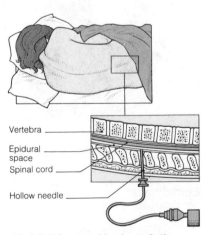

Vertebra
Epidural space
Spinal cord
Hollow needle

Administering an epidural anesthetic
The anesthetic is injected into the epidural space (the region surrounding the spinal cord within the spinal canal).

epidural space to allow further anesthetic doses to be given as necessary without more needle puncture.

Epidural *analgesia* is pain relief achieved by injecting narcotics or dilute local anesthetic solutions into the epidural space. Its applications include postoperative analgesia, pain relief during childbirth, and the control of cancer pain that is unresponsive to all other measures.

Epiglottiditis
A rare but serious and sometimes fatal infection that mainly affects children between 2 and 6. Caused by the bacterium HEMOPHILUS INFLUENZAE, it results in sudden inflammation and swelling of the epiglottis (the flap of cartilage at the back of the tongue that closes off the windpipe during swallowing). The swollen epiglottis obstructs breathing. If the condition is not recognized and treated promptly, it can cause death by suffocation.

SYMPTOMS
The illness comes on suddenly. The child becomes feverish, breathing becomes noisy (stridor), swallowing is painful, and the child drools because he or she cannot swallow saliva. Breathing becomes increasingly difficult and the child prefers to sit upright in an attempt to make breathing easier. Within a few hours of the onset of the illness, the child may become semiconscious and cyanotic (bluish) due to lack of oxygen.

DIAGNOSIS AND TREATMENT
The symptoms and signs of epiglottiditis resemble those of *croup* (inflammation of the airways); expert assessment by an experienced pediatrician may be necessary to distinguish between them. For this reason, any child who becomes feverish and in whom noisy breathing develops should be seen by a physician as soon as possible. If he or she suspects epiglottiditis, the child will be admitted to a hospital. In the hospital, neck X rays are usually taken to help confirm the diagnosis. A tube is almost always passed through the nose or mouth and into the trachea so breathing can be maintained; often a ventilator is needed. Intravenous antibiotics (usually ampicillin and/or chloramphenicol) are needed to cure the infection. With prompt treatment the prognosis is good; recovery usually takes place within two weeks.

The bacterium H. INFLUENZAE is highly contagious; family members should be screened or treated with antibiotics to prevent its spread.

Epiglottis
The flap of cartilage lying behind the tongue and in front of the entrance to the larynx (voice box). At rest, the epiglottis is upright and allows air to pass through the larynx and into the rest of the respiratory system. During swallowing it folds back to cover the entrance to the larynx, preventing food and drink from being inhaled.

Epilepsy
A tendency to recurrent seizures or temporary alteration in one or more brain functions.

Seizures are defined as transient neurological abnormalities caused by abnormal electrical activity in the brain. Human activities, thoughts, perceptions, and emotions are normally the result of the regulated and orderly electrical excitation of nerve cells in the brain. During a seizure, a chaotic and unregulated electrical discharge occurs. In some cases, a stimulus such as a flashing light sets off this abnormal sequence, but often seizures appear spontaneously.

CAUSES
Seizures are a symptom of brain dysfunction and, like symptoms in other parts of the body, can result from a wide variety of disease or injury. Seizures may occur in association with *head injury*, birth trauma, brain infection (such as *meningitis* or *encephalitis*), *brain tumor*, *stroke*, drug intoxication, drug or alcohol withdrawal states, or metabolic imbalance in the body. A tendency to seizures may develop for no obvious reason or there may be an inherited predisposition.

INCIDENCE
About one person in 200 suffers from epilepsy. The number of epileptics in the US is estimated to be close to 1 million. The disorder usually starts in childhood or adolescence. Many people outgrow epilepsy and do not require medication.

TYPES AND SYMPTOMS
Epileptic seizures can be classified into two broad groups—generalized and partial seizures. The form a seizure takes depends on the part of the brain in which it arises and on how widely and rapidly it fans out from its point of origin. Generalized seizures, which cause loss of consciousness, affect the whole body and may arise over a wide area of the brain. *Temporal lobe epilepsy* is a type of partial seizure. Partial seizures, in which consciousness may be retained, are usually caused by damage to a more limited area of the brain. Though partial seizures begin

in a limited area, the electrical disturbance may spread and affect the whole brain, causing a generalized seizure.

Many people with epilepsy lead normal lives and have no symptoms between seizures. Some can tell when an attack is imminent by experiencing an aura (a restless, irritable, or uncomfortable feeling).

GENERALIZED SEIZURES

There are two main types of generalized seizure—grand mal and petit mal (absence) seizures.

GRAND MAL During a grand mal seizure the person falls down unconscious and the entire body stiffens and then twitches or jerks uncontrollably. There may be an initial cry; breathing is then absent or very irregular during the seizure. Following the seizure, the muscles relax, and bowel and bladder control may be lost. The person may feel confused and disoriented and perhaps have a headache; often he or she will want to sleep. These effects usually clear in several hours. The person usually has no memory of the event. Prolonged seizures, referred to as status epilepticus, can be fatal without emergency treatment.

ABSENCE SEIZURES These seizures, in which there is a momentary loss of consciousness without abnormal movements, occur mainly in children. There is a blank period lasting from a few seconds to up to half a minute or so, during which the sufferer is unaware of anything. To the onlooker, it may appear that the person is simply daydreaming or inattentive, and the attack may even pass unnoticed. Absence seizures may occur hundreds of times daily and can markedly impair school performance.

PARTIAL SEIZURES

Partial seizures are divided into simple seizures (in which consciousness is maintained) and complex seizures (in which it is lost). In simple partial seizures an abnormal twitching movement, tingling sensation, or even hallucination of smell, vision, or taste, occurs without warning and lasts several minutes. When the twitching occurs and spreads slowly from one part of the body to another on the same side, it is referred to as jacksonian epilepsy. Sufferers retain awareness during the event and can recall the details.

During complex partial seizures, the person becomes dazed and may not respond if addressed. Sometimes involuntary actions, such as fumbling with buttons or lip smacking, occur.

These actions are called automatisms and can (rarely) take more bizarre forms. The person typically remembers little, if any, of the event.

Both types of partial seizure can sometimes spread to involve the entire brain, in which case generalization is said to have occurred. The symptoms then become the same as those of a grand mal seizure.

PREVENTION

Many epileptics experience seizures at times of extreme fatigue or stress. Infectious illnesses, especially if fever is present, also lower the seizure threshold. By avoiding these situations and taking prescribed medication regularly, epileptics can reduce seizure frequency. Occasionally, epileptics discover a distracting technique that can abort a seizure once the aura has begun.

DIAGNOSIS

In making the diagnosis, the physician seeks as much information as possible about the attacks. Since patients frequently do not have recall, information may be obtained from witnesses. After a complete neurological examination, the physician usually orders an *EEG* to help with the diagnosis. It is important to realize that the EEG cannot always absolutely confirm or refute the diagnosis of seizures, and that the results must be weighed in light of other clinical findings. Sometimes tests of heart function (such as an *ECG* or *Holter monitor*) are obtained to exclude cardiac irregularities as a cause of loss of consciousness in an adult. Patients thought to have seizures are usually given *CT scanning* of the brain and *blood tests* to check for the conditions associated with epilepsy. Opinion is divided on whether a single seizure should be treated; physicians agree that people with recurrent seizures should take *anticonvulsant drugs*.

TREATMENT

Anticonvulsant drugs are the first line of treatment for epilepsy, and, in almost all cases, they lessen the frequency of seizures. The drugs may have unpleasant side effects, including drowsiness and impaired concentration. The physician will attempt to find the one drug that works best, but, with very severe epilepsy, a combination may be needed to control seizures. If no seizures occur for two to three years (depending on their cause), the physician may suggest reducing or stopping drug treatment.

Rarely, surgery may be considered if it is thought that a single area of

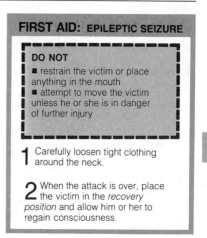

brain damage (usually in the temporal lobe) is causing the seizures and medication is ineffective.

OUTLOOK

If epilepsy develops during childhood and there is a strong family history of the disease, the chances are good that the problem will decrease after adolescence; it may even disappear altogether. However, seizure control is likely to be more difficult in temporal lobe epilepsy or if the disorder has been brought about by severe brain damage.

One third of those in whom epilepsy develops eventually grow out of the condition and experience no further seizures. Another third find that the seizures become less frequent in response to drug treatment. The conditions of the remaining third remain the same.

Sufferers from epilepsy usually are able to work, but the disorder may limit their choice of jobs. There are restrictions on obtaining a driver's license (generally an applicant is required to have been seizure-free for several years). It is advisable, unless the seizures are very well controlled, to avoid high-risk jobs involving heights or dangerous machinery and sports such as skiing.

Many epileptics carry a special card, tag, or bracelet that states they have epilepsy. Epileptics are recommended to advise colleagues on what to do if a seizure occurs.

DEALING WITH AN EPILEPTIC SEIZURE

Most major epileptic seizures last only a minute or two and demand little of the bystander. All that is necessary is to let the attack run its course and to ensure that the person is in no physical danger and can breathe while he or she is unconscious.

The person should not be held down, nor should his or her movements be restrained. Any tight clothing around the neck should be loosened and something soft should be placed beneath the head. The mouth should not be forced open and no object should be wedged between the teeth. Once the convulsions have ceased, the victim should be put into the *recovery position*.

An ambulance should be called if the seizure continues for more than five minutes, if another seizure immediately follows the first one, or if consciousness is not regained a few minutes after the epileptic seizure has come to an end.

Epiloia

See *Tuberous sclerosis*.

Epinephrine

| ALLERGY BRONCHODILATOR |
| GLAUCOMA DECONGESTANT |

Injection Inhaler Eye drops Nose drops

| 📄 Prescription needed |
| 🔲 Available as generic |

A naturally occurring hormone, also called adrenaline. Epinephrine has been produced synthetically as a drug since 1900.

Epinephrine is one of two chemicals (the other is *norepinephrine*) released by the adrenal gland in response to signals from the sympathetic division of the *autonomic nervous system*. These signals are triggered by stress, exercise, or by an emotion such as fear.

Epinephrine increases the speed and force of the heart beat and thereby the work that can be done by the heart. It dilates the airways to improve breathing and narrows blood vessels in the skin and intestine so that an increased flow of blood reaches the muscles, allowing them to cope with the demands of exercise.

USE AS A DRUG

Epinephrine is sometimes given by injection as an emergency treatment for *cardiac arrest* (stopped heart beat) and is used to treat *anaphylactic shock* (a severe allergic reaction) and acute *asthma* attacks.

During surgery, it is injected into tissues to reduce bleeding. When combined with a local anesthetic, epinephrine prolongs the effect by slowing down the rate at which the anesthetic spreads into the surrounding tissues.

Epinephrine eye drops are used to treat *glaucoma* and they are used during eye surgery because they reduce pressure in the eyeball. Epinephrine is also used to stop nosebleeds and reduce *nasal congestion*.

POSSIBLE ADVERSE EFFECTS

Regular use of epinephrine as eye drops may cause a burning pain and, occasionally, blurred vision or pigment deposits on the eye's surface.

In nose-drop form, epinephrine may cause palpitations, restlessness, and nervousness; newer *decongestant drugs* are now usually preferred.

Epiphora

See *Watering eye*.

Epiphysis

Either of the two growing ends of the long bones (femur, tibia, humerus, ulna, radius, and fibula) of the limbs. The epiphysis is separated from the diaphysis (shaft of the bone) by a layer of cartilage, called the epiphyseal plate or growth plate.

During childhood and adolescence, bones grow as the result of *ossification*, a process in which cartilage cells multiply and absorb calcium to develop into bone. In this way, the cartilage in the epiphyseal plate is gradually replaced by new bone.

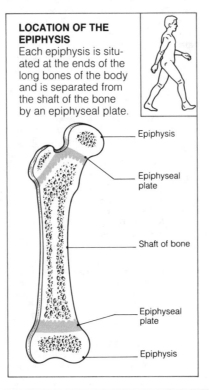

LOCATION OF THE EPIPHYSIS
Each epiphysis is situated at the ends of the long bones of the body and is separated from the shaft of the bone by an epiphyseal plate.

Epiphysis

Epiphyseal plate

Shaft of bone

Epiphyseal plate

Epiphysis

Epiphysis, slipped

See *Femoral epiphysis, slipped*.

Episcleritis

A localized patch of inflammation affecting the outermost layers of the sclera (the white of the eye) immediately under the conjunctiva (outer covering layer of the eye).

Episcleritis usually occurs for no known reason and usually affects middle-aged men. It may be a complication of rheumatoid arthritis. The purplish patch of inflammation is oval, slightly raised, and only a fraction of an inch across. It may cause a deep, dull, aching pain that tends to be worse at night. During the day there may be photophobia.

The condition usually disappears by itself within a week or two but may recur. Symptoms may be relieved by corticosteroid eye drops or ointment.

Episiotomy

A surgical procedure in which an incision is made in the perineum (the tissue between the vagina and the anus) to facilitate the delivery of a baby. After delivery, the cut tissues are stitched back together.

WHY IT IS DONE

Episiotomy is used to enlarge the vaginal opening. Some medical practitioners advocate its use almost routinely on the theory that a surgical cut will heal better than a tear, and that women who have had episiotomies will experience less "vaginal relaxation" (stretching of the vagina) later in life. Other practitioners rarely perform episiotomies on the theory that the naturally elastic vagina should not have to be cut to allow a normal delivery, and that small tears cause less damage and pain than does an episiotomy.

If the perineum fails to stretch up over the baby's head and/or a large perineal tear looks likely, an episiotomy is advisable. It prevents a ragged tear that is more painful, more difficult to repair, and more easily leads to complications. When the woman has had a previous vaginal repair (for *prolapse* of the uterus or urinary incontinence), an episiotomy prevents damage to the repair by increasing the size of the vaginal opening. Episiotomy is usually necessary in forceps deliveries because the instruments occupy additional space in the vaginal opening; it is likewise necessary in a breech delivery, when there is little opportunity for gradual stretching of the perineal tissues to occur.

Indications for episiotomy that concern the baby directly include *fetal distress* (when the baby is not receiving enough oxygen during labor), because episiotomy speeds delivery. An episiotomy also reduces pressure on the head of a premature baby.

HOW IT IS DONE
As the baby's head descends through the maternal pelvis and begins to distend the perineum, local anesthetic is injected into the area (unless the woman has already been given an epidural or another anesthetic).

Scissors or a scalpel are used to make a cut extending from the back wall of the vagina through the perineal skin and muscles. This cut may be directed to the side of the anus (mediolateral) or in a direct vertical line with the anus (midline).

HOW IT IS REPAIRED
An episiotomy is usually repaired shortly after delivery of the baby. The woman lies on her back with her feet in stirrups. The perineum is thoroughly cleaned and more local anesthetic is injected if necessary. The vagina is then inspected to assess the size of the incision and to see whether further tears have occurred. The wound is repaired in layers, usually with absorbable sutures.

RECOVERY PERIOD
The woman can walk as soon as she wishes. Perineal washes and/or showers are advised. Occasionally, ice packs and analgesics are required. Care is taken to avoid constipation. The sutures dissolve after about 10 days (if catgut is used) and thus do not require removal. In most cases, healing is straightforward. Discomfort in the scar is sometimes noted for up to three months.

Epispadias
A rare congenital abnormality in which the opening of the urethra is not in the glans (head) of the penis, but on the upper surface of the penis. The penis may also curve upward.

Surgery is carried out in infancy, using tissue from the foreskin to reconstruct the urethra and to create a penis that will allow satisfactory sexual intercourse in adult life. Sometimes more than one operation is needed to correct the condition.

Epistaxis
The medical term for a *nosebleed*.

Epithelium
The cells, occurring in one or more layers, that cover the entire surface of the body and that line most of the hollow structures within it. (The blood vessels, lymph vessels, and the inside of the heart are lined with *endothelium*, and the chest and abdominal cavities are lined with mesothelium.)

Epithelium varies in cell type and thickness of layer according to the function it performs. There are three basic cell shapes: squamous (thin and flat), cuboidal, and columnar. These structures may vary further. In the respiratory tract, for example, epithelial cells bear whiplike filaments called cilia that propel dust particles from inhaled air back up the tracheobronchial tree.

Most internal organs lined with epithelium are covered with only one layer of cells, but the skin, which is subjected to more trauma, consists of many layers with a dead outer layer of cells that is constantly being shed.

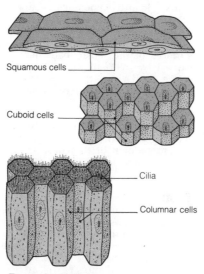

Squamous cells

Cuboid cells

Cilia

Columnar cells

Types of epithelium
The cells of the epithelium vary in shape and size according to function. The three basic types are squamous, cuboidal, and columnar.

Epstein-Barr virus
A virus that causes infectious *mononucleosis* and is associated with *Burkitt's lymphoma* and nasopharyngeal cancer.

ERCP
The abbreviation for endoscopic retrograde cholangiopancreatography, an X-ray procedure for examining the biliary system and the pancreatic duct. It is used mainly when *ultrasound scanning* or *CT scanning* fails to provide a sufficiently detailed image.

HOW IT IS DONE
ERCP is usually an outpatient procedure and takes 20 to 40 minutes. No food or drink is taken for eight hours before the examination. A sedative and a local anesthetic of the throat are usually given.

An *endoscope* (a flexible viewing tube with a lens and light attached) is passed down the esophagus, through the stomach, and into the duodenum (the upper part of the small intestine). After identifying the ampulla of Vater (the entrance within the duodenum to both the common bile duct and the pancreatic duct), the endoscope operator passes a catheter (fine, flexible tube) through the endoscope and into the ampulla. He or she then passes a radiopaque dye (one that shows up on X-ray film) through the catheter to fill the pancreatic duct and all the ducts of the biliary system. X-ray pictures are then taken to show any abnormalities in the ducts.

If disease is detected, it can sometimes be treated at the same time. For example, stones obstructing the lower end of the common bile duct can be removed by using an attachment on the endoscope to widen the duct. If there is a suspected tumor at the ampulla, the endoscope can be used to perform a *biopsy* (removal of a small sample of tissue for analysis) and/or brushing of cells for cytologic examination (see *Cytology*).

Erection
Hardness, swelling, and elevation of the *penis*. Usually caused by sexual arousal or physical stimulation, it also occurs regularly during sleep and may occur for no obvious reason in very young boys.

The penis contains three cylinders of erectile tissue with a network of blood vessels controlled by the spinal nerves. During an erection, the penis becomes filled with blood as the vessels dilate (widen) to allow increased blood flow. Muscles around the vessels contract and prevent blood from leaving to maintain the erection.

Erection, disorders of
Conditions in which there is total or partial failure to attain or maintain erection (see *Impotence*), persistent erection without any sexual desire (see *Priapism*), or a painfully bowed erection (see *Chordee*).

Ergocalciferol
An alternative name for vitamin D$_2$ (see *Vitamin D*), also called calciferol.

E

Ergometer

A machine that measures the amount of physical work done and the body's response to a controlled amount of exercise. It makes continuous recordings, during and immediately after activity, of heart rate and rhythm (using an *ECG*), blood pressure, the rate of breathing, and the volume of oxygen that is taken up from the surrounding air.

The physician-supervised exercise is done on a fixed bicycle, rowing machine, or treadmill, and the effort required is adjusted to suit the particular test being performed. In *fitness testing*, the exercise is vigorous enough to require maximum effort; in a *cardiac stress test*, the exercise is adjusted to a level sufficient to produce a certain predetermined level of heart rate. Symptoms that occur during the exercise, such as chest pain, breathing difficulty, or a fall in blood pressure, terminate the test.

Ergonovine

A drug that is injected after childbirth or termination of pregnancy to control the loss of blood from the uterus. Ergonovine works by causing the muscles of the uterus to contract, which compresses the blood vessels and thus reduces bleeding.

If blood loss remains heavy after the injection and there is no underlying cause (such as a retained placenta or infection) requiring treatment, ergonovine may be prescribed as a tablet for one or two days to help control bleeding.

Ergot

A product of *CLAVICEPS PURPUREA*, a fungus that grows on rye and other grains. Ergot contains several *alkaloids* (nitrogen-containing substances) with medicinal and poisonous effects.

The most important drugs produced from ergot are *ergotamine*, used to treat migraine, and *ergonovine*, used to control blood loss from the uterus following childbirth or an abortion.

Before it was known that ergot was a poison, bread made with contaminated rye caused outbreaks of ergot poisoning. The effects included gangrene of the toes and fingers, seizures, mental disorders, and, in some cases, death.

Ergotamine

A drug used in the prevention and treatment of *migraine*. It works by con-

stricting the dilated blood vessels surrounding the brain and is used as an alternative to *analgesics* (painkillers).

Ergotamine is most effective if taken during the very early warning stages of a migraine attack. Once the headache and nausea of migraine are present, it is less likely to be effective and may even increase the nausea.

Erosion, dental

Loss of enamel from the surface of a tooth as a result of attack by chemicals or acids, such as from gastric juices brought through the mouth in vomiting or from tobacco juice. The first sign of enamel loss is a dull, frosted appearance. As the condition progresses, smooth, shiny, shallow cavities form.

Erosion affecting the outer surfaces of the front teeth is most often caused by excessive consumption of citrus fruits, fruit juices, or carbonated drinks; it also sometimes occurs in workers using acid in industrial processes (such as battery construction). Erosion that mainly affects the inner surfaces of the molar teeth may be caused by frequent regurgitation of acidic fluid from the stomach—for example, in people suffering from *acid reflux* or *bulimia*.

Erosion may be combined with, and also accelerate, *abrasion* (mechanical wearing away of teeth) and attrition (wearing down of the chewing surfaces), leading to extensive damage to many teeth.

Eroticism

A state of sexual excitement. People are usually most easily stimulated by thoughts, but this stimulation may be augmented by touching of the erogenous zones—the breasts, genitals, mouth, and anus. Sexual arousal can also be produced by a variety of other sensations and stimuli (i.e., the look and feel of certain clothes, the scent of a perfume, or the sound of a piece of music).

In *psychoanalytic theory*, eroticism (named for Eros, the Greek god of physical love) is contrasted with *narcissism* (self love). Eroticism is a mature love that can be fulfilled only when the loved one is also satisfied. Narcissism is typical of immature personalities and is a love that merely wishes to satisfy itself.

Eruption

Breaking out or appearing, as in the development of a skin rash or the appearance of a new tooth.

Eruption of teeth

The process by which developing *teeth* move through the bone of the jaws and the covering gum to project into the mouth.

DECIDUOUS DENTITION

Deciduous (primary) teeth (the milk teeth) usually begin to appear at around 6 months of age, with the lower front teeth erupting first, but the timing may vary. Occasionally a baby is born with one or two of these teeth already visible, while in other babies no teeth appear until about 9 months of age. All 20 deciduous teeth usually erupt by age 3. Infants may suffer a mild general upset at the time of eruption (see *Teething*).

PERMANENT DENTITION

Permanent teeth (the secondary teeth) generally begin erupting at 6 years. The first permanent molars erupt toward the back of the mouth, behind the existing deciduous teeth rather than replacing any of them. Children and parents are often unaware that these are permanent teeth. The later eruption of permanent teeth nearer the front of the mouth is preceded by reabsorption of the roots of the deciduous teeth, which become loose and detach. The succeeding permanent tooth emerges a few weeks after its deciduous predecessor falls out. Wisdom teeth (the last molar teeth) usually erupt between the ages of 17 and 21, but in some people never appear. Frequently, wisdom teeth are impacted (blocked from erupting) because of lack of available space in the jawbone (see *Impaction, dental*).

Erysipelas

An infection of the face caused by streptococcal bacteria, which are thought to enter the skin through a small wound or sore. Young children and elderly people are the groups mainly affected.

SYMPTOMS AND TREATMENT

The disorder starts abruptly with malaise, fever, headaches, and vomiting. Itchy, red patches appear on the face and spread across the cheeks and bridge of the nose to form an inflamed area with raised edges. Within this area, pimples develop that first blister, then burst, and then crust over.

Treatment is with penicillin, which usually clears the condition within a week. (See also *Cellulitis*.)

Erythema

Redness of the skin. Disorders of which skin redness is one symptom include *erythema multiforme*, *erythema*

TOOTH ERUPTION

The top diagrams show the approximate ages at which particular deciduous teeth usually appear. The ages at which specific types of permanent teeth usually appear are shown in the lower diagrams. Red denotes erupting teeth; gray denotes erupted deciduous teeth; white denotes erupted permanent teeth.

Deciduous teeth
The full deciduous set (left) consists of eight incisors, four canines, and eight molars. They usually start erupting at 6 months.

Permanent teeth
The full set of permanent teeth (below) consists of eight incisors, four canines, eight premolars, and 12 molars. They usually start erupting at 6 years.

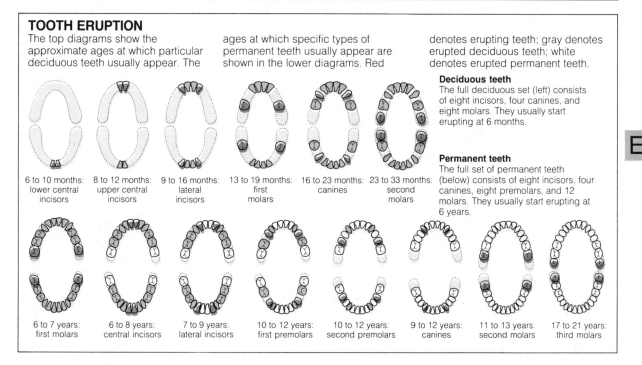

6 to 10 months: lower central incisors

8 to 12 months: upper central incisors

9 to 16 months: lateral incisors

13 to 19 months: first molars

16 to 23 months: canines

23 to 33 months: second molars

6 to 7 years: first molars

6 to 8 years: central incisors

7 to 9 years: lateral incisors

10 to 12 years: first premolars

10 to 12 years: second premolars

9 to 12 years: canines

11 to 13 years: second molars

17 to 21 years: third molars

---

nodosum, *lupus erythematosus*, and erythema infectiosum (*fifth disease*).

Facial erythema can have many causes, including *blushing*, *hot flashes*, *sunburn*, raised temperature, and skin conditions such as *acne*, *dermatitis*, *eczema*, *erysipelas*, *rosacea*, and *urticaria* (hives).

Erythema ab igne

Red skin that may also be dry and itchy, caused by exposure to strong direct heat. It occurs most commonly in elderly women—on the shins, as the result of sitting too close to a fireplace in cold weather, or on the abdomen, due to hugging a heating pad or a hot-water bottle.

Dryness and itching of the skin can often be relieved by an *emollient* (soothing cream). The redness usually fades in time, although it rarely disappears completely.

Erythema infectiosum

See *Fifth disease*.

Erythema multiforme

An acute inflammation of the skin, and sometimes of the internal mucous membranes (the thin moist tissue that lines bodily cavities). Erythema multiforme is sometimes accompanied by generalized illness. Erythema multiforme means literally "skin redness of many varieties."

CAUSES AND INCIDENCE
The disease can occur as a reaction to certain drugs (including penicillin, sulfonamides, salicylates, and barbiturates), or may accompany certain viral infections (including cold sores) or bacterial infections (such as streptococcal throat infection). Pregnancy, vaccination, and radiation therapy are other possible causes. However, half of all cases occur for no apparent reason. The disease is most common in children and young women.

SYMPTOMS
A symmetrical rash of red, often itchy spots, similar to the rash of measles, erupts on the limbs and sometimes on

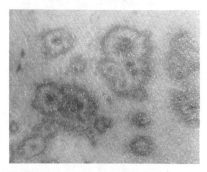

The rash of erythema multiforme
The spots of this rash are usually itchy and have a bull's-eye appearance, with concentric rings of different shades of red around a pale center.

the face and the rest of the body. The spots may blister or may progress to urticaria (hives), in which there are raised, red, pale-centered wheals. Those affected may have fever, sore throat, headache, and/or diarrhea.

In a severe form of erythema multiforme, called Stevens-Johnson syndrome, the mucous membranes of the mouth, eyes, and genitals become inflamed and ulcerated.

TREATMENT
If treatment for some other disorder is believed to be the cause of the erythema, the treatment will be withdrawn. Similarly, any possible causative illness will be treated. Corticosteroid drugs are sometimes given to reduce inflammation and irritation. Patients suffering from Stevens-Johnson syndrome are given analgesics (painkillers), plenty of fluids (sometimes intravenously), sedatives, and sometimes corticosteroid drugs.

Erythema multiforme usually clears within five to six weeks, although it may recur. The Stevens-Johnson syndrome normally responds to treatment, but in some cases the patient may become seriously ill as a result of shock or of inflammation spreading within the body.

Erythema nodosum

A condition characterized by an eruption of red-purple swellings on the legs in association with another illness. It is most common between the ages of 20 and 50 and affects women more than men.

CAUSES AND INCIDENCE

The most common cause of erythema nodosum is a throat infection with streptococcal bacteria, but it is also associated with other diseases, most commonly *tuberculosis* and *sarcoidosis*, and may occur as a reaction to certain drugs, including sulfonamides, penicillin, and salicylates. In about one third of cases of erythema nodosum no cause can be discovered.

SYMPTOMS AND TREATMENT

The swellings, which range from 0.5 to 4 inches in diameter, are shiny and tender and occur on the shins, thighs, and, less commonly, the arms. They are usually accompanied by fever and joint and muscle pains.

Effective treatment of any underlying condition clears the swellings. Otherwise, the only treatment that is necessary is bed rest, analgesics (painkillers), and, occasionally, *corticosteroid drugs* to reduce inflammation. The condition usually subsides within a month.

Erythrocyte

The medical name for a red blood cell. See *Blood cells*.

Erythroderma

See *Exfoliative dermatitis*.

Erythromycin

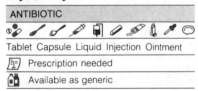

ANTIBIOTIC				
Tablet	Capsule	Liquid	Injection	Ointment
℞ Prescription needed				
Available as generic				

A drug used to treat infections of the skin, chest, throat, and ears. Erythromycin is particularly useful in the treatment of *pertussis* (whooping cough) and *legionnaires' disease*. In children under 8 years old, this drug is a useful alternative to tetracycline, an antibiotic that can cause permanent staining of developing teeth.

Erythromycin is destroyed by the acid in the stomach. To overcome this problem, the drug is prepared as a specially coated tablet or as compounds, such as erythromycin estolate and erythromycin stearate, which are more resistant to acid.

POSSIBLE ADVERSE EFFECTS

Adverse effects include nausea, vomiting, abdominal pain, diarrhea,

and an itchy rash. Certain brands of erythromycin can be taken with food to reduce the likelihood of irritation of the stomach.

Eschar

A scab on the surface of the skin formed to cover damage caused by a burn, abrasion, severe scratching, or some skin diseases and infections.

Esmarch's bandage

A broad, rubber bandage wrapped around the elevated limb of a patient to force blood out of the blood vessels toward the heart; this enables surgery to be performed more easily in a blood-free area. The Esmarch's bandage is wrapped from the toes or fingers upward, and a pneumatic (inflatable) tourniquet is then applied to the thigh or upper arm to stop blood from returning to the limb. The Esmarch's bandage is removed, leaving the inflated tourniquet in position during surgery.

Esophageal atresia

A rare birth defect caused by a failure of the esophagus to form correctly during embryonic development. A short section of the esophagus is absent, so that its upper part comes to a dead end, and the upward projection of the esophagus from the stomach is also blind-ending. In most cases, there is also an abnormal channel (known as a *tracheoesophageal fistula*) between one of these sections of esophagus and the trachea (windpipe). This abnormality occurs in about one live-born baby in 3,500.

SYMPTOMS, DIAGNOSIS, AND TREATMENT

The infant cannot swallow saliva or milk, and continuous regurgitation from the mouth occurs. If there is an upper tracheoesophageal fistula, milk may be sucked into the lungs; as a result, attempts at feeding provoke attacks of coughing and cyanosis (a blue-purple skin coloration).

A soft tube inserted into the nose can normally be passed down the esophagus; in cases of esophageal atresia, it cannot be passed. The diagnosis is confirmed by a chest X ray.

Immediate surgery is necessary. Using a general anesthetic, the baby's chest is opened, the blind ends of the esophagus are joined, and any tracheoesophageal fistula is closed.

Complications can be prevented by skilled nursing care. Some affected babies do not survive, but usually the operation is successful and the baby is able to lead a normal, healthy life.

Esophageal dilatation

Stretching of the esophagus after it has become narrowed by disease (see *Esophageal stricture*), which prevents normal swallowing. The usual cause of the narrowing is swelling and scarring from *esophagitis* (inflammation of the esophagus), but the narrowing may also be due to cancer (see *Esophagus, cancer of*) or *achalasia* (inability of the muscles in the lower esophagus to relax).

HOW IT IS DONE

The patient must not eat for at least eight hours before the esophageal dilatation, which is usually carried out under sedation.

First, an *endoscope* (a fine, flexible viewing tube) is passed through the mouth and down the esophagus to permit identification of the obstruction. The patient then swallows a length of thread, which anchors in the intestine, and a metal guide is passed over the string.

The next step is to pass a series of *bougies* (cylindrical rods with olive-shaped tips) of increasing size down over the guide wire to stretch the narrowed area. Bougies are being replaced by the *balloon catheter* (a fine tube with a balloon at the end). After being inflated, the balloon is kept in position for three minutes, then deflated and withdrawn; the same procedure is repeated later with a larger balloon. Guide wires are not always used with balloons.

Esophageal diverticulum

A saclike outward protrusion of part of the wall of the esophagus.

TYPES

There are two types of esophageal diverticulum—a pharyngeal pouch (Zenker's or pulsion diverticulum) and a mid-esophageal diverticulum (traction diverticulum).

PHARYNGEAL POUCH This type lies at the top of the esophagus, at its entrance from the pharynx (throat). It usually projects backward. The cause is a failure of the sphincter (circular muscle) at the entrance to the esophagus to relax during the act of swallowing, due to muscular incoordination. Instead, the sphincter resists the passage of food. As the powerful throat muscles used for swallowing work against this resistance, part of the lining of the esophagus is forced through the esophageal wall, thus forming the diverticulum.

Once the diverticulum is formed, it gradually enlarges, and food becomes trapped in it, causing irritation,

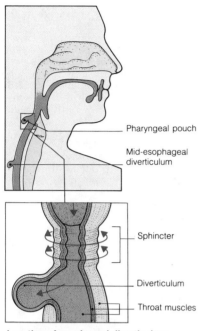

Location of esophageal diverticulum
The pharyngeal pouch forms at the top of the esophagus as a reaction to the sphincter's failure to relax during swallowing. The usually symptomless mid-esophageal diverticulum is a pouch that forms further down the esophagus.

Labels on illustration:
Pharyngeal pouch
Mid-esophageal diverticulum
Sphincter
Diverticulum
Throat muscles

difficulty swallowing, *halitosis* (bad breath), and regurgitation. The diagnosis is made by an *esophagogram* and the diverticulum is treated by removal after the surgeon has made an incision in the neck. The sphincter muscle is partly cut at the same time to weaken it and prevent recurrence.

MID-ESOPHAGEAL DIVERTICULUM This disorder consists of a pouch formed further down the esophagus. It rarely causes symptoms and usually requires no treatment.

Esophageal spasm
Uncoordinated contractions of the muscles in the esophagus that fail to propel food effectively down into the stomach. The contractions may be caused by some other esophageal disorder, such as reflux *esophagitis*, but in many cases they occur for no apparent reason. Women are affected more often than men. Pain is felt in the chest or upper abdomen and there is difficulty swallowing, but symptoms are intermittent and do not worsen.

An *esophagogram* will show the irregular contractions of the esophagus and, along with *endoscopy* (passage of a viewing tube down the

esophagus) and esophageal *manometry*, can rule out the possibility of a more serious condition, such as a cancer. There is no treatment unless an underlying cause, such as esophagitis, can be treated.

Esophageal stricture
Narrowing of the esophagus, which may cause swallowing difficulty.
CAUSES AND SYMPTOMS
Narrowing may be due to a cancer (see *Esophagus, cancer of*) or to any of numerous noncancerous causes. These include persistent reflux *esophagitis*, in which constant irritation from gastric acid causes inflammation and swelling followed by the formation of fibrous scar tissue and narrowing. Prolonged use of a *nasogastric tube* may inflame the esophagus, leading to a stricture, as may the accidental swallowing of a corrosive liquid.

The symptoms of a stricture are difficulty swallowing, pain, weight loss, and regurgitation of food.
DIAGNOSIS AND TREATMENT
A barium swallow (see *Barium X-ray examinations*) shows a smooth narrowing of the esophagus. *Endoscopy* (passage of a viewing tube down the esophagus) is used to look at the narrowed area, and a *biopsy* (removal of a small piece of tissue for analysis) is performed to exclude cancer.

In most cases, the narrowed area is widened by *esophageal dilatation*. In cases of very severe narrowing over a long segment of the esophagus (usually due to swallowing corrosives), the affected area may require surgical removal. A loop of colon may be substituted for the removed section, or the ends of the esophagus may be joined and the stomach brought up into the chest. These operations are rarely required.

Patients too old or frail for surgery may be treated by the insertion of a soft, pliable, plastic tube through the stricture or by a feeding *gastrostomy*.

Esophageal varices
Dilated, incompetent veins in the walls of the lower part of the esophagus and, at times, the upper part of the stomach. They arise as a consequence of *portal hypertension* (increased blood pressure in the portal vein due to liver disease). Blood passing from the intestines to the liver via the portal vein meets increased resistance and is instead diverted through the veins in the walls of the esophagus and stomach, where the pressure causes the veins to balloon outward.

SYMPTOMS, DIAGNOSIS, AND TREATMENT
The affected veins are thin-walled and contain blood at high pressure; they may rupture, causing recurrent episodes of torrential hematemesis (vomiting of blood) and melena (tarry, black feces). Most patients also have other symptoms of chronic liver disease.

Endoscopy (passage of a viewing tube down the esophagus) or a barium swallow (see *Barium X-ray examinations*) shows the affected veins bulging from the esophageal walls.

Acute bleeding may be controlled by means of a specially designed *balloon catheter*, which is passed into the esophagus and stomach; the balloon is blown up to press on the bleeding varices. Later, the varices may be treated with intravenous pitressin and/or by injection of a sclerosant—a solution that clots the blood and permanently hardens and seals off the affected veins. Surgery may be performed to lower the pressure in the blood supply to the liver. Recurrent bleeding can also sometimes be controlled by drugs such as propranolol.

Esophagitis
Inflammation of the esophagus.
TYPES
There are two main types—corrosive esophagitis, caused by the swallowing of caustic chemicals (acid or lye) accidentally or in a suicide attempt, and reflux esophagitis, caused by regurgitation of the stomach contents into the esophagus.

CORROSIVE ESOPHAGITIS The severity of the inflammation depends on the amount, concentration, and type of caustic chemical swallowed. Chemicals likely to cause very severe corrosive esophagitis include cleaning or disinfectant solutions.

Immediately after swallowing such a chemical, there is severe pain with *shock* and *edema* (swelling) in the throat and mouth. Antidotes are of limited value and gastric lavage (washing out the stomach) must be avoided as this may only increase the damage. Treatment consists mainly of reducing pain and providing nursing care until the esophagus heals. Sometimes a severe *esophageal stricture* (narrowing of the esophagus) develops, requiring prolonged dilatation and/or extensive surgery later.

REFLUX ESOPHAGITIS This is a very common condition. The cause is poor function of the musculature of the lower esophageal segment, which permits reflux of the stomach's con-

E

tents. Poor lower esophageal segment function may be associated with a *hiatal hernia*, in which the top part of the stomach slides back and forth between the chest and the abdomen. Symptoms may be worsened by alcohol, smoking, and obesity.

The stomach content is usually acid but, after certain operations, such as partial *gastrectomy*, the stomach contains bile. If this bile flows backward into the esophagus, it causes an alkaline type of esophagitis, which tends to be more severe and difficult to treat. Severe, chronic esophagitis can cause an esophageal stricture.

The main symptom of reflux esophagitis is heartburn—a burning pain in the chest—which worsens on bending over.

Barrett's esophagus is a complication of reflux esophagitis in which stomach lining is found in the esophagus. It may lead to cancer.

DIAGNOSIS AND TREATMENT
A barium swallow (see *Barium X-ray examinations*) will show reflux of stomach contents, and *endoscopy* (passage of a viewing tube down the esophagus) will show inflammation. In doubtful cases, special tests may be required. A small tube may be swallowed and a probe positioned in the lower esophagus to record the acidity over a 24-hour period; alternatively, a dilute acid solution may be introduced into the stomach to see if it reproduces the symptoms.

The treatment for most cases of persistent esophagitis is for the sufferer to change his or her life-style—to reduce weight and alcohol consumption, stop smoking, and avoid heavy meals. *Antacid drugs* may be given to reduce the acidity of the stomach contents. Elevation of the head of the bed with blocks may be employed. Sometimes, surgical treatment may be needed for a hiatal hernia.

Esophagogastroscopy
See *Gastroscopy*.

Esophagogram
A type of barium swallow of the esophagus (see *Barium X-ray examinations*) that is documented by still or motion X-ray films. The films show alterations in function and motility (muscular activity) of the esophagus. In addition, the pictures can reveal structural anatomic disorders such as a tumor, stricture, ulcer, diverticulum, or hernia. (See also *Esophagus, cancer of*; *Hiatal hernia*; *Esophageal diverticulum*.)

Esophagoscopy
Examination of the esophagus by means of an *endoscope*, a thin, flexible viewing instrument with a light and lenses attached. (See *Gastroscopy*.)

Esophagus
The muscular tube that carries food from the throat to the stomach.

STRUCTURE
The top end of the esophagus is the narrowest part of the entire digestive tract and is encircled by a sphincter (circular muscle) that is normally closed but can open to allow the passage of food. There is a similar sphincter at the point where the esophagus enters the stomach. The walls of the esophagus consist of strong muscle fibers arranged in bundles, some circular and others longitudinal. The inner lining of the esophagus consists of smooth, squamous epithelium (flattened cells).

FUNCTION
The esophagus acts as a conduit by which liquids and food (once it has

---

ANATOMY OF THE ESOPHAGUS
A muscular tube that propels food to the stomach from the throat. The upper and lower ends are bounded by sphincters – muscular valves that open to allow food to pass through.

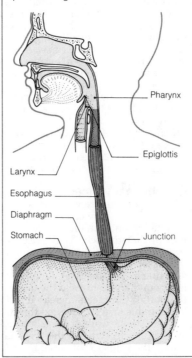

Pharynx

Epiglottis

Larynx

Esophagus

Diaphragm

Stomach

Junction

---

been chewed) are conveyed to the stomach and intestines for digestion. Food is propelled downward toward the stomach by a peristaltic action, powerful waves of contractions passing through the muscles in the esophageal wall. Gravity plays little part in getting food into the stomach—making it possible to drink while upside down. (See also *Swallowing*.)

Esophagus, cancer of
A malignant tumor of the esophagus, which ultimately causes difficulty in swallowing. Most esophageal cancers develop in the middle or lower sections of the esophagus.

CAUSES AND INCIDENCE
The causes of esophageal cancer are mainly unknown, but a high alcohol consumption and smoking are thought to play a role.

The incidence varies throughout the world, but there are about seven to 10 new cases diagnosed per 100,000 population in the US each year, mainly in people over 50. The cancer is more common in men than women and more common in blacks than whites. There is a particularly high incidence in parts of the Far East and Iran, where the cancer is linked to chemicals in certain foods.

SYMPTOMS
Difficulty in swallowing is noticed first with solids and later with fluids (even saliva) and becomes progressively worse. If food cannot pass it is immediately regurgitated. Rapid weight loss occurs, but no pain develops until the cancer is well advanced. Respiratory infections are common, because regurgitated fluid spills over into the trachea.

DIAGNOSIS
A barium swallow (see *Barium X-ray examinations*) can indicate the site and often the nature of the obstruction of the esophagus. Definite diagnosis is provided by examination of a *biopsy* sample (small piece of tissue) obtained through an *endoscope* (viewing tube with a tissue-collecting attachment).

TREATMENT AND OUTLOOK
Esophagectomy (removal of the esophagus) provides the best hope of cure but is a major undertaking. Incisions are made in the abdomen, chest, and sometimes in the neck. Most of the esophagus is then removed and the stomach or sometimes a portion of the colon is pulled up into the chest and joined to the upper esophagus.

For older patients who might not survive this operation, *radiation therapy*, sometimes combined with

DISORDERS OF THE ESOPHAGUS

Despite its apparently simple structure, the esophagus is prone to a number of disorders, most of which lead to difficulty, or completely prevent, swallowing and/or cause a pain in the chest.

CONGENITAL DEFECTS

Esophageal atresia is an absence from birth of a section of the esophagus, with the remaining sections ending in dead ends. It requires urgent surgical correction. Rarely, babies are born with weblike constrictions of the esophagus. These are rarely serious enough to require treatment, but may, if necessary, be broken down with a rubber dilator.

INFECTION AND INFLAMMATION

Infections of the esophagus are uncommon, but can occur in severely immunosuppressed patients whose defenses against infection are weakened. The most common infections are *herpes simplex* infection or *candidiasis* (thrush) extending downward from the mouth. Both cause pain on swallowing.

Esophagitis (inflammation of the esophagus) is usually due to reflux of the contents of the stomach, causing heartburn (a burning sensation in the chest). A more severe form—corrosive esophagitis—can occur as a result of swallowing caustic chemicals. Either of these types of esophagitis may lead to formation of an *esophageal stricture* (narrowing of the esophagus).

INJURY

Apart from the damaging effects of swallowing corrosive chemicals, the most common cause of injury to the esophagus is severe vomiting and retching, which occasionally tear the esophageal lining (and result in bleeding) or in extreme cases lead to rupture. A hard, swallowed *foreign body* can also cause injury and sometimes perforation if it lodges in the esophageal wall.

TUMORS

Tumors of the esophagus are not rare. About 90 percent are malignant (see *Esophagus, cancer of*); the remainder are benign. With both types, the initial symptom is usually difficulty swallowing.

OTHER DISORDERS

An *esophageal diverticulum* is an outwardly protruding sac, formed usually at the top end of the esophagus, in which food may collect and cause halitosis (bad breath) and sometimes difficulty swallowing. *Esophageal spasm* consists of uncoordinated and uncontrollable contractions of the esophagus, which may make swallowing difficult. In *achalasia*, the sphincter muscle at the junction between esophagus and stomach fails to relax to allow the passage of food, causing pain on swallowing and sometimes regurgitation of food. (See also *Swallowing difficulty*.)

INVESTIGATION

Esophageal disorders are investigated by barium swallow (see *Barium X-ray examinations*) and by *endoscopy*. Occasionally, a *biopsy* (tissue sample) may be taken for pathologic examination.

---

chemotherapy (particularly cisplatin), can sometimes provide a significant regression of the cancer, relief from symptoms, and even an occasional cure. Some relief from starvation can also be achieved by intubation—the insertion of a rigid tube through the tumor to allow swallowing of liquid or semiliquid food.

The overall outlook is poor, with only about 5 percent of patients surviving for five years; if the cancer is diagnosed early, the outlook is better.

Esotropia

Convergent squint, or "cross-eye," in which only one eye looks directly at the object while the other turns inward. (See also *Strabismus*.)

ESR

The abbreviation for erythrocyte sedimentation rate, measurement of the rate at which red blood cells sink toward the bottom of a test tube. Because the ESR is increased in certain disorders, it is a useful aid to diagnosis and can also be used to monitor the effect of treatment.

HOW IT IS DONE

Whole blood from the patient is mixed with anticoagulant (which prevents the blood from clotting) in a test tube and left undisturbed at a constant temperature for one hour.

The red blood cells, which can be seen as a dark red clump, settle toward the bottom of the tube, leaving the clear, straw-colored plasma at the top. The ESR is the number of millimeters the red cells fall in one hour.

RESULTS

The ESR is high when the red cells are sticky due to abnormal levels of fibrinogen or *globulins* (types of protein) in the blood. Globulins are usually produced in response to serious infection, inflammation of blood vessels (as in *temporal arteritis*), and some types of cancer, such as *myeloma*. Fibrinogen is produced in response to inflammation.

Estradiol

ESTROGEN

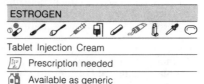

Tablet Injection Cream
📋 Prescription needed
🔒 Available as generic

The most important of the *estrogen hormones* (female sex hormones). They are essential for the healthy functioning of the reproductive system and for breast development.

In its synthetic form, estradiol is prescribed as a tablet to treat symptoms of the *menopause* (see *Hormone replacement therapy*), to treat *osteoporosis*, and to stimulate sexual development in *hypogonadism* (underdeveloped ovaries). Estradiol is also prescribed as a cream to treat atrophic *vaginitis* (dryness of the vagina).

Estriol

One of the *estrogen hormones* (female sex hormones).

Estrogen drugs

COMMON DRUGS

Conjugated estrogens Diethylstilbestrol Dienestrol Estradiol Estrone Ethinyl estradiol

WARNING

Tobacco smoking while taking estrogen drugs significantly increases the risk of abnormal blood clotting, which may cause myocardial infarction, pulmonary embolism, or stroke.

E

A group of drugs produced synthetically for use in the birth-control pill (see *Oral contraceptives*) and to supplement or replace the naturally occurring estrogen hormones in the body (see *Ovary*). Estrogen drugs are often used in conjunction with *progesterone drugs*.

Estrogens suppress the production of *gonadotropin hormones* (hormones that stimulate cell activity in the ovaries). High doses of estrogens may be given as postcoital contraception (see *Contraception, postcoital*).

Synthetic estrogens are used to treat, and in some cases to prevent, symptoms and disorders related to the *menopause*, including atrophic *vaginitis* (dryness of the vagina) and *osteoporosis* (a bone disorder).

Estrogens may also be used to treat certain forms of infertility, *hypogonadism* (underdeveloped ovaries), menstrual disorders in which there is abnormal bleeding from the uterus, prostate cancer, and certain types of breast cancer.

POSSIBLE ADVERSE EFFECTS
Estrogen drugs may cause breast tenderness and enlargement, bloating, weight gain, nausea, reduced sex drive, depression, migraine, and bleeding between periods. Side effects often settle after two or three months, but, if they persist or are troublesome, a different estrogen drug may be prescribed. Vaginal creams containing estrogen should be used sparingly and usually only for a short time to reduce the risk of adverse effects throughout the body.

Estrogen drugs increase the risk of abnormal blood clotting and are therefore not recommended for people with a history (or family history) of *stroke*, *pulmonary embolism*, or deep-vein *thrombosis*, or for people about to undergo surgery. Estrogen drugs may increase a person's susceptibility to *hypertension* (high blood pressure) and are not usually prescribed if a person has suffered from this disorder in the past. Estrogens should not be taken during pregnancy as they may adversely affect the fetus.

Estrogen hormones

A group of hormones essential for normal female sexual development and for the healthy functioning of the reproductive system. In women, they are produced mainly in the ovaries. Estrogen hormones are also formed in the placenta during pregnancy and, in both men and women, in small amounts in the adrenal glands. In men, estrogens have no known specific function. (See also *Ovary*.)

Estrone

One of the *estrogen hormones*. Estrone is also prepared synthetically and given by injection or as a tablet in the treatment of symptoms of the menopause (see *Hormone replacement therapy*) and osteoporosis. It is also prescribed as a cream for the treatment of atrophic *vaginitis* (dryness of the vagina).

ESWL

Extracorporeal shock wave lithotripsy. See *Lithotripsy*.

Ethambutol

A drug used in conjunction with other drugs in the treatment of *tuberculosis*. Ethambutol rarely causes side effects, although occasionally it may cause inflammation of the optic nerve, resulting in blurred vision.

Ethanol

The chemical name for the *alcohol* in alcoholic drinks; it is also sometimes called ethyl alcohol.

Ether

The first general anesthetic. Ether was commonly used for surgery until the 1930s, but has now largely been replaced by other anesthetic agents. Ether (full name, diethyl ether) is a colorless liquid administered on a gauze mask placed over the patient's nose and mouth. When inhaled, ether fumes produce unconsciousness.

Ether is among the safest of all anesthetics, but it is so flammable that even static electricity can cause it to explode. Ether has therefore been superseded by other agents (see *Anesthesia, general*), although these require more skill to administer.

Ethical drug

A drug that requires a physician's prescription for purchase.

Ethics, medical

A code of behavior that addresses the relationships between the patient and physician, and among physicians.

The characteristic that distinguishes a profession, such as medicine, from a trade, such as repairing automobiles, is that the members establish and maintain standards of training, competence, and professional behavior. These standards are enforced by professional organizations, such as the American Medical Association, which has a Council on Ethical and Judicial Affairs.

Traditionally, medical ethics covers a wide range of behavior, including the physician's involvement with patients and their families, and his or her competence, public image, and commercial behavior.

Physicians must not abuse the relationship of trust they develop with patients. In particular, they must not enter into sexual relationships with patients and they must maintain in confidence information learned from patients. They must give clear priority to their patients' interests.

Physicians are expected to maintain their skills and to update their knowledge to the standard of their colleagues. They should not refer patients to unlicensed practitioners of alternative medicine. Fees should conform to recognized schedules; all forms of fee splitting or rebates are unacceptable. In addition, it is against ethical standards for a physician to be dependent on alcohol or drugs.

The physician should ensure that the patient not only consents to all procedures, investigations, and treatments, but that this consent is based on an unbiased and full explanation of any risks, drawbacks, and alternatives that might be considered.

Any time a patient is asked to enroll in a research study, the investigator should see that consent is full and free, and that patients do not feel pressured to agree because of a sense of gratitude owed to the physician for previous treatment. Research on children or on patients with mental handicap should, in general, be considered only when there is a reasonable prospect that the person concerned will benefit from the investigation and that the risks and any discomfort inherent in the research are minimal.

Ethical considerations are also important in the care of the dying, in termination of pregnancy, in the care of children born with major physical and mental handicaps, and in the care of patients with mental disorders.

Ethinyl estradiol

ESTROGEN

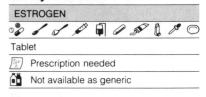

Tablet

Prescription needed

Not available as generic

A synthetic form of the female sex hormone estradiol. It is most commonly used in *oral contraceptives*, where it is combined with a *progesterone drug*.

Ethinyl estradiol is also prescribed to stimulate sexual development in female *hypogonadism* (underdeveloped ovaries) and in the treatment of symptoms caused by the *menopause*, such as hot flashes and sweating (see *Hormone replacement therapy*). It is also used to treat menstrual disorders.

Ethosuximide

An *anticonvulsant drug* used to treat petit mal (a form of *epilepsy*). Ethosuximide is often prescribed in preference to other anticonvulsant drugs because, unlike some of them, it rarely causes drowsiness or liver damage. Ethosuximide may, however, cause nausea and vomiting and in rare cases affects the production of blood cells in the bone marrow and causes aplastic anemia (see *Anemia, aplastic*).

Ethyl alcohol

Another name for ethanol, the *alcohol* in alcoholic drinks.

Ethyl chloride

A colorless, flammable liquid once used as a general anesthetic and now as a local anesthetic.

WHY IT IS USED

Applied to the skin as a spray, ethyl chloride quickly evaporates and, as a result, makes the skin feel so cold that any pain or irritation is reduced. It may be used to numb an area of skin before a minor surgical procedure, such as lancing a boil, and is sometimes used to alleviate the pain that arises from sprained or strained muscles or ligaments.

Ethyl chloride is also used in the treatment of *larva migrans*, a hookworm infection acquired from cats and dogs. (See also *Anesthetics, local*.)

Etiology

The study of the causes of disease. In some cases a specific cause may be found. For example, the cause of *meningitis* may be identified as tuberculosis bacillus after examining a sample of cerebrospinal fluid under a microscope. Many disorders have a multifactorial etiology. The causative factors of degenerative arthritis, for example, include genetic susceptibility, being overweight, and repeated joint injuries. Many disorders, such as osteoarthritis and cancer of the intestine, are of unknown etiology.

Eunuch

A man whose testicles have been removed or destroyed so that he is sterile. The term was used especially to describe boys who were castrated before puberty to preserve their high-pitched singing voices or to make them suitable for guarding harems. A male castrated before puberty has eunuchoid body proportions (i.e., undeveloped male secondary sexual characteristics with a small penis, sparse body hair, broad hips, narrow shoulders, and a feminine distribution of body hair).

Euphoria

A state of confident well-being. A normal reaction to personal success, it can also be induced by drugs.

Feelings of euphoria with no rational cause may indicate the presence of brain disease or damage caused by *head injury* (particularly damage to the frontal lobes), *dementia*, *brain tumors*, or *multiple sclerosis*. In these cases, the euphoria results from the victim's general lack of awareness.

Eustachian tube

The passage that connects the middle ear and the back of the nose. It acts as a drainage passage from the middle ear and maintains hearing by opening periodically to regulate air pressure.

STRUCTURE

The tube is about 1.33 inches (36 mm) long in an adult. From the middle ear it runs forward, downward, and in toward the middle of the head; it ends in the space at the back of the nose just above the soft *palate* (part of the roof of the mouth). A smooth, wet, mucous membrane lines the tube.

FUNCTION

The lower end of the eustachian tube opens during swallowing and yawning, thus allowing air to flow up to the middle ear and equalizing air pressure on both sides of the eardrum. If a change in external pressure is large and rapid, pressure may build up on one side of the eardrum, pushing it inward or outward; this is uncomfortable and dulls hearing. Most people have experienced this sensation when taking off in a plane (reduced pressure) or going into a tunnel in a car or train (increased pressure). Symptoms can usually be relieved by swallowing hard to open the tube.

A person with a blocked eustachian tube who is subjected to rapid changes in pressure may suffer from *barotrauma* (pressure damage to the eardrum or other structures).

When a head cold blocks the eustachian tube, equalization cannot occur, which may cause severe pain. Because the displaced eardrum cannot vibrate properly, hearing may be temporarily impaired.

DISORDERS

Persistent *middle-ear effusion* (chronic accumulation of secretions in the middle ear) or chronic *otitis media* (middle-ear infection) may occur if the eustachian tube becomes blocked, preventing adequate drainage from the middle ear. These conditions, which often cause partial hearing loss, are more common in children because their adenoids are larger and more likely to block the tube if they become infected. Children's eustachian tubes are shorter, making it easier for bacteria to travel from infected areas in the throat to the middle ear.

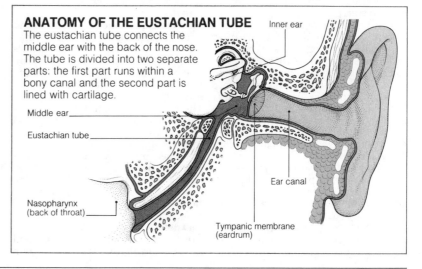

ANATOMY OF THE EUSTACHIAN TUBE
The eustachian tube connects the middle ear with the back of the nose. The tube is divided into two separate parts: the first part runs within a bony canal and the second part is lined with cartilage.

Inner ear

Middle ear

Eustachian tube

Ear canal

Nasopharynx (back of throat)

Tympanic membrane (eardrum)

Euthanasia

The act of killing a person painlessly to relieve suffering. Even when it is requested by a patient with incurable disease, euthanasia (the literal meaning is "easy death") is against the law in most Western countries. There are groups attempting to change the law to allow patients to ask physicians to give a fatal dose of drugs.

Euthanasia is distinct from nonintervention, which is the physician's recognition that, if a patient has an advanced or incurable disease, he or she has a right to refuse medical treatment that would simply prolong the process of dying.

Euthyroid

The term used to describe a person whose *thyroid gland* is functioning normally, or to describe a person who has been successfully treated for *hypothyroidism* (underactive thyroid) or *hyperthyroidism* (overactive thyroid) so that the gland functions normally.

Eversion

A turning outward. The term is commonly applied to a type of ankle injury or deformity in which the foot is turned outward.

Evoked responses

The tracing of electrical activity in the brain in response to a specific external stimulus. The responses are much smaller than the impulses recorded by electroencephalography (see *EEG*) and are a refinement of that technique. Evoked responses were first demonstrated in 1947. Today, with the increased sophistication of computerized electronic technology, it is a widely used diagnostic tool.

WHY IT IS DONE

The functioning of various sensory systems—for example, sight, hearing, and touch—can be checked by this technique. The information obtained can be used to reveal abnormalities in the system caused by inflammation, pressure from a tumor, or other pathological changes, and to confirm the diagnosis of *multiple sclerosis*. The test is extremely sensitive and can often pinpoint the location of a fault.

HOW IT IS DONE

The method for testing each sensory system is similar, painless, and takes 30 to 60 minutes, depending on whether more than one system is being assessed.

A set of small disk electrodes is attached to the scalp in the same way as in electroencephalography. The electrodes are attached to different parts of the scalp, depending on which sensory system is being tested. The output from the brain is linked to a computer, which produces a printout after a specific period of stimulation (e.g., 100 flashes from a light).

Analysis is based on the time lapse between stimulus and response; the computer is used to extract this information from the background brain activity that shows up on an EEG.

For testing the visual system, a series of flashes from a stroboscopic light may be used. An example of a more demanding stimulus for the brain, which gives more consistent results, is a board made up of black and white squares constructed so that the colors alternate every second.

To test hearing, the ears are subjected to different sounds. To test touch and pain sensations, small electrical stimuli are applied, for example, to a nerve at the wrist.

RESULTS

This test does not necessarily give an unequivocal diagnosis and is used as a supplement to other tests of the nervous system (e.g., EEG or *EMG*), other investigations, and radiological tests such as *CT scanning*.

Ewing's sarcoma

A rare malignant tumor of bone. The sarcoma (cancer of connective tissue) arises in a large bone, most commonly the femur (thigh bone), tibia (shin), humerus (upper arm bone), or one of the pelvic bones, and spreads to other parts of the body at an early stage.

The condition is most common in children between 10 and 15; it affects twice as many boys as girls and is rarely seen in black children.

SYMPTOMS

The affected bone is painful and tender and part of it may swell. It may also become weakened and fracture easily (called a pathologic fracture). Other possible symptoms include weight loss, fever, and anemia.

DIAGNOSIS

The sarcoma is diagnosed by X rays and a bone *biopsy* (removal of a small piece of bone for analysis). If cancer is found, the complete skeleton is examined by X rays and *radionuclide scanning*, and the lungs by *CT scanning*, to determine if, and how far, the cancer has spread. Spreading by the time of diagnosis is found in 15 to 20 percent of cases.

TREATMENT

Treatment is by *radiation therapy* and *chemotherapy*. Before the introduction of chemotherapy, death usually occurred within two to three years of diagnosis. Today, the chances of survival have improved considerably; 65 percent of those affected are still alive five years after diagnosis and most of those remain well.

Examination, physical

The inspection, palpation, percussion, and auscultation of the various body parts and organs. Physical examination is the second stage of most medical consultations; it follows history-taking, in which the physician listens to the patient's complaints and then asks questions. Aside from history-taking, the physical examination is the physician's most important means of making a diagnosis or of finding the clues that aid him or her in selecting the appropriate diagnostic studies. If there are generalized symptoms, such as loss of energy, the physician examines the patient's entire body. The physician also performs a complete physical examination during the patient's initial visit and usually annually thereafter. Examination may be limited to a certain part of the body (such as when a patient has a localized injury).

Excision

Surgical cutting out of diseased tissue from surrounding healthy tissue, such as the removal of a breast lump or gangrenous skin.

Excoriation

Injury to the surface of the skin or of a mucous membrane (the thin, moist tissue that lines parts of the body, such as the mouth) caused by physical abrasion (such as scratching) or chemical action. The loss of surface cells causes a raw area to develop. (See also *Ulcer*.)

Excretion

The discharge of waste material from the body. To maintain health, the body must dispose of the by-products of digestion (such as food residues and an excess of salt or other substances), waste products from the repair of body tissues, medication or its breakdown products, poisonous substances, and water (to maintain the correct volume of fluid and to remove solid wastes in solution).

ORGANS OF EXCRETION

The *kidneys* excrete excess nitrogen in the urine in the form of urea, along with excess water, salts, some acids, and most prescribed drugs.

TYPES OF PHYSICAL EXAMINATION

Examination may include looking for skin changes and feeling organs for size, consistency, and shape. Assessment is made of muscle strength, coordination, joint mobility, and skin sensation. The state of the eyes, ears, mouth, throat, and teeth is checked.

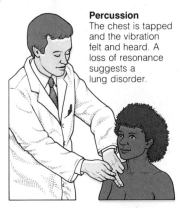

Percussion
The chest is tapped and the vibration felt and heard. A loss of resonance suggests a lung disorder.

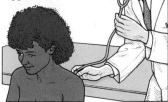

Auscultation
The physician uses a stethoscope to listen to lung and heart sounds. Abnormal sounds suggest disease.

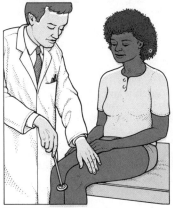

Tendon reflexes
One test of the nervous system is to tap a stretched tendon. If the reflex is normal, the muscle should contract.

The *liver* excretes bile, which, as well as containing salts that help emulsify fats in the small intestine, consists of waste products and bile pigments formed from the breakdown of red blood cells. Part of the bile is passed from the body in the feces, which it colors brown.

The large *intestine* excretes undigested food, some salts, and some excess water in the form of feces.

The *lungs* discharge carbon dioxide and water vapor into the atmosphere.

Sweat glands excrete salt and water onto the surface of the skin as a method of regulating the body's temperature.

Exenteration

The surgical removal of all organs and soft tissue in a body cavity in the hope of arresting a cancerous process. Exenteration is an operation that is occasionally performed for cancer in the orbit (the bony structure surrounding the eye) or the pelvis.

Exercise

The performance of any physical activity that improves health or that is used for recreation or correction of physical injury or deformity (see *Physical therapy*). Different types of exercise affect the body in one or more of the following ways: some improve flexibility, some improve muscular strength, some improve physical endurance, and some improve the efficiency of the cardiovascular and respiratory systems. (See illustrated box, next page.)

BENEFITS OF EXERCISE

There is an established association between high levels of aerobic exercise and low incidence of *coronary heart disease*. Regular exercise usually leads to a reduction in blood pressure. It also increases the amount of high-density lipoprotein in the blood, which is thought to help protect against *atherosclerosis* (fat deposits in arteries) and *myocardial infarction* (heart attack). Exercise has also been shown to be valuable in relieving the symptoms of peripheral vascular disease and of some psychological disorders such as depression.

Vigorous work with a muscle or a group of muscles, even if it is of short duration, leads to an increase in the size, strength, and possibly the number of the muscle cells, and an increase in the strength of their ligamentous attachment to bones. Improving the strength of muscles in the back and abdomen can help prevent or ease

lower back pain. The increased strength of the muscles and tendons is also an insurance against damage due to an unexpected strain.

Elderly people are especially inclined to become inactive and lose joint mobility. Regular, gentle, rhythmic movements can help maintain the range of movement of important joints. Coordination and balance deteriorate with age; exercise helps maintain muscle strength and reduce the risk of falls. (See also *Aerobics; Fitness; Fitness testing.*)

Exfoliation

Flaking off, shedding, or peeling from a surface in scales or thin layers, as in *exfoliative dermatitis*.

Exfoliative dermatitis

Inflammation, marked redness, and scaling of the skin of most of the body, also called erythroderma.

Exfoliative dermatitis may be the result of a drug reaction (an allergic response to a particular drug) or may be caused by the worsening of a skin condition, such as *psoriasis* or *eczema*. Sometimes, exfoliative dermatitis occurs in *lymphoma* and *leukemia*.

There is a widespread rash with severe flaking of the skin. The loss of surface skin, with exposure of its deeper layers, results in increased loss of water and protein from the body surface. Water loss may result in a rise in body temperature; protein loss may cause *edema* (a buildup of fluid in tissues) and muscle wasting. Further complications are infection and *heart failure* (reduced pumping efficiency of the heart).

The treatment and outlook depend on the cause. About 60 percent of sufferers recover within two to three months, but about 30 percent die as a result of complications; in the remainder the disease takes a chronic form unresponsive to treatment.

Exhibitionism

The habit of deliberately exposing the genitals to strangers.

This form of behavior is almost always confined to men. The exhibitionist displays his penis to a female passerby, usually in a secluded spot (such as a side street) or from a car or house window with the aim of surprising or frightening the victim.

In 80 percent of cases, a single court appearance puts an end to the exhibitionist's behavior. *Psychotherapy* can help those who relapse; the outlook is poor for persistent offenders.

E

THE EFFECTS OF EXERCISE

There are many changes in different body organs during exercise. Muscles require an increase in blood flow because of their greater energy requirements; the heart and lungs work faster and more efficiently. These changes are controlled by the release of the chemicals epinephrine and norepinephrine from the sympathetic nervous system.

The lungs
The rate and depth of breathing increase to ensure sufficient flow of oxygen from the lungs into the blood. This also aids in the removal of additional carbon dioxide produced by muscle cells during exercise.

The joints
Regular exercise helps maintain the mobility of joints. Increased strength in the muscles and tendons around joints makes them more resistant to injury.

The muscles
There is a rise in the chemical activity within muscle cells. The rate of consumption of oxygen and glucose increases.

Flexed muscles

Relaxed muscles

The heart and circulation
The heart beats more rapidly and more powerfully to provide an increased flow of blood to the working muscles. Blood vessels in the stomach and beneath the skin are narrowed to compensate for the increased requirements of the muscles.

ECG printouts
Resting heart rate (above) and during exercise (below).

COMMON TYPES OF EXERCISE

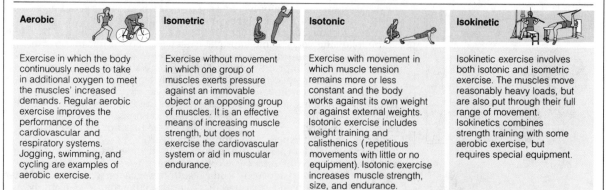

Aerobic

Exercise in which the body continuously needs to take in additional oxygen to meet the muscles' increased demands. Regular aerobic exercise improves the performance of the cardiovascular and respiratory systems. Jogging, swimming, and cycling are examples of aerobic exercise.

Isometric

Exercise without movement in which one group of muscles exerts pressure against an immovable object or an opposing group of muscles. It is an effective means of increasing muscle strength, but does not exercise the cardiovascular system or aid in muscular endurance.

Isotonic

Exercise with movement in which muscle tension remains more or less constant and the body works against its own weight or against external weights. Isotonic exercise includes weight training and calisthenics (repetitive movements with little or no equipment). Isotonic exercise increases muscle strength, size, and endurance.

Isokinetic

Isokinetic exercise involves both isotonic and isometric exercise. The muscles move reasonably heavy loads, but are also put through their full range of movement. Isokinetics combines strength training with some aerobic exercise, but requires special equipment.

Exocrine gland
A gland that secretes substances through a duct onto the inner surface of an organ or onto the outer surface of the body. Examples include the *salivary glands*, which release saliva into the mouth, *lacrimal* glands, which release tears, and *sweat glands*. The release of exocrine secretions can be triggered by a hormone or by a neurotransmitter, released by nerve endings. (See also *Endocrine gland*.)

Exomphalos
A rare birth defect in which a part of the intestines, covered by a thin membrane, protrudes through the umbilicus (navel). In mild cases only one or two loops of intestine protrude, but in severe cases most of the abdominal organs are exposed.

Also called omphalocele, exomphalos is associated with other birth defects, especially *anencephaly*. Many babies with the condition are stillborn or die soon after birth. Exomphalos is treated by surgery.

Exophthalmos
Protrusion of one or both eyeballs caused by a swelling of the soft tissue in the bony orbit (eye socket). The eye-ball is pressed forward, exposing an abnormally large amount of the front of the eye, forcing the eyelids apart and causing a staring appearance.

CAUSE
The most common cause of exophthalmos is *thyrotoxicosis* (overactive thyroid gland). Other causes include an *eye tumor*, an *aneurysm* (swelling of an artery) behind the eye, or inflammation of eye tissues; in these cases only one eye is affected.

SYMPTOMS AND SIGNS
Exophthalmos may restrict eye movement and cause double vision. In severe cases, the pressure in the orbit

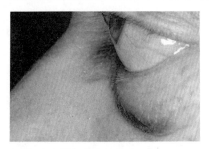

Appearance of exophthalmos
An affected eye protrudes markedly compared with a normal eye. In most cases, both eyes are affected.

may be so high that the blood supply to the optic nerve may be restricted; blindness results. The lids may be prevented from closing, and vision may become seriously blurred due to drying of the cornea.

TREATMENT AND OUTLOOK
In thyroid exophthalmos, treatment of the thyroid disorder may sometimes relieve the exophthalmos, but often it does not. Early treatment usually returns the vision to normal. Surgery to decompress the orbit may be required to relieve pressure on the optic nerve.

Exostosis
A type of benign *bone tumor* in which there is an outgrowth of bone. It occurs most commonly at the end of the femur (thigh bone) or tibia (shin).

Exostoses account for 90 percent of all bone tumors; they affect twice as many men as women. In about 65 percent of cases the condition is due to hereditary factors; another cause is prolonged pressure on a bone.

SYMPTOMS AND TREATMENT
In most cases, exostosis produces no symptoms and goes unnoticed. Often it is recognized (as a hard swelling) only after an injury. Occasionally the bony outgrowth presses on a nerve, causing pain or weakness in the affected area (usually when it is beneath a fingernail or toenail).

A preliminary diagnosis of the condition is confirmed by X ray. Treatment may be surgical removal of the growth, but usually surgery is performed only if the exostosis causes symptoms or is unsightly.

Exotoxin

A poison released by some types of bacteria into the bloodstream, from where it causes widespread effects throughout the body. Exotoxins are among the most poisonous

substances known. They are produced by bacteria such as tetanus bacilli, which enter the body through a wound and produce an exotoxin that affects the nervous system to cause muscle spasms (lockjaw) and paralysis, and diphtheria bacilli, which initially infect the throat, but release an exotoxin that damages the heart and nervous system.

Immunization with vaccines consisting of detoxified exotoxins can prevent dangerous symptoms from bacterial diseases that are potentially fatal due to the effects of exotoxins. If such an infection occurs, treatment usually includes antibiotics and an antitoxin to neutralize the exotoxin. (See also *Endotoxin*; *Enterotoxin*.)

Exotropia
Divergent squint, in which one eye is used for detailed vision; the other is directed outward. (See *Strabismus*.)

Expectorants
A group of *cough remedies* used to promote the coughing up of phlegm.

Expectoration
The coughing up and spitting out of sputum (phlegm). See also *Cough*.

Expiration
The act of breathing out air from the lungs. See *Breathing*.

Exploratory surgery
Any operation to investigate or thoroughly examine part of the body to discover the extent of known disease or to establish a diagnosis. Exploratory thoracotomy is performed on the chest and exploratory laparotomy on the abdomen.

Explosive disorder
A mental condition characterized by uncontrolled violent behavior that is completely out of proportion to any known cause. There may be several separate acts of aggression or a single violent outburst; in any case, the resulting damage to people or property may be very serious.

Similar behavior may occur in people with *epilepsy*, *brain damage*, *schizophrenia*, or an *antisocial personality disorder*, but in these cases there are also other symptoms.

Exposure
The effects on the body from being subjected to very low temperatures, or to a combination of cold, wet, and high winds. The primary danger

comes from the lowering of body temperature in these conditions (see *Hypothermia*). The term also applies to being subjected to radiation or a variety of environmental pollutants.

Expressing milk
A technique used by breast-feeding women for removing milk from the

EXPRESSING MILK BY HAND
Wash your hands thoroughly before starting, then follow the method below. Repeat the sequence twice on each breast, alternating between breasts. If the breasts are engorged, bathe them in hot water first to help milk flow.

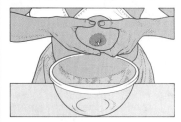

1 Cup the breast in both hands, thumbs on top and fingers underneath. Squeeze the outer part of the breast firmly. Repeat 10 times, moving around the breast.

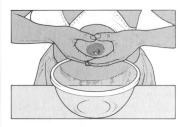

2 Move hands closer to the nipple area and repeat the squeezing movement 10 more times.

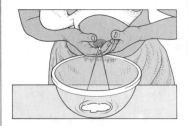

3 Hold the breast in one hand. With the thumb and forefinger of the other hand, squeeze the edge of the areola in and up so that milk squirts out. Move your hand around the areola, squeezing gently and rhythmically for about five minutes.

breasts. Expressing milk may be necessary when the breasts are engorged (overfull), which often happens several days after delivery when the milk supply arrives quickly and forcibly. Not only is engorgement painful for the mother, but the tightly swollen nipples are impossible for the baby to suckle.

A woman may also want to express milk from her breasts so that the milk can be given to the baby in her absence. In this case, the milk should be expressed into a sterilized container and sealed and stored in the refrigerator; it will keep for 48 hours. When properly prepared, milk may be frozen and stored in a freezer. Milk may be kept up to six months in the back or bottom of a deep freeze unit. Most women find it easier to express milk by hand, but a *breast pump* can also be used.

Exstrophy of the bladder
A rare birth defect in which the bladder is turned inside out and is open to the outside of the body through a space in the lower abdominal wall.

Usually, there are also other defects, such as *epispadias* (emergence of the urethra through a hole in the shaft of the penis) in males, and failure of the pubic bones to join at the front.

Untreated, an affected child constantly leaks urine. Surgical treatment consists of reconstructing the bladder and closing the abdominal wall.

Extraction, dental
The removal of one or more teeth.
WHY IT IS DONE
Extraction may be performed when a tooth is severely decayed, when an abscess has formed, or when a tooth is too badly broken to be repaired by crowning or root-canal treatment. Teeth that are causing crowding or malocclusion (incorrect bite), teeth that are loose because of advanced gum disease, or teeth that are preventing another tooth from erupting may also require extraction.
HOW IT IS DONE
For most extractions, local anesthesia is used. General anesthesia may be used to extract badly impacted wisdom teeth, to extract several teeth at once, or for extremely anxious patients or young children.

Most teeth are extracted with dental forceps, which are designed to grasp the root of the tooth. When gentle but firm pressure is applied, the blades cut through the periodontal ligaments (the tough fibrous membranes sup-

porting the tooth in its socket), the socket is gradually expanded, and the tooth is removed. Occasionally the root of the tooth fractures during this procedure, especially if the bone is dense (as in older people) and may need to be removed separately.

If the tooth is especially difficult to remove—for example, if it is impacted, the crown is missing, or the roots are very curved—it may be necessary to cut a small flap into the gum and remove a small amount of bone nearby. The tooth is then extracted and the gum sewn up.
COMPLICATIONS
Most extractions take place without complications. Occasionally, if a blood clot fails to form in the empty tooth socket, or if the blood clot is dislodged, *dry socket* (infection in the tooth socket) develops. Dislodging a clot can also cause bleeding from the wound to begin again; this can be eased by placing a tightly folded handkerchief or a gauze pad on the wound and biting on it gently for about 30 minutes. If bleeding continues, suturing of the tissue around the socket may be necessary.

Extradural hemorrhage
Bleeding into the space between the inner surface of the skull and the external surface of the dura mater, the outer layer of the meninges (protective covering of the brain).
CAUSES AND SYMPTOMS
An extradural hemorrhage usually results from a blow to the side of the head that fractures the skull and ruptures an artery running over the surface of the dura mater. The person may momentarily lose consciousness and then apparently recover.

A hematoma (collection of clotted blood) forms and rapidly enlarges, increasing pressure within the skull (which is the main cause of symptoms occurring a few hours to days after the injury). A headache that gradually increases in severity develops in the affected person; other symptoms include drowsiness, vomiting, seizures, and paralysis on one side of the body. The patient eventually lapses into a coma and, without treatment, may die.
DIAGNOSIS AND TREATMENT
CT scanning confirms the diagnosis. Surgical treatment consists of drilling burr holes in the skull (see *Craniotomy*), draining the blood clot, and clipping the ruptured blood vessel. If the bleeding is diagnosed early (before serious symptoms develop), the

outlook is excellent; hence the importance of seeking medical advice and investigation following even a moderate blow to the head (see *Head injury*).

Extrapyramidal system
A network of nerve pathways that links nerve nuclei in the surface of the *cerebrum* (the main mass of the brain), the *basal ganglia* deep within the brain, and parts of the *brain stem*. The system influences and modifies electrical impulses that are sent from the brain to the skeletal muscles.

Damage or degeneration of components in the extrapyramidal system can cause a disturbance in the execution of voluntary (willed) movements and in muscle tone, and can also cause the appearance of involuntary (unwanted) movements such as tremors, jerks, or writhing movements. Such disturbances are seen in *Huntington's chorea, Parkinson's disease*, some types of *cerebral palsy*, and can also occur as a side effect of taking phenothiazine drugs, which are used to treat some psychiatric disorders.

Extrovert
A person whose interests are constantly directed outward, to other people and the environment. Extroverts are active, energetic, sociable, easy to talk to, and have many outside interests and concerns. (See also *Personality*.)

Exudation
The discharge of fluid from blood vessels into a tissue or onto the tissue's surface. An exuded fluid (called an exudate) contains cells, pus, and/or a large amount of protein (or a combination of these) and is usually produced as a result of *inflammation*. When tissue is inflamed, its small blood vessels become wider and the tiny pores in the vessel walls become enlarged, which allows fluid and cells (mainly white blood cells) to escape.

Eye
The organ of sight. It consists of structures that focus an image onto the retina at the back of the eye and a network of nerves that convert this image into electrical impulses recorded in a region of the brain.

The two eyes work in conjunction under the control of the brain, aligning themselves on an object so that a clear image is formed on each *retina*. If necessary, the eyes sharpen images by altering focus in an automatic process known as *accommodation*.

ANATOMY OF THE EYE

The eye is a complex organ that focuses light rays to form an image on the retina, which then converts this image into a pattern of nerve impulses that are transmitted to the brain. The cornea and lens focus the light, the pupil controls the amount of light entering the eye, the ciliary body alters the shape of the lens to adjust the focus, and the retina contains millions of nerve cells that respond to light.

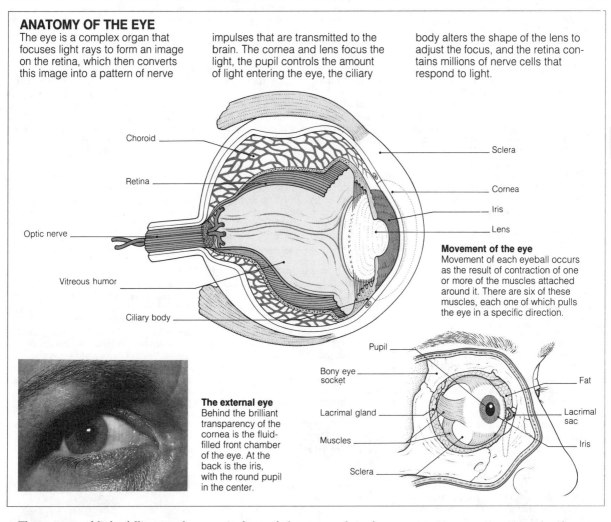

Choroid

Retina

Optic nerve

Vitreous humor

Ciliary body

Sclera

Cornea

Iris

Lens

Movement of the eye
Movement of each eyeball occurs as the result of contraction of one or more of the muscles attached around it. There are six of these muscles, each one of which pulls the eye in a specific direction.

Pupil

Bony eye socket

Lacrimal gland

Muscles

Sclera

Fat

Lacrimal sac

Iris

The external eye
Behind the brilliant transparency of the cornea is the fluid-filled front chamber of the eye. At the back is the iris, with the round pupil in the center.

The pattern of light falling on the retina stimulates a complex flow of impulses along the optic nerves to the brain. The two optic nerves pass into the skull, meet, partially cross over, and run back, at first on the underside of the brain, and then through its substance to the visual cortex—the area of the back surface of the brain concerned with vision.

STRUCTURE

EYEBALL The eyeball lies in pads of fat within the orbit, the bony eye socket that provides protection from injury. Each eyeball is moved by six delicate muscles, the action of these muscles for both eyes being coordinated by a nerve network in the brain stem.

The eyeball has a tough outer coat, the *sclera* (the white of the eye). The front, circular part of the outer coat, the *cornea*, is transparent and protrudes slightly. The cornea is the main lens of the eye and performs most of the focusing. Behind the cornea is a shallow chamber full of aqueous humor (watery fluid), at the back of which is the *iris* (colored part) with its *pupil* (central hole). The pupil appears black and its size is altered with changes in light intensity to control the amount of light entering it.

Immediately behind the iris, and in contact with it, is the crystalline *lens*, suspended by delicate fibers from a circular muscle ring called the ciliary body. Contraction of the ciliary body alters the shape of the lens to allow focusing power. Behind the lens is the main cavity of the eyeball, filled with a clear gel called the vitreous humor.

On the inside of the back of the eye is the retina, a complex structure of nerve tissue on which the image formed by the cornea and the crystalline lens falls. The retina requires a constant supply of oxygen and sugar. To meet this need, a thin network of branching blood vessels, the choroid plexus, lies immediately under it. The *choroid* is continuous at the front with the ciliary body and the iris. These three parts constitute the uveal tract.

CONJUNCTIVA The eyeball is sealed off from the outside by a flexible membrane called the *conjunctiva*, which is firmly secured around the margin of the cornea but lies freely on the sclera over the front third of the globe. It is attached to the skin at the corners of the eye and forms the inner lining of the lids, with a deep cul-de-sac above and below. This arrangement provides a permanent seal while allowing free mobility of the eyeball.

The conjunctiva contains many tiny tear-secreting and mucus-producing glands. They, along with an oily secretion from the meibomian glands in the eyelids, provide the important, three-layer tear film that must constantly cover the cornea and conjunctiva to protect them from damage due to drying out of the cells.

EYELIDS Each lid contains about 30 meibomian glands, with their openings along the lid margin just behind the roots of the lashes. The glands secrete an oil that prevents lid margin adhesion during sleep and forms the outer layer of the tear film—a layer that retards evaporation and helps maintain the continuity of the tear film. The blink reflex is protective and helps to spread the tear film evenly over the cornea. This is essential for clear vision. Should the tear film dry out, corneal abrasion is more likely.

Just under the skin of the lid is a flat but powerful muscle that can, in an emergency, contract to push the globe back into the orbit and interpose a bunched-up mass of tissue to protect the eye; this occurs as a rapid, reflex response to danger. (See also *Vision*.)

Eye, artificial

A prosthesis to replace an eye that has been removed. It is worn for cosmetic and psychological reasons.

Often wrongly called a "glass eye," the ocular prosthesis is actually a slim plastic shell. The artificial iris behind the transparent artificial cornea may be produced by hand painting or by a photograph.

The eye fits neatly behind the eyelids within the cavity left when the

natural eye has been removed. Movement is achieved by attaching the eye-moving muscles to the conjunctiva, or by using a buried magnetic implant.

Eye drops

Medication in solution for the treatment of eye disorders or to aid in diagnosis. To use eye drops, the lower lid is held away from the eye and the drop allowed to fall behind it. Care should be taken to avoid touching the skin or eye with the dropper to reduce the risk of contamination.

Common examples of drugs given in this form are antibiotics, corticosteroids, antihistamines, drugs to control glaucoma (raised pressure in the eye), and drugs to dilate or constrict the pupil.

Eye, examination of

An inspection of the external and internal appearance of the eyes either as part of a standard vision test or to make a diagnosis.

WHY IT IS DONE
Eye examinations are performed to determine the cause of vision disturbance or other symptoms relating to the eye, and to assess whether or not glasses or contact lenses are necessary. Some serious eye disorders, such as glaucoma, are symptomless in the early stages and can be detected only by an eye examination.

HOW IT IS DONE
The examination begins with an inspection of the external appearance of the eyes, the lids, and the surrounding skin. A check of eye movements is usually performed. The examiner looks for *strabismus*, using the cover test to demonstrate that a squinting eye will move to align itself when the other eye is covered. A check of the visual acuity (sharpness of vision) in each eye using a Snellen's chart (the standard eye testing wall chart) follows. Refraction testing (using lenses of different strengths) may be done to determine the requirement for glasses or contact lenses.

A test of the visual fields (extent of the peripheral vision) may also be performed, especially in suspected glaucoma or neurological conditions. Color vision may also be checked because it is disturbed in certain conditions affecting the retina.

To check for abrasions or ulcers, the cornea and conjunctiva may be stained with fluorescein (a yellow dye); any abrasions or ulcers are then revealed as green areas under light.

Applanation tonometry (measurement of the pressure within the eye) is an essential test for glaucoma. It is done using a slit lamp microscope.

EQUIPMENT
The retina can be examined with an *ophthalmoscope*. The slit lamp microscope, with its brilliant illumination and lens magnification, allows meticulous examination of the conjunctiva, cornea, front chamber of the eye, iris, and crystalline lens.

By means of special corneal contact lenses, the magnified view may be extended to include the vitreous gel behind the lens and the retina. These contact lenses incorporate mirrors to allow examination of structures at the base of the iris and the front edge of the retina. For a full view of the crystalline lens and the structures behind it, the pupil must be widely dilated with drops, such as tropicamide or phenylephrine.

CONDUCTING AN EYE EXAMINATION

During an eye examination, the physician checks external appearance, eye movement, visual acuity, visual field, and color vision. The eyes are checked for the presence of strabismus, abrasions, and ulcers. Applanation tonometry and a refraction test are also done.

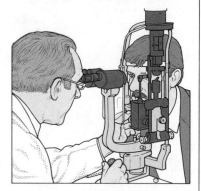

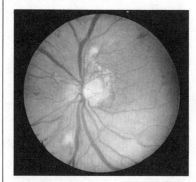

View of retina through ophthalmoscope
The retina (inner back surface of the eye) is examined to assess conditions such as hypertensive *retinopathy*, as seen here.

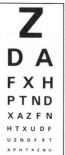

Applanation tonometry
Measurement of the pressure within the eye is a routine test for glaucoma.

Snellen's chart
The chart is used to check visual acuity of each eye; the patient's ability to read letters of different sizes from the same distance is assessed.

DISORDERS OF THE EYE

Many eye disorders are minor, but some lead to serious complications unless treated. (See also *Cornea* disorders box; *Retina* disorders box; *Eye, painful red*.)

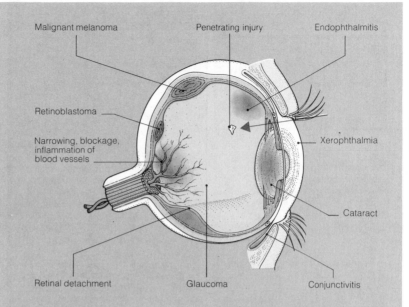

Malignant melanoma
Penetrating injury
Endophthalmitis
Retinoblastoma
Narrowing, blockage, inflammation of blood vessels
Xerophthalmia
Cataract
Retinal detachment
Glaucoma
Conjunctivitis

CONGENITAL DEFECTS

Strabismus (squint or malalignment of the eyes) is often congenital (present at birth). *Cataracts* (opacity of the lens of the eye) can occur in infants, when the cause may be maternal *rubella* infection early in pregnancy. Very rarely, babies are born with microphthalmos (abnormally small eye) on one or both sides. Vision in a microphthalmic eye is usually very poor. *Nystagmus* (rapid, uncontrollable movement in the eyes) can be congenital.

Retinoblastoma is a malignant tumor of the retina that appears in early life and may occur in one or both eyes. Other congenital disorders affecting the eye include *albinism* (absence of pigment) and abnormalities of development of the cornea and retina.

INFECTION

Conjunctivitis, the most common infection, rarely affects vision. In the late stages of neglected conjunctival infection, such as *trachoma* or severe bacterial conjunctivitis, vision can be impaired.

Corneal infections are more serious and can lead to blurred vision or corneal perforation if not treated early. Endophthalmitis (infection within the eye), which may make it necessary to remove the eye surgically, can occur after a penetrating injury, after severe ulceration, in rare cases after major eye surgery, or from infections elsewhere in the body.

IMPAIRED BLOOD SUPPLY

Narrowing, blockage, inflammation, or other abnormalities of the blood vessels of the retina may cause partial or total loss of vision.

TUMORS

Malignant *melanoma* of the choroid (middle layer of the eye) is the most common primary malignant eye tumor. It can be found in the eyes of people who do not have symptoms (during routine examinations) or it can cause a decrease in vision.

NUTRITIONAL DISORDERS

Various vitamin deficiencies (particularly vitamin A deficiency) can affect the eye. This may lead to xerophthalmia (dryness of the cornea and conjunctiva), night blindness, or, ultimately, *keratomalacia* (corneal softening and destruction) and total loss of vision.

AUTOIMMUNE DISORDERS

Uveitis (inflammation of the uveal tissues—iris, choroid, and/or ciliary body), when not caused by an infectious agent, may have an autoimmune basis (when the defense mechanisms of the body attack its own tissues). It is commonly encountered in people with *ankylosing spondylitis* (crippling and deforming arthritis of the spine) and *sarcoidosis*.

DEGENERATION

Macular degeneration of the retina is common in the elderly. It causes loss of fine, detailed vision, although peripheral vision remains.

Cataract is also common in elderly people; although the exact cause of the condition is unknown, the process is thought to be degenerative.

OTHER DISORDERS

Glaucoma (a condition in which the pressure in the fluid that maintains the normal shape of the eye is raised) may take various forms. If untreated, glaucoma can lead to permanent loss of vision.

In *retinal detachment*, the retina lifts away from the underlying layer of the eye; this may have various causes. *Ametropia* is a general term that means the eye has a refractive error (an error in focusing), such as *myopia* (nearsightedness), *hyperopia* (farsightedness), *astigmatism*, or *anisometropia*. None of these is a disease in the ordinary sense of the word; they are caused simply by variations of shape and focusing ability of the eye. *Presbyopia* is the progressive loss of accommodation (ability to focus at near range) with age. *Amblyopia* (poor vision in one eye without any obvious structural abnormality) is often due to strabismus.

INVESTIGATION

Because of the transparency of its structures, the eye is particularly accessible for examination. Many of the disease processes affecting it can be viewed directly by use of the *ophthalmoscope* and *slit lamp*. Photography of the retina and *fluorescein* angiography are also used. (See also *Eye, examination of*.)

FIRST AID: FOREIGN BODY IN THE EYE

> **WARNING**
> Never attempt to remove a particle embedded in the eyeball. Do not remove a foreign body if it is resting on the iris (colored part of the eye).

LOWER LID

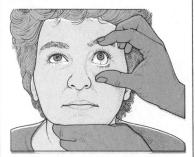

1 Wash your hands. Ask the victim to look up while you separate the lids and examine the eye.

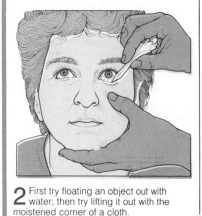

2 First try floating an object out with water; then try lifting it out with the moistened corner of a cloth.

UPPER LID

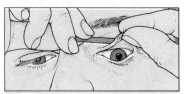

1 Grasp the lashes and carefully draw the upper lid outward and downward. If this does not dislodge the object, try floating it off by having the victim blink under water.

2 If these measures fail, ask the victim to look down while you place a matchstick across the upper lid and fold the lid up over it. Then pick off the object with a clean cloth.

CORROSIVES IN THE EYE

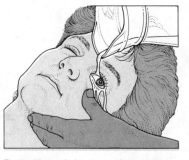

Flush with continuously running water – some alkalis penetrate deeply and take longer to wash out.

Eye, foreign body in

Any material on the surface of the eye or under the eyelid, or an object that penetrates the eyeball.

INCIDENCE AND CAUSES

Most people get something in their eye at least once in their lives. Usually it is a particle of dust; occasionally it is a metal, plastic, or wood fragment that has been deflected into the eye while doing some home or car maintenance. Rarely, an object traveling at high speed actually penetrates the eyeball—for example, a piece of metal in an industrial accident.

SYMPTOMS

A foreign body under the eyelid or on the cornea or conjunctiva irritates the eye, causing pain, redness, and tearing. It usually causes blepharospasm (uncontrollable eyelid contractions). These symptoms may improve even if the foreign body remains. Occasionally, there will not be any symptoms, especially if the eye has been penetrated.

COMPLICATIONS

Some foreign bodies left within the eyeball may dissolve to release pigment into the substance of the eye, causing blindness. Other foreign bodies may remain whole but cause infection, again leading to blindness.

DIAGNOSIS

If a foreign body is suspected, a physician should be consulted. He or she will examine the eye and both eyelids. Fluorescein (a yellow stain) is used to show up abrasions or sites of penetration. Imaging procedures are used if a penetrating injury is suspected.

TREATMENT

Superficial foreign bodies may be removed at home. Use the corner of a clean cloth, or pull the upper lid down over the lower lid or irrigate the eye using an eyecup.

Objects on the iris or pupil or embedded in the eye should be removed by a physician. A sharp spatula is often used after the surface of the eye has been anesthetized with local anesthetic eye drops. The eye is then stained with fluorescein to assess the area of damage to the cornea. Antibiotics as drops or ointment will be prescribed and the eye is then protected with a patch (see also *Corneal abrasion*). Metallic objects that have penetrated the eye can sometimes be extracted using a powerful magnet.

Eye injuries

The greatest danger to the eye arises from objects of relatively small size traveling at high speed, such as BB gun pellets, slingshot missiles, or small stones sometimes thrown up by rotary lawnmowers. Many industrial activities, such as drilling, sawing, hammering, or grinding, can cause objects from high-speed machinery to penetrate the eye. Penetrating injuries also can occur from windshield glass in automobile accidents. Foreign bodies within the eye can cause serious problems.

The serious injuries are generally those that damage both the cornea and the crystalline lens. Central corneal wounds impair vision by causing scarring (see *Corneal abrasion*). Damage to the lens may cause a *cataract* to form, with resultant loss of vision in that eye. The most serious injuries also extend to the back of the eye to include the retina and posterior sclera (outer lining).

Blunt trauma to the eyeball, such as a blow from a stick, may cause tearing of the iris or may cause rupture of the sclera, with collapse of the eyeball and permanent blindness. Lesser degrees of injury that do not cause penetration may lead to a vitreous hemorrhage (bleeding behind the lens), *hyphema*

E

(bleeding into the front chamber of the eye), retinal detachment, or injury to the trabeculum (fluid outflow drain of the eye), which can lead to glaucoma. Hyphema affects vision until the blood is reabsorbed, unless other vision-threatening damage occurred with it. (See also *Eye, foreign body in*.)

Eyelashes, disorders of

Eyelashes are arranged in two rows at the front edge of each lid and curve outward. Growth in an abnormal direction may be due to injury to the lid or, more commonly, infection. Occasionally, lashes grow in an abnormal direction for no obvious reason. With age, the lashes become finer.

Severe *blepharitis* (eyelid infection) may cause the lid margins to be so damaged that lash roots are destroyed. *Trachoma*, an eye infection in which the lid is distorted by scarring, may lead to trichiasis, a condition in which the lashes turn inward. They may rub against the cornea, causing corneal abrasion.

Eye, lazy

A popular term for *amblyopia*, in which normal vision has failed to develop, usually in one eye.

Eyelid

One of a pair of complex structures that lies on the upper and lower edges of the eye socket. The eyelids are held in position by ligaments attached to the socket's bony edges. They consist of thin fibrous tissue, called the tarsal plate, covered by muscle and a very thin layer of skin. The inner layer is covered by part of the *conjunctiva*.

Along the edge of the eyelid are two rows of eyelashes, which are strong, curved hairs. Immediately behind the eyelashes are the openings of the ducts leading from the meibomian glands, which secrete the oily part of the tear film from within the tarsal plate (see also *Tears*).

The eyelids act as protective shutters, closing very rapidly as a reflex action in response to anything approaching the eye. A squeezing action of the eyelids pushes the eyeball back into the socket as an additional protective measure. The eyelids also act as wipers to smear the tear film across the cornea.

DISORDERS

Disorders include a *chalazion* (a swelling of a meibomian gland), *blepharitis* (inflammation of the edge of the eyelid), and a *stye* (an abscess at the root of one of the eyelashes).

The shape and position of the eyelids are abnormal in a number of disorders, including *entropion* (the eyelid margin turning inward), *ectropion* (the eyelid margin turning outward), *ptosis* (a drooping eyelid covering all or part of the eye), and baggy eyelids due to dermatochalasis (excess lid skin) or blepharochalasis (excess fat under the lid skin).

Myokymia (twitching of the eyelid) is a common phenomenon usually due to fatigue. *Blepharospasm* (rapid contractions of the eyelid) is usually caused by a foreign body in the eye.

The skin of the eyelid is a common site for a *basal cell carcinoma*.

Eyelid, drooping

See *Ptosis*.

Eyelid surgery

See *Blepharoplasty*.

Eye, painful red

A very common combination of eye symptoms that can be due to several different eye disorders. The presence of pain and redness in one or both eyes requires examination and treatment by a physician.

The most common eye disorder that causes pain and redness is *conjunctivitis*. The redness is due to dilation of the superficial (conjunctival) blood vessels. The pain is similar to that caused by grit in the eye. Conjunctivitis can be due to viral or bacterial infections, irritants (such as chemicals), or allergies. Viral conjunctivitis usually eventually affects both eyes and precautions should be taken to prevent infecting others.

Uveitis (inflammation of all or a portion of the uvea, such as the iris) is another common cause. The dull, aching pain may be due to swelling within the front of the eye and spasm in muscles around the iris. The redness is caused by widening of blood vessels around the iris.

A serious cause of pain and redness in one eye is acute closed-angle *glaucoma* (sudden, highly increased pressure within the eyeball). The pain is severe and may be accompanied by nausea, vomiting, halos, and blurred vision. There is redness of the white of the eye due to increased blood flow in the surrounding vessels.

Other important causes of painful, red eye include a *corneal ulcer*, *keratitis* (inflammation of the outer protective layer of the eye), or the presence of a foreign body on the surface of the eye or under one of the eyelids.

Eyestrain

A term often used to describe aching or discomfort in the eye. Eyestrain is not a medical term, and physicians do not accept the popular belief that the eyes can be damaged by being used.

Eye teeth

A common name for canine *teeth*.

Eye tumors

Tumors of the eye are rare. When eye tumors do occur, they are usually malignant and painless.

TYPES AND TREATMENT

RETINOBLASTOMA This is a *congenital* malignant tumor of the retina that occurs in one or both eyes. If the central vision in only one eye is affected, the child may have strabismus (squint). If the tumor is not discovered in its early growth, it may be seen as a white or yellowish reflection in one pupil. Retinoblastoma may sometimes be treated by *radiation therapy*, *laser treatment*, or freezing, but the eye may require removal to prevent spread of the tumor.

MALIGNANT MELANOMA A form of skin cancer, this is a tumor of the choroid layer that usually affects the middle-aged and elderly. It is the most common eye tumor. Often there are no early symptoms, but the tumor eventually causes detachment of the retina and distortion of vision. Small malignant melanomas can be destroyed by laser treatment, but removal of the eye is often advised to avoid spread of the tumor to the brain or elsewhere.

SECONDARY EYE TUMORS These occur when cancer in another part of the body spreads to the eye, where it produces effects similar to those of the primary tumor. If the secondary tumors grow behind the eyeball, they may cause bulging of the eye. Their effect on vision varies, depending on the location and growth rate. Secondary tumors may sometimes be controlled by radiation therapy; separate treatment is necessary for the primary tumor.

BASAL CELL CARCINOMA This is the most common eyelid tumor. Like other basal cell carcinomas, it is related to excessive exposure to sunlight. The tumor usually has a small crusty central crater and a hard rolled edge. Although it may grow large, it very rarely spreads to other parts of the body. In the early stages, basal cell carcinoma of the lids may be treated by surgery, radiation therapy, or freezing. Extensive plastic surgery or removal of the eye may be necessary.

E

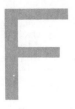

F

Face-lift

A cosmetic operation to smooth out wrinkles and lift sagging skin on an aging face to make it look younger. A face-lift is usually performed as an outpatient procedure using a local anesthetic. The two sides of the face are treated during the same operation.

OUTLOOK

Some bruising of the face is common, but there is usually no pain. The stitches are removed three to five days after the operation. In most cases, the scars, which fade within a year, are hidden by natural crease lines or by the hair. The effect of a face-lift usually lasts about five years.

Occasionally, satisfactory healing does not occur as a result of *hematoma* (bleeding under the skin) or infection, leading to severe scarring; in the worst cases, a *skin graft* may be necessary.

Facial nerve

The seventh *cranial nerve*. It arises from the pons and medulla oblongata (parts of the brain stem) and sends branches to the face, neck, salivary glands, and outer ear.

LOCATION OF THE FACIAL NERVE

Arising from the brain stem, the facial nerve has branches that connect to the outer ear, tongue, salivary glands, and muscles of the neck and face.

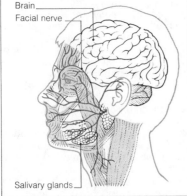

Brain
Facial nerve
Salivary glands

FACE-LIFT

A face-lift is really a skin-lift. It is a serious surgical operation and its effects are not always permanent. There is some discomfort after a face-lift and the cosmetic effects are not immediately apparent. Care should be taken in choosing a highly reputable surgeon.

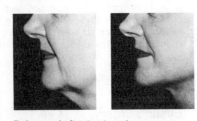

Skin removed
Line of incision

Before and after treatment
The results of most face-lifts are excellent. However, it should be realized that the outcome may not be exactly as expected, and there is always some risk associated with any operation.

How it is done
An incision is made where shown. The skin is undercut as far as the crease running from the nose to the corner of the mouth. It is then pulled upward and backward, and its margins are sewn near the hairline.

The facial nerve performs both motor and sensory functions. It controls the muscles of the neck and of facial expression (including muscles in the forehead); it also stimulates secretion by the submandibular and sublingual salivary glands. In addition, the facial nerve conveys taste sensations from the front two thirds of the tongue and carries sensations from the outer ear.

Damage to the facial nerve causes weakness of the facial muscles (see *Facial palsy*) and, in some cases, loss of taste. Such damage is most commonly due to a virus infection. It may also be a feature of a *stroke*; more rarely, it may occur as a result of surgery (typically for a tumor) to the parotid gland (one of the salivary glands).

Facial pain

Pain in the face may be caused by injury, infection, or a nerve disorder, may be referred from elsewhere in the body (see *Referred pain*), or may occur for no known reason.

INJURY

In addition to pain in the face from a direct injury, pain may be caused indirectly by *teething* problems in a baby, wisdom tooth problems in an adult (see *Impaction, dental*), or partial dislocation of the jaw.

INFECTION

Sinusitis (inflammation of the air spaces around the nose) can cause pain around the eyes and in the cheek bones. The onset of *mumps* also can cause pain in the cheeks before any swelling appears in front of and/or below the ears. Pain from a boil in the nose or ear may radiate to the face, as may pain from a tooth abscess (see *Abscess, dental*) or dental *caries*.

NERVE DISORDERS

Damage to a nerve that supplies the face can result in severe pain. Examples include the knifelike pain that precedes the one-sided rash in *herpes zoster* (shingles), and the intermittent shooting pain of *trigeminal neuralgia* (tic douloureux), which usually affects only one side of the face and is often brought on by touching the face or chewing.

REFERRED PAIN

In *angina pectoris* (pain in the chest due to lack of oxygen to the heart), pain may be felt in the jaw. With *migraine* headaches, pain may occur on one side of the face. When facial pain or headache occurs for no reason, it may be a symptom of *depression*.

TREATMENT

Analgesics (painkillers) can provide temporary relief, but, if the pain is severe or persistent, a physician or dentist should be consulted.

Facial palsy

Also known as Bell's palsy (for the Scottish surgeon Sir Charles Bell), paralysis of the facial muscles, usually one-sided and temporary, due to inflammation of a facial nerve. Facial palsy is common and usually comes on suddenly. The cause is unknown, although, rarely, it may be associated with *herpes zoster* (shingles).

SYMPTOMS
The eyelid and corner of the mouth droop on one side of the face and there may be pain in the ear on that side. It may be impossible to wrinkle the brow or to close the eye, and smiling is distorted. Depending on which branches of the nerve are affected, taste may be impaired or sounds may seem unnaturally loud.

TREATMENT
Corticosteroid drugs or *ACTH* is sometimes given to reduce inflammation of the nerve, along with analgesics (painkillers) if the ear is painful. Exercising the facial muscles may facilitate recovery. Electrostimulation of the nerve is of unproved value. It may be necessary to tape the eyelid shut at bedtime to avoid corneal abrasion. In most cases, the condition clears up with or without treatment.

Facial spasm
An uncommon disorder in which there is frequent twitching of facial muscles supplied by the *facial nerve*. (This condition is often called a tic, but, in fact, tic is a general term that can refer to spasmodic twitching in any part of the body.) The disorder, which affects mainly middle-aged women, is of unknown cause.

Facies
A medical term for the appearance of the face, as in adenoid facies, the dull, open-mouthed expression seen in many children whose nasal passages are blocked due to enlarged adenoids.

Factitious disorders
A group of disorders in which symptoms mimic a true illness, but actually have been invented and are under the control of the patient. This is done willingly and for no apparent reason other than the wish to receive the attention given to a patient.

The most common type of factitious disorder is characterized by real physical symptoms and is known as *Munchausen's syndrome*. In a second form, called *Ganser's syndrome*, there is a psychological disturbance.

These disorders differ from malingering, in which the person claims to be ill for a particular purpose, such as obtaining time off from work or claiming compensation.

Factor VIII
One of the blood proteins (coagulation factors) that takes part in the "coagulation cascade"—an important process in *blood clotting*. Some people with the inherited condition *hemophilia* have a reduced level of factor VIII in their blood and, consequently, have a tendency to abnormal bleeding and prolonged bleeding when injured.

Freeze-dried concentrates of factor VIII are given to hemophiliacs by regular intravenous injection (some hemophiliacs administer the treatment themselves at home), which reduces the bleeding tendency and improves the quality of life.

Fahrenheit scale
A temperature scale in which the melting point of ice is 32° and the boiling point of water is 212°. On this scale, normal body temperature is 98.6°F (37°C). The scale is named for the German physicist Gabriel Fahrenheit.

To convert Fahrenheit to Celsius, subtract 32 and then multiply by 0.56 (or 5/9). To convert a Celsius temperature to a Fahrenheit temperature, multiply by 1.8 (or 9/5) and then add 32. (See also *Celsius scale*.)

Failure to thrive
Lack of expected growth in an infant, usually assessed by comparing the rate at which a baby gains weight with a standardized growth chart. Babies who fail to thrive are not growing enough in relation to birth weight.

The undernourishment may be due to some problem at home, often an unsatisfactory relationship between parent and child. In some cases, the child is actually neglected. Deprived children often have delayed emotional and intellectual development as well as failure to thrive.

If a baby fails to gain weight despite receiving an adequate diet and having a stable family background, other conditions may be responsible. Failure to thrive can indicate a serious problem, such as congenital *heart disease*, *renal failure*, or *malabsorption*.

A baby who fails to thrive is often observed (along with a parent) for a week or two to see how the parent feeds and handles the baby. The baby's diet and weight are carefully monitored. If there are social problems, support for the family can be initiated. (See also *Short stature*.)

Fainting
Temporary loss of consciousness due to insufficient oxygen reaching the brain. A fainting attack, known medically as syncope, is often preceded by dizziness, nausea, or a feeling of extreme weakness.

CAUSES
One common cause of fainting is a vasovagal attack, overstimulation of the *vagus nerve* (which helps control breathing and blood circulation). Usually such an attack is due to severe pain, stress, or fear; more rarely it may be caused by prolonged coughing, or by straining to defecate, urinate, or blow a wind instrument. In such cases, unconsciousness is usually accompanied by profuse sweating or

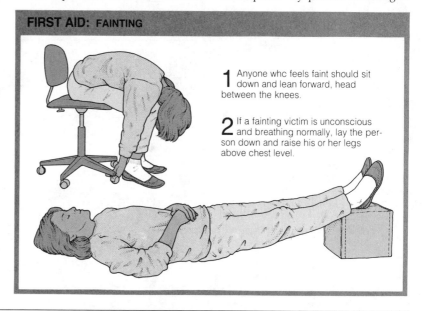

FIRST AID: FAINTING

1 Anyone who feels faint should sit down and lean forward, head between the knees.

2 If a fainting victim is unconscious and breathing normally, lay the person down and raise his or her legs above chest level.

paleness of the skin. A common cause of fainting is being in a stuffy atmosphere that has little oxygen.

Standing still for a long time, or standing up suddenly, can cause fainting. This is due to blood pooling in veins in the legs and reducing the amount available for the heart to pump to the brain, with a resultant drop in blood pressure (postural *hypotension*). It is common in the elderly, in sufferers from *diabetes mellitus*, and in people taking *antihypertensive* or *vasodilator drugs*.

In some people, episodes of fainting may be associated with temporary difficulty in speaking or weakness in the limbs; this may indicate a disorder called *vertebrobasilar insufficiency*, in which there is an obstruction to the blood flow in vessels that pass through the neck to the brain. This is one form of a *transient ischemic attack*.

Fainting may be a symptom of *Stokes-Adams syndrome*, in which the blood flow to the brain temporarily is inadequate due to an *arrhythmia* (irregularity of the heart beat) usually associated with a form of *heart block* (interruption of electrical impulses in the heart).

TREATMENT
Recovery from syncope takes place when normal blood flow to the brain is restored. This usually happens within minutes because falling to the ground places the head at the same level as the heart. To ensure another attack does not occur, the person should remain lying down for 10 to 15 minutes after regaining consciousness.

A person who experiences warning signs of a faint can sometimes prevent fainting by sitting with the head between the knees or, if possible, lying flat with the legs raised.

If a person fails to regain consciousness within a minute or two of fainting, medical help should be obtained promptly and appropriate first aid given (see *Unconsciousness*) until help arrives. Repeated attacks require investigation by a physician.

Faith healing
The supposed ability of certain people to cure disease by their possession of a healing force inexplicable to science. The healer usually transmits this supposed force to the sufferer by direct contact, placing his or her hands on the body ("laying on of hands"). Often the healer and patient have a deep religious faith and believe the force to be divine, but in many cases no religious faith is involved—only a firm

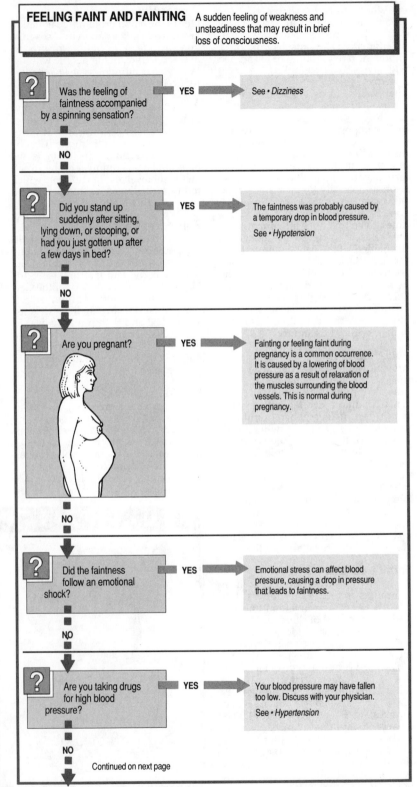

FEELING FAINT AND FAINTING A sudden feeling of weakness and unsteadiness that may result in brief loss of consciousness.

Was the feeling of faintness accompanied by a spinning sensation?
YES → See • *Dizziness*
NO ↓

Did you stand up suddenly after sitting, lying down, or stooping, or had you just gotten up after a few days in bed?
YES → The faintness was probably caused by a temporary drop in blood pressure. See • *Hypotension*
NO ↓

Are you pregnant?
YES → Fainting or feeling faint during pregnancy is a common occurrence. It is caused by a lowering of blood pressure as a result of relaxation of the muscles surrounding the blood vessels. This is normal during pregnancy.
NO ↓

Did the faintness follow an emotional shock?
YES → Emotional stress can affect blood pressure, causing a drop in pressure that leads to faintness.
NO ↓

Are you taking drugs for high blood pressure?
YES → Your blood pressure may have fallen too low. Discuss with your physician. See • *Hypertension*
NO ↓

Continued on next page

F

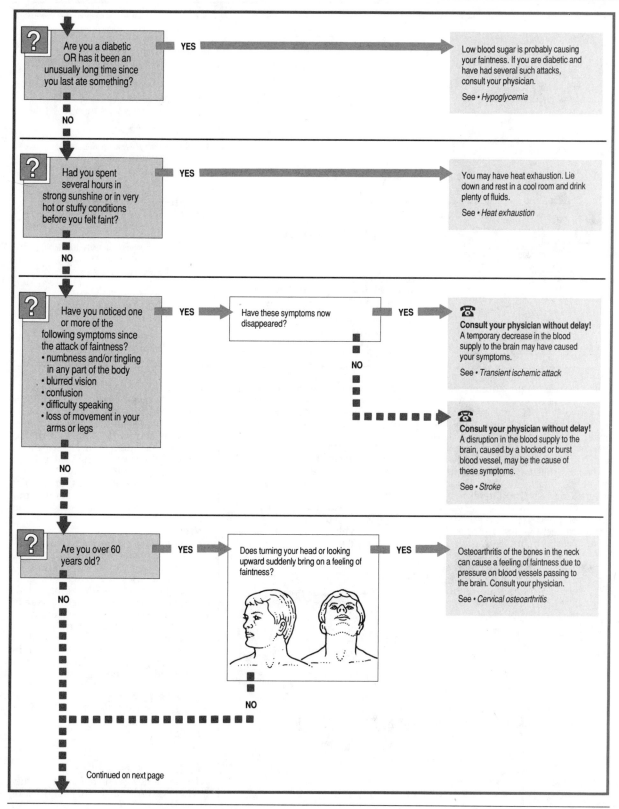

? Are you a diabetic OR has it been an unusually long time since you last ate something?

YES → Low blood sugar is probably causing your faintness. If you are diabetic and have had several such attacks, consult your physician.

See • *Hypoglycemia*

NO

? Had you spent several hours in strong sunshine or in very hot or stuffy conditions before you felt faint?

YES → You may have heat exhaustion. Lie down and rest in a cool room and drink plenty of fluids.

See • *Heat exhaustion*

NO

? Have you noticed one or more of the following symptoms since the attack of faintness?
• numbness and/or tingling in any part of the body
• blurred vision
• confusion
• difficulty speaking
• loss of movement in your arms or legs

YES → Have these symptoms now disappeared?

YES → ☎ **Consult your physician without delay!** A temporary decrease in the blood supply to the brain may have caused your symptoms.

See • *Transient ischemic attack*

NO

☎ **Consult your physician without delay!** A disruption in the blood supply to the brain, caused by a blocked or burst blood vessel, may be the cause of these symptoms.

See • *Stroke*

NO

? Are you over 60 years old?

YES → Does turning your head or looking upward suddenly bring on a feeling of faintness?

YES → Osteoarthritis of the bones in the neck can cause a feeling of faintness due to pressure on blood vessels passing to the brain. Consult your physician.

See • *Cervical osteoarthritis*

NO

NO

Continued on next page

F

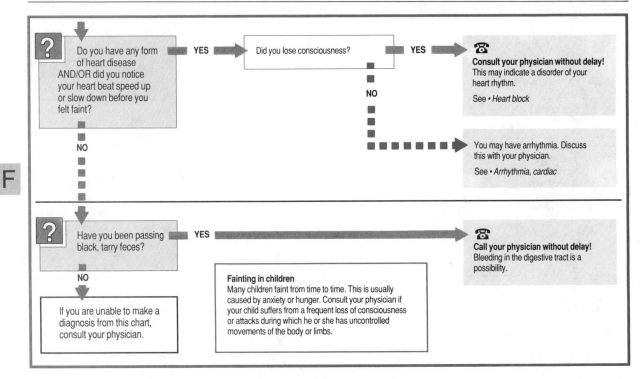

Do you have any form of heart disease AND/OR did you notice your heart beat speed up or slow down before you felt faint?

YES → Did you lose consciousness? **YES** →

☎ **Consult your physician without delay!** This may indicate a disorder of your heart rhythm.

See • *Heart block*

NO

You may have arrhythmia. Discuss this with your physician.

See • *Arrhythmia, cardiac*

NO

Have you been passing black, tarry feces? **YES** →

☎ **Call your physician without delay!** Bleeding in the digestive tract is a possibility.

NO

If you are unable to make a diagnosis from this chart, consult your physician.

Fainting in children
Many children faint from time to time. This is usually caused by anxiety or hunger. Consult your physician if your child suffers from a frequent loss of consciousness or attacks during which he or she has uncontrolled movements of the body or limbs.

---

belief, by healer and sufferer alike, in the healer's powers.

The existence of cures by faith healing is not in doubt—they have been demonstrated many times to the satisfaction of medical observers; in addition, the cures do not involve any of the risks that may accompany medical or surgical treatment. However, the medical profession tends to argue that most such cures are due not to a divine or otherwise inexplicable force, but to the fact that the disorders were hysterical in origin (see *Hysteria*) and therefore susceptible to *autosuggestion*. Physicians also believe that people who turn to faith healing rather than seek medical advice are depriving themselves of effective treatment of the underlying problem.

Fallen arches
A cause of *flatfoot*, which can develop as a result of weakness of the muscles that support the arches of the foot.

Fallopian tube
The tube that extends from the *uterus* to the *ovary*. The fallopian tube transports eggs and sperm and is where *fertilization* takes place.
STRUCTURE
The funnel-shaped tube is about 3 inches long. The narrow end opens into the uterus and the free, expanded end, divided into fimbriae (fingerlike projections), lies close to the ovary. Its muscular wall is lined by cells with cilia (hairlike projections).

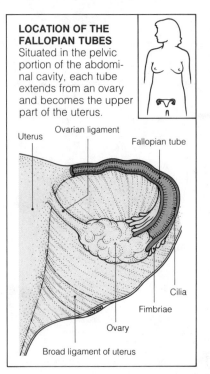

LOCATION OF THE FALLOPIAN TUBES
Situated in the pelvic portion of the abdominal cavity, each tube extends from an ovary and becomes the upper part of the uterus.

Uterus
Ovarian ligament
Fallopian tube
Cilia
Fimbriae
Ovary
Broad ligament of uterus

FUNCTION
The fimbriae sweep up the egg after it is expelled from the ovary. The beating cilia and waves of muscular contractions propel the egg toward the uterus. After intercourse, sperm swim up the fallopian tube from the uterus. The lining of the tube and its secretions sustain the egg and sperm. They also encourage fertilization and nourish the egg until it reaches the uterus.
DISORDERS
Salpingitis is inflammation of the fallopian tube, usually following bacterial infection. It accounts for almost 15 percent of cases of *infertility*.

Ectopic pregnancy (development of an embryo outside the uterus) usually occurs in the fallopian tube. A delay in the transport of the fertilized egg along the tube results in implantation within the tube wall, which is too thin to sustain growth. The tube then ruptures and may hemorrhage.

Fallot's tetralogy
See *Tetralogy of Fallot*.

Fallout
See *Radiation hazards*.

Falls in the elderly
The tendency to fall increases steadily with age. Although the majority of

falls produce no permanent injury, a significant number of the injuries that do result are ultimately fatal.

CAUSES AND INCIDENCE

Reflex actions in the elderly are much slower than in the young, and an elderly person who trips or stumbles is often too slow to prevent a fall.

Half of all falls are accidental and half have a medical cause. Poor sight, walking disorders, arrhythmias (see *Arrhythmia, cardiac*), *hypotension* (reduced blood pressure), dizziness for various reasons, and the effect of drugs are causes. Falls sometimes herald the onset of serious illness such as pneumonia, stroke, myocardial infarction (heart attack), or internal hemorrhage. Epilepsy, Parkinson's disease, alcohol consumption, the hangover effects of some sleeping tablets, and use of daytime tranquilizers may also increase the likelihood of a fall.

RISKS AND COMPLICATIONS

Broken bones as a result of falls are particularly common in the elderly. Women are more vulnerable to broken bones than men. Not only do women have more falls, they are also more likely to suffer fractures because their bone strength is reduced as a result of calcium loss after the menopause (see *Osteoporosis*). The incidence of fractures of the neck of the femur (thigh bone) doubles approximately every seven years after the age of 65, and, by the age of 90, one woman in four has suffered this type of fracture.

Apart from injuries, there may be serious indirect consequences of the fall. The outlook is particularly grave for those who fall and lie on the floor for more than an hour, particularly if it is cold. This may lead to *hypothermia* (low body temperature) or pneumonia. In this group, 50 percent die within three months of the fall.

A serious fall, or fear of such a fall and the helplessness and dependence it could bring, can have bad psychological effects on an elderly person, sometimes causing a previously active person to become demoralized and housebound.

ACTION AFTER A FALL

Immediate medical help should be obtained if the person is unconscious, is in severe pain, is bleeding profusely, is burned, has suspected broken bones, or is showing signs of shock. First-aid measures (for bleeding, burns, or fractures) and *cardiopulmonary resuscitation* (if the heart and/or breathing have stopped) may be necessary.

PREVENTION AND OUTLOOK

These measures can be taken to guard against falls: ensure that handles in bathrooms and on stairs are secure, good lighting is available, suitable footwear is worn, floor coverings and wiring are safe, and that there is minimal clutter on the floor. Elderly people who live alone can arrange for an alarm system to be installed or for a regular visit by a neighbor. It is also helpful to teach the elderly person several different ways of getting up from the floor.

False teeth

See *Denture*.

Familial

A term applied to a characteristic or disorder that runs in families (that is, it occurs in more members of a particular family than would be expected from the occurrence in the population as a whole). An example of a familial characteristic is male pattern baldness (see *Alopecia*); an example of a familial disorder is *hyperlipidemia* (abnormally high levels of fat in the blood).

Familial Mediterranean fever

An inherited condition that affects certain Sephardic Jewish, Armenian, and

F

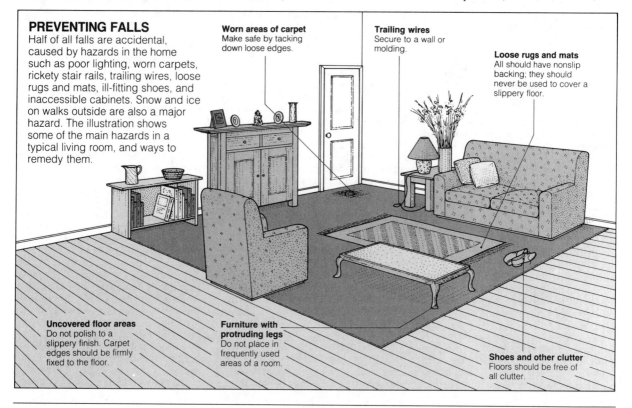

PREVENTING FALLS

Half of all falls are accidental, caused by hazards in the home such as poor lighting, worn carpets, rickety stair rails, trailing wires, loose rugs and mats, ill-fitting shoes, and inaccessible cabinets. Snow and ice on walks outside are also a major hazard. The illustration shows some of the main hazards in a typical living room, and ways to remedy them.

Worn areas of carpet
Make safe by tacking down loose edges.

Trailing wires
Secure to a wall or molding.

Loose rugs and mats
All should have nonslip backing; they should never be used to cover a slippery floor.

Uncovered floor areas
Do not polish to a slippery finish. Carpet edges should be firmly fixed to the floor.

Furniture with protruding legs
Do not place in frequently used areas of a room.

Shoes and other clutter
Floors should be free of all clutter.

Arab families. Its cause is unknown. Symptoms usually begin between the ages of 5 and 15 years. The main symptoms are recurrent episodes of fever, abdominal pain, arthritis, and chest pain. Red swellings in the skin sometimes occur, and affected people may also suffer psychiatric problems.

Attacks usually last between 24 and 48 hours, but may last longer. Between attacks there are usually no symptoms. There is no specific treatment, but known sufferers are able to reduce the incidence of attacks by taking colchicine, a drug usually used to treat gout. Death may eventually occur from *amyloidosis*, which is a complication of the condition.

Family planning

Limitation of the number or spacing of children through choices made by sexually active people. In some countries, financial and taxation incentives are used by the state to encourage couples to have more or fewer children; in other countries, penalties are imposed on those who do not conform to government recommendations.

In most countries the factors governing family size are economic and social. In many developing countries few older people have pensions, and those too frail to work rely on support from their adult children. Under these circumstances, having many children is seen as a provision for care in old age. In the past 20 years, however, most nations have experienced the economic ill effects of rapid population growth and large families are no longer encouraged.

The number of children born to a couple may be limited by social factors—late marriage for both men and women reduces the reproductive period, and economic barriers to marriage may restrict childbearing to a fraction of the population.

Strategies for restricting family size include contraceptive techniques (see *Contraception*) and elective abortion (see *Abortion, elective*).

Family practitioner

A physician who provides comprehensive medical services for individuals, regardless of sex or age, on a continuing basis. The family practitioner (FP) often cares for all members of a family.

Emphasis is placed on treatment of all problems experienced by the person and on coordination of care, with referrals to specialists as necessary. Care by an FP may range from stitches

and sniffles to management of long-term conditions (e.g., terminal cancer, congestive heart failure, or diabetes mellitus), including the delivery of a baby and care afterward. Family practitioners have replaced the former general practitioner (GP), but the training for the FP is broader.

Family therapy

Treatment of the family, as a whole rather than individual treatment of one or more members. Family therapy is based on the belief that a troubled or mentally ill person cannot be seen in isolation from the family unit. Disturbed children may merely reflect parental conflicts. This approach has become popular in recent years for dealing with the problems of children and adolescents.

Usually the therapist arranges regular meetings with the family to find out what feelings lie behind the way parents and children deal with each other. Through discussion and confrontation, these feelings can gradually be changed, leading to greater harmony and understanding.

Famotidine

A recently released (1986) *ulcer-healing drug* related to the *antihistamine drugs*. Famotidine reduces the secretion of acid in the stomach and, by doing so, promotes healing of *peptic ulcers* and reduces *esophagitis* (inflammation of the esophagus).

Fanconi's anemia

A rare type of aplastic *anemia*, characterized by a severely reduced production of all types of blood cells by the bone marrow.

Fanconi's syndrome

A rare kidney disorder, occurring mainly in childhood, in which various important nutrients and chemicals such as amino acids, phosphate, calcium, and potassium are lost in the urine; this leads to failure to thrive, stunting of growth, and bone disorders such as *rickets*.

Fanconi's syndrome has a wide variety of possible causes, including a number of rare inherited abnormalities of body chemistry; it may also occur as a side effect of some drugs, such as the ingestion of outdated tetracycline. In some cases there is no obvious cause.

The child may resume normal growth if an underlying chemical abnormality can be corrected. Alternatively, he or she may benefit from a

kidney transplant. In some cases, neither of these measures is possible or beneficial and kidney function progressively worsens, leading to death in childhood or early adolescence. Fanconi's syndrome in adults has a much brighter outlook.

Fantasy

The process of imagining events or objects that are not actually occurring or present. The term also refers to the mental image itself. Fantasy can give the illusion that wishes have been met. In this sense, it provides satisfaction and can be a means of helping people to cope when reality becomes too unpleasant. Fantasy can also be creative, stimulating ideas and activities by presenting mental images in new combinations.

Psychoanalysts believe that some fantasies are unconscious and represent certain primitive instincts; these fantasies are always presented to the conscious mind in symbols. For example, the fantasy of returning to the womb might be represented by the image of a cave deep within the earth.

Farmers' lung

 An occupational disease affecting the lungs of farm workers in whom *hypersensitivity* (an excessive allergic reaction) develops when exposed to certain molds or fungi that grow on hay, grain, or straw.

CAUSES AND INCIDENCE

Farmers' lung is an example of an allergic *alveolitis*—a reaction of the lungs to inhaled dust containing fungal spores. The causative fungi grow on hay or grain that has been stored in warm, damp conditions. Outbreaks of farmers' lung often occur toward the end of a winter following a wet summer in areas with a high rainfall.

SYMPTOMS

Typical symptoms develop about six hours after exposure to dust containing fungal spores. The symptoms may include shortness of breath and flulike symptoms of fever, headache, and muscle aches. In single acute attacks, the symptoms persist for one or two days. Repeated exposure to the molds or fungi that provoked the attack may lead to a chronic form of the disease, causing permanent scarring of the lung tissues.

DIAGNOSIS AND TREATMENT

The physician takes a full occupational history and listens through a stethoscope for crackles. A chest X ray may show abnormalities; *pulmonary func-*

tion tests show that the efficiency of the lungs is reduced. Specific blood tests, indicating that the patient has antibodies to the fungus, can confirm the diagnosis.

The sufferer should avoid further exposure to moldy hay or grain; if symptoms persist, *corticosteroid drugs* may be prescribed. Complete recovery can be expected, provided the disease is diagnosed before permanent lung damage has occurred.

PREVENTION

Farmers can reduce their own and their workers' chances of developing the condition by reducing the water content of hay and grain before storage and by ensuring that storage conditions are cool and dry (to discourage growth of fungi). Well-ventilated work areas help prevent a buildup of fungal spores in the air; wearing protective masks may help.

Farsightedness

See *Hyperopia*.

Fascia

Fibrous *connective tissue* that surrounds many structures in the body. One layer of the tissue, known as the superficial fascia, envelopes the entire body just beneath the skin. Another layer, the deep fascia, encloses muscles, forming a sheath for individual muscles and separating them into groups. The deep fascia also holds in place soft organs, such as the kidneys. Thick fascia in the palm of the hand and sole of the foot have a cushioning, protective function.

Fasciculation

Spontaneous, irregular, and usually continual contractions of a muscle apparently at rest. Unlike *fibrillation*, a similar condition, fasciculation is visible under the skin and is described as fine or coarse.

A minor degree of fasciculation is common and is no cause for concern. However, persistent fasciculation with weakness in the affected muscle indicates damage to (or disease of) nerve cells in the spine that control the muscle or nerve fibers that connect the spinal nerves to the muscle; *motor neuron disease* is one such disorder.

Fasciitis

Inflammation of a layer of *fascia* (fibrous connective tissue), causing pain and tenderness. Fasciitis is usually the result of straining or injuring the fascia surrounding a muscle; it most commonly affects the sole of the

foot (a condition called plantar fasciitis). It may occur in people who suffer from *ankylosing spondylitis* (rheumatism of the spine) or *Reiter's syndrome* (inflammation of the urethra with conjunctivitis and arthritis).

Treatment consists of resting the affected area and protecting it from pressure (i.e., by wearing cushioned pads in the shoes if the foot is affected). In some cases, injections of *corticosteroid drugs* have been given in an attempt to relieve pain.

Fasciotomy

An operation to relieve pressure on muscles by making an incision in the fascia (connective tissue) that surrounds them.

WHY IT IS DONE

Fasciotomy is usually performed to treat *compartment syndrome*, a painful condition in which a group of muscles is constricted with consequent obstruction of their blood flow. The condition can result in damage to, or even the death of, affected muscles. Fasciotomy gives the muscles space in which to expand.

The operation is also sometimes performed as a surgical emergency to treat a crush injury in which the muscle group has swollen or there is bleeding into the muscle compartment, raising the pressure within it.

HOW IT IS DONE

Fasciotomy is performed using a general anesthetic. An incision is made in the skin over the affected muscle group and then in the underlying fascia to allow the muscles to bulge through. For compartment syndrome, only a small incision is usually required; in an emergency procedure, a much larger incision may be needed.

Once the muscles have expanded through the opening, the wound is sewn up. In some cases, the muscle bulges out so much that a *skin graft* is required to repair the incision.

Fasting

Abstaining from all food and drinking only water. In temperate conditions and at moderate levels of physical activity, a person can survive on water alone for more than two months; without food or drink, death usually occurs within about 10 days (survival times are shorter in hot or cold conditions and at high levels of activity).

EFFECTS ON THE BODY

Without food, the energy needed to maintain essential body processes, such as *metabolism*, is supplied by substances stored in the body.

About six hours after the last meal, the body starts to use glycogen (a carbohydrate stored in the liver and muscles). This continues for about 24 hours, after which, while the body adapts to obtaining energy from stored fat, protein from the breakdown of muscles is also used as an energy source.

After a few days, most energy is obtained from fat, although some continues to come from muscle breakdown. If fasting continues, the body's metabolism slows to conserve energy. As a result of this slowdown, the fat and protein from muscles is consumed more slowly.

In the initial stages of fasting, weight loss is rapid. Later it slows, not only because metabolism slows down, but also because the body starts to conserve its salt supply, which causes water retention. Water that would normally be excreted in the urine is absorbed by the tissues. The accumulated fluid causes edema (swelling), mainly of the legs and abdomen.

In prolonged fasting, the ability to digest food may be impaired or lost entirely because the stomach gradually stops secreting digestive juices. If this occurs, medical supervision may be necessary when eating resumes. Prolonged fasting also halts the production of sex hormones, causing *amenorrhea* (absence of periods) in women. In addition, the body's ability to fight infection deteriorates, which, along with degeneration of the heart muscle, may be fatal.

FASTING TO REDUCE WEIGHT

Omitting a main meal each day for a limited period, or occasionally not eating anything for up to 24 hours, may be an effective means of losing weight. However, nobody should go without any food for more than a day without consulting a physician.

Fatigue

See *Tiredness*.

Fats and oils

Nutrients that provide the body with its most concentrated form of *energy*; 1 gram of fat provides nine Calories, whereas 1 gram of carbohydrate produces only four to five Calories.

Fats are compounds containing *carbon* and hydrogen with very little *oxygen*. Chemically, they consist mostly of *fatty acids* combined with an oily alcohol, *glycerol*. They are divided into two main groups, saturated and unsaturated, depending on the proportion of hydrogen atoms. If the fatty

F

F

acids contain the maximum quantity possible of hydrogen, they are said to be saturated. If there are some sites on the carbon atom unoccupied by hydrogen, they are unsaturated; when many sites are vacant, they are polyunsaturated. Animal fats, such as those found in meat and dairy products, are highly saturated with hydrogen, while vegetable fats tend to be unsaturated to varying degrees.

There is no difference between fats and oils except in consistency. Saturated fats are solid at room temperature (but liquid when heated); oils are liquid at room temperature.

TYPES

Dietary fats are sources of the fat-soluble vitamins A, D, E, and K and of essential fatty acids. They are mainly triglycerides (combinations of glycerol and three fatty acids) but also contain other types of fats. Sources in the diet include not only the visible fats (such as butter, margarine, and vegetable oils) but also the so-called invisible fats found in meat, fish, poultry, and dairy products. The oils of certain cold-water ocean fish are being investigated for their potential ability to protect against coronary heart disease.

Structural fats (referred to as lipids) include triglycerides, phospholipids, and sterols. Triglycerides are the main form of fat found in stores of body fat. These stores act as an energy reserve as well as providing insulation and a protective layer for delicate organs. Phospholipids are structural fats found in cell membranes. Sterols, such as *cholesterol*, are found in animal and plant tissues; they have a variety of functions within the body, often being converted by chemical actions into hormones or vitamins.

FAT METABOLISM

Dietary fats are first dissolved by the action of bile salts and then broken down into fatty acids and glycerol by lipase, a pancreatic enzyme. They are absorbed via the lymphatic system before entering the bloodstream.

The lipids are carried in the blood bound to a protein, when they become known as lipoproteins. There are four classes of lipoprotein—chylomicrons, very low-density lipoproteins (VLDLs), high-density lipoproteins (HDLs), and low-density lipoproteins (LDLs). LDLs and VLDLs contain large amounts of cholesterol, which they carry through the bloodstream and deposit in cells. The HDLs pick up cholesterol and carry it back to the liver for processing and excretion. (See also *Nutrition*.)

Fatty acids

Organic acids, containing *carbon*, hydrogen, and *oxygen*, that are constituents of fats. There are over 40 different fatty acids found in nature, distinguished by their number of carbon atoms.

Certain fatty acids cannot be synthesized by the body and must be provided by the diet. These fatty acids are linoleic, linolenic, and arachidonic acids, sometimes referred to collectively as the essential fatty acids. (See also *Nutrition*.)

Favism

 A disorder characterized by an extreme sensitivity to the broad bean *VICIA FABA* (fava). If an affected person eats these beans, a chemical in the bean causes rapid destruction of his or her red blood cells, leading to a severe type of anemia (see *Anemia, hemolytic*).

Favism is uncommon except in some areas of the Mediterranean, especially lowland Greece, where up to 10 percent of the population is affected. Favism is an inherited condition caused by a sex-linked *genetic disorder*. Affected people have a defect in a chemical pathway within their red blood cells that helps to protect the cells from injury. This defect is called glucose-6-phosphate dehydrogenase deficiency or *G6PD deficiency*.

Children in any family with a history of favism should be screened for the condition at an early age. If the disorder is found, they must avoid broad beans and certain drugs (including some antimalarials and antibiotics) that can have a similar destructive effect on their red blood cells. A list of drugs to avoid can be obtained from a physician when the disorder is diagnosed. With these precautions, affected people are able to remain in good health.

FDA

See *Food and Drug Administration*.

Febrile

Feverish or related to *fever*, as in febrile seizures—convulsions that occur mainly in young children who have high temperatures.

Fecal impaction

A large mass of hard feces that cannot be evacuated from the rectum. The condition usually is associated with long-standing *constipation*, along with dehydrated feces. Fecal impaction is most common in very young children

and the elderly, especially those who are bedridden.

The main symptoms are an intense desire to have a bowel movement, pain in the rectum, anus, and center of the abdomen, and, in some instances, watery feces (which may be mistaken for diarrhea) that are passed around the impacted mass.

To diagnose the condition, the physician inserts a gloved finger into the rectum. Treatment consists of giving enemas (see *Enema*). If this is ineffective, the fecal mass may require removal manually.

Fecalith

A small, hard, almost stonelike piece of impacted feces that occasionally forms in a diverticulum (an outpouching, usually in the large intestine). A fecalith is harmless unless it blocks the entrance to the appendix, causing *appendicitis*, or a diverticulum, causing diverticulitis (see *Diverticular disease*).

Feces

Waste material from the digestive tract that is expelled through the anus. Solidified in the large intestine, feces consists of indigestible food residue (roughage, or dietary *fiber*), dead bacteria (which may account for as much as half the weight of the feces), dead cells shed from the intestinal lining, secretions from the intestine (such as mucus), bile from the liver (which colors the feces brown), and water.

Examination of the feces—for color, odor, consistency, or the presence of blood, pus, fat, parasites, or unusual microorganisms—is important in the diagnosis of digestive tract disorders. (See also *Feces, abnormal*.)

Feces, abnormal

Feces that differ from normal in color, odor, consistency, or content. The changes may be the result of a harmless condition, but in some cases they are due to a disorder of the digestive tract or a disorder of a related organ, such as the liver.

Liquid or very loose feces, passed frequently (see *Diarrhea*), may be due simply to anxiety but may also be caused by an intestinal infection (see *Gastroenteritis*); by an intestinal disorder such as *ulcerative colitis* or *Crohn's disease*; or by the *irritable bowel syndrome*. Loose stools may also reflect various states of *malabsorption*. At the other extreme, feces may be very hard and infrequently passed (see *Constipation*). Constipation is usually harmless but may be associated with rumbling and gurgling (*borborygmi*), bloating, and abdominal discomfort attributable to an irritable colon.

Pale feces may be due to diarrhea, to a lack of bile in the intestine as a result of *bile duct obstruction*, or to a disease that causes malabsorption (such as *celiac sprue*). In malabsorption, the paleness of the feces is due to the high fat content. Such feces may be oily, frothy, foul-smelling, and difficult to flush away.

Dark feces may simply be the result of unusually large amounts of iron or red wine in the diet. However, if feces are black, there may be bleeding in the stomach, duodenum, small intestine, or cecum.

Slimy feces, which contain excessive mucus, may be passed normally, but are sometimes associated with constipation or the irritable bowel syndrome. *Enteritis*, *dysentery*, or a tumor of the intestine (see *Intestine, tumors of*) may also cause slimy feces, often accompanied by blood.

Blood in the feces varies in appearance according to the site of bleeding. When blood is in the stomach or duodenum, it usually shows only as black, tarry feces; blood from a disease of the colon, such as ulcerative colitis or a tumor, is red and can usually be seen separate from the feces. Bleeding from the rectum, which occurs with *hemorrhoids* or rectal tumors, often streaks the feces, is visible only on toilet paper, or drips into the toilet bowl. This blood is usually bright red.

INVESTIGATION

Blood in the feces and any other persistent abnormality should be reported immediately to a physician, who may ask for a sample of the feces. (See also *Rectal bleeding*.)

Feces, blood in the

See *Feces, abnormal*; *Rectal bleeding*.

Feeding, artificial

Administration of nutrients other than by mouth, usually through a tube inserted into the stomach or small intestine. Occasionally, a tube is inserted directly into the stomach or jejunum (upper part of the small intestine) by surgical means. This is called enteral nutrition. If the gastrointestinal tract is not functioning, food must be sent into the bloodstream by *intravenous infusion*. This technique is known as total parenteral nutrition.

WHY IT IS DONE

Tube feeding may be necessary for people with disorders of the gastro-

intestinal tract, *malabsorption*, or neurological or renal disorders. Premature babies often require tube feeding if their sucking reflexes are undeveloped, as do burn or fever patients because of their increased nutritional requirements.

Intravenous feeding is usually necessary when there has been damage to the small intestine as a result of disease or surgical removal of large areas of the absorbing surface.

HOW IT IS DONE

TUBE FEEDING Suitable food mixtures or preparations of predetermined levels of nutrients are administered via a narrow plastic tube. The tube is passed through the patient's nose (guided via the nasopharynx to the esophagus) and into either the stomach or the duodenum.

If tube feeding is the sole means of nutrition, it must provide all of the essential nutrients (and adequate fluids) to meet the person's daily needs, which can vary markedly. There are two alternative methods of tube feeding—bolus feeding and continuous drip feeding.

Bolus feeding involves the rapid administration of a set amount of nutrients at intermittent periods throughout the day. Continuous drip feeding is, however, more widely preferred because it is tolerated better by the patient. In both methods the rate of flow can be controlled by a pump. The tube is left in place for adults and older children, but, for infants and young children, it is removed and reinserted for each feeding.

INTRAVENOUS FEEDING This method is generally used only when tube feeding is impractical or ineffective; its main drawback is the risk of introducing infection directly into the bloodstream or of blocking a blood vessel. Some problems with the liver or gallbladder have occurred.

The nutrient preparations are given directly into a large central vein near the heart via a catheter (thin, flexible tube) inserted using an anesthetic and strict *aseptic techniques*. Intravenous feeding is sometimes used to supplement feeding by mouth, but can if necessary provide all the nutrients needed to meet a patient's requirements. Essential vitamins and minerals are included.

Feeding, infant

During a baby's first year, it grows more rapidly than at any other time in its life. A good diet is essential for healthy growth.

BREAST- OR BOTTLE-FEEDING

NUTRITIONAL REQUIREMENTS During the first four to six months, most babies' nutritional requirements are met by milk alone, whether by *breast-feeding* or *bottle-feeding*. Both human milk and artificial milk (modified dried cow's milk) contain carbohydrate, protein, fat, vitamins, and minerals in similar proportions (see *Milk* for components), but human milk is the food of choice because it provides these nutrients in the perfect blend as well as containing antibodies and white blood cells that protect the baby against infections.

After the baby is 6 months old, vitamin D supplements should be given to breast-fed babies and to bottle-fed babies whose locations or backgrounds pose a risk of rickets. At 6 months a baby can safely be taken off artificial milk and fed with natural cow's milk. Supplementary vitamin D should be given until the baby is established on a mixed diet. Drops containing vitamins A, C, and D, although often given, are usually not required by most infants.

If a baby seems unable to tolerate milk of any kind (see *Food allergy*; *Food intolerance*), the pediatrician should be consulted; he or she may recommend a preparation based on soybeans, vegetable oils, sucrose, corn sugar, modified meat protein, and other substances. Babies should not be fed skim milk, which has relatively too much protein and minerals and insufficient calories compared with whole milk.

EMOTIONAL REQUIREMENTS For healthy emotional development, a baby requires warmth, security, and contentment; the act of feeding plays an important part in meeting these needs. Breast-feeding is again preferable in this respect because it establishes an intimate bond between mother and child, but bottle-feeding is a perfectly satisfactory alternative if the baby is cuddled and talked to while he or she is fed.

INTRODUCING SOLIDS

Solid foods, initially in the form of purees and cereals, should be introduced into an infant's diet at some time between the ages of 3 and 6 months, depending on the baby's birth weight and rate of growth. By 6 months the baby should be eating some true solids, such as chopped up meat and vegetables. The accompanying chart gives the optimum times for the introduction of solids, but a baby's general contentment also provides some guide. A rapidly growing baby

F

who is unable to drink enough milk to satisfy his or her hunger needs the more concentrated calories found in solid food.

Many parents prefer to give their infants home-prepared purees rather than prepared foods. In this case, salt and other additives should not be used, since an overconcentration of salt and other minerals can dangerously overburden a baby's kidneys. Sugar, too, should be kept to a minimum in the diet; a baby easily learns to have a "sweet tooth," which will lead to future dental decay; for the same reason, babies should not be given bottles of sweetened drinks to comfort them.

A baby can live healthily on a vegetarian diet (one that contains no meat or fish) provided eggs are included, but a baby fed on a vegan diet (one that also excludes all animal products, such as dairy produce and eggs) runs the risk of severe malnutrition. A vegan diet makes it very hard to obtain enough calories, essential fatty acids, vitamins (especially B_{12}), and protein. Overall, it is a very bad diet for infants and growing children whose nutrient requirements are much greater than adults.

FEEDING PROBLEMS
Any difficulties associated with milk usually appear within the first month.

Some babies have an intolerance to certain foods; reactions can include vomiting, diarrhea, or allergic rashes. For this reason, solids should be introduced one by one so that any that cause problems can be identified.

Prolonged crying after feedings may mean that the baby needs help bringing up gas, that artificial milk is not being digested properly, or that the baby has colic (see *Colic, infantile*). See also *Nutritional disorders*.

Fee for service
The traditional financial arrangement between patient and physician. The patient is charged for each service he or she receives; the physician is compensated for each service he or she provides. (See also *Health maintenance organization*.)

Femoral epiphysis, slipped
Displacement of the upper *epiphysis* (growing end) of the femur (thigh bone). Such displacement is rare, usually affects those between the ages of 11 and 13, and occurs more often in boys, in obese children with delayed sexual and physical development, and in children who grow rapidly.

APPROXIMATE AGES FOR INTRODUCING SOLIDS

Age		
4 months	At second breast- or bottle-feeding offer one or two	teaspoons of vegetable or fruit puree or cereal.
4½ months	At second breast- or bottle-feeding offer two teaspoons of cereal. At third breast- or bottle-	feeding offer two teaspoons of vegetable or fruit puree.
5 to 6 months	*Early morning* Breast- or bottle-feeding. *Breakfast* Two teaspoons of cereal and lightly boiled egg yolk, followed by breast- or bottle-feeding. *Lunch* One teaspoon of meat or fish puree with three teaspoons	of strained vegetables. Offer water or well-diluted fruit juice instead of milk. *Mid-afternoon* Mashed banana or other soft fruit followed by usual milk feeding. *Dinner* Breast- or bottle-feeding if the baby is still hungry.
6 to 7 months	*Early morning* Breast- or bottle-feeding. *Breakfast* Two teaspoons of cereal with lightly scrambled egg. Offer cow's milk from a cup.	*Lunch* Offer minced or mashed food instead of pureed. Give meat or fish with some vegetables, then offer yogurt and fruit. Give a drink of water or well-diluted fruit juice.
7 to 8 months	*Early morning* Offer a drink of water or diluted juice instead of the milk. *Breakfast* Cereal and boiled egg with whole-grain bread and butter. A drink of cow's milk. *Lunch* Cheese, fish, or minced	meat with mashed vegetables. Pudding or fresh fruit. A drink of water or well-diluted fruit juice. *Late afternoon/dinner* Whole-grain bread and butter with peanut butter or cheese. Fresh fruit and a drink of cow's milk.
9 to 12 months	*Early morning* A drink of water or well-diluted fruit juice. *Breakfast* Cereal, then egg or fish with whole-grain toast and butter. A drink of cow's milk. *Lunch* Chopped meat or fish, or	cheese, with vegetables. Pudding or fresh fruit. A drink of water or well-diluted fruit juice. *Late afternoon/dinner* Meat or cheese sandwiches. A drink of cow's milk.

While the bone is still growing, the epiphysis is separated from the shaft of the bone by a plate of cartilage. This constitutes a zone of relative weakness in the bone, so that a fall or other injury, even a minor one, can cause the epiphysis to slip out of position.

SYMPTOMS
A limp develops and the child feels pain in the knee rather than in the hip. The leg tends to turn outward and hip movements are restricted.

TREATMENT
An operation is performed using general anesthetic to manipulate the displaced parts of bone and fix them together with metal pins. To prevent possible damage to the other thigh, it, too, may be strengthened with pins during the same operation.

OUTLOOK
Surgery usually provides an effective repair and prevents further accidents of the same type. However, after the injury, the hip tends to be more susceptible than normal to *osteoarthritis*. In rare cases, the hip becomes stiff and painful, sometimes permanently so.

Femoral nerve
One of the primary nerves of the leg. It is made up of fibers from nerves in the second, third, and fourth segments of the lumbar spinal cord. The nerves emerge from the lower back region of the spine and run down into the thigh, where they branch to supply the skin and muscles of the front of the thigh. The nerve branches that supply the skin convey sensation; the branches that supply the muscles stimulate contraction of the *quadriceps muscle* of the thigh, causing the knee to straighten.

Damage to the femoral nerve (which impairs the ability of the knee to straighten) is usually caused by a slipped disk in the lumbar region of the spine (see *Disk prolapse*). Damage may also occur as the result of a backward dislocation of the hip or, rarely, as a result of a *neuropathy*.

Femur

The medical name for the thigh bone, the longest bone in the body. The lower end hinges with the tibia (shin) to form the knee joint. The upper end is rounded into a ball (head of the femur) that fits into a socket in the pelvis to form the hip joint. The head of the femur is joined to the bone shaft by a narrow piece of bone called the neck of the femur. While it gives the hip joint a wide range of movement, the neck of the femur is a point of structural weakness and a common fracture site (see *Femur, fracture of*).

The femur can be felt through the skin at two sites. At the lower end, the bone is enlarged to form two lumps (the condyles) that distribute the weight-bearing load on the knee joint. On the outer side of the upper end of the femur is a protuberance (called the greater trochanter).

The shaft of the femur is surrounded by powerful muscles whose principal functions are to move the hip and knee joints. The shaft is also well supplied with blood vessels; because of this, a fracture can result in considerable blood loss.

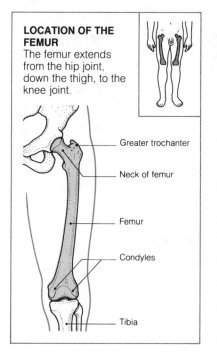

LOCATION OF THE FEMUR
The femur extends from the hip joint, down the thigh, to the knee joint.

Greater trochanter

Neck of femur

Femur

Condyles

Tibia

Femur, fracture of

The nature, symptoms, treatment, and possible complications of a fractured femur (thigh bone) depend on whether the bone has broken across its neck (the short section between the top of the shaft and the hip joint) or across the shaft.

NECK OF FEMUR

This type of fracture is very common in elderly people suffering from *osteoporosis* (thinning of the bone) and is usually associated with a fall. The broken ends of the bone are often considerably displaced; in such cases there is usually severe pain in the hip and groin (made worse by movement) and the leg cannot bear any weight. Occasionally, the broken ends of bone become impacted (wedged together). In this case there is less pain and walking is often still possible, which may delay reporting of the injury and detection of the fracture.

DIAGNOSIS AND TREATMENT Diagnosis of a suspected fracture is confirmed by X ray. If the bone ends are displaced, an operation using general anesthesia is necessary, either to realign the bone ends (a procedure called reduction) and to fasten them together with metal screws, plates, or nails, or to replace the entire head and neck of the femur with a metal or plastic substitute (see *Hip joint replacement*). Both procedures produce a stable repair, and hip and knee movement can be resumed immediately.

If the bone ends are impacted, the person is kept in bed for a few weeks to prevent any jarring movement that might dislodge the bones. The fracture heals naturally without surgery, but supervised exercise is necessary to maintain hip and knee mobility. X rays are taken periodically to determine how well the fracture is healing.

With either type of repair, walking is started with the aid of crutches, progresses to walking with a walker, walking with a cane, and, finally, walking without aid.

COMPLICATIONS These depend on the site of the fracture. A break at the union of the neck and shaft may result in hip deformity (see *Coxa vara*). A fracture across the neck itself may damage the blood supply to the head of the femur, causing the head to crumble (osteonecrosis). As a result, the bone ends may fail to fuse, or *osteoarthritis* may develop. In either case, more surgery (usually hip joint replacement) is required. Osteoarthritis may also develop even if avascular necrosis does not occur.

SHAFT OF FEMUR

This type of fracture usually occurs when the femur is subjected to extreme force, such as in an automobile accident. In most cases, the bone ends are considerably displaced, causing severe pain, tenderness, and swelling.

DIAGNOSIS AND TREATMENT Diagnosis of this injury is confirmed by X rays. With a fractured femoral shaft there is often substantial blood loss from the bone. In most cases, the fracture is repaired by an operation (using general anesthesia) in which the two ends of the bone are realigned and fastened together with a long metal pin. However, sometimes the bone ends can be realigned by manipulation, and surgery is not necessary. After realignment of the bones, the leg is supported with a *splint* and put in *traction* to hold the bone together while it heals.

Following both types of treatment, supervised exercise and massage of the knee, ankle, and foot is started to prevent the joints from becoming stiff. The progress of healing is checked regularly by X rays; when it is complete, weight bearing and walking is started gradually.

COMPLICATIONS These include failure of the bone ends to unite or successful fusion of the broken ends at the wrong angle, infection of the bone, or damage to a nerve or artery. All of these complications usually require more surgery. A fracture of the lower end of the shaft can result in permanent stiffness of the knee.

Fenoprofen

A *nonsteroidal anti-inflammatory drug* (NSAID). Fenoprofen is used to relieve pain and stiffness caused, for example, by *rheumatoid arthritis*, *osteoarthritis*, and *gout*. Fenoprofen is also used in the treatment of muscle and ligament sprains; it reduces pain and helps speed recovery.

Ferrous sulfate

An alternative name for iron sulfate (see *Iron*).

Fertility

The ability to reproduce children without undue difficulty.

MALE FERTILITY

A man's fertility depends on the production of normal quantities of healthy *sperm* in the testes, and on the ability to achieve *erection* and to ejaculate *semen* into the vagina during *sexual intercourse*.

F

THE PROCESS OF FERTILIZATION

Fertilization occurs when the head of a sperm penetrates a mature ovum in a fallopian tube. After penetration, the nuclei (which contain the genetic material) of the sperm and ovum fuse, and the body and tail of the sperm drop off. The newly fertilized ovum, called a zygote, then forms an outer layer that is impenetrable to other sperm. The zygote undergoes repeated cell divisions as it passes down the fallopian tube, so that, by the time it reaches the uterus, it has grown into a solid ball of cells called a morula. It then develops an inner cavity with a small cluster of cells to one side; this is called a blastula.

FERTILE PERIOD

Ovulation occurs about halfway through the menstrual cycle (14 to 16 days before the start of a period), after which the released ovum is available for fertilization for about two days. Sperm can also live for approximately two days, so the actual fertile period is about four days.

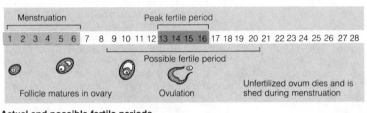

Actual and possible fertile periods
Although the actual fertile period is about four days, the possible fertile period may last seven to 12 days, due to variations in how long the ovum and sperm can survive and the timing of ovulation. The illustration shows the actual and maximum possible fertile periods in a 28-day cycle.

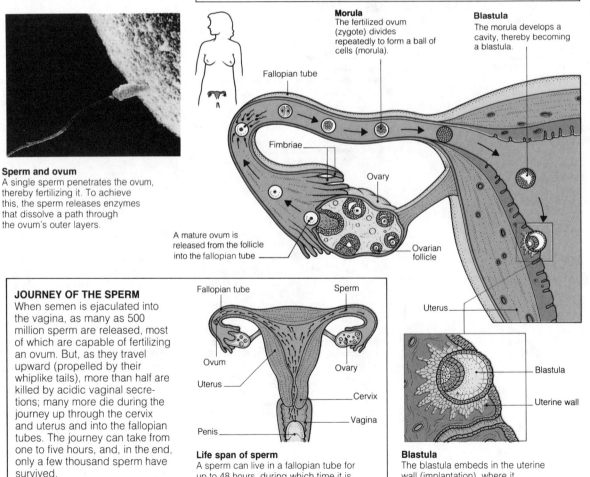

Sperm and ovum
A single sperm penetrates the ovum, thereby fertilizing it. To achieve this, the sperm releases enzymes that dissolve a path through the ovum's outer layers.

Morula
The fertilized ovum (zygote) divides repeatedly to form a ball of cells (morula).

Blastula
The morula develops a cavity, thereby becoming a blastula.

Fallopian tube

Fimbriae

Ovary

A mature ovum is released from the follicle into the fallopian tube

Ovarian follicle

Uterus

Blastula
The blastula embeds in the uterine wall (implantation), where it develops into an embryo and also forms the placenta.

Blastula

Uterine wall

JOURNEY OF THE SPERM

When semen is ejaculated into the vagina, as many as 500 million sperm are released, most of which are capable of fertilizing an ovum. But, as they travel upward (propelled by their whiplike tails), more than half are killed by acidic vaginal secretions; many more die during the journey up through the cervix and uterus and into the fallopian tubes. The journey can take from one to five hours, and, in the end, only a few thousand sperm have survived.

Fallopian tube

Sperm

Ovum

Ovary

Uterus

Cervix

Vagina

Penis

Life span of sperm
A sperm can live in a fallopian tube for up to 48 hours, during which time it is capable of fertilizing an ovum.

The testes—under the influence of *gonadotropin hormones* from the pituitary gland—produce hundreds of millions of sperm. The large output is necessary for normal fertility because only about one in 80,000 sperm ejaculated into the vagina reaches a fallopian tube (see *Fertilization*).

Normal fertility also requires a large proportion of the sperm to be healthy. After ejaculation, the sperm must be able to pass through the hostile environment of acid secretions in the vagina, penetrate a barrier of mucus around the cervix, and swim upward into the fallopian tubes.

Men become fertile at puberty and usually remain so (although to a lesser degree) well into old age.

FEMALE FERTILITY
The ability of a woman to conceive depends on normal *ovulation* (the monthly production of a healthy *ovum* by one of the ovaries) and the egg's unimpeded passage down a fallopian tube toward the uterus, on thinning of the mucus surrounding the mouth of the cervix to enable sperm to penetrate more easily, and on changes in the lining of the uterus that prepare it for the implantation of a fertilized ovum. These processes are in turn dependent on normal production of gonadotropins by the pituitary, and on production of the sex hormones *estrogen* and *progesterone* by the ovaries.

Women become fertile at puberty and remain so until *menopause*, which usually occurs during a woman's 40s or 50s. (See also illustrated box, left; *Fertility drugs*; *Infertility*.)

Fertility drugs
A diverse group of hormonal or hormone-related drugs used to treat female and male *infertility*. In women, fertility drugs may be prescribed when abnormal hormone production by the pituitary gland or ovaries disrupts *ovulation* or causes mucus around the cervix to become so thick that sperm cannot penetrate it. In men, fertility drugs may be used when abnormal hormone production by the pituitary gland or the testes interferes with normal sperm production. (See also *Clomiphene*; *Gonadotropin hormones*; *Infertility*.)

Fertilization

The union of a *sperm* and an *ovum*. In natural fertilization, this occurs after *sexual intercourse* (see box). Fertilization may also occur as a result of semen being artificially introduced into the cervix (see *Artificial insemination*), or may take place in the laboratory (see *In vitro fertilization*).

Fetal alcohol syndrome
A combination of birth defects resulting from high alcohol consumption by the mother during pregnancy.

Even small amounts of alcohol may be harmful in pregnancy, since (like tobacco) alcohol seems to affect fetal growth. The risks of miscarriage and congenital physical defects may also be increased. Fetal alcohol syndrome, however, normally occurs only if there is persistent alcohol consumption during pregnancy. Fetal alcohol syndrome has been reported in babies of women who consistently drank 30 milliliters of alcohol per day (equal to two mixed drinks or two to three bottles of beer or glasses of wine). While there is no evidence that an occasional glass of wine or beer is dangerous, it is best to abstain completely from alcohol during pregnancy.

The affected baby is abnormally short, has small eyes with epicanthic folds (vertical folds of skin extending from the upper eyelid to the side of the nose), and a small jaw. He or she may have a small brain, a cleft palate, heart defects, a dislocated hip, and other joint deformities. As a newborn, the baby sucks poorly, sleeps badly, and is irritable. In effect, he or she is suffering from alcohol withdrawal.

Almost one fifth of affected babies die during the first few weeks of life; many who survive are physically and mentally retarded to some degree. (See also *Alcohol dependence*.)

Fetal circulation
Blood circulates differently in the fetus than it does after birth (see *Circulatory system*). The fetus neither breathes nor eats, so oxygen and nutrients are obtained—via the *placenta* and *umbilical cord*—from the mother's blood. The other fundamental difference in circulation is that blood bypasses the lungs in the fetus.

Oxygen and nutrients enter the fetal blood in the placenta, an organ embedded in the inner lining and wall of the uterus and connected to the fetus by the umbilical cord. The oxygenated blood flows to the fetus along a vein in the umbilical cord, then enters the right atrium (right upper chamber) of the heart, after which, instead of flowing to the lungs, it bypasses them. It does this by passing into the left atrium through a hole called the foramen ovale.

The blood then passes to the left ventricle (left lower chamber), from where it is pumped to the upper parts of the body to provide the tissues with oxygen. It then returns to the heart, flowing into the right atrium and from there into the right ventricle. (After birth, blood pumped from this ventricle passes via the pulmonary artery to the lungs for reoxygenation and elimination of carbon dioxide and other wastes.) However, in the fetus, the blood is only partly deoxygenated at this stage and has more tissues to supply with oxygen. Bypassing the lungs again, it flows from the pulmonary artery into the aorta; it does this through a channel called the ductus arteriosus which, like the foramen ovale, closes after birth.

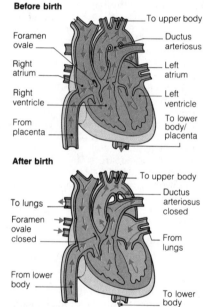

Fetal heart circulation
In the fetus, blood passes from the right atrium of the heart to the left atrium through the foramen ovale. Another channel, the ductus arteriosus, allows blood to pass from the pulmonary artery to the aorta. Both channels close after birth.

The aorta carries the blood to the lower parts of the body, from where, completely deoxygenated, it is carried by two arteries in the umbilical cord to the placenta. There, carbon dioxide and other waste products diffuse into, and are carried away by, the mother's blood and are excreted by the mother.

In rare cases, the foramen ovale or ductus arteriosus fails to close after birth, causing a congenital heart disorder (see *Heart disease, congenital*).

F

Fetal distress

Physical stress experienced by a fetus during labor as the result of not receiving enough oxygen. The most stressful period of labor for a baby is during a contraction, when the uterus tightens to squeeze it out and thus reduces its supply of oxygen from the placenta. If, in addition, there are problems with the labor, such as the mother losing blood or having a pelvis too small for the size of the baby's head, the amount of oxygen reaching the baby may be inadequate.

MONITORING

Fetal distress causes the baby's heart rate to slow, which can be seen as a dip on a cardiotocograph (see *Fetal heart monitoring*). Alternatively, a distressed baby may show no variability in heart rate. This is in contrast to a healthy baby, whose heart rate varies within a normal range of from 120 to 160 beats per minute. The obstetrician keeps a close watch on the heart rate and, if necessary, may obtain a blood sample from the baby's scalp for analysis. High acidity indicates that the baby is not getting enough oxygen. In addition, the fluid around the baby is examined for signs of meconium (fetal feces), which a distressed baby often passes.

DELIVERY

A fetus in distress needs to be delivered promptly—by *cesarean section* if oxygen shortage occurs during the first stage of labor, and by *forceps delivery* or *vacuum extraction* during the second stage.

Fetal heart monitoring

Use of an instrument to record and/or listen to an unborn baby's heart beat during pregnancy and labor. Some form of monitoring of fetal well-being is performed during labor in all hospitals. In its simplest form the nurse or obstetrician uses a special fetal stethoscope to listen to the baby's heart beat. A more sophisticated version is the electronic fetal heart monitor, which is used to make a continuous paper or sound recording of the heart beat.

WHY IT IS DONE

In pregnancy, monitoring is carried out at intervals if tests indicate that the placenta is not functioning normally or if the baby's growth has been slow. Uterine contractions or other stimuli, such as the baby kicking, increases the heart rate in a healthy fetus; the obstetrician can detect this using a fetal heart monitor.

During labor, monitoring can detect *fetal distress*, caused by the baby not receiving enough oxygen. A fetus deprived of oxygen has an abnormal heart rate. Fetal monitoring can detect this abnormality and, at an early stage, allows the attending physician to take appropriate action.

HOW IT IS DONE

An electronic fetal monitor is used to make a continuous recording of the baby's heart beat. The beat is picked up either externally by an ultrasound transmitter strapped to the mother's abdomen or, as an alternative during labor, internally by an electrode attached to the baby's head and linked to the recording device by a wire inserted through the mother's vagina. The fetal heart beat is amplified and heard as a beeping noise or printed as a paper trace. Electronic monitors also have a pressure gauge for measuring and recording contractions. Contractions of the uterus can also be measured by an external gauge that is strapped to the mother's abdomen or by an internal plastic tube that is inserted through the vagina into the amniotic fluid.

ADVANTAGES AND DISADVANTAGES

Electronic fetal monitoring has the advantage of giving the physician a minute-by-minute assessment of the baby's condition. Many obstetricians are convinced that babies are less likely to become hypoxic (deprived of oxygen) during labor with continuous monitoring and therefore feel that the monitoring results in healthier babies.

However, routine electronic fetal monitoring has been controversial for a number of reasons. Critics have claimed that it limits maternal mobility during labor and that it leads to over-diagnosis of fetal distress and therefore to unnecessary cesarean sections. Critics also claim that external monitoring unnecessarily exposes the healthy baby to ultrasound and that internal monitoring may increase the risk of infection during labor without resulting in improvement in the outcome of low-risk pregnancies.

Fetishism

Reliance on special objects for achieving sexual arousal. Fetishism is thought to be rare and restricted to men; because of the nature of the practice, there are no reliable statistics.

The objects need not have an obvious sexual meaning; they include shoes, gloves, rubber or leather garments, and parts of the body such as the feet or ears. It seems that once a particular fetish has led to successful orgasm, it becomes increasingly difficult to obtain sexual satisfaction without it. Nevertheless, many fetishists are able to have a stable sexual relationship, provided their partners join in the practice.

CAUSES

Fetishism usually has no obvious cause, although it may, rarely, result from certain forms of brain damage. According to psychoanalysts, the origin may be a childhood *fixation* of sexual interest upon some aspect of the mother's body or appearance.

TREATMENT

As long as fetishism does not impair sexual or social life, there is no reason for any form of medical interference. Treatment is needed only if the behavior is causing distress or if there are persistent criminal acts, such as stealing underwear.

Fetoscopy

A procedure for directly observing a fetus inside the uterus by means of a fetoscope, a type of *endoscope* (flexible viewing tube). The fetoscope can also be used to take samples of fetal blood and tissue for *biopsy* and to permit treatment of some fetal disorders.

WHY IT IS DONE

Fetoscopy is used to diagnose various congenital abnormalities and genetic defects before the baby is born. Because the technique carries some risks, it is attempted only if there is a higher-than-normal chance that the baby will have some abnormality (for example, if the mother has already had an abnormal baby or if there is a family history of genetic defects).

Fetoscopy allows a close-up look at the developing fetus, particularly the face, limbs, genitals, and spine, and can detect abnormalities, such as spinal column defects, facial clefts, and limb defects. By attaching additional instruments, the fetoscope can also be used to surgically correct some defects, such as certain urinary system disorders. (See also *Amniocentesis*; *Chorionic villus sampling*.)

Fetus

The unborn child from the end of the eighth week after fertilization until birth. For the first eight weeks, the unborn child is called an *embryo*.

The fetus develops in the mother's uterus in a sac filled with *amniotic fluid*, which cushions it against injury. The oxygen and nutrients the fetus needs are supplied through the *placenta*, an organ embedded in the inner wall of the uterus and attached to the fetus by the umbilical cord (see box).

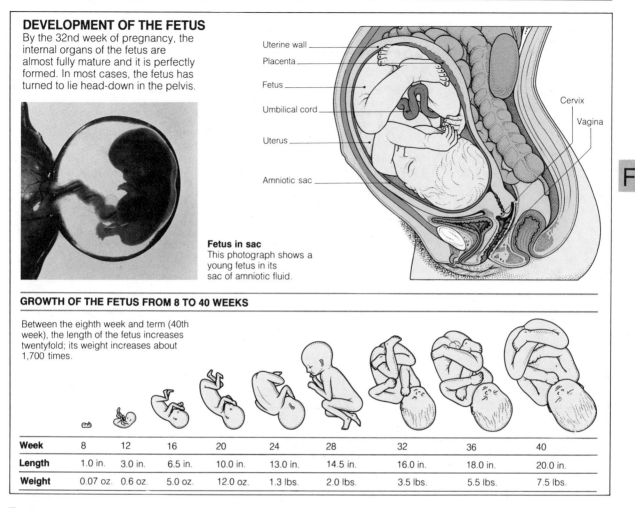

DEVELOPMENT OF THE FETUS

By the 32nd week of pregnancy, the internal organs of the fetus are almost fully mature and it is perfectly formed. In most cases, the fetus has turned to lie head-down in the pelvis.

Fetus in sac
This photograph shows a young fetus in its sac of amniotic fluid.

Uterine wall
Placenta
Fetus
Umbilical cord
Uterus
Amniotic sac
Cervix
Vagina

GROWTH OF THE FETUS FROM 8 TO 40 WEEKS

Between the eighth week and term (40th week), the length of the fetus increases twentyfold; its weight increases about 1,700 times.

Week	8	12	16	20	24	28	32	36	40
Length	1.0 in.	3.0 in.	6.5 in.	10.0 in.	13.0 in.	14.5 in.	16.0 in.	18.0 in.	20.0 in.
Weight	0.07 oz.	0.6 oz.	5.0 oz.	12.0 oz.	1.3 lbs.	2.0 lbs.	3.5 lbs.	5.5 lbs.	7.5 lbs.

Fever

Known medically as pyrexia, a fever is defined as a body temperature above 98.6°F, measured in the mouth, or 99.8°F, measured in the rectum.

A fever may be accompanied by other symptoms, such as shivering, headache, sweating, thirst, a flushed face, hot skin, and faster than normal breathing. In some cases there may be rigors (attacks of severe shivering followed by drenching sweats and a sudden fall in body temperature). Confusion or delirium sometimes occurs with fever, especially in the elderly; a very high fever may also cause seizures or coma.

CAUSES

Most fevers are caused by bacterial or viral infections, such as typhoid, tonsillitis, influenza, or measles. In these cases, proteins called pyrogens are released when the white blood cells of the body's defense system fight the microorganisms responsible for the illness. These pyrogens act on the temperature-controlling center in the brain, causing it to raise body temperature in an attempt to destroy the invading microorganisms.

Fever may also occur in noninfectious conditions, such as dehydration, thyrotoxicosis (a condition that results from overactivity of the thyroid gland), myocardial infarction (heart attack), and tumors of the lymphatic system. Its function is not understood in such cases. (See also *Fever* chart, next page.)

TREATMENT

A physician should be consulted if a fever lasts longer than three days or if there are atypical accompanying symptoms, such as severe headache with stiff neck, abdominal pain, or painful urination. Medical advice is also necessary if the sufferer is a baby less than 6 months old, a child with a history of febrile seizures (see *Seizures, febrile*), or an elderly person.

Antipyretic (temperature-lowering) drugs may be given to treat fevers due to infections; such drugs also help relieve any aches and pains accompanying the fever. Otherwise, treatment is directed toward the underlying cause (for example, giving the appropriate antibiotics for a bacterial infection).

Febrile seizures can often be prevented by cooling the entire body as soon as the fever starts, either in a lukewarm bath or by sponging with lukewarm water.

Fever blister

Also known as a cold sore, a blister caused by the *herpes simplex* virus, usually on the face. The term dates from the preantibiotic era, when such blisters would often appear during feverish infectious illnesses.

F

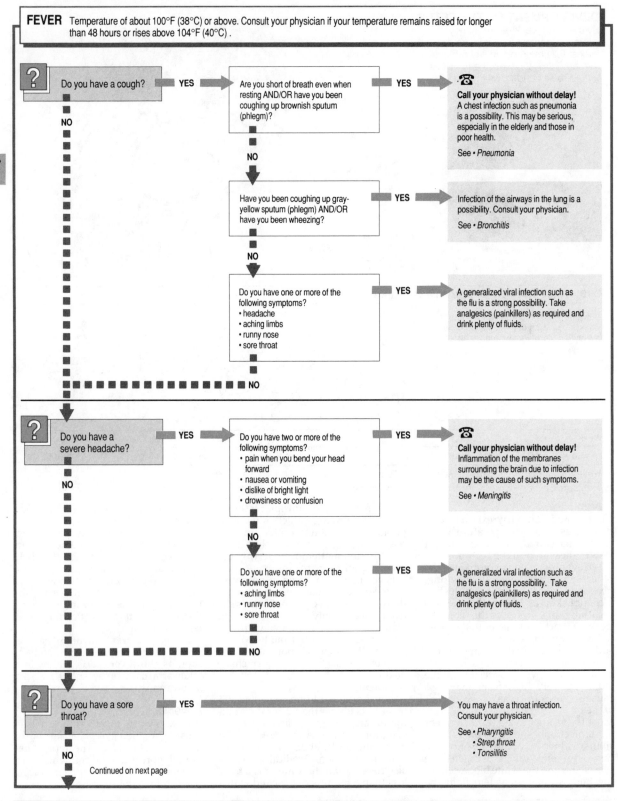

FEVER Temperature of about 100°F (38°C) or above. Consult your physician if your temperature remains raised for longer than 48 hours or rises above 104°F (40°C) .

Do you have a cough? — YES → Are you short of breath even when resting AND/OR have you been coughing up brownish sputum (phlegm)? — YES → ☎ **Call your physician without delay!** A chest infection such as pneumonia is a possibility. This may be serious, especially in the elderly and those in poor health.

See • *Pneumonia*

NO → Have you been coughing up gray-yellow sputum (phlegm) AND/OR have you been wheezing? — YES → Infection of the airways in the lung is a possibility. Consult your physician.

See • *Bronchitis*

NO → Do you have one or more of the following symptoms?
• headache
• aching limbs
• runny nose
• sore throat
— YES → A generalized viral infection such as the flu is a strong possibility. Take analgesics (painkillers) as required and drink plenty of fluids.

NO

Do you have a severe headache? — YES → Do you have two or more of the following symptoms?
• pain when you bend your head forward
• nausea or vomiting
• dislike of bright light
• drowsiness or confusion
— YES → ☎ **Call your physician without delay!** Inflammation of the membranes surrounding the brain due to infection may be the cause of such symptoms.

See • *Meningitis*

NO → Do you have one or more of the following symptoms?
• aching limbs
• runny nose
• sore throat
— YES → A generalized viral infection such as the flu is a strong possibility. Take analgesics (painkillers) as required and drink plenty of fluids.

NO

Do you have a sore throat? — YES → You may have a throat infection. Consult your physician.

See • *Pharyngitis*
• *Strep throat*
• *Tonsillitis*

NO

Continued on next page

F

Do you have one or more of the following symptoms?
• pain in the small or side of the back
• abnormally frequent urination
• pain when passing urine
• pink or cloudy urine

YES →

☎
Consult your physician without delay!
An acute infection of the kidney or bladder may be the cause of this.

See • *Cystitis*
• *Glomerulonephritis*
• *Pyelonephritis*

NO ↓

Have you recently returned from a stay in a hot country?

YES →

☎
Consult your physician without delay!
A tropical disease that is rare in this country is a possibility.

See • *Malaria*
• *Typhoid fever*

NO ↓

Fever in children
A fever is usually caused by infection from a virus or bacterium. However, a child may also become feverish if allowed to become overheated. Do not give aspirin; use an aspirin substitute. A raised temperature causes a child's forehead to feel hot and causes increased sweating and a general feeling of being sick. Normal temperature may vary from 97 to 99°F (36 to 37.5°C). Minor fluctuations within this range are no cause for concern if your child seems otherwise well.

If your baby's temperature rises above 102°F (39°C), whatever the suspected cause, call your physician at once. High temperatures can lead to seizures in some babies.

Have you spent most of the day in strong sunlight or in very hot conditions?

YES →

Exposure to heat may have caused your temperature to rise. In most cases your temperature will return to normal after you have rested for an hour or so in a cool room. Drink plenty of fluids. Call your physician at once if the fever continues to rise.

NO ↓

Are you a woman?

YES →

Have you had a baby within the past two weeks?

YES →

☎
Call your physician without delay!
Puerperal infection, although rare today, is a possible cause of fever after childbirth. It occurs when the uterus and/or vagina become infected after delivery. If, however, you also have pain or redness of the breast, you may have a breast infection.

See • *Breast-feeding*
• *Mastitis*
• *Puerperal sepsis*

NO ↓ (Are you a woman?)

NO ↓ (Have you had a baby...)

Do you have pain in the lower abdomen AND/OR have you had an unusually heavy or unpleasant-smelling vaginal discharge?

YES →

An infection of the uterus AND/OR fallopian tubes is a possible cause of such symptoms.
Consult your physician.

See • *Salpingitis*

NO ↓

If you are unable to make a diagnosis from this chart, consult your physician.

Fiber, dietary

The indigestible components of plants, some of which are fibrous. Dietary fiber includes certain types of polysaccharides, cellulose, hemicelluloses, gums, and pectins, and also lignin (see *Carbohydrates*).

STRUCTURE

Cellulose, hemicelluloses, and lignin form the main structural components of plant cell walls. Pectins and gums are viscous substances in plant sap. Together, these five substances provide the plant with a structure that is stable and partially rigid. Humans do not possess the necessary enzymes to digest these substances. They pass through the digestive system virtually unchanged and are unable to be used as a source of energy. Some of them are fermented by bacteria in the large intestine to produce acids and gas.

FUNCTION

Some components of dietary fiber have the capacity to bind water and add bulk to the feces, which then pass through the intestines more easily, aiding normal bowel function. For this reason, dietary fiber can be effective in treating *constipation* and such disorders as *diverticular disease*. It may also be valuable in the treatment of *irritable bowel syndrome*.

The easiest way to increase the amount of fiber in the diet is to increase the intake of unrefined carbohydrate foods such as whole-grain bread, cereals, and grains, root vegetables, and fruits. (See also *Nutrition*.)

Fiberoptics

The transmission of images through bundles of thin, flexible, glass or plastic threads that propagate light by total internal reflection. This means that all the light from a powerful external source travels the full length of the fiber without losing its intensity.

Fiberoptics has led to the development of *endoscopes*, instruments that enable structures deep within the body to be viewed directly. One bundle of fibers carries light to the far end of the instrument and another bundle transmits the image to the viewer's eye or to a still or video camera. The flexibility of the fibers allows them to be passed through the loops of the large intestine or down through the curve of the stomach and into the duodenum without distorting the image. (See also *Endoscopy*.)

Fibrillation

Localized, spontaneous, rapid contractions of individual muscle fibers.

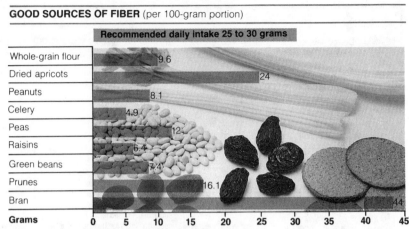

GOOD SOURCES OF FIBER (per 100-gram portion)

Recommended daily intake 25 to 30 grams	Grams
Whole-grain flour	9.6
Dried apricots	24
Peanuts	8.1
Celery	4.9
Peas	12
Raisins	6.4
Green beans	7.4
Prunes	16.1
Bran	44

Essential for the efficient working of the digestive system, fiber is usually eaten as fruit or grains. Among the best sources are bran, apricots, prunes, and whole-grain bread. Eating sufficient fiber in food can reduce constipation.

Unlike *fasciculation* (a similar muscular "quivering"), fibrillation cannot be seen under the skin. It is detected by tests such as an electromyogram (*EMG*) or electrocardiogram (*ECG*).

Fibrillation usually occurs after a nerve that supplies a muscle is destroyed, in which case the affected muscle becomes weak and wastes away. Fibrillation of the heart muscle is caused by disruption of the spread of nerve impulses through the muscle wall of a heart chamber. As a result, the chamber no longer contracts as a single unit; instead, it produces a rapid, irregular rhythm (see *Atrial fibrillation*; *Ventricular fibrillation*).

Fibrinolysis

The breakdown or dissolution of fibrin, the principal component of any blood clot. Fibrin is a stringy protein that is formed in blood from a precursor substance, fibrinogen, as the end product of coagulation. Along with platelets and red blood cells, fibrin forms the final clot that plugs and seals a damaged blood vessel (see *Blood clotting*).

In addition to the coagulation system, blood contains a fibrinolytic system, the end product of which is an enzyme called plasmin, formed from a precursor called plasminogen. Plasmin acts directly to break up fibrin filaments and thus dissolve clots.

The fibrinolytic system is activated in parallel with the coagulation system when a blood vessel is damaged. It helps restrain clot formation in blood vessels (thus helping to prevent clots from blocking blood vessels) and eventually dissolves a clot once a broken blood vessel wall has healed. *Thrombosis* (i.e., the formation of undesirable, persistent blood clots) occurs only if there is a disturbance in the balance between mechanisms that encourage clot formation, such as sluggish blood flow, and those, such as fibrinolysis, that restrain clot formation or dissolve clots.

Fibrinolytic drugs

Drugs used to dissolve blood clots. (See *Thrombolytic drugs*.)

Fibroadenoma

A benign, fibrous tumor found commonly in the breast. Fibroadenomas of the breast are painless, firm, round lumps, usually 0.5 to 2 inches (1 to 5 cm) in diameter, and movable. Fibroadenomas occur most often in women under 30 and are more common in black women. Multiple fibroadenomas may develop in one or both breasts.

Removal is accomplished using either a local or a general anesthetic. After removal, the lump is examined by a pathologist to rule out the small chance of breast cancer.

Fibrocystic breast disease

See *Breast lump*.

Fibrocystic disease

A term that may refer either to the inherited disorder *cystic fibrosis*, characterized by the secretion of abnormal mucus by various glands and by recurrent respiratory infection, or to the presence of single or multiple benign tumors or cysts in the breast (see *Breast lump*; *Mastitis*).

Fibroid

A benign tumor of the uterus. Fibroids consist of smooth muscle bundles and connective tissue that grow slowly within the uterine wall. As the fibroid enlarges, it may grow within the muscle so that the uterine cavity is distorted, or it may protrude from the uterine wall into the uterine cavity but remain attached by a stalk. Fibroids vary from the size of a pea to that of a grapefruit, and several of them may develop simultaneously.

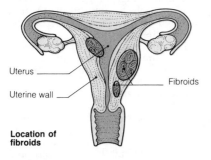

Uterus

Uterine wall

Fibroids

Location of fibroids

INCIDENCE AND CAUSE

Fibroids are one of the most common tumors, occurring in about 20 percent of women over 30. They appear most often in women aged 35 to 45 and seldom before age 20.

The cause of fibroids is unknown, but it is thought to be related to an abnormal response to estrogens. Pregnancy and estrogen hormone replacement therapy can cause fibroids to enlarge; decreased estrogen production after the menopause usually causes them to shrink.

SYMPTOMS

In many cases there are no symptoms, especially if the fibroid is small. If the fibroid grows and erodes the lining of the uterine cavity, it may cause heavy or prolonged menstrual periods; if severe, the bleeding can lead to iron-deficiency *anemia*. Large fibroids may exert pressure on the bladder, causing discomfort or urinary frequency, or on the bowel, causing backache or constipation. Occasionally, a fibroid attached to the uterine wall becomes twisted and causes a sudden pain in the lower abdomen. Fibroids that distort the uterine cavity may cause recurrent miscarriage or infertility.

DIAGNOSIS

Symptomless fibroids are often discovered during a routine pelvic examination. When fibroids are thought to be the cause of menstrual disturbances or responsible for other symptoms, *ultrasound scanning* can confirm the diagnosis.

TREATMENT

Small, symptomless fibroids usually require no treatment, but regular examinations may be necessary to determine if they are growing. Surgery is required for fibroids causing serious symptoms or complications. A *hysterectomy* (removal of the uterus) is sometimes considered if there are large numbers of fibroids. Myomectomy (shelling out the fibroid from its capsule) saves the uterus and is another alternative. Fibroids tend to shrink after the menopause.

Fibroma

A benign tumor of the cells that make up connective tissues (tissues that surround and support specialized structures). For example, a neurofibroma is a tumor of the cells that surround nerve fibers (see *Neurofibromatosis*). An ovarian fibroma is a tumor of the cells that surround the follicles from which ova (eggs) develop. If the tumor is not causing symptoms, treatment is not required.

Fibrosarcoma

A rare, malignant (cancerous) tumor of the cells that make up connective tissue (any tissue that surrounds and supports specialized structures). A fibrosarcoma may develop from a fibroma (a benign tumor) or it may be malignant from the start.

A fibrosarcoma is usually found in the tissues around the muscles in a limb but it can also affect a bone or the cells around nerve fibers. It can spread to damage nearby structures.

A fibrosarcoma causes a localized swelling, which may not be noticed at first, depending on its site and how deep it is. Occasionally, widened veins appear on the skin over the growth; the fibrosarcoma may feel warm or may pulsate.

Treatment is by surgical removal or *radiation therapy*; this may be only temporarily successful if cells from the tumor have spread via the blood to start growths elsewhere.

Fibrosis

An overgrowth of scar or connective tissue (any tissue that surrounds and supports specialized structures). Fibrous tissue may be formed as an exaggerated healing response to injury, infection, or inflammation. It can also result from a lack of oxygen in a tissue, usually due to inadequate blood flow through it—for example, in heart muscle damaged by myocardial infarction (heart attack).

As fibrous tissue replaces specialized structures (such as kidney cells or muscle cells) the function of the organ concerned is impaired and its structure modified.

An overgrowth of fibrous tissue can compress and thus block hollow structures. An example is *retroperitoneal fibrosis*, in which the tubes draining urine from the kidneys (ureters) into the bladder become blocked.

Fibrous tissue formed within a muscle after a tear shortens the muscle and disrupts the normal contraction of fibers. This increases the likelihood of further tears unless the muscle is stretched and exercised.

Fibrositis

Pain and stiffness in the muscles around joints and sometimes in the back. Fibrositis is not a medical term, and some physicians refuse to recognize the condition because investigation usually fails to reveal any inflammation of the muscles. In addition, there is no other detectable reason for the pain in most cases.

Tension and bad posture may cause the condition. It seems to occur more often in anxious people and in those who spend time sitting in a cramped position. Sometimes, an attack occurs after an infection or new exercise. Fibrositis is most common in middle-aged and elderly people.

SYMPTOMS

Pain and stiffness may be felt in the neck, shoulders, chest, buttocks, and knees, as well as in the back. There is usually no restriction of movement. Trigger zones may be felt in the affected muscles and are tender to the touch. In some cases, attacks (which are generally worse in cold, damp weather) are accompanied by exhaustion and disturbed sleep.

TREATMENT

Analgesics (painkillers), hot baths, massage, and relaxation exercises can usually relieve the pain and stiffness.

It is likely that exercises to improve posture, starting with a gradual program to tone the muscles, can help prevent attacks. (See also *Back pain*.)

Fibula

The outer and thinner of the two long bones of the lower leg. The fibula is much narrower than the other bone, the *tibia* (shin), to which it runs parallel and to which it is attached at both ends by ligaments. The top end of the fibula does not reach the knee, but the lower end extends below the tibia and forms part of the ankle.

F

LOCATION OF THE FIBULA
The fibula lies beside the tibia on the outside of each lower leg.

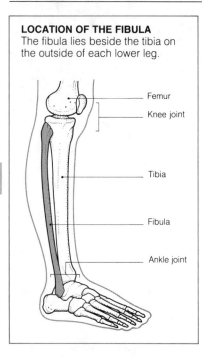

- Femur
- Knee joint
- Tibia
- Fibula
- Ankle joint

The main function of the fibula is to provide an attachment for muscles. It provides little supportive strength to the lower leg, which is why bone can safely be taken from it for grafting elsewhere in the body.

FRACTURE
The fibula is one of the most commonly broken bones. The usual site of fracture is just above the ankle as the result of a violent twisting movement, which can occur in a severe ankle sprain. Rarely, such a fracture of the fibula occurs with dislocation of the ankle, with or without fracture of the tibia (see *Pott's fracture*).

A suspected fracture of the fibula is X rayed; if the diagnosis is confirmed, the lower leg is immobilized in a plaster cast to allow the bone to heal, but, if the fracture occurs in the middle portion of the fibula, no immobilization is necessary for healing. With a severe fracture (especially accompanied by dislocation), surgery may be necessary to fasten together broken pieces of bone with metal pins.

A fractured fibula may take up to six weeks to heal, depending on the severity of the break and the age of the person.

Fifth disease
An infectious childhood disease characterized by a widespread rash. It is also known as slapped cheeks' disease (because it often starts as a dramatic rash on the cheeks) or as erythema infectiosum. Fifth disease is the least well known of five common childhood infections, the other four being *measles*, *mumps*, *chickenpox*, and *rubella* (German measles).

Fifth disease affects young children, usually occurring in small outbreaks in the spring. The cause is a virus known as parvovirus.

SYMPTOMS AND TREATMENT
The rash starts on the cheeks as separate, rose-red, raised spots, which subsequently converge. Within a few days the rash spreads in a lacy pattern over the trunk, buttocks, and limbs. It is often accompanied by mild fever.

The only treatment required is bed rest, plenty of clear fluids, and acetaminophen to reduce any fever. The rash usually clears within 10 days.

Fight or flight response
The physical response when the sympathetic division of the *autonomic nervous system* is aroused. The features are common to all animals, including man, and are a reaction to sensing a threat of any kind. Epinephrine, norepinephrine, and other hormones are released from the adrenal glands and the nervous system, leading to a raised heart rate, dilation of the pupils, the hair standing on end, and increased flow of blood to the muscles. All these responses make the body more efficient in either fleeing or fighting the apparent danger. These physiological changes occur in fear and also in *anxiety* and its disorders.

Filariasis
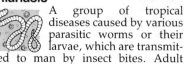
A group of tropical diseases caused by various parasitic worms or their larvae, which are transmitted to man by insect bites. Adult females, which vary in length from three quarters of an inch (2 cm) to 20 inches (50 cm), produce thousands of microfilariae (larvae) that are carried throughout the body in the bloodstream. Blood-sucking insects (primarily certain species of mosquito, fly, and midge) ingest the microfilariae while feeding on blood from infected people and transmit them by biting others.

Filariasis is prevalent in tropical Africa, Indonesia, the South Pacific, coastal Asia, southern Arabia, southern Mexico, and Guatemala.

TYPES AND SYMPTOMS
Some species of worm live in the lymphatic vessels, which they block. This results in localized *edema* (an accumulation of fluid in the tissues, causing swelling). Following repeated infections, the affected area—commonly a limb or the scrotum—becomes enormously enlarged and the skin becomes thick, coarse, and fissured, leading to a condition known as *elephantiasis*.

The larvae of another type of worm invade the eye, causing blindness (see *Onchocerciasis*). A third type, which may sometimes be seen and felt moving just beneath the skin, produces irritating, sometimes painful areas of edema called Calabar swellings.

THE CYCLE OF FILARIASIS
Filariasis is caused by parasitic worms and/or their larvae. There are several stages in the development of this infection as it spreads through the body.

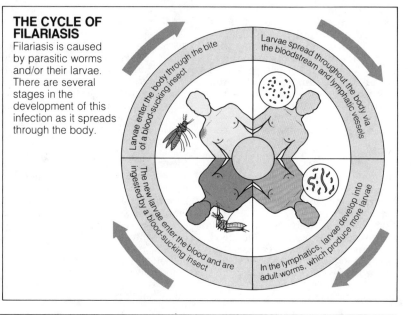

- Larvae enter the body through the bite of a blood-sucking insect
- Larvae spread throughout the body via the bloodstream and lymphatic vessels
- In the lymphatics, larvae develop into adult worms, which produce more larvae
- The new larvae enter the blood and are ingested by a blood-sucking insect

DIAGNOSIS AND TREATMENT

The diagnosis of filariasis is confirmed by microscopic examination of blood or lymph fluid for the presence of microfilariae.

A three-week course of the drug diethylcarbamazine usually cures the infection, but may cause a reaction marked by fever, sickness, and muscle and joint pains.

PREVENTION

Where resources are available, filariasis can be controlled by all persons taking diethylcarbamazine preventively and by the use of insecticides, repellents, nets, and protective clothing to help avoid insect bites. (See also *Roundworms; Guinea worm disease; Insects and disease.*)

Filling, dental

The process of replacing a chipped or decayed area of a tooth with an inactive material. The term is also used to describe the restorative (filling) material itself. Amalgam, a hardwearing mixture of silver, mercury, and other metals, is generally used for back teeth, where the filling will not show. Tooth-colored plastic material, porcelain, or acrylic is more likely to be used for front teeth. Other substances, such as gold, also are used.

WHY IT IS DONE

When enamel is damaged, bacteria can invade the dentin beneath and eventually attack the pulp (blood vessels and nerves), causing the tooth to die. It is therefore preferable to repair teeth at as early a stage as possible—ideally when only the enamel is affected. Filling also restores a tooth to its original shape, which is important not only for appearance but for maintaining a correct bite.

HOW IT IS DONE

If the filling required is large or in a sensitive area, the dentist will numb the surrounding gum with a local anesthetic. Any soft, decayed material is scooped out with sharp instruments. A high-speed drill is used to remove harder material and to shape a hole that will hold the filling securely. While the dentist works, a suction tube placed in the patient's mouth draws away saliva; the cavity is kept as dry as possible with occasional bursts of compressed air.

If the pulp is exposed, the bottom of the cavity is lined with a sedative paste to protect the sensitive pulp from pressure and temperature changes. If one or more of the walls of the tooth is missing because of extensive decay, a matrix (steel band) may be placed around the tooth to support the filling. The dentist then mixes the amalgam (or other filling material), which at first has a gummy consistency, and packs it into the cavity, contouring the surface so that it is smooth. The filling sets sufficiently to allow the matrix to be removed after a few minutes. The amalgam hardens completely over the next 24 hours.

If a front tooth is chipped, the dentist may use a *bonding* technique in which the surface of the tooth is etched with a mild acid solution and plastic or porcelain tooth-colored material is then attached to the roughened surface, shaped, polished, and finished.

OUTLOOK

Amalgam fillings have a limited longevity and may need to be replaced after about 10 years. Occasionally, a filling needs to be replaced earlier—for example, if decay has continued to spread underneath the filling, either because of leakage at the filling margins or due to recurrent decay. Occasionally, fillings are dislodged, usually by chewing on sticky candy, or they fracture as a result of biting.

Film badge

A device that enables hospital staff members to monitor their exposure to radiation. Film badges are worn by those who perform X-ray procedures and radiation therapy to keep their exposure within safe levels.

The badge consists of a piece of photographic film in a holder that is worn on the clothing. The film has a fast (sensitive) emulsion on one side and a slow emulsion on the other. Small doses of radiation blacken the fast emulsion only; higher dosages start to blacken the slow emulsion and make the fast emulsion opaque.

Finger

One of the digits of the hand. Each finger has three phalanges (bones), except for the thumb, which has two. The phalanges join at hinge joints moved by muscle tendons that flex (bend) or extend (straighten) the finger. The tendons are covered by synovial sheaths that contain fluid, to enable the muscles to work without friction. A small artery, vein, and nerve run down each side of the finger. The entire structure is enclosed in skin with a nail at the tip.

DISORDERS

Congenital disorders include *polydactyly* (extra fingers), *syndactyly* (fused

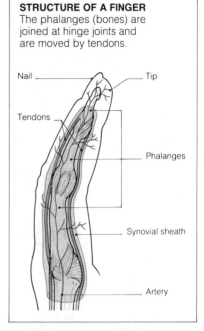

STRUCTURE OF A FINGER
The phalanges (bones) are joined at hinge joints and are moved by tendons.

Nail — Tip

Tendons

Phalanges

Synovial sheath

Artery

fingers), or missing fingers. Sometimes the skin membrane between the fingers is very long and deep, giving an appearance of *webbing.*

Injuries to the finger are common, particularly *lacerations, fractures,* and tendon ruptures. *Baseball finger* occurs when the extensor tendon that runs along the back of the finger is pulled from its attachment following a blow to the fingertip.

Inflammation due to *rheumatoid arthritis* or *osteoarthritis* may affect the finger joints, causing stiffness, pain, swelling, and deformity. The flexor tendons, which run along the front of the fingers, may become inflamed and stuck in the tendon sheath, causing *trigger finger.*

Infections commonly occur in the finger pulp at the tip; *paronychia* (infection of the tissue around the nail) usually follows a minor cut.

Altered control of the muscles in the walls of the vessels and impaired blood supply to the hands and fingers may cause *Raynaud's disease.*

Dactylitis is a term for a spindle-shaped swelling of the fingers that occurs in *sickle cell anemia.* Dactylitis is also an uncommon feature of tuberculosis and syphilis.

Clubbing of the fingers may occur as a sign of chronic lung disease, lung cancer, and some forms of congenital heart disease, especially *tetralogy of Fallot.*

F

Tumors of the finger are rare but may be due to chondromas, which are benign cartilage tumors. (See also *Hand; Nail.*)

Finger joint replacement

A surgical procedure in which artificial joints made of metal, plastic, or silicone rubber are used to replace finger joints destroyed by disease.

WHY IT IS DONE

The main use of the operation is to relieve pain and restore some degree of movement to hands that have been crippled by *rheumatoid arthritis*, which destroys the cartilage, bone, and lining of finger (and other) joints, leaving them weak and unstable.

Less commonly, surgery is performed to relieve pain and improve mobility in joints in which *osteoarthritis* has destroyed the cartilage and created new bone.

HOW IT IS DONE

The operation is performed using an anesthetic. Several joints are usually treated simultaneously.

An incision is made to expose the joint; the ends of the two diseased bones in the joint are cut away, along with diseased cartilage. An artificial joint is then inserted into the bone ends. The tissue covering the joint and the overlying skin are sewn up and the finger is immobilized in a splint until the wound has healed.

RECOVERY PERIOD

The hand is bandaged and held high in a sling to prevent swelling. The stitches are removed after about 10 days, after which the patient is encouraged to move the fingers and return to normal activities. Exercises for the fingers may be required later to maintain function in them.

RESULTS

The procedure is usually successful in relieving pain and enabling the patient to use his or her hands again. However, it can rarely restore normal movement to the hand because joint diseases affect not only bones and cartilage in the joints, but also surrounding tissue that contributes to the flexibility of joints.

Fingerprint

An impression left on a surface by the pattern of fine curved ridges on the skin of the fingertips. The impression is made by minute amounts of sweat from pores in the skin or by ink or some other substance applied to the fingertips. The ridges occur in four main patterns—loops, arches, whorls, and compounds (combinations of the other three). It is on these ridges that fingerprint classification is based.

In law, fingerprints are accepted as a means of identification, since no two people—not even identical twins—have the same fingerprints.

First aid

The treatment of any injury or sudden illness given before professional medical care can be provided.

MINOR INJURIES

Most first aid consists of treating minor injuries, such as small *wounds*, *sprains*, foreign bodies in the eye (see *Eye, foreign body in*), minor *burns*, and *fractures*. Coping with these injuries requires proficiency with *bandages* and *splints*, and in applying *dressings*.

EMERGENCY FIRST AID

The aims of first-aid treatment in an emergency are to preserve life, to prevent the condition from worsening and protect the individual from further harm, to aid recovery, to provide reassurance to victim and family, and to make the ill or injured person as comfortable as possible.

The role of the person giving first aid is to assess the situation, to give immediate and appropriate treatment, and to arrange for the ill or injured person to be seen by a physician or taken to the hospital without delay. Additionally, the person administering first aid should find out as much as possible about the events surrounding the accident or injury from the victim or from bystanders.

If the person is unconscious or losing consciousness, the person giving first aid must first ensure that the airway is clear, that breathing is satisfactory (by checking respiratory rate), and that the circulation is good (by checking pulse and skin color). Airway, breathing, and circulation are easily remembered by the letters ABC.

The *recovery position* helps maintain an open airway in an unconscious person who is breathing. *Artificial respiration* is necessary if a patient is not breathing. *Cardiopulmonary resuscitation* is essential if the person is not breathing and has no heart beat. Any significant *bleeding* must be controlled by the rescuer applying pressure at the appropriate *pressure point*.

No severely injured or ill person should be moved without trained help

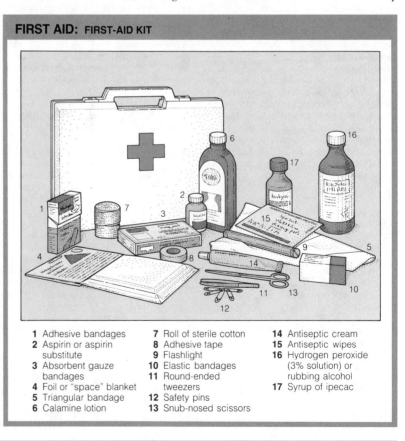

FIRST AID: FIRST-AID KIT

1 Adhesive bandages	**7** Roll of sterile cotton	**14** Antiseptic cream
2 Aspirin or aspirin substitute	**8** Adhesive tape	**15** Antiseptic wipes
3 Absorbent gauze bandages	**9** Flashlight	**16** Hydrogen peroxide (3% solution) or rubbing alcohol
4 Foil or "space" blanket	**10** Elastic bandages	**17** Syrup of ipecac
5 Triangular bandage	**11** Round-ended tweezers	
6 Calamine lotion	**12** Safety pins	
	13 Snub-nosed scissors	

unless life is in immediate danger. This especially applies to anyone with a suspected *spinal injury*. The person should be covered to keep him or her warm, and any tight or constricting clothing should be loosened.

If there are many people injured, the person giving first aid must establish an order of priority for their care. Highest priority is for those who have no pulse, are breathing with difficulty or not at all, are unconscious, or bleeding severely. Such people may die unless immediate treatment is given.

First-aid training is provided by various organizations, which award certificates to those who have attended courses and passed an examination. (See also *Childbirth emergency box; Choking; Drowning; Frostbite; Heat stroke; Hypothermia; Poisoning*. First-aid treatment for specific conditions appears under the appropriate heading—for example, *Epilepsy; Nosebleeds*.)

Fistula

An abnormal passage from an internal organ to the body surface or between two organs.

Fistulas may be congenital (present from birth) or may be acquired as a result of tissue damage. Congenital types include *tracheoesophageal fistulas*, branchial fistulas (see *Branchial disorders*), and thyroglossal fistulas (see *Thyroglossal disorders*). Acquired fistulas may result from injury, infection, or cancer. Some types of arteriovenous fistula (between an artery and a vein) are constructed artificially to provide ready access to the blood circulation, which may be necessary in *dialysis* patients.

Fistulas of the urinary tract, which open from the urethra or bladder to the perineum (the area between the anus and the genitals) usually occur as a complication of radiation therapy to the pelvis or damage caused by a difficult childbirth. Such fistulas may cause urinary *incontinence* or infection.

Fistulas between the intestine and the skin may occur in people with *Crohn's disease* and may also occur as complications of abdominal surgery. The intestinal contents may escape through an opening to the skin or through a surgical wound.

Some types of fistula close spontaneously, but most need to be cut and repaired surgically.

Fitness

Having the capacity for physical work so that normal daily activities can be performed without exhaustion. Fitness depends on strength (the ability to exert force for pushing, pulling, lifting, and other bodily functions), flexibility (the ability to bend, stretch, and twist through a full range of movements), and endurance (the ability to maintain a certain amount of effort for a certain period of time).

HOW FITNESS IS ACHIEVED

Because cardiovascular fitness is the precondition for all other forms of fitness, aerobic exercise, which increases the efficiency of the body's use of oxygen, is the basis for any fitness program. Exercises to develop flexibility and strength should be combined with aerobic exercise for a total fitness program. Although fitness training has cumulative effects that build up over many months (providing there is a sustained increase in activity levels), the effects are specific to the muscles used and the ways in which they are used. A variety of activities is necessary to achieve a general training effect.

BENEFITS OF FITNESS

A person who is fit has a better chance of avoiding *coronary heart disease* and preventing the effects of age and chronic disease. When the body is fit, the maximum work capacity is increased, endurance is increased, and a particular task utilizes a smaller proportion of the work capacity.

The strength, endurance, and efficiency of the heart is also increased by exercise. A fit heart pumps 25 percent more blood per minute when at rest and over 50 percent more blood per minute during physical exertion than an unfit heart. A fit person's heart normally beats 60 to 70 times a minute; an unfit person's heart beats 80 to 100 times per minute. The heart of a fit person works more efficiently than that of an unfit person and is therefore less subject to strain. (See also *Aerobics; Exercise*.)

Fitness testing

A series of exercises designed to determine an individual's level of fitness, primarily cardiovascular fitness and muscle performance.

WHY IT IS DONE

Fitness testing is usually performed to determine a person's level of fitness before starting an exercise program. It also determines whether or not a person will be at risk when starting to exercise, particularly following a heart attack. Fitness testing is also done periodically to assess and monitor progress during an exercise program.

HOW IT IS DONE

The tests are usually carried out by a physician in his or her office or in the outpatient department of a hospital. A physical examination is usually performed, including taking measurements of height, weight, and body fat. Blood and urine tests may be done, including an analysis of blood cholesterol and high-density and low-density lipoprotein content, since high cholesterol levels are related to *atherosclerosis*.

One test involves measuring the performance of the heart during physical work. The heart's efficiency at pumping blood is measured using the pulse rate (number of heart beats) per minute. The more efficient the heart, the slower it works during exercise and the quicker it returns to normal afterward. The pulse is taken at rest, and then the heart performance is measured during exercise at one or more intensities. This exercise may include step climbing, riding a stationary bicycle, or walking or running on a treadmill. After a specific period, the exercise is stopped and the pulse is taken to determine how hard the heart is working at its maximum level. The pulse is usually taken again after a minute to determine how long it takes for the heart beat to return to normal. The blood pressure response to exercise also provides useful information to the physician and patient.

Another type of exercise test involves measuring the overall performance in a standard exercise. This is most suitable for monitoring progress through an exercise program and for setting goals. The test may be based on measuring the distance covered in a fixed time or on the time needed to cover a fixed distance. (See also *Aerobics; Exercise; Fitness*.)

Fixation

A term used by Sigmund Freud to describe the attachment of a person's libido (sexual drive or interest) to real or imagined events during early childhood. Freud suggested that young children go through various stages related to certain parts of the body. In modern psychoanalysis, the stages are viewed within the context of the child's early relationships, starting with the mother. The major stages Freud called the oral, anal, and phallic, because putting things in the mouth, concern about feces, and playing with the penis or clitoris seemed to be prominent forms of behavior (because they are zones of pleasure).

F

EFFECTS

Fixations are unconscious and exist to some extent in all human beings; experiences from childhood are seen as permanently affecting the adult's thoughts and feelings. However, when the fixations are very powerful, resulting from especially traumatic relationships or series of events (experiences), they lead to the sort of repetitive behavior that would be expected from an immature child. Regression (going back) to one of these early stages is thus regarded by some analysts as the underlying cause of certain emotional disorders.

The type and severity depend on the stage regressed to. For example, fixation at the anal stage may be associated with concerns about control (*obsessive-compulsive behavior*), whereas fixation at the phallic stage may be associated with other deviations. Because these fixations are unconsciously repressed, the task of *psychoanalysis* is to uncover them so that patients become aware of the reason for their feelings and reactions.

Flail chest

A type of chest injury, usually resulting from a traffic accident or from violence. In flail chest, multiple rib fractures, usually at the front and side of the chest, produce an isolated portion of the chest wall. This portion moves in when the victim breathes in and moves out when he or she breathes out; this motion is opposite to the normal direction.

The injury may severely impair the efficiency of breathing and result in collapse due to *respiratory failure* and *shock*. It makes breathing and coughing very painful, which can predispose to chest infection and collapse of the lung (see *Atelectasis*).

Emergency treatment consists of turning the person onto the affected side or supporting the flail segment by firm strapping. In the most severe cases, the patient may need immediate admission to an intensive-care unit, where artificial *ventilation* will be performed. This treatment is continued for about 10 days until the ribs are sufficiently healed.

Flatfoot

Lack of an arch in the foot, resulting in the sole resting flat on the ground. The condition, known medically as pes planus, usually affects both feet.

CAUSES

Almost everyone is born with flatfeet. The arches, which then begin to develop from the formation of supportive ligaments and muscles in the soles of the feet, are not fully formed until the age of 6. In some people, however, the ligaments and muscles are weak and the feet remain flat (for unknown reasons). Less commonly, the arches do not form because of a hereditary defect in the structure of the small bones of the foot.

Flatfeet can also be acquired in adult life due to fallen arches, sometimes as a result of a rapid increase in weight. Flatfeet may also be caused by a weakening of the muscles and ligaments that support the arch, which sometimes occurs in a neurological or muscular disease such as *poliomyelitis*.

SYMPTOMS AND TREATMENT

Most flatfeet—due to ligaments and muscles never having developed fully—are usually painless and require no treatment. When the condition is caused by a defect in the foot bones or develops in adult life, the feet may ache when walking or standing. Affected children infrequently require an operation to correct the bones in the feet. In adults, treatment consists of wearing arch supports in the shoes and performing exercises to strengthen the weakened ligaments and muscles.

Flatulence

Expulsion of *flatus* (intestinal gas formed by swallowed air or fermentation) through the anus, sometimes accompanied by abdominal discomfort, which is relieved by the passage of flatus.

In an upright position, most swallowed air passes back up the esophagus to be expelled through the mouth. However, when in a prone position, the air may pass through the intestine and anus instead. Gas formed in the intestine is always passed through the anus.

Flatus

Gas or air in the intestines. Gas is formed in the large intestine as a result of the action of bacteria on carbohydrates and amino acids in digested food; the gas consists of hydrogen, carbon dioxide, and methane. Air in the stomach or intestine is swallowed usually while eating, but also (in anxious people) in times of stress.

Large amounts of flatus do not, as many believe, cause abdominal discomfort; such discomfort is usually due to intestinal sensitivity to normal amounts of flatus (see *Irritable bowel syndrome*; *Flatulence*).

Flatworm

Any species of worm that has a flattened shape—as opposed to a *roundworm* or nematode, which has a cylindrical shape. Flatworms are also sometimes called platyhelminths.

Two types of flatworm are parasites of humans—cestodes (tapeworms) and trematodes (flukes and schistosomes). (See also *Tapeworm infestation*; *Liver fluke*; *Schistosomiasis*.)

Flavoxate

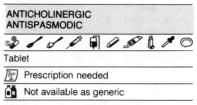

ANTICHOLINERGIC ANTISPASMODIC
Tablet
📄 Prescription needed
🔒 Not available as generic

A drug used to treat the urinary symptoms of *cystitis*, *prostatitis*, and *urethritis*. The underlying disorder is treated with other drugs, usually *antibiotic drugs*.

HOW IT WORKS

Flavoxate works by suppressing muscular activity in the bladder by blocking the action of acetylcholine. As a result, the muscles that control urination relax and the volume of urine that can be held by the bladder increases. The drug also has an analgesic (painkilling) effect.

POSSIBLE ADVERSE EFFECTS

Adverse effects are rare, but may include dry mouth, blurred vision, and constipation.

Flea bites

See *Insect bites*.

Flies

See *Insects and disease*.

Floaters

Semitransparent bodies perceived to be floating in the field of vision. Floaters move rapidly with eye movement but drift slightly when the eyes are still. They do not affect vision.

Most floaters are shadows cast on the retina by microscopic structures in the *vitreous humor*, a jellylike substance that lies behind the lens. In older people, the vitreous humor tends to shrink slightly and detach from the retina, often causing conspicuous floaters, which usually decrease with time.

The sudden appearance of a cloud of dark floaters, especially if accompanied by bright light flashes, suggests *retinal detachment*. A large red floater that obscures vision is usually due to a *vitreous hemorrhage*.

Floppy infant syndrome

A condition in which a baby's muscles lack normal tension or tone. (See *Hypotonia in infants*.)

Floppy valve syndrome

See *Mitral valve prolapse*.

Floss, dental

Soft nylon or silk thread, waxed or unwaxed, used to remove plaque and food particles from between the teeth and around the gum line.

Flow cytometry

An automated test that reveals the arrangement and amount of deoxyribonucleic acid (DNA), or genetic material, within cells as a means of diagnosing malignancy. The pattern of DNA in cancer cells is different from that of normal cells.

The test is helpful in distinguishing benign from malignant cells, and also in monitoring the effects of *anticancer drug* treatment. (See also *Cytology*.)

Flu

See *Influenza*.

Fluctuant

A medical term for the sensation of fluid moving within a swelling as it is palpated (examined by touch). It is a sign that the swelling contains liquid (such as pus in an abscess).

Fluke

A type of flattened worm, also called a trematode, that may infest humans or animals. The two main diseases caused by flukes are *liver fluke* infestation, which occurs worldwide, and *schistosomiasis*, a common and debilitating disease in the tropics.

Fluocinolone

A *corticosteroid drug*. Fluocinolone is prescribed as an ointment to relieve symptoms of skin inflammation, such as itching and redness, caused by *eczema* or another skin disorder.

Fluorescein

A harmless orange-red dye used mostly in ophthalmology. Fluorescein drops are useful for showing up corneal ulcers, which stain bright green. The dye is also used in fluorescein *angiography*, a method of highlighting the details of blood circulation in the

HOW TO USE DENTAL FLOSS

Floss should be used as an adjunct to toothbrushing to remove plaque and food particles from gaps between teeth and around gums. Care should be taken to avoid damaging the gum margins.

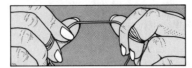

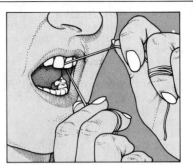

1 Break off a generous length of floss (about 18 inches) and wrap the ends around one finger of each hand. Do not use the same length of floss twice.

2 Holding the floss taut, guide it gently into the gap between the teeth until it reaches the gum line. Then rub the sides of each tooth with the floss using an up-and-down motion.

inside of the back of the eye. For this procedure, a sterile solution of fluorescein is injected into a vein. While the dye is passing through the eye in the bloodstream, photographs are taken of the retina (the innermost layer of the eye) using blue light and a green filter on the camera.

Fluoridation

The addition of fluoride to the water supply as a means of reducing the incidence of dental *caries* (tooth decay). Fluoridation began in the US in the 1940s; since then, water supplies serving 60 percent of the population have been fluoridated.

WHY IT IS DONE

Fluoride has been shown to be effective in helping to prevent dental caries, particularly if the fluoride is ingested while the teeth are forming. Children drinking fluoridated water from birth have up to 65 percent fewer

FLUORIDE AND DENTAL CARIES

Controlled water fluoridation is an effective means of reducing dental caries. Today, 60 percent of the US population drinks from a fluoridated water supply.

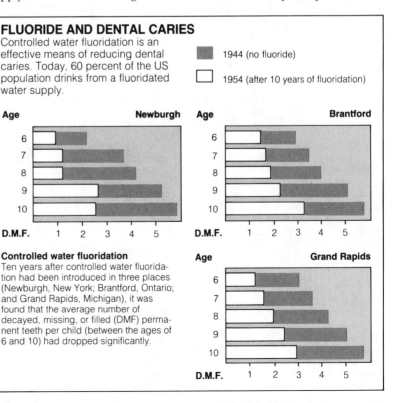

Controlled water fluoridation
Ten years after controlled water fluoridation had been introduced in three places (Newburgh, New York; Brantford, Ontario; and Grand Rapids, Michigan), it was found that the average number of decayed, missing, or filled (DMF) permanent teeth per child (between the ages of 6 and 10) had dropped significantly.

cavities and 90 percent fewer extractions during childhood than their counterparts who have drunk water with less than the recommended fluoride level.

Some areas have naturally high levels of fluoride in the drinking water; in other areas fluoride is added to bring levels up to the recommended standard of 0.7 to 1.2 parts per million, depending on the climate.

SAFETY

Although considerable controversy has surrounded fluoridation programs, there is no evidence that fluoridation at the recommended level has any harmful effects.

Fluoride

A mineral that is useful in helping prevent dental caries (tooth decay). Fluoride is thought to work by strengthening the mineral composition of the tooth enamel, making it more resistant to acid attacks; it may also affect plaque directly, reducing the acid-producing ability of the organisms plaque contains.

Fluoride is most effective when ingested during the formation of teeth, when it becomes incorporated into the tooth substance. It is most beneficial when taken from birth and has a lifelong effect. The water supply may naturally provide adequate amounts of fluoride (the recommended level is 0.7 to 1.2 parts per million) or provide fluoride as a result of *fluoridation*. If the level is inadequate, children can be given fluoride drops or tablets.

Fluoride is also beneficial to both children and adults when applied directly to the teeth. The dentist may treat children's teeth by painting on a fluoride solution or by holding a fitted tray filled with fluoride gel against the teeth for a few minutes. Fluoride mouthwashes and toothpastes are available for daily use at home.

Ingestion of excess fluoride during tooth formation may lead to *fluorosis*, mottling of the teeth that sometimes causes brown discoloration.

Sodium fluoride has been used without FDA approval to treat certain cases of osteoporosis.

Fluorosis

Mottling of the tooth enamel caused by ingestion of excess fluoride during tooth formation. In the most severe cases, mottling is so great that the enamel develops unsightly brown stains. Severe cases usually occur only in people living in areas where the natural level of fluoride in water is many times greater than the recommended level of 0.7 to 1.2 parts per million. Fluorosis can occur in other areas if excessive additional fluoride is consumed—for instance, via the unsupervised use of fluoride tablets.

Mild white mottling of the teeth may occur in a small percentage of children ingesting water at the recommended level, but this form of fluorosis does not cause discoloration or impair appearance.

Fluorouracil

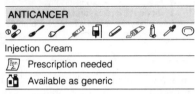

ANTICANCER
Injection Cream
Prescription needed
Available as generic

An anticancer drug used in the treatment of cancers of the breast, bladder, ovary, stomach, and intestine.

Fluorouracil in cream form is used to treat some types of skin tumor, such as *keratosis* and *basal cell carcinoma*. It is used especially when several tumors occur together, making surgical removal difficult.

POSSIBLE ADVERSE EFFECTS

Fluorouracil may cause nausea, vomiting, diarrhea, hair loss, and impaired production of blood cells. Applied as a cream, it can cause inflammation of the skin.

Fluphenazine

One of the phenothiazine group of *antipsychotic drugs* used to relieve the symptoms of disorders such as *schizophrenia*, *mania*, and *dementia*. Fluphenazine (given as a tablet, liquid, or by injection) suppresses confused or abnormal behavior and has a tranquilizing effect.

Flurazepam

A *benzodiazepine drug* used in the treatment of *insomnia*.

Flush

See *Blushing*.

Foam, contraceptive

See *Spermicide*.

Folic acid

A vitamin essential to the production of red blood cells by the bone marrow. Folic acid is contained in a variety of foods, particularly liver and raw vegetables; adequate amounts are usually obtained from a well-balanced diet.

During pregnancy, folic acid plays an important part in fetal growth—in the development of the nervous system and in the formation of blood cells. During the last three months of pregnancy, folic acid tablets may be necessary to supplement the diet.

Folic acid deficiency is a cause of megaloblastic *anemia*, which causes symptoms such as fatigue, depression, and pallor.

Folk medicine

Any form of medical treatment based on the beliefs of a particular society. Examples include the charming of warts, the use of copper bracelets for the treatment of rheumatism, and the piercing of ears to improve the eyesight. What these remedies have in common is their support by belief within the culture and their lack of reliance on a practitioner. By contrast, the diagnostic and healing techniques used by a witch doctor are known as traditional medicine; those used by a chiropractor or a homeopathist are known as *alternative medicine*.

Follicle

A small cavity in the body. One example is a hair follicle, a pit on the surface of the skin from which a hair grows. Another is an ovarian follicle, one of the many fluid-filled cavities in the female ovary from which an ovum (egg) develops.

Follicle-stimulating hormone

A *gonadotropin hormone* (one that stimulates the gonads—the ovaries and testes) produced by the anterior part of the pituitary gland; also known by its initials, FSH.

Folliculitis

 Inflammation of one or more hair follicles as a result of infection with *STAPHYLOCOCCUS* bacteria. Folliculitis may occur almost anywhere on the skin. It commonly is found on the neck, thighs, buttocks, or armpits, causing a boil, or it may affect the bearded area of the face, which leads to the development of pustules (see *Sycosis vulgaris*).

Treatment is with antibiotics. The infection often spreads from an infected person to the rest of the family. To prevent this or to control an outbreak, each person should shower frequently and use a separate washcloth and towel; clothes worn next to the skin should be washed daily in boiling water.

Fomites

Inanimate objects, such as clothing, books, bed linen, or a telephone receiver, that are not harmful in themselves, but which may be capable of harboring bacteria, viruses, parasites, or other harmful organisms and thus may convey an infection from one person to another.

Fomites mainly transmit respiratory infections, such as influenza.

Fontanelle

One of the two soft areas on a baby's scalp, a membrane-covered gap between the bones of the skull. At birth the skull bones are not yet fully fused and there are spaces between them. The only gaps of any size are the anterior (front) fontanelle, which is diamond-shaped, about 1 inch (2.5 cm) across, and usually closes up by the age of 18 months, and the posterior (rear) fontanelle, which is triangular, about 0.25 inch (0.6 cm) across, and closes within about two months of birth.

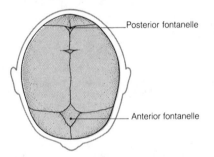

Location of the fontanelles
Two soft areas on the baby's skull—the anterior fontanelle is diamond-shaped, the posterior fontanelle is triangular.

DISORDERS

It is normal for the fontanelles to bulge and become tense when a baby cries. However, persistent tension at other times may indicate an abnormality, particularly *hydrocephalus* (an accumulation of fluid within the baby's skull). A sunken fontanelle may be a sign of *dehydration*. If a fontanelle is abnormally large or takes a long time to close, it may be due to *rickets* or a brain abnormality. Early closure of the fontanelles results in a deformity called *craniosynostosis*.

Occasionally, a third fontanelle is present between the other two; this occurs most commonly in *Down's syndrome*. Some babies have extra bones in the anterior fontanelle; this is normal. The extra bones fuse into the skull when the gap closes.

Food additives

Any substance that is added to food to perform a technological function. Contrary to popular belief, not all additives are artificial; sugar and salt are probably the most common.

Before any additive is accepted for use in food processing, the need for the additive must be proved and its safety assessed by the *Food and Drug Administration* (FDA).

TYPES AND USES

Additives fall into four main groups: those that preserve food and affect its "keeping" quality, those that affect texture, those that affect appearance and taste, and miscellaneous additives, such as rising and glazing agents, flour "improvers," and antifoaming agents.

Preservatives, such as sodium nitrate, are added to food to control the growth of bacteria, molds, and yeasts, especially those that might contaminate the food after it has left the manufacturer. Other additives, such as antioxidants, improve the keeping quality of the food by preventing undesirable changes (such as by stopping rancidity in foods containing fat).

Additives that improve food texture include emulsifiers, stabilizers, thickeners, and gelling agents. They alter the "mouth feel" and consistency of food. Lecithin, which occurs naturally in all animal and plant cells, is an emulsifier added to margarine to prevent separation.

Appearance and taste are often improved by the use of colorings, flavorings, sweeteners, and flavor enhancers. Colors and flavors are used mainly to compensate for losses during processing, to strengthen existing colors or flavors, and to ensure standardization in products. *Artificial sweeteners*, such as saccharin and aspartame, are used in place of sugar, especially in products designed for diabetics and weight control.

RISKS

All food additives are carefully monitored and regulated; there is no evidence that any additives in general use can harm the population as a whole. However, even though an additive may be harmless to most people, it may produce an allergic reaction in others. The best known flavor enhancer, *monosodium glutamate* (MSG), often causes *Chinese restaurant syndrome*, with reactions similar to a migraine. Tartrazine, a widely used yellow food coloring, produces an allergic reaction in a significant number of people.

Additives are often blamed for causing hyperactivity in children, but most physicians believe that, although this is true for a very small number of children, the majority of hyperactive children are not allergic to food additives. Foods containing nitrites and nitrates have been alleged to be involved with causing certain cancers (e.g., stomach cancer).

Food allergy

An inappropriate or exaggerated reaction of the *immune system* to a food. Sensitivity to cow's milk protein is a common food allergy in young children. Other foods most commonly implicated in food allergy include wheat, fish, shellfish, and eggs.

Food allergy is more common in people who suffer other forms of allergy or hypersensitivity, such as asthma, allergic rhinitis (hay fever), and dermatitis.

Immediate reactions, occurring within an hour or sometimes minutes of eating the trigger food, include lip swelling, tingling in the mouth or throat, vomiting, abdominal distention, *borborygmi* (audible bowel sounds), and diarrhea.

The only effective treatment of food allergy is to strictly avoid eating the offending food.

Food and Drug Administration

Part of the US Department of Health and Human Services, the Food and Drug Administration (FDA) monitors the safety of foods and cosmetics, and the radiation hazards of TV sets and microwave ovens. Most important, it determines, before general distribution, the safety and effectiveness of drugs and medical devices (such as insulin pumps).

Food-borne infection

Any infectious illness caused by eating food that has been contaminated with viruses, bacteria, worms, or other organisms.

CAUSES

There are two main mechanisms by which food can become infected.

First, many animals that are kept or caught for food may harbor disease organisms in their tissues or internal organs. If meat or milk from such an animal is eaten without being thoroughly cooked or pasteurized, the organisms may cause illness in their human host. In the US, the only common infection of this type is *food poisoning* from improperly cooked poultry, meat, fish, or shellfish.

F

Second, food may be contaminated with disease organisms spread from an infected person or animal—usually from their excrement (such as by flies moving from feces to food).

PREVENTION

In developed countries, food-borne infections are controlled or prevented by adequate sanitation and sewage treatment; by multiple laws and regulations that govern animal husbandry, the production of food in farms and factories, and its subsequent storage and distribution; and by generally high standards of personal hygiene with regard to handling and eating of food.

In some less affluent parts of the world, many of these controls do not exist and the chances of a food-borne infection are thus much higher. When visiting such countries, it is wise to avoid certain foods, particularly salads, any meat or fish that looks suspect or not thoroughly cooked, shellfish, milk, butter, cream, and ice cream. Raw fruits and vegetables are generally safe once the exterior peel or skin has been removed.

Immunization is available against certain food-borne and water-borne infections, such as typhoid and cholera, but it usually provides only partial protection and is no substitute for good food hygiene. (See also *Water-borne infection*.)

Food fad

A like or dislike of a particular food or foods that is carried to extremes. It may lead to an undue reliance on, or avoidance of, a particular foodstuff.

Fads are particularly common in toddlers and adolescents and in those under stress. For most people, food fads are not serious since they are either short-lived or restricted to a limited number of foods. However, when food fadism or food aversion has an obsessional quality about it, or is persistent, it may be indicative of a more serious eating disorder. (See also *Anorexia nervosa*; *Bulimia*.)

Food intolerance

A reproducible, adverse reaction to a food or food ingredient that is not caused either psychologically or by *food poisoning*.

CAUSES AND INCIDENCE

Food intolerance is mainly of unknown cause, but is sometimes due to various unknown irritants, toxins,

INFECTED ANIMAL PRODUCTS

Some animals harbor disease organisms (e.g., bacteria, worms, and parasites) in their tissues and these may cause infection if meat or milk is consumed raw or improperly cooked. Beef, pork, and fish tapeworm infestations, salmonella poisoning, and (rarely) brucellosis can be transmitted in this way.

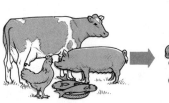

1 Cows, pigs, poultry, fish, and particularly shellfish are sources of bacterial, viral, or worm infection or infestation.

2 Adequate milk pasteurization and inspection of meat and fish before sale prevents most infections and infestations of this type.

3 Thorough thawing, preparation, and cooking of meats, fish, shellfish, and poultry further reduces the risk of infection.

FOOD CONTAMINATION

Intestinal infections may be spread from person to person if organisms in feces contaminate food, directly or indirectly. This can occur if vegetable crops are sprayed with sewage, if flies settle on feces and then on food, or if food is handled by a person who has not washed his or her hands.

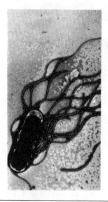

Contaminating organism
The photograph (left) taken through an electron microscope shows a typical SALMONELLA bacterium. The organism uses its many flagellae (whiplike structures) to move. SALMONELLA is a common contaminant of poultry, eggs, and egg products and causes severe food poisoning.

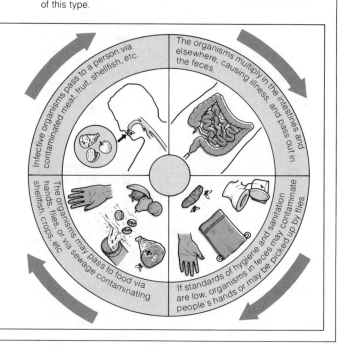

or *food additives*. It may be associated with an adverse reaction to foods such as green peppers, fried foods, or onions. Food intolerance can be caused by an inborn or acquired biochemical defect, such as *lactase deficiency* (an inability to digest milk sugar found more commonly in blacks, Asians, Indians, and people of Mediterranean origin).

Food poisoning

A term used for any illness of sudden onset, usually with stomach pain, vomiting, and diarrhea, suspected of being caused by food eaten within the previous 48 hours. Most cases are the result of contamination of food by bacteria or viruses.

Food poisoning is usually suspected when, for example, several members of a household (or customers at a restaurant) become ill after eating the same food.

TYPES AND CAUSES

Food poisoning can be classified, according to cause, into infective and noninfective types. Some foods can cause poisoning of either type. For example, shellfish such as mussels, clams, and oysters can become contaminated by viruses or bacteria, by toxins acquired from poisonous plankton (tiny marine animals and plants), or by chemical pollutants in the water.

BACTERIAL CAUSES The bacteria most commonly responsible for food poisoning belong to a group called salmonella, certain strains of which are able to multiply rapidly in the intestines to cause widespread inflammation. Some farm animals, especially poultry, commonly harbor such bacteria. If frozen poultry is not completely thawed before being cooked, it is liable to cause poisoning.

Salmonella bacteria may also be transferred to food from the excrement of infected animals or people, either by flies or by the handling of food by an infected person—especially if the hands have not been washed after using the toilet. If contaminated food is left for any time in warm conditions, a large colony of bacteria may develop without obvious food spoilage.

Other bacteria cause the formation of toxins that may be difficult to destroy even with thorough cooking. Toxin-forming strains of staphylococcal bacteria, for example, may spread to food from a septic abscess on a food-handler's skin. *Botulism* is a rare, life-threatening form of food poisoning

caused by a bacterial toxin and associated with home preservation of food.

VIRAL CAUSES The viruses that most commonly cause food poisoning are Norwalk virus (a common contaminant of shellfish) and rotavirus. They cause food poisoning when raw or partly cooked foodstuffs have been in contact with water contaminated by human excrement.

NONINFECTIVE CAUSES include poisonous mushrooms and toadstools (see *Mushroom poisoning*), and fresh fruit and vegetables that have been accidentally contaminated with high doses of insecticide. Chemical poisoning can also occur if food has been stored in an unsuitable container—for example, if a container that has previously held a poison is used to store food, or if acidic fruit juice is kept in a metal container made partly of zinc.

Various exotic foods (for example, the puffer fish, considered a delicacy in Japan, or cassava, a staple food in many tropical countries) can also cause moderate to lethal poisoning if improperly prepared and cooked.

SYMPTOMS

The onset of symptoms varies according to the cause of poisoning. The symptoms usually develop within 30 minutes in the case of chemical poisoning, between one and 12 hours in the case of bacterial toxins, and between 12 and 48 hours with virus and salmonella infections. Symptoms vary considerably according to how heavily the food was contaminated, but usually include nausea, vomiting, diarrhea, stomach pain, and, in severe cases, *shock* and collapse.

The symptoms of botulism are markedly different, with nervous system symptoms such as difficulty speaking, visual disturbances, muscle paralysis, and vomiting.

DIAGNOSIS

The diagnosis of bacterial food poisoning can usually be made from a culture of a sample of the person's vomit or feces. Chemical food poisoning can often be diagnosed from a description of what the person has eaten within the previous few hours, and from analysis of a sample of the suspect food, if available.

FIRST AID AND TREATMENT

If severe vomiting and diarrhea suddenly develop (or if a person collapses), medical assistance should be sought. Samples of any food left from a recent meal should be kept; they may help pinpoint the cause and possibly prevent a widespread outbreak of food poisoning.

If poisoning by a chemical or bacterial toxin is suspected, gastric *lavage* (washing out the stomach) may be carried out. Otherwise, treatment in a hospital is directed primarily toward preventing dehydration by replacing fluids intravenously.

Milder cases can be treated at home. The affected person should eat no solid food but should drink plenty of fluids, which should include some salt and sugar to replace what is being lost (see *Rehydration therapy*).

Except for botulism and some cases of mushroom poisoning, most food poisoning is not serious. Recovery generally occurs within three days.

PREVENTION

Some simple measures can virtually eliminate the chances of food poisoning. Hands should always be washed before handling food, and fresh vegetables and fruit rinsed in clean water. Cutting boards and implements used on raw meat should also be rinsed before they are used on other food. Frozen poultry should always be completely thawed before cooking and then should be well cooked.

Ask for advice on the preparation of any food unfamiliar to you at the point of sale. Suspect items—such as mussels that do not open when boiled, bulging tin cans, or any food that smells or looks obviously spoiled—should be rejected. Finally, people who preserve food at home should take care to sterilize food thoroughly by heating it in a pressure cooker at 250°F (120°C) for 30 minutes.

Foot

The foot has two vital functions—to support the weight of the body in standing or walking and to act as a lever to propel the body forward.

STRUCTURE

One of the bones of the foot is the calcaneus (heel bone); it is jointed with the talus, the second largest bone of the ankle. In front of the talus and calcaneus is a series of smaller bones—the navicular, cuboid, and cuneiform. These in turn are jointed with five long bones called the metatarsals. The phalanges are the bones of the toes; the big toe has two phalanges, all the other toes have three.

Tendons passing around the ankle connect the muscles that act on the various bones of the foot and toes. The main blood vessels and nerves pass in front of and behind the inside of the ankle joint to supply the foot. The undersurface of the normal foot forms a natural arch that is supported by

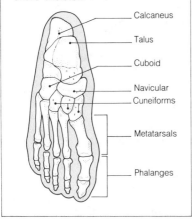

SKELETON OF THE FOOT
The calcaneus is attached to the talus above. In front are the navicular, cuboid, and cuneiform bones, which are attached to the metatarsals. Phalanges form the toes. An adult has 26 bones in each foot—one eighth of the total number in the entire skeleton.

Calcaneus

Talus

Cuboid

Navicular

Cuneiforms

Metatarsals

Phalanges

ligaments and muscles. Fascia (fibrous tissue) and fat form the sole of the foot, which is covered by tough skin.
DISORDERS
Injuries to the foot commonly result in *fracture* of the metatarsals and phalanges. The calcaneus may fracture following a fall from a height onto a hard surface.

Deformities of the foot are fairly common and include *talipes* (clubfoot), *flatfoot*, and *clawfoot*. Another common deformity is a *bunion*, which is a *bursa* (fluid-filled pad) overlying the joint at the base of the big toe.

A number of disorders can affect the skin of the foot. *Corns*, small areas of thickened skin on a toe, are usually caused by tight-fitting shoes. *Plantar warts* appear on the skin on the sole, while *athlete's foot*, a fungal infection, mainly affects the skin between the toes, causing it to become itchy, sore, and cracked.

Gout, a fairly common type of arthritis, often affects the joint at the base of the big toe or one of the joints in the foot. *Ingrown toenail* commonly affects the nail of the big toe, causing inflammation of the surrounding tissue and *paronychia* (infection of these tissues). *Footdrop*, the inability to raise the foot properly, is due to damage to the muscles in the leg that perform this movement or the nerves that supply these muscles.

Footdrop
A condition in which the foot cannot be raised properly. It hangs limp from the ankle joint, causing it to catch on the ground when walking.
CAUSES
Neuritis (inflammation of a nerve) affecting the nerves that supply muscles that move the foot is a common cause of footdrop; it may be due to *diabetes mellitus*, *multiple sclerosis*, or certain neuropathies (see *Neuropathy*). Pressure on a nerve root as it leaves the spinal cord due to *disk prolapse* or, rarely, a tumor can also cause weakness in the foot muscles.
TREATMENT
The underlying cause is treated, but in many people the weakness persists. A footdrop splint (see *Brace, orthopedic*) can keep the foot fixed in position when walking.

Foramen
A natural hole or passage in a bone or other body structure, usually to allow the passage of nerves or blood vessels. The foramen magnum is the large opening in the base of the skull through which the spinal cord passes.

Forceps
A tweezerlike instrument used for handling tissues or equipment during surgical procedures. Various types of forceps are designed for specific purposes. For example, forceps used for holding or removing wound dressings have scissor handles to make manipulation easier. Tissue forceps have fine teeth at the tip of each blade so that tissues can be handled delicately during operations. (See also *Forceps delivery*; *Forceps, obstetric*.)

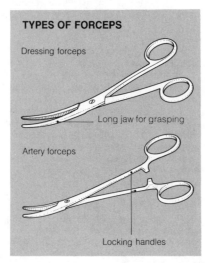

TYPES OF FORCEPS

Dressing forceps

Long jaw for grasping

Artery forceps

Locking handles

Forceps delivery
The use of forceps (see *Forceps, obstetric*) by an obstetrician to ease out the baby's head during a difficult birth (see also *Childbirth*). *Vacuum extraction* may be used as an alternative.
WHY IT IS DONE
Forceps delivery is used if the mother is overtired or unable to push out her baby unaided, or if the baby is showing signs of *fetal distress*. (If fetal or maternal distress occurs before the second stage of labor begins, a *cesarean section* rather than a forceps delivery is necessary.)

Forceps are used to control the head in *breech delivery* (with the baby's buttocks first) to prevent a too-rapid delivery. Forceps are also used if the baby's head is stuck in the middle of the mother's pelvis and needs to be rotated before delivery is possible. Called a midforceps delivery, this requires extreme skill on the part of the obstetrician; a cesarean section may be performed instead.
HOW IT IS DONE
The mother is given an analgesic (painkiller) and either local or *epidural anesthesia*. She then lies on her back, with her legs raised in stirrups, and her bladder is emptied with a catheter. The obstetrician then examines the mother. Forceps can be applied only if the cervix (neck of the uterus) is fully dilated and the baby's head is engaged in the pelvis. An *episiotomy* (making of a small cut in the perineum) is usually performed before a forceps delivery.

The forceps blades are placed on either side of the infant's head, just in front of the ears. If the baby's chin points downward, gentle traction is applied to the forceps and the baby delivered. If the chin is pointing sideways or upward, rotation of the head is necessary before traction can be applied; in such cases, rotation forceps are used.
RECOVERY PERIOD
After a forceps delivery, care is similar to that following a spontaneous (unassisted) vaginal delivery. Sometimes there is greater bruising of the perineum, but this usually heals rapidly and can be eased by the application of ice packs. After a forceps delivery, the baby may have forceps marks on the face. They disappear after a few days. The length of stay in the hospital is usually the same as after a delivery without forceps.

Forceps, obstetric
Surgical instruments used to deliver the head of a baby in a difficult labor.

OBSTETRIC FORCEPS
The two wide, blunt blades are designed to fit around the baby's head. The handles lock together so that the blades are held apart.

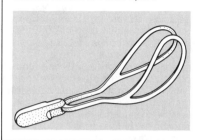

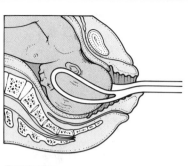

Positioning
The forceps blades lie along the sides of the baby's head, just in front of the ears.

The first obstetric forceps were invented about 300 years ago by the obstetrician Peter Chamberlen. They were kept as a family secret for use on private patients, and were not in common use until about 100 years later.

Obstetric forceps consist of two blades that cup the baby's head. Each blade is joined to a separate handle and the two handles are fitted together; when assembled, the blades are separated by a fixed distance (see illustrated box).

Foreign body
Any object in an organ, opening, or passage of the body that should not be there. It may enter accidentally (by inhalation or swallowing, for example) or it may be deliberately introduced. Common sites include the airways (see *Choking*), ear (see *Ear,*

foreign body in), eye (see *Eye, foreign body in*), rectum, urethra, and vagina. A metallic, glass, or wood splinter that embeds in the subcutaneous tissue is also a foreign body.

Foreign medical graduate
Graduates of non-US medical schools, even if US citizens. Foreign medical graduates (FMGs) may qualify for training in US residency programs and for subsequent licensing after successfully passing a test of language and medical skills.

Forensic medicine
The branch of medicine concerned with the law, especially criminal law. The forensic pathologist is a physician who specializes in the examination of bodies when circumstances suggest death was unnatural (i.e., suicide, homicide, or an accident). The examination usually includes an assessment of the time of death (from data such as the temperature of the corpse and its state of decomposition), deduction of the likely nature of any weapon used (from study of the injuries), and matching of blood, hair,

F

COMMON FOREIGN BODIES IN CHILDREN
Children constantly experiment with objects in the environment. They frequently place small objects into their mouths, noses, or ears. As a result, a swallowed or stuck foreign body is a common occurrence. It is wise to keep all small objects well out of reach of children.

Ear and nose
Attempting to remove a foreign body from the ear can be dangerous because of the risk of pushing the object further in. The physician uses a syringe, suction, or forceps. A foreign body in the nose may be taken out with tweezers by the physician; an older child may be able to blow it out while the other nostril is blocked.

Lungs
Inhaled objects such as peanuts or teeth may become lodged in the bronchi and cause obstruction of air flow, resulting in pneumonia or lung collapse. Symptoms may include choking, coughing, and breathing difficulty. The child should *not* be inverted, slapped on the back, or made to vomit, but should be taken to the hospital immediately.

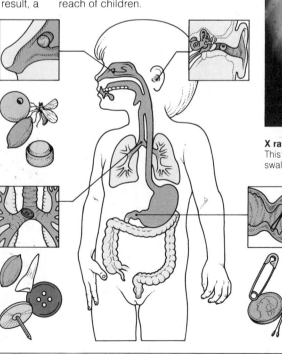

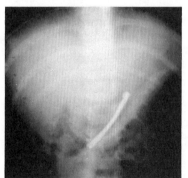

X ray of foreign body
This X ray shows that the child has swallowed a closed hair barrette.

Stomach
Foreign bodies in the stomach include coins, batteries, marbles, and buttons. Most small, smooth objects pass safely out of the body in feces, but an object that has failed to pass through the body after seven to ten days usually requires removal. Batteries should be removed surgically because they release acid that seriously damages the digestive tract.

F

and skin from the victim with those on any weapons, on the clothing of suspects, or on parts of an automobile.

Forensic pathologists may also be asked to examine victims of alleged sexual assault or child abuse. They also consult in cases of attempted poisoning and possible drug deaths.

Forensic scientists use laboratory methods to study body fluids (such as blood, semen, and saliva) found on or near the victim and compare the fluids with those from suspects. They are also trained in ballistics and the identification of fibers from clothing.

In addition, forensic scientists may advise on blood grouping (see *Blood groups*) in cases of disputed paternity.

Foreskin

The popular name for the prepuce, the loose fold of skin that covers the glans (head) of the penis when it is flaccid and which retracts during erection.

At birth, the foreskin is attached to the glans, but, after the age of 6 months, it gradually separates from the glans. In some boys, the foreskin remains tight until the age of 3 or 4, making retraction difficult or impossible. However, unless this causes recurrent infection (by preventing adequate cleaning of the glans) or prevents normal urination, there is no need to consult a physician and no attempt should be made to force the foreskin back.

In some societies, the foreskin is routinely removed from newborn boys, an operation called *circumcision*, usually for religious or hygienic reasons. Circumcision may be performed at any age as a treatment for disorders of the foreskin.

DISORDERS

In *phimosis*, the foreskin remains persistently tight after the age of 5, causing difficulty in urination and ballooning of the foreskin. There may be recurrent *balanitis* (infection and inflammation of the glans and foreskin). Erection is often painful, which is why the condition is frequently discovered only at puberty.

In the related disorder *paraphimosis*, the foreskin becomes stuck in the retracted position, causing painful swelling of the glans.

Forgetfulness

See *Memory*.

Formaldehyde

A colorless, pungent, irritant gas. In medicine, a solution of formaldehyde and a small amount of alcohol in water—a preparation known as formalin—is used to preserve tissue specimens or to harden them (a procedure called fixation) before they are stained and examined. Formalin is also used as a *disinfectant*.

Formication

An unpleasant sensation, as if ants were crawling over the skin. It is an uncommon symptom, most often resulting from abuse of cocaine or similar drugs. Formication should be distinguished from a paranoid *delusion* in which people falsely believe they are infested by ants or worms. In either case, a rash may result from excessive scratching and lead in rare cases to a misleading diagnosis of a skin disease.

Formula, chemical

A way of expressing the constituents of a chemical in symbols and numbers. Every known chemical substance has a formula. Water, for example, has the formula H_2O, indicating that it is composed of two hydrogen atoms (H_2) and one oxygen atom (O).

Fracture

A break in a bone, most commonly caused by a fall. A bone is usually broken directly across its width, but can also be fractured lengthwise, obliquely, or spirally.

TYPES OF FRACTURE

Fractures are divided into two main types: closed (or simple) and open (or compound). In a closed fracture the broken bone ends remain beneath the skin and little or no surrounding tissues are damaged; in an open fracture one or both bone ends project through the skin.

Fractures may also be classified according to the shape or pattern of the break (see box).

If the two bone ends have moved apart, the fracture is termed displaced; in an undisplaced fracture the ends remain in alignment and there is simply a crack in the bone.

CAUSES AND INCIDENCE

Most fractures are caused by a sudden injury that exerts more force on the bone than it can withstand. The force may be direct, as when a finger is hit by a hammer, or indirect, as when twisting the foot exerts severe stress on the tibia (shin).

Some diseases, such as *osteoporosis* and certain forms of cancer, weaken bone so much that it takes only a minor injury—or none at all—for the bone to break. This type of fracture is termed pathological.

Common sites of fracture include the hand, the wrist (see *Colles' fracture*), the *ankle joint*, the *clavicle* (collarbone), and the neck of the *femur* (thigh bone), usually as the result of a fall.

Elderly people are the most prone to fractures because they fall more and because their bones are fragile.

SYMPTOMS AND SIGNS

There is usually swelling and tenderness at the site of the fracture and, in some cases, deformity or projecting bone ends. The pain is often severe and is usually made worse by any movement of the area.

FIRST-AID TREATMENT

Anyone suffering a suspected or known fracture should be taken to the hospital; if the injured person cannot walk, medical help should be summoned. Do not try to force back a displaced bone yourself.

Treat severe bleeding (see *Bleeding, treatment of*), covering any open wounds with a clean dressing. Move the patient as little as possible. *Splinting* is usually necessary, especially if the injured person needs to be moved or if there is a long delay before help arrives. If an injured arm can be bent comfortably across the chest, splint it first and then apply a *sling*. If *spinal injury* is suspected, do not move the person at all unless his or her life is in immediate danger or he or she is choking on vomit.

Do not give the injured person any food or liquid in case an operation requiring a general anesthetic must be carried out.

PROFESSIONAL TREATMENT

X rays are taken to confirm the diagnosis and to provide a clear picture of the type of fracture and the degree of displacement or malalignment.

Bone begins to heal immediately after it has broken. The first aim of treatment is therefore to ensure that the bone ends abut each other and are in alignment so that, when the fracture heals, the bone will retain its previous shape. Bone ends that have been displaced are maneuvered back into position—a procedure known as reduction. The bone may be manipulated through the skin (closed reduction) using a local or general anesthetic. Alternatively, the bone may be repositioned by means of an operation using anesthetic in which the site is opened (open reduction).

Once the fracture has been reduced, the bone is immobilized to allow the broken pieces to reunite firmly.

FRACTURES: TYPES AND TREATMENT

There are two main types of fractures: simple (closed) and compound (open). Within these two categories are several other types, three of which are illustrated here.

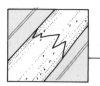

Simple fracture
The broken bone does not break the skin. Because organisms do not come into contact with the fracture, infection is rare.

Compound fracture
A sharp piece of bone punctures the skin and is therefore exposed to organisms. There is a high risk of infection.

Transverse fracture
The result of a sharp, direct blow or a stress fracture caused, for example, by prolonged running.

Greenstick fracture
This type usually occurs in children. Sudden force causes only the outer side of the bent bone to break.

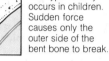

Comminuted fracture
The bone shatters into more than two pieces. This fracture usually is caused by severe force, such as in a car accident.

F

REPAIR OF FRACTURES

There are various ways of repairing fractures, depending on the particular bone, the severity of the fracture, and the age of the patient.

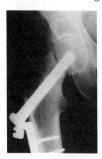

Internal fixation
The photograph at left shows immobilization of an unstable hip fracture by the insertion of metal screws across the bone ends.

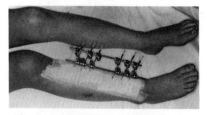
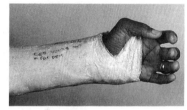
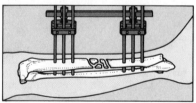

External fixation
Immobilization may be achieved by means of a plaster cast (above) or, in cases such as an unstable fracture of the tibia (left and above left), through the use of metal pins inserted into the bone on either side of the break and locked into position on an external metal frame.

THE BONE HEALING PROCESS

After a fracture, the bone starts to heal immediately. Any displacement of the bone ends must therefore be corrected without delay to minimize deformity.

1 A blood clot forms between the bone ends, sealing off the ends of the damaged vessels.

2 Macrophages invade the fracture site to remove wound debris. Fibroblasts then create a mesh to form a base for new tissue.

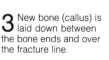

3 New bone (callus) is laid down between the bone ends and over the fracture line.

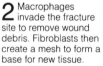

4 Remodeling takes place, with more dense, stronger bone laid down.

5 Over a period of weeks, the bone returns to its former shape.

F

In some cases the ends of the fractured bone may be fixed together by metal pins inserted through the skin and into the bone and kept in position by attachment to an external frame (external fixation); once the fracture has healed, the pins and frame are removed. In other cases an operation is done to open up the injury site and fasten together the bone pieces with metal screws, nails, plates, rods, or wires (internal fixation).

RECOVERY PERIOD

The time taken for fractures to heal varies considerably and depends on many factors. Fractures mend much more easily in children than in adults, and in babies they can heal in as little as two weeks. In an adult a weight-bearing bone, such as the tibia, may take up to six months to knit together completely; bones that do not bear weight, such as the radius and clavicle (collarbone), generally take no longer than eight weeks.

COMPLICATIONS

Most fractures heal without problem. Healing is sometimes delayed because the blood supply to the affected bone is inadequate (as a result of damaged vessels) or because the bone ends are not close enough together. If the fracture fails to unite, internal fixation or a *bone graft* may be required.

Occasionally, bone ends reunite at the wrong angle. If this causes deformity, an operation may be necessary to refracture the bone, set it correctly, and fix it with nails. *Osteomyelitis* is a danger of open fractures and may be difficult to eradicate.

REHABILITATION

Complete immobility of a bone for a prolonged period can cause loss of muscle bulk, stiffness in nearby joints, and *edema* (accumulation of fluid in the tissues) with the risk, especially in the elderly, of permanent disability. For this reason the patient is encouraged to begin gradually using the affected part as soon as is safely possible and is given exercises to perform to restore flexibility to the joints and strength to the muscles (see *Physical therapy*).

Fracture, dental

A break in a tooth. Although tooth enamel is hard, it is also brittle and can easily be fractured by suddenly striking a hard surface, as may occur in a sports injury or a fall.

If the fracture is confined to the tooth's enamel or to the enamel and dentin, it can usually be repaired by bonding, in which the surface of the tooth is etched with a mild acid solution and a plastic resin material is attached to the roughened surface. If the pulp is affected, *root-canal treatment* may be necessary. Fractures of the root are most damaging if they occur in the lower two thirds of the tooth because the remaining fragment does not offer sufficient support for a replacement crown. A tooth fractured vertically usually cannot be saved.

Front teeth that project more than normal are vulnerable to accidental fracture. They should be repositioned by orthodontic treatment. (See also *Orthodontics; Bonding, dental*.)

Fragile X syndrome

An inherited defect of the X *chromosome* that causes mental retardation. Fragile X syndrome is the most common cause of mental retardation in males after *Down's syndrome*.

The disorder occurs within families according to an X-linked recessive pattern of inheritance (see *Genetic disorders*). Although males are mainly affected, women are able to carry the genetic defect responsible for the disorder and pass it on to some of their sons, who are affected, and some of their daughters, who in turn become carriers of the defect.

Approximately one in 1,500 men is affected by the condition; one in 1,000 women is a carrier. In addition to being mentally retarded, affected males are generally tall, physically strong, have a prominent nose and jaw, increased ear length, large testicles, and are prone to epileptic seizures. About one third of female carriers show some degree of intellectual impairment.

There is no treatment for the condition. If a woman has a history of the syndrome in her family, it is useful to seek *genetic counseling* regarding the risk of a child being affected.

Freckle

A tiny patch of pigmented skin, often round or oval in shape. Freckles occur on sun-exposed areas of skin and tend to become more numerous as a result of continued exposure. The tendency to freckling is inherited and most often occurs in fair and red-haired people.

Freckles are harmless, but people with highly freckled complexions should avoid excess sunlight and should use sunscreens.

Free-floating anxiety

Vague feelings of apprehension and tension associated with *generalized anxiety disorder*.

Frequency

See *Urination, frequent*.

Freudian slip

Also known as a slip of the tongue, a minor error in speech or action that turns out to be what the person really wanted to say or do. The term, also called a parapraxia, is derived from Sigmund Freud's book "The Psychopathology of Everyday Life." As the error tends to be laughed off, Freud saw the process as a compromise between the fulfillment of an unconscious wish and the conscious effort to repress it.

Freudian theory

A discipline of psychology developed by Sigmund Freud (1856-1939), a Viennese neurologist. The theory developed out of his treatment of neurotic patients using hypnosis and formed the basis of his technique of *psychoanalysis*. Freud believed that feelings, thoughts, and behavior were controlled by unconscious wishes and conflicts and that problems occurred when these desires were not fulfilled or the conflicts remained unresolved.

According to Freud, the conflicts originated in childhood and persisted into adulthood. The essence of his theory concerns early psychological development, particularly sexual development, which now is seen to encompass much more than just the "sexual" to include the early relationship with the parent. Freud defined a number of stages—oral, anal, and genital (representing the areas of the body on which an infant's attention becomes fixed at different ages)—and three components of personality—the id, ego, and superego (based on pleasure, reality, and moral and social constraints, respectively). The classic Freudian model sees all behavior as having its roots in unconscious instincts, but ultimately being determined by the interplay between the id, ego, and superego.

Psychoanalysis aims to treat mental disorders by encouraging the patient to allow thoughts to flow in any conscious direction without censorship. Freud believed that important information would emerge from the unconscious mind. (See also *Psychoanalytic theory; Psychotherapy*.)

Friedreich's ataxia

A very rare inherited disease in which degeneration of nerve fibers in the spinal cord causes *ataxia* (loss of coordinated movement and balance). The disease is the result of a genetic defect, usually of the autosomal recessive type (see *Genetic disorders*). It affects about two people per 100,000.

SYMPTOMS

Symptoms first appear in late childhood or adolescence. The main symptoms are unsteadiness when walking, clumsy hand movements, slurred speech, and rapid, involuntary eye movements. In many cases there are also abnormalities of bone structure and alignment.

TREATMENT AND OUTLOOK

There is as yet no cure for the disease. Once it has developed, it becomes progressively more severe, and, within 10 years of onset, more than half the sufferers are confined to wheelchairs. If *cardiomyopathy* (heart muscle disease) develops, it may contribute to an early death. People who have blood relatives with Friedreich's ataxia should seek *genetic counseling* before starting a family.

Frigidity

A term used to describe the inability to want or enjoy sexual intercourse (see *Sexual desire, inhibited*). The term has been used almost exclusively with reference to women and is now being discouraged because of its negative connotations—blaming a woman for something that may exist only in the mind of her partner.

In the past, the term frigid was also used to describe a woman who does not achieve orgasm. This condition is now called inhibited sexual excitement; the terms anorgasmia, and foreorgasmy are also sometimes used (see *Orgasm, lack of*).

Frostbite

Damage to tissues caused by extremely cold temperatures—below 32°F (0°C). Frostbite can affect any part of the body that is not properly covered, but the nose, ears, fingers, and toes are most susceptible. If only the skin and underlying tissues are damaged, recovery may be complete. If blood vessels are affected, the damage is permanent and *gangrene* can follow, which may necessitate amputation of the affected part.

The lower the temperature, the shorter the time required to cause damage; wind and blizzard conditions also cause damage more quickly.

The first symptoms are a pins and needles sensation, followed by complete numbness. The skin appears white, cold, and hard, and then becomes red and swollen. After the

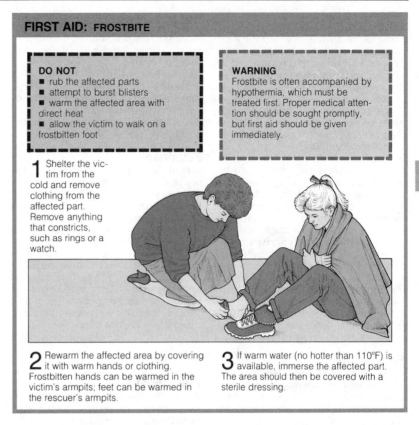

FIRST AID: FROSTBITE

DO NOT
- rub the affected parts
- attempt to burst blisters
- warm the affected area with direct heat
- allow the victim to walk on a frostbitten foot

WARNING
Frostbite is often accompanied by hypothermia, which must be treated first. Proper medical attention should be sought promptly, but first aid should be given immediately.

1 Shelter the victim from the cold and remove clothing from the affected part. Remove anything that constricts, such as rings or a watch.

2 Rewarm the affected area by covering it with warm hands or clothing. Frostbitten hands can be warmed in the victim's armpits; feet can be warmed in the rescuer's armpits.

3 If warm water (no hotter than 110°F) is available, immerse the affected part. The area should then be covered with a sterile dressing.

tissue has thawed, blisters form and some areas of skin are black, indicating that the tissue is dead.

Frostbite must be treated promptly. The person should be sheltered from the cold and the affected parts warmed as quickly as possible by immersing them in lukewarm water at 110°F (44°C). Movement of the affected parts should be avoided; massage is not helpful.

Frottage

The act of rubbing against another person to achieve sexual arousal. Also called frotteurism, it is usually carried out in a densely packed crowd where a man rubs his (clothed) genitals against a woman's buttocks or thigh. Such men commonly indulge in other sexual deviations, may have a fetishist interest in buttocks, and are unable to form successful sexual relationships.

Frozen section

A rapid technique for preparing *biopsy* specimens (small pieces of tissue) for microscopic examination.

WHY IT IS DONE

Frozen section is carried out during surgical procedures to determine

whether tissue is malignant, so that the surgeon knows whether to remove more tissue before completing the operation. It is primarily used in diagnosing a breast lump as benign or malignant, but can also be useful in excluding malignancy as a diagnosis in growths of the thyroid or intestine or in diagnosing a lymphoma.

In many instances, diagnosis is made before surgery, obviating the need for frozen section. Diagnosis may be by percutaneous (through the skin) needle biopsy.

HOW IT IS DONE

A small piece of tissue is removed by the surgeon and sent to the histology laboratory. After being frozen quickly in liquid nitrogen, the specimen is cut into very thin sections, placed on a glass slide, and stained so that the cells can be examined under the microscope. The entire process takes about 20 minutes.

Frozen shoulder

Stiffness and pain in the shoulder, making normal movement of the joint impossible. In severe cases, the shoulder may be completely rigid and pain may be extremely intense.

Frozen shoulder is caused by inflammation and thickening of the lining of the capsule in which the joint is contained. The problem usually develops for no known reason, but in some cases it follows a minor injury to the shoulder, a *stroke*, chronic *bronchitis*, or *angina pectoris*.

The condition mainly affects middle-aged people, and there is a higher-than-average incidence among people with *diabetes mellitus*.

TREATMENT

Moderate symptoms can be eased by taking analgesics (painkillers) and anti-inflammatory drugs, and by applying ice packs to the shoulder or using a heat lamp on it. A severe case may require injections of *corticosteroid drugs* into the joint to relieve pain and exercises to restore movement. Manipulation of the joint using a general anesthetic can also restore mobility, but carries the risk of initially increasing pain in the joint.

Whatever the severity and treatment of the condition, recovery is usually slow and may be prolonged.

Frustration

A deep feeling of discontent and tension because of unresolved problems, unfulfilled needs, or because the path to a goal is blocked. In a person who is mentally healthy, frustration can be dealt with in a socially acceptable way. In less well-adapted people, it may lead to *regression* (going back to childlike behavior) and, in particular, *aggression* or *depression*.

There has been much research into the relationship between frustration and violent and criminal behavior. Some people believe that all aggressive acts are related to exposure to violence while growing up or are an indication of prior frustration.

FSH

Abbreviation for *follicle-stimulating hormone*, a *gonadotropin hormone* (one that stimulates the gonads—the ovaries and testes) produced by the anterior part of the pituitary gland.

Fugue

An episode of altered consciousness that causes the sufferer to wander (e.g., from home or work). It may last hours or days and the subject does not remember it afterward.

In a fugue of long duration, behavior may appear normal but certain symptoms (e.g., hallucinations, feeling unreal, or an unstable mood) may accompany it. In a fugue that lasts only for a matter of hours, the patient may be confused and agitated. A fugue is not common, but causes great alarm among relatives and friends because of its sudden onset and strange quality.

Causes include *dissociative disorders*, the *automatism* of certain types of *epilepsy* (especially temporal lobe or psychomotor epilepsy), *depression*, *head injury*, and *dementia*.

Fulminant

A medical term used to describe a disorder that develops and progresses suddenly and with great severity. The term is usually applied to an infection that has spread rapidly through the bloodstream to affect several organs and cause a high fever.

The term may also be applied to types of arthritis in which many joints are painful and stiff and deformities appear soon after the onset of symptoms, or to a cancer that has spread rapidly to cause dramatic weight loss and debility.

Fumes

See *Pollution*.

Functional disorders

A term for illnesses in which there is no evidence of organic disturbance even though performance is impaired.

Fungal infections

Diseases of the skin or other organs caused by the multiplication and spread of fungal organisms. Infections range from mild and unnoticed to severe and sometimes fatal. Fungal infections are also called mycoses. Fungi can also cause *asthma* and allergic *alveolitis* but these are allergic disorders not infections.

CAUSES

Some fungi are harmlessly present all the time in areas of the body such as the mouth, skin, intestines, and vagina, but are prevented from multiplying through competition from bacteria. Other fungi are dealt with by the body's *immune system* (defenses against infection).

Fungal infections are more common and serious in people who are taking long-term antibiotics (which destroy the bacterial competition) and in those who are taking *corticosteroid drugs* or *immunosuppressant drugs* (used to suppress the immune system). These infections more commonly involve people with an immune deficiency disorder, such as *AIDS*. Fungal infections are described as opportunistic because they take advantage of the victim's lowered defenses.

Some fungal infections are also more common in people with *diabetes mellitus*. A warm, moist atmosphere encourages the development of fungal skin infections.

TYPES

Fungal infections can be broadly classified into superficial infections (those that affect the skin, hair, nails, genital organs, and the inside of the mouth); subcutaneous infections (those beneath the skin); and "deep" infections (those affecting internal organs, such as the lungs or, more rarely, the liver, bones, lymph nodes, brain, heart, or urinary tract).

SUPERFICIAL INFECTIONS The main superficial fungal infections are *candidiasis* (thrush) and *tinea* (including ringworm and athlete's foot), both of which are very common. Candidiasis is caused by the yeast CANDIDA ALBICANS and usually affects the genitals or inside of the mouth. Tinea affects external areas of the body.

SUBCUTANEOUS INFECTIONS These are rare. The most common is called *sporotrichosis* and may follow contamination of a scratch. Most other conditions of this type occur mainly in tropical countries. The most important example of this type is *mycetoma*, or Madura foot.

DEEP INFECTIONS These are rare or uncommon (although becoming more common), but can be a serious threat to people who have an immune deficiency disorder or are taking immunosuppressive drugs. In the US, fungal infections of this sort include *aspergillosis*, *histoplasmosis*, *cryptococcosis*, and *blastomycosis*, all caused by different fungi. The fungal spores enter the body by inhalation into the lungs. Candidiasis can also spread from its usual sites to infect the esophagus, urinary tract, and numerous other internal sites.

Fungi

 Simple parasitic life-forms including molds, mildews, yeasts, mushrooms, and toadstools. There are more than 100,000 different species of fungi worldwide. Of these, most are either harmless or positively beneficial to human health, including various yeasts used in baking and brewing, some molds that are the source of certain *antibiotic drugs*, and various edible mushrooms and truffles that are considered gastronomic delicacies in many parts of the world. There are,

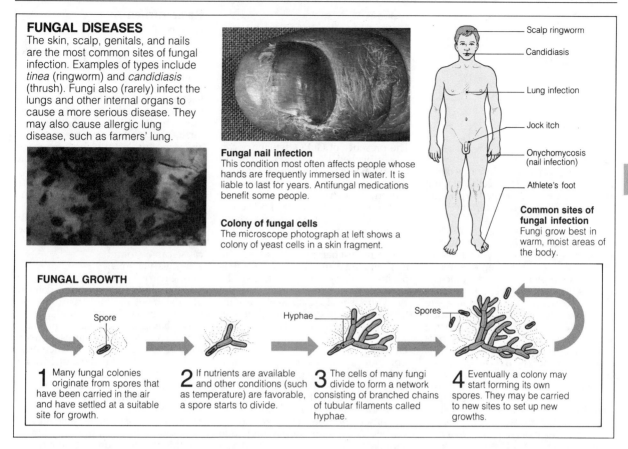

FUNGAL DISEASES
The skin, scalp, genitals, and nails are the most common sites of fungal infection. Examples of types include *tinea* (ringworm) and *candidiasis* (thrush). Fungi also (rarely) infect the lungs and other internal organs to cause a more serious disease. They may also cause allergic lung disease, such as farmers' lung.

Fungal nail infection
This condition most often affects people whose hands are frequently immersed in water. It is liable to last for years. Antifungal medications benefit some people.

Colony of fungal cells
The microscope photograph at left shows a colony of yeast cells in a skin fragment.

Scalp ringworm
Candidiasis
Lung infection
Jock itch
Onychomycosis (nail infection)
Athlete's foot

Common sites of fungal infection
Fungi grow best in warm, moist areas of the body.

FUNGAL GROWTH
Spore
Hyphae
Spores

1 Many fungal colonies originate from spores that have been carried in the air and have settled at a suitable site for growth.

2 If nutrients are available and other conditions (such as temperature) are favorable, a spore starts to divide.

3 The cells of many fungi divide to form a network consisting of branched chains of tubular filaments called hyphae.

4 Eventually a colony may start forming its own spores. They may be carried to new sites to set up new growths.

---

however, also a number of types of fungi that can cause illness and sometimes fatal disease in humans. The study of fungi and fungal diseases is known as *mycology*.

Some fungi, notably the yeasts, occur as colonies of individual cells. In others, the cells divide to form chains of tubular filaments called hyphae, which are organized into a complex network called a mycelium. With some soil-living fungi, parts of the mycelium form into large fruiting bodies, seen as mushrooms or toadstools. Many fungi form minute bodies called spores, which are like seeds. These spores can be carried in the air and, if they settle in a suitable location with nutrients available, they divide to form a new mycelium; the molds that eventually form on exposed food are a type of mycelium. Fungal spores are ever-present in the air and soil.

FUNGI AND DISEASE
Fungi can cause illness and disease in a variety of ways.

First, the fruiting bodies of some soil-living fungi contain toxins that

can produce direct poisoning if eaten (see *Mushroom poisoning*).

Second, certain fungi that infect food crops produce dangerous toxins that can cause a type of food poisoning if contaminated food is eaten. The best known of these are a fungus that infects rye and other cereals and produces a toxin called *ergot*, and another that grows on groundnuts and produces the poison *aflatoxin*. Ergot poisoning is rare today, but chronic aflatoxin poisoning from eating moldy groundnuts is a suspected cause of liver cancer in some regions of Asia and Africa.

Third, the inhaled spores of some fungi can cause a persistent allergic reaction in the lungs, known as allergic *alveolitis*. Farmers' lung, caused by spores from moldy hay, is an example of such a reaction. Fungal spores are also sometimes responsible for other allergic disorders such as *asthma* and allergic *rhinitis* (hay fever).

Fourth, some fungi are able to invade and form colonies or mycelia within the lungs, in the skin, beneath the skin, or sometimes in various

tissues throughout the body, leading to conditions ranging from mild skin irritation to severe, or even fatal, widespread infection and illness (see *Fungal infections*).

Fungicidal
See *Antifungal drugs*.

Funny bone
Popular term for the small area at the back of the *elbow* where the ulnar nerve passes over a prominence of the humerus (upper arm bone). A blow to the nerve causes acute pain and sometimes numbness of the forearm.

Furosemide
A *diuretic drug* commonly used to treat *edema* (fluid retention) and *hypertension* (high blood pressure). When given by injection, furosemide has a rapid effect. It is therefore often used in emergencies to treat pulmonary *edema* (fluid in the lungs).

Furuncle
Another name for a *boil* that usually involves a hair follicle.

G

G6PD deficiency

An inherited disorder that affects the chemistry of red blood cells, making them prone to damage during an infectious illness or from certain drugs or foods.

CAUSES AND INCIDENCE

G6PD deficiency is caused by the production within red blood cells of abnormal molecules of an enzyme (a type of protein) called glucose-6-phosphate dehydrogenase. Because the molecules of this substance are defective, they cannot carry out their normal function, which is to help in a chemical process that protects the cells from damage.

The disorder is the result of an abnormality in the affected person's genetic material and is inherited in an X-linked recessive pattern (see *Genetic disorders*). This means that most of those affected are male, but women may carry the defective gene in a hidden form and pass it on to some of their sons.

The disorder is much more common among blacks than whites, affecting about 15 percent of black males in the US. A variant of the disorder, called *favism*, affects a small number of whites of Mediterranean origin.

The particular drugs that can precipitate hemolysis (red cell destruction) in affected people are shown below. Individuals with favism are, in addition, extremely sensitive to a chemical in broad beans, which they must avoid eating.

SYMPTOMS

A few days after taking an incriminated drug or food, or during the course of an infectious illness, symptoms of hemolytic *anemia* (such as jaundice, fatigue, headaches, shortness of breath on exertion, and sometimes darkening of the urine due to the destruction of red blood cells) may develop in affected people.

DIAGNOSIS AND TREATMENT

The presence of G6PD deficiency can be established by a blood screening test. The deficiency cannot be treated but any episode of hemolytic anemia caused by a drug can be halted by stopping use of the drug. Full recovery then takes place within a few days.

Anyone with a history of G6PD deficiency in the family should ask for a screening test before taking any of the incriminated drugs. If the test result is positive, these drugs should be avoided. Anyone known to have the condition should also seek prompt treatment for any infectious illness to prevent a hemolytic crisis.

GABA

Common abbreviation for gamma-aminobutyric acid, a *neurotransmitter* (chemical released from nerve endings). GABA controls the flow of nerve impulses by blocking the release of other neurotransmitters (e.g., *norepinephrine* and dopamine) that stimulate nerve activity. The activity of GABA is increased by *benzodiazepine drugs* and by *anticonvulsant drugs*.

It has been suggested that people with *Huntington's chorea* (a hereditary disease characterized by mental retardation and involuntary movement) have insufficient GABA-producing nerve cells in the brain centers that coordinate movement.

Gait

The style or manner of *walking*. Some neuromuscular disorders are evaluated on the basis of altered gait.

Galactorrhea

Spontaneous, persistent production of milk by a woman who is not pregnant or lactating (producing milk after childbirth), or, very rarely, production of milk by a man.

CAUSES

Lactation is initiated by a rise in the level of prolactin (a hormone produced by the pituitary gland). Galactorrhea is caused by an excessive amount of prolactin being secreted as a result of a *pituitary tumor*, or due to other endocrine diseases, such as *hypothyroidism*. Certain *antipsychotic drugs* (such as chlorpromazine) and some brain diseases (for example, *meningitis*) may be associated with increased prolactin production. However, in about 50 percent of cases, no cause can be found.

SYMPTOMS AND SIGNS

The breast secretion is obviously milklike. If it is of any other color or bloodstained, another cause (such as a breast tumor) should be suspected. Excessive levels of prolactin may also adversely affect the ovaries, causing *amenorrhea* (absence of menstrual periods) or *infertility*. If the underlying cause is a pituitary tumor, the symptoms may include headache and visual disturbances.

TREATMENT

Surgery or *radiation therapy* may be required if there is a pituitary tumor, but the symptoms are often controlled and the size of the tumor is decreased by treatment with *bromocriptine*.

In addition to treating the underlying cause, hormone or drug therapy may be used to suppress prolactin and prevent milk production. Bromocriptine, which suppresses prolactin production, can successfully treat galactorrhea when the cause is unknown, and also may regulate periods and fertility.

Galactosemia

An extremely rare inability of the body's biochemical system to break down galactose (a sugar derived from the milk sugar lactose) into glucose because of the absence of an enzyme in the liver. Galactosemia is caused by an autosomal recessive genetic defect (see *Genetic disorders*).

SYMPTOMS

Galactosemia causes no symptoms at birth, but jaundice, diarrhea, and vomiting soon develop and the baby fails to gain weight. If untreated, the condition results in liver disease, *cataract* (opacity in the lens of the eye), and *mental retardation*.

DRUGS TO BE AVOIDED BY PEOPLE WITH G6PD DEFICIENCY

Class	Drugs to avoid
Antimalarial drugs	Primaquine, chloroquine, quinine, dapsone
Antibacterial and antibiotic drugs	Nitrofurantoin, sulfonamides (such as sulfisoxazole and sulfacetamide), chloramphenicol,* nalidixic acid
Analgesics (painkillers)	Aspirin*
Miscellaneous	Vitamin K (water-soluble form), probenecid, quinidine*

*These drugs do not usually cause problems in the type of G6PD deficiency that affects blacks in the US.

DIAGNOSIS AND TREATMENT

The diagnosis is confirmed from urine and blood tests. Feeding with a special lactose-free milk leads to dramatic improvement; normal milk must be avoided throughout life.

Gallbladder

A small, pear-shaped sac situated underneath the liver, to which it is attached by fibrous tissue. Bile produced by the liver passes to the gallbladder by means of a small tube, the cystic duct. This duct branches off from the bile duct, which carries bile from the liver to the duodenum.

Within the gallbladder, bile is stored and concentrated (by absorption of its water content through the gallbladder walls). When food passes from the stomach to the duodenum, secretin and cholecystokinin (gastrointestinal hormones) cause the gallbladder to contract and expel its content of bile into the duodenum, where the bile emulsifies fats contained in the food. (See also *Biliary system*.)

ANATOMY OF THE GALLBLADDER

A small, muscular sac that lies under the liver. The gallbladder expels bile via the common bile duct into the duodenum.

- Mucosa
- Gallbladder
- Cystic duct
- Serous coat
- Common bile duct

Gallbladder cancer

A rare cancer of unknown cause, occurring mainly in old age. It usually occurs in gallbladders with *gallstones*, but affects only a minute number of gallstone sufferers. The incidence of this cancer is less than three new cases per 100,000 population per year.

The cancer may cause *jaundice* and tenderness in the upper right abdomen but is sometimes symptomless. It is diagnosed by *ultrasound scanning*; occasionally, the cancer is discovered during surgery on the gallbladder.

Cancer of the gallbladder is treated by removal of as much of the tumor as possible. The cancer often has invaded the liver by the time it is detected, making the outlook poor.

Gallium

A metallic element whose radioactive form is used in *radionuclide scanning* (a technique for obtaining images of internal organs). Gallium is injected into the bloodstream and, about 72 hours later, scanning is performed.

G

DISORDERS OF THE GALLBLADDER

The gallbladder rarely causes problems in childhood or early adulthood but, from middle age onward, the increasing occurrence of gallstones can sometimes give rise to symptoms.

Because the digestive system can function normally without a gallbladder, its removal has little known long-term effect.

CONGENITAL AND GENETIC DEFECTS

Abnormalities present from birth may include no gallbladder, an oversized gallbladder, or two gallbladders; these defects rarely cause problems.

METABOLIC DISORDERS

The principal disorder of the gallbladder, with which most other problems are associated, is the formation of *gallstones*. Gallstones are common, but only about 20 percent of people with gallstones have symptoms requiring *cholecystectomy* (surgical removal of the gallbladder). Attempts by the gallbladder to expel the stone or stones can cause severe *biliary colic* (abdominal pain). There are three main types of gallstones: cholesterol gallstones, pigment gallstones, and mixed gallstones. The great majority are cholesterol or

mixed gallstones, and women are affected four times as often as men. Every year about 1 million Americans develop gallstones. Many people carry "silent" gallstones, which produce no symptoms.

INFECTION AND INFLAMMATION

If a gallstone becomes stuck in the outlet from the gallbladder, the trapped bile may irritate and inflame the gallbladder walls and the bile itself may become infected. This is called acute *cholecystitis*. The first symptom may be biliary colic, which is followed by fever and abdominal tenderness.

Repeated attacks of biliary colic and acute cholecystitis can lead to chronic cholecystitis, in which the gallbladder becomes shrunken and thick-walled and ceases to function. Rarely, the gallbladder may become inflamed without the presence of gallstones—a condition that is called acalculous cholecystitis.

Occasionally, cholecystitis proceeds to a condition in which the gallbladder fills with pus, called *empyema* of the gallbladder. This can cause a high fever and severe abdominal pain.

TUMORS

Gallbladders harboring *gallbladder cancer* usually contain gallstones. However, this cancer is extremely

uncommon compared to the high prevalence of gallstones.

OTHER DISORDERS

In rare cases where a gallbladder is empty when a stone obstructs its outlet, it may fill with mucus secreted by the gallbladder walls, resulting in a distended, mucus-filled gallbladder known as a *mucocele*.

INVESTIGATION

Gallbladder problems are investigated by physical examination and techniques such as *ultrasound scanning*, *radionuclide scanning*, or *cholecystography* (X rays of the gallbladder after it has been filled with a contrast medium). Blood tests may also be carried out.

Gallium tends to accumulate in tumors and pus cells; its main uses in scanning are to detect malignant diseases, such as *Hodgkin's disease*, and abscesses or areas of *osteomyelitis*.

Gallstones

Round or oval, smooth or faceted lumps of solid matter found in the gallbladder (the sac under the liver where bile is stored and concentrated). Gallstones are sometimes found in the bile ducts (which connect the gallbladder and liver to the duodenum). In these cases, the symptoms can be severe. There may be between one and 10, or sometimes more, stones varying in size from about 0.05 inch to 1 inch (1 to 25 mm) across. Gallstones composed principally of cholesterol are the most common type, but some contain a high content of bile pigments and other substances, such as chalk.

CAUSES AND INCIDENCE

Gallstones develop when an upset occurs in the chemical composition of bile. When the liver makes bile, it can put too much cholesterol into it (which occurs in obesity) or it may fail to put in enough of the detergent substances that normally keep cholesterol, a fatty substance, in solution.

Once the bile is overloaded with cholesterol, a tiny particle can form that gradually grows as more material solidifies around it, eventually forming a stone. Something else in the bile (its nature is unknown) actually triggers this process. Fasting for long periods may help gallstones develop by causing bile to stagnate in the gallbladder.

Gallstones are rare in childhood and become progressively more common with age. Two to three times more women than men are affected (autopsies show that 20 percent of all women have gallstones when they die).

Risk groups include overweight people and women who have had many children. Use of the birth-control pill may cause gallstones to form earlier than they would otherwise.

PREVENTION

People should avoid becoming overweight and should eat as little sugar and fat as possible. Some experts believe a high intake of fiber helps and that drinking one alcoholic drink a day has a protective value.

SYMPTOMS

Only about 20 percent of gallstones cause symptoms or complications. Symptoms commonly begin only when a gallstone gets stuck in the duct leading from the gallbladder. This causes *biliary colic* (intense pain in the upper right side of the abdomen or between the shoulder blades) and may make the sufferer feel sick and possibly vomit. Indigestion made worse by fatty foods often seems to be associated with gallstones. Other potential complications include *cholecystitis* (inflammation of the gallbladder) and *bile duct obstruction* leading to jaundice.

DIAGNOSIS AND TREATMENT

Ultrasound scanning can detect 95 percent of gallstones and is therefore the first test to be performed. An older and slightly less sensitive method is X-ray *cholecystography*, which utilizes an iodinated dye that is taken either by mouth or injected into a vein. Blood tests may also be performed. If the physician suspects the stones have escaped into the bile ducts, *cholangiography* may be carried out.

Stones that do not cause symptoms can safely be left alone, as they are unlikely to cause trouble. When symptoms are severe, *cholecystectomy* (surgical removal of the gallbladder) is carried out; this cures the problem in 95 percent of cases.

In some cases drug treatment may be used, especially if the stones are small and noncalcified. Tablets containing chenodiol or ursodeoxycholic acid can dissolve stones over several months. X rays or ultrasound scans of the gallbladder are done to check progress. Stones recur in about half the cases when the drug is stopped, so ultrasound scans are carried out over the following few years.

OUTLOOK

New treatments are being developed. Extracorporeal shock-wave *lithotripsy* uses shock waves to shatter the stones. In another technique a tube is inserted into the gallbladder and a strong solution that dissolves cholesterol is flushed through. The safety and long-term value of these treatments is still being investigated.

Gambling, pathological

Chronic inability to resist impulses to gamble, resulting in personal or social problems. Most gamblers can stop at a given point; pathological or "compulsive" gamblers seem unable to control the amount they spend and are unable to stop even when they continue to lose. The urge to gamble is so great that tension can be relieved only by more gambling. Family problems, bankruptcy, and crime may follow.

Gamma globulin

A substance prepared from human blood that contains *antibodies* against most common infections. (See *Immune serum globulin*.)

Ganglion

A cystic swelling associated with the sheath of a tendon. It is a common condition and usually occurs on the wrist, although a finger or foot may sometimes be affected. The cyst, which contains thick fluid derived from the synovial fluid that lubricates tendons and joints, can vary from the size of a small pea to, rarely, the size of a golf ball.

A ganglion may disappear spontaneously; if it does not, treatment is usually necessary only if it is painful or unsightly. The fluid may be sucked out with a needle and syringe. The cyst commonly recurs after such treatments, however. The best approach is to remove the cyst surgically, after which recurrence is rare.

Gangrene

Death of tissue, usually as a result of loss of blood supply. It may affect a small area of skin, a finger, or a substantial portion of a limb.

SYMPTOMS

Pain is felt in the dying tissues, but once they are dead they become numb. The affected skin and underlying tissue turn black. Bacterial infection may develop, causing the gangrene to spread and give off an unpleasant smell. There may be redness, swelling, and oozing pus around the blackened area.

There are two types of gangrene (dry and wet). In dry gangrene there is usually no bacterial infection; the deprived area dies because its blood supply is blocked. This type of gangrene does not spread to other tissues. It may be caused by *arteriosclerosis*, *diabetes mellitus*, *thrombosis*, an *embolism*, or *frostbite*.

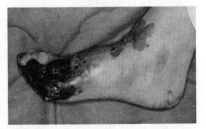

Gangrene of the foot
This photograph shows a foot with an extensive area of dead tissue, with blackening of the overlying skin.

G

Wet gangrene develops when dry gangrene or a wound becomes infected by bacteria. A particularly virulent type—known as gas gangrene—is caused by a dangerous strain of bacteria that destroys muscles and produces a foul-smelling gas. Gas gangrene has caused millions of deaths in war.

TREATMENT

Treatment of dry gangrene consists of improving circulation to the affected body part before it is too late. If the tissue becomes infected, the patient is given antibiotics to prevent wet gangrene from setting in.

If wet gangrene is diagnosed, *amputation* of the affected part is unavoidable. Usually, some of the adjacent living tissue must be removed as well.

Ganser's syndrome

A rare, *factitious disorder* in which a person seeks, consciously or unconsciously, to mislead others regarding his or her mental state. Ganser's syndrome occurs most often in prisoners. A characteristic of the disorder is the giving of "approximate answers" (for example, 2x2=5); the choice of an answer near the correct one suggests that the person knows the real response. The sufferer also displays symptoms that simulate *psychosis*, such as episodes of intense agitation or stupor.

Gardnerella vaginalis

A bacterium found in increasing numbers in the vaginal discharge of women with *vaginitis* (inflammation of the vagina).

Gargle

A liquid preparation to wash and freshen the mouth and throat, usually not meant to be swallowed. Gargles may contain mouth fresheners, flavorings, *antiseptics*, or local anesthetics (see *Anesthesia, local*). Those containing antiseptics and local anesthetics relieve the irritation associated with sore throats, but do not cure the underlying cause. The home remedy of gargling with salt water is equally effective in most circumstances.

Gastrectomy

Removal of the whole stomach (total gastrectomy) or, more commonly, a part of the stomach (partial gastrectomy). Gastrectomy is a major operation requiring hospitalization and extensive postoperative care.

WHY IT IS DONE

Total gastrectomy is a rare operation used to treat some stomach cancers. Partial gastrectomy is fairly common; it is usually performed to deal with a *peptic ulcer* (gastric ulcer or duodenal ulcer), ulcers that have failed to heal after changes in diet or drug treatment, ulcers that bleed very badly or perforate (break through the stomach

or duodenal wall), and some cancers located closer to the stomach's outlet. In treating duodenal ulcers, removal of part of the stomach may be combined with *vagotomy* (cutting of the nerves to the acid-secreting part of the stomach) to prevent more ulcers.

HOW IT IS DONE

A general anesthetic is given and the stomach emptied by means of a *nasogastric tube* (a tube passed through the nose down the esophagus into the stomach). The entire stomach is removed in a total gastrectomy; the risk of complications or death from this procedure is high. Smaller portions of stomach are removed with less danger.

RECOVERY PERIOD

After the operation, the nasogastric tube is left in position to allow digestive system secretions to drain. When the volume of these secretions diminishes and normal *peristalsis* (the rhythmic contractions that force food through the digestive system) returns, the patient is given small amounts of water. If these do not cause abdominal pain or nausea, the nasogastric tube is removed. Intake of fluids is gradually increased and, within a few days, a light diet can be started.

COMPLICATIONS

Because removal of the stomach disturbs normal digestion, post-gastrectomy syndromes (side effects after gastric surgery) can develop

G

TYPES OF GASTRECTOMY

There are several different types of gastrectomy operations. In total gastrectomy, the whole stomach is removed; in partial gastrectomy, between one half and two thirds of the stomach is removed. There are two common types of partial gastrectomy operation—the Billroth I and the Billroth II.

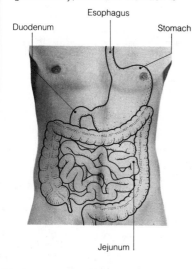

Duodenum · Esophagus · Stomach · Jejunum

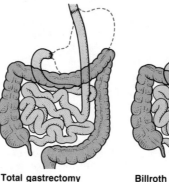

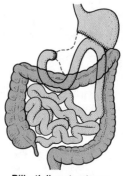

Total gastrectomy
The whole stomach is removed and the esophagus is joined directly to the jejunum (the middle section of the small intestine).

Billroth I gastrectomy
The remaining part of the stomach is joined to the duodenum (the first part of the small intestine).

Billroth II gastrectomy
The surgeon performs a *gastrojejunostomy* (a procedure in which the stomach is joined to the jejunum) and seals the end of the duodenum to form a blind loop.

in some patients. The most troublesome are fullness and discomfort after meals; formation of an ulcer at the new junction between stomach and small intestine; regurgitation of bile, which may lead to *gastritis* (inflammation of the stomach), *esophagitis* (inflammation of the esophagus), and vomiting of bile; diarrhea; and the *dumping syndrome* (sweating, nausea, dizziness, and weakness felt soon after eating a meal because food leaves the stomach too quickly). These side effects usually disappear in time, but diet and drug treatment or another operation may be necessary.

Other complications include *malabsorption* (a reduced ability to absorb food, minerals, and vitamins), which may lead to *anemia* or *osteoporosis* (thinned bones). After total gastrectomy, patients cannot absorb vitamin B_{12} and are therefore given monthly injections for the rest of their lives.

OUTLOOK
Only about 10 percent of patients suffer complications requiring further treatment. Ulcer recurrence is infrequent, but there is a small risk of cancer of the stomach developing after partial gastrectomy.

Gastric bubble
A balloon, about 2 inches (5 cm) in diameter and 3.5 inches (9 cm) long, that is inserted through the mouth and into the stomach as a means of weight control in people who are dangerously obese.

The gastric bubble was approved in 1985 by the US Food and Drug Administration (FDA) only for people who are 100 percent overweight. The procedure is not without risk. In addition, no studies have been performed to evaluate whether or not weight is regained after removal of the balloon.

Gastric erosion
A break in the innermost layer (mucosa) of the membrane that lines the stomach. If a break extends deeper than this layer, it is called a gastric ulcer (see *Peptic ulcer*). Gastric erosion occurs in some cases of *gastritis* (inflammation of the stomach lining).

The causes of gastric erosions are not clear, but many cases are the result of the ingestion of alcohol, iron tablets, aspirin, or other nonsteroidal anti-inflammatory drugs (NSAIDs), such as phenylbutazone or indomethacin. The stress of serious illness, such as septicemia (blood poisoning), burns, or renal failure, may also bring on a gastric erosion.

Often there are no symptoms, although erosions may bleed, resulting in hematemesis (see *Vomiting blood*) or *melena* (black feces containing blood). The blood loss, on the other hand, may be small but persistent, eventually causing *anemia*. The condition is diagnosed by *gastroscopy* (direct examination of the stomach through a flexible viewing tube), which reveals the small bleeding points in the stomach lining.

Gastric erosions usually heal completely in a few days when treated with *antacid drugs* and *ulcer-healing drugs*, such as cimetidine, ranitidine, or famotidine.

Gastric ulcer
A raw area in the wall of the stomach caused by a breach of its inner surface lining. (See *Peptic ulcer*.)

Gastritis
Inflammation of the mucous membrane that lines the stomach. The illness may be acute, occurring as a sudden attack, or chronic, developing gradually over a long period.

CAUSES
Gastritis may be caused by irritation of the stomach lining by a drug, most commonly aspirin or alcohol; by infection of the stomach by *CAMPYLOBACTER* bacteria; or, in some people, by extreme physical stress such as head injury, severe burns, or the development of liver failure.

Chronic gastritis may be caused by prolonged irritation of the stomach by alcohol, tobacco smoke, or bile; damage of the lining by an *autoimmune disorder*, as in pernicious anemia (see *Anemia, megaloblastic*); or degeneration of the lining with age.

Acute gastritis may cause erosions in the lining that bleed easily. In the chronic form, blood may ooze continually from the lining.

SYMPTOMS
Gastritis produces many of the same symptoms as a gastric ulcer, with which it may be confused. Symptoms include discomfort in the upper abdomen (often aggravated by eating), nausea, and vomiting. In acute erosive gastritis, the feces may be black with blood lost from the stomach; in the chronic condition, slow blood loss may cause anemia (see *Anemia, iron-deficiency*), resulting in pallor, tiredness, and breathlessness.

DIAGNOSIS
The diagnosis is made by examining the stomach lining through a gastroscope, a viewing tube passed down

the esophagus to the stomach (see *Gastroscopy*). A *biopsy* (removal of a tiny sample of tissue for analysis) may be performed at the same time, using an attachment at the end of the gastroscope. Microscopic examination of the sample indicates the type of inflammation. The correlation between the microscopic findings and the symptoms is not always clear.

TREATMENT
A person with gastritis should take acetaminophen rather than aspirin for pain relief, avoid alcohol, and not smoke. *Ulcer-healing drugs* may help heal the inflamed lining.

Gastroenteritis
Inflammation of the stomach and intestines, often causing sudden and sometimes violent upsets. The illness does not usually last for more than two or three days and the sufferer tends to recover without any specific treatment other than replacement of lost fluid and salt. *Dysentery, typhoid fever, cholera, food poisoning*, and travelers' diarrhea—as well as many milder stomach upsets—are all forms of gastroenteritis.

CAUSES AND INCIDENCE
Gastroenteritis is an extremely common cause of mild illness in developed countries and a major cause of death in some developing ones.

The illness may be caused by any of a variety of viruses, bacteria, and other small organisms that have contaminated food or water supplies. There are also a number of noninfectious causes of gastroenteritis—for example, *food intolerance*, very spicy foods, certain drugs, toxic substances, and excessive intake of alcohol. In many people, *antibiotic drugs* cause symptoms similar to those of gastroenteritis because the drugs can upset the balance of bacteria that occur naturally in the intestines.

SYMPTOMS
The onset and severity of symptoms depends on the type and concentrations of the microorganisms, food, or toxic substance causing the illness. Appetite loss, nausea, vomiting, cramps, and diarrhea are the symptoms; these may come on gradually, but more often appear suddenly. The combination of symptoms may be so mild that they cause little disruption to daily routine, or the attack may be so severe and persistent that it is disabling, causing dehydration, *shock*, and collapse. In babies and the very old, this may warrant intravenous fluid treatment.

DIAGNOSIS

In mild attacks, the symptoms alone are sufficient to make a diagnosis, but in more serious cases the physician may ask about contact with infected people, food that has been eaten recently, and recent travel abroad.

TREATMENT AND OUTLOOK

Mild cases are treated at home. The affected person should rest, preferably in bed, and take plenty of fluids, which should include salt and sugar if much fluid is being lost by vomiting and diarrhea—4 level teaspoons of sugar and a quarter of a teaspoon of salt for each pint of liquid (see *Rehydration therapy*). No solid food should be eaten until symptoms subside.

In severe cases where shock and collapse occur, the person will be taken to the hospital. Patients are given intravenous fluids to replace the vital body salts lost by vomiting and diarrhea. After the acute phase, water and then other clear fluids are given; if these fluids do not cause further upset, a bland diet is introduced. Antibiotic treatment is reserved for specific bacterial infections such as typhoid.

In most cases the illness subsides gradually without any special measures; recovery is usually complete with no complications.

PREVENTION

Care taken in food preparation and hygiene can substantially reduce the chances of gastroenteritis (see *Food poisoning; Food-borne infection*). Some protection against typhoid and cholera can be acquired by vaccination before traveling to countries where these diseases are still common. Avoidance of substances known to cause upset helps minimize noninfectious attacks of gastroenteritis.

Those caring for a person with the symptoms of gastroenteritis should be scrupulous about personal hygiene to prevent the illness from spreading.

Gastroenterologist

A physician specially trained in the management of disorders of the digestive system. His or her work is concerned with the treatment of *peptic ulcers* of the stomach and duodenum, conditions affecting the gastrointestinal tract from mouth to anus, and diseases of the liver and gallbladder.

The work of the gastroenterologist has been revolutionized in recent years by the development of fiberoptic *endoscopes*. Much of the gastrointestinal tract can now be visualized directly by these instruments and samples can be taken for laboratory examination.

HORMONES IN THE DIGESTIVE TRACT

Hormones released from endocrine cells in the stomach, pancreas, and intestine aid digestion by stimulating the release of bile from the gallbladder and enzymes from the pancreas into the duodenum.

Cholecystokinin
Released by the duodenum in response to fats and acid. It causes the gallbladder to squeeze bile into the duodenum and stimulates the production of pancreatic enzymes, which pass into the duodenum through the pancreatic duct.

Secretin
Secreted by the lining of the duodenum in response to acid entering from the stomach. It acts on the pancreas to increase the output of bicarbonate, which neutralizes acid from the stomach. It also increases the release of enzymes from the pancreas.

Gastrin
Secreted mainly by cells in the stomach in response to eating food (especially protein). It causes the stomach to produce more acid and stimulates contraction of muscle in the wall of part of the stomach, ileum, and colon. This contraction propels food through the digestive tract.

Food enters the stomach
Gallbladder
Esophagus
Stomach
Pancreas
Duodenum

The gastroenterologist, whenever possible, treats patients by advising on diet and life-style and/or by prescribing medication; if necessary, the gastroenterologist refers patients for surgical treatment.

Gastroenterology

The study of the digestive system and the diseases and disorders affecting it. The major organs involved include the mouth, esophagus, stomach, duodenum, small intestine, colon, and rectum. Diseases of the liver, gallbladder, and pancreas are also included in this specialty.

Gastrointestinal hormones

A group of hormones released from specialized endocrine cells in the stomach, pancreas, and intestine that controls various functions of the digestive organs. Gastrin, secretin, and cholecystokinin are probably the best documented of these hormones. (See illustrated box, above.)

Various other gastrointestinal hormones released by the intestine include motilin, neurotensin, and enteroglucagon; their precise functions are still being studied.

DISORDERS

Disorders that are produced by gastrointestinal hormones are relatively rare. The most notable example is a tumor of gastrin-secreting cells in the pancreas or the wall of the intestine, a condition called *Zollinger-Ellison syndrome*.

Gastrointestinal tract

The part of the *digestive system* that consists of the *mouth, esophagus, stomach,* and *intestine*; it excludes the liver, gallbladder, and pancreas.

Gastrojejunostomy

A surgically created connection between the stomach and the jejunum (the middle two thirds of the small intestine). It is sometimes combined with partial *gastrectomy* (removal of the lower part of the stomach).

WHY IT IS DONE

The operation is performed as part of the treatment of a duodenal ulcer (see *Peptic ulcer*). The purpose of the procedure is to allow food to pass directly from the stomach to the small intestine, thereby avoiding the faulty emptying encountered when *vagotomy* alone is performed, and permitting a bypass around a scarred, obstructed duodenum.

HOW IT IS DONE

The preparation of the patient is the same as for gastrectomy. If the gastrojejunostomy is to be combined with partial gastrectomy, some of the lower part of the stomach is removed. The surgeon then pulls up the first part of the jejunum and stitches it to the lower part or remnant of the stomach; a new opening is made through which food will pass.

RECOVERY PERIOD AND OUTLOOK

Complications, recovery, and outlook are the same as for gastrectomy.

Gastroscopy

Examination of the lining of the esophagus, stomach, and duodenum (first part of the small intestine) by means of a long, flexible viewing tube, called an esophagogastroduodeno-scope, inserted through the mouth (see *Endoscope*).

WHY IT IS DONE

Gastroscopy is used to investigate symptoms (such as severe pain or bleeding in the upper abdomen) and to look for disorders of the esophagus, stomach, and duodenum. The procedure may also be used to assess how these disorders are responding to treatment. Gastroscopy is used to identify the source of bleeding and sometimes to treat bleeding sites in the stomach and duodenum.

Attachments at the end of the instrument enable the physician to remove *biopsy* samples (small amounts of tissue for inspection).

Other procedures may be carried out using a gastroscope, such as injecting *esophageal varices* (abnormally enlarged veins in the esophagus) or dilatation (opening up) of an *esophageal stricture*. The gastroscope is also used to facilitate passage of a gastric feeding tube through the skin (percutaneous gastrostomy).

HOW IT IS DONE

The stomach should be empty for gastroscopy, so patients are asked to fast for at least six hours beforehand.

The procedure is usually performed using a local anesthetic sprayed onto the back of the throat and a sedative to relax the patient. A general anesthetic is used if elaborate investigations or treatments are required or if the patient is particularly anxious.

A diagnostic examination usually lasts for between five and 20 minutes. Some discomfort may be felt as the tube passes down the throat; there may be a sore throat afterward.

Complications from gastroscopy are rare. Most are caused by inhalation of vomit or reactions to the sedatives.

Gastrostomy

A surgically produced opening in the stomach, usually connecting the stomach to the outside so that a feed-ing tube can be placed into the stomach or passed into the small intestine. (*Gastroscopy* utilizes a flexible viewing tube to examine the lining of the stomach and other organs.)

People who are starving because of cancer of the esophagus (see *Esophagus, cancer of*) or who are unable to chew and swallow due to stroke or other neurologic disease may be candidates for gastrostomy. (See also *Feeding, artificial*.)

Gauze

An absorbent, open-weave fabric, usually made of cotton. For medical purposes it is usually sterilized and sealed in a package.

Gauze is often used as a *dressing* for wounds. It can be applied dry or can be immersed in an antiseptic fluid or cream; a bandage is used to hold it in place. The gauze absorbs blood and other fluids oozing from the wound. Gauze is usually not used to dress skin ulcers because it tends to stick to moist surfaces and, when removed, dislodges new tissue.

Surgeons sometimes insert pieces of gauze into wounds during surgery to keep the operative site relatively free of blood, which otherwise might obscure structures.

Gavage

The process of feeding liquids through a *nasogastric tube* (one passed into the stomach through the nose). See *Feeding, artificial*.

Gavage also refers to hyperalimentation (treatment of a patient by excessive feeding beyond the requirements of appetite).

Gay bowel syndrome

A group of conditions affecting the anus, rectum, and colon that occurs most frequently, but not exclusively, in male homosexuals.

Most of the conditions in gay bowel syndrome result from various forms of sexual contact, including penile-anal contact, oral-anal contact, and fisting (insertion of the fist into the rectum). If carried out regularly, these activities are likely to cause structural abnormalities (such as *hemorrhoids*, *anal fistulas*, and rectal ulcers) or inflammatory anal-rectal conditions (such as *proctitis*). They may also cause the spread of *AIDS*, *hepatitis*, and intestinal infections (such as *shigellosis* and *amebiasis*) or other infections (such as genital *warts*, *gonorrhea*, *syphilis*, and *lymphogranuloma venereum*) that can also be spread by vaginal intercourse.

Gemfibrozil

A *lipid-lowering drug* used in the treatment of certain types of *hyperlipidemia* (raised levels of fats such as cholesterol in the blood). Gemfibrozil works mainly by reducing the production of lipoproteins (fats combined with protein) in the liver.

Gender identity

The inner feeling of maleness or femaleness. Gender identity is not necessarily the same as biological sex. Gender identity is fixed within the first two to three years of life and is reinforced during puberty; once established, it usually cannot be changed. Gender role is the public declaration of gender identity—that is, the image people present outwardly that confirms their inner feelings about their gender.

Gender identity problems occur when a person has persistent feelings of discomfort about his or her sexual identity. *Transsexualism* is the most common example of this problem.

Gene

 A unit of the material of heredity. In physical terms, a gene consists of a short section of the substance deoxyribonucleic acid (DNA) contained within the nucleus of a cell (see *Nucleic acids*). In functional terms, a particular gene has a specific influence on the workings of a cell; the activities of the same gene in many different cells specifies a particular physical or biochemical feature of the whole body (for example, hair color or a chemical step in the digestion of food).

Every human cell holds, within its nucleus, more than 50,000 different genes. Through the sum of their effects, genes influence and direct the development and functioning of all organs and systems within the entire body. In short, they provide an instruction manual or program for growth, survival, reproduction, and possibly also for aging and death.

Each of a person's cells (with the exception of egg and sperm cells) contains an identical set of genes. This is because all the cells are derived, by a process of division, from a single fertilized egg, and with each division the genes are copied to each offspring cell. Within any cell, however, some genes are active and others are idle, according to the specialized nature of the cell (e.g., different sets of genes are active within liver cells and nerve cells).

WHERE DO YOUR GENES COME FROM?

A person's genes are inherited from his or her parents. Half come from the mother and half from the father via the egg and sperm cells. Each parent provides a different selection, or "mix," of his or her genes to each child; this accounts for the marked differences in appearance, health, and personality among most brothers and sisters. Everyone holds a copy of his or her genes within each body cell.

Gene transmission
In this diagram, only eight genes are shown—in reality, each cell in the body contains about 50,000 genes. Half of them come from the mother and half from the father—thus a quarter of the genes originate from each of the four grandparents.

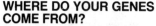
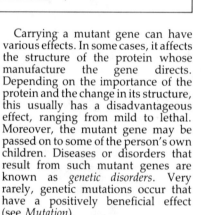

G

If the genes from any two people (other than identical twins) are compared, they always show a number of differences. These differences account for all or much of the variation among people in such aspects as gender, height, skin, hair and eye color, and body shape, and in susceptibility to certain diseases and disorders (see *Inheritance*; *Genetic disorders*). Genes also influence intelligence, personality, physical and mental talents, and behavior, although the extent of their contribution here is less clear-cut because environment and learning also play an important role.

GENE STRUCTURE AND FUNCTION

The physical material of inheritance, DNA, is an extremely long, chainlike structure. Along with some protein, it is what makes up the 23 pairs of *chromosomes* in the nuclei of all cells. A gene corresponds to a small section of DNA within a chromosome.

All genes fulfill their function, or exert an influence in cells or in the body at large, by directing the manufacture of particular proteins. (See illustrated box, next page.)

Although many proteins have a particular structural or catalytic role in the body, others are synthesized solely for the purpose of influencing the activity of other genes, which they are able to switch "on" or "off." The genes responsible for making these proteins are termed "control" genes. The whole process of development and growth can be thought of as being programmed by the sequential switching "on" or "off" of particular genes; this control program is exceedingly complex.

The activities of control genes help differentiate, for example, between nerve and liver cells, where quite different sets of genes are active or idle. If the control genes are disrupted, cells may lose their specialist abilities and begin to multiply out of control; this is the probable mechanism by which cancers and other tumors are started (see *Carcinogenesis*; *Oncogenes*).

MUTANT GENES

Whenever a cell divides, copies of all of its genetic material are made for the two daughter cells by the process of DNA replication (see *Nucleic acids*) and chromosomal division. However, the copying process is not perfect, and very occasionally a fault occurs, leading to a small change (mutation) in the nucleic acid sequence; this, in turn, alters the structure of the DNA in one of the daughter cells—and thus leads to a change in one of its genes. This mutant gene is then passed on each time the cell subsequently divides. If a gene mutation occurs during the formation of an egg or sperm cell that later takes part in fertilization, the person who develops from the fertilized egg will have the mutant gene in each of his or her cells.

Carrying a mutant gene can have various effects. In some cases, it affects the structure of the protein whose manufacture the gene directs. Depending on the importance of the protein and the change in its structure, this usually has a disadvantageous effect, ranging from mild to lethal. Moreover, the mutant gene may be passed on to some of the person's own children. Diseases or disorders that result from such mutant genes are known as *genetic disorders*. Very rarely, genetic mutations occur that have a positively beneficial effect (see *Mutation*).

ALLELES, DOMINANCE, AND RECESSIVENESS

The consequences of inheriting a mutant gene are influenced by further factors. For every protein in the body, there are normally two genes capable of directing the manufacture of that protein—one inherited from the mother and one from the father. These may or may not be identical. The two genes are carried at the same location on each of a pair of chromosomes. If one of the genes mutates, leading to production of an altered protein, it can often be "masked" by the presence of a normal gene on the other chromosome of the pair.

In fact, the gene at any particular location on a chromosome can exist in any of various forms, called alleles, consisting usually of a normal form and one or more mutant forms, which

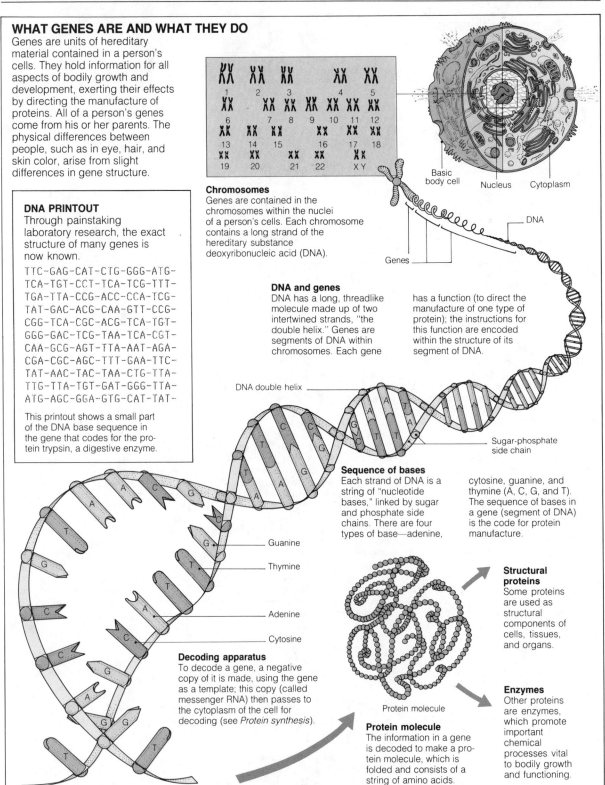

WHAT GENES ARE AND WHAT THEY DO

Genes are units of hereditary material contained in a person's cells. They hold information for all aspects of bodily growth and development, exerting their effects by directing the manufacture of proteins. All of a person's genes come from his or her parents. The physical differences between people, such as in eye, hair, and skin color, arise from slight differences in gene structure.

G

DNA PRINTOUT

Through painstaking laboratory research, the exact structure of many genes is now known.

TTC–GAG–CAT–CTG–GGG–ATG–
TCA–TGT–CCT–TCA–TCG–TTT–
TGA–TTA–CCG–ACC–CCA–TCG–
TAT–GAC–ACG–CAA–GTT–CCG–
CGG–TCA–CGC–ACG–TCA–TGT–
GGG–GAC–TCG–TAA–TCA–CGT–
CAA–GCG–AGT–TTA–AAT–AGA–
CGA–CGC–AGC–TTT–GAA–TTC–
TAT–AAC–TAC–TAA–CTG–TTA–
TTG–TTA–TGT–GAT–GGG–TTA–
ATG–AGC–GGA–GTG–CAT–TAT–

This printout shows a small part of the DNA base sequence in the gene that codes for the protein trypsin, a digestive enzyme.

Basic body cell
Nucleus
Cytoplasm

Chromosomes
Genes are contained in the chromosomes within the nuclei of a person's cells. Each chromosome contains a long strand of the hereditary substance deoxyribonucleic acid (DNA).

DNA

Genes

DNA and genes
DNA has a long, threadlike molecule made up of two intertwined strands, "the double helix." Genes are segments of DNA within chromosomes. Each gene has a function (to direct the manufacture of one type of protein); the instructions for this function are encoded within the structure of its segment of DNA.

DNA double helix

Sugar-phosphate side chain

Sequence of bases
Each strand of DNA is a string of "nucleotide bases," linked by sugar and phosphate side chains. There are four types of base—adenine, cytosine, guanine, and thymine (A, C, G, and T). The sequence of bases in a gene (segment of DNA) is the code for protein manufacture.

Guanine

Thymine

Adenine

Cytosine

Decoding apparatus
To decode a gene, a negative copy of it is made, using the gene as a template; this copy (called messenger RNA) then passes to the cytoplasm of the cell for decoding (see *Protein synthesis*).

Protein molecule

Protein molecule
The information in a gene is decoded to make a protein molecule, which is folded and consists of a string of amino acids.

Structural proteins
Some proteins are used as structural components of cells, tissues, and organs.

Enzymes
Other proteins are enzymes, which promote important chemical processes vital to bodily growth and functioning.

cause the production of altered proteins. If the effects of a particular allele mask or override those of the allele carried at the same location on its partner chromosome, it is said to be dominant. The masked allele is said to be recessive.

Dominant genetic traits, such as brown eyes and blood group A, are those in which the allele producing the trait needs to be present only in a single dose for it to have an outwardly apparent effect. Recessive traits, such as blue eyes and blood group O, are those in which an allele for the trait must usually be present in a double dose for it to have an outward effect.

The patterns by which various traits and disorders are passed on from parents to children, including the further complication of sex-linked and multifactorial inheritance and disorders, are discussed under *Inheritance* and *Genetic disorders*. Medical advice on genetic matters—for example, to parents on the chances of an intended child being affected by a particular genetic disorder—is the province of *genetic counseling*.

Generalized anxiety disorder

A neurotic illness in which the main symptoms are chronic and persistent apprehension and tension about nothing in particular ("free-floating anxiety"). There may also be many unspecific physical reactions such as trembling, jitteriness, sweating, lightheadedness, and irritability.

Symptoms may be so severe that they interfere with everyday living and require medical attention. *Psychotherapy* and drugs are the treatment, although sedatives and tranquilizers are kept to a minimum because dependence can result.

General paralysis of the insane

The common term for the mental and physical deterioration that occurs in the late stage of untreated *syphilis* when it affects the brain substance.

Generic drug

A medicinal drug marketed under its official, chemical name (its generic name) rather than under a patented brand name. Generic names are chosen by appointed drug experts and approved by governmental agencies.

Genetic code

The inherited instructions, contained in chemical form within the nuclei of cells, that specify the activities of cells and thus the development and func-

tioning of the whole body. The term "genetic code" is also used more widely to include the system by which the instructions are copied from a cell to its offspring, the chemical basis by which the instructions are encoded, and the "key" by which the coded instructions are translated.

The basis of the genetic code is contained within molecules of the long, chainlike substance deoxyribonucleic acid (DNA). DNA, along with some protein, makes up the *chromosomes* present in the nuclei of cells. A particular *gene*, or unit of inheritance, corresponds to a section of DNA within a chromosome. Each gene contains the coded instructions for a cell to manufacture a particular protein, which may be an *enzyme* with a vital role in the cell's activities or may have some other function or structural use in the body. Most activity in the body stems from the manufacture of proteins under the guidance of genes.

Little was known about how bits of DNA could specify the manufacture of proteins until the chemical structure of DNA was worked out in 1953. It was found that DNA consists of two long intertwined strands (the "double helix"), each consisting of a sequence of simple chemicals called nucleotide bases. Four different types of base, labeled A, C, G, and T, occur in DNA. The sequence of these bases along particular sections of one of the strands provides the instructions for protein manufacture.

The bases A, C, G, and T can be thought of as the letters of the code. Their sequence along a section of DNA (for example, CGGATCCTAGT-TGATCATGAC) would be completely meaningless without the key to the code, employed by the cell's decoding apparatus. This decoder reads the bases three at a time, and each triplet of bases codes for a particular amino acid, the chemical unit from which proteins are made. For example, the base sequence ACG in a section of DNA codes for the amino acid cysteine and the sequence TGA codes for threonine. As triplets of nucleotide bases are read in turn, the corresponding amino acids are brought together and linked, and, as a complete sequence of bases is read, a chain of amino acids (a polypeptide chain) is formed. This may be a protein molecule itself or may form part of a larger protein structure. Certain base triplets, found at the end of gene sequences, code for termination of protein synthesis.

A complication of the system is that the decoding apparatus does not read directly from DNA but from an intermediary substance, messenger ribonucleic acid (RNA). The DNA acts as a template for RNA manufacture (see *Protein synthesis*). See *Nucleic acids* for the process by which DNA is copied and passed on from each cell to its offspring (and via egg and sperm cells to a new individual).

Genetic counseling

Guidance given to a person or persons (usually by a physician who has experience in genetics) who are considering having a child but are concerned because there is a blood relative (including perhaps a previous child) with an inheritable disorder, or because they are at risk for some other reason of bearing a child with such a disorder.

In most cases, genetic counseling entails predicting the chances of recurrence of a condition that has already affected one or more members of a family. Such counseling depends first on a precise diagnosis of the disorder; the counselor must be able to explain why the disorder occurred and how it is inherited.

Genetic counseling may also include discussion of the prognosis (outlook) for an affected child, advising couples about contraception if, after counseling, they decide not to have children or more children, and sometimes discussing the alternative routes to parenthood.

WHO IS COUNSELED?

Counseling is important for parents of a child with a *genetic disorder*, such as cystic fibrosis or hemophilia, or a *chromosomal abnormality*, such as Down's or Turner's syndrome. It may be useful if a child is born with *birth defects*, such as a cleft lip or congenital heart disease, and may be helpful in many other conditions, such as epilepsy, mental retardation, or abnormal sexual development. It may also be useful for prospective parents if there is a history of any of these conditions in a blood relative.

Genetic counseling may also help in relation to first-cousin marriages and advanced maternal age.

HOW IT IS DONE

Genetic counseling may be provided by a clinical geneticist, by a pediatrician, or by the family practitioner.

The counselor makes a pedigree (family tree) of the family. This includes details of any diseases in the family, any blood relationship

G

G

between partners, or any history of miscarriages. Information from death certificates or postmortem reports of relatives may also be needed.

When a couple has already had a child with abnormalities, the counselor will ask if there was any exposure to radiation or drugs during pregnancy, or if there was any injury to the child at birth, as these can cause abnormalities in otherwise healthy families. The counselor also examines the affected child (and his or her parents) and arranges for any necessary tests, such as *chromosome analysis*, to be done. The parents' chromosomes may sometimes need to be studied as well, because certain conditions, such as Down's syndrome, sometimes result from abnormalities in the parents' chromosomes.

For many genetic disorders, it is now possible to establish with some certainty whether or not the parents of an affected child are "carriers" of a defective gene, which can significantly affect the chances of recurrence. Although the actual genes are not identified, DNA markers (fragments of genetic material known to be close to the defective gene on a chromosome) have been identified, and these can be looked for on the parents' chromosomes by advanced laboratory techniques (see *Genetic probe*). Such techniques are becoming more readily available.

Virtually every case investigated by a genetic counselor is unique. Several factors may influence the chances of a disorder recurring and, in some cases, complex mathematical calculations must be carried out to estimate the risk for a couple.

WHAT IT CAN OFFER

When a couple has had a child with abnormalities, an important aspect of counseling is the explanation of how it occurred and how the child will fare, including the chances of the child having children and whether they, too, will be affected.

Otherwise, advice consists mainly of an estimate of the risk of occurrence or recurrence of the disorder in question. The couple's decision to have children or more children of their own depends partly on the risk estimate, but also on other factors, such as the severity of the disorder, the burden an affected child would place on the family, and the availability of alternative routes to parenthood.

The decision on the best course of action is left to the parents after they have had detailed discussions with the counselor and feel satisfied that they understand the condition in question and its implications.

When there is a significant risk of producing an abnormal child, the parents may choose to try for a healthy child (but may allow the pregnancy to continue to term only if no abnormality is found during prenatal testing). This applies only to certain conditions, such as spina bifida, Down's syndrome, hemophilia, and muscular dystrophy, in which prenatal diagnosis by *amniocentesis* or *chorionic villus sampling* is able to reveal (with reasonable accuracy) an abnormality early in pregnancy. In such cases, an elective abortion may be chosen if an abnormality is found.

If a couple decides against having children, options for parenthood include adoption and *artificial insemination* by donor (the mother's egg is fertilized by a donor sperm). The latter is worth considering if both parents are carriers of a rare inherited condition or if the father has a dominant or X-linked genetic disorder.

Test-tube fertilizaton of a donor egg by the father's sperm, in cases where the mother carries an abnormal gene, is not yet widely available but is a possibility for the future.

Genetic disorders

Any disorder caused, wholly or in part, by a fault or faults in the inherited, genetic material within a person's cells—that is, in the *genes* formed from the substance deoxyribonucleic acid (DNA), which make up the *chromosomes* in a person's cells. A large number of diseases have, wholly or in part, a genetic cause.

Many genetic disorders are apparent at birth and are thus also *congenital*. However, the terms genetic and congenital are not synonymous; many genetic defects do not become apparent until many years after birth, and many congenital abnormalities are not genetic in origin.

Most people with a genetic disorder have one or more relatives affected by the same disorder—that is, the disorder is also *familial*. However, there are also occasions when a child is born unexpectedly with a genetic disorder (that is, with no previous family history). There are a number of mechanisms by which this can occur.

CAUSES AND TYPES

The reason abnormal genetic material can lead to disorders or disease is that genes control the manufacture in cells of *enzymes* and other proteins that play roles of varying importance in cells and in the body as a whole. If the genetic material is defective, abnormal proteins (or abnormal amounts of proteins) may be produced, causing disturbances in body chemistry that lead to disease.

For a person to exhibit a genetic disorder, the abnormality in the genetic material must usually be present in each of his or her cells, which means that it must also have been present in either the egg or the sperm cell (or both) from which the individual was derived. There are two ways in which this can happen. The first is that one or both parents carried a defect in their own genetic material; the second is that a *mutation* (a change in the genetic material) occurred during the formation of egg or sperm cell. Mutations are one of the mechanisms by which a child affected by a genetic disorder can be born into a family that has never had a known history of genetic disorders. With some of the more common genetic disorders, such as hemophilia, about one third of cases are due to new mutations.

Genetic disorders fall into three broad classes: chromosome abnormalities, unifactorial defects, and multifactorial defects. In the first, a child is born with an abnormal number of whole chromosomes, or extra or missing bits of chromosomes, in the cells. Since chromosomes contain many genes, this can lead to multiple disturbances and disorders. (See *Chromosomal abnormalities*.)

Unifactorial disorders are caused by a single defective gene or pair of genes; these disorders are distributed among the members of an affected family according to relatively simple laws of inheritance. Multifactorial disorders are caused by the additive effects of several genes, along with environmental factors; the pattern of inheritance is less straightforward.

UNIFACTORIAL DISORDERS

These disorders are rare, but there are many, and in total they cause a considerable amount of disability.

All unifactorial genetic disorders are the result of defects in a gene, or in a pair of genes, controlling the production of a particular protein. They can be divided into two groups—called sex-linked and autosomal disorders—according to whether the affected gene or genes are located on the sex chromosomes (nearly always the X chromosome) or on any of the other 22 pairs of chromosomes, which are called autosomes (see *Chromosomes*).

UNIFACTORIAL GENETIC DISORDERS

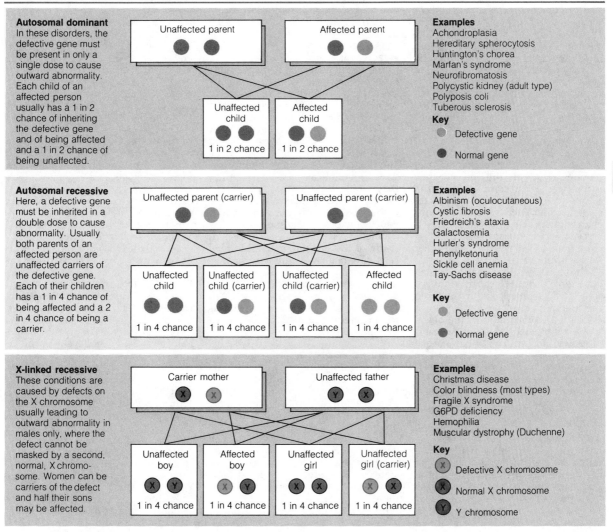

Autosomal dominant
In these disorders, the defective gene must be present in only a single dose to cause outward abnormality. Each child of an affected person usually has a 1 in 2 chance of inheriting the defective gene and of being affected and a 1 in 2 chance of being unaffected.

Unaffected parent

Affected parent

Unaffected child — 1 in 2 chance

Affected child — 1 in 2 chance

Examples
Achondroplasia
Hereditary spherocytosis
Huntington's chorea
Marfan's syndrome
Neurofibromatosis
Polycystic kidney (adult type)
Polyposis coli
Tuberous sclerosis

Key
Defective gene
Normal gene

Autosomal recessive
Here, a defective gene must be inherited in a double dose to cause abnormality. Usually both parents of an affected person are unaffected carriers of the defective gene. Each of their children has a 1 in 4 chance of being affected and a 2 in 4 chance of being a carrier.

Unaffected parent (carrier)

Unaffected parent (carrier)

Unaffected child — 1 in 4 chance

Unaffected child (carrier) — 1 in 4 chance

Unaffected child (carrier) — 1 in 4 chance

Affected child — 1 in 4 chance

Examples
Albinism (oculocutaneous)
Cystic fibrosis
Friedreich's ataxia
Galactosemia
Hurler's syndrome
Phenylketonuria
Sickle cell anemia
Tay-Sachs disease

Key
Defective gene
Normal gene

X-linked recessive
These conditions are caused by defects on the X chromosome usually leading to outward abnormality in males only, where the defect cannot be masked by a second, normal, X chromosome. Women can be carriers of the defect and half their sons may be affected.

Carrier mother

Unaffected father

Unaffected boy — 1 in 4 chance

Affected boy — 1 in 4 chance

Unaffected girl — 1 in 4 chance

Unaffected girl (carrier) — 1 in 4 chance

Examples
Christmas disease
Color blindness (most types)
Fragile X syndrome
G6PD deficiency
Hemophilia
Muscular dystrophy (Duchenne)

Key
X Defective X chromosome
X Normal X chromosome
Y Y chromosome

G

Autosomal disorders generally affect both sexes equally and are further divided into two groups, called autosomal dominant and autosomal recessive, according to whether the defective gene need be present in a single or double dose to cause an outward abnormality.

The sex-linked disorders show a bias in their incidence among the sexes. Most are of one type—called X-linked recessive disorders—and primarily males are affected.

Some examples of these three varieties of unifactorial disorder are shown in the table.

AUTOSOMAL DOMINANT DISORDERS With these disorders, a person need carry the defective gene in only a single dose for it to have an outwardly apparent effect. Such individuals are termed *heterozygotes* with respect to the gene, which means they carry one normal copy and one defective copy of the gene. Because the defective gene is dominant—that is, it overrides the normal gene—its presence usually leads to an outward abnormality (but not always a severe one).

Some affected people have inherited the defective gene from one of their parents. In other cases there is no family history of the condition; the defect has usually arisen as a result of a mutation.

If an affected individual has children, each one has a 50 percent chance of inheriting the defective gene and thus also the chance of being affected. Often these disorders appear in each of several generations, finally disappearing only when the affected individuals in a generation have no affected children or no children at all.

AUTOSOMAL RECESSIVE DISORDERS People who manifest these disorders have always acquired the particular gene defect in a double dose—they are said to be *homozygotes* with respect to the defective gene. In most cases, both parents of an affected person are heterozygotes—they carry the defective gene in a single dose along with a normal gene. But, because the defective gene is recessive and "masked" by the normal gene, they display no outward abnormality.

With all autosomal recessive defects, the number of such carriers in the population always outnumbers those who are actually affected. For example, with *cystic fibrosis* (the most common disorder of this type), one in 22 of the population is a carrier of the defective gene, but only one person in 2,000 is born with the condition. The majority of carriers are unaware of the fact and have no family history of the condition—the defective gene has been passed on to them silently over many generations. When two carriers have children and one is born with an autosomal recessive condition, the manifestation of the defect thus usually comes as a complete surprise.

If both parents are carriers, any subsequent child will have a one in four chance of also being affected.

X-LINKED RECESSIVE DISORDERS In these conditions, the defective gene is on the X chromosome. Women have two X chromosomes in their cells; men have only one, which they inherit from their mothers and pass on to their daughters.

When a woman inherits the defective gene in a single dose, because it is recessive, it is masked by the normal gene on her other X chromosome, so she displays no outward abnormality. She is a heterozygote carrier of the defective gene. However, when a male inherits the defective gene, there is no normal gene on a second X chromosome to mask it, and he will display the abnormality.

The familial pattern of these disorders is as follows. Affected males far outnumber affected females and in all cases have inherited the genetic defect from their mother (who is a carrier). They pass the defective gene to none of their sons but to all of their daughters, who become carriers in turn. Carrier females transmit the defective gene on average to half their sons, who are affected, and to half their daughters, who become carriers in turn. Thus, the pattern is for some of the males in an affected family to have the disorder, while the females in the family are either known or possible carriers.

MULTIFACTORIAL DISORDERS
A large number of disorders fall into this category—including *asthma*, insulin-dependent *diabetes mellitus*, *schizophrenia*, and a number of conditions present at birth, such as clubfoot and *cleft lip and palate*.

In each case, susceptibility to the disorder is thought to be determined by a number of different genes that,

along with environmental influences, have an additive effect. The degree to which susceptibility to each of these various disorders is determined by genes has been estimated and is termed its *heritability*.

AFFECTED FAMILIES
The underlying cause of genetic disorders (defects in genes) cannot be treated. However, there are a number of methods by which the chances of a child being born with a genetically based disorder can be reduced.

If a couple is considering having children and any parents or close blood relatives (or they themselves) have a genetically based disorder, they would be wise to obtain *genetic counseling*. This is especially important if the couple has had a child with a genetically based condition.

Once a pregnancy is established, study of the genetic material in fetal cells obtained by techniques such as *chorionic villus sampling* and *amniocentesis* can establish whether or not certain genetic disorders are present. In cases where a serious disorder is found, a termination of the pregnancy may be chosen.

Genetic engineering
A branch of *genetics* concerned, in its broadest sense, with the alteration of the inherited, genetic material carried by a living organism to produce some desired change in the characteristics of the organism.

In practice, the main application of genetic engineering to date has been to mass-produce a variety of substances—all proteins of various sorts—that have uses in medical treatment and diagnosis. The function of any *gene* is to control the production of a particular protein in a living cell. If the gene responsible for synthesizing a useful protein can be identified, and if such a gene can be inserted into another cell that can be made to reproduce rapidly, then a colony of cells containing the gene can be grown. The colony will then produce the protein in large amounts.

WHY IT IS DONE
Genetic engineering has been used for producing some human hormones (notably *insulin* and *growth hormone*), some proteins for use in vaccines (against hepatitis, for example), and *interferon*, a substance with potential for treating viral infections. Other valuable aids to treatment are genetically engineered *factor VIII* (a protein used for the treatment of hemophilia), TPA (*tissue plasminogen*

activator), a substance that dissolves blood clots, and many other medically useful substances.

HOW IT IS DONE
The main technique for mass-producing useful proteins by genetic engineering is called recombinant deoxyribonucleic acid (DNA) technology. DNA is the substance in cells that consists of strings of genes, which control the manufacture of different proteins.

The first step is to identify the gene in the DNA of a cell that controls the manufacture of a particularly useful protein. This involves a number of highly sophisticated laboratory techniques. The next step is either to extract the gene from the cell or, if the exact chemical structure of the gene can be worked out, to synthesize it.

The final step is to introduce the gene into the DNA of a suitable recipient cell. By the use of *enzymes* that can split a molecule of the recipient cell's DNA at certain sites, a gap can be produced into which the additional gene can be spliced (hence the term recombinant DNA).

The types of cells or organisms suitable for such genetic alteration are those that can subsequently be made to reproduce rapidly and indefinitely. The most popular organisms to date have been the common intestinal bacterium *ESCHERICHIA COLI* and various yeasts, but cells of other organisms, including human cancer cells, have also been used with success.

OUTLOOK
In view of the ease with which some of the bacteria and other organisms used for genetic engineering can reproduce, and the possibility of accidentally creating and liberating highly dangerous microorganisms, doubts have frequently been expressed about the dangers of "tampering with nature" in this way. These dangers are real but are well recognized by researchers in the field, who have produced stringent codes of practice and regulations to ensure safety.

In the future, it may be possible to extend genetic engineering to the manipulation of human genetic material for purposes of treating *genetic disorders*.

Genetic probe
A specific fragment of deoxyribonucleic acid (*DNA*) used to determine whether particular defects or genetic "markers" are present in a person's or a fetus's genetic material—that is, in the DNA that, along with some pro-

tein, makes up the *chromosomes* in his or her cells.

Genetic probes are used primarily in the prenatal diagnosis of certain genetic disorders and to determine whether or not certain people are "carriers" of gene defects. Often, there is no technique for detecting the defective gene itself. However, for certain gene defects (e.g., the one responsible for *cystic fibrosis*) markers (sections of DNA with a specific base sequence) have been identified that very commonly occur on particular chromosomes in association with the defect. Hence, if the marker can be found, it provides strong evidence that the gene defect is also present. This has particular implications for *genetic counseling*.

In one technique, the chromosome under test (obtained from a cell of the person or the fetus under investigation) is first broken up using *enzymes* (the probe) in a test tube; the fragments are then fixed onto a filter. A radioactively labeled sequence of DNA that will bind to the "marker" sequence of DNA in the chromosome (if present) is then added, and sophisticated techniques are performed to see whether such binding has occurred.

Genetics

The study of *inheritance*—that is, how the characteristics of living organisms are passed from one generation to another, the chemical basis by which such characteristics are determined, and the causes of the similarities and differences among individuals of one species (for example, the human species) or among different species. More particularly, genetics includes the study of deoxyribonucleic acid (*DNA*), the substance in cells that determines the characteristics of an organism, and of *genes*, which are units of inheritance corresponding to specific bits of DNA.

Particular branches of human genetics include population genetics, which studies the relative frequency of various genes in different human races; molecular genetics, which is concerned with the structure, function, and copying of DNA from one cell to another, and also how *mutations* (changes) occur in DNA; and medical or clinical genetics, which is concerned with the study and prevention of *genetic disorders*.

Genital herpes

See *Herpes, genital*.

Genitalia

The reproductive organs, especially the external ones. The male genitalia include the *penis*, *testes* (within the *scrotum*), *prostate gland*, seminal vesicles, and associated ducts, such as the *epididymis* and *vas deferens*. The female genitalia include the *ovaries*, *fallopian tubes*, *uterus*, *vagina*, *clitoris*, *vulva*, and *Bartholin's glands*.

Genital ulceration

An eroded area of skin on the *genitalia*. In men the ulcer may be on the skin of the penis or scrotum; in women it may be on the vulva or within the vagina.

CAUSES

The most common cause of genital ulceration is a *sexually transmitted disease*. The early stages of *syphilis* are characterized by a hard *chancre*, a painless ulcer where the bacteria penetrated the skin. This may be followed by shallow, elongated ulcers once the chancre has healed. The *herpes simplex* virus causes painful, fluid-filled blisters to develop on the genitalia; if these blisters become infected by bacteria they may ulcerate. Both *chancroid* and *granuloma inguinale* are bacterial infections that cause genital ulcers; they are common in tropical countries. In the former the ulcers are painful, in the latter they are painless. *Lymphogranuloma venereum* is a viral infection in which the resulting blisters occasionally ulcerate.

Other causes of genital ulceration include *herpes zoster*, *tuberculosis*, or a tumor of the testis, which can erode the scrotum to cause an ulcer.

Genital ulceration may also be a side effect of drugs. It can be caused by solutions applied to genital warts in high concentrations. It can also be a reaction to a drug taken by mouth; sulfonamide antibacterial drugs, for example, can cause mouth and genital ulcers (see *Stevens-Johnson syndrome*).

Behçet's syndrome is a rare condition that causes tender, recurrent ulcers in the mouth and on the genitals. Cancer of the penis or vulva may cause a single, painless ulcer with raised, rolled edges that turn outward.

DIAGNOSIS

The diagnosis of the underlying cause is made from the appearance of the ulcer and the presence of other signs, such as enlarged lymph glands or a skin rash. Swabs from the ulcer are taken and the material examined and cultured to look for a specific bacterium or virus. Blood tests to detect antibodies to a specific type of infection may be performed.

Genital warts

See *Warts, genital*.

Gentamicin

ANTIBIOTIC			
Injection	Ointment	Cream	Eye drops
📄 Prescription needed			
🆔 Available as generic			

A drug given by injection, sometimes in combination with another antibiotic, to treat serious infections. For example, gentamicin is used to treat *meningitis*, *septicemia* (blood poisoning), and *endocarditis* (inflammation of the heart lining). Gentamicin cannot be given by mouth because it is inactivated during digestion.

During treatment, blood tests are taken to determine gentamicin levels to monitor dosage and thus reduce the risk of toxic damage to the kidneys or inner ear.

The drug is used in eye drops to treat *conjunctivitis* caused by infection.

Gentian violet

A purple dye used mainly by biologists to make bacteria visible under the microscope. Gentian violet also has antiseptic properties and can be applied to the skin to treat burns, boils, carbuncles, and fungal infections. It is occasionally used to relieve soreness in the mouth caused by *candidiasis* (thrush).

Genu valgum

The medical term for *knock-knee*.

Genu varum

The medical term for *bowleg*.

Geriatrician

A physician who specializes in treating elderly patients and the special conditions related to aging.

Geriatric medicine

The medical specialty concerned with care of the elderly. Many diseases and disorders that affect the elderly may occur in patients of all ages, but older people tend to respond differently to sickness and treatment. For example, *aging* is associated with a progressive decline in the functioning of major organs—the heart, lungs, kidneys, liver, and brain. Consequently, an infection in one of these organs or elsewhere in the body that would cause only minor illness in a young adult might be life-threatening in an

G

older person. Any illness in an elderly person may cause a temporary but marked slowing of thought processes, and may even lead to confusion and other features that may be mistaken for dementia. This is due to the added stress placed on the brain during the illness. Furthermore, many medicinal drugs are eliminated from the body by the liver or kidneys and, if these organs are affected by aging, dosages of drugs used in treatment may need to be modified to avoid dangerous side effects.

A physician who specializes in geriatrics is expert at assessing the health of patients and in assessing the complex features of their disease. He or she takes particular care not to give excessive doses of drugs and tries also to avoid moving the patient away from familiar surroundings unless hospital admission is essential. Geriatricians are also skilled at rehabilitation; they usually make the contacts (with social services and voluntary agencies) that are necessary to arrange a comprehensive rehabilitation program.

Germ

The popular term for any microorganism that causes disease. Examples include a *virus* or bacterium (see *Bacteria*). In medicine, the term is used to describe simple, undifferentiated cells that are capable of developing into specialized tissues, such as the cells of the early embryo.

German measles

Another name for *rubella*.

Germ cell tumor

A localized proliferation of cells that are the immature forms of either sperm in the male testis or ova (eggs) in the female ovary. (See *Seminoma*.)

Gerontology

The study of *aging* in all its aspects (developmental, biological, medical, sociological, and psychological). The specialty that treats the medical problems of the elderly is called geriatrics (see *Geriatric medicine*).

Gestalt theory

Ideas based on the notion that the whole is more than the sum of its parts; a school of psychology based on the idea that a sense of wholeness is more important than the individual bits and pieces of perception and behavior. It was founded in Germany

early this century by a group that adopted the name gestalt, meaning "form," "pattern," or "configuration." In studying emotional states and social issues, Gestalt theory emphasizes viewing things as a whole rather than breaking them down into collections of stimuli and responses. Gestalt therapy became popular as a means of coping with personal problems and is still practiced today by some therapists; this type of therapy aims to increase self-awareness by looking at all aspects of an individual within his or her environment.

Gestation

The period from conception to birth, during which the developing fetus is carried in the uterus.

Gestation normally lasts around 270 days, about nine months. Because of the difficulty in determining the precise date of conception, physicians time pregnancies from the first day of the last normal menstrual period, giving a gestation period of 284 days.

Giardiasis

An infection of the small intestine, caused by the protozoan (single-celled) parasite *GIARDIA LAMBLIA*. Giardiasis is most common in tropical areas and in travelers to the tropics. Recently it has become more common in developed countries, affecting especially homosexual men, people living in institutions, and preschool children. The infection is particularly

common where large numbers of young children gather together—for example, in day-care centers and preschools. The disease is spread by contaminated food or water or by direct personal contact (e.g., by hand-to-mouth contact).

SYMPTOMS

About two thirds of those infected have no symptoms. When symptoms do occur they begin one to three days after the parasite has entered the body. The person has violent attacks of diarrhea accompanied by flatus (gas); the feces are foul-smelling, may be greasy, and tend to float in the toilet bowl. Abdominal discomfort, cramps, or swelling, loss of appetite, and nausea may also occur. In some cases, the infection becomes chronic.

DIAGNOSIS AND TREATMENT

The infection is diagnosed from microscopic examination of a sample of feces for the presence of the parasites. If there is any doubt, a jejunal *biopsy* (removal of a small sample of tissue for microscopic analysis) may be carried out.

Acute giardiasis usually clears up without treatment. However, treatment incorporating the antibiotic metronidazole or quinacrine relieves symptoms quickly and prevents the spread of infection.

PREVENTION

Infection can be prevented by thorough hand washing before handling food and by avoiding eating food or drinking water that could possibly be contaminated.

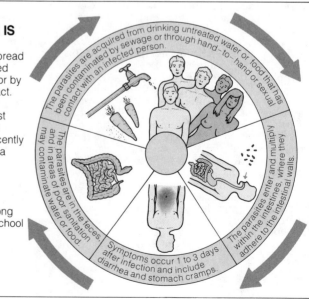

HOW GIARDIASIS IS SPREAD

Giardiasis is spread by contaminated water or food, or by personal contact. This parasitic infection is most common in the tropics, but recently it has become a more frequent occurrence in developed countries, especially among groups of preschool children.

The parasites are acquired from drinking untreated water or food that has been contaminated by sewage or through hand-to-hand or sexual contact with an infected person.

The parasites enter and multiply within the intestine, where they adhere to the intestinal walls.

Symptoms occur 1 to 3 days after infection and include diarrhea and stomach cramps.

The parasites are in the feces and in areas of poor sanitation may contaminate water or food.

Giddiness
See *Dizziness*.

Gigantism
Excessive growth (especially height) resulting from overproduction, during childhood or adolescence, of growth hormone by a tumor of the pituitary gland. Untreated, the tumor eventually destroys the pituitary gland and results in death during early adult life. If the tumor develops after growth has stopped, the result is *acromegaly* rather than gigantism.

Oversecretion of growth hormone from early life can result in an individual attaining an immense height. The tallest documented giant in medical history, Robert Wadlow, reached a height of 8 feet 11 inches and a weight of 475 pounds before he died at age 22. Such instances are rare, however. By far the most common reason for a child being tall is that his or her parents are tall. Other rare causes of excessive height in childhood are *Marfan's syndrome* and *thyrotoxicosis*.

DIAGNOSIS AND TREATMENT
The diagnosis of gigantism is made when *brain imaging* and blood tests confirm the presence of a pituitary tumor and excessive growth hormone. The condition may be treated with bromocriptine, a drug that blocks the release of growth hormone, or by surgery or radiation therapy to destroy or remove the tumor.

Gilbert's disease
An inherited disorder that affects the way bilirubin is processed by the liver and that may cause mild jaundice. Sufferers are otherwise healthy.

Gilbert's disease is common, affecting about 2 percent of the population. Usually there are no symptoms. When there are symptoms, they may include malaise, anorexia, upper abdominal pain, and mild jaundice.

Usually no treatment is necessary, but the drug phenobarbital can relieve jaundice and other symptoms.

Gilles de la Tourette's syndrome
A rare disorder of movement, named for the French neurologist who first described it in 1885. It starts in childhood with repetitive grimaces and tics, usually of the head and neck, sometimes of the arms, legs, and trunk. Involuntary barks, grunts, or other noises may appear as the disease progresses. In about half the cases, the sufferer has episodes of coprolalia (using foul language).

The syndrome is more common in males, partially inherited, and is probably underdiagnosed because of its strange symptoms. It is usually of lifelong duration but *antipsychotic drugs*, such as haloperidol, can often provide effective relief.

Gingiva
The Latin name for the *gum* that surrounds the base of the teeth.

Gingivectomy
Surgical removal of part of the gum margin. Gingivectomy may be used to treat severe cases of gingival *hyperplasia* (thickening of the gums), a condition usually caused by anticonvulsant treatment with phenytoin. Gingivectomy also is used to remove pockets of infected gums formed during advanced stages of gum disease (*periodontitis*).

Gingivectomy is performed in the dentist's office using local anesthetic. After surgery, the newly exposed area around the base of the teeth may initially be sensitive; the exposure also gives the teeth a longer appearance. There are no complications as long as scrupulous *oral hygiene* is maintained after surgery.

Gingivitis
Inflammation of the gingiva (gums), often due to infection. Gingivitis is a reversible stage of gum disease.

CAUSES
Gingivitis is usually caused by the buildup of plaque (a sticky deposit of bacteria, mucus, food particles, and other irritants) around the base of the teeth. It is thought that toxins produced by bacteria within the plaque irritate the gums, causing the gums to become infected, tender, and swollen. Gingivitis can result from injury to the gums, usually from overvigorous toothbrushing or careless flossing.

INCIDENCE
Mild gingivitis is very common in young adults. Pregnant women and diabetics are susceptible because of changes in their hormone levels.

SYMPTOMS
Healthy gums are pink or brown and firm; in people with gingivitis, they become red-purple, soft, shiny, and swollen. The gums bleed easily, especially during toothbrushing, and are often tender.

PREVENTION AND TREATMENT
Good *oral hygiene* is the main means of preventing and treating gingivitis. Teeth should be thoroughly brushed with a fluoride dentifrice (toothpaste)

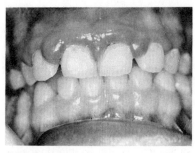

Example of gingivitis
The gums around the bases of the upper teeth are puffy, shiny, and tender. They overhang the teeth margins. Affected gums often bleed when brushed.

at least once a day and after meals, if possible; dental floss should be used at least once a day. It is also important to visit your dentist at least once a year (or more often if he or she recommends) so that teeth can be cleaned to remove calculus (mineralized plaque) and accumulated plaque through a procedure known as scaling. The dentist may prescribe an antibacterial mouthwash for use at home.

COMPLICATIONS
Untreated gingivitis may damage gum tissue around the base of the teeth, leading to the formation of pockets in which plaque and calculus can collect. Bacteria within the plaque may cause inflammation to spread, eventually leading to *periodontitis*, an advanced stage of gum disease in which the supporting tissues of the teeth and the surrounding bone become eroded, loosening the teeth.

Acute necrotizing ulcerative gingivitis may develop due to invasion of tissue by *anaerobic* bacteria in people with chronic gingivitis, especially those with lowered resistance to infection. Also called trench mouth or Vincent's disease, acute necrotizing ulcerative gingivitis is a serious condition resulting in destruction of gum tissue; it requires a course of antibiotic treatment.

Gland
A group of specialized cells that manufactures and releases chemical substances, such as hormones and *enzymes*, for use in the body.

There are two main types of glands: endocrine and exocrine. *Endocrine glands* do not have ducts and thus release their secretions directly into the bloodstream; examples include the pituitary, thyroid, and adrenal glands. Target organs may be quite distant from the endocrine glands.

Exocrine glands have ducts and release their secretions either onto the surface of the skin or into a hollow structure such as the mouth or digestive tract; examples include the sebaceous glands, which secrete sebum onto the skin, and the salivary glands.

Collections of cells in the *lymphatic system*, the lymph nodes, are sometimes referred to as glands. Strictly speaking, this is incorrect usage because they do not secrete chemical substances. However, they do release white blood cells, which play an important role in fighting infections and allergic reactions.

Glanders

An infection of horses and donkeys that is rarely transmitted to humans. It occurs in Asia, Africa, and South America and is caused by the bacterium PSEUDOMONAS MALLEI, which enters the body through a cut or abrasion or by being breathed in.

Initially, symptoms (mild fever, headache, general aches and pains, and possibly some generalized swelling of the lymph nodes) are vague. If bacterial entry was through a wound, ulcers or abscesses may then appear at the site; if entry was through the lungs, *pneumonia* may develop. In severe cases, *septicemia* (blood poisoning) may then follow.

DIAGNOSIS AND TREATMENT

The disease is diagnosed by identifying the bacteria in a sample of pus or sputum (phlegm) or by detecting antibodies to the bacteria in a blood sample. Early treatment with an appropriate antibiotic usually clears the infection.

Glands, swollen

Known medically as lymphadenopathy, enlargement of the lymph nodes (glands) as a result of inflammation and/or proliferation of white blood cells within them.

CAUSES

Swollen glands are a very common symptom and are usually due to an infection or allergic reaction (see *Allergy*). Children are especially prone to swollen glands as a result of infection, partly because the lymphatic system plays a more important part in combating infections in childhood than in adult life.

Rarer causes of swollen glands include *lymphoma*, *Hodgkin's disease*, *leukemia* (cancer of the white blood cells), or a *metastasis* (secondary cancer that has spread from elsewhere in the body).

When the underlying cause is localized, swollen glands also tend to be confined to a limited area; for example, a throat infection may result in swelling only of the lymph glands in the neck.

Swollen glands near the surface of the skin—in the groin or neck, for example—are usually felt as tender, slightly warm lumps. However, swelling of deeper glands, such as those in the lungs or abdomen, is almost invariably unnoticeable.

INVESTIGATION AND TREATMENT

In many cases, the cause of swollen glands is obvious from the presence of a localized infection or a bee sting that has caused an allergic reaction. In other cases, the accompanying symptoms usually indicate the cause; for example, swollen glands with a sore throat, fever, and tiredness suggest infectious *mononucleosis* (glandular fever).

If swollen glands persist or there is no obvious cause, tests may be necessary. These may include a blood count, chest X rays to look for swollen glands in the lungs, or a *biopsy* (removal of tissue for microscopic analysis) of an affected gland.

Treatment depends on the underlying cause. Antibiotics may be given for a bacterial infection, antihistamines for an allergy, or *radiation therapy* or *chemotherapy* (or both) may be used to treat a tumor.

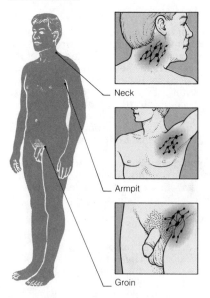

Common sites of swollen glands
The three most common sites where swollen glands can be felt are in the neck, armpit, and groin.

Glandular fever

See *Mononucleosis, infectious.*

Glasses

Simple optical devices used to correct focusing errors in the eyes so that clear vision is achieved. The lenses are made of glass or plastic and the shape and thickness are chosen during an eye test (see *Vision tests*).

TYPES OF LENSES

Lenses may be convex (outwardly curved), concave (inwardly curved), or cylindrical. Most are single-vision lenses, but bifocal or trifocal lenses, with smaller areas differing in power from the main lens, are common. Varifocal lenses, with power increasing gradually from the center to one edge, are becoming popular. Lenses may have a permanent tint or may incorporate chemicals that produce darkening on exposure to light.

Glass eye

See *Eye, artificial.*

Glaucoma

A condition in which the pressure of the fluid in the eye is so abnormally high that it causes damage. A minimal pressure is required to maintain the shape of the eyeball, but excessive pressure may result in the compression and obstruction of the small internal blood vessels and/or the fibers of the optic nerve. The result is nerve fiber destruction and partial or complete loss of vision.

TYPES AND CAUSES

The most common form is chronic open-angle glaucoma, which rarely occurs before the age of 40 and often causes no symptoms until blindness is advanced. It is due to a gradual blockage of the outflow of aqueous humor (fluid in the front compartment of the eye) over a period of years, causing a slow rise in pressure. This type tends to run in families.

In acute closed-angle glaucoma, there is a sudden obstruction to the outflow of aqueous humor from the eye and the pressure rises suddenly. Subacute angle-closure glaucoma is similar to acute glaucoma, but develops more slowly or occurs intermittently.

Congenital glaucoma is due to a structural abnormality in the drainage angles of the eyes.

Glaucoma can also be caused by injury to the eye, or by a serious eye disease such as *uveitis*, dislocation of the lens, or adhesions between the iris and the cornea.

WHY GLASSES ARE USED

For *hyperopia* (farsightedness), convex (or plus) lenses are needed. Sufferers of *presbyopia* also need plus (magnifying) lenses. Myopia (nearsightedness) requires concave (or minus) lenses.

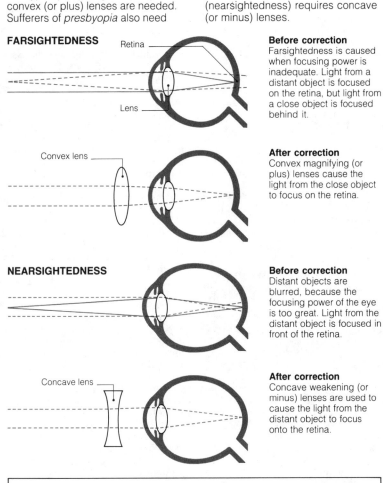

FARSIGHTEDNESS

Retina

Lens

Before correction
Farsightedness is caused when focusing power is inadequate. Light from a distant object is focused on the retina, but light from a close object is focused behind it.

Convex lens

After correction
Convex magnifying (or plus) lenses cause the light from the close object to focus on the retina.

NEARSIGHTEDNESS

Before correction
Distant objects are blurred, because the focusing power of the eye is too great. Light from the distant object is focused in front of the retina.

Concave lens

After correction
Concave weakening (or minus) lenses are used to cause the light from the distant object to focus onto the retina.

ASTIGMATISM

The surrounding surfaces of the cornea are steeper in one direction than in the other. The correcting lenses are designed with additional curvature in one meridian. The lenses are then set accurately in the frame of the glasses so that the steepest curves correspond to the flattest meridian of the cornea. Both concave lenses for myopia and convex lenses for hyperopia and presbyopia can be designed in this way to correct astigmatism.

Vertical plane in focus

Lens

Horizontal plane out of focus

Retina

INCIDENCE

Glaucoma is one of the most common major eye disorders in people over 60; it is responsible for 15 percent of blindness in adults in the US. Nearly 2 percent of people over the age of 40 have chronic glaucoma. The incidence rises with age and about 10 percent of people over 70 have abnormally raised pressure within the eye.

SYMPTOMS AND SIGNS

Chronic glaucoma often causes no symptoms because the gradual loss of peripheral vision is not apparent to the affected person. Only late in the disease, when there is severe, irreversible damage, may the person be aware of some visual loss.

G

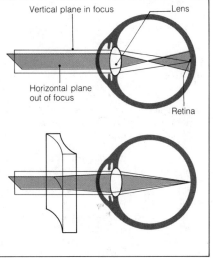

Ciliary body

Blocked drainage channel

Cornea

Iris

Aqueous humor

Lens

Acute closed-angle glaucoma
This type of glaucoma is caused by an unduly narrow angle between the iris and the back of the peripheral cornea. Dilation of the pupil may therefore lead to a sudden complete blockage of the outflow, causing a rapid increase in pressure in the eyeball.

The symptoms of acute glaucoma include a dull, severe, aching pain in and above the eye, some fogginess of vision, and the perception of rainbow rings around lights at night (halos). Nausea and vomiting can occur and the eye can become red and have a partly dilated pupil and a hazy cornea. Subacute glaucoma can cause similar mild, brief episodes.

DIAGNOSIS

Chronic glaucoma often causes no symptoms and is usually detected only by regular, routine eye examina-

G

tions. Applanation tonometry (by which eye pressure is measured) is an essential check for glaucoma (see *Eye, examination of*), especially if there is a family history of the disorder. Use of an *ophthalmoscope* to examine the back of the eye may show an abnormal optic nerve. Visual field testing and gonioscopy (examination of the drainage angle) can also be important.

TREATMENT

Chronic open-angle glaucoma can usually be controlled with eye drops, which reduce the pressure in the eye. Repeated tonometry and visual field testing may be carried out to ensure that the pressure is being controlled; if necessary, other eye drops will be given. If drops fail to control the pressure, tablets or long-acting capsules may also be prescribed. The medications for treatment of chronic glaucoma usually are prescribed for life since, if stopped, the pressure generally rises. If medications fail to reduce the pressure in chronic glaucoma, and if there is a continuing loss of visual field or vision, laser surgery or cutting surgery may be necessary to open up the drainage channel or to create an artificial channel for the aqueous humor.

Acute closed-angle glaucoma is a medical emergency calling for urgent treatment. Various treatments (i.e., eye drops, pills, liquids, and/or intravenous fluids) are given to try to reduce the very high eye pressure. Usually, after the pressure is controlled, laser surgery or cutting surgery is necessary for the treatment of acute glaucoma and subacute glaucoma to try to prevent a recurrent attack. Usually a peripheral *iridectomy* is done. A small opening is made in the periphery of the iris so that aqueous humor can drain more easily. The iridectomy is often curative but, if the drainage angle was damaged by the attack, medications may be needed to control the pressure after surgery. If the iris is scarred at the drainage angle, other types of surgery, such as creating an artificial drainage channel, may be necessary.

OUTLOOK

The pressure rise of glaucoma can be prevented by treatment, but early diagnosis and treatment are needed to prevent any impairment of vision. Regular eye examinations are important for early detection.

Glioblastoma multiforme

A fast-growing and highly malignant type of *brain tumor*. Glioblastoma multiforme is a type of *glioma*, a tumor arising from glial (supporting) cells within the brain. Most glioblastomas develop within the cerebrum (the main mass of the brain).

There are about five to 10 new cases of glioblastoma multiforme per million population per year in the US. The cause is unknown.

Symptoms, diagnosis, and treatment are as for other types of brain tumor. Despite treatment, the outlook is poor, with few patients surviving beyond two years.

Glioma

A type of *brain tumor* arising from the supporting glial cells within the brain.

Gliomas make up about 60 percent of all primary brain tumors (growths originating from the brain itself rather than spread from elsewhere). There are about two to four new cases of glioma per 100,000 people annually in the US.

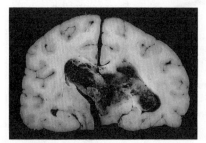

Cross section of a brain
This photograph (taken from an autopsy specimen) shows a large area of brain infiltrated by a glioma (dark color).

Types of glioma include *astrocytoma*, *glioblastoma multiforme* (a highly malignant variety of astrocytoma), *ependymoma* and *medulloblastoma* (more common in children), and *oligodendroglioma*. Symptoms, diagnosis, and treatment are as for other types of brain tumor.

Glipizide

An oral *hypoglycemic drug* used in the treatment of non-insulin-dependent *diabetes mellitus*. Glipizide stimulates the pancreas to produce *insulin*, which promotes glucose uptake into muscle and fat, thereby lowering the blood glucose level.

Globulin

Any of a group of proteins characterized by being insoluble in water but soluble in dilute salt solutions; *antibodies* (also known as *immunoglobulins*) are an example.

TYPES

Globulins can be divided into three main groups, known as alpha-, beta-, and gamma-globulins.

Alpha-globulins include alpha$_1$-antitrypsin and haptoglobin. The former is an enzyme produced by the lungs and liver; deficiency is associated with *hepatitis* in children and *emphysema* (a lung disorder) in young adults. Haptoglobin is found in the blood, where it binds together *hemoglobin* (the oxygen-carrying protein in red blood cells) and prevents it from being excreted in the urine by the kidneys. Various other alpha-globulins are produced as a result of inflammation, tissue damage, *autoimmune disorders* (when the immune system attacks the body's own tissues), or certain cancers.

Beta-globulins consist mainly of low-density lipoproteins (LDLs), substances involved in the transport of fats in the blood circulation, and transferrin, which carries iron in the blood. The amount of beta-globulins is increased in certain types of *hyperlipidemia* (abnormally high levels of fats in the blood).

All of the gamma-globulins are antibodies, proteins produced by the immune system in response to infection, during allergic reactions, and after organ transplants. Gamma-globulins may also be produced in any disorder that causes persistent inflammation of an organ, such as *rheumatoid arthritis* or *cirrhosis* of the liver. In addition, certain conditions, such as *multiple myeloma*, result in the production of large amounts of a specific gamma-globulin.

Globus hystericus

A form of hysteria in which there is an uncomfortable feeling of a "lump in the throat." This lump is felt to interfere with swallowing and breathing, sometimes so much so that the sufferer is convinced that he or she cannot breathe. Respiration comes in sighs or gasps, anxiety increases, and *hyperventilation* (rapid breathing) and symptoms of a *panic attack* often ensue. Some patients insist that their Adam's apple has become larger or displaced in some way.

There is no true physical basis for these attacks, which occur in anxious or depressed people. The condition is not life-threatening. Breathing in and out of a small paper bag fitted tightly around the nose and mouth will alleviate the symptoms brought on by hyperventilation. Treatment is by reassurance, breath-control training, and, in some instances, psychotherapy. Use of *antianxiety drugs* or *antidepressant drugs* to treat the condition is rarely helpful.

Glomerulonephritis
Inflammation of the glomeruli (filtering units of the kidney). Both kidneys are affected, although not all the glomeruli are affected simultaneously. Damage to the glomeruli hampers the removal of waste products, salt, and water from the bloodstream, which may cause serious complications.

CAUSES AND INCIDENCE
The incidence of glomerulonephritis varies markedly among different parts of the world, mainly because some common tropical diseases (such as malaria and schistosomiasis) are important causes. Although these diseases rarely are responsible for glomerulonephritis in developed countries, glomerulonephritis is still the most common cause of chronic *renal failure* (loss of kidney function) in the US and Europe.

Some types of the disease are caused by the patient's *immune system* making antibodies to eliminate microorganisms—usually the bacteria responsible for a minor infection, such as streptococcal sore throat infections. Particles called immune complexes, formed from antibodies and bacterial antigens, circulate in the bloodstream and become trapped in the glomeruli; this triggers an inflammatory process that may damage the glomeruli and prevent them from working normally. Glomerulonephritis also occurs in some *autoimmune disorders*, systemic *lupus erythematosus* (a chronic disease of connective tissues), and the immunoglobulin A (IgA) glomerulonephritis known as Berger's disease.

SYMPTOMS
Mild forms of glomerulonephritis may produce no symptoms and the disease may be noted only when a urine sample is tested for some other reason. Sometimes a mild puffiness of the soft tissues surrounding the eyeballs (periorbital edema) may be apparent. Other times it comes to light only when renal failure has reached an advanced stage and symptoms arise because of the accumulation of waste products and fluid that are usually eliminated in the urine.

High blood pressure may develop and some sufferers experience a dull ache in the loins. Damaged glomeruli may allow the escape of red blood cells

into the urine, which can become blood-stained. When protein is continually lost in the urine, the result is *edema* (swelling of parts of the body; see illustration). The combination of proteinuria (large amounts of protein in the urine), low albumin (protein) in the blood, and edema is called the *nephrotic syndrome*.

In some cases, glomerulonephritis is severe and sudden, so that kidney failure develops over a few days; patients often notice that they are passing very small quantities of urine.

DIAGNOSIS
There are numerous types of glomerulonephritis; one cause may produce a different type in different individuals. Urinalysis and examination of the urine sediment (after centrifugation) is helpful in diagnosis. Kidney *biopsy* (removal of a small amount of tissue for laboratory analysis) is also important for diagnosis. Other tests that may be performed are blood and urine sampling to measure how well the kidney is removing waste products and to measure how much protein is being lost in the urine. These tests may be repeated during treatment to see how the kidneys are responding.

TREATMENT AND OUTLOOK
Treatment depends on the type and severity of the disease, as revealed by biopsy. Affected children usually have mild forms characterized by the nephrotic syndrome; they usually recover completely after treatment. Children who experience acute glomerulonephritis after a streptococcal infection usually recover even without specific treatment of the glomerulonephritis.

Adults tend to respond less well to treatment, but drugs may be prescribed to control hypertension and a special diet given to reduce the kidneys' load. This may prevent or delay eventual renal failure. A minority of people with severe glomerulonephritis may be given *immunosuppressant drugs* (to dampen the body's defense system), or *plasmapheresis* to remove substances and particles from the bloodstream that trigger the inflammation (i.e., substances released as a result of the immune response).

Glomerulosclerosis
Scarring that occurs as a result of damage within the glomeruli (filtering units) of the kidney.

G

THE EFFECTS OF GLOMERULONEPHRITIS
The glomeruli are damaged as a result of inflammation. Red blood cells and protein leak into the urine.

Protein loss from the circulation causes fluid to accumulate in body tissues, causing edema.

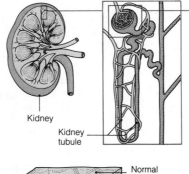

Kidney

Kidney tubule

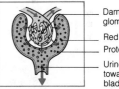

Damaged glomerulus
Red blood cells
Protein
Urine travels toward the bladder

Cross section of a damaged glomerulus
Damage to the glomerulus causes red blood cells and protein to pass into the urine, which may be blood-stained.

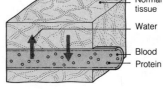

Normal tissue
Water
Blood
Protein

Healthy tissue
Through osmotic pressure, protein molecules in the blood draw back water lost to surrounding tissues.

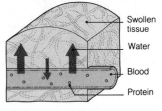

Swollen tissue
Water
Blood
Protein

Edema
If protein is lost into the urine, there is a fall in osmotic pressure and more water escapes into surrounding tissues, causing swelling.

Mild glomerulosclerosis occurs normally with age; a 10 percent decrease in renal function is common each decade after age 30. However, even a 75 percent reduction in renal function is compatible with a normal life.

Glomerulosclerosis may occur in some severe types of *glomerulonephritis* that are difficult to treat and in which damage progresses to destroy the kidneys. Typically, sufferers develop heavy *proteinuria* (the presence of protein in the urine) and severe *edema* (swelling of parts of the body due to fluid collection).

Glomerulosclerosis is also found in some people with *diabetes mellitus*. It is seen in reflux nephropathy (backflow of urine from bladder to kidney sometimes associated with infection) and in some people with hypertension. Intravenous drug abuse may cause glomerulosclerosis. The condition has also been found in some people who have AIDS.

Glomus tumor
A small, painful, bluish swelling in the skin, usually on a finger or toe near or under the nail, that is tender to touch and more painful if the limb is hot or cold. The tumors result from an overgrowth of glomus bodies, structures with numerous nerve endings that normally control blood flow and temperature in the skin. Glomus tumors are surgically removed.

Glossectomy
Removal of all or part of the tongue. Glossectomy may be performed in the treatment of cancer of the tongue, but more usually such cancers are treated by radiation therapy. If a large part of the tongue is removed, speech is impaired and eating is difficult. A liquid diet is then necessary.

Glossitis
Inflammation of the tongue. The tongue feels sore and swollen and looks red and smooth; adjacent parts of the mouth may also be inflamed.

Glossitis occurs in iron deficiency anemia, in pernicious and megaloblastic anemias, and in other vitamin B deficiencies. Other causes include infection (especially *herpes simplex*) of the mouth, irritation by dentures, and excessive use of alcohol, tobacco, or spices. A congenital form of glossitis affects the middle portion of the back of the tongue.

Treatment is for the underlying cause. Self-help measures include maintaining good oral hygiene, not smoking, and avoiding acidic or spicy foods that aggravate the soreness. Regular rinsing of the mouth with a salt solution may help.

Glossolalia
Speaking in jargon or an imaginary language that has no actual meaning or syntax. Today it occurs almost exclusively at religious meetings. Some Christians regard glossolalia as a sign of possession by the Holy Spirit; scientists tend to view it as a form of *hypnosis* or *hysteria*.

Glossopharyngeal nerve
The ninth *cranial nerve*, the glossopharyngeal nerve performs both sensory and motor functions. It conveys sensations, especially taste, from the back of the tongue, regulates secretion of saliva by the parotid gland, and controls movement of the throat muscles.

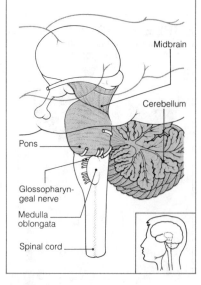

LOCATION OF THE GLOSSOPHARYNGEAL NERVE
The nerve arises from the medulla oblongata and branches to the tongue, parotid gland, and pharynx.

Midbrain

Cerebellum

Pons

Glossopharyngeal nerve

Medulla oblongata

Spinal cord

Glottis
The part of the *larynx* (voice box) that consists of the vocal cords and the slitlike opening between them.

Glucagon
A hormone produced by the pancreas. Glucagon stimulates the breakdown of glycogen (a carbohydrate stored in the liver and muscles) into glucose (sugar). The glucose is then released into the bloodstream, where it is available as a source of energy for cells anywhere in the body. Glucagon therefore regulates the level of glucose in the blood; when the level falls, glucagon is released from the pancreas. Glucagon opposes the action of *insulin*.

USE AS A DRUG
Glucagon is extracted from the pancreas of pigs or cows for use as a drug. It is given by subcutaneous (under the skin) injection in the emergency treatment of sufferers of *diabetes mellitus* who are unconscious as a result of hypoglycemia (low blood sugar). Glucagon produces recovery within 15 to 20 minutes; the patient is then given glucose by mouth to prevent a relapse. Nausea and vomiting are occasional adverse effects.

Glucocorticoids
Hormones produced by the cortex (outer layer) of the adrenal glands that affect carbohydrate metabolism by increasing the blood sugar level and the amount of glycogen in the liver. The principal glucocorticoid is *hydrocortisone* (also called cortisol), which also has a milder *mineralocorticoid* (affecting sodium and potassium balance) effect.

Glucose
The body's chief source of energy for cell *metabolism*. A monosaccharide (simple sugar) *carbohydrate*, it comes principally from the digestion of other carbohydrates, although a small amount is also produced in cells by the metabolism of fats and proteins.

BLOOD SUGAR LEVELS
Despite wide variation in carbohydrate intake (and, therefore, large fluctuations in the amount of glucose in the body), the concentration of glucose in the blood—the blood sugar level—is normally kept within narrow limits. This is achieved by the actions of several hormones, notably *insulin, glucagon, epinephrine, corticosteroids,* and *growth hormone*. If the blood sugar level is abnormally high (known as *hyperglycemia*), it may cause *glycosuria* (glucose in the urine). An abnormally low blood sugar level is called *hypoglycemia*.

Insulin, released by the pancreas in response to increased blood sugar levels, lowers the level by stimulating the uptake of glucose by cells. Inside the cells, glucose may be "burned" to produce energy, converted to *glycogen* for storage (mainly in the liver and

G

muscles), or used in the production of triglycerides and fats.

Glucagon is released by the pancreas when the blood sugar level is low. It stimulates the breakdown of stored glycogen to glucose, which is then released into the bloodstream.

Epinephrine (released by the adrenal glands at times of stress) and corticosteroids (also released by the adrenals in response to factors such as infection) have the same basic effect as glucagon. That is, they stimulate the release of glucose to increase the blood sugar level.

Glue sniffing
See *Solvent abuse*.

Gluten

One of the proteins of wheat and certain other grains that gives dough its tough, elastic character. *Celiac sprue*, a sensitivity to gluten, is thought to affect between 0.1 and 0.2 percent of the population.

Gluten enteropathy
See *Celiac sprue*.

Gluten intolerance
See *Celiac sprue*.

Gluteus maximus
The large, powerful muscle in each of the buttocks that helps give them their rounded shape. The gluteus maximus is responsible for moving the thigh sideways and backward.

Glyburide
An oral *hypoglycemic drug* used to treat non-insulin-dependent *diabetes mellitus*. Glyburide stimulates the pancreas to produce insulin, which promotes the uptake of glucose (sugar) into muscle and fat tissue, thereby lowering the level of glucose in the blood.

Glycerin
A colorless syrup made from *glycerol* (an essential constituent of fats) and used in several drug preparations. Glycerin has a high water content, evaporates slowly, is easily absorbed, and has a softening effect.
WHY IT IS USED
Glycerin is used in moisturizing creams to help prevent dryness and cracking of the skin (for example, it is used to protect the nipples during breast-feeding).

Glycerin is used in ear drops to help soften *earwax* prior to syringing of the ears, and in *cough remedies* to help soothe a dry, irritating cough. Taken as a suppository or an enema, glycerin relieves constipation by softening hard feces.

Glycerol
An essential constituent of fats. Glycerol is released during digestion and absorbed either alone or in combination with fatty acids. When one molecule of glycerol combines with three molecules of fatty acids, the result is a type of fat known as a triglyceride.

Most of the glycerol is deposited in the body's fat stores; the remainder is taken up by the liver, where it may be converted into *glucose* (sugar) to provide energy.

Glycogen
The principal *carbohydrate* storage material in the body. It is a polysaccharide, consisting of many saccharide (sugar) molecules linked to form a long chain, and is found mainly in the liver and muscles.

Glycogen plays an important role in controlling blood sugar levels. When there is too much sugar (glucose) in

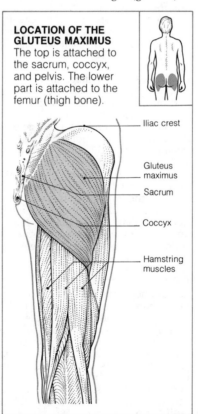

LOCATION OF THE GLUTEUS MAXIMUS
The top is attached to the sacrum, coccyx, and pelvis. The lower part is attached to the femur (thigh bone).

Iliac crest

Gluteus maximus

Sacrum

Coccyx

Hamstring muscles

the blood, the excess is converted to glycogen. This conversion (controlled by *insulin* and *corticosteroid hormones*) takes place chiefly in the liver and muscles. When the blood sugar level is low, glycogen is converted back to glucose (a process regulated by the hormones *glucagon* and *epinephrine*) and released into the bloodstream.

Glycosuria
The presence of glucose (a type of sugar) in the urine.
CAUSES
Glucose is normally filtered from the bloodstream by the kidneys (along with many other normal blood constituents and unwanted waste products). The filtered fluid passes down the many tubules of the kidneys, where all except the unwanted substances are reabsorbed and returned to the bloodstream (see *Kidney*). Glucose is one of the substances that the tubules almost completely reabsorb.

The kidney may fail to reabsorb all the glucose because of *hyperglycemia* (a high level of glucose in the blood) or if the tubules have been damaged and are unable to reabsorb even normal amounts of glucose. Hyperglycemia occurs in *diabetes mellitus*. Damage to the kidney tubules may be a result of rare metabolic disorders present from birth or be a consequence of drug or heavy metal poisoning.

Glycosuria can also sometimes occur in people with healthy kidneys that are unable to reabsorb all of the glucose filtered out of the bloodstream. This condition tends to run in families. Glycosuria often occurs during pregnancy because of hormonal changes, a condition that is usually not serious if it is not accompanied by other symptoms and if the blood glucose level is normal.
DIAGNOSIS AND TREATMENT
Glycosuria by itself does not necessarily indicate a serious condition. It may be found during a routine examination or if the physician is performing specific tests because diabetes mellitus is suspected. Urine can be tested for glucose by using a chemically impregnated strip that changes color when it comes in contact with glucose. Treatment depends on the underlying cause.

Gnat bites
See *Insect bites*.

Goiter
Enlargement of the thyroid gland, visible as a swelling on the neck.

G

CAUSES

The thyroid gland may enlarge (without any disturbance of its function) at puberty, during pregnancy, or as a result of taking the birth-control pill. In many parts of the world the main cause of a goiter is lack of sufficient iodine in the diet. The thyroid requires this mineral to produce the hormone thyroxine; a deficiency causes the gland to swell.

A toxic goiter is one that develops in *Graves' disease* or with other types of overactivity of the thyroid gland in which there is excessive production of thyroid hormones. This leads to *thyrotoxicosis*, characterized by symptoms such as increased appetite, warm, dry skin, weight loss, tremor, insomnia, and occasional muscle weakness and agitation. A goiter also usually is found in *Hashimoto's thyroiditis*, an autoimmune disorder, and de Quervain's *thyroiditis*, an inflammatory condition, both of which damage the gland; it may also be caused by a tumor or nodule in the gland and, in rare cases, by cancer (see *Thyroid cancer*). A goiter can also be caused by taking antithyroid drugs for overactivity of the thyroid gland.

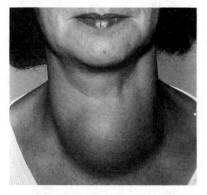

Appearance of goiter
The thyroid may become enlarged for any of various reasons, including dietary deficiency of iodine, inflammation, or an autoimmune disorder affecting the gland.

SYMPTOMS

A goiter can range in size from a barely noticeable lump to an enormous swelling, depending on the cause. Large swellings may press on the esophagus or the trachea, making swallowing or breathing difficult. Any accompanying symptoms must be verified with X-ray pictures.

DIAGNOSIS AND TREATMENT

Diagnosis is based on the nature of the swelling, along with accompanying symptoms and the results of blood

tests or *radionuclide scanning* carried out to determine the activity of the thyroid gland.

A goiter not caused by disease may eventually disappear naturally or may be so small that it does not require treatment. However, a large or unsightly goiter, or one that is causing difficulties with swallowing or with breathing may require total or partial removal (see *Thyroidectomy*).

If iodine deficiency is identified as the cause, the patient will be advised to eat more fish and iodized salt, which are rich in the mineral. When a goiter is the result of disease, treatment will be for the underlying disorder. If a drug is the cause, the goiter usually disappears once the course of treatment is over.

Gold

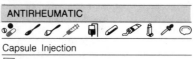

ANTIRHEUMATIC
Capsule Injection
📋 Prescription needed
🔒 Not available as generic

Gold is used to treat *rheumatoid arthritis* and arthritis arising as a complication of *psoriasis*. It is usually prescribed in severe active cases when a *nonsteroidal anti-inflammatory drug* (NSAID) has been ineffective.

HOW IT WORKS

Gold has an anti-inflammatory action that relieves joint pain and stiffness and can prevent more damage.

POSSIBLE ADVERSE EFFECTS

A common adverse effect of gold is *dermatitis* (inflammation of the skin); if itching occurs, the drug is usually withdrawn. Gold may damage the kidneys, liver, and bone marrow. Tests are performed during treatment to check the function of these organs.

Gold may cause loss of appetite, nausea, diarrhea, abdominal pain, and, occasionally, *anaphylactic shock* (a serious allergic reaction that requires emergency treatment).

Golfers' elbow

A condition caused by inflammation of the bony prominence (epicondyle) on the inner side of the elbow, to which certain forearm muscles are attached. It is caused by overuse of these muscles, which act to bend the wrist and fingers. Activities that can cause the condition include gripping and twisting (such as using a screwdriver) or playing golf with a faulty grip or swing.

SYMPTOMS AND TREATMENT

The inflammation causes pain and tenderness at the inner side of the elbow and sometimes in the forearm. Treatment consists of resting the elbow, applying ice packs, and taking analgesics (painkillers) and/or anti-inflammatory tablets. If the pain is severe or persistent, injection of a *corticosteroid drug* may be helpful.

If the pain has occurred after participation in a sport, it is wise to take a break from the sport for a week or two to prevent recurrence and to seek advice about playing technique.

Gonadotropin hormones

Hormones that stimulate cell activity in the gonads (ovaries and testes). Gonadotropins are essential for female and male fertility. The most important gonadotropins, follicle-stimulating hormone (FSH) and *luteinizing hormone* (LH), are secreted by the *pituitary gland*. Another gonadotropin, HCG (see *Gonadotropin, human chorionic*), is produced by the placenta.

GONADOTROPIN HORMONE THERAPY

Synthetic HCG is used in the treatment of recurrent *miscarriage* and certain types of female and male *infertility*. Menotropin (a gonadotropin extracted from the urine of women past the menopause) contains both FSH and LH and is used in the treatment of female infertility due to a failure to ovulate.

Gonadotropinlike substances are currently being evaluated as contraceptives and as a treatment for cancer of the prostate gland.

Gonadotropin, human chorionic

A hormone produced by the placenta in early pregnancy. Human chorionic gonadotropin (HCG) stimulates the ovaries to produce *estrogen* and *progesterone*, hormones needed to maintain a healthy pregnancy.

HCG is excreted in the urine; its measurement forms the basis of most pregnancy tests (a high level confirming pregnancy).

HCG THERAPY

HCG extracted from the urine of pregnant women is given by injection to treat certain types of *infertility*. Along with clomiphene tablets it may induce ovulation in women who have not been ovulating. In men, it may be used to increase sperm production.

HCG is occasionally given to prevent *miscarriage* in women whose production of progesterone is deficient.

HCG is also prescribed for the treatment of cryptorchidism (see *Testis, undescended*) in young boys, although surgical correction is usually required.

Gonads

The sex glands—the *testes* in men and the *ovaries* in women. The testes, situated in the scrotum, produce sperm and secrete the hormone *testosterone*. The ovaries, situated in the abdomen, release usually one ovum (egg) between them each month and secrete the hormones *estrogen* and *progesterone*. The activities of the gonads—both male and female—are regulated by *gonadotropin hormones* released by the pituitary gland.

Gonorrhea

A sexually transmitted disease, commonly known as "the clap." It is one of the most common infectious diseases in the world.

CAUSES AND INCIDENCE

Gonorrhea, caused by the bacterium *NEISSERIA GONORRHOEAE*, is most frequently transmitted during sexual intercourse, including oral or anal sex. An infected woman may also transmit the disease to her newborn baby during childbirth.

Gonorrhea is the second most common sexually transmitted disease, after *nonspecific urethritis*, and is most prevalent among young adults who have had multiple sexual partners. There are approximately 1 million cases of gonorrhea reported annually in the US. Since many cases are not reported, the true annual incidence may be closer to 3 million cases.

SYMPTOMS AND SIGNS

Gonorrhea has a short incubation period of two to 10 days. In men, symptoms usually include a urethral discharge and pain on urination. About 60 percent of infected women have no symptoms; if symptoms are present, they usually consist of a vaginal discharge or a burning sensation when urinating.

Infection acquired through anal sex causes gonococcal *proctitis* (inflammation of the rectum and anus). It causes pain and anal discharge in only about 10 percent of infected people. Oral sex with an infected person may lead to gonococcal *pharyngitis*, causing soreness in the throat but, again, most people have no symptoms. A baby exposed to infection in the mother's reproductive tract during childbirth may acquire gonococcal *ophthalmia*, a severe inflammation affecting one or both eyes.

COMPLICATIONS

Untreated gonorrhea may spread to other parts of the body. In men, it may cause *prostatitis* (inflammation of the prostate) or *epididymo-orchitis* (inflammation of the testes), affecting fertility. In women, untreated gonorrhea involves the fallopian tubes, causing *pelvic inflammatory disease* (PID). If the fallopian tubes are damaged, the woman is very likely to become infertile as a result.

Gonococcal bacteria may spread through the bloodstream to cause gonococcal *arthritis*, with pain and swelling of joints around the body. Multiplication of bacteria in the bloodstream causes *septicemia*, with generalized symptoms and signs, including fever and malaise; it can even spread to the brain or heart and cause death.

DIAGNOSIS

Many disorders can cause urethral or vaginal discharge. To confirm a diagnosis of gonorrhea, laboratory tests are necessary. Tests are carried out on a sample of the discharge or on swabs taken from the urethra or cervix.

TREATMENT

Gonorrhea is treated with antibiotics, usually *penicillin* or ampicillin. If the infection is caused by penicillin-resistant *NEISSERIA GONORRHOEAE* or if the infected person is allergic to penicillin, other antibiotics, such as tetracycline, ceftriaxone, or spectinomycin, may be used. Tests are performed to ensure that the infection has been cured.

OUTLOOK

Treatment for gonorrhea is effective but does not protect against reinfection. Sexual partners must be told that they might have gonorrhea even if they have no symptoms; many clinics have counselors (known as contact tracers) who identify and inform all people who might have been infected by the patient.

Goodpasture's syndrome

A rare condition characterized by *glomerulonephritis* (inflammation of the filtering units of the kidney), *coughing up blood* (hemoptysis), and *anemia*. Goodpasture's syndrome is a serious disease; unless treated at an early stage, it may lead to life-threatening bleeding into the lungs and progressive *renal failure*.

Goodpasture's syndrome is an *autoimmune disorder* (one in which the body's *immune system* attacks its own tissues). Antibodies are formed that attack the capillaries (tiny blood vessels) in the lungs and kidneys, eventually resulting in inflammation and disruption of the normal functioning of the lungs and kidneys.

The disease usually affects young men, but can develop at any age. Mild forms may be treated with *immunosuppressant drugs* (drugs that hamper the normal working of the body's immune system) and plasma exchange (*plasmapheresis*). The outlook is not good for people with severe and repeated attacks; they are treated by *dialysis* (a technique for removing waste products from the blood) and, eventually, *kidney transplant*.

Good Samaritan laws

Statutes (in most states) that legally protect a physician who voluntarily aids an injured or unconscious person at the scene of an accident.

Gout

A metabolic disorder that causes attacks of *arthritis*, usually in a single joint. Gout may be associated with kidney stones and ultimately may lead to kidney failure.

SYMPTOMS AND SIGNS

An acute attack of gout usually affects a single joint, most commonly the joint at the base of the big toe, but it can affect other joints, including the knee, ankle, wrist, foot, and small joints of the hand.

The affected joint is red, swollen, and extremely tender; the pain reaches a peak level of intensity within 24 to 36 hours. The redness and swelling may spread and be confused with *cellulitis* (inflammation of the connective tissue). The intensity of the pain is such that the person may not be able to stand on an affected foot or even tolerate the pressure of bedclothes on it. Sometimes there is a mild fever.

The first attack usually involves only one joint and lasts a few days. Some people never have another attack, but most have a second attack between six months and two years after the first. After the second attack, more and more joints may be involved, and there may be constant pain due to damage to the joint from chronic inflammation.

TREATMENT

Pain and inflammation in gout can be controlled with large doses of a *nonsteroidal anti-inflammatory drug* (NSAID). If use of an NSAID is contraindicated, *colchicine* may be prescribed. For maximal benefit, treatment should start as soon as an attack begins; patients prone to recurrent attacks should carry their gout medication. As the inflammation subsides, usually within two to three days, the dose of medication is reduced and finally stopped. If an attack of gout is not responding to treatment with NSAIDs or colchicine, a *corticosteroid drug* may be injected into the affected joint.

Increased levels of purine (a product of DNA) can raise the level of uric acid in the blood. Although a strict low-purine diet is not necessary, people with gout should avoid foods that are high in purine, such as liver and other organ meats, legumes, and poultry. Excess alcohol consumption should also be avoided because it may precipitate an acute attack in a susceptible individual.

Many people never have more than a few attacks of gout, and further treatment is usually unnecessary. If attacks are recurrent, the frequency can be reduced by lowering the urate levels with drugs that either inhibit the formation of uric acid (such as allopurinol) or increase the excretion of uric acid by the kidneys with uricosuric drugs (such as probenecid and sulfinpyrazone). If the serum urate is very high, these drugs will need to be taken for life, as untreated hyperuricemia may lead to hypertension or kidney disease.

Grafting

The process of transplanting healthy tissue from one part of the body to another (autografting), from one person to another (allografting or homografting), or from an animal to a person (xenografting).

Grafting is used to repair or replace diseased or otherwise defective tissue. The primary tissues transplanted are skin (see *Skin graft*); bone (see *Bone graft*); bone marrow (see *Bone marrow transplantation*); the cornea of the eye (see *Corneal graft*); the kidney, the heart, and the liver (see *Kidney transplant; Heart transplant; Liver transplant; Transplant surgery*); heart valves (see *Heart valve surgery*); and blood vessels and nerves (see *Microsurgery*).

COMPLICATIONS

With autografting, the grafted tissue is usually assimilated at the new site without any trouble and soon grows into the surrounding tissue to provide a good repair.

Problems occur, however, with allografting (homografting) and xenografting, both of which are usually carried out to replace rather than repair tissue. Xenografting is not performed clinically except for the use of porcine (pig) heart valves. The major drawback to allografting is that the recipient's defense system automatically attempts to reject the foreign cells of the donor's tissue and to destroy them in the same way that it would invading microorganisms. The only exceptions are in the case of identical twins (because their tissue matches exactly) and in that of corneal grafting, since the cornea has no blood supply (and therefore no white blood cells and antibodies to act as a defense system).

To overcome rejection, as close a match as possible between the tissues of the recipient and donor is sought (see *Tissue-typing*). *Immunosuppressant drugs* (especially *cyclosporine*) are given to suppress the body's defense system—though this can cause other problems, such as decreased kidney function. Cyclosporine, the immunosuppressant drug introduced in 1984, has been particularly effective in the control of organ rejection and *graft-versus-host disease*.

GOUT

Gout is a common joint disease, affecting 10 times more men than women. In men it occurs at any time after puberty; in women it usually occurs only after the menopause. There is often a family history of the disorder. Hyperuricemia (excess uric acid in the blood) leads to formation of uric acid crystals in joints; crystals may also be deposited in soft tissues in the ears and around tendons.

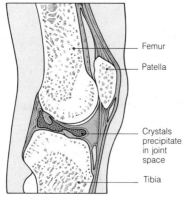

Crystal precipitation
Crystals of uric acid precipitate into the joint space and surrounding tissues of the knee, causing intense inflammation and extreme pain.

Femur
Patella
Crystals precipitate in joint space
Tibia

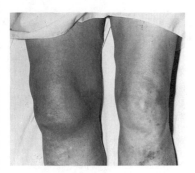

Appearance of gout
Deposition of uric acid crystals in the joint space have caused inflammation and obvious swelling of the affected right knee.

DIAGNOSIS
Gout is considered as a diagnosis whenever an attack of arthritis affects a single joint. A blood test is usually performed; a high level of uric acid suggests gout.

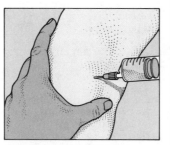

Aspiration
Fluid is aspirated (removed through a needle into a syringe) from the swollen knee joint and examined under a microscope.

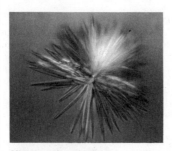

Microscopic evidence
The presence of uric acid crystals confirms the diagnosis.

Graft-versus-host disease

A common complication of *bone marrow transplantation*. It is caused by cells called cytotoxic T-*lymphocytes*, present in the transplanted marrow, attacking the transplant recipient's tissues. Lymphocytes form part of the *immune system* and normally play a beneficial role by attacking cells recognized as foreign. However, in transplant procedures, it is just this activity of the lymphocytes that causes disease.

Graft-versus-host (GVH) disease may occur soon after any organ transplantation or may appear some months later. The first sign of the disease is usually a skin rash. Then there may also be diarrhea, abdominal pain, jaundice, inflammation of the eyes and mouth, and breathlessness. Most patients recover within a year, but some gradually get weaker and thinner and about one third die.

Graft-versus-host disease can be prevented by giving *immunosuppressant drugs*, such as cyclosporine, to all transplant recipients. If the disease develops, it is treated with *corticosteroid drugs* and with other immunosuppressants. It may be possible to prevent GVH disease in bone marrow transplants by removing cytotoxic T cells from the donor marrow before the transplant is done.

Gramicidin

An *antibiotic drug* used in combination with other drugs of this class to treat bacterial infections of the eye or skin. It is prescribed in the form of eye drops or an ointment.

Gram's stain

An iodine-based stain widely used in bacteriology to help differentiate among various types of bacteria. It is also known as Gram's iodine.

There are several different methods of Gram staining. Basically, the specimen is stained with gentian violet, followed by Gram's solution, and then treated with a decolorizing agent such as acetone. Finally, the specimen is counterstained with a red dye. Bacteria that retain the dark violet stain are known as gram-positive; those that lose the violet stain after decolorization but take up the counterstain (causing them to appear pink) are gram-negative. Examples of gram-positive bacteria include several species of streptococcus, staphylococcus, and clostridium; gram-negative bacteria include VIBRIO CHOLERAE (which causes cholera) and various species of salmonella.

Grand mal

A type of epileptic seizure in which the person, sometimes after warning symptoms, cries out, falls to the ground unconscious, and suffers generalized jerky muscle contractions. The seizure may last for a few minutes. The person usually remains unconscious for a time and may have no recall of the seizure on awakening. (See also *Epilepsy*.)

Granulation tissue

A mass of red, moist, granular tissue that develops on the surface of an ulcer or open wound during the process of healing. The tissue consists mainly of fibroblasts (which make collagen) and numerous small blood vessels. (See also *Healing*; *Wound*.)

Granuloma

An aggregation of cells, of a type associated with chronic inflammation, anywhere in the body.

CAUSES AND TYPES

Granulomas usually occur as a reaction to the presence of certain infectious agents or to a foreign body, but may occur in conditions of unknown cause.

Certain infections, such as *tuberculosis*, *brucellosis*, *leprosy*, and *syphilis*, although caused by different bacteria, give rise to infective granulomas in many different organs of the body. *Sarcoidosis*, a condition of unknown cause, is also characterized by granulomas in different organs. Granulomas may also occur in parasitic and fungal infections.

A foreign body granuloma can occur as a reaction to inorganic material, such as dust, talcum powder, dirt, or a suture. A pyogenic granuloma is a common benign skin tumor that develops on exposed areas following minor injury. It is frequently found on the hands of gardeners. The swellings are raised, moist, and tender and often disappear gradually without treatment. They can be excised surgically, or by *electrocoagulation* or *cryosurgery*.

Many other, largely unrelated, conditions are described as granulomas. For example, a dental granuloma is a swelling arising from poorly fitting false teeth; a granuloma may also form a benign growth on the iris. (See also *Granuloma annulare*; *Granuloma inguinale*; *Granuloma, lethal midline*.)

Granuloma annulare

A harmless skin condition characterized by a circular, raised area of skin, occurring most commonly in children on the knuckles or fingers, or less commonly on the upper part of the feet or on the elbows or ears. The raised area spreads slowly outward to form a ring, 1 to 3 inches in diameter, with raised edges and a flattened center. Rarely, several of these ringlike plaques occur over a wider area. The cause of the condition is unknown.

The diagnosis of granuloma annulare is by means of a skin *biopsy* (removal of a small sample of tissue for microscopic investigation). No treatment is necessary. In most cases, the affected skin heals completely over several months or years.

G

Granuloma inguinale

A sexually transmitted disease that causes ulceration of the genitals. The infection is caused by bacterialike organisms called Donovan's bodies. Granuloma inguinale is common in the tropics, especially Papua, New Guinea, although it is very rare in developed countries. There are about 100 cases in the US per year, usually occurring in homosexual men.

The first symptoms are painless, raised nodules on the penis or labia or around the anal area. The nodules gradually ulcerate and then form bright red, raised areas that are usually painless. These areas sometimes become purulent (contain pus) and, if left untreated, may eventually heal with extensive scarring.

Diagnosis is based on finding Donovan's bodies in a *biopsy* sample (tissue removed from a sore). The antibiotics tetracycline or gentamicin provide effective therapy.

Granuloma, lethal midline

A rare disorder of unknown cause in which the nose and other facial structures become inflamed and eventually destroyed by progressive damage to the skin and underlying tissues.

Patients with midline granuloma are usually in their 40s or 50s; women are affected more often than men. The first symptoms are usually caused by ulceration within the nose. Tissue destruction may spread to the facial sinuses, the gums, and the eye orbits.

The most effective treatment is *radiation therapy*, which usually halts the progression of the disease and may improve symptoms for years.

Graves' disease

A disorder characterized by toxic *goiter* (an overactive and enlarged thyroid gland), excessive production of thyroid hormones leading to *thyrotoxicosis*, and sometimes *exophthalmos* (bulging eyeballs). It is a type of *autoimmune disorder* (disturbance in the body's immune system).

Gravida
The medical term for a pregnant woman. The term is often combined with a prefix to indicate the total number of pregnancies (including the present one). For example, primigravida is a woman who is pregnant for the first time, and secundigravida is one who is pregnant for the second time; multigravida is a general term for a woman who has been pregnant at least once before.

Gray
An SI (International System of Units) unit of radiation dosage (see *Radiation units box*).

Gray matter
Regions of the central nervous system (brain and spinal cord) consisting principally of closely packed and interconnected nuclei of nerve cells, rather than their filamentous projections or axons, which make up the white matter.

In the brain, gray matter is primarily found in the outer layers of the *cerebrum* (the main mass of the brain and the region responsible for advanced mental functions) and in some regions deeper within the brain. Gray matter also makes up the inner core of the spinal cord.

Grief
An intensely unhappy and painful emotion caused by the loss of a loved one. (See *Bereavement*.)

Grip
The *hand* is particularly well adapted for gripping, with an opposable thumb (that is, able to touch all the other fingers), specialized skin on the palm and fingers to provide adhesion, and a complex system of muscles, tendons, joints, and nerves that enables precise movements of the digits.

The hand can perform two basic grips: grasping, which is a strength hold that involves the whole hand, and pinching, a precision hold using the thumb and a finger. Both grips are controlled by a combination of long muscles in the forearm and short muscles in the hand itself.

Gripping ability can be reduced by any condition that causes muscular weakness or impairment of sensation

in the palms or fingers (e.g., a stroke or nerve injury) or by disorders that affect the bones or joints of the hand or wrist, such as arthritis or a fracture.

Grippe
A term of French origin for any influenzalike illness (see *Influenza*). The term was once used commonly in English-speaking as well as French-speaking countries.

Griseofulvin

ANTIFUNGAL

Tablet Capsule Liquid
℞ᵀ Prescription needed
🔲 Available as generic

A drug given by mouth to treat *tinea* infections (a group of fungal infections) that have not responded to creams and lotions. Griseofulvin is particularly useful in the treatment of infections affecting the scalp, beard, palms, soles of the feet, and nails.

Common side effects are headache, loss of taste, dry mouth, abdominal pain, and increased sensitivity of the skin to sunlight. During long-term treatment, griseofulvin may cause liver or bone marrow damage; blood tests are usually carried out to check organ function.

Groin
The hollow between the lower abdomen and top of the thigh. (See also *Groin, lump in the*; *Groin strain*.)

Groin, lump in the
The most common cause of a swelling in the groin is enlargement of a lymph gland as a result of an infection (see *Glands, swollen*). Another common cause is a *hernia*, a protrusion of intestine through a weak area in the abdominal wall.

Other possible causes of a lump in the groin include an *abscess* (a pus-filled sac), a *lipoma* (a painless benign tumor of fat cells), or an undescended testis (see *Testis, undescended*). Rarely, a lump in the groin may be due to a *varicose vein* or an *aneurysm* (a balloonlike swelling in an artery).

INVESTIGATION
Examination of the swelling by a physician usually reveals its cause.

Groin strain
Pain and tenderness in the groin due to overstretching a muscle, typically while running or participating in

sports. The muscles commonly affected are the adductors on the inside of the thigh, which rotate and flex the thigh and pull it inward, and the rectus femoris (at the front of the thigh), which also flexes the thigh.

Pain and tenderness in the groin that mimic pain due to muscle strain may sometimes be caused by *osteoarthritis* in the hip or lower spine, pubic *osteitis* (inflammation of the pubic bones, situated at the front and base of the spine), or an inguinal *hernia* (a protrusion of intestine through a weak area in the abdominal wall).

INVESTIGATION AND TREATMENT
When the cause is obviously a simple muscle strain, treatment is with physical therapy. However, if another cause is suspected, or if what was thought to be a muscle strain does not respond to physical therapy, tests such as X rays may be required. An X ray may show that a muscle has pulled a small piece of bone away from the pelvis; surgery to wire the bone back into position may be necessary.

Ground substance
The thick, gellike material, sometimes called tissue matrix, in which the cells, fibers, and blood capillaries of cartilage, bone, and connective tissue are embedded. Ground substance consists principally of a large amount of water chemically linked to complex carbohydrate and protein molecules. The water enables nutrients and gases essential for metabolism and respiration to pass easily from the blood capillaries to the cells. Because of its gellike consistency, ground substance also protects the cells, fibers, and capillaries from damage.

Excess ground substance is produced in *hypothyroidism* (underactivity of the thyroid gland). This results in a condition called myxedema, in which ground substance accumulates in the skin, leading to thickening of the skin and coarsening of the facial features.

Group therapy
Any treatment of emotional or psychological problems in which groups of patients meet regularly with a therapist. Interaction among members of the group is thought to be therapeutic and for certain problems is considered to be more effective than the traditional patient-therapist relationship. The group setting is also useful for job-related therapy.

The group may range in number from three to 40 people, but eight to 10 people is the usual size. Members meet for an hour or more once or twice a week to discuss their problems openly with one another under the guidance of the therapist.

Group therapy is most useful for people with personality problems and for sufferers from *alcohol dependence, drug dependence, anxiety disorders*, eating disorders (such as *anorexia nervosa* and *bulimia*), and depressive illnesses (see *Depression*).

Growing pains

Vague aches and pains that occur in the limbs of children. The pains usually are felt at night and most often affect children between 6 and 12 years old. Their cause is unknown, although they do not seem to be related to the process of growth itself.

Growing pains are of no medical significance and require no treatment, though the pains may interfere with the child's sleep and may alarm the parents. If pain is severe or associated with other symptoms, such as joint swelling or malaise, a pediatrician should be consulted.

Growth

An abnormal proliferation of cells within a localized area (see *Tumor*); the increase in height and weight as a child develops (see *Growth, childhood*).

Growth, childhood

The period of most rapid growth occurs before birth, during embryonic and fetal development. After birth, the growth rate decreases steadily, although it is still very rapid in the first few years of life, especially the first year. At the onset of *puberty* there is another major period of growth and development that continues until full adult height is reached, usually at about the age of 18. As a general rule, increase in weight follows the same pattern as increase in height.

Significant variations occur within the typical overall growth pattern. For example, baby boys grow faster than girls until the age of about 7 months, when girls grow faster than boys. Girls continue to grow more rapidly until about 4 years, when the rate of growth becomes the same, and remains so until puberty. However, in overall height, girls tend to be shorter than boys at all ages until puberty, when they become taller for a few years because they enter the pubertal growth spurt earlier than boys. But because puberty occurs later in boys, their final height is greater.

Growth is not simply a process of becoming taller and heavier. The body shape also changes because different areas grow at different rates. At birth, the head is already about three quarters of its adult size; the head grows to almost full size during the first year. Thereafter, it becomes proportionately smaller because the body grows at a much faster rate. The limbs grow faster than the trunk during early childhood but more slowly during puberty.

Different tissues also grow at different rates. For example, lymphatic tissue grows rapidly until just before adolescence, when it begins to shrink. The brain also grows quickly during the early years, but reaches about nine tenths of its adult weight by the age of 5, after which its growth rate decreases markedly.

FACTORS THAT INFLUENCE GROWTH

Growth can be influenced by heredity and by environmental factors, such as nutrition, general health, and emotional welfare. Hormones also play an important role, particularly *growth hormone*, thyroid hormone, and, at puberty, the sex hormones.

A child with taller-than-average parents also tends to grow to above-average height because of the effects of heredity. However, this may be counteracted by poor health or inadequate nutrition. In infancy, weight is the best indicator of health and the state of nutrition. Thereafter, height is equally important. Regular measurement of height, weight, and, in babies, head circumference, provides an invaluable record of a child's growth rate.

A chronic illness, such as *asthma*, will retard growth if it is undetected. Even a minor, short-lived illness can slow growth, although the growth rate usually catches up again when the child recovers. In some cases, slow growth may be the only indication that a child is ill, malnourished, or emotionally distressed or deprived. However, there is wide individual variation in the rate at which children grow and *short stature* does not necessarily indicate poor health. Each case of slow growth requires assessment by a pediatrician.

Abnormally rapid growth is rare. Usually, it is a familial trait but occasionally it may indicate an underlying disorder, such as a pituitary gland tumor. (See also *Age; Child development; Gigantism*.)

G

CHANGES IN BODY PROPORTIONS BETWEEN BIRTH AND ADOLESCENCE

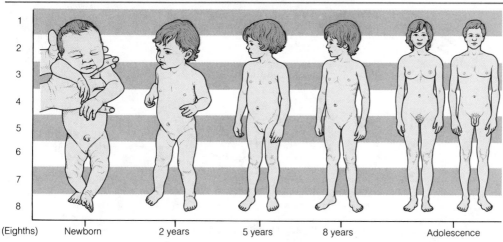

(Eighths)   Newborn   2 years   5 years   8 years   Adolescence

If the body is divided into eight equal parts, it can be seen that proportions change radically in relation to the body's overall length. For example, a newborn baby's legs account for only three eighths of his or her height while an adolescent's legs account for one half. A newborn's head accounts for as much as one fourth of his or her height while an adolescent's head accounts for only one eighth.

GROWTH CHART: BOYS 1 TO 18 YEARS

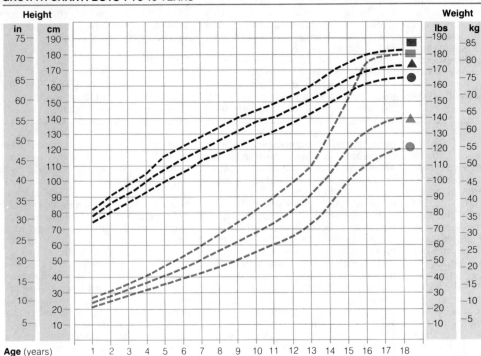

Age (years)

G

Growth in boys

Normally, there is a steady increase in weight until the end of puberty. Height increases steadily until a sudden spurt occurs during puberty (between the ages of 13 and 16). This chart was constructed using the height and weight of thousands of children; it is used by physicians to check whether growth of a particular boy is significantly above or below average.

Key

Height

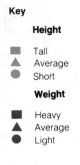

■ Tall
▲ Average
● Short

Weight

■ Heavy
▲ Average
● Light

GROWTH CHART: GIRLS 1 TO 18 YEARS

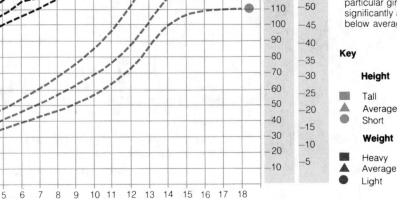

Age (years)

Growth in girls

Normally, there is a steady increase in weight that levels out by age 14. Height increases steadily until a sudden spurt occurs during puberty (between the ages of 11 and 14). This chart was constructed using the height and weight of thousands of children; it is used by physicians to check whether growth of a particular girl is significantly above or below average.

Key

Height

■ Tall
▲ Average
● Short

Weight

■ Heavy
▲ Average
● Light

Growth hormone

A substance produced by the *pituitary gland* that stimulates normal body growth and development by altering chemical activity in cells. Growth hormone stimulates the production of protein in muscle cells and the release of energy from the breakdown of fats.

GROWTH HORMONE THERAPY

In the past, growth hormone was extracted from human corpses; it is now prepared synthetically. Growth hormone therapy is used to treat *short stature* when the underlying cause is a pituitary gland disorder. Treatment is usually started in early childhood. Growth hormone is sometimes given with an anabolic *steroid*, which also promotes tissue growth.

POSSIBLE ADVERSE EFFECTS

There is a slight risk that *diabetes mellitus* may develop during treatment. Some people produce *antibodies* to growth hormone, but this does not seem to reduce its effectiveness.

Guanethidine

An *antihypertensive drug* used to treat severe *hypertension* (high blood pressure) that has not responded to other drugs. Adverse effects of guanethidine include dizziness or fainting, diarrhea, and impotence.

Guanethidine is currently under investigation as a treatment for *glaucoma* (raised pressure in the eyeball) in combination with *epinephrine*, in the form of eye drops.

Guar gum

A high-fiber plant substance used to help control the blood glucose (sugar) level in people with *diabetes mellitus*. Guar gum granules are either sprinkled on food or dissolved in water to form a thick gel for drinking.

HOW IT WORKS

Guar gum forms a sticky solution in the stomach and slows the movement of nutrients from there into the small intestine. This action slows the rate at which glucose is absorbed from the small intestine into the bloodstream, thus preventing a sudden rise in blood glucose after a meal.

POSSIBLE ADVERSE EFFECTS

Guar gum has an unpleasant taste and may cause flatulence, nausea, and abdominal discomfort.

Guillain-Barré syndrome

A rare form of damage to the peripheral nerves (see *Peripheral nervous system*) that causes weakness of the limbs. The nerves become inflamed, particularly where their roots leave the spine, impairing both movement and sensation. The disease is also known as acute polyneuritis and ascending paralysis.

CAUSES AND INCIDENCE

The cause of the disease is believed to be an allergic reaction to an infection, usually viral; the nerves are inflamed by antibodies produced by the reaction. In most cases the disease develops two or three weeks after the onset of an infection, usually an infection of the upper respiratory tract, such as a sore throat or influenza, or a gastrointestinal upset. In 1976, an epidemic occurred in the US following mass vaccination against swine flu. The incidence is about 15 cases per million population per year in the US.

SYMPTOMS

Weakness, often accompanied by numbness and tingling, usually starts in the legs and spreads to the arms. It becomes progressively worse and may develop into paralysis. The muscles of the face and those that control speech, swallowing, and breathing may also be affected, causing difficulty with all three activities.

DIAGNOSIS

The diagnosis is made from the patient's symptoms and signs, from the results of electrical tests to measure how fast nerve impulses are being conducted, and from a *lumbar puncture*, in which a sample of cerebrospinal fluid is taken from the spinal canal for analysis.

TREATMENT AND OUTLOOK

Patients are treated in the hospital, where their condition (particularly any breathing difficulty) can be closely monitored. If it becomes severe, *intubation* (inserting a breathing tube down the throat) and mechanical *ventilation* are carried out. *Plasmapheresis* (in which blood plasma is withdrawn from the patient, treated to remove antibodies, and replaced) may be employed in severe cases.

Most people recover completely without specific treatment, but some are left with permanent weakness in affected areas and/or suffer from further attacks of the disease.

Guilt

A painful feeling that arises from the awareness of having broken a moral or legal code. Guilt is self-inflicted, unlike shame, which depends on others knowing about the transgression. Some psychoanalysts see guilt as a result of the prohibitions of the *superego* (conscience) instilled by parental authority in early life. Others see guilt as a conditioned response to actions that in the past have led to punishment.

Feeling guilty from time to time is normal. However, feeling very guilty for no reason or experiencing guilt at an imagined crime is one of the main symptoms of psychotic *depression*.

Guinea worm disease

 A tropical disease caused by a female parasitic worm more than 3 feet (1 meter) long. Infection is the result of drinking water containing the crustacean water flea CYCLOPS, which harbors larvae of the worm. The larvae pass through the intestinal wall of the infected person and mature in connective tissue. After about a year, the adult female worm, now pregnant, approaches the surface of the skin, and creates an inflamed blister that bursts, exposing the end of the worm.

The disease occurs in Africa, South America, the Caribbean, the Middle East, and India.

SYMPTOMS AND TREATMENT

Urticaria (hives), nausea, vomiting, and diarrhea often develop while the blister is forming.

The traditional remedy is to wind the worm gently from the skin onto a small stick. Once the worm is out, the condition usually clears up.

The drugs niridazole and thiabendazole are given to reduce inflammation and make extraction of the worm safer, antibiotics are given to control secondary infection, and the patient is immunized against tetanus.

Gum

Also called the gingiva, the soft tissue surrounding the teeth that protects underlying structures and helps keep the teeth tightly in position in the jaw. The gingival margin, a cuff of gum about 2 mm thick, fits tightly around the base of the teeth and is anchored within the bony socket by the periodontal ligaments.

Normal, healthy gums are pink or brown and firm. Careful *oral hygiene*, including daily brushing and flossing, is needed to avoid gum disease, especially on reaching middle age.

DISORDERS

Gingivitis (an early, reversible stage of gum disease characterized by inflammation of the gums) may occur if plaque, which contains bacteria, is allowed to collect around the base of the teeth. Bleeding gums are nearly always a symptom of gingivitis; rarely, they are due to *leukemia* (blood cell cancer) or *scurvy* (vitamin C deficiency). Bruised gums are more likely to be caused by a *bleeding disorder*. Gingival *hyperplasia* (fleshy thickening of the gums) is most commonly a side effect of *anticonvulsant drug* treatment with phenytoin.

Untreated gingivitis may lead to *periodontitis*, the advanced stage of gum disease, in which infected pockets form between the gums and the teeth.

Gumma
A soft tumor that is characteristic of the late stages of untreated *syphilis*.

Gut
Popular name for the *intestine*.

Guthrie test
A blood test performed routinely on babies between the eighth and fourteenth day after birth to check for *phenylketonuria*. This is an inherited disorder in which the amino acid phenylalanine accumulates in the blood and tissues, usually leading to severe brain damage unless treated. The Guthrie test measures the amount of phenylalanine in the blood.

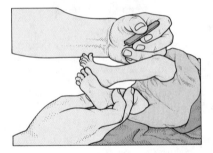

Carrying out a Guthrie test
A few drops of blood are taken from the baby's heel and sent to the laboratory to be tested for phenylalanine content.

HOW IT IS DONE
The baby's heel is pricked with a needle and a few drops of blood are soaked onto a piece of absorbent filter paper. The paper is then placed onto a nutrient medium containing bacteria whose growth is activated by phenylalanine. The size of the area of bacterial growth that appears is directly related to the concentration of phenylalanine in the blood.

RESULTS
A concentration of phenylalanine above 20 mg/ml indicates that phenylketonuria may be present; other, more accurate tests are performed to confirm the diagnosis.

Gynecologist
A physician who specializes in diagnosing and treating problems of the female reproductive tract, including disorders relating to *menstruation* and *menopause* and sexual dysfunctions that may have a physical cause. A gynecologist also offers advice on *contraception* and treats *infertility*.

From the time a woman starts menstruating, she should see a gynecologist every one to three years for a *pelvic examination* and a *cervical smear* (Pap test). These tests are often performed on a preventive basis, because cervical smears can detect cancer of the cervix at an early stage. A gynecologist also investigates and treats menstrual disorders, such as *amenorrhea* (lack of menstruation), *menorrhagia* (excessive menstrual bleeding), *dysmenorrhea* (painful menstruation), and *premenstrual syndrome* as well as structural disorders, including uterine *fibroids*, cervical *polyps*, and ovarian *cysts*.

Although an *obstetrician* deals with the management of pregnancy, the gynecologist treats disorders of early pregnancy, including recurrent *miscarriage*. Many gynecologists are also obstetricians.

Gynecology
The study of the female *reproductive system* and the diagnosis and treatment of disorders affecting it. Gynecology involves both medical treatment, using drugs including hormones, and surgical procedures, such as *D and C* (dilatation and curettage) and *hysterectomy* (removal of the uterus). The specialty also involves the investigation and treatment of *infertility*, including *artificial insemination* and *in vitro fertilization*, and advice on *contraception*, including *sterilization*. (See also *Gynecologist*.)

Gynecomastia
Enlargement of one or both breasts in the male, almost always due to an excess of the female sex hormone *estrogen* in the blood.

CAUSES
Estrogen, which is responsible for female secondary sexual characteristics, is produced in large quantities in women, but is also produced in small amounts in all men (just as all women produce small amounts of male sex hormones). In some males, however, an abnormal amount of estrogen is produced, usually for reasons that are not fully understood, but sometimes because of disease.

Gynecomastia is quite common at puberty, taking the form of a slight swelling in one or both breasts, often accompanied by some tenderness. A young boy with gynecomastia is likely to be worried and embarrassed; he should be reassured that his masculinity is not threatened and that the problem will soon pass. Gynecomastia of this mild, temporary kind can also occur at birth.

If the condition develops later— most commonly when a man is over the age of 50—the enlargement may be greater, especially in an already obese man. Such cases are usually not serious, but investigation is necessary to rule out the possibility of an underlying disease. This disease could be *cirrhosis* of the liver, in which the liver is unable to break down estrogen; a tumor of the testis (see *Testis, cancer of*), which can raise the level of estrogen in the blood; or, if only one breast is affected, *breast cancer*, in which case the swelling is caused by a tumor.

Adult gynecomastia can also occur when any one of a number of drugs changes the balance of sex hormones in the blood.

DIAGNOSIS
The physician may arrange for blood tests. If cancer is suspected, a *biopsy* (removal of the entire nodule or a piece of tissue for analysis) will be performed; early treatment is essential for breast cancer.

TREATMENT
The treatment depends on the underlying cause. If a drug is responsible, an alternative drug will be prescribed if possible; otherwise, the gynecomastia must be weighed against the effects of withdrawing drug treatment.

If there is no underlying disease, the swelling usually subsides without treatment, although it may take a few years. A man who is embarrassed by enlarged breasts may prefer to have cosmetic surgery.

If the swelling is moderate or bothersome, an operation can be performed that leaves only a small, unnoticeable scar around part of the areola (the dark skin surrounding the nipple). In many cases, this operation can be carried out as an office procedure using a local anesthetic. *Mammoplasty*, an operation more frequently performed on women, is used when breast enlargement is severe. This operation takes longer, requires a general anesthetic, and leaves extensive and obvious scarring.

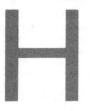

H-2 receptor antagonists

See *Histamine-2 receptor antagonists*.

Habituation

The effect of becoming accustomed to an experience. In general, the more a person is exposed to a stimulus, the less he or she is aroused by it. Experiments have shown that frightening pictures make the pulse rate rise less the more they are seen. Likewise, people can become habituated to drugs (see *Tolerance*).

Habsburg jaw

An inherited prominence of the lower jaw named for the European royal house of Habsburg.

Hair

A threadlike structure composed of dead cells filled with *keratin*, the protein that makes up nails and the outer skin layer.

STRUCTURE

The root of each hair is embedded in a tiny pit in the skin called a hair follicle. Each shaft of hair consists of a spongy semihollow core (the medulla), a surrounding layer of long, thin fibers (the cortex), and, on the outside, several layers of overlapping cells (the cuticle). During the growing phase of a hair the root is firmly enclosed by live tissue called a bulb, which supplies the hair with keratin; the bulb is the pale swelling that sometimes can be seen when a hair is pulled out. The upgrowth of dead cells and keratin from the root forms the hair.

TYPES

There are three types of human hair. From the fourth month of gestation, the fetus is covered with downy hair called lanugo, which is shed during the ninth month. After birth and until puberty, vellus hair, which is fine, short, and colorless, covers most of the body. The third type, terminal hair, is thicker, longer, and often pigmented; it grows on the scalp, the eyebrows, and the eyelashes. At puberty, terminal hair replaces vellus in the pubic area and the armpits. In

THE STRUCTURE OF A HAIR

The hair shaft contains dead cells and keratin (a type of protein). The root is embedded in the skin.

Cuticle
Medulla
Cortex
Hair shaft
Sebaceous gland

Follicle   Root   Bulb   Erector pili muscle

Cross section through hairs
The central medulla, cortex, and outer cuticle can all be clearly differentiated in this microscope photograph.

most men and some women the process continues on the face, limbs, and trunk (see *Hirsutism*).

COLOR AND TEXTURE

Hair color is determined by the amount of pigment called *melanin* in the hair shaft. Melanin is produced by special pigment-producing cells called melanocytes at the base of the hair follicle. Red melanin is responsible for red and auburn hair, black melanin for all other colors. If cells receive no pigment, the cortex of each hair becomes transparent and the resulting hair appears white.

The degree of curliness of a hair depends on the shape of its follicle (see box, overleaf).

DISORDERS

Many hair disorders appear to be purely cosmetic, but they can also be a symptom of a more serious underlying disorder.

Brittle hair, which breaks easily and splits at the ends, is usually due to excessive shampooing, combing, or blow-drying. Occasionally, it can be a sign of severe vitamin or mineral deficiency, or may indicate *hypothyroidism*. Very dry hair is often the result of excessive use of hot rollers or curling irons, or frequent perming, tinting, or bleaching; it can also be caused by malnutrition.

Ingrown hairs occur primarily in blacks or people with very curly hair. The free-growing end of the hair penetrates the skin near the follicle, often causing severe inflammation.

Hairball

A ball of hair in the stomach. Also known as a trichobezoar, it is found in people who nervously pull, suck, or chew their hair. (See *Bezoar*.)

Hairiness, excessive

See *Hirsutism*; *Hypertrichosis*.

Hair removal

Hair is usually removed from different parts of the body for cosmetic reasons. It may also be shaved from around an incision site to allow thorough cleansing before surgical operations.

HOW IT IS DONE

The method used depends on the part of the body involved and the degree of permanency required.

Shaving removes hair at skin level and is suitable for the legs, for armpit and pubic hair, and for the facial beard in men. Shaving is quick and safe, but the hair soon grows back.

Depilatory creams dissolve the hair just below the skin surface, creating a smoother effect than shaving. However, depilatories may irritate sensitive areas and their use is generally best restricted to the legs.

Waxing, a method often used in beauty salons, is suitable for the legs and face. The wax is applied to the area and peeled off, pulling out the hair with it. Plucking with tweezers is suitable for small areas. After each of these methods, hair takes several weeks to regrow.

Permanent removal of hair requires *electrolysis*, in which an electric current is used to destroy the growing part of

HAIR GROWTH

Hair on the scalp grows about half an inch per month. There are about 300,000 hairs on the scalp at any given time, though there is considerable individual variation. The exact number of hairs depends on the number of hair follicles, which is established before birth. Each hair goes through alternating periods of growth and rest. On average, each person sheds 100 to 150 hairs a day from the scalp.

Growth phase
At the start of a growth phase (which, on the scalp, lasts about three years for each hair), the hair root stimulates the growth of a bulb and then a shaft.

Hair shaft
Root
Bulb

Rest phase
During the rest phase (which lasts about three months on the scalp), the bulb retracts from the root and eventually the hair falls out. A new hair begins to grow in the same follicle.

Old hair falls out
New hair forms

TYPES OF HAIR
There are three types of hair—straight, curly, and wavy.

Straight hair
Grows from a more or less round follicle and is round in cross section.

Curly hair
Oval in cross section and grows from a highly curved follicle.

Wavy hair
Kidney-shaped in cross section; the extent of the curl depends on the curve of the follicle.

the hair. Electrolysis requires expertise, is very time-consuming, and is expensive, so it is usually used only for small areas.

Hair transplant

A cosmetic operation in which hairy sections of scalp are removed and transplanted to hairless areas as a treatment of baldness.

HOW IT IS DONE

One or a combination of the following techniques may be employed.

PUNCH GRAFTING This is the most common method of hair transplantation; it is performed using a local anesthetic and is an outpatient procedure. A punch is used to remove small areas of bald scalp, about 0.25 inch (0.6 cm) across, which are replaced with areas of hairy scalp. The grafts are taped into position until the natural healing process takes effect.

STRIP GRAFTING This requires a general anesthetic and is carried out in the hospital. Strips of bald skin are cut from the top of the head; strips of hairy scalp are then stitched in position to replace them.

FLAP GRAFTING This is often used to form a new hairline. It is similar to strip grafting, except that flaps of hairy skin are lifted, swiveled, and stitched to replace areas of bald skin.

MALE PATTERN BALDNESS REDUCTION This relatively new technique consists of cutting out areas of bald skin and then stretching surrounding areas of hair-bearing scalp to replace the bald areas.

RESULTS

The success of hair transplantation varies. The hair in punch grafts often falls out after transplantation, leaving unsightly patches for several months until new hair grows. Also, hair does not always grow properly in the areas from which graft skin is taken. Even successful transplants do not last indefinitely; as time passes, the transplanted areas also become bald.

Half-life

The time taken for the activity of a substance to reduce to half its original level. The term is usually used to refer to the time taken for the level of radiation emitted by a radioactive substance to decay to half its original value. This is useful in *radiation therapy* to assess the length of time radioactive material will remain in the body.

The term half-life is also used in pharmacology to refer to the time the body takes to eliminate enough of a drug so that the amount remaining in the bloodstream is halved.

Halitosis

The medical term for bad breath. Halitosis is occasionally a sign of illness, but is usually simply a result of smoking, drinking alcohol, eating garlic or onions, or poor oral and dental hygiene. Contrary to popular belief, neither constipation nor indigestion is a cause.

If bad breath is persistent and is not due to any of the above causes, it may be a symptom of a mouth infection, *sinusitis*, or certain lung disorders, such as *bronchiectasis*.

Hallucination

A perception that occurs when there is no external stimulus (for example, hearing voices or seeing faces when there is no one there). Hallucination differs from an *illusion*, in which a real stimulus is present but has been misinterpreted (thinking that the ticking of a clock is a bomb, for example).

TYPES AND CAUSES

Auditory hallucinations (the hearing of voices) are the most common type. They are a major symptom of *schizophrenia*, but may also be caused by *manic-depressive illness* and certain brain disorders. Visual hallucinations (seeing visions) are most often found in states of *delirium* brought on either by a physical illness (such as pneumonia) or by alcohol withdrawal (see *Delirium tremens*). *Hallucinogenic drugs*, such as mescaline, are another common cause. Hallucinations of smell are often a sign of *temporal lobe epilepsy*, especially when the epilepsy is caused by a tumor. Hallucinations of touch and taste are uncommon; they probably occur primarily in people with schizophrenia.

There is evidence that people subjected to *sensory deprivation* or to overwhelming physical stress hallucinate temporarily.

Hallucinogenic drug

A drug that causes a *hallucination*. Hallucinogens include drugs of abuse, also called psychedelic drugs, such as

LSD, marijuana, mescaline, and *psilocybin.* Alcohol may also have a hallucinogenic effect if taken in large amounts; hallucinations also occur during alcohol withdrawal. Certain prescription drugs, including *anticholinergic drugs, levodopa,* and *timolol,* may cause takers to have hallucinations in rare instances.

Hallux

The medical name for the big toe.

Hallux rigidus

Loss of movement in the large joint at the base of the big toe due to *osteoarthritis.* The condition often follows an injury and is aggravated by sports that involve running and jumping. The joint is usually tender and swollen, and pain is worse during walking or running.

Hallux rigidus, which may be mistaken for *gout,* is diagnosed if X rays reveal degeneration of the joint. Treatment consists of resting the toe and wearing an insert in the shoe to support the front of the foot and to reduce movements of the toe during walking. If severe symptoms persist, surgery may be required.

Hallux valgus

A deformity of the big toe in which the joint at the base projects outward and the top of the toe turns inward. The condition (which is more common in women) is usually caused by wearing narrow, pointed shoes with high heels, but is sometimes caused by an inherited weakness in the joint. A hallux valgus often results in a *bunion* (a firm, fluid-filled, sometimes painful swelling over the joint) or *osteoarthritis* in the joint.

Treatment is required only if the bunion becomes very large or persistently inflamed or if the osteoarthritis causes pain and limits foot movement. In these cases, the toe may be straightened by means of *osteotomy* (removing part of a bone and realigning its ends) or *arthrodesis* (fusing the bones of a joint).

Haloperidol

An *antipsychotic drug* used in the treatment of mental illnesses such as *schizophrenia* and *mania.* Haloperidol is also given to control the symptoms of *Gilles de la Tourette's syndrome* (a rare neurological disorder) and is used to sedate aggressive or hostile people with *dementia.* Because haloperidol has a powerful *antiemetic* effect, it is sometimes used to relieve nausea and

vomiting caused by *narcotic drugs, anesthesia, anticancer drugs,* and *radiation therapy.*

POSSIBLE ADVERSE EFFECTS
Adverse effects include drowsiness, lethargy, weight gain, dizziness, and, more seriously, *parkinsonism* (a neurological disorder that causes symptoms such as abnormal involuntary movements and stiffness of the face and limbs).

Halothane

A colorless liquid inhaled as a vapor to induce and help maintain general anesthesia (see *Anesthesia, general*). In rare cases it may cause *arrhythmia* (irregular heart beat) or liver damage.

Hamartoma

A benign, tumorlike mass consisting of an overgrowth of tissues that are normally found in the affected part of the body. Hamartomas are most frequent in the skin (the most common is a *hemangioma,* an overgrowth of blood vessels in the skin), but also occur in the lungs, heart, or kidneys.

Hammer toe

A deformity of the toe (usually the second toe) in which the main toe joint is bent upward like a claw. There is often a painful *corn* on this joint due to pressure from the overlying shoe. The deformity is caused by an abnormality of the tendons in the toe.

A protective felt pad usually eases pressure on the joint and thus relieves pain. If pain persists, the deformity may require surgical correction.

Hamstring muscles

A group of muscles at the back of the thigh that bends the knee and swings the leg backward from the thigh.
DISORDERS
Tearing of the muscles is common in sports, particularly in sprinting. The injury happens suddenly and is very painful. Bruising over the area develops several days later. Repeated strenuous exercise may cause a sprain of the muscles, with pain coming on gradually (see *Overuse injury*). Both types of injury can often be prevented by warm-up exercises.

Sciatica (pain down the back of the leg caused by pressure on the sciatic nerve) may be particularly severe in the hamstring muscles. Painful spasms of the muscles may also occur as a protective response to a knee injury. By restricting movement of the damaged knee joint, the spasms limit further injury.

Hand

The most flexible part of the skeleton, the hand allows humans (and other primates) to hold and manipulate objects. This movement is primarily due to the ability of the thumb and fingers to move independently of, and oppose, each other (see *Grip*).
STRUCTURE
The hand is made up of the wrist, palm, and fingers (see next page).

Movements of the hand are achieved mainly by tendons that attach the muscles of the forearm to the bones of the hand. These tendons are surrounded by synovial sheaths containing a lubricating fluid to prevent friction. Other movements are controlled by short muscles in the palm of the hand, some of which make up the prominent areas along the sides of the hand from the bases of the thumb and little fingers to the wrist.

Blood is supplied to the hand by two arteries (the radial on the thumb side of the wrist and the ulnar on the little finger side) and is carried away by veins prominent on the back of the hand. Sensation and movement in the hand are controlled by the radial, ulnar, and median nerves.
DISORDERS
Because they are so frequently used, the hands are susceptible to injury, including cuts, burns, bites, fractures,

---

ANATOMY OF THE HAMSTRING MUSCLES

The upper ends of these muscles are attached by tendons to the pelvis, and the lower ends by tendons called hamstrings to the tibia and fibula.

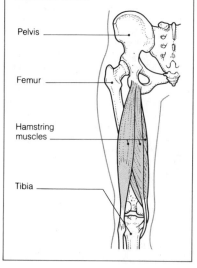

Pelvis

Femur

Hamstring muscles

Tibia

and, occasionally, tendon injuries. *Dermatitis* is also common, since the hands are exposed to a variety of irritating agents.

The hand may be affected by contracture, a deformity caused by shrinkage of tissues in the palm of the hand (see *Dupuytren's contracture*) or damage to muscles in the forearm (see *Volkmann's contracture*). Degeneration of a synovial sheath on the upper side of the wrist may cause a harmless swelling known as a *ganglion*.

Osteoarthritis commonly attacks the joint at the base of the thumb, rendering it painful and immobile. *Rheumatoid arthritis* may cause deformity by attacking the joints at the base of the fingers and rupturing tendons.

Handedness

Preference for using the right or left hand. Some 90 percent of healthy adults use the right hand for writing; two thirds favor the right hand for most activities requiring coordination and skill. The remainder are either left-handed or ambidextrous (able to use both hands equally) to a varying degree. There is no male-female difference in these proportions.

It is uncertain why all humans are not simply ambidextrous. Up to the age of about 12, it is possible to switch handedness if a person's dominant hemisphere of the brain is damaged.

CAUSES

Inheritance is probably the most important factor in determining handedness. Studies have shown a greater number of nerves going to one side of the brain even in the newborn. A child made to use the right hand despite natural preference, however, may "become" right-handed. In earlier times, left-handed people were considered to be unlucky or evil (the word sinister is derived from the Latin word for left), so children were trained to be right-handed. Even today, so many people are naturally right-handed that the pressure to conform is high, especially in some cultures where the left hand is reserved for wiping the anus after defecation. Some left-handed people have been known to rebel subconsciously when forced to use the right hand.

Handedness is related to the division of the human brain into two hemispheres, each of which controls movement and sensation on the opposite side of the body. In most right-handed people, the speech center is in the left hemisphere, so that a *stroke* affecting this side of the brain

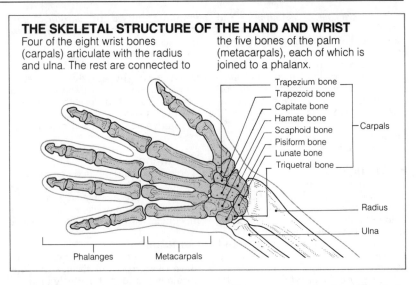

THE SKELETAL STRUCTURE OF THE HAND AND WRIST

Four of the eight wrist bones (carpals) articulate with the radius and ulna. The rest are connected to the five bones of the palm (metacarpals), each of which is joined to a phalanx.

Trapezium bone
Trapezoid bone
Capitate bone
Hamate bone — Carpals
Scaphoid bone
Pisiform bone
Lunate bone
Triquetral bone

Radius

Ulna

Phalanges   Metacarpals

causes *aphasia* (speech impairment) as well as paralysis and weakness of the right arm and leg. In 70 percent of left-handed people, the speech center is on the right, and left hemisphere damage does not cause aphasia.

EFFECTS OF HANDEDNESS

It is not clear whether handedness is related to special abilities. Left-handed tennis players or "southpaw" pitchers seem to succeed because their shots or balls come from an unusual angle. While the left brain is related to verbal ability and logical reasoning, and the right to emotional and spatial awareness, there is no evidence that more artists are left-handed or more philosophers are right-handed.

Hand-foot-and-mouth disease

A common infectious disease of toddlers, caused by a type of virus called coxsackievirus. Hand-foot-and-mouth disease often occurs in small epidemics in nursery schools, usually in the summer months.

The illness is usually mild and lasts only a few days. Symptoms include blistering of the palms, soles, and inside of the mouth, reluctance to eat, and a slight fever.

There is no treatment other than mild *analgesics* (painkillers) to relieve the discomfort of the blisters. The illness is unrelated to foot-and-mouth disease in cattle.

Handicap

The extent to which a physical or mental *disability* (loss or permanent impairment of a faculty) prevents a person from performing everyday activities such as walking or dressing.

The management and treatment of a handicap involves assessment of the specific disability, the provision of suitable aids, and, in severe cases, institutional care.

Hangnail

A strip of skin torn away from the side or base of a fingernail, exposing a raw, painful area. It usually occurs after frequent immersion in water has dried the skin on the fingers. Biting the nails is another common cause. The raw area may become infected and develop into a *paronychia*.

A hangnail should be trimmed with scissors and covered until it heals. The condition may be prevented by applying a moisturizing cream.

Hangover

The unpleasant effects sometimes experienced on waking after overindulgence in *alcohol*. Characterized by headache, nausea, vertigo, and depression, the severity of a hangover is determined by the amount and type of alcohol consumed. Brandy, bourbon, and red wine have high concentrations of congeners (secondary products of alcohol fermentation) and usually produce bad hangovers.

Alcohol has a diuretic effect and some of the symptoms of a hangover are due to mild dehydration; drinking a large quantity of water before going to sleep may help. Recovery from a hangover is usually just a matter of time, but, in alcoholics (see *Alcohol dependence*) there may be withdrawal symptoms or the hangover may be more severe and persistent. (See also *Alcohol intoxication*.)

Hansen's disease

See *Leprosy*.

Hardening of the arteries

The popular term for *arteriosclerosis*, the most common form of which is *atherosclerosis*.

Hare lip

A common term for the congenital defect in which there is a split in the upper lip due to failure of the two halves to fuse during fetal development. Also called cleft lip, it is often associated with a similar failure of the two halves of the palate to join. (See *Cleft lip and palate*.)

Hashimoto's thyroiditis

An *autoimmune disorder* in which the body's immune system develops antibodies against its own thyroid gland cells. As a result, the thyroid gland becomes unable to produce enough hormones, a condition called *hypothyroidism*.

The principal symptoms are tiredness, muscle weakness, and weight gain. Enlargement of the thyroid gland (goiter) is present.

The condition is diagnosed by blood tests to measure the level of thyroid hormones and detect the presence of thyroid antibodies. Treatment consists of thyroid hormone replacement therapy, which is continued for life. It does not always cure the goiter, which may require surgery.

Hay fever

The popular name for allergic *rhinitis*.

Headache

One of the most common types of pain; a headache is very rarely a sign of some underlying, serious disorder. The pain of a headache comes from outside the brain (the brain tissue itself does not contain sensory nerves). Pain arises from the *meninges* (the outer linings of the brain) and from the scalp and its blood vessels and muscles. It is produced by tension in, or stretching of, these structures.

The pain may be felt all over the head or may occur in one part only—for example, in the back of the neck, the forehead, or one side of the head. Sometimes the pain moves to another part of the head during the course of the headache. The pain may be superficial or deep, throbbing or sharp, and there may be accompanying or preliminary symptoms, such as nausea, vomiting, and visual or sensory disturbances.

TYPES

Many headaches are simply the body's response to some adverse stimulus, such as hunger or a change in the weather. These headaches usually clear up in a few hours and leave no aftereffects.

Tension headaches, caused by tightening in the muscles of the face, neck, and scalp as a result of stress or poor posture, are also common. They may last for days or weeks and can cause variable degrees of discomfort.

Some types of headaches are especially painful and persistent, but, despite these symptoms, do not indicate any progressive disorder. *Migraine* is a severe, incapacitating headache preceded or accompanied by visual and/or stomach disturbances. Cluster headaches cause intense pain behind one eye and may wake the sufferer nightly for periods of weeks or months.

CAUSES

Common causes of headache include *hangover*, irregular meals, prolonged travel, poor posture, a noisy or stuffy work environment, excitement, and excessive sleep. Recent research has shown that certain foods (such as cheese, chocolate, and red wine) trigger migraine attacks in susceptible people. *Food additives* may also cause headache. Other causes include *sinusitis*, toothache, ear infection, head injury, and *cervical osteoarthritis*. (See also chart, overleaf.)

Among the rare causes of headache are *brain tumor*, *hypertension* (high blood pressure), *temporal arteritis* (inflammation of the arteries of the brain and scalp), *aneurysm* (localized swelling of a blood vessel), and increased pressure within the skull.

INVESTIGATION

If headaches are persistent, without obvious cause, and do not respond to self-help treatment, medical advice should be sought. The physician will ask about the nature and site of the pain and at what intervals the headaches occur. A careful general physical and neurological examination will be performed. *CT scanning* or *MRI* (magnetic resonance imaging) may be carried out if a neurological cause is suspected.

TREATMENT

Prevention is more important than treatment; many of the known causes can easily be avoided, particularly if the sufferer knows what triggers the headaches. Once a headache has started, however (if it is not a migraine or cluster headache), one or more of

the following measures should ease the pain: relaxing in a hot bath, lying down, avoidance of aggravating factors (such as excessive noise or a stuffy room), stretching and massaging the muscles in the shoulders, neck, face, and scalp, taking a mild analgesic, such as acetaminophen, and, if convenient, sleeping for a few hours.

Head injury

Injury to the head may occur as the result of traffic accidents, sports injuries, falls, assault, accidents at work and at home, or bullet wounds. Most people have a head injury at least once in their lives, but very few of the injuries are severe enough to require treatment by a neurosurgeon. One percent of all deaths are caused by head injury, half of them as a result of traffic accidents.

A head injury can damage the scalp, skull, or brain in any combination. Minor injuries cause no damage to the underlying brain. Even when there is a *skull fracture*, or the scalp is split, the brain may not be damaged. However, a blow may severely shake the brain, sometimes causing *brain damage*, even when there are no signs of external injury (closed head injury).

A blow often bruises the brain tissue, causing death of some of the brain cells in the injured area. When an object actually penetrates the skull, foreign material and dirt may be implanted into the brain and lead to infection. A blow or a penetrating injury may tear blood vessels and cause *brain hemorrhage* (bleeding in or around the brain). Head injury may cause edema (swelling) of the brain; this is particularly notable after bullet wounds because their high velocity causes extensive damage. If the skull is fractured, bone may be driven into the underlying brain.

SYMPTOMS AND SIGNS

If the head injury is mild, there may be no symptoms other than a slight headache. In some cases there is *concussion*, which may cause confusion, dizziness, and blurred vision (sometimes persisting for several days). More severe head injuries, particularly blows to the head, may result in unconsciousness that lasts longer than a few minutes, or *coma*, which may be fatal.

Postconcussive *amnesia* (loss of memory of events that occurred after an accident) may occur, especially if the skull has been fractured. It usually lasts more than an hour after consciousness is regained. There may also

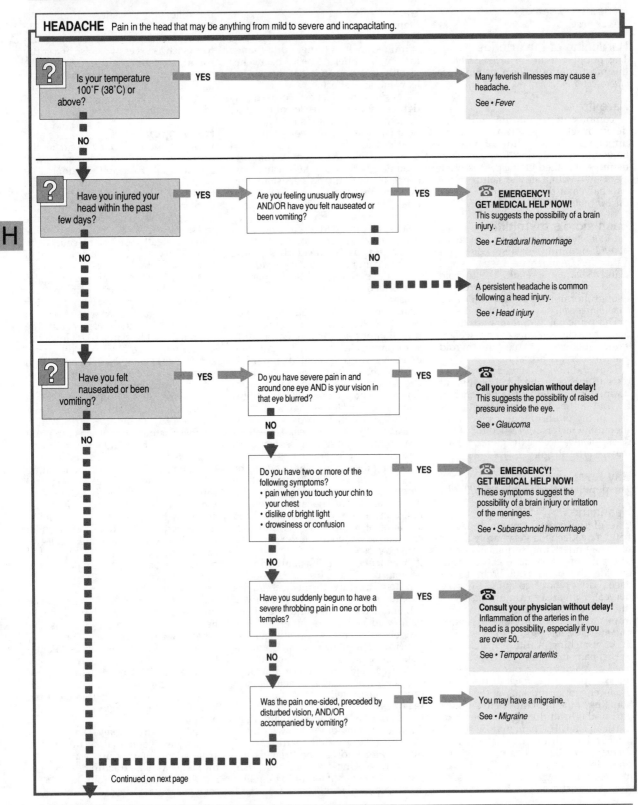

HEADACHE Pain in the head that may be anything from mild to severe and incapacitating.

? Is your temperature 100°F (38°C) or above?

YES → Many feverish illnesses may cause a headache.

See • *Fever*

NO

? Have you injured your head within the past few days?

YES → Are you feeling unusually drowsy AND/OR have you felt nauseated or been vomiting?

YES → ☎ **EMERGENCY!**
GET MEDICAL HELP NOW!
This suggests the possibility of a brain injury.

See • *Extradural hemorrhage*

NO

NO → A persistent headache is common following a head injury.

See • *Head injury*

? Have you felt nauseated or been vomiting?

YES → Do you have severe pain in and around one eye AND is your vision in that eye blurred?

YES → ☎
Call your physician without delay!
This suggests the possibility of raised pressure inside the eye.

See • *Glaucoma*

NO

Do you have two or more of the following symptoms?
• pain when you touch your chin to your chest
• dislike of bright light
• drowsiness or confusion

YES → ☎ **EMERGENCY!**
GET MEDICAL HELP NOW!
These symptoms suggest the possibility of a brain injury or irritation of the meninges.

See • *Subarachnoid hemorrhage*

NO

Have you suddenly begun to have a severe throbbing pain in one or both temples?

YES → ☎
Consult your physician without delay!
Inflammation of the arteries in the head is a possibility, especially if you are over 50.

See • *Temporal arteritis*

NO

Was the pain one-sided, preceded by disturbed vision, AND/OR accompanied by vomiting?

YES → You may have a migraine.

See • *Migraine*

NO

NO

Continued on next page

H

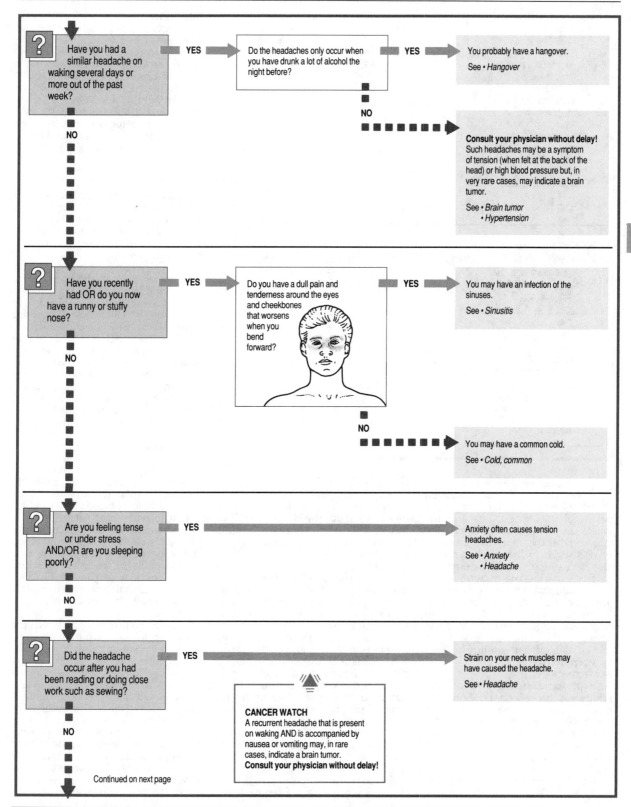

H

Have you had a similar headache on waking several days or more out of the past week?

YES → Do the headaches only occur when you have drunk a lot of alcohol the night before?

YES → You probably have a hangover.

See • *Hangover*

NO → **Consult your physician without delay!**
Such headaches may be a symptom of tension (when felt at the back of the head) or high blood pressure but, in very rare cases, may indicate a brain tumor.

See • *Brain tumor*
• *Hypertension*

NO

Have you recently had OR do you now have a runny or stuffy nose?

YES → Do you have a dull pain and tenderness around the eyes and cheekbones that worsens when you bend forward?

YES → You may have an infection of the sinuses.

See • *Sinusitis*

NO → You may have a common cold.

See • *Cold, common*

NO

Are you feeling tense or under stress AND/OR are you sleeping poorly?

YES → Anxiety often causes tension headaches.

See • *Anxiety*
• *Headache*

NO

Did the headache occur after you had been reading or doing close work such as sewing?

YES → Strain on your neck muscles may have caused the headache.

See • *Headache*

CANCER WATCH
A recurrent headache that is present on waking AND is accompanied by nausea or vomiting may, in rare cases, indicate a brain tumor.
Consult your physician without delay!

NO

Continued on next page

H

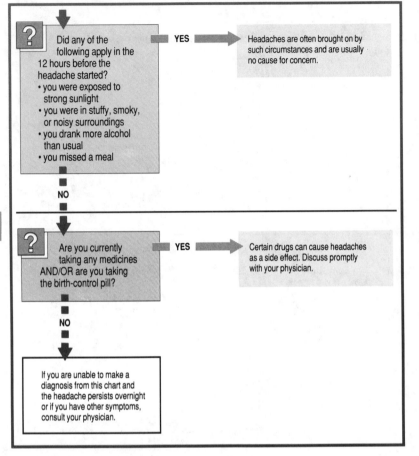

Did any of the following apply in the 12 hours before the headache started?
• you were exposed to strong sunlight
• you were in stuffy, smoky, or noisy surroundings
• you drank more alcohol than usual
• you missed a meal

YES → Headaches are often brought on by such circumstances and are usually no cause for concern.

NO

Are you currently taking any medicines AND/OR are you taking the birth-control pill?

YES → Certain drugs can cause headaches as a side effect. Discuss promptly with your physician.

NO

If you are unable to make a diagnosis from this chart and the headache persists overnight or if you have other symptoms, consult your physician.

Head lag
The backward flopping of the head that occurs when an infant is placed in a sitting position. Head lag is notable in the newborn because the neck muscles are still weak, but, by 4 months of age, the baby can hold the head upright in line with the trunk. The disappearance of head lag is a measure of motor development (see *Child development*); good control of the head is essential before a baby can learn to sit.

Healing
The process by which the body repairs bone, tissue, or organ damage caused by injury, infection, or disease. In popular usage, the term means simply "restoring to health."

THE HEALING PROCESS
The initial stages of healing are the same for all parts of the body. After injury, the blood clots in damaged areas of tissue, and white blood cells and various chemicals (including *histamine, enzymes,* and proteins from which new cells can be made) accumulate at the site of damage. Fibrous tissue is laid down within the blood clot to form a supportive structure; any dead cells are broken down and absorbed by the white blood cells.

Some tissues, such as bone, are then able to regenerate by proliferation of the cells that remain around the damaged area. In such cases, the original structure and function are fully restored. In other cases, however, the cells may be unable to proliferate (nerve cells, for example) or there may be an inadequate blood supply or persistent infection that prevents tissue regeneration. If this occurs, the fibrous tissue that forms in the blood clot may develop into tough scar tissue that keeps the tissue structure intact, but may impair its function (e.g., the restriction of movement that may occur after a muscle tear).

WOUND HEALING
There are two processes by which the body repairs skin wounds—healing by first intention and healing by second intention.

Healing by first intention occurs when the edges of the wound are close together and there has been minimal loss of tissue. If the wound is deep, the edges of the skin may need to be held together with stitches or a butterfly bandage. The blood that seeps from the edges of the wound forms a clot that becomes the base on which scar tissue is laid down. When healing is complete, only a fine scar remains.

be preconcussive amnesia (loss of memory of events that occurred before the accident). The longer the period of unconsciousness and the longer the period of amnesia, the more serious the injury to the brain.

After severe brain injury the person may have some muscular weakness or paralysis and loss of sensation.

Symptoms such as persistent vomiting, pupils of unequal size, double vision, or a deteriorating level of consciousness suggest progressive brain damage. The symptoms may begin immediately after the injury or after apparent recovery.

INVESTIGATION
Any person suffering loss of consciousness, however brief, should see a physician. The person may be hospitalized for observation; skull X rays are performed to identify any fracture. If brain hemorrhage is suspected, *CT scanning* is carried out.

TREATMENT
Cuts to the scalp may require stitching using local anesthesia. People whose consciousness is deteriorating may be kept in a neurosurgical unit for close observation. If a blood clot forms inside the skull, the clot may be life-threatening and requires surgical removal; severe skull fractures may also require surgery.

OUTLOOK
Recovery from a minor head injury may be delayed due to persistent symptoms of concussion, but these symptoms usually improve within a few days. Survival following a major head injury has improved due to advances in nursing and medical care, but permanent physical or mental disability (including changes in personality) has been observed if there has been permanent damage to the brain. Epileptic seizures sometimes occur after severe head injury (usually after penetrating injuries, a severe skull fracture, or serious brain hemorrhage). Recovery from a major head injury is very slow, and victims may continue to show signs of progressive recovery for as long as five years.

Healing by second intention occurs when the edges of the wound are not brought together. In this slower type of healing, pink *granulation tissue* grows from the exposed tissue. It is eventually covered by skin that grows over the wound from the cut edges. By the time healing is complete, the granulation tissue has developed into tough scar tissue.

Health

At its simplest, health is the absence of physical and mental disease. However, the wider concept promoted by the World Health Organization is that all people should have the opportunity to fulfill their genetic potential. This includes the ability to grow and develop physically and mentally without the impediments of inadequate nutrition or environmental contamination, and to be protected as much as possible against infectious diseases. (See also *Diet and disease; Health hazards*.)

Health food

 A term applied to products that are meant to promote health, including unprocessed and whole grains, organically grown fruits and vegetables, and dietary supplements. The term is misleading because it suggests that only "health foods" are good for people. In fact, a healthy diet is based on sound *nutrition*.

Health hazards

Environmental factors that are known or suspected to cause disease. Some health hazards are obvious, such as contamination of water supplies with sewage or other effluents, and pollution of the air with smoke or poisonous chemicals. Others are less apparent—for example, radioactivity (which is detectable only with special instruments) and sunlight.

TYPES

For people in developing countries (the majority of the world's population), the main hazards come from lack of access to safe, pure water, from inadequate means of disposal of sewage and domestic refuse, and from insufficient or contaminated food. Foods contaminated with microorganisms (such as bacteria and molds) present far greater health hazards than those associated with the additives that are used in developed countries to combat such contamination (see *Food additives; Food-borne infection; Food poisoning*).

There are four other main types of health hazard, all of which are present worldwide. First, there are many *infectious diseases* transmitted by contact or by insects or other animals. (See *Bacteria; Fungal infections; Insects and disease; Viruses; Zoonoses*.)

The second type comprises work-related hazards (such as industrial accidents) and the wide variety of occupational disorders—for example, *asbestosis, pneumoconiosis, lead poisoning*, and cancers associated with exposure to chemicals. (See *Accidents; Occupational disease and injury*.)

The third category of hazards includes those associated with domestic and social life, such as *accidents* in the home or on the road, and injuries and other hazards (such as drowning) from sports activities. In many developed countries, domestic and traffic accidents are the most important risks to health in early adult life. Alcohol and tobacco are other primary hazards to health.

Finally, there are many types of global environmental hazards, ranging from sunlight and cosmic radiation to air *pollution* and background radioactivity. (See *Radiation hazards*.)

Health Maintenance Organization

A form of prepaid hospital and medical insurance that first received attention in about 1970. A person or family enrolling in a Health Maintenance Organization (HMO) pays the same monthly premium regardless of the amount of services needed. Care may be provided by HMO staff physicians (closed panel) or by members of an outside group (independent practice association).

According to original theory, HMOs would limit costs by encouraging preventive medicine. Since the HMO's financial performance would depend on premium income exceeding the cost of services, the HMO theoretically would have a financial incentive to keep patients healthy through periodic checkups and screenings. Recent studies indicate that HMOs do reduce medical costs. But the reason appears to be reduced rates of hospitalization rather than preventive care.

Hearing

The sense that enables sound to be perceived. The *ear* (the organ of hearing) transforms the sound waves it receives into nerve impulses that pass to the brain.

MECHANISM OF HEARING

Almost all sound is heard by a mechanism known as air conduction (see box, next page). This process, in which sound waves are channeled down the ear, is supplemented by a secondary form of hearing called bone conduction. Some sound waves set up vibrations in the skull bones that pass directly to the inner ear. This form of hearing affects the way a person hears his or her own voice.

HEARING DISORDERS

Problems with hearing (from minor sound distortions to total deafness) result when any part of the sound-transmitting and analyzing mechanism is damaged. (See also *Deafness*.)

Hearing aids

Electronic devices that improve hearing in people with certain types of *deafness*. A hearing aid consists of a tiny microphone (to pick up sounds), an amplifier (to increase their volume), and a tiny speaker (to transmit sounds to the ear).

HOW IT WORKS

A tiny microphone collects sound and transforms it into electric current. The amplifier increases the strength of the current and feeds it along a tube to an earpiece, which fits into the outer-ear canal and converts the current back to (now amplified) sound.

A volume control on the aid, usually operated by turning a tiny wheel, enables the level of incoming sound to be adjusted. The aid is designed at the factory to amplify those pitches for which the user has the most loss. Further modifications of this sort may be made by the hearing aid dispenser.

TYPES

The most common types of hearing aids are inconspicuous. The mechanical parts, along with a battery to power them, are contained in a small plastic case that fits comfortably behind the ear, in the side piece of an eyeglass frame, or entirely within the ear canal. Aids that fit entirely in the ear are most popular today.

More powerful aids that amplify sound to a greater degree are also available, but rarely used anymore. In these aids, the microphone, amplifier, and battery are contained in a larger case worn on the body; the current is carried to the earpiece by a thin wire.

Most modern hearing aids include switches that enable normal reception of sound by the microphone to be replaced by a process known as electromagnetic induction. This process picks up transmitted speech in

H

HEARING

The ears are the organs of hearing. Each ear has three separate regions—the outer ear, middle ear, and inner ear. Sound waves are channeled into the ear canal to the middle ear, where a complex system of membranes and tiny bones conveys the vibrations to the inner ear. A part of the auditory nerve converts the vibrations to nerve impulses, which are then transmitted to the brain.

To function properly, the eardrum must have equal air pressure on each side so that it can vibrate freely. Pressure is equalized via the eustachian tube, which runs from the back of the throat to the middle ear.

ROUTE TO THE BRAIN

Auditory sensations are picked up by nerve fibers in the cochlea and travel along the auditory nerve to the medulla. From there, they pass via the thalamus to the superior temporal gyrus—the part of the cerebral cortex involved in receiving and perceiving sound.

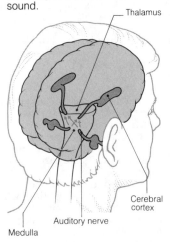

Thalamus

Cerebral cortex

Auditory nerve

Medulla

Outer ear
The pinna (the visible part of the ear) channels sound waves into the outer-ear canal (auditory canal) toward the eardrum. Hairs and waxy cerumen line the canal.

Malleus (hammer) and incus (anvil)
The malleus, attached to the eardrum, transmits vibration to the incus.

Stapes (stirrup) and oval window
The incus in turn transmits vibration to the stapes and the oval window membrane.

Eardrum
The tympanic membrane (eardrum) is a taut membrane between the outer and middle ears. Sound waves of different frequencies cause the eardrum to vibrate at different speeds.

Cochlea
The cochlea consists of a hollow spiral passage in the temporal bone. The cochlear duct, a fluid-filled membranous tube, virtually divides the cochlea lengthwise; it is full of microscopic hairs that stimulate nerve cells in response to sound vibrations, transmitted through the oval window.

Cochlea

Oval window

Basilar membrane

Nerve fibers

Function of cochlea
Inside the cochlea (shown uncoiled), the first part of the basilar membrane responds most to high-frequency vibrations; the far end registers only lower frequencies.

COMPARISON OF FREQUENCY RANGES

Different animals are able to hear different ranges of sound frequencies. The diagram shows the normal ranges of sound, in hertz (cycles per second), that can be heard by a human, a bat, a dolphin, and a dog.

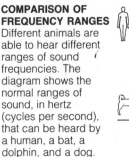
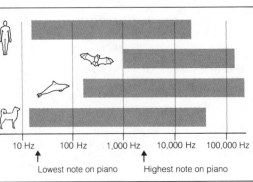

10 Hz 100 Hz 1,000 Hz 10,000 Hz 100,000 Hz

Lowest note on piano Highest note on piano

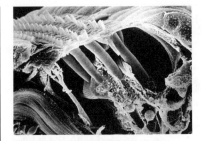

Electron micrograph of inner ear
The section shows four rows of hair cells, which convert sound waves into electrical impulses to be sent to the brain.

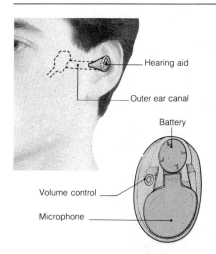

Labels: Hearing aid, Outer ear canal, Battery, Volume control, Microphone

Hearing aids
Hearing aids amplify sound waves for people who are hearing impaired. Many hearing aids include an earpiece, a microphone, an amplifier, volume control, and a battery.

telephones and in many public buildings that have been equipped for the purpose. The greatest advantage of electromagnetic induction is that it obscures amplified background noise.

Other devices are available for the hard-of-hearing. They include amplified telephone receivers, flashing lights instead of doorbells and telephones that ring, vibrators that respond to sound, headphones for television sets, and teletypewriters. Exciting developments include the *cochlear implant* and temporal bone implant, which aid nerve and bone conduction deafness, respectively.

Hearing loss
See *Deafness*.

Hearing tests
Tests performed to determine whether a person has a hearing loss, how bad the hearing loss is, and what part of the ear may be causing the loss. The tests may be done routinely as part of a general assessment of *child development* or during a general medical examination. The tests may be used for a person who complains of impaired hearing or in whom hearing loss is suspected (such as a child with poor speech development or an elderly person suffering from apparent *dementia*). Hearing tests may be carried out regularly as a safeguard for people who are exposed to high noise levels in their work. A hearing test can also help determine the cause of *tinnitus* and dizziness.

AIMS OF TESTING
The physician attempts to establish the extent and pattern of any hearing deficit by testing the ability to hear sounds of different frequencies and volumes; the physician also tries to ascertain whether any hearing loss is conductive or sensorineural.

Conductive hearing loss is caused by a defect in sound conduction through the outer-ear canal or middle ear. Sensorineural loss is caused by damage to the inner ear, acoustic nerve, or hearing centers in the brain; the inner ear is isolated for testing by placing a speaker directly on the mastoid bone behind the ear.

The lowest level at which a person can hear and repeat words (the speech reception threshold) is tested, as is the ability to hear words clearly (speech discrimination).

The results of hearing tests (see box, below) enable the physician and patient to decide on treatment, usually a *hearing aid* or surgery.

TYPES OF HEARING TEST

Tests	Function	
Tuning fork tests	These tests are used to determine whether hearing loss is conductive or sensorineural. In the Rinne test, the patient is asked whether the sound is louder with the vibrating tines held near the opening of the ear canal (air conduction) or with the base of the fork held against the mastoid bone (bone conduction). In a normal ear or in one with sensorineural loss,	air conduction is greater than bone conduction. In conductive loss, bone conduction is greater than or equal to air conduction. Weber's test, in which the base of the fork is placed on the forehead, is useful for diagnosing unilateral hearing loss. If hearing loss is conductive, the patient hears the tuning fork better in the ear with the poorer hearing.
Pure-tone audiometry	This is a test in which an audiometer is used to generate sounds of varying frequency and intensity. The audiometer is an electrical instrument that measures a person's ability to hear sounds of different frequencies and intensities. Hearing is first assessed by transmitting the sounds through one earphone while the other ear is prevented from hearing them. The sound frequencies range from 250 to 8,000 hertz (cycles per second); for each	frequency, the sound is decreased in intensity until it can no longer be heard. The person whose hearing is being tested gives a signal at the moment when he or she detects each sound, and the results are recorded on a graph called an audiogram. Bone conduction hearing is then assessed using a rubber rod connected to the audiometer (the rod is placed against the mastoid bone behind the ear and kept in place by a headband).
Auditory evoked response	In this form of testing, the brain's response to sound stimulation by the audiometer is analyzed by means of electrodes placed on the scalp. This test attempts to evaluate the presence of hearing in a person who is unable to cooperate with other	tests (because of mental handicap, for example). Auditory evoked response is commonly used to assess hearing in very young babies. The test can also help rule out acoustic neuroma (a benign tumor within the auditory canal).
Impedance audiometry	This test is used to determine the type of middle-ear damage occurring in cases of conductive deafness. A probe is fitted tightly into the entrance to the outer-ear canal, sealing it off from outside air pressure and sound. The probe emits a continuous sound. Air is pumped through the probe at varying pressures and, at the same time, a microphone in the probe registers the differing	reflections of sounds from the eardrum as pressure changes in the ear canal. The reflections are recorded on a graph known as a tympanogram. The pattern of differing reflections reveals the extent of elasticity in the eardrum and middle-ear bones, thus indicating the type of disease that is causing the deafness. This device can also measure the air pressure in an air-filled middle ear.

H

H

THE HEART

The heart is positioned centrally in the chest, with its right margin directly underneath the right side of the sternum (breastbone). The rest of the heart points to the left, with its lowest point (the apex) located directly underneath the left nipple.

The heart acts as a dual pump. Deoxygenated blood from the body arrives, via the vena cava, in the right atrium (upper heart chamber), is transferred to the right ventricle (lower chamber), and is then pumped via the pulmonary artery to the lungs. There it is reoxygenated and returns, via the pulmonary veins, to the left side of the heart. It enters the left atrium, is transferred to the left ventricle, and is then pumped, via a large vessel (the aorta) to all parts of the body.

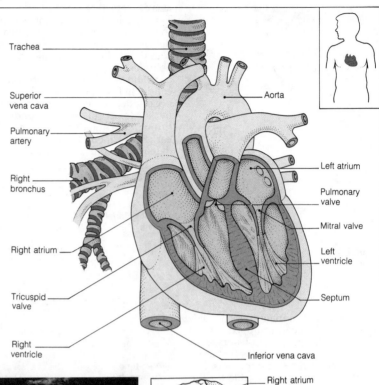

Trachea

Superior vena cava

Pulmonary artery

Right bronchus

Right atrium

Tricuspid valve

Right ventricle

Aorta

Left atrium

Pulmonary valve

Mitral valve

Left ventricle

Septum

Inferior vena cava

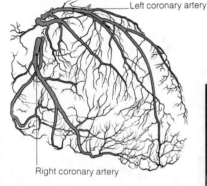

Left coronary artery

Right coronary artery

Blood supply
Although the heart muscle is continually pumping blood, it cannot obtain much oxygen from this flow, so it needs its own blood supply. This is furnished by the two coronary arteries, which arise from the aorta. With their branches, these arteries supply the entire heart muscle.

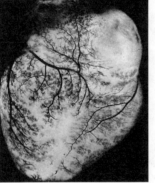

Right atrium

Left coronary artery

Circumflex branch of left coronary artery

Right coronary artery

Right ventricle

Left ventricle

Angiogram of coronary arteries
The image at left gives a view of the heart from the rear and shows clearly the coronary arteries. The image was achieved by angiography—an X ray of the heart was taken after injecting the coronary arteries with a contrast medium.

Heart

The muscular pump in the chest that, throughout life, beats continuously and rhythmically to send blood to the lungs and to the rest of the body. During an average lifetime, the heart contracts more than 2.5 billion times.

STRUCTURE

Much of the heart consists of a special type of muscle, called myocardium. The myocardium, given sufficient oxygen and nutrients, contracts rhythmically and automatically without any other stimulation.

The interior of the heart consists of four distinct chambers. A thick central muscular wall (the septum) divides the cavity into right and left halves. Each half consists of an upper chamber (atrium) and a larger lower chamber (ventricle). Various large blood vessels emerge from the top and sides of the heart; they deliver blood to the atria or carry blood pumped out by the ventricles.

The internal surface of the heart is lined with a smooth membrane (the endocardium) and the entire heart is enclosed in a tough, membranous bag (the pericardium).

FUNCTION

The two sides of the heart have distinct, although interdependent, functions. The right side receives deoxygenated blood from the entire body via two large veins called the vena cava. This blood arrives in the right atrium and, after transfer to the right ventricle, is pumped to the lungs via the pulmonary artery to be oxygenated (receive oxygen from the *alveoli*) and to lose carbon dioxide. The left side receives oxygenated blood from the lungs (via the pulmonary veins, which drain into the left atrium); this blood is first transferred to the left ventricle and then pumped to all tissues in the body. The heart can thus be viewed as a dual pump.

Nonreturn (one-way) valves situated at the exits from each heart chamber guarantee that blood can flow through the circuit in one direction only (see *Heart valves*).

THE CARDIAC CYCLE

The pumping action of the heart consists of three phases, which together make up a cycle corresponding to one heart beat. These phases are called diastole, atrial systole, and ventricular systole (see illustration).

To work efficiently, the different parts of the heart must contract in a precise sequence. This sequence is brought about by electrical impulses that emanate from the sinoatrial node, the heart's own pacemaker situated at the top of the right atrium. The electrical impulses are carried partly by the heart muscle itself and partly by specialized nerve fibers.

To avoid bottlenecks developing in the blood circulation, the volume pumped at each stroke by the two sides of the heart must exactly balance each other. However, resistance to blood flow through the general circulation is much greater than resistance to flow through the lungs; this means that the left side of the heart must contract much more forcibly than the right side. Hence, the muscular bulk of the left side of the heart is considerably greater than that of the right side.

FACTORS AFFECTING HEART RATE AND OUTPUT

The rate at which the heart beats, and the amount of blood it puts out with each contraction, can vary considerably according to the demands of the body's muscles for oxygen, and thus blood. At rest, the heart contracts at 60 to 80 beats per minute and puts out about one sixth of a pint of blood at each stroke, thus pumping about 12 pints per minute. However, during extreme exercise, the heart rate may increase to 200 contractions per minute and the output may increase to almost half a pint per beat, thereby increasing the total output to 100 pints per minute.

Such changes in heart rate and output are brought about in two ways. First, the heart muscle is able to respond automatically to any increase in the amount of blood returned to it from active muscles by increasing its output. This occurs because the more the ventricles are filled with blood during the filling phase of the heart's cycle, the more forcibly they contract during ventricular systole to expel the blood. Second, the heart rate is under external control of the *autonomic nervous system* (the part of the nervous

HEART CYCLE

The pumping action of the heart has three main phases for each heart beat. Each beat is brought about by electrical waves that emanate from the heart's own pacemaker, the sinoatrial node. The electrocardiogram tracing also shows the phases of the cycle.

Diastole
During this resting phase, the heart fills with blood. Deoxygenated blood flows into the right side of the heart; at the same time, oxygenated blood flows into the left side.

Atrial systole
In this second phase, the two atria (upper chambers of the heart) contract simultaneously, squeezing more blood into the two ventricles, which become fully filled.

Ventricular systole
The ventricles contract to pump deoxygenated blood into the pulmonary artery and oxygenated blood into the aorta. When the heart is emptied, diastole begins again.

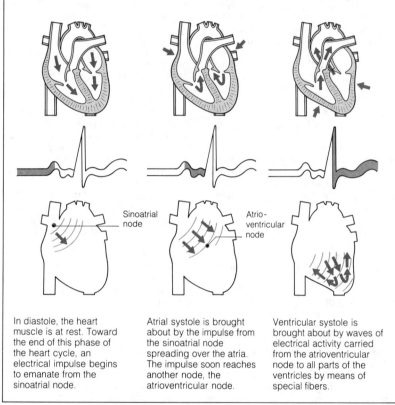

In diastole, the heart muscle is at rest. Toward the end of this phase of the heart cycle, an electrical impulse begins to emanate from the sinoatrial node.

Atrial systole is brought about by the impulse from the sinoatrial node spreading over the atria. The impulse soon reaches another node, the atrioventricular node.

Ventricular systole is brought about by waves of electrical activity carried from the atrioventricular node to all parts of the ventricles by means of special fibers.

system concerned with automatic control of body functions). The parts of the autonomic nervous system concerned with heart action are a nucleus of nerve cells called the cardiac center in the brain stem, and two sets of nerves (parasympathetic and sympathetic) whose activities, controlled by the cardiac center, exert opposite effects on the heart.

At rest it is the parasympathetic nerves—particularly the *vagus nerve*—that are active. Signals carried along the vagus nerve act on the sinoatrial node to slow the heart rate from its inherent rate of about 140 impulses per minute to a rate closer to 70 per

minute. This phenomenon is called vagal inhibition. During or in anticipation of muscular activity, the vagal inhibition lessens, the heart rate speeds up, and may speed up even more when the sympathetic nerves come into action. The nerves release norepinephrine, which increases the heart rate and the force of contraction.

The switch from parasympathetic to sympathetic activity is triggered by any influence on the cardiac center that signals an extra need for increased blood output from the heart. Such influences may include fear or anger, low blood pressure, or a reduction of oxygen in the blood.

Heart, artificial

An implantable mechanical device that takes over the heart's action in pumping blood to maintain the circulation. First used in humans in 1985 after years of research in animals, the presently available artificial heart is now seen as a temporary measure to keep a patient alive from a few days to weeks until heart transplant surgery can be performed.

HOW IT WORKS

The type of artificial heart used most frequently, but not exclusively, to date (the Jarvik 7) is a metal and plastic device installed in the patient's chest in place of the diseased heart. During installation, the device is sewn to parts of the two atria (upper chambers) remaining from the original heart and to the pulmonary artery and aorta (main blood vessels carrying blood out of the heart).

The device is powered by an external machine connected to the device by air lines passing through the chest wall. Pulses of pressure sent through these lines operate the device's pumping action. The patient's movements are restricted by the need to be continuously connected to the machine.

LIMITATIONS AND RISKS

As a temporary measure, the artificial heart has a place in the treatment of life-threatening heart disease, but medical opinion is, at present, strongly against attempts to employ it on a permanent basis. The complications of its use have included *renal failure*, infection, internal bleeding, mental confusion, and *stroke* from blood clots being formed in the heart and carried to the brain. Up to early 1987, all four US patients in whom an artificial heart had been installed on a permanent basis had died. Several of these people experienced strokes and serious infection, which contributed to their deaths.

ALTERNATIVES

A device known as the intra-aortic balloon pump has been in use since the middle 1970s; it has been found helpful as an alternative method of maintaining the circulation when the heart is grossly diseased. The balloon is inflated automatically between each heart beat to provide extra force to the circulation. It has the extra advantage of increasing the pressure in the arteries that supply blood to the heart muscle and of relieving the strain on the heart.

Heart attack

See *Myocardial infarction*.

Heart beat

A contraction of the heart to pump blood to the lungs and rest of the body. The heart beat is readily felt on the left side of the chest, where the apex of the left ventricle (lower heart chamber) lies close beneath the skin (see *Heart*). The rate at which contractions occur is called the *heart rate*. The term *pulse* refers to the character and rate of the heart beat when felt (at the wrist, for example).

Heart block

A disorder of the heart beat that may lead to episodes of dizziness, fainting attacks, or strokes. Heart block is caused by an interruption to the passage of impulses through the specialized conducting system of the heart. Consequently, although the atria beat normally, the ventricles lag behind or contract less often than the atria. This is a completely different problem from the blockage of vessels associated with atherosclerosis.

TYPES

There are several grades of heart block. In the least severe form, the delay between the contractions of the atria and ventricles is just slightly longer than normal (called a prolonged P-R interval from its appearance on an *ECG*). Sometimes the delay lengthens with successive beats, until eventually a ventricular beat is dropped. In more severe cases, only a half, a third, or a quarter of the atrial beats is conducted to the ventricles. In complete heart block, the atria and ventricles beat independently. Thus, while the rate of atrial contraction varies according to the patient's activity, the ventricles contract at a fairly constant rate of about 40 beats per minute.

CAUSES AND INCIDENCE

Heart block may occur as a result of *coronary heart disease*, in active *myocarditis* (inflammation of heart muscle), with an overdose of a *digitalis drug*, in *rheumatic fever*, or in syphilitic *aortitis*. In about half the cases, the patient has no history of heart disease.

Heart block is a common disorder. It develops in about 30 persons per 100,000 annually in the US.

SYMPTOMS

A prolonged P-R interval causes no symptoms even though it can be detected on an *ECG*. Dropped beats may also be symptomless.

In other cases, the rate of the ventricular beat is slower than normal; in complete heart block, the rate does not increase in response to exercise. Sometimes the ventricles are able to compensate by expelling more blood with each contraction. In other cases, the blood output from the ventricles is inadequate, and the patient may become breathless due to *heart failure*, may develop the chest pains of *angina pectoris*, or may faint.

If the ventricular beat becomes very slow, or stops altogether for a few seconds, the patient may black out and have a seizure due to insufficient blood reaching the brain. However, the ventricular beat usually restarts within a few seconds. If the delay is prolonged and cerebral *atherosclerosis* exists, *stroke* may result.

DIAGNOSIS

Heart block may be diagnosed by a physician who finds a slow regular heart beat (below 50 beats per minute) that does not accelerate during exercise and is confirmed by an ECG.

TREATMENT

Some cases of heart block do not require treatment (e.g., when there are no symptoms or in the case of an elderly person whose only symptom is slight uneasiness). If the heart block is causing fainting attacks, it usually is treated by fitting an artificial *pacemaker*, which overrides the natural pacemaker and faulty electrical conducting system in the heart.

Less commonly, the condition may be treated with drugs (such as isoproterenol), although usually only in emergencies or as a temporary measure until an artificial pacemaker can be fitted.

Heartburn

A burning pain in the center of the chest that may travel from the tip of the breastbone to the throat.

Heartburn may be caused by overeating, eating rich or spicy food, or drinking alcohol. Recurrent heartburn is a symptom of *esophagitis*, which is usually caused by *acid reflux* (backflow of stomach acid). This backflow of acid is associated with the inability of the lower esophageal segment to close completely (sometimes accompanied by a *hiatal hernia*). Heartburn is often brought on by lying down or bending forward.

Occasionally, heartburn may cause chest pain that is mistaken for the pain of heart disease.

DISORDERS OF THE HEART

Heart disorders are by far the most common cause of death in developed countries. They also impair the quality of life of millions of people, restricting activity by causing pain, breathlessness, fatigue, fainting spells, and anxiety. A wide range of conditions can affect the heart by ultimately interfering with the pumping action of the heart.

GENETIC DISORDERS
In general, inherited or genetic factors do not play a large part in the causation of heart disorders. However, they do contribute to the *hyperlipidemias* that predispose a person to *atherosclerosis* and *coronary heart disease.*

CONGENITAL DEFECTS
Structural abnormalities in the heart are among the most common birth defects, but are usually treatable. They result from errors of development in the fetus and include such conditions as *septal defects* ("holes in the heart") and some types of abnormal *heart valves.* (See *Heart disease, congenital.*)

INFECTION
Endocarditis is an infection of the heart valves, usually occurring in people whose hearts have already been damaged by *rheumatic fever* or are abnormal because of some congenital or degenerative disorder. It may also affect drug addicts who inject themselves intravenously with nonsterile needles. The infection may cause deformity and malfunctioning of any of the heart valves, leading to, for example, *mitral insufficiency* or *aortic insufficiency* (although heart valve disease can also have other causes). Some types of cardiomyopathy are triggered by viral infection.

TUMORS
Tumors arising from the heart tissues are rare, the most common being the benign *myxoma* (which grows inside one of the chambers of the heart and may interfere with blood flow or valve action). Occasionally a malignant *sarcoma* develops. Secondary tumors, spreading from cancer elsewhere in the body (such as the breast or lung) are several times more common than primary tumors.

These *metastases* usually grow within the heart muscle or the pericardium (sac that surrounds the heart), but seldom affect the valves. The tumors may produce electrocardiographic (see *ECG*) abnormalities and, if extensive, result in congestive *heart failure.*

MUSCLE DISORDERS
Cardiomyopathy is a general term for disease of the heart muscle itself. One type of cardiomyopathy is inherited; others may be caused by vitamin deficiency or alcohol poisoning, or may be triggered by a viral infection.

Myocarditis is inflammation of the heart muscle. It may be caused by a viral infection or by toxins released during a bacterial infection. Rarely, it results from drugs or radiation therapy.

INJURY
Blunt injury to the heart usually occurs in car accidents through impact with the steering wheel. The heart is compressed between the sternum (breastbone) and the spine and may suffer injury ranging from mild bruising to complete rupture. In immediately fatal car accidents, up to two thirds of the victims have suffered rupture of a heart chamber. Seat belt use could probably prevent some of these deaths.

Stab wounds to the heart are often fatal within minutes, but, of patients who reach the hospital, the great majority survive. Bullet wounds are more serious; about 10 percent of people shot in the heart reach the hospital alive.

NUTRITIONAL DISORDERS
The heart muscle is sensitive to severe nutritional deficiency and may become thin and flabby from simple lack of protein and calories. Thiamine (vitamin B_1) deficiency, which is common in chronic alcoholics, causes *beriberi* with congestive heart failure. *Obesity* is another important factor in causing heart disease, probably through its effect on other risk factors such as *hypertension, diabetes,* and *cholesterol.*

IMPAIRED BLOOD SUPPLY
The major cause of heart disease in developed countries is impaired blood supply. The coronary arteries (which supply blood to the heart) become narrowed due to *atherosclerosis* and parts of the heart muscle are deprived of oxygen. The result of coronary heart disease may be *angina pectoris* or, eventually, a *myocardial infarction.*

POISONING
The most common toxic substance affecting the heart is alcohol. A large intake for many years may cause a type of cardiomyopathy in which the heart becomes enlarged and heart failure develops. If alcohol intake is stopped, recovery is possible.

DRUGS
Certain drugs may disturb the heart beat or even cause permanent damage to the heart muscle. These drugs include the anticancer drug doxorubicin, the tricyclic antidepressants, and even many drugs used to treat heart disease.

OTHER DISORDERS
Many common and important heart disorders may result from some other underlying condition, such as coronary heart disease, cardiomyopathy, or a congenital defect. Such disorders include cardiac *arrhythmia* (a disturbance in the rhythm of the heart beat), some cases of *heart block* (in which contractions of the upper and lower parts of the heart are not synchronized), and heart failure (inability of the heart to keep up with its work load). *Cor pulmonale* is a failure of the right side of the heart; it is a consequence of lung diseases (such as *emphysema*), which increase resistance to blood flow.

H

INVESTIGATION
Heart disease and disorders are investigated by such techniques as auscultation (listening to the heart sounds) and *ECG* (electrocardiography); heart *imaging techniques* such as chest X ray, echocardiography, coronary angiography, *CT scanning,* and *MRI*; cardiac catheterization; blood tests; and, in rare cases, by a *biopsy* of the heart muscle (removal of a small sample of tissue for analysis).

TYPES OF CONGENITAL HEART DISEASE

The major malformations are *septal defects*, *coarctation of the aorta*, *transposition of the great vessels*, *patent ductus arteriosus*, *tetralogy of Fallot*, *hypoplastic left heart syndrome*, *pulmonary stenosis*, and *aortic stenosis*. The bars (right) show the incidence of each type of malformation among affected babies.

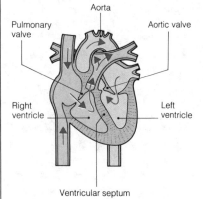

Aorta
Pulmonary valve
Aortic valve
Right ventricle
Left ventricle
Ventricular septum

How blood circulates
Deoxygenated blood (gray) is pumped from the right ventricle into the lungs, where it exchanges carbon dioxide for oxygen. The newly oxygenated blood (pink) enters the left side of the heart and is then pumped out of the left ventricle to all body tissues.

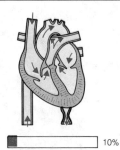

5%

Pulmonary stenosis
Narrowing of the pulmonary valve, or (rarely) of the upper right ventricle, which reduces blood flow to the lungs.

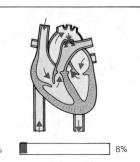

10%

Coarctation of the aorta
In this disorder, localized narrowing of the aorta reduces the supply of blood to the lower part of the body.

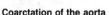

8%

Patent ductus arteriosus
The ductus arteriosus fails to close after birth and blood from the aorta continues to flow through it into the pulmonary artery.

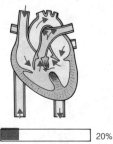

20%

Ventricular septal defect
A hole in the ventricular septum, causing blood to flow from the left ventricle to the right and into lungs.

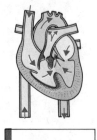

7%

Tetralogy of Fallot
A hole in the ventricular septum, displacement of the aorta, pulmonary stenosis, and thickening of the right ventricle.

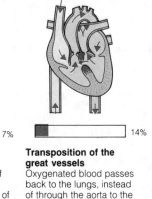

14%

Transposition of the great vessels
Oxygenated blood passes back to the lungs, instead of through the aorta to the tissues.

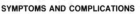

Heart disease, congenital

Any heart abnormality that has been present from birth. Congenital heart defects are the most common major malformations compatible with life.

CAUSES AND INCIDENCE

About 700 babies per 100,000 are born with a congenital heart defect. The errors of development leading to defects arise early in the life of the embryo. In most cases, there is no known cause. Of known causes, the most significant is *rubella* in the mother during the first three months of pregnancy. This can be prevented by vaccination. About one third of babies with *Down's syndrome* have a congenital heart defect, and congenital heart disease often accompanies other birth defects.

Hereditary factors do not seem to play a significant role. If a couple has an affected child, there is little increased risk of a second child being affected. People born with heart defects have little increased risk of having an affected child.

SYMPTOMS AND COMPLICATIONS

The symptoms of congenital heart disease arise from insufficient or excessive circulation of blood to the lungs or to the body. The defects in heart anatomy can also mean that some deoxygenated blood is pumped to the body instead of to the lungs or some oxygenated blood to the lungs instead of to the body. These anomalies can result in *cyanosis* (blueness caused by a reduced oxygen level in the general blood circulation), breathlessness, or both.

Symptoms may first appear at any time over a wide range of ages, according to the defect. Similarly, recognition of a defect may occur any time from before birth to adulthood.

Apart from cyanosis and breathlessness, an untreated heart defect can cause stunted growth and underdeveloped limbs and muscles. Colds repeatedly lead to pneumonia. With prolonged cyanosis, *clubbing* (thickening and broadening) of the tips of fingers and toes may develop. If there is insufficient capacity of the heart to increase blood flow during exercise, the child may rapidly tire and be unable to take part in physical exercise. In some untreated cases, a serious complication called *Eisenmenger complex* (in which there is increased resistance of the lungs to blood flow) develops.

DIAGNOSIS

A heart defect may be diagnosed by procedures such as *chest X rays*, *ECG*, *echocardiography*, and, less commonly, cardiac *catheterization*.

TREATMENT

Rest, oxygen, and various drugs to assist the circulation and lung function may improve matters for a limited time or sometimes indefinitely. Some conditions, such as small septal defects, may get smaller or disappear on their own. Other defects are likely to worsen, and surgical correction often is a consideration.

Today, surgical correction is available for most affected children; the risk of death from unsuccessful surgery lessens every year. One condition—hypoplastic left heart syndrome (in which the left side of the heart is severely underdeveloped)—can be treated only by performing a *heart transplant* operation.

Narrowed heart valves can now frequently be treated by balloon *valvuloplasty*, in which a special catheter is introduced into the heart to widen the narrowed valve.

In other cases, *open heart surgery* is necessary. Sometimes, any of a range of *prostheses* (artificial spare parts), such as replacement heart valves or blood vessels, may be used. In some cases, a heart transplant or *heart-lung transplant* may be necessary.

OUTLOOK
Following successful heart surgery, recovery to good health with resumption of growth, increased activity, and better appetite follow rapidly, and the child usually has a near-normal life expectancy. Full activities, including sports, are generally possible after three to six months.

Children with heart defects (corrected or uncorrected) are at an increased risk of bacterial *endocarditis*, a potentially dangerous infection of the lining of the heart. Preventive antibiotics may be prescribed.

Heart disease, ischemic
The most common form of heart disease, in which there is a reduced blood supply resulting from narrowing or obstruction of the coronary arteries. (See *Coronary heart disease*.)

Heart failure
A medical term that describes an inability of the heart to keep up its work load of pumping blood to the lungs and to the rest of the body. Although it sounds life-threatening, heart failure is usually a treatable condition and compatible with survival for many years.

TYPES AND CAUSES
Failure of the heart is conventionally divided into left- or right-sided failure.
LEFT-SIDED FAILURE Left-sided heart failure may be due to *hypertension, anemia,* or *hyperthyroidism,* to a heart valve defect (such as *aortic stenosis* or *aortic insufficiency*), or to a congenital heart defect (such as *coarctation of the aorta*). In all these conditions, the left side of the heart must work harder to pump the same amount of blood. Sometimes, the extra load can be compensated for by an increase in the size of the left side of the heart and in the thickness of its muscular walls, or by

an increase in heart rate. Compensation is only temporary, however, and heart failure follows.

Other causes of left-sided heart failure include heart *arrhythmias, myocardial infarction* (death of part of the heart muscle due to interruption of its blood supply), and *cardiomyopathy* (intrinsic muscle disease). In cardiomyopathy, the pumping power of the heart is reduced and it can no longer deal with its normal load.

Whatever the cause, the left side of the heart fails to empty completely with each contraction or has difficulty accepting blood returning from the lungs. The retained blood creates a back pressure that causes the lungs to become congested with blood. This in turn leads to pulmonary *edema* (excess fluid in the lungs), of which the main symptom is shortness of breath.
RIGHT-SIDED FAILURE Right-sided failure most often results from *pulmonary hypertension* (raised pressure and resistance to blood flow through the lungs)—itself caused by left-sided failure or by lung disease (such as chronic *bronchitis* or *emphysema*). Right-sided failure can also be due to a valve defect (such as *tricuspid insufficiency*) or a congenital heart defect (such as a *septal defect, pulmonary stenosis,* or *tetralogy of Fallot*).

In all types of right-sided failure, there is a back pressure in the blood circulation from the heart into the venous system, causing distended neck veins, enlarged liver, and *edema* (fluid in the tissues).

SYMPTOMS
Fatigue is an early symptom of heart failure. Breathing difficulty is the most frequent symptom of left-sided heart failure caused by fluid in the lungs. Breathlessness may first be noticed only during or after exercise, but worsens and is eventually apparent even at rest. The patient may be able to breathe easily only when well propped up in bed. Sometimes he or she may awaken at night with an attack of breathlessness, wheezing, and sweating. Such paroxysms may subside on their own or may require urgent, lifesaving treatment.

Right-sided heart failure produces less breathlessness and more swelling of the ankles and legs, often with enlargement of the liver and congestion of the intestines, causing discomfort and indigestion.

TREATMENT
Immediate treatment of the heart failure is followed by treatment of its underlying cause.

Immediate treatment consists of bed rest, with the patient sitting up. The patient is given *diuretic drugs* (which increase the output of urine from the kidneys), thus ridding the body of excess fluid and reducing blood volume. In some cases, *vasodilator drugs* (which ease the work load of the heart) or digitalis (which strengthens the contractions of the heart beat) may also be given. Morphine is sometimes given as an emergency treatment in acute left-sided failure. These measures usually bring about a significant improvement within a few days.

Once the heart failure is treated, attention is directed to treating the underlying cause. If a defective heart valve is responsible, it may be treated by *heart valve surgery* (although, ideally, defective heart valves should be corrected surgically before severe heart failure develops).

Many other causes of heart failure are also treatable; hypertension and arrhythmias are treated through drug treatment and congenital septal defects are treated by open heart surgery. However, when the cause is a long-standing disease of the heart muscle (a cardiomyopathy) or chronic lung disease, the outlook is generally not as good.

Heart imaging
Techniques that provide images of the heart and its structure. Imaging is performed to detect structural abnormality, disease, or impaired function.

TYPES
A *chest X ray* is the simplest and most widely used method of obtaining an image of the heart. It can show the heart size and shape, and whether or not abnormal calcification is present in the valves, major blood vessels, or the pericardium. Pulmonary *edema* (accumulation of fluid in the lungs) and engorgement of the vessels connecting the heart and lungs are usually detectable on a chest X ray, which may indicate the presence of *heart failure*. Pacemakers and artificial heart valves show up clearly on X ray and can be checked for position.

Angiography may be performed to show the heart chambers. Children with complex forms of congenital heart disease (such as *tetralogy of Fallot*) may benefit from this procedure. Angiography is also performed to evaluate the state of the coronary arteries in patients with *coronary heart disease* and helps with decisions about valve replacement.

H

Echocardiography (cardiac ultrasound) is most useful as the first step in investigating congenital heart abnormalities or in evaluating valvular or heart wall abnormalities. *Doppler* techniques enable the physician to measure blood flow across valves. *Radionuclide scanning* produces images that give less anatomical detail but some information about heart function. For example, radionuclide scanning can show how well the heart wall moves and how effectively it empties.

A new generation of extremely fast CT scanners has been developed with heart imaging in mind; previous scanners were too slow to "freeze" a heart beat (see *CT scanning*).

Magnetic resonance imaging (*MRI*) techniques are also capable of producing high quality cardiac images. These techniques are sometimes used to test graft efficiency after a *coronary artery bypass*. They eliminate the need for angiography and for other techniques used previously to investigate congenital heart disease.

Heart-lung machine

A machine that temporarily takes over the function of the heart and lungs to facilitate certain operations in the chest. A heart-lung machine consists principally of a pump (to replace the heart) and an oxygenator (to replace the lungs). The machine is sometimes called a cardiopulmonary bypass or pump oxygenator.

Once the machine is connected and working, the patient's heart and lungs are effectively bypassed and the heart can be stopped. The surgeon can then operate unhurriedly in a blood-free surgical field to perform *open heart surgery*, a *heart transplant*, or a *heart-lung transplant*.

HOW IT WORKS
Blood is taken via cannulas (tubes) inserted into the inferior and superior venae cavae (the main veins draining blood into the heart) and pumped through the oxygenator, which acts as an artificial lung, putting oxygen into the blood and removing carbon dioxide from it. The freshly oxygenated blood is then returned to the arterial circulation via a cannula inserted into the aorta (the main artery carrying blood from the heart) or the femoral artery (a large artery in the leg).

There are two main types of oxygenator. In one type, the blood is passed up a column, through which a gas mixture with a high oxygen content is bubbled. This adds oxygen and removes carbon dioxide. The blood is

then treated with a defoaming agent and held in a reservoir until it is returned to the patient. In the second type, called a membrane oxygenator, the blood and gas flow on either side of a thin, semipermeable membrane, through which oxygen passes from gas into blood; carbon dioxide passes in the opposing direction. This method more closely mimics the function of the lungs.

A heat exchanger is another component of the machine. Generally, it is used to rewarm blood before returning it to the patient (otherwise, blood cools in the machine); sometimes the blood is intentionally cooled to cause a drop in the patient's temperature (see *Hypothermia, surgical*), giving surgeons more time for the operation.

PRECAUTIONS AND LIMITATIONS
The main difficulty with heart-lung machines is they tend to damage red blood cells and cause the blood to clot. To minimize these problems, the patient is given the anticoagulant drug heparin before the bypass is started. During operation of the machine, the supply of blood to the patient's vital organs is less efficient than normal. A patient can thus be kept on a heart-lung machine only for a few hours.

Heart-lung transplant

A radical procedure in which both the heart and lungs of a person are removed and replaced with organs from a donor who has been declared brain dead. (See illustrated box for how and why the operation is done.)

RISKS AND COMPLICATIONS
The early attempts at heart-lung transplant were unsuccessful. In the early 1980s the risk of donor organ rejection was reduced by the introduction of the drug cyclosporine. Some centers are now obtaining very good results. Nevertheless, the operation carries substantial risks. Problems may arise from airway obstruction and other lung complications (including *bronchiolitis*) in addition to the risks of organ rejection. Patients face the long-term problems associated with receiving any form of organ transplant (see *Transplant surgery*).

Heart rate

The rate at which the heart beats—that is, contracts to pump blood around the body.

Most people have a heart rate of between 60 and 100 beats per minute at rest. This rate remains fairly constant throughout life, although it tends to be faster in childhood and to

slow slightly with age. Some athletes have a resting rate below 60 beats per minute. Their hearts are very well developed and can pump blood around the body as efficiently at a slow rate as the normal heart can pump it at a faster rate.

Exercise or stress causes an increase in heart rate. In either case, the increase is due to the release of the hormones epinephrine and norepinephrine by the adrenal glands and of norepinephrine by the sympathetic nerves around the sinoatrial node, the heart's own pacemaker. A small decrease in heart rate occurs during total relaxation and sleep.

Many people have a harmless irregularity of heart rhythm in which the rate is more rapid during breathing in than breathing out.

MEASURING HEART RATE
A physician uses one of two methods to measure heart rate and rhythm (the regularity of the beat). One is to feel the pulse (the expansion of an artery in response to contractions of the heart). The other method, which can be more accurate, is to listen with a stethoscope placed just below the left nipple (see *Heart sounds*).

An even more accurate record is provided by an *ECG* (electrocardiogram), which registers the pattern of electrical activity from the heart muscle that precedes each beat.

DISORDERS OF HEART RATE
A resting heart rate above 100 beats per minute is termed a *tachycardia* and a rate below 60 beats per minute a *bradycardia*. Tachycardias and bradycardias are considered abnormal when the cause is a condition affecting nerve conduction pathways through the heart or the activity of the sinoatrial node, rather than a response of the heart to exercise or relaxation. Irregularities may also occur in the rhythm of the heart's contractions. (See also *Arrhythmia, cardiac*.)

Heart sounds

The sounds made by the heart with each beat. The two main sounds can be heard simply by putting an ear to someone's chest. Classically, the sounds are said to sound like "lubb" followed by a higher-pitched "dupp." A pause follows each lubb-dupp. These sounds are caused by the slamming shut of the heart valves in each heart cycle, and are sometimes called the first and second heart sounds.

Using a stethoscope, a physician can hear the heart sounds much more clearly (and may sometimes hear

H

HEART-LUNG TRANSPLANT

In this procedure, both the heart and lungs of a patient are removed and replaced with organs taken from a brain-dead donor. The removed heart can sometimes be given to another patient.

HOW IT IS DONE

Heart and lungs must be removed from both donor and patient; the donor organs then are inserted into the patient.

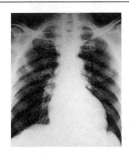

1 The donor heart and lungs must be healthy, and the lungs must match the size of the patient's chest, as measured by chest X rays.

2 In both donor and patient, the heart and lungs are reached via an incision made in the breastbone, and the chest is opened up.

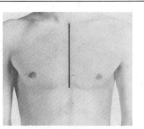

Site of incision

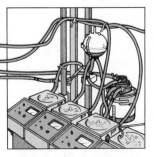

3 The patient is connected to a heart-lung machine. It takes over the function of heart and lungs, oxygenating blood taken from the venae cavae and pumping it back to the body via the aorta.

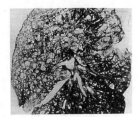

Trachea

Aorta

Right atrium/Vena cava

4 In both patient and donor, heart and lungs are removed through cuts in the trachea, aorta, and where the heart connects to the venae cavae. The blood vessels linking donor heart and lungs are left intact.

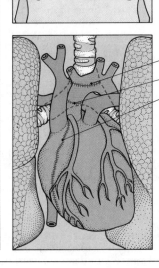

Tracheal reconnection

Aortic reconnection

Right atrium/Vena cava reconnection

5 Insertion of the donor organs into the patient is, in some respects, easier than in the heart transplant, since fewer reconnections have to be made. The main reconnections are between the patient's and donor's tracheas and aortas and between the right atrium of the donor heart and the patient's venae cavae.

WHY IT IS DONE

Subject to availability of a donor, a heart-lung transplant can offer hope to someone who is dying of an end-stage chronic lung disease, whether or not he or she is also suffering from heart disease. Diseases treated include *emphysema*, *cystic fibrosis*, *sarcoidosis*, or *interstitial pulmonary fibrosis*. The heart-lung transplant operation has a better success record than that of lung transplant alone.

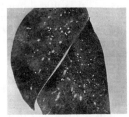

These sections were taken from a healthy lung (at left) and an emphysematous lung; transplanting of heart and lungs may give an emphysema patient new hope.

abnormal additional sounds or an abnormality of one of the two main sounds). Interpretation of these sounds can be important in the diagnosis of heart valve disorders and other heart abnormalities.

FIRST AND SECOND SOUNDS

The first sound (lubb) results from the closure of the tricuspid and mitral valves at the exits from the upper chambers of the heart. This occurs when the ventricles (lower chambers) begin contracting to pump blood out of the heart. The second heart sound (dupp) is caused by closure of the pulmonary and aortic valves at the exits from the ventricles when they have finished contracting.

Through a stethoscope, the second heart sound is heard to consist of a double sound, especially in children and young adults. This is due to a slight time gap between the closure of the aortic and pulmonary valves, and is normal.

ADDITIONAL SOUNDS

In children and young adults, there is often a normal low-pitched third heart sound after the second sound. It is thought to be caused by vibration of muscle fibers in the ventricles as they begin to refill. In people over age 40, this sound is abnormal and a sign of heart failure.

A fourth sound, preceding the first sound and also low-pitched, is occasionally heard; it always indicates an abnormality of heart muscle. The sound is often present after a *myocardial infarction* (heart attack) or in someone with a *cardiomyopathy*.

An opening "snap" is an abnormal sound that may occur during opening of the mitral valve. It is high pitched, heard shortly after the second heart sound, may be accompanied by a presystolic *murmur*, and is associated with *mitral stenosis*.

Ejection sounds or "clicks" are high-pitched sounds caused by the abrupt halting of valve opening. They can occur in *hypertension* (high blood pressure) or in the heart valve defects *mitral valve prolapse, aortic stenosis,* or *pulmonary stenosis.*

Heart *murmurs* are abnormal sounds caused by turbulent blood flow. They may occur as a result of any of various heart valve defects or types of congenital heart disease.

Heart surgery

Any operation performed on the heart. Heart surgery was a rare and hazardous undertaking until the early 1950s, when an operation called mitral valvotomy, performed to correct a narrowed heart valve (by means of a finger passed into the beating heart to stretch open the tight valve), became a standard and successful procedure.

Such "closed" operations on the heart are still occasionally performed, but have largely been superseded in developed countries by *open heart surgery*, in which the heart beat is deliberately stopped and the heart opened to make repairs. Open heart surgery became possible through developments such as controlled surgical *hypothermia* (cooling of the patient before surgery) and the *heart-lung machine*, introduced in the middle 1950s. The machine allows the circulation of oxygenated blood to the brain and other tissues to be maintained with the heart stopped, considerably prolonging the time during which the surgeons can work.

Open heart surgery allows the treatment of many previously serious or fatal conditions, including most types of congenital *heart disease* (heart defects present at birth) and various disorders of the heart valves (see *Heart valve surgery*). *Coronary artery bypass* (for the treatment of obstructed arteries supplying the heart muscle) was first performed in 1967, and, within five years, was being done all over the world. In the same year, the first *heart transplant* was performed in South Africa; the results have since improved largely because of advances in preventing organ rejection.

Another significant development was the introduction in 1979 of balloon *angioplasty*. In this procedure, a fine catheter with an inflatable segment is carefully passed along a narrowed coronary artery and then inflated to stretch the constriction. The results are excellent and many lives have been saved because of it. Angioplasty balloons are also being used to open up narrowed heart valves.

Balloon angioplasty is not without risk; the vessel may fracture or the fatty plaque narrowing the vessel may rupture, permitting cholesterol-rich material to travel down the vessel, thus plugging it. The procedure is most safely performed at centers where facilities for emergency open heart surgery are available.

Experimental work using lasers to open up more stubborn narrowing in arteries is also being done.

Heart transplant

Replacement of a person's damaged or diseased heart by a healthy human heart taken from a donor in whom *brain death* has been certified.

HISTORY

Heart transplantation was first achieved in animals in 1959, but it was not until 1967 that Professor Christiaan Barnard in South Africa carried out the first human heart transplant. Early results were disappointing, with few patients surviving beyond a month or two, but, in 1969, the Stanford University team led by Professor Norman Shumway began its program, which, in 1984, showed that as many as 85 percent of patients could be expected to survive for at least a year after surgery.

WHY IT IS DONE

Heart transplantation is considered for the treatment of patients with progressive, irremediable heart disease, but who are otherwise in good health. Many such patients have advanced *coronary heart disease*; most of the others have *cardiomyopathy* (disease of the heart muscle). If the heart disorder is associated with lung disease, a *heart-lung transplant* may be performed.

HOW IT IS DONE

Heart transplantation poses some special problems compared with the more common procedure of kidney transplantation. First, there can be a problem of timing. Whereas the condition of a patient with kidney failure can be maintained in health by *dialysis* until a donor kidney becomes available, there is no equivalent method for maintaining the condition of someone with a nonfunctioning heart for a prolonged period. Hence, heart transplantation is possible only when a suitable donor heart is available at the right time. Furthermore, heart transplantation has no "fall back" system; if the heart is rejected (attacked by the body's *immune system*), the only hope for the patient is another transplant.

The mechanical, artificial heart is a possible solution to these problems, though in practice the best it seems able to offer is a temporary respite for a patient until the desperately needed new heart becomes available (see *Heart, artificial*).

A further limitation of heart transplantation is that the heart must be removed from the donor while it is still beating for the operation to have the best chance of success. One reason for the success of the Stanford heart transplant program was that California was the first state to allow physicians to certify death with the heart still beating (provided the brain was irreversibly destroyed by disease or accident). Certification of brain death in a patient connected to an artificial ventilator is now permitted in most developed countries, allowing the heart to be removed in optimum condition. The donor heart can then be chilled in saline at 40°F (4°C) and transported many miles by air before being implanted in the recipient.

The actual heart transplant operation is no more or less difficult than other major heart surgery. The first step is to connect the patient's major blood vessels to a *heart-lung machine*, which pumps oxygenated blood to the brain and other vital organs while the surgeon operates. Once the bypass is working, the surgeon removes the diseased heart, leaving the back walls of the atria (upper heart chambers) in place, and then inserts the donor heart, which is kept cooled in saline after its removal. The major blood vessels are reconnected and the new heart is ready to function. The nerves that help control the heart rate are severed during the procedure, but the heart functions without them.

OUTLOOK

Once the immediate postoperative period is over, the outlook is good, with better than 80 percent of patients surviving the first year at certain centers; there is a death rate of around 5 percent per year thereafter. These results are much better than for the surgical treatment of lung or stomach cancer. The main problems are rejection (countered by *immunosuppressant drugs* such as cyclosporine, prednisone, and cyclophosphamide) and infection, which is always a hazard for people taking immunosuppressives, since these drugs weaken the body's natural defenses.

Heart valve

A structure at the exit of a heart chamber that allows blood to flow out of the chamber, but which prevents backwash. There are four heart valves (one at the exit of each heart chamber). Their correct functioning is vital to the efficiency of the heart as a pump. (See *Heart* illustration.)

The opening and, more particularly, the closing of heart valves during the cycle of a heart beat are responsible for *heart sounds*.

DISORDERS

Any of the four heart valves may be affected either by stenosis (narrowing)—so that it takes more work for the heart to force blood through the

HEART VALVE REPLACEMENT

Any one of the four heart valves (aortic, pulmonary, mitral, or tricuspid) may require replacing (see diagram below right). Replacement of the aortic heart valve is described in the steps below.

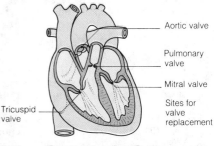

Sternum
Line of incision
Heart

Aortic valve
Pulmonary valve
Mitral valve
Sites for valve replacement
Tricuspid valve

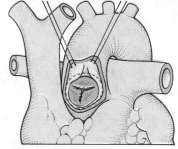

Oxygenated blood returned to circulation
Site of incision
Deoxygenated blood to machine

1 In nearly all surgery on the heart valves, the incision into the chest cavity is made through the sternum (breastbone). The patient is put on a *heart-lung machine*, the beating of the heart is stopped, and the heart is opened.

2 The valve is first examined to determine whether it can be repaired or whether it requires replacement. If the latter is necessary (as here), the valve is excised (dotted line indicates where the incision is made).

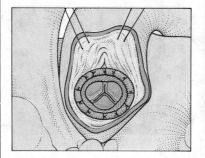

3 A prosthesis is sutured into position and the aorta is closed. The patient is disconnected from the machine and the chest wall is sewn up. The operation takes between two and four hours.

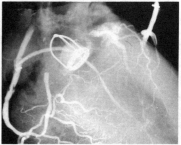

Artificial heart valve in place
This chest X ray shows the metal components of an artificial heart valve. A ball-and-socket valve has been used to replace the patient's diseased valve.

valve—or by insufficiency or incompetence (inability to prevent backwash of blood). With these valve defects, characteristic murmurs are heard by the physician.

Valve defects may be present at birth, either alone or with other defects (see *Heart disease, congenital*), or may be acquired later in life. The most common congenital valve defects are *aortic stenosis* and *pulmonary stenosis*.

Acquired heart valve disease is usually the result of degenerative changes or ischemia (diminished blood supply) affecting part of the heart and leading to aortic stenosis or *mitral insufficiency*.

Rheumatic fever was once the main cause of *mitral stenosis* and insufficiency, aortic valve defects, and, less commonly, *tricuspid stenosis* and *tricuspid insufficiency*. Rheumatic fever is now rare in developed countries, but still prevalent in poorer countries.

Valves are also destroyed by bacterial *endocarditis*, seen often among intravenous drug users. Bacterial endocarditis is, however, a possible complication of any valve disorder.

The symptoms and signs of valve disorders vary, but generally they lead to *heart failure*, rhythm irregularities, or symptoms resulting from reduced blood supply to body tissues.

Valve defects may be diagnosed by *auscultation* (listening to the heart sounds), *chest X ray*, *ECG*, *echocardiography*, *Doppler* echocardiography, and cardiac *catheterization*. They may be corrected by *heart valve surgery*.

Heart valve surgery

An operation to correct a *heart valve* defect or, in many cases, to remove the diseased or damaged valve. The valve is replaced by a mechanical valve (made from metal and plastic), a valve fashioned from human or bovine tissue, a pig valve, or a human valve taken from a corpse.

WHY IT IS DONE

A heart valve may need to be corrected or replaced either because it is stenotic (narrowed) or insufficient (leaky). The mitral and aortic valves (on the left side of the heart) are the ones that most often need correction or replacement, followed by the tricuspid; pulmonary valve surgery is performed only rarely in adults.

In general, heart valve surgery is considered only when the potential effects of the malfunctioning valve on the heart and on general health are so severe that they will soon be a threat to the patient.

The timing of the operation is crucial; it is based on the patient's symptoms and on the results of tests (such as *ECG*, *chest X rays*, *echocardiography*, and cardiac *catheterization*).

HOW IT IS DONE

The illustration on the previous page shows how an aortic valve is replaced.

Valvuloplasty, a new technique, uses a balloon catheter that is inserted into the circulatory system through the skin without opening the chest. It can be used in the treatment of some cases of stenotic valves.

RECOVERY AND OUTLOOK

After the operation, the patient is usually kept in an intensive-care unit for 24 hours, followed by a few days in the hospital. However, a longer hospital stay may result if complications develop or if the patient had been suffering from severe heart failure before the operation.

Symptoms such as breathlessness may take many weeks to improve and may require continuing medication to maintain the improvement. Some people (those with a mechanical replacement valve and those with heart rhythm abnormalities, for example) require long-term treatment

---

TYPES OF REPLACEMENT HEART VALVES

The three main types
There are three main types of replacement valve—biological, mechanical, and homograft. Biological valves are taken from pigs or made from bovine tissue or the patient's own tissue; examples include the Carpentier-Edwards and Ionescu-Shiley valves. Mechanical valves are made from metal, plastic, and carbon fiber. There are two main types—ball-and-cage valves (such as the Starr-Edwards valve) and those with one or more tilting disks (such as the Bjork-Shiley and St. Jude valves). Homografts are human valves that have been removed from people who have died of a disease that does not affect the heart.

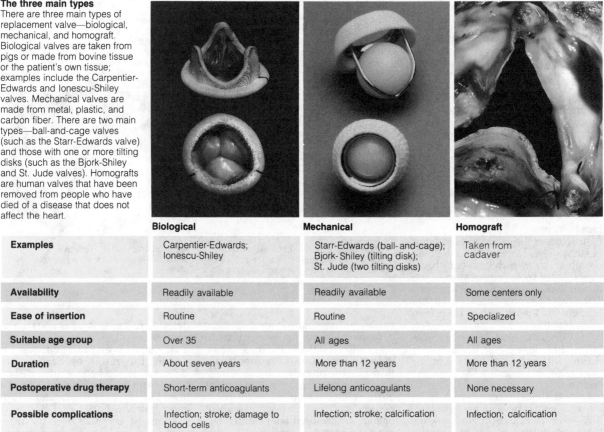

	Biological	Mechanical	Homograft
Examples	Carpentier-Edwards; Ionescu-Shiley	Starr-Edwards (ball- and-cage); Bjork- Shiley (tilting disk); St. Jude (two tilting disks)	Taken from cadaver
Availability	Readily available	Readily available	Some centers only
Ease of insertion	Routine	Routine	Specialized
Suitable age group	Over 35	All ages	All ages
Duration	About seven years	More than 12 years	More than 12 years
Postoperative drug therapy	Short-term anticoagulants	Lifelong anticoagulants	None necessary
Possible complications	Infection; stroke; damage to blood cells	Infection; stroke; calcification	Infection; calcification

H

with anticoagulant drugs. This treatment prevents blood clots from forming around the new valve, prevents them from becoming detached, and prevents them from being carried to the brain or other organs. All patients need long-term follow-up examinations to ensure that the corrected or replaced valve is working well. In addition, most need to take antibiotics before any dental and certain other operative procedures to reduce the risk of the valve becoming infected.

Most heart valve surgery is successful; the death rate is low and is continuing to decline. If a replacement valve malfunctions, it is often possible to insert a new one.

Heat cramps

Painful spasms in a muscle caused by excessive salt loss due to profuse sweating. Heat cramps are usually brought on by strenuous physical activity in extreme heat. The condition may occur by itself or as a symptom of *heat exhaustion* or *heat stroke*.

Treatment (and prevention) consists of the use of salt tablets or drinking enough of a weak salt solution (0.25 level teaspoon of salt to a pint of cold water) to keep the urine pale.

Heat disorders

The body functions most efficiently at a temperature of 98.6°F (37°C); any major deviation disrupts the body processes. Malfunctioning or overload of the body's mechanisms for keeping its temperature constant may lead to a heat disorder. For example, poor adaptation to heat may lead to *heat cramps*, *heat exhaustion*, or *heat stroke*; excessive environmental heat may result in *prickly heat*. In addition, excessive heat production by the body due to a very high fever-producing infection may be damaging.

HEAT REGULATION

The mechanisms by which the body loses unwanted heat to maintain the optimum internal temperature are controlled by the *hypothalamus* (part of the brain). When the hypothalamus is disrupted (for example, by drugs or a fever) the body may overheat progressively, which may lead to fatal heat stroke if emergency treatment is not given.

When the temperature of the blood rises, the hypothalamus sends nerve impulses to stimulate the sweat glands and dilate blood vessels in the skin. Sweating itself does not cool the body; the cooling effect is caused by the evaporation of sweat from the

FIRST AID: HEAT EXHAUSTION

1 Offer plenty of saltwater to drink (about 0.25 teaspoon to a glass) and seek medical help immediately.

2 Lay the victim down in a cool place and raise the feet about 12 inches off the ground.

skin. However, excessive sweating can result in an imbalance of salts and fluids in the body, which can lead to heat cramps or heat exhaustion. Dilation of the blood vessels increases the blood flow near the surface of the skin, thereby increasing the amount of heat that is lost by convection and radiation.

ACCLIMATION

Most heat disorders can be prevented by gradual acclimation to hot conditions. Full acclimation takes one to three weeks. It involves spending gradually longer periods in the heat, alternating with rest periods in cool conditions. Strenuous exercise should be avoided. Frequent cool baths or showers should be taken and salt tablets or dilute salt solution used (0.25 level teaspoon of salt dissolved in a pint of cold water) to replace salt lost by sweating. It is also helpful to eat a light diet, avoid alcohol, and wear loose, lightweight clothes.

Heat exhaustion

Fatigue, sometimes culminating in collapse, caused by overexposure to heat. It is most common in people unaccustomed to working in a hot environment. Unless treated, heat exhaustion may develop into *heat stroke*, which is a life-threatening condition.

CAUSES

There are three principal causes of heat exhaustion—insufficient water intake, insufficient salt intake, and a deficiency in the production of sweat, the evaporation of which helps to cool the body (see *Heat disorders*).

SYMPTOMS AND SIGNS

Heat exhaustion causes fatigue, faintness, dizziness, nausea, restlessness, headache, and, when salt loss is heavy, *heat cramps* in the legs, arms, back, or abdomen. The skin is usually

pale and clammy, breathing is fast and shallow, and the pulse is rapid and weak. There may also be vomiting, and the victim may faint.

TREATMENT

The victim should lie down in a cool place and, if conscious, should take 1 to 2 grams of sodium chloride (salt) tablets or continual sips of weak salt solution made up of 0.25 level teaspoon of salt to a pint of cold water. If the victim is unconscious, he or she should be placed in the *recovery position* until consciousness returns, when salt can be administered.

With rest and replacement of lost water and salt, a full recovery usually takes place. However, the victim should consult a physician because of the risk of heat stroke.

Heat stroke

A life-threatening condition in which overexposure to extreme heat and a consequent breakdown of the body's heat-regulating mechanisms cause the body to become overheated to a dangerous degree. In some cases, body temperature may reach 107°F (41.5°C) or more. Without emergency treatment, the victim lapses into a coma and death soon follows.

CAUSES

Heat stroke is most commonly brought on by prolonged, unaccustomed exposure to the sun in a hot climate. It is more likely to occur in humid conditions, which reduce the body's ability to cool itself by the evaporation of sweat.

Heat stroke can also be caused by working in an extremely hot environment or, very rarely, by a severe fever. Susceptibility is greater in those with a disorder of the skin or sweat glands, those taking *anticholinergic drugs* (which reduce sweating), and in older people in poor health. Overstrenuous

H

H

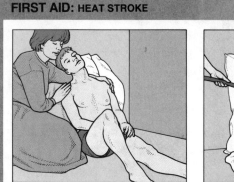

1 Move the victim to a cool, shady place and remove clothing. Place him or her in a half-sitting position and support the head and shoulders (for example, using pillows).

2 Cover the victim with a wet sheet and keep it wet. Fan him or her with a magazine or use an electric fan until the temperature drops to 101°F. Seek medical help immediately.

activity, unsuitable clothing, overeating, and drinking too much alcohol are sometimes contributory factors.

SYMPTOMS AND SIGNS

Heat stroke is often preceded by *heat exhaustion*, with fatigue, weakness, faintness, and profuse sweating. However, with the onset of heat stroke itself, sweating diminishes markedly and often stops completely. The skin becomes hot, dry, and flushed, breathing is shallow, and the pulse is rapid and weak. As the condition progresses, body temperature rises dramatically, and, without treatment, the victim may quickly lose consciousness and die.

TREATMENT

Emergency medical help should be summoned as soon as possible. The victim should be wrapped naked in a cold, wet sheet; the material should be kept continuously wet. Alternatively, the victim should be constantly sponged with cold water. Cooling should be increased by fanning. If the victim is unconscious, he or she should be placed in the *recovery position* while being cooled.

The above treatment should be continued until the victim's rectal temperature falls to 101°F (38.3°C) or until the body feels cool to the touch. If the victim is conscious, he or she may be given sodium chloride (salt) tablets or a weak salt solution to sip (0.25 level teaspoon of salt dissolved in a pint of water).

If heat stroke is treated early, the victim usually recovers fully.

PREVENTION

The key to preventing heat stroke is acclimation (see *Heat disorders*).

Heat treatment

The use of heat to treat disease or aid recovery from injury.

Moist heat may be administered by soaking the affected part in a warm bath or by applying a hot *compress* or *poultice*. Dry heat may take the form of a heating pad, hot-water bottle, or heat lamp that produces *infrared* rays. More precise methods of administering heat to tissues deeper in the body include *ultrasound treatment* and shortwave *diathermy*.

WHY IT IS USED

Heat is used to aid recovery from injury, such as a muscle tear or ligament sprain; by stimulating blood flow, it is thought to help tissues heal more rapidly. Heat is also useful in relieving pain and stiffness in joints and muscles caused by excessive exercise or by rheumatic disorders, such as osteoarthritis. A hot compress is effective in encouraging the formation and drainage of pus from skin infections.

To avoid the risk of internal bleeding and swelling, heat usually should not be used within 48 hours after an injury. This allows time for the blood vessels to heal.

Heel

The part of the foot below the ankle and behind the arch. The heel consists of the *calcaneus* (heel bone), an underlying pad of fat (which acts as a protective cushion), and a layer of skin that usually has thickened (especially on the ball of the heel) as a result of pressure from walking.

Heimlich maneuver

A first-aid treatment for *choking*.

Heliotherapy

Treatment by exposure to sunlight; a form of *phototherapy*.

Helminth infestation

An infestation by any species of parasitic worm (see *Worm infestation*).

Hem-

A prefix indicating blood, as in *hemoglobin* (an important protein in red blood cells).

Hemangioblastoma

A rare type of brain tumor that consists of blood-vessel cells. It usually develops in the form of cysts in the *cerebellum* and affects mainly children and young adults. The principal symptoms include headache, vomiting, *ataxia* (incoordination), and *nystagmus* (rapid, involuntary eye movements).

The tumor, which is slow-growing, is normally clearly differentiated from the surrounding brain tissue so it can usually be removed surgically. In most cases, such treatment completely cures the condition.

Hemangioma

A red-purple birthmark caused by an abnormal distribution of blood vessels in the skin.

TYPES

There are two types of hemangioma— flat and raised. Large, flat, purple-red marks are known as port-wine stains. They are permanent and can be unsightly. In rare cases, they are associated with abnormalities in the blood vessels of the brain (see *Sturge-Weber syndrome*). Small, flat marks are common in newborn babies, particularly on the back of the neck (where they are called stork bites); they fade about three weeks after birth.

Raised marks may be bright red and protuberant (when they are known as strawberry marks) or may be tinged with blue, caused by the presence of blood from a vein. They usually enlarge rapidly for the first few weeks after birth. After the age of about 6 months, the redness gradually fades and the lump subsides. By the age of about 7 years, the mark may have disappeared altogether.

COMPLICATIONS AND TREATMENT

Hemangiomas do not usually require treatment unless they are causing a particular problem. If a hemangioma starts to bleed, medical advice should be sought; meanwhile, the bleeding can be controlled by firm pressure with a clean handkerchief.

A hemangioma that bleeds persistently may require removal, especially if it is on the lip or tongue, where it may easily be bitten, or if it is on the vulva (external female genitalia) or anus, where it is subject to repeated pressure. It may also be necessary to remove a hemangioma from the eyelid because it interferes with vision and threatens blindness in the affected eye. A hemangioma on the face may need to be removed if it is causing psychological distress.

Removal is carried out by *laser treatment* (most successful in young people), *cryosurgery* (destroying tissue by extreme cold), or plastic surgery. If removal is not possible, the marks can be disguised with cosmetics.

Hemarthrosis

Bleeding into a joint, causing the capsule that encloses the joint to swell.

CAUSES

Hemarthrosis is usually the result of severe damage to a joint, such as a torn capsule, torn ligaments, or fracture of a bone forming part of the joint. The most common cause is a sports injury to the knee.

A rarer cause is a *bleeding disorder*, such as *hemophilia* (in which failure of the blood-clotting mechanism causes all bleeding to persist). Any joint may be affected and bleeding into the joint may occur spontaneously or be caused by even the slightest knock. Overuse of *anticoagulant drugs* can cause hemarthrosis.

SYMPTOMS AND SIGNS

Hemarthrosis causes a joint to swell immediately after injury; swelling that occurs 12 to 24 hours later is probably caused by *synovitis* (inflammation of the lining of the joint). In addition to swelling and pain, hemarthrosis may cause the joint to stiffen into a fixed position as a result of spasm in surrounding muscles.

DIAGNOSIS AND TREATMENT

As a first-aid measure, *ice packs* may be used to reduce swelling and pain. After a sports injury, *aspiration* (withdrawing fluid from the joint through a needle) is used to diagnose the condition and to relieve pain; X rays may be necessary if fracture is suspected. Hemophiliacs are given *factor VIII* to promote blood clotting.

To prevent further bleeding, the physician will bandage the joint and advise resting it in an elevated position; cells in the joint capsule gradually absorb any remaining blood. Surgery (such as *ligament* repair) is sometimes necessary.

Repeated hemarthrosis may damage the surfaces of the joint, causing *osteoarthritis* (characterized by persistent pain and stiffness).

Hematemesis

The medical term for *vomiting blood*.

Hematologist

A physician who specializes in diagnosing and treating disorders of the *blood* and blood-forming organs.

Hematology

The study of *blood* and disorders of the blood. Measurements of blood constituents are used in the diagnosis of a wide range of disorders, not only those of the blood. Microscopic examination and the counting of blood and bone marrow cells are essential procedures in diagnosing different types of blood disorders, such as *anemia* or *leukemia*.

Hematoma

A localized collection of blood (usually clotted) caused by bleeding from a ruptured blood vessel. A hematoma may occur almost anywhere in the body and, depending on the site and amount of accumulated blood, may vary in seriousness from a minor to a potentially fatal disorder.

TYPES

Less serious types include subungual hematoma (under a fingernail or toenail), hematoma auris (in the tissues of the outer ear, better known as *cauliflower ear*), and perianal hematoma (under the skin around the anus). The accumulated blood presses on the surrounding tissues, which may cause considerable pain. In such cases, a physician may lance and drain the hematoma to relieve the pressure and alleviate the pain. Most hematomas disappear on their own within a few days.

Among the more serious types are those that press on the brain, notably extradural and subdural hematomas (see *Extradural hemorrhage; Subdural hemorrhage*). They usually are due to an injury that ruptures a blood vessel just under the skull and may be fatal unless treated promptly. (See also *Intracerebral hemorrhage*.)

Hematoma auris

The medical term for *cauliflower ear*.

Hematuria

Red blood cells in the urine. Blood in the urine may be readily visible or small amounts may give the urine a smoky appearance. However, sometimes the blood is not visible to the naked eye. Hematuria can be caused by blood entering the urine at any point along the urinary tract, from the kidney to the urethral opening.

CAUSES

Almost any disorder of the urinary tract can cause hematuria. Infection (including *cystitis*, *urethritis*, and *pyelonephritis*) is one of the most common causes; *prostatitis* often causes hematuria in men. Cysts, tumors, and kidney or bladder stones may cause blood in the sufferer's urine, as can *glomerulonephritis*, in which the glomeruli (the filtering units of the kidney) become inflamed. *Bleeding disorders* may also cause hematuria.

INVESTIGATION

If the blood is not visible to the naked eye, it may be discovered during a urine test when the urinary sediment is examined under the microscope. Urine dip sticks have a small patch that is impregnated with a dye at one end; when dipped in urine containing blood, the patch turns blue.

To determine the cause of blood in the urine, it may be necessary to obtain images of the urinary tract by *ultrasound scanning*, *CT scanning*, or intravenous *pyelography*. These tests usually detect conditions such as cysts, stones, and tumors. If bladder disease is thought to be the cause, a *cystoscopy* (direct examination of the bladder through a viewing tube passed through the urethra) is performed. If a kidney tumor seems likely, *angiography* may be performed to show the blood vessels of the affected kidney.

Hemianopia

Loss of one half of the field of vision in each eye. Hemianopia may be homonymous (affecting the same side of each eye) or heteronymous (affecting opposite sides of each eye). In either case the visual loss may be temporary or permanent.

Hemianopia is not caused by any disorder of the eyes themselves; it is caused by damage to the nerve tracts or brain. Transient homonymous hemianopia in young people is usually caused by *migraine*. In older people it occurs in *transient ischemic attacks* (symptoms of *stroke* lasting less than 24 hours). Permanent homonymous hemianopia is usually caused by stroke, but may be caused by damage to the back of the brain from tumor, injury, or infection. Hemianopia may also be caused by a tumor of the pituitary gland pressing on the optic nerve. In this case, the outer half of the field of vision in each eye is lost.

Hemiballismus

Irregular, uncontrollable, flinging movements of the arm and leg on one side of the body, caused by disease of the *basal ganglia* (part of the brain). The movements are unpredictable in timing and strength, and may be so severe that they cause injury to the afflicted person or others. (See also *Athetosis*; *Chorea*.)

Hemicolectomy

Surgical removal of half or a major portion of the *colon*. The surgeon may remove either the portion between the beginning of the colon and a point two thirds of the way across the transverse colon, or the portion between this point of the colon and the end, including (or excluding) the rectum. (See also *Colectomy*.)

Hemiparesis

Muscular weakness or partial paralysis affecting one side of the body only. (See *Paralysis*.)

Hemiplegia

Paralysis or weakness in the arm, leg, trunk, and sometimes the face on one side of the body only. One or more sites may be involved at the same time. When the affected muscles are stiff, the disorder is known as spastic hemiplegia; when the muscles are limp and wasted, the term flaccid hemiplegia is used.

CAUSES AND SYMPTOMS

A common cause of hemiplegia is a *stroke* (associated with *hypertension* or *diabetes mellitus*). Others are *head injuries*, *brain tumor*, *brain hemorrhage*, *encephalitis* (inflammation of the brain), *multiple sclerosis*, complications of *meningitis*, or a *conversion disorder* (a type of psychological illness).

TREATMENT AND OUTLOOK

Treatment is directed at the underlying cause and is carried out in conjunction with *physical therapy* to exercise the unused muscles. The prospects for a person with hemiplegia depend on how successfully the underlying cause can be treated and on how motivated the person is to recover.

Hemochromatosis

An inherited disease (also known as "bronze diabetes") in which too much dietary iron is absorbed. Over the

years the excess iron accumulates in the liver, pancreas, heart, testes, and, to a lesser extent, in other organs.

CAUSES

The disease is confined almost entirely to men. Women are very rarely affected because they regularly lose iron in their menstrual blood. Although the disease is known to be genetic in origin, the exact mode of inheritance is unclear. Male relatives of an affected person are at risk.

SYMPTOMS, COMPLICATIONS, AND DIAGNOSIS

Hemochromatosis rarely causes problems until middle age. A loss of sexual drive and a reduction in the size of the testes are often the first signs. Eventually the iron overload causes liver enlargement and *cirrhosis* (chronic liver damage), deficient insulin production by the pancreas leading to *diabetes mellitus*, bronzed skin coloration due to iron pigment deposition under the skin (hence the alternative name), cardiac *arrhythmia* and other heart disorders, and, during the late stages of the disease, *liver failure* and *liver cancer*.

The diagnosis is based on *blood tests* that reveal a high level of iron in the blood and a *liver biopsy* (removal of a small sample of tissue for analysis).

TREATMENT

The disease is treated by *venesection* (removing blood) in the same way that blood is removed during blood donation. Initially, venesection is performed once or twice a week. Once the iron level has returned to normal, the procedure is required only three or four times a year.

For young men, treatment can prevent the development of complications; for those who have the fully developed disease, regular venesection can prolong life. *Chelating agents* (such as deferoxamine) have been investigated as an alternative to venesection. (See also *Hemosiderosis*.)

Hemodialysis

One of the two means of *dialysis* (purification of the blood by means of blood filtration to treat *renal failure*).

Hemoglobin

The oxygen-carrying pigment found in red blood cells. Hemoglobin binds with oxygen to form oxyhemoglobin, a compound that gives oxygenated blood its bright red color. There are 350 million hemoglobin molecules in the average blood cell, and each can carry four molecules of oxygen.

STRUCTURE

Hemoglobin is a large molecule made in the bone marrow from two components, heme and globin.

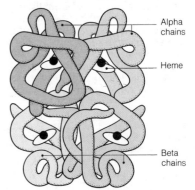

Alpha chains

Heme

Beta chains

Structure of hemoglobin
Each molecule contains four globin chains—two alpha and two beta. Each chain carries a heme component capable of binding oxygen.

The composition of the globin chains can vary, giving rise to several different normal and abnormal forms of hemoglobin. Hemoglobin F is the normal form in fetal life and infancy. It is replaced by the normal adult forms, hemoglobin A and A_2.

FUNCTION

The principal function of hemoglobin is to combine with and transport oxygen from the lungs and deliver it to all body tissues, where it is required to provide energy for the chemical reactions of all living cells. Carbon dioxide, which is produced as the waste product of these reactions, is transported to the lungs for excretion during breathing out.

Defects in hemoglobin production may be either genetic in origin (for example, *sickle cell anemia*) or acquired (see *Anemia, iron-deficiency*; *Anemia, megaloblastic*). The genetic defects are subdivided into errors of heme production known as *porphyria* and those of globin production known collectively as the *hemoglobinopathies*.

Hemoglobinopathy

A term used to describe a variety of genetic (inherited) disorders in which there are errors in the production of globin chains (one of the main components of *hemoglobin*, the oxygen-carrying substance in the blood).

There are two primary categories of hemoglobinopathy. In the first category, abnormal globin chains are produced, giving rise to abnormal hemoglobin molecules. This is the underlying defect in *sickle cell anemia*.

In the second category, normal globin chains are produced in abnormal amounts (known as the *thalassemias*). Combined forms also occur.

The hemoglobinopathies cause anemia and chronic sickness in millions of people in Asia, Africa, and the Caribbean, and in many blacks and Hispanics in the US.

Hemoglobinuria

The presence of hemoglobin in the urine. *Hemoglobin* (the oxygen-carrying pigment in the blood) is mainly contained within red blood cells, although a small amount is free in plasma. Excessive *hemolysis* (breakdown of red cells), which may be caused by heavy exercise, cold weather, falciparum *malaria* (blackwater fever), and hemolytic *anemia*, increases the concentration of hemoglobin in the plasma.

Hemolysis

The destruction of red blood cells, a process that releases iron (which is repackaged into new red cells), bilirubin (which is excreted by the liver in bile), and other breakdown products of the red cell.

Hemolysis is usually a normal process, occurring when red cells age and lose their elasticity; it takes place mainly in the spleen. When red cells are destroyed prematurely, the hemolysis is considered abnormal and may cause anemia and jaundice (see *Anemia, hemolytic*).

Hemolytic anemia

See *Anemia, hemolytic*.

Hemolytic disease of the newborn

Excessive destruction of red blood cells (hemolysis) in the fetus and newborn infant by antibodies produced by the mother. Hemolytic disease of the newborn is typically caused by *Rh incompatibility* factor (a blood group incompatibility between mother and baby, named after the Rhesus monkey in which the Rh factor was discovered), although a milder form of the disease may result from ABO and more rare blood group incompatibilities.

CAUSE
Hemolytic disease may occur if the woman's blood is Rh negative, if she is carrying a baby whose blood is Rh positive, and if she has previously had a baby whose blood was Rh positive. A previous miscarriage, elective abortion, or *amniocentesis* in which the

fetus's blood was Rh positive can also sensitize the woman. In each of these situations, blood has passed at some stage from the fetus to the woman. This causes the woman to produce Rh antibodies (directed against the Rh-positive blood cells) because her *immune system* recognizes the fetal blood cells as "foreign." The Rh antibodies have not formed sufficiently to harm the first baby, but, during a subsequent pregnancy, they cross the placenta and attack the fetal blood cells. A mismatched *blood transfusion* (giving Rh-positive blood to a woman who is Rh negative) also sensitizes the woman so that she produces Rh antibodies.

DIAGNOSIS
All pregnant women have their blood groups tested at the first prenatal check. Rh-negative women are tested for Rh antibodies at this visit and again at 32 and 38 weeks' gestation. They are tested more frequently if there has been a previous pregnancy.

If the pregnant woman shows rising levels of Rh antibodies, amniocentesis is performed at intervals to measure *bilirubin* levels in the *amniotic fluid*. Bilirubin is a breakdown product of red blood cells, so the bilirubin level indicates the severity of blood cell destruction in the fetus.

SYMPTOMS AND SIGNS
In mild cases, the newborn baby becomes mildly jaundiced during the first 24 hours of life (due to excess bilirubin in the blood) and slightly anemic. In more severe cases, the blood level of bilirubin may increase to a dangerous level, risking a form of brain damage known as *kernicterus*. The most severely affected babies have marked anemia in the uterus, become very swollen (hydrops fetalis), and are often stillborn.

TREATMENT
If the condition is very mild, no treatment is required. In other cases, the aim is to deliver the baby before anemia becomes very severe. This usually means *induction of labor* between 35 and 39 weeks' gestation. If the baby is severely affected before he or she is mature enough to be delivered safely (about 30 weeks' gestation), fetal blood transfusions may be necessary. Rh-negative blood is injected into the fetal abdominal cavity at 30 to 32 weeks' gestation, with the procedure being monitored by *ultrasound scanning*.

After the baby is born, frequent blood tests are performed to assess jaundice and anemia. *Phototherapy*

(light treatment that breaks down bilirubin in the skin) and plenty of fluids help reduce the jaundice. However, if the bilirubin level becomes dangerously high, exchange transfusion is performed (blood is removed from the baby and replaced by Rh-negative blood).

PREVENTION AND OUTLOOK
The disorder is far less common since the introduction and use of $Rh_o(D)$ *immune globulin* (anti-D serum) in the early 1970s. It is given by injection to any Rh-negative woman within 72 hours of childbirth, miscarriage, or elective abortion, destroying Rh-positive blood cells from the fetus before they have had time to sensitize the woman's immune system.

Improved general obstetric and pediatric care have also resulted in a reduction in the severity of the cases that still occur.

Hemolytic-uremic syndrome

A rare disease in which red blood cells are destroyed prematurely and the kidneys are severely damaged, causing *renal failure*. Hemolytic-uremic syndrome occurs mostly in infants and young children.

CAUSES
The precise cause of the disorder is unknown. It is thought that the lining of small blood vessels in the kidneys becomes damaged, causing small clots to form. These clots cause *hemolysis* (breakdown of red cells) as blood flows past them, leading to anemia. The resultant damage to the kidneys causes them to fail; this often occurs in epidemics and appears to be triggered by a bacterial or viral infection.

SYMPTOMS AND SIGNS
The onset of the disease is sudden, with headache, fatigue, shortness of breath, and sometimes jaundice. Little urine is passed and what is passed may contain blood. Severe *hypertension* (high blood pressure) is common and may cause *seizures*.

DIAGNOSIS AND TREATMENT
Blood and urine tests are performed to determine the degree of kidney damage. *Dialysis* (artificial removal of waste products from the blood) is necessary until the kidneys have recovered. *Antihypertensive drugs* are given to lower the blood pressure and transfusions of red blood cells may be given to control the anemia. In severe cases, transfusion of plasma (the fluid in which blood cells are suspended) may be required to prevent continual blood clotting and red cell breakdown. Most children make a full recovery.

H

Hemophilia

An inherited *bleeding disorder* caused by a deficiency of a particular blood protein. Hemophiliacs (who are almost exclusively male) suffer recurrent bleeding, most often into their joints. Bleeding may occur spontaneously and/or after injury. In recent years, the problems of hemophiliacs have been compounded by the very high incidence of *AIDS* among their numbers as a direct result of the treatment of their condition.

INCIDENCE AND CAUSES

About one male in 10,000 is born with hemophilia. The blood protein lacking is called *factor VIII*; it is one of a series of proteins essential to the process of *blood clotting*.

The lack of factor VIII is due to a defective gene, which shows a sex-linked pattern of inheritance (see *Genetic disorders*). Affected males pass the defective gene on to none of their sons but to all of their daughters, who are carriers of the condition. Some of the sons of carrier females may be affected, and some of the daughters of carriers may themselves be carriers. Many hemophiliacs have an uncle, brother, or grandfather who is affected, but, in about one third of the cases, there is no family history.

SYMPTOMS

The severity of the disorder varies markedly among affected individuals. Hemorrhage into joints and muscles makes up the majority of the bleeding episodes. The episodes often start when an affected child reaches weight-bearing age as a toddler. The bleeding episodes are painful and, unless treated promptly, can lead to crippling deformities of the knees, ankles, and joints.

Injury and even minor operations such as tooth extraction may lead to profuse bleeding. Internal bleeding can give rise to symptoms such as *hematuria* (blood in the urine) or extensive bruises.

DIAGNOSIS AND TREATMENT

Hemophilia is diagnosed by *blood-clotting tests* that reveal factor VIII activity is abnormally low.

Fifty years ago, most hemophiliacs did not survive to adulthood; today, bleeding episodes can be controlled by infusions of concentrates of factor VIII. Infusions must be given as soon as possible after the start of bleeding. Alternatively, the person can take regular doses of factor VIII as a preventive treatment. Patients can be trained to administer the treatment themselves. However, for more serious or unusual bleeding, the patient may require hospitalization.

Although the use of factor VIII concentrates has considerably improved the quality of life for many hemophiliacs, in recent years problems have arisen because of the AIDS virus. Factor VIII must be made from large pools of donor blood (2,000 to 5,000 individual donations). During the first few years of the AIDS epidemic (before its cause was recognized) large numbers of hemophiliacs became infected with HIV (the virus responsible for AIDS) through factor VIII infusions. Consequently, a percentage of hemophiliacs (and their sexual partners) have been exposed to the virus and some have died of AIDS.

Blood donations are now screened for evidence of the AIDS virus to prevent transmission of the virus by transfusion. Work is also under way to produce a genetically engineered factor VIII, which would prevent all problems of blood-borne transmission for hemophiliacs.

OUTLOOK

A child with hemophilia should avoid activities that expose him or her to a risk of injury, including contact sports such as judo and football; activities such as swimming and walking should be encouraged.

Hemophiliacs who test positive for the HIV antibody should take the usual precautions against transmitting the virus (see *AIDS*) and are advised not to have children.

Hemophiliacs who do not test positive for the HIV antibody (as well as the female relatives of hemophiliacs) should obtain *genetic counseling* before starting a family to discuss concerns about children or grandchildren being affected. Any female relative is a possible carrier of the condition; carrier status can now be ascertained with high accuracy by means of a blood test. The diagnosis can sometimes be determined prenatally.

Hemoptysis

The medical term for *coughing up blood*.

Hemorrhage

The medical term for *bleeding*.

Hemorrhoidectomy

The surgical removal of hemorrhoids.

WHY IT IS DONE

Hemorrhoidectomy is carried out if other, simpler methods of treatment (see *Hemorrhoids*) fail to resolve the problem. The procedure therefore tends to be reserved for people who have large, prolapsing, bleeding hemorrhoids.

HOW IT IS DONE

Stages in a hemorrhoidectomy are shown in the illustrated box.

RECOVERY PERIOD

Laxatives such as mineral oil are given after the operation to soften the stools and make them easier to pass. Non-narcotic analgesics (painkillers) and warm baths ease discomfort. Complete healing occurs after three to six weeks. Avoidance of constipation can frequently prevent recurrences.

COMPLICATIONS

Bleeding is a possible complication. There may be a slight loss of sensation in the anal area that may impair the ability to control release of gas.

Hemorrhoids

Distended veins in the lining of the anus. Hemorrhoids may be near the beginning of the anal canal (internal hemorrhoids) or at the anal opening (external hemorrhoids). Hemorrhoids sometimes protrude outside the anus (prolapsing hemorrhoids).

CAUSES AND INCIDENCE

Hemorrhoids are very common, particularly during pregnancy and immediately after childbirth. Some people have a congenital weakness of the veins in the anus that makes them more likely to develop hemorrhoids. Hemorrhoids occur because of increased pressure in the veins of the anus, usually due to straining during attempts to move hard feces that are difficult to pass. Modern diets consisting of too many highly refined foods fail to provide enough fiber and bulk, which is what produces normal stools.

SYMPTOMS

Rectal bleeding and increasing discomfort, even pain, on defecation are the most common features. Prolapsed hemorrhoids often produce a mucous discharge and itching around the anal opening. A complication of prolapse is thrombosis and strangulation (in which a clot forms in the vein, the vein does not spring back into position in the anus, and its blood supply is reduced); this can cause extreme pain. Iron deficiency *anemia* may result from prolonged bleeding.

DIAGNOSIS AND TREATMENT

Proctoscopy (examination of the rectum through a viewing tube) is usually performed to exclude cancer.

REMOVING HEMORRHOIDS
In both procedures shown below, the patient is first usually given a laxative so that the lower bowel is clear of feces. General or epidural anesthesia is given before a hemorrhoidectomy is performed.

BANDING HEMORRHOIDS

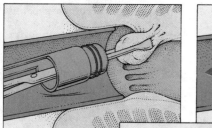

1 This common, simple, and effective procedure is usually painless (causing no more than a mild ache afterward) and no anesthesia is required. The patient lies on his or her side, the proctoscope is positioned and the hemorrhoid is grasped with the forceps.

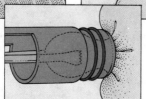

2 Gentle traction is applied to draw the mass into the drum and the banding instrument is pressed into the anal wall.

3 The trigger mechanism of the banding instrument is fired and the bands are squeezed off onto the neck of the hemorrhoid. The proctoscope is withdrawn, leaving the hemorrhoid with its base tightly constricted by the bands. The hemorrhoid then withers and drops off painlessly.

HEMORRHOIDECTOMY

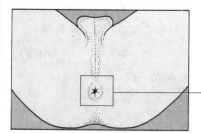
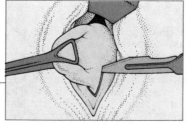

Using general or epidural anesthesia, the patient is examined with a proctosigmoidoscope to exclude a diagnosis of tumor. The patient is then placed in the *lithotomy position*. The hemorrhoid is clamped, placed under traction, secured with a suture, and then removed with a knife.

Mild cases are controlled by drinking fluids, eating a high-fiber diet, and having regular toilet habits. Rectal suppositories and creams containing *corticosteroid drugs* and local anesthetics help reduce swelling and pain.

Internal hemorrhoids can be treated during proctoscopy on an outpatient basis. If the hemorrhoids are very distended, tiny, tight rubber bands may be slipped onto the end of each vein, causing them to wither within a few days. Alternatively, *cryosurgery* may be used to shrink the veins. Prolapsing hemorrhoids require a *hemorrhoidectomy*.

Hemosiderosis
A general increase in iron stores. It may occur after repeated blood transfusions or, more rarely, as a result of excessive ingestion of iron. Hemosiderosis does not usually cause organ dysfunction.

Hemospermia
The medical term for blood in the semen (see *Semen, blood in the*).

Hemostasis
The arrest of bleeding. There are three main natural mechanisms by which bleeding is stopped after injury. First, small blood vessels constrict when damaged, thus lessening the "gaps" through which blood can flow. Second, blood cells called platelets aggregate (clump) and plug the bleeding points. Third, the blood plasma coagulates, forming filaments of a substance called fibrin. These filaments enmesh blood cells at the bleeding points and contract to form a solid clot that seals the damaged blood vessel (see *Blood clotting*). Defects in any of the three natural mechanisms of hemostasis can cause a *bleeding disorder*. (See also *Bleeding, treatment of*.)

Hemostatic drugs
A group of drugs used in the treatment of *bleeding disorders*.

Preparations of coagulation factors are an important type of hemostatic drug. Coagulation factors are present naturally in the body to aid *blood clotting* but are deficient in certain disorders. Preparations of factor VIII, for example, are used to treat *hemophilia*; factor IX is used in the treatment of *Christmas disease*. The coagulation factor is injected after abnormal bleeding to allow clotting, or before surgery to reduce the risk of excessive bleeding.

Other commonly prescribed hemostatic drugs include *vitamin K* preparations (used to treat an overdose of certain *anticoagulant drugs*) and aminocaproic acid, which disrupts *fibrinolysis* (the body's mechanism for dissolving blood clots).

Hemostatic preparations of gelatin and cellulose may be applied to the skin or gums to stop bleeding (e.g., following tooth extraction).

Hemothorax
A collection of blood in the pleural cavity (the space between the chest wall and the lung). Hemothorax is most commonly caused by chest injury, but it may arise spontaneously in people with defects of blood coagulation or, occasionally, as the result of cancer.

Symptoms include pain in the affected side of the chest and the upper abdomen, breathlessness, and an increased pulse. If extensive, hemothorax may compress the lung and cause it to partially collapse. Blood in the pleural space tends to remain in a fluid state and can be drawn off by a needle.

Heparin
An *anticoagulant drug* used to prevent and treat abnormal *blood clotting*. Heparin is given by injection and is

particularly useful as an immediate treatment for deep-vein *thrombosis* or pulmonary *embolism*.

POSSIBLE ADVERSE EFFECTS

Bruising around the injection site is common. Other adverse effects include rash, aching bones, and abnormal bleeding in different parts of the body. Long-term use may cause *osteoporosis* (a bone disorder).

Hepatectomy, partial

Surgical removal of part of the liver. The liver has remarkable powers of regeneration; up to three quarters of the organ can be removed before it ceases to function.

WHY IT IS DONE

Severe injury to the liver sometimes occurs in automobile accidents, causing serious bleeding of and death to the damaged area. Treatment is to remove the dead tissue.

Benign liver tumors and sometimes *hydatid disease* require partial hepatectomy; rarely, *liver cancer* is also treated in this way.

Hepatectomy, total

Surgical removal of the liver. Hepatectomy is performed as the first stage in a *liver transplant* operation.

Hepatic

Related to the liver. For example, the hepatic vein is the vessel that drains blood from the liver.

Hepatitis

An inflammation of the liver, with accompanying liver cell damage or death, caused most frequently by viral infection, but also by certain drugs, chemicals, or poisons. Hepatitis may be either acute (of limited duration) or chronic (continuing).

ACUTE HEPATITIS

This form is a common condition, with about 20 to 30 cases per 100,000 population per year in the US. The most frequent cause is infection with a virus, such as viral hepatitis, type A or type B or non-A, non-B virus (see *Hepatitis, viral*). Other causes include overdose with drugs (such as acetaminophen), exposure to certain chemicals (such as dry-cleaning agents), or, rarely, a reaction to certain drugs in normal dosage. Acute hepatitis may also affect heavy drinkers who have progressive liver disease (see *Liver disease, alcoholic*).

SYMPTOMS

The most obvious sign of acute hepatitis is *jaundice*. In many cases, it is preceded by a flulike illness, accompanied by nausea, vomiting, loss of appetite, tenderness in the right upper abdomen, aching muscles, and sometimes joint pain.

In uncommon, severe cases, jaundice may be intense and *liver failure* may develop, with possible effects on other organs (including the brain), resulting in coma.

DIAGNOSIS AND TREATMENT

A physician may strongly suspect acute hepatitis from the symptoms alone, particularly if the patient is in a risk group for exposure to one of the causative viruses, chemicals, or drugs. *Ultrasound scanning* of the liver may help rule out bile duct obstruction (another cause of jaundice), and *liver function tests* can aid in diagnosis.

There is no specific treatment of acute hepatitis. However, if drug or chemical poisoning is suspected, the physician must determine the causative substance and stop the patient's exposure to it (for example, by withdrawing a drug). Sometimes, detoxification may be possible using an antidote to the substance. In all cases, rest and a nourishing diet are usually recommended; recovery usually occurs after a few weeks. Abstinence from alcohol after the illness aids in liver regeneration.

In severe cases leading to liver failure, intensive care is required. Acute hepatitis causes several hundred deaths in the US each year.

CHRONIC HEPATITIS

Occasionally, a person may fail to recover fully from an episode of acute hepatitis, leading to continued liver cell damage and inflammation. This occurs most commonly, but not exclusively, with certain types of viral hepatitis. Chronic hepatitis may also develop insidiously over a number of years without any acute episodes. Heavy alcohol consumption may again be responsible. In some cases the cause is an *autoimmune disorder* (in which the body's defenses attack its own tissues), a reaction to a medication, or a metabolic disorder affecting the liver.

Several types of chronic hepatitis are recognized, although generally they can be distinguished only by taking a *liver biopsy* (tissue sample) and looking at the liver cells under a microscope. In the type affecting heavy drinkers, damaged liver cells with areas of inflammation around them are scattered throughout the liver, and fat droplets can be seen within the cells. In another type, called chronic active hepatitis, there is obvious liver cell destruction and scarring that can lead to liver *cirrhosis* if untreated. In a third type, called chronic persistent hepatitis, there is a lesser degree of inflammation and little risk of progression to cirrhosis.

SYMPTOMS AND DIAGNOSIS

The symptoms of chronic hepatitis are usually no worse than a vague feeling of being sick. Often the disease remains undetected until the patient has a medical examination and the liver is found to be enlarged, a causative virus or specific antibody is found in the blood, or the results of *liver function tests* are abnormal. Liver biopsy helps the physician establish the type of chronic hepatitis.

TREATMENT

For hepatitis caused by alcohol consumption, total abstinence is the only cure. If strictly observed, it allows complete restoration of liver function. For chronic persistent hepatitis, treatment is not usually needed. For the chronic active form, therapy depends on the precise cause of the disease (see *Hepatitis, chronic active*).

Hepatitis A

See *Hepatitis, viral*.

Hepatitis B

See *Hepatitis, viral*.

Hepatitis, chronic active

A type of chronic *hepatitis* in which there is intense and progressive inflammation and destruction of cells surrounding certain structures within the liver. Scar tissue forms and leads to liver *cirrhosis*.

CAUSES

Chronic active hepatitis may be caused in any of four ways—as a result of an autoimmune reaction (immune system disturbance), a viral infection, a reaction to a medication (rare), or to a metabolic disorder (rare).

In the autoimmune type, antibodies (proteins with a defense role) that inappropriately attack liver cells are formed. This is the most common cause of hepatitis in Northern Europe and one of the most common causes in the US. Women are affected more often than men. Primary biliary cirrhosis may fall into this category.

Viral infection is the most common cause in the US, most often due to viral hepatitis, type B, or non-A, non-B virus (see *Hepatitis, viral*). Men are affected more often than women.

Medications are a rare cause of chronic active hepatitis. Drugs that have been implicated include

MAIN TYPES OF VIRAL HEPATITIS

	Viral hepatitis type A (infectious hepatitis)	Viral hepatitis type B (serum hepatitis)
Transmission of infection	Virus is present in feces of infected people and transmitted to others by fecal contamination of food (e.g., through infected people handling food). Feces are infective from two to three weeks before until eight days after onset of jaundice. Local epidemics can occur.	Virus is present in blood and other body fluids of infected people. In the US, virus is spread mainly sexually and by needle-sharing among drug abusers. Health workers are at risk from infected blood. In Africa and Asia, spread from mother to baby is common.
Incidence	Worldwide. In the US, about 40 percent of young adults have been exposed to the virus. In some parts of the world where hygiene is poor, almost everyone has been exposed to this type of hepatitis.	Worldwide. In parts of Africa and Asia, up to 20 percent of the population has been carrying the virus without symptoms for years. In the US, carrier rate is much lower (less than 1 percent).
Groups at particular risk	Travelers to areas where hygiene standards are poor and prevalence of the virus is high (i.e., parts of Asia, Africa, or South America).	Homosexuals, people with multiple sexual partners, intravenous drug abusers, health care personnel, or children born to carrier mothers.
Incubation period	Three to six weeks after virus has entered the body.	A few weeks to several months after infection.
Illness	In many cases there is no illness. Otherwise, typical acute hepatitis (flulike illness with jaundice), usually mild and never progressing to chronic hepatitis.	Typical acute hepatitis, often more severe than with type A virus. Progression to chronic hepatitis and other liver disease may occur. Sometimes, no illness.
Prevention	For nonimmune travelers at risk, passive immunization with immunoglobulin plus good hygiene and care in selection of food and drink. A vaccine has also recently been developed.	Observance of "safe" sex with possibly infected sexual partners and avoidance of blood exchange. Vaccine and/or passive immunization for groups at high risk.

oxyphenisatin, nitrofurantoin, and isoniazid. Metabolic disorders that may cause the disease include *hemochromatosis* and *Wilson's disease*.

SYMPTOMS, DIAGNOSIS, AND TREATMENT
The disease may cause vague feelings of tiredness, or no symptoms at all. It is diagnosed by *liver biopsy*.

The autoimmune type is treated with *corticosteroid drugs*, which usually bring some improvement. Antiviral agents have been tried unsuccessfully against viral infections. In the drug-induced type, withdrawal of the medication can lead to recovery. For metabolic disturbances, treatment depends on the underlying disorder.

Hepatitis, viral
Any type of *hepatitis* (inflammation of the liver) caused by a viral infection.

TYPES AND CAUSES
A number of viruses may secondarily infect the liver, but, for certain viruses, the liver is a primary target. These are called hepatotropic viruses and include hepatitis viruses type A, type B, and delta viruses. Tests are available for detecting any of these in the blood or tissues. Sometimes, a person has obvious symptoms of viral hepatitis, but the type A, type B, and delta viruses cannot be detected; in such cases the illness is called non-A, non-B hepatitis. A few viruses may cause this type, which is a common form among people who contract hepatitis from blood transfusions.

The different viruses have varying incidences in different parts of the world and different modes of transmission (see table).

Hepatitis, type A (formerly called infectious hepatitis), is thought to be spread by virus from an infected person's feces directly or indirectly contaminating food, drinking water, or someone else's fingers. In most parts of the world, a high proportion of the population has been infected with the virus, often without symptoms, and is immune to further attack. Many cases occur among travelers who have recently returned from an area where the virus is prevalent and standards of hygiene are low.

Viral hepatitis, type B, used to be spread mainly by blood transfusions and blood products (and was referred to as serum hepatitis), but the development of tests for the virus has removed this risk. Today hepatitis B is mainly sexually transmitted (being particularly common among male homosexuals) or spread by mechanisms in which an infected person's blood is inoculated into someone else (i.e., by needle sharing among drug abusers, razor sharing, or ear piercing). These are precisely the same mechanisms by which *HIV* (the virus responsible for *AIDS*) is spread.

Viral hepatitis, type B, is in many respects more serious than viral hepatitis, type A. In a proportion of cases, the virus persists for years after the initial infection and may lead to a chronic form of hepatitis (see *Hepatitis, chronic active*) and eventually to liver *cirrhosis* and/or *liver cancer*. Carriers of the virus may have few or no symptoms during this time, but can infect others. The non-A, non-B hepatitis virus is the cause of most transfusion-associated hepatitis cases.

Hepatitis delta virus can exist only in someone who is already carrying or has recently been infected with hepatitis, type B. In the US, it seems to be spread mainly by needle sharing among drug abusers.

SYMPTOMS, DIAGNOSIS, AND TREATMENT
Infection with any of the causative viruses may be symptomless or may cause a typical acute *hepatitis* with a flulike illness followed by jaundice. About 10 percent of patients infected with the hepatitis, type B; delta; or non-A, non-B viruses go on to acquire chronic hepatitis. This rarely, if ever, happens with hepatitis, type A.

Diagnosis is made by identification of the virus (or by identification of antibodies to the virus) in the blood or, in the case of non-A, non-B hepatitis, by exclusion of the other types. Treatment is as for other causes of hepatitis.

PREVENTION

Vaccines are available against viral hepatitis, type B. However, vaccination is generally offered or recommended only to those who are at high risk of infection. For viral hepatitis, type B, it includes health care workers, children born to carrier mothers, male homosexuals, and drug addicts.

Passive immunization with immunoglobulins (antibodies) directed against viral hepatitis, type A and type B, is also available and can provide some protection. It is recommended for people who will be traveling to high incidence areas on vacation or on short business trips. Hepatitis, type B, immunoglobulin is also given immediately after birth to babies who had carrier mothers, to prevent infection while the vaccine (given at the same time) is beginning to build up.

Avoidance of viral hepatitis, type A, is further helped by observing good hygiene, especially food hygiene, in parts of the world where sanitary standards are low (see *Food-borne infection*). The chances of getting viral hepatitis, type B, can be reduced through use of a condom, by not sharing needles, and by avoiding activities such as ear piercing or tattooing unless the equipment used is sterile. These precautions are broadly the same as for the avoidance of *AIDS*.

Hepatoma

The most common form of malignant tumor arising within the liver. (See *Liver cancer*.)

Hepatomegaly

Enlargement of the liver, which may occur as a result of virtually any type of liver disorder. Enlargement of the liver may cause tenderness just beneath the ribs and can be detected by a physician during the course of a physical examination. (See *Liver disorders* box.)

Herbal medicine

 Systems of medicine in which various parts of different plants are used to treat symptoms and promote health. Herbal medicine was the most common medical treatment in most cultures for many centuries.

Heredity

 The transmission of traits and/or disorders through genetic mechanisms. Each person inherits a combination of *genes* (units of inheritance)—half paternal, half maternal—via the sperm and egg cells from which he or she is derived. The interaction of these genes determines the person's inherited characteristics, including, in some cases, disorders or susceptibility to disorders. Half of an individual's genes are passed on, in turn, to each of his or her children. (See also *Genetic disorders*; *Inheritance*.)

Heritability

A measure of the extent to which a disease or disorder is the result of inherited (genetic) factors as opposed to environmental influences, such as diet and climate.

Certain disorders (such as *hemophilia* or *cystic fibrosis*) are known to be caused entirely by hereditary factors. Others (such as occupational disorders) are caused entirely by environmental factors. Between these two extremes lies a large number of disorders in which both inheritance and environment probably play a part.

Pinpointing hereditary factors is notoriously difficult. A rough estimate of heritability can be obtained from the known incidence of a disorder in the first-degree relatives (i.e., parents, siblings, and offspring) of affected people and by comparing it to the incidence in a population exposed to similar environmental influences. Other estimates of heritability are obtained from studies of identical twins who have been reared apart.

Such studies suggest a relatively high heritability for *schizophrenia*, *asthma*, *coronary heart disease*, non-insulin-dependent *diabetes mellitus*, *ankylosing spondylitis*, and some birth defects, such as *cleft lip and palate*, *pyloric stenosis*, and *talipes* (clubfoot). The heritability for congenital *heart disease* and *peptic ulcer* is low.

Estimates of heritability are useful in *genetic counseling*. (See also *Genetic disorders*; *Histocompatibility antigens*.)

Hermaphroditism

A congenital disorder in which both male and female gonads (testes and ovaries) are present and the external genitalia are not clearly male or female. True hermaphroditism is extremely rare and its cause unknown. The majority of affected children are raised as males because

the external genitalia usually appear more male than female.

A more common condition is pseudohermaphroditism, in which the external genitalia may be ambiguous, but the gonads of only one sex are present. Pseudohermaphroditism is caused by a hormonal imbalance (such as in congenital *adrenal hyperplasia*) and can usually be treated by plastic surgery and hormone therapy.

Hernia

The protrusion of an organ or tissue through a weak area in the muscle or other tissue that normally contains it. The term is usually applied to a protrusion of the intestine through a weak area in the abdominal wall. In *hiatal hernia*, the stomach protrudes through the diaphragm into the chest. Very rarely, other organs or tissue (e.g., the brain) may herniate.

CAUSES

Abdominal hernias are usually caused by a *congenital* weakness in the abdominal wall. They may appear following surgery or after damage caused by lifting heavy objects, substantial weight gain, persistent coughing, or straining to defecate.

SYMPTOMS

The first symptom of a hernia is usually a bulge in the abdominal wall. There may also be abdominal discomfort. In some people, the protruding intestine can be pushed back through the abdominal wall.

Severe pain occurs when the hernia bulges out and cannot be replaced. If the blood supply to a twisted, trapped intestine becomes impaired (a condition known as a strangulated hernia), the bowel may become gangrenous. This requires urgent treatment.

DIAGNOSIS AND TREATMENT

Hernias are diagnosed by physical examination. If the hernia is causing only slight discomfort and is readily pushed back, a supportive garment, or truss, may be recommended. Hernias that are painful or impossible to push back are usually treated surgically (see *Hernia repair*).

Hernia repair

Surgical correction of a *hernia*. The procedure is performed to treat a hernia of the abdominal wall that is painful or cannot be pushed back. A strangulated hernia requires an emergency operation.

HOW IT IS DONE

Many hernias are repaired on an outpatient basis unless an underlying

MAIN TYPES OF ABDOMINAL HERNIA

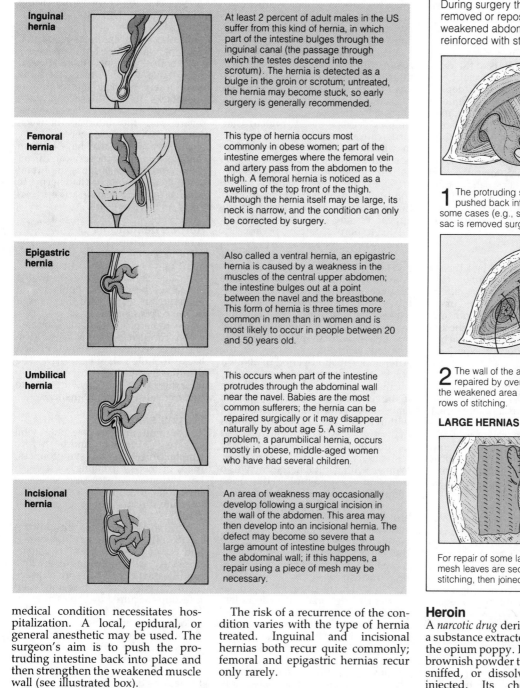

Inguinal hernia

At least 2 percent of adult males in the US suffer from this kind of hernia, in which part of the intestine bulges through the inguinal canal (the passage through which the testes descend into the scrotum). The hernia is detected as a bulge in the groin or scrotum; untreated, the hernia may become stuck, so early surgery is generally recommended.

Femoral hernia

This type of hernia occurs most commonly in obese women; part of the intestine emerges where the femoral vein and artery pass from the abdomen to the thigh. A femoral hernia is noticed as a swelling of the top front of the thigh. Although the hernia itself may be large, its neck is narrow, and the condition can only be corrected by surgery.

Epigastric hernia

Also called a ventral hernia, an epigastric hernia is caused by a weakness in the muscles of the central upper abdomen; the intestine bulges out at a point between the navel and the breastbone. This form of hernia is three times more common in men than in women and is most likely to occur in people between 20 and 50 years old.

Umbilical hernia

This occurs when part of the intestine protrudes through the abdominal wall near the navel. Babies are the most common sufferers; the hernia can be repaired surgically or it may disappear naturally by about age 5. A similar problem, a parumbilical hernia, occurs mostly in obese, middle-aged women who have had several children.

Incisional hernia

An area of weakness may occasionally develop following a surgical incision in the wall of the abdomen. This area may then develop into an incisional hernia. The defect may become so severe that a large amount of intestine bulges through the abdominal wall; if this happens, a repair using a piece of mesh may be necessary.

HERNIA REPAIR
During surgery the hernia is removed or repositioned and the weakened abdominal wall is reinforced with stitching or mesh.

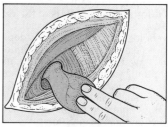

1 The protruding sac of intestine is pushed back into the abdomen or, in some cases (e.g., strangulation), the sac is removed surgically.

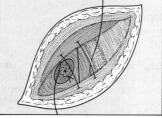

2 The wall of the abdomen may then be repaired by overlapping the edges of the weakened area and securing with rows of stitching.

LARGE HERNIAS

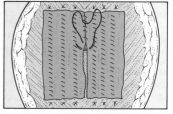

For repair of some large hernias, two mesh leaves are secured by rows of stitching, then joined at the center.

medical condition necessitates hospitalization. A local, epidural, or general anesthetic may be used. The surgeon's aim is to push the protruding intestine back into place and then strengthen the weakened muscle wall (see illustrated box).

RECOVERY AND OUTLOOK
The speed of recovery depends on the patient's underlying medical condition and on the type of hernia repaired. Lifting heavy objects should be avoided for three to six months.

The risk of a recurrence of the condition varies with the type of hernia treated. Inguinal and incisional hernias both recur quite commonly; femoral and epigastric hernias recur only rarely.

Herniated disk
See *Disk prolapse.*

Herniorrhaphy
Surgical correction of a hernia. (See *Hernia repair.*)

Heroin
A *narcotic drug* derived from *morphine,* a substance extracted from the pods of the opium poppy. Heroin is a white or brownish powder that can be smoked, sniffed, or dissolved in water and injected. Its chemical name is diacetylmorphine.

Heroin abuse is a major health problem in many countries. It has many adverse effects on the user and is a sociological and economic problem of immense proportions.

EFFECTS

In addition to having an analgesic (painkilling) effect, heroin produces sensations of warmth, calmness, drowsiness, and a loss of concern for outside events.

Long-term use causes *tolerance* (the need for greater amounts of the drug to have the same effects) and psychological and physical dependence (see *Drug dependence*). Sudden withdrawal of the drug produces symptoms such as shivering, abdominal cramps, diarrhea, vomiting, sleeplessness, and restlessness.

Other common problems of heroin addiction include injection scars, skin abscesses, weight loss, and impotence. Infections, such as *hepatitis B* and *AIDS*, are spread by sharing needles. Death commonly occurs from accidental overdose.

Herpangina

A throat infection caused by a type of virus called coxsackievirus. Herpangina most commonly affects young children, although it occurs in adults. The virus is usually transmitted via infected droplets coughed or sneezed into the air. Many people harbor the virus but do not experience any symptoms.

SYMPTOMS

After an incubation period of two to seven days, there is a sudden onset of fever, loss of appetite, and sore throat. There may also be headache, abdominal discomfort, and vague muscular aches and pains. The throat becomes red and a few small blisters appear, which enlarge and burst, forming shallow ulcers. The condition usually clears up within a week.

TREATMENT

Usually no treatment is required other than simple *analgesics* (painkillers). There is no specific antiviral therapy available. Antibiotics are generally of no therapeutic value unless a bacterial infection develops as a secondary complication. Recurrent attacks of herpangina may result from infection with different strains of the virus.

Herpes

Any of a variety of conditions characterized by an eruption of small, usually painful, blisters on the skin.

When a person is said to be suffering from herpes, it usually refers to an infection with the *herpes simplex* virus. Forms of the virus are responsible for *cold sores* (painful blisters around the lips) and for the sexually transmitted infection genital herpes, which is characterized by blisters on the sex organs (see *Herpes, genital*). The virus can also cause a number of other conditions affecting the skin, mouth, eyes, brain, or, in rare cases, the whole body.

A closely related virus, the varicella-zoster virus, is responsible for two more conditions in which skin blisters are a feature—*chickenpox* (also known as varicella) and *herpes zoster* (also known as shingles). Like the herpes simplex virus, the varicella-zoster virus can affect the eyes or, rarely, may infect the brain or cause an infection throughout the body.

Herpes gestationis and *dermatitis herpetiformis* are among various other conditions in which "herpetiform" (herpeslike) groups of blisters may appear on the skin, but neither is related to herpes simplex or varicella-zoster virus infections.

Herpes, genital

A sexually transmitted disease that produces a painful rash on the genitals. Caused by the *herpes simplex* virus (*HERPESVIRUS HOMINIS*, type 2), genital herpes is transmitted by sexual intercourse with an infected person.

SYMPTOMS AND SIGNS

After an incubation period of about a week, the virus produces itching, burning, soreness, and small blisters in the genital area. The blisters burst to leave small, painful ulcers, which heal within 10 to 21 days. The lymph nodes in the groin may become enlarged and painful, and the affected person may feel sick, with headache and fever. Women with genital herpes may find urination very painful if the urine comes into contact with the sores. Occasionally, there may be cold sores around the mouth.

TREATMENT

Genital herpes cannot be cured, but the earlier treatment is given, the more likely the treatment will prevent or reduce the severity of an attack. An antiviral medication (such as acyclovir) helps make the ulcers less painful and encourages them to heal more quickly. Additional soothing measures include taking analgesics (painkillers) and warm baths with a tablespoon of salt added.

Subsequent attacks tend to occur after sexual intercourse, after sunbathing, or when the affected person is run down; these recurrent attacks often clear up quickly with or without treatment. Sexual activity should be avoided until the symptoms have disappeared. If a pregnant woman has an attack of genital herpes when the baby is due, a cesarean section is performed to prevent the baby from being infected during delivery.

OUTLOOK

Once the virus enters the body, it stays there for the rest of the person's life. About 40 percent of those affected never have another attack after the first. Others, however, suffer four or five attacks annually for several years. Gradually, the attacks become less severe and the intervals between recurrences become longer.

The herpes virus may have a role in the development of cervical cancer (see *Cervix, cancer of*); it is important for any woman who has had herpes to have a *cervical smear test* (Pap test) every one to two years.

Herpes gestationis

A rare skin disorder, characterized by crops of blisters on the legs and abdomen, that occurs only in pregnancy. The cause is not known and, despite its name, herpes gestationis is not related to any of the disorders caused by the *herpes simplex* viruses.

Severe herpes gestationis is treated with *corticosteroid drugs* in tablet form and may require hospital admission because of the risk of *miscarriage*. The disorder usually clears up completely after the birth of the baby, but tends to recur in subsequent pregnancies.

Herpes simplex

A common and troublesome viral disease. Although most herpes simplex infections are symptomless, mild, or merely irritating, others can be extremely distressing (notably infections affecting the genitals) and even life-threatening.

TYPES

The virus exists in two forms, known as HSV1 (herpes simplex virus, type 1) and HSV2 (type 2). HSV1 is usually associated with infections of the lips, mouth, and face. HSV2 is often associated with infections of the genitals and infections acquired by babies at birth. However, there is a considerable amount of overlap. Some conditions usually caused by HSV1 are sometimes caused by HSV2 and vice versa. Both virus types are contagious. Infection is spread by direct contact with the lesions themselves or by the fluid contained therein.

TYPE 1 VIRUS Most people have been infected with HSV1 by the time they reach adulthood; most of the remainder are infected during adulthood. The initial infection may cause no symptoms or may cause a sometimes severe flulike illness with mouth ulcers. Thereafter, the virus remains in the nerve cells within the facial area. In many people, however, the virus is occasionally reactivated, causing recurrent *cold sores* that always erupt in the same site (usually around the lips), but are not serious. They often recur at times when there is an elevated temperature at the affected site (such as with fever or prolonged sun exposure).

Rarely, the virus may infect the fingers, causing an eruption of very painful blisters known as a herpetic *whitlow*. Sometimes it may cause an extensive rash of blisters (known as eczema herpeticum) in someone with a preexisting skin condition such as dermatitis.

If a person with an *immunodeficiency disorder* (such as *AIDS*) or someone who is taking *immunosuppressant drugs* is infected with the virus, it may cause a severe, generalized infection that is occasionally fatal.

If the virus gets into an eye, it may cause *conjunctivitis* (which usually lasts only a few days) or, more seriously, a *corneal ulcer*.

Very rarely, the type 1 virus may spread to the brain, leading to a serious *encephalitis*.

TYPE 2 VIRUS This form of the virus is the usual cause of sexually transmitted genital herpes, in which painful blisters erupt on the sex organs (see *Herpes, genital*). As with cold sores, the blisters recur in some people.

TREATMENT
Treatment of herpes simplex depends on its type, site, and severity. Antiviral drugs, such as acyclovir, are sometimes helpful. Lesions may also become infected with bacteria. If so, antibiotics (topical or oral) and tepid soaks may be helpful.

Herpes zoster
The medical term for shingles. Herpes zoster is an infection of the nerves that supply certain areas of the skin. It causes a painful rash of small, crusting blisters. After the rash heals, pain may persist for months or, rarely, years.

TYPES
Herpes zoster often affects a strip of skin over the ribs on one side or, less commonly, a strip on one side of the neck and arm or the lower part of the body. Sometimes it involves the upper half of the face on one side; in this case, the eye may also be affected. Shingles in this area is known as herpes zoster ophthalmicus.

CAUSES
Herpes zoster is caused by the varicella-zoster virus, which also causes *chickenpox*. During an attack of chickenpox, most of the viral organisms are destroyed, but some survive and lie dormant in certain sensory nerves, remaining there for many years. In some people, a decline in the efficiency of the *immune system* (the body's defenses against infection) allows the viruses to reemerge and cause shingles.

The competence of the immune system declines with age; this decline is probably accelerated by stress and by the use of *corticosteroid drugs*. Herpes zoster commonly follows a stressful episode.

INCIDENCE
Herpes zoster is a common disease. Every year in the US, a few hundred people per 100,000 suffer an attack. It mainly affects people over 50 and the incidence rises with age. Herpes zoster is very common in people whose immune systems have been weakened either by diseases such as *lymphoma* or *Hodgkin's disease*, or by treatment with *immunosuppressant* or *anticancer drugs*.

SYMPTOMS AND SIGNS
The first indication is excessive sensitivity in the area of skin to be affected; this is soon followed by pain, which is sometimes severe and which may, until the rash appears, be mistaken for pleurisy or appendicitis.

After about five days, the rash appears, starting as small, slightly raised, red spots that quickly turn to tense blisters, teeming with viruses. Within three days the blisters have turned yellowish and soon dry, flat-

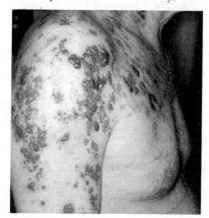

Example of herpes zoster
An extensive rash of crusting blisters over one side of the neck that spreads over the shoulder and onto the front of the chest.

ten, and crust over. During the next two weeks or so these crusts drop off, often leaving small pitted scars.

The most serious feature of herpes zoster is pain following the attack. The pain is a consequence of damage to the nerves, causing strong nerve impulses to be constantly produced and passed upward to the brain. The pain, which affects about one third of sufferers, may be severe and may last for months or years. The older the patient and the more pronounced the rash, the more likely the pain will be severe and persistent.

Ophthalmic herpes zoster may be confined to the skin of the lids and the forehead and need not affect the eye, but, if it does, it may cause a *corneal ulcer* or *uveitis*, both of which are potentially serious.

TREATMENT
Once the rash is fully established, little can be done to influence the course of the disease or the likelihood of postherpetic pain. Only palliative measures and *analgesics* (painkillers) are of value. It is, however, possible to reduce the severity of the active stage and to minimize nerve damage by the prompt use of *antiviral drugs* (such as acyclovir).

Many different measures have been advocated, in addition to analgesics, for the relief of postherpetic pain. They include skin stimulation by intermittent rubbing, the passage of alternating electric currents through the skin, local heat, cold spraying, injection of local anesthetics, and even surgical cutting of the nerves. None of these measures has been shown to be consistently effective.

Heterosexuality
Sexual attraction to members of the opposite sex. (See also *Bisexuality*; *Homosexuality, male*; *Lesbianism*.)

Heterozygote
A term used to describe a person whose cells contain two different *genes* controlling a specified inherited trait, in contrast to a *homozygote* who has identical genes controlling that trait. (See also *Inheritance*; *Genetic disorders*.)

Hiatal hernia
A condition in which part of the stomach protrudes upward into the chest through a hiatus (opening) in the diaphragm (the sheet of muscle involved in respiration that separates the chest from the abdomen).

H

CAUSES AND INCIDENCE

The underlying cause of this common condition is unknown, but it tends to occur more frequently in obese people (and especially in upper middle-aged women) and in those who smoke. In some cases it is present at birth.

SYMPTOMS

Many people have no symptoms, but in some people hiatal hernia affects the efficiency of the muscle at the end of the esophagus (esophagogastric junction), permitting *acid reflux* (regurgitation of acidic juices from the stomach into the esophagus). This reflux may in turn cause *heartburn*, which is often made worse by bending over or lying down, and peptic *esophagitis* (inflammation of the esophagus). The pain of esophagitis or esophagospasm may mimic the pain of *coronary heart disease*.

DIAGNOSIS

Esophagoscopy (passage of a viewing tube down the throat into the esophagus) may be performed to determine the severity of esophagitis and to check for stricture (narrowing) of the esophagus (see *Esophageal stricture*). If there is any suspicion of esophageal cancer, a *biopsy* (removal of a small sample of tissue for examination) is carried out. Manometric studies (pressure measurements, see *Manometry*) can confirm the reduced pressure at the esophagogastric junction. A barium swallow (see *Barium X-ray examinations*) is performed with the patient tilted headdown. If the barium is seen on X ray to cause reflux into the esophagus, it indicates incompetence at the esophagogastric junction.

TREATMENT

To alleviate symptoms, the patient should avoid eating large, heavy meals and should never lie down or bend over immediately after a meal. The head of the bed should be raised to prevent reflux during the night. People who are obese need to lose weight and smokers should stop smoking. *Antacids* may be given to reduce stomach acidity and to protect the esophagus against acid juices.

In severe cases, an operation may be required to return the protruding part of the stomach to the abdomen and to prevent further reflux of acid gastric contents into the esophagus.

Hiccup

A sudden, involuntary contraction of the diaphragm followed by rapid closure of the vocal cords (which causes the characteristic sound); also called hiccough. Hiccups usually occur at brief intervals and attacks last for only a few minutes.

CAUSES AND TREATMENT

Attacks of hiccups are extremely common; in almost all cases, they occur without obvious cause and are not medically significant. Such minor attacks often stop of their own accord. There are also numerous popular remedies, the effectiveness of which varies from one person to another.

Rarely, hiccups may be due to a condition that causes irritation of the diaphragm or of the phrenic nerves that supply it. Known causes include pleurisy, pneumonia, certain disorders of the stomach or esophagus, pancreatitis, alcoholism, and hepatitis. Most bouts are of unknown cause.

Frequent, prolonged attacks of hiccups, which are extremely rare, may lead to severe exhaustion. In such cases, when medication has failed, surgery may be recommended. It may involve either crushing or injecting a drug around one of the phrenic nerves to paralyze half the diaphragm; this measure is sometimes unsuccessful.

Hip

The joint between the pelvis and the upper end of the femur (thigh bone). The hip is an extremely stable ball-and-socket joint; the smooth, rounded head of the femur fits securely into the acetabulum, a deep, cuplike cavity in the pelvis. Tough ligaments attach the femur to the pelvis, further stabilizing the joint and providing it with the necessary strength to support the weight of the upper body and to take the strain of running, jumping, and other vigorous leg movements. In addition, the ball-and-socket structure of the joint allows the leg a considerable range of movement that is available only because of the unique design of this joint.

DISORDERS

ARTHRITIS *Osteoarthritis* of the hip, one of the most common of all disorders, causes stiffness and pain in the joint, particularly during movement. Occasionally, *ankylosing spondylitis* and *rheumatoid arthritis* of the hip cause similar problems.

FRACTURE What is commonly called fracture of the hip (most common in elderly people as the result of a fall) is in fact fracture of the head or neck of the femur (see *Femur, fracture of*).

DISLOCATION Congenital dislocation of the hip usually clears up of its own accord or is remediable (see *Hip, congenital dislocation of*). Dislocation of the hip by injury is rare and usually results only from extreme force, such as that from an automobile accident. Such dislocation may cut off the blood supply to the head of the femur, causing the bone to die (aseptic necrosis), or may injure the sciatic nerve, leading to weakness in the leg.

Hip, congenital dislocation of

A disorder present at birth in which the ball-like head of the femur (thigh bone) fails to fit into the cuplike socket in the pelvis to form a joint but instead lies outside. One or both of the hips may be affected.

CAUSES AND INCIDENCE

The cause of congenital dislocation of the hip is not known, but it is more common in babies born by *breech delivery* and following pregnancies in which there was *oligohydramnios* (an abnormally small amount of amniotic fluid in the uterus).

About 400 in every 100,000 babies born are affected; in most cases the condition soon corrects itself. Only about 125 in 100,000 suffer from persistent dislocation. The disorder runs in families and affects many more girls than boys.

DIAGNOSIS

Shortly after birth and at intervals until walking starts, all babies are given a routine physical examination of the hip to check its stability and range of motion. If the condition is not

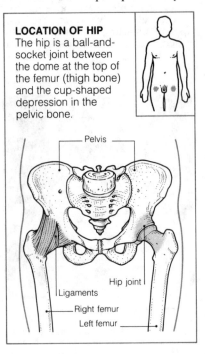

LOCATION OF HIP
The hip is a ball-and-socket joint between the dome at the top of the femur (thigh bone) and the cup-shaped depression in the pelvic bone.

Pelvis

Hip joint

Ligaments

Right femur

Left femur

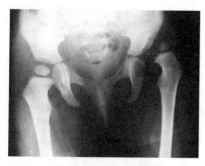

X ray showing congenital dislocation
The left femur (thigh bone) is displaced
upward and backward from its socket.

detected in infancy it may be diagnosed when a limp develops when the
child is learning to walk.

TREATMENT
If the condition is found in early
infancy, light splints are applied to the
thigh to maneuver the ball of the joint
into the socket and keep it in position.
The splints are worn for two to four
months and usually aid in correcting
the problem.

If the condition is not discovered
until later in infancy, traction is used.
The head of the femur is moved into
the correct position and kept there by
a system of weights and pulleys
attached to the leg.

If the dislocation is not detected
until childhood, surgery using a
general anesthetic may be required to
correct it. The child usually must stay
in the hospital for several weeks and
wear a plaster cast for a few months.

OUTLOOK
Provided the disorder is treated in
infancy, the child usually walks normally and there are no aftereffects.
When treatment is delayed until childhood, there may be lifelong problems
with walking. If the condition remains
untreated, the dislocation often leads
to shortening of the leg, limping, and
early *osteoarthritis* in the joint.

Hippocratic oath
A part of the writings attributed to
Hippocrates, a fifth century BC Greek
physician. The oath has served as a
widely used ethical guide for the
medical profession ever since. It
pledges the physician to work for the
good of the patient, to do him or her
no harm, to prescribe no deadly
drugs, to give no advice that could
cause death, and to keep confidential
medical information regarding the
patient. The oath is often administered as a part of the graduation
ceremonies at medical schools.

Hip replacement
A surgical procedure to replace all or
part of a diseased hip joint with an
artificial substitute.

WHY IT IS DONE
Hip replacement is most often carried
out in older people whose joints are
stiff and painful as a result of
osteoarthritis. It may also be needed if
rheumatoid arthritis has spread to the
hip joint, making walking difficult, or
if the top end of the femur is badly
fractured (see *Femur, fracture of*).

The operation is not usually advised
for young patients, since their greater
activity puts more strain on the joints
and it is unknown how long any artificial replacement is likely to last.

PERFORMING A HIP REPLACEMENT
In this operation, the surgeon
pushes aside or cuts through the
surrounding muscles to expose the
hip joint. The femur (thigh bone) is
cut and the pelvis is drilled to make
room for the two components of the
artificial joint. These parts are
secured in place, the femur is
repaired, and the muscles and
tendons are replaced and repaired.

Sites of incision
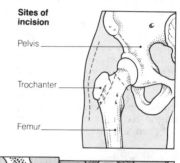
Pelvis
Trochanter
Femur

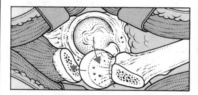
1 The trochanter at the top of the femur is detached, and the hip joint is dislocated to separate the femur and the pelvis. The ball at the top of the femur is then cut away.

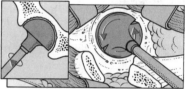
2 An instrument known as a reamer is used to make the hollow in the pelvis large enough to make room for the cup-shaped socket (one of the two components of the artificial hip joint).

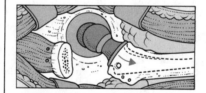
3 A coarse file is used to cut a shaft in the femur, and the ball part of the artificial joint is inserted. The components are fixed in place with a special cement, which binds them to the bone.

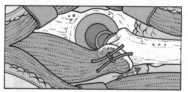
4 The ball is placed in the socket and the trochanter is reattached to the femur with wires. The muscles and tendons are replaced and repaired, and the incision is then closed.

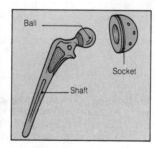
Before
This X ray shows a hip joint that has been badly damaged by arthritis.

Components
The ball and shaft are made of metal; the socket may be metal or plastic.
Ball
Socket
Shaft

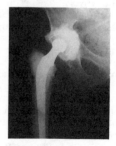
After
This X ray shows the artificial hip joint in position after surgery.

H

RECOVERY PERIOD

The joint remains unstable for a week or two after the operation, and patients must take care not to dislocate the new joint during this time. Patients are advised to sleep on their backs and not to cross their legs, and are taught how to get in and out of a bathtub without disturbing the joint.

OUTLOOK

Hip joint replacement is a remarkably successful operation that has transformed the lives of many people who suffered from severe pain and stiffness. However, with time, a substantial proportion of artificial joints show signs on X ray of loosening at the cemented union between bone and metal. Surgeons and engineers are continuing to develop newer joint designs that do not rely on cement to hold them in place.

Hip, snapping

A fairly common condition in adults in which a characteristic clicking is heard and felt during certain movements of the joint. Snapping hip is generally harmless and does not indicate disease of the hip joint.

The noise and sensation are caused by a tendon slipping over the bony prominence on the outside of the femur when the hip is bent upward.

Snapping hip should not be confused with a hip that clicks when a newborn baby is being examined, which is a sign that there may be congenital dislocation of the hip (see *Hip, congenital dislocation of*).

Hirschsprung's disease

Also known as congenital megacolon, a congenital disorder in which a segment of intestine (sometimes near the anus) lacks the ganglion cells that control the rhythmic motion of the bowel. This segment becomes narrowed and blocks the movement of fecal material. The bowel above becomes dilated and tortuous (twisted). Hirschsprung's disease is uncommon and tends to run in families. It occurs about four times more often in boys than girls.

SYMPTOMS

Symptoms usually appear in infancy or early childhood; they include marked constipation and bloating. The child usually has a poor appetite and may fail to grow properly.

DIAGNOSIS

A barium enema (see *Barium X-ray examinations*) can show the narrowed rectal segment of the intestine. A *biopsy* sample taken from the involved area during *proctoscopy* or surgical biopsy confirms the lack of ganglion cells and establishes the diagnosis.

TREATMENT

Treatment involves removing the narrowed intestinal segment and rejoining the normal colon to the normal colonic or rectal segments. Before surgery, a temporary *colostomy* (making an artificial outlet for the colon on the abdominal wall) may be necessary if the child is considerably underweight or to facilitate treatment for severe anemia.

Hirsutism

Excessive hairiness, particularly in women. The additional hair is coarse, like a man's, and grows in a male pattern on the face, trunk, and limbs.

CAUSES AND INCIDENCE

Hirsutism occurs in some conditions in which the level of male hormones in the blood is abnormally high (e.g., in *polycystic ovary* syndrome and congenital *adrenal hyperplasia*).

Much more commonly, hirsutism is not a sign of any underlying disorder; it occurs in many normal women, especially after the menopause. The condition tends to run in families. Dark-haired women, particularly those of Hispanic or Indian extraction, are particularly likely to be hirsute.

TREATMENT

Hair can be bleached or removed in various ways (see *Hair removal*); the only method of permanent removal is by *electrolysis* (destruction of hair roots by an electric current). See also *Hypertrichosis*.

Histamine

A chemical present in cells (mainly *mast cells*) throughout the body that is released during an allergic reaction (see *Allergy*); histamine is one of the substances responsible for the symptoms of *inflammation*. It also stimulates production of acid by the stomach and narrows the bronchi (airways) in the lungs.

The effects of histamine can be counteracted by *antihistamine drugs*; its action on the gastric acid-forming glands is blocked by *histamine-2 receptor antagonists*.

Histamine-2 receptor antagonists

A group of *ulcer-healing drugs* related to the *antihistamine drug* group. Histamine-2 (or H-2) receptor antagonists work by blocking the action of the chemical histamine at specific *receptors* (sites on a cell's surface), preventing release of acid in the stomach. Acid reduction promotes the healing of *peptic ulcers* and relieves symptoms of *esophagitis*. (See also *Cimetidine; Ranitidine; Famotidine*.)

Histiocytosis X

A rare childhood disease in which there is an overgrowth of a type of tissue cell called a histiocyte. The cause is unknown, but it probably results from a disturbance of the *immune system*.

In the mildest form of the disease, rapid cell growth occurs in one bone only, usually affecting the skull, clavicle, or a rib or vertebra, causing swelling and pain. The chances of recovery are good in these cases.

The most severe, and least common, form of the disease affects infants. This form of the disease behaves like advanced *leukemia*, leading rapidly to death.

Histocompatibility antigens

A group of proteins that is naturally present within tissues and has a role in the *immune system* (body's defenses against infection). The main group of histocompatibility antigens is known as the HLA (human leukocyte antigen) system. The particular set or types of HLAs in a person's tissues (called his or her tissue type) is inherited. These antigens have an influence on the outcome of organ transplantation (see *Transplant surgery*) and also seem to affect susceptibility to certain diseases. However, these are probably just side effects of the primary immunologic (defense) function of the antigens.

TYPES AND STRUCTURE

Like all proteins, histocompatibility antigens are synthesized in cells under the control of genes. The genes controlling their production are called the major histocompatibility complex; they give rise to several series of antigens called HLA-A, HLA-B, HLA-C, HLA-D, and HLA-DR.

Each histocompatibility antigen is composed of two parts, a constant region (which is the same for all people) and a variable region (which differs among people). The structure of this region is genetically determined (inherited from one of the parents) and can take any of several forms, which have been given numbers. Thus, a particular antigen has a letter (the series it belongs to) and a number corresponding to the form within the series—for example, HLA-A3, HLA-B13, or HLA-C5 types. The number of possible combinations of antigens from the different series is vast, and, apart from identical twins, each person has a unique combination. By a technique called *tissue-typing*, every person can be immunologically "fingerprinted."

IMMUNOLOGICAL FUNCTION
Histocompatibility antigens within the series HLA-A, B, and C are present on virtually all living cells in the body. They are essential for the function of certain *lymphocytes* (white blood cells with an immunological function) called killer T cells. The antigens act as a guide for killer T cells to recognize and kill abnormal cells (i.e., virus-infected and tumor cells).

Histocompatibility antigens within the HLA-D series are present on the surfaces of various other cells with a defense role; they influence the interactions of these cells in fighting infection and tumors.

EFFECT IN TRANSPLANTATION
When an organ is transplanted from one person to another, the histocompatibility antigens in the donor organ are generally recognized as foreign and are attacked by the recipient's immune system, leading to rejection. However, if a donor can be found whose HLA types are very similar to those of the recipient (often a blood relative and ideally an identical twin), the chances of rejection occurring are minimized.

DISEASE ASSOCIATION
Certain HLA types occur more frequently in patients with particular diseases than in the rest of the population. For example, *multiple sclerosis* is associated with HLA-A3, *celiac sprue* with HLA-B8, and *ankylosing spondylitis* with HLA-B27.

It is suspected that susceptibility to these diseases is influenced by the HLA types, presumably as a result of their immunologic actions. The associations are of interest because they allow identification of individuals at risk and can help in the confirmation of disease.

LEGAL USES
An individual's HLA types are inherited (half from the father and half from the mother); blood relatives in general have similar types. Study of HLA types is thus sometimes of use in *paternity testing* and other situations in which there is a dispute as to whether two people are related. For example, if two people both have a highly unusual combination of HLA types, it may provide very strong evidence (although it can never be proven absolutely) that they are related.

Histologist
A specialist in *histology*, the study of the microscopic appearance of tissues.

Histology
The study of tissues, including their cellular structure and function. Its main practical use in medicine is in the diagnosis of disease. This often involves obtaining a tissue sample by *biopsy* and examining it for abnormalities. The histologist's skill lies in his or her familiarity with the range of normal appearances of tissues and the recognition of the abnormal appearances in different diseases.

Histopathology
The branch of *histology* (the study of tissues) concerned with the effects of disease on the microscopic structure of tissues.

Histoplasmosis
An infection caused by inhaling the spores of HISTOPLASMA CAPSULATUM, a fungus found in soil, particularly areas contaminated with droppings from birds or bats. Histoplasmosis occurs in the central and southern US and in parts of South America, the Far East, and Africa.

Most people who inhale the spores are not affected by them. The rare cases of infection occur either in people who are exposed to large quantities of the spores (such as pigeon handlers) or in people whose resistance to infection has been lowered—for example, by an *immunodeficiency disorder*, such as *AIDS*.

SYMPTOMS AND TREATMENT
The most common form of histoplasmosis is an acute illness (marked by breathlessness, cough, and joint pains) that usually clears up on its own. However, in some people (mainly in those with a low resistance to infection) the disease takes a chronic form and spreads throughout the body, resulting in fever, loss of weight, mouth ulcers, enlargement of the spleen, liver, and lymph nodes, failure of the adrenal glands, and anemia. Treatment with the antifungal drugs amphotericin B or ketoconazole is usually effective. In severe, untreated cases, the disease may be fatal (it causes about 50 to 100 deaths in the US each year).

History-taking
The process by which a physician learns from patients the symptoms of their illnesses and any previous disorders. (See *Diagnosis*.)

HIV
Human immunodeficiency virus. HIV belongs to the class of retroviruses (see *Virus*) and is the cause of *AIDS* and *AIDS-related complex*.

HIV gains access to the body by entering the bloodstream via blood transfusions, nonsterile needles, or sexual intercourse. A fetus can be infected by its mother. HIV has an affinity for the T-*lymphocytes* (part of the *immune system*), in which the virus multiplies and, in some cases, destroys function. HIV also attacks the brain and may cause severe damage with *dementia*; most infected people are likely to succumb to AIDS before this happens.

HIV is an organism of low infectivity; infected people present no threat to the health of their contacts at work or home, except for sexual partners and needle sharers.

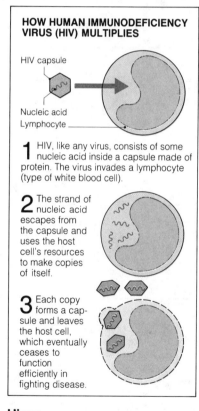

HOW HUMAN IMMUNODEFICIENCY VIRUS (HIV) MULTIPLIES

HIV capsule

Nucleic acid
Lymphocyte

1 HIV, like any virus, consists of some nucleic acid inside a capsule made of protein. The virus invades a lymphocyte (type of white blood cell).

2 The strand of nucleic acid escapes from the capsule and uses the host cell's resources to make copies of itself.

3 Each copy forms a capsule and leaves the host cell, which eventually ceases to function efficiently in fighting disease.

Hives
The popular name for *urticaria*.

HLA types
See *Histocompatibility antigens*.

HMO
See *Health Maintenance Organization*.

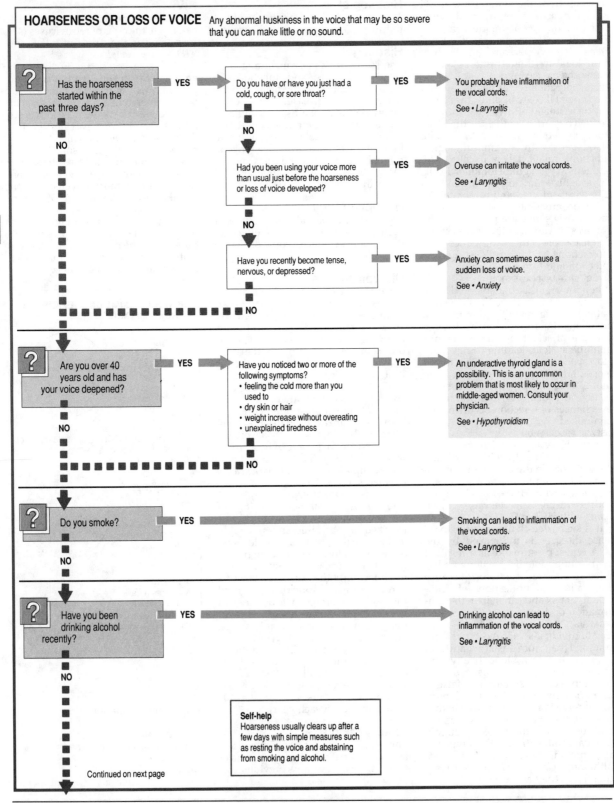

HOARSENESS OR LOSS OF VOICE
Any abnormal huskiness in the voice that may be so severe that you can make little or no sound.

Has the hoarseness started within the past three days?

YES → Do you have or have you just had a cold, cough, or sore throat?
- YES → You probably have inflammation of the vocal cords. See • *Laryngitis*
- NO ↓

Had you been using your voice more than usual just before the hoarseness or loss of voice developed?
- YES → Overuse can irritate the vocal cords. See • *Laryngitis*
- NO ↓

Have you recently become tense, nervous, or depressed?
- YES → Anxiety can sometimes cause a sudden loss of voice. See • *Anxiety*
- NO →

NO ↓

Are you over 40 years old and has your voice deepened?

YES → Have you noticed two or more of the following symptoms?
- feeling the cold more than you used to
- dry skin or hair
- weight increase without overeating
- unexplained tiredness

- YES → An underactive thyroid gland is a possibility. This is an uncommon problem that is most likely to occur in middle-aged women. Consult your physician. See • *Hypothyroidism*
- NO →

NO ↓

Do you smoke?

YES → Smoking can lead to inflammation of the vocal cords. See • *Laryngitis*

NO ↓

Have you been drinking alcohol recently?

YES → Drinking alcohol can lead to inflammation of the vocal cords. See • *Laryngitis*

NO ↓

Self-help
Hoarseness usually clears up after a few days with simple measures such as resting the voice and abstaining from smoking and alcohol.

Continued on next page

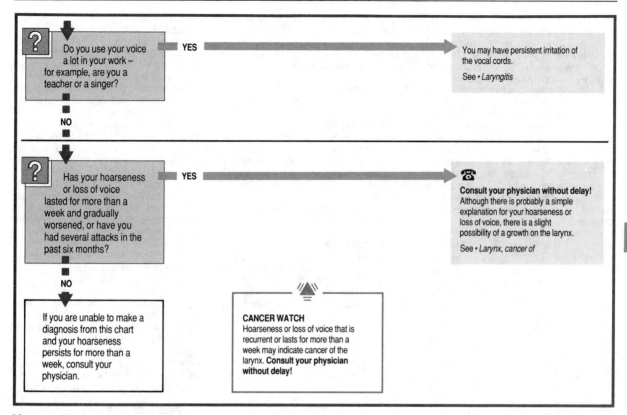

Do you use your voice a lot in your work – for example, are you a teacher or a singer?

YES → You may have persistent irritation of the vocal cords.

See • *Laryngitis*

NO ↓

Has your hoarseness or loss of voice lasted for more than a week and gradually worsened, or have you had several attacks in the past six months?

YES → ☎ Consult your physician without delay! Although there is probably a simple explanation for your hoarseness or loss of voice, there is a slight possibility of a growth on the larynx.

See • *Larynx, cancer of*

NO ↓

If you are unable to make a diagnosis from this chart and your hoarseness persists for more than a week, consult your physician.

CANCER WATCH
Hoarseness or loss of voice that is recurrent or lasts for more than a week may indicate cancer of the larynx. **Consult your physician without delay!**

H

Hoarseness

A rough, husky, or croaking voice, usually caused by interference with the normal working of the vocal cords in the *larynx* (voice box). Most attacks do not last long and clear up of their own accord, but persistent hoarseness needs investigation to exclude the possibility of serious disease.

CAUSES

Hoarseness of limited duration is often due to overuse of the voice (for example, in teachers or singers), which strains small muscles in the larynx. It is also commonly caused by inflammation of the vocal cords as part of acute *laryngitis*, which is usually due to an upper respiratory tract infection such as a cold or sore throat.

Persistent hoarseness has many possible causes. It may be due to chronic irritation of the larynx (which can be caused by smoking or excessive consumption of alcohol) or chronic *bronchitis*. Irritation can also be caused by mucus constantly dripping on the larynx, as may occur in nasal *polyps* (harmless growths in the nose), allergic *rhinitis* (hay fever), *sinusitis*, or a deviated *nasal septum* (crookedness of the cartilage wall that separates the two nostrils).

Polyps on the vocal cords may also cause hoarseness, as may any accidental damage to them as the result of thyroid gland surgery. In *hypothyroidism* (underactivity of the thyroid gland), hoarseness can result from tissue forming on the vocal cords.

In young children, hoarseness is one of the symptoms of *croup* (inflammation and narrowing of the airways).

Occasionally, persistent hoarseness in adults has a more serious cause—including cancer of the larynx (see *Larynx, cancer of*). Less commonly, persistent hoarseness is caused by *thyroid cancer*.

SELF-HELP

Anyone suffering from hoarseness believed to be brought on by straining the voice should rest his or her voice until it has returned to normal; otherwise, permanent damage may eventually occur in the vocal cords. Voice training may reduce the chance of recurrence. Resting the voice, along with not smoking or drinking alcohol, also helps clear up laryngitis.

INVESTIGATION

If hoarseness persists for more than two weeks in anyone over the age of 40, it is essential to consult a physician. The physician will perform a *laryngoscopy* (examination of the larynx with a viewing tube) to exclude the possibility of cancer, which can be completely cured if diagnosed early.

Hodgkin's disease

Also known as Hodgkin's lymphoma, a malignant disorder of lymphoid tissue (found mainly in the *lymph nodes* and *spleen*) in which there is proliferation of its constituent cells and a resultant enlargement of the lymph nodes. The lymphoid tissues constitute an important part of the immune system and frequently do not function normally. The cause of Hodgkin's disease is unknown.

INCIDENCE

Hodgkin's disease is rare; about three new cases per 100,000 are diagnosed annually in the US. It is more common in men than women, and occurs with a peak incidence in people in their 20s and in people between 55 and 70 years of age.

SYMPTOMS AND SIGNS

The most common symptom is painless enlargement of a group of lymph nodes, typically those in the neck or armpits. Most other symptoms are caused by the presence of the enlarged nodes, invasion of other organs by proliferating lymphoid tissue, or impairment of the body's immune system. Thus, there may be a general feeling of illness, with fever, loss of appetite, weight loss, and night sweats. There may also be generalized itching and, rarely, pain after drinking alcohol. Involvement of other organs may cause a diverse range of symptoms (such as breathlessness if the lungs are involved or paralysis if the spine is affected). As the disease progresses, the immune system becomes increasingly impaired and the patient may suffer life-threatening complications from an infection that would be trivial in a healthy person.

DIAGNOSIS

For a positive diagnosis of Hodgkin's disease, it is necessary to identify cells (called Reed-Sternberg cells) having a characteristic appearance in a sample of tissue (obtained by *biopsy*) from an enlarged lymph node or from another organ affected by the Hodgkin's disease. In addition, the relative proportions of other surrounding cells—including plasma cells, eosinophils, lymphocytes, and granulocytes (all types of white blood cell)—are usually determined. This enables the disease to be classified according to its histological type, which is one factor that affects the chances of a cure.

The extent of the disease (known as its *stage*) is also assessed in terms of the number of groups of lymph nodes affected and in terms of any other organs that are involved. This process, called staging, is important for the planning of treatment. Typically, this assessment includes a *chest X ray*, *CT scanning* of the abdomen, and a *bone marrow biopsy*. Other tests may include *laparotomy* (surgical exploration of the abdomen) sometimes with node biopsies, liver biopsy, *splenectomy*, or *lymphangiography* (X-ray imaging of the lymphatic system) of the abdomen.

TREATMENT AND OUTLOOK

Treatment varies according to the stage of the disease. In an early stage, *radiation therapy* is usually curative. If the disease has progressed to involve many organs, however, *chemotherapy* with *anticancer drugs* is usually recommended; this treatment may need to be continued for several months. In some cases, both radiation therapy and chemotherapy are used to increase the chances of a cure.

The outlook depends on the stage to which the disease has progressed and on the histological type. However, after treatment, some 70 to 80 percent

of patients survive for at least five years. The condition is apparently cured in most people who receive treatment at an early stage. (See also *Lymphoma, non-Hodgkin's*.)

Hole in the heart

The common name for a *septal defect*.

Holistic medicine

A form of therapy aimed at treating the whole person—body and mind—not just the part or parts in which symptoms occur. A holistic approach is claimed to be emphasized by practitioners of *alternative medicine*, such as homeopathists, acupuncturists, and herbalists.

Holter monitor

A portable (worn by the patient), 24-hour electrocardiographic (see *ECG*) monitoring device used to detect paroxysmal *arrhythmias* (intermittent, irregular heart beats or palpitations). See also *Monitor*.

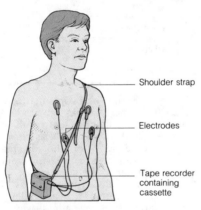

Shoulder strap

Electrodes

Tape recorder containing cassette

The Holter monitor
The patient wears the Holter monitor over one shoulder; electrodes attached to the chest transmit the heart rhythms to a slow-running cassette tape in the monitor.

Homatropine

An *anticholinergic drug* that is similar to, but less powerful than, *atropine*.

Homeopathy

A system of *alternative medicine* that seeks to treat patients by administering small doses of medicines that would bring on symptoms similar to those of the patient in a healthy person. For example, the homeopathic treatment for diarrhea would be a miniscule amount of a laxative.

Homeostasis

The dynamic processes by which an organism maintains a constant inter-

nal environment despite external changes. It is a major function of most organs. Examples of homeostatic mechanisms include the regulation of blood pressure, body temperature, and blood sugar levels.

Homeostasis plays a vital role in the body because tissues and organs can function efficiently only within a narrow range of conditions such as temperature and acidity. The homeostatic mechanisms regulate such conditions by negative feedback. When a certain factor varies from its optimum set point, automatic regulatory mechanisms act to counterbalance the disturbance and reestablish the internal equilibrium. For example, when the body overheats, sweating is stimulated until the temperature returns to normal. Similarly, when the level of oxygen in the blood is low, breathing is stimulated; when blood pressure falls, the heart rate increases.

Homeostatic mechanisms sometimes malfunction. For example, in malignant *hyperthermia*, the body's thermostat is somehow reset to a higher temperature than normal. In *diabetes mellitus*, blood sugar levels can no longer be regulated because of a malfunction of insulin production.

Homocystinuria

A rare, inherited condition caused by an *enzyme* deficiency. Homocystinuria is a type of inborn error of *metabolism* in which there is an abnormal presence of a particular *amino acid* (homocystine) in the blood and urine. Affected people resemble those with *Marfan's syndrome*—very tall and long-limbed with long, spindly fingers, and sometimes skeletal deformities (such as curvature of the spine).

The disease cannot be cured, but can be improved by vitamin B_6 and a special diet.

Homosexuality, female

See *Lesbianism*.

Homosexuality, male

Sexual attraction to other men. According to Alfred Kinsey's studies of sexuality carried out in the 1940s, about 5 to 10 percent of men are completely homosexual; up to one third of men have had sexual contact with another man at some time.

CHARACTERISTICS

Homosexuals are no more effeminate than heterosexuals, despite the popular stereotype. Each partner may adopt a particular role in the relationship (either active or passive) that may be reflected in styles of dress and behavior; more often, however, roles are interchangeable. Homosexuals achieve orgasm in various ways, including oral sex, mutual masturbation, and anal penetration.

Some male homosexuals have monogamous relationships. Others have multiple partners, high rates of sexual activity, and are consequently at high risk of venereal disease. It was in male homosexuals that the *AIDS* virus was first identified.

Homosexuality is more openly considered than it once was, but some homosexuals feel guilty about their sexual orientation. This may cause them to mask their feelings behind a cloak of apparent heterosexuality or to seek a medical cure.

CAUSES

Various theories have been put forward to explain homosexuality. Some studies have shown an increased incidence of homosexuality among men who had absent or weak fathers and who formed close emotional relationships with their mothers. Evidence for either a genetic tendency or a hormone imbalance is lacking.

The prevalence of homosexuality appears to be much the same in all cultures, with no change over thousands of years—suggesting that homosexuality is a consistent variation in behavior. (See also *Bisexuality*.)

Homozygote

A term used to describe a person whose cells contain two identical *genes* controlling a specified inherited trait, in contrast to a *heterozygote*, whose cells contain two different genes controlling that trait. (See also *Inheritance; Genetic disorders*.)

Homunculus

From the Latin for "a little man." It may refer to a perfectly proportioned person of *short stature*; a fetus, by extension of the archaic theory that human germ cells contained minute human beings; a small model of a person, particularly one created by magic or alchemy; and, in psychiatry, a little man created by the imagination.

Hookworm infestation

An infestation of the small intestine by small, round, blood-sucking worms of the species NECATOR AMERICANUS or ANCYLOSTOMA DUODENALE. The worms are about half an inch long and have hooklike teeth.

HOOKWORM LIFE CYCLE

Infestation begins with larvae that penetrate the skin or are ingested and enter the bloodstream. They migrate throughout the body, particularly to the small intestine. Adult worms develop and lay eggs, which leave the body in feces and eventually hatch into larvae.

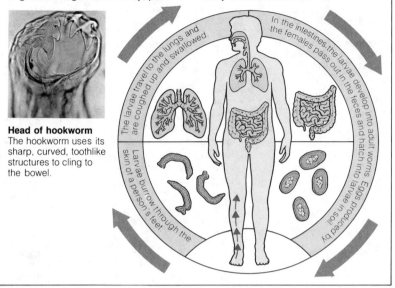

Head of hookworm
The hookworm uses its sharp, curved, toothlike structures to cling to the bowel.

INCIDENCE AND CAUSES

Hookworms infest about 700 million people worldwide, mainly those living in poor countries in the tropics. There is very little risk of contracting a hookworm infestation in the US.

The illustration above shows how hookworms can enter and multiply in the body. In a heavy infestation, there may be several hundred worms in the intestine, consuming up to one tenth of a pint of blood every day.

SYMPTOMS AND COMPLICATIONS

When the larvae penetrate the skin, a red and intensely itchy rash may develop on the feet. This is called ground itch and may last for several days. In light infestations, no symptoms may be felt. In heavier infestations, migration of the larvae through the lungs may produce cough and pneumonia; the presence of adult worms in the intestines may cause vague abdominal discomfort.

By far the most important problem caused by a heavy infestation is iron-deficiency *anemia* due to loss of blood.

DIAGNOSIS AND TREATMENT

Diagnosis is made by microscopic examination of feces, which can reveal hookworm eggs. *Antihelmintic drugs*, such as mebendazole, kill the worms. Treatment also involves improving nutrition with a high-protein diet and correcting anemia with iron tablets or

blood transfusion, if necessary. Elimination of the disease from a community depends on efficient sanitation. (See also *Larva migrans*.)

Hormonal disorders

See *Endocrine system*.

Hormonal methods of contraception

See *Contraception, hormonal methods*.

Hormone antagonist

A drug that blocks the action of a hormone. *Tamoxifen*, for example, blocks the effects of *estrogen hormones* and is used in the treatment of some types of breast cancer.

Hormone replacement therapy

The use of a synthetic or natural hormone to treat a hormone deficiency. In its broadest sense, the term describes the replacement of any deficient hormone, such as giving thyroxine to treat *hypothyroidism* or *insulin* to treat *diabetes mellitus*. More commonly, however, the term hormone replacement therapy refers to the use of *estrogen hormones* to treat symptoms accompanying the *menopause*.

WHY IT IS DONE

Estrogen replacement therapy is given to relieve menopausal symptoms such as hot flashes and excessive sweating at night. Estrogen hormones help prevent atrophic *vaginitis* (dryness of the vagina) and shrinkage of the genitals, which may make sexual intercourse painful and difficult. Estrogen hormones also help prevent the development of *osteoporosis* (a bone disorder) and *atherosclerosis* (narrowing of the arteries causing impaired blood flow).

HOW IT IS DONE

In hormone replacement therapy, estrogen drugs are usually prescribed in combination with a *progesterone drug* (which can result in monthly spotting in place of menstruation) because estrogen drugs given alone may increase a woman's susceptibility to cancer of the uterus.

THE SOURCES AND MAIN EFFECTS OF SELECTED HORMONES

Section of body	Hormone secreted	Effects
Hypothalamus	Releasing hormones	Stimulate hormone secretion by pituitary gland
Pituitary gland	Growth hormone	Stimulates growth and metabolism
	Prolactin	Stimulates milk production after childbirth
	ACTH (adrenocorticotropic hormone)	Stimulates hormone production by adrenal glands.
	TSH (thyroid-stimulating hormone)	Stimulates hormone production by thyroid gland
	FSH (follicle-stimulating hormone); LH (luteinizing hormone)	Stimulate gonads (ovaries or testes)
	ADH (antidiuretic hormone)	Acts on kidneys to reduce urine production.
	Oxytocin	Stimulates contractions of uterus during labor and ejection of milk during breast-feeding
	MSH (melanocyte-stimulating hormone)	Acts on the skin to promote production of skin pigment (melanin)
Brain	Endorphins; enkephalins	Alleviate pain
Thyroid gland	Thyroid hormone	Increases metabolic rate; affects growth
	Calcitonin	Controls level of calcium in blood
Parathyroid glands	Parathyroid hormone	Controls level of calcium in blood
Thymus	Thymic hormone	Stimulates lymphocyte development
Adrenal glands	Epinephrine; norepinephrine	Prepare body for stress
	Hydrocortisone	Affects metabolism
	Aldosterone	Regulates sodium and potassium excretion by kidneys
	Androgens	Affect growth and, in women, sex drive
Kidneys	Renin	Regulates blood pressure
	Erythropoietin	Stimulates erythrocyte production
	Vitamin D	Controls calcium and phosphorus metabolism
Pancreas	Insulin; glucagon	Regulate blood sugar level
Placenta	Chorionic gonadotropin; estrogens; progesterone	Maintain pregnancy
Gastrointestinal tract	Gastrin; secretin; cholecystokinin	Regulate secretion of some digestive enzymes
Testes	Testosterone	Affects development of male secondary sexual characteristics and genital organs
Ovaries	Estrogens; progesterone	Affect development of female secondary sexual characteristics and genital organs; control menstrual cycle; maintain pregnancy

The various glands that make up the hormonal system constitute a control and communications network that is complementary to the nervous system. However, instead of using nerve impulses, the glands secrete chemical messengers (hormones) to affect other glands and tissues in various parts of the body. Hormones are carried in the bloodstream to their targets, where they exert their specific effects. This table lists the hormones secreted by different parts of the body and gives a description of their wide-ranging actions.

The drugs are usually taken orally in a three-stage cycle repeated each month—estrogen for the first 11 to 14 days, estrogen and progesterone for the next seven to 10 days, and no drugs for the last seven days.

Alternatively, an implant containing estrogen is placed under the skin of the abdomen. The estrogen is released slowly and progesterone is taken in tablet form.

Therapy is usually continued for between two and five years. Regular tests, including weight and blood pressure checks, breast and pelvic examinations, and cervical smears, are carried out to monitor the effects of the therapy. Occasionally, a *biopsy* of the lining of the uterus may be carried out to test for cancer.

POSSIBLE ADVERSE EFFECTS

Minor adverse effects include nausea, breast tenderness, fluid retention, and leg cramps. In some women, estrogen replacement therapy may increase the risk of abnormal blood clotting. It is therefore not usually given to women who smoke heavily or have suffered from *thrombosis*, *stroke*, liver disease, or severe *hypertension* (raised blood pressure). Women who have had cancer of the breast or uterus are also not usually given hormone replacement therapy because estrogen may increase the risk of recurrence.

Hormones

A group of chemicals (such as *cortisol*, *estrogen*, *insulin*, and *epinephrine*), each of which is released into the bloodstream by a particular gland or tissue to have a specific effect on tissues elsewhere in the body. Hormones control numerous body functions, including the *metabolism* (chemical activity) of cells, growth, sexual development, and the body's response to stress or illness.

Glands that primarily produce hormones make up the *endocrine system*, which comprises the *adrenal glands*, gonads (*ovaries* or *testes*), *pancreas*, *parathyroid glands*, *pituitary gland*, *placenta* (in pregnant women), and *thyroid gland*. Hormones are also secreted by other organs, including the kidneys, intestines, and brain.

Horn, cutaneous

A hard, noncancerous protrusion occasionally found on the skin (usually the face) of elderly people. Horns are slow growing and vary in color from yellow to brown to black. They may develop where there was previously a wart on normal skin.

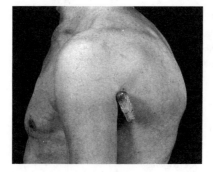

Appearance of cutaneous horn
The horny protuberance that has developed under the arm results from an overgrowth of keratin (a skin protein).

Left untreated, they can grow to a considerable size and may protrude as much as 0.75 inch (2 cm). Surgical removal is usually recommended.

Horner's syndrome

A group of physical signs that affects one side of the face and indicates damage to part of the sympathetic nervous system (see *Autonomic nervous system*). The signs are narrowing of the pupil of the eye (miosis), drooping of the lid (ptosis), and absence of sweating (anhidrosis). They are caused by damage to or destruction of sympathetic nerve fibers, usually in the lower part of the neck, and may be the first sign of disease in the area.

Hornet stings

See *Insect stings*.

Horseshoe kidney

A congenital abnormality in which the two kidneys are joined at the base, forming a horseshoe shape, rather than being separate. Horseshoe kidney affects about one person in 600; it is twice as common in men.

The joined kidneys usually function normally and cause no problems.

Hospice

A hospital or part of a hospital devoted to the care of patients who are dying, often from one specified cause. One hospice may thus care only for AIDS patients, another for cancer patients, and another for those dying of old age (see *Dying, care of the*).

Hospitals, types of

The roughly 7,000 hospitals in the US, which maintain about 1.3 million beds, can be classified in many ways. There are government hospitals—federal, state, county, and municipal.

Many hospitals are owned and run by religious orders. Though graduate medical education is conducted in many hospitals, teaching hospitals generally have a close affiliation with universities and medical schools. A growing number of hospitals are owned by for-profit corporations. Far more are community hospitals that depend on community-generated contributions. By far the largest number of hospitals are classified as short-term acute care general hospitals.

Hot flashes

Reddening of the face, neck, and upper trunk usually facilitated by decreased *estrogen hormone* production by the ovaries during or after the *menopause*. A hot flash typically lasts one to two minutes and is accompanied by a sensation of heat; it is often followed by sweating. Hot flashes are aggravated when the sufferer is under stress.

Hot flashes may also occur after a total *hysterectomy*, in which the uterus and the ovaries are removed. Occasionally, men experience hot flashes after *orchiectomy* (removal of a testis), which causes a reduction in testosterone levels. If hot flashes are severe, they can usually be alleviated by *hormone replacement therapy*.

Housemaid's knee

Inflammation of the *bursa* that acts as a cushion over the kneecap. The inflammation is usually caused by prolonged kneeling, but may develop after a sharp blow to the front of the knee. (See also *Bursitis*.)

HTLV III

Human T-cell lymphotropic virus, strain III, a name once used for the virus that causes *AIDS*. The organism is now called *HIV*.

Human chorionic gonadotropin

See *Gonadotropin, human chorionic*.

Humerus

The bone of the upper arm. The smooth, dome-shaped head of the bone lies at an angle to the shaft and fits into a shallow socket in the scapula (shoulder blade) to form the shoulder joint. Below the head, the bone narrows to form a cylindrical shaft. It flattens and widens at its lower end, forming a prominence on each side called an epicondyle. At its base, the humerus articulates with the ulna and radius (the bones of the lower arm) to form the elbow.

H

LOCATION OF HUMERUS

The humerus is the bone of the upper arm, located between the shoulder and elbow joints.

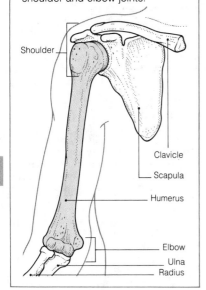

Shoulder

Clavicle
Scapula
Humerus
Elbow
Ulna
Radius

A spiral groove in the shaft of the humerus carries the *radial nerve*, the major nerve of the arm.

Humerus, fracture of

The most usual site of fracture of the humerus (the bone of the upper arm), especially in the elderly, is at the neck of the bone, just below the head. Fracture of the lower end of the bone (a supracondylar fracture) occurs most commonly in children. The fracture may be accompanied by damage to the brachial artery. If injury to this artery goes undetected, it may impair circulation to the arm, resulting in *Volkmann's contracture*, a deformity of the forearm and hand due to muscle damage caused by *ischemia* (insufficient blood supply).

Any suspected fracture of the humerus is first X rayed. If the neck of the bone is found to be fractured, it usually requires only a sling to keep the bone immobilized; a supracondylar fracture usually needs to be put in a plaster cast.

A fractured humerus normally takes six to eight weeks to heal. However, supracondylar fractures sometimes fail to mend properly, resulting in deformity of the elbow.

Humors

Liquid or jellylike substances in the body. The term usually refers to the aqueous humor (the watery fluid in the front chamber of the *eye*) and vitreous humor (the jellylike substance in the rear chamber of the eye).

According to early medical theory, there were four humors—blood, phlegm, black bile, and yellow bile—that permeated the entire body and determined its state of health. This theory was generally discarded in the 17th century.

Hump back

See *Kyphosis*.

Hunch back

See *Kyphosis*.

Hunger

A disagreeable feeling caused by the need for food (as opposed to *appetite*, a pleasant sensation felt in anticipation of a meal).

Hunger occurs when the stomach is empty and when the blood sugar level is low. In response to these stimuli, the hypothalamus in the brain indirectly causes the muscular wall of the stomach to contract rhythmically, signaling the need for food; if pronounced, these contractions produce hunger pains.

Hunger caused by a low blood sugar level is usually the result of strenuous exercise. However, it can also occur in certain diseases (notably *thyrotoxicosis*, which is marked by a speeding-up of body processes) and insulin-dependent *diabetes mellitus* if an incorrect balance between insulin and carbohydrate intake causes *hypoglycemia*.

Huntington's chorea

An uncommon disease in which degeneration of the basal ganglia (paired nerve cell clusters in the brain) results in *chorea* (rapid, jerky, involuntary movements) and *dementia* (progressive mental impairment). Symptoms do not usually appear until the age of 35 to 50; in rare cases the condition is apparent in childhood.

Huntington's chorea is a *genetic disorder* with an autosomal pattern of inheritance. Because the age of onset of symptoms is generally so late, an affected person may bear children before realizing that he or she has the disease. Each child has a 50 percent chance of the condition developing. The disease develops in about 5 persons per 100,000 in the US.

SYMPTOMS

The chorea usually affects the face, arms, and trunk, resulting in random grimaces and twitches and general clumsiness. Dementia takes the form of personality and behavior changes, irritability, difficulty making decisions, memory loss, and apathy.

When the disease starts in childhood, it may be marked by loss of movement and muscle rigidity.

DIAGNOSIS

Until recently there was no way of detecting whether a child of a person with Huntington's chorea had inherited the abnormal gene responsible for the condition. As a result of recent advances in genetics, young adults with parents who have the condition can now learn, with 95 percent accuracy, whether or not they have the abnormal gene and thus have the disorder. This may affect their decisions on whether to have children themselves (see *Genetic counseling*).

TREATMENT AND OUTLOOK

There is no known cure. Treatment is aimed at lessening the chorea with drugs, such as chlorpromazine (which was investigational in 1987), and alleviating the effects of dementia with good nursing care.

Most sufferers survive for about 15 years after the onset of symptoms; some live for up to 30 years afterward.

Hurler's syndrome

A rare, inherited condition caused by an *enzyme* defect. Hurler's syndrome is a type of inborn error of *metabolism* in which there is an abnormal accumulation of substances called mucopolysaccharides in the tissues.

Affected children may appear normal at birth, but, between 6 and 12 months of age, cardiac abnormalities, umbilical hernia, skeletal deformities, and enlargement of the tongue, liver, and spleen develop. Physical growth is limited and mental development slows, leaving the child mentally retarded. The strange features of affected children gave the condition its former name of gargoylism.

Hydatid disease

 A rare infestation caused by the larval stage of the small tapeworm ECHINO-COCCUS GRANULOSUS. The larvae settle in the liver, lungs, or brain or other organs and cause the development of slowly growing cysts.

CAUSE AND INCIDENCE

The illustration on the next page shows how eggs or larvae can enter the body.

Hydatid disease is prevalent only in areas of the world where sheep are reared with the aid of dogs, including some parts of California and Utah. About 200 cases of hydatid disease are diagnosed in the US each year.

SYMPTOMS AND TREATMENT

Although the infestation is usually acquired in childhood, the cysts grow very slowly, so symptoms, if any, occur mainly in adults. In many cases there are no symptoms. However, a cyst in the liver may cause a tender, localized lump or lead to *bile duct obstruction* and jaundice. In the lungs, a cyst may press on an airway, causing *bronchitis*. Rupture of a cyst can cause chest pain, hemoptysis (coughing up blood), wheezing (if present in the lung), or *anaphylactic shock* (a severe allergic reaction). Cysts in the brain can cause seizures or other symptoms similar to those of a brain tumor.

Hydatid cysts are diagnosed by *CT scanning*. Treatment of cysts that are causing symptoms consists of surgical removal, or sterilization followed by drainage. Newer antiparasite drugs are under investigation.

Hydatidiform mole

An uncommon benign tumor that develops from placental tissue during an early pregnancy in which the embryo has failed to develop normally. A hydatidiform mole, which resembles a bunch of small grapes, is caused by degeneration of the chorionic villi, minute fingerlike projections in the placenta. The cause of the degeneration is unknown.

INCIDENCE

A hydatidiform mole is the most common form of *trophoblastic* disease. It occurs in about one in 2,000 pregnancies in developed countries; the incidence is much higher in developing areas. In about 3 percent of affected pregnancies the growth develops into a *choriocarcinoma*, a malignant tumor that can invade the walls of the uterus if left untreated.

SYMPTOMS AND DIAGNOSIS

There is usually vaginal bleeding and excessive morning sickness. The diagnosis is made by *ultrasound scanning* and from urine and blood tests. The mole produces excessive amounts of the hormone human chorionic *gonadotropin* (HCG), which can be detected in urine and blood.

TREATMENT

The tumor can be removed either by suctioning out the contents of the uterus or by a *D and C*. A *hysterectomy* may be considered.

OUTLOOK

There is a small risk that a malignant tumor may develop later; for this

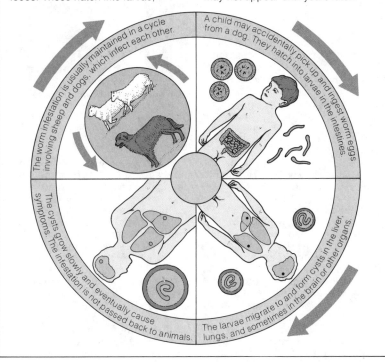

ORIGINS OF HYDATID DISEASE
The infestation is generally confined to dogs and sheep, but occasionally a child swallows eggs from dog feces. These hatch into larvae, which migrate through the body, especially to the liver or lungs, to form slow-growing cysts. Symptoms may not appear until years later.

A child may accidentally pick up and ingest worm eggs from a dog. They hatch into larvae in the intestines.

The worm infestation is usually maintained in a cycle involving sheep and dogs, which infect each other.

The cysts grow slowly and eventually cause symptoms. The infestation is not passed back to animals.

The larvae migrate to and form cysts in the liver, lungs, and sometimes in the brain or other organs.

reason, tests are performed regularly for several years to determine the levels of HCG in the blood and urine.

A woman should not become pregnant again until her HCG levels have returned to normal for at least a year. There is a one in 75 risk of the growth recurring in a future pregnancy.

Hydralazine

An *antihypertensive drug* that is particularly useful as an emergency treatment for *hypertension*. Hydralazine is often also used when the combination of *diuretic* and *beta-blocker drugs* fails to control high blood pressure.

Hydralazine may cause nausea, vomiting, headache, dizziness, and irregular heart beat. Less common adverse effects include loss of appetite, rash, and joint pain. When prescribed in high doses over a prolonged period, hydralazine may cause *lupus erythematosus*.

Hydramnios

Excess *amniotic fluid* in the uterus during pregnancy. Hydramnios occurs in about one in 250 pregnancies.

CAUSES

In many cases, there is no known cause for hydramnios. It sometimes occurs if the fetus has a malformation (particularly *anencephaly* or *esophageal atresia*) that makes normal swallowing impossible. Hydramnios may also occur if the pregnant woman has *diabetes mellitus*. It occurs in about 10 percent of multiple pregnancies.

SYMPTOMS AND SIGNS

An excess of amniotic fluid usually accumulates slowly during the second half of the pregnancy, producing symptoms from about week 32. The main symptom is abdominal discomfort. Other possible symptoms are breathlessness and edema of the legs. The uterus is larger than usual for the duration of the pregnancy.

Less commonly, the fluid accumulates rapidly, causing abdominal pain, breathlessness, nausea, and vomiting. The abdomen becomes tense, the overlying skin is stretched and shiny, and the legs swell. Hydramnios may cause premature labor and the baby may not be in the usual delivery position (see *Malpresentation*).

H

DIAGNOSIS

Hydramnios is usually evident from the patient's history and a physical examination. *Ultrasound scanning* is needed to detect fetal abnormality or multiple pregnancy.

TREATMENT

In the case of severe fetal abnormality, a therapeutic *abortion* may be performed. Mild cases without fetal abnormality require no treatment other than extra rest. Withdrawal of amniotic fluid via a needle inserted through the abdominal wall can provide relief in severe cases although the procedure may cause premature labor. If the pregnant woman has diabetes mellitus, careful attention must be paid to her diabetic control. If symptoms occur in late pregnancy, *induction of labor* may be performed to deliver the baby early.

Hydrocele

A soft, painless swelling in the scrotum caused by the space around the testis filling with fluid. A hydrocele is sometimes caused by inflammation, infection, or injury to the testis. Occasionally, a tumor may cause fluid to accumulate, but in most cases there is no apparent cause. Hydroceles occur very commonly in middle-aged men.

Treatment is rarely necessary. If the swelling is large enough to be uncomfortable or painful, the fluid may be aspirated (drawn off through a hollow needle) using local anesthetic. The most common surgical method of dealing with recurrent swelling is to remove the lining around the testis.

Hydrocephalus

An excessive amount of *cerebrospinal fluid*, usually under increased pressure, within the skull. The term "water on the brain" is sometimes used to describe the condition. Hydrocephalus is often associated with other congenital abnormalities, particularly *spina bifida*.

CAUSES

The condition may be *congenital* (present at birth) or may develop as a result of major head injury, brain hemorrhage, infection (*meningitis*, for example), or a tumor.

Hydrocephalus is caused by excessive formation of cerebrospinal fluid, by a block in the circulation of this fluid, or both.

SYMPTOMS

When the condition is congenital, the main feature is an enlarged head that continues to grow at an abnormally

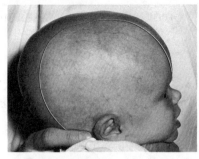

Infant with hydrocephalus
Skull enlargement is due to pressure from excess fluid within the cavities of the brain. To prevent brain damage, the fluid must be drained by means of a tube inserted through a hole made in the skull.

fast rate because the bones are not rigid and expand to accommodate the fluid. Other features are rigidity of the legs, *epilepsy*, irritability, lethargy, vomiting, and the absence of normal reflex actions. If the condition is not treated, it progresses to extreme drowsiness, severe brain damage, and seizures, which may lead to the baby's death within a matter of weeks.

When the condition occurs later in childhood or in adulthood, the skull is no longer flexible and symptoms are caused by raised pressure within the skull. Symptoms include headache, vomiting, loss of coordination, and deterioration of mental function.

DIAGNOSIS AND TREATMENT

CT scanning or *MRI* show the location and nature of any obstruction.

In most cases, treatment aims to drain excess fluid away from the brain to another part of the body, such as the lining of the abdomen or chest wall, where it can be absorbed. Drainage is achieved by means of a *shunt* (tube), which is inserted into the brain through a hole made in the skull. In some cases, the shunt must be left in position indefinitely. In older children and adults, treatment is sometimes for the underlying cause only.

Hydrochloric acid

A strong acid released by the stomach lining. It forms part of the stomach juices and is important in the digestion of proteins. Excessive acid production, which may be stimulated by stress or tobacco smoking, is an important factor in the development of *peptic ulcers*. *Acid reflux* (regurgitation of stomach acid into the esophagus) resulting in *esophagitis* and heartburn is another problem created by hydrochloric acid secretion. (See also *Digestive system*.)

Hydrochlorothiazide

A thiazide *diuretic drug* used to reduce *edema* (fluid retention) in people with *heart failure* (reduced pumping efficiency), *nephrotic syndrome* (a kidney disorder), *cirrhosis* of the liver, and breast tenderness before menstruation. Hydrochlorothiazide is also given to treat *hypertension* (high blood pressure), and is occasionally used to prevent the recurrence of certain types of kidney stones.

POSSIBLE ADVERSE EFFECTS

Adverse effects include leg cramps, lethargy, dizziness, rash, and impotence. Hydrochlorothiazide may (rarely) cause *gout* and may aggravate *diabetes mellitus*.

Hydrocortisone

CORTICOSTEROID
Tablet Injection Rectal suppository Cream Eye drops
📋 Prescription sometimes needed
🔒 Available as generic

A *corticosteroid drug* sometimes used to treat inflammatory and allergic disorders, such as *dermatitis*, *uveitis*, *ulcerative colitis*, types of *arthritis*, and *asthma*. Hydrocortisone is chemically identical to *cortisol*, a hormone produced by the adrenal glands. Hydrocortisone is therefore given to replace this hormone when the amount produced by the body is insufficient, as in *Addison's disease*.

POSSIBLE ADVERSE EFFECTS

Hydrocortisone creams used in excess may cause thinning of the skin. Taken by mouth over a prolonged period, high doses of hydrocortisone may cause *diabetes mellitus*, *glaucoma*, *osteoporosis*, *peptic ulcer*, fluid retention, weight gain, acne, muscle weakness, mood changes, and retarded growth in children.

Hydrogen peroxide

An *antiseptic* solution used to treat infections of the skin or mouth and to bleach hair. Hydrogen peroxide combines with catalase, an enzyme present in the skin and mouth, to release oxygen. This effect kills bacteria and cleanses infected areas. Hydrogen peroxide occasionally causes soreness and irritation.

Hydronephrosis

A condition in which the kidney becomes distended with urine due to a blockage or narrowing of the *ureter*. If left untreated, hydronephrosis can severely damage the kidney and, if bilateral, cause *renal failure*.

CAUSES
Obstruction of a ureter is usually caused by a stone (see *Calculus, urinary tract*), a *kidney tumor*, or sometimes by a blood clot. Alternatively, the urine in the bladder may be under pressure caused by obstruction of its outflow from an enlarged prostate gland. In some cases, constriction of the ureter is present from birth.

SYMPTOMS AND SIGNS
Acute hydronephrosis, with sudden blockage of the ureter, results in severe pain in the small of the back. Chronic hydronephrosis, in which the obstruction develops slowly, may, however, cause no symptoms until the ureter has become completely blocked and renal failure occurs. There is also a risk that the kidney may become infected, resulting in pyonephrosis (pus-filled kidney).

DIAGNOSIS AND TREATMENT
Ultrasound scanning can provide an image of the kidneys and ureter. If it reveals obstruction and the kidney is still relatively healthy, the blockage is removed or relieved by surgery; the kidney soon resumes normal functioning. Occasionally, however, the kidney is so badly damaged that it requires removal (see *Nephrectomy*). In this case, the remaining kidney compensates for the loss of the other.

Hydrophobia
A popular term—now almost obsolete—for *rabies*. Meaning "fear of water," hydrophobia refers to the inability to drink that is one of the characteristic symptoms of rabies.

Hydrops
An abnormal accumulation of fluid in the body tissues or in a sac (such as the gallbladder). Hydrops fetalis is marked generalized *edema* (fluid collection causing tissue swelling) affecting the fetus. It may occur in pregnancy as a result of severe *hemolytic disease of the newborn*.

Hydrotherapy

The external use of water to treat patients recovering from injury or suffering from lack of mobility. It includes the use of exercise pools, whirlpool baths, and showers.
People who are unable to bear full weight on a limb (because of arthritis or after a fracture, for example) often can exercise more fully and effectively

in a hydrotherapy pool. The buoyant effect of the water allows a greater range of movement and permits fuller use of the limb with little discomfort.
Warm whirlpool baths provide a gentle massage to stimulate areas of the body and relieve stiffness. Cold baths or showers can reduce blood flow, swelling, and bruising after injury and minimize tissue damage. (See also *Heat treatment*; *Ice packs*.)

Hydroxocobalamin
A long-acting synthetic preparation of *vitamin B$_{12}$*.

Hydroxyprogesterone
A *progesterone drug* given by injection to treat cancer of the uterus (see *Uterus, cancer of*) and certain types of *breast cancer*.

Hydroxyzine
An *antihistamine drug* commonly used in the treatment of *urticaria* (hives) and other allergic rashes. Hydroxyzine is also used as a *premedication* before surgery, in the management of alcohol withdrawal, and, occasionally, in the short-term treatment of mild anxiety. It is also used to relieve nausea and vomiting in *motion sickness, vertigo*, and following a general anesthetic.
Possible adverse effects include drowsiness, dry mouth, and tremor.

Hygiene
The science and practice of preserving health. Today the word is commonly equated with cleanliness. However, in the early years of this century the term hygiene was widely used as an equivalent to *public health*—the scientific study of environmental influences on health (especially the provision of pure water supplies, safe sanitation, good housing, and safe conditions in the workplace).

Hygiene, oral
See *Oral hygiene*.

Hygienist, dental
A licensed professional who is qualified to carry out *scaling* (the removal of calculus from the teeth) and to demonstrate methods of keeping the teeth and gums healthy (see *Oral hygiene*). Keeping the teeth and gums healthy is especially important in preventing or controlling gum disorders occurring in middle life, such as *gingivitis* and *periodontitis*.

Hygroma, cystic
A type of *lymphangioma*.

Hymen
The thin fold of membrane surrounding the vaginal opening. The hymen has a central perforation that is usually stretched or torn by the use of tampons or during first sexual intercourse. Once torn, the hymen becomes an irregular ring of tissue around the vaginal opening.

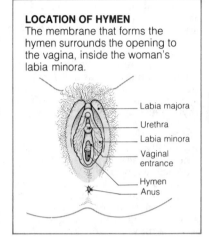

LOCATION OF HYMEN
The membrane that forms the hymen surrounds the opening to the vagina, inside the woman's labia minora.

Labia majora
Urethra
Labia minora
Vaginal entrance
Hymen
Anus

Imperforate hymen is a rare condition in which the hymen has no perforation; at the onset of menstruation, menstrual blood collects in the vagina, causing lower abdominal pain. It is corrected by minor surgery.

Hyoid
A small, U-shaped bone situated deep in the muscles at the back of the tongue. It is not joined to any other bone but is suspended by ligaments

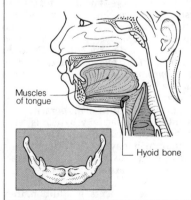

LOCATION OF HYOID BONE
The U-shaped hyoid bone provides an anchor for the muscles at the back of the tongue.

Muscles of tongue
Hyoid bone

from the base of the skull. Its function is to provide an anchor point for the muscles of the tongue and for those in the upper part of the front of the neck.

The hyoid is commonly fractured in homicidal strangulation.

Hyoscyamine

An *anticholinergic drug* used to treat the spasm of the bladder muscle that occurs with an *irritable bladder* and the spasm of the intestinal wall that accompanies *irritable bowel syndrome*.

Hyper-

A prefix meaning above, excessive, or greater than normal, as in *hypertension* (raised blood pressure) and *hyperthyroidism* (overactivity of the thyroid gland).

Hyperacidity

A condition in which an excessive amount of acid is produced by the stomach. Hyperacidity is commonly confused with *acid reflux* (which causes a burning sensation in the upper abdomen or lower chest) or a sudden filling of the person's mouth with a fluid (water brash). Most people with a duodenal ulcer (see *Peptic ulcer*) produce more acid than normal, and those with *Zollinger-Ellison syndrome* produce vast amounts.

Hyperactivity

A behavior pattern of certain children who are constantly overactive and have difficulty concentrating on one activity. Also known as hyperkinetic syndrome, the condition may affect as many as 5 to 10 percent of children in the US. It is four to five times more common in boys than girls.

CAUSES

It has been suggested that some hyperactive children, especially those who are clumsy, may have a subtle form of "minimal" brain damage. However, there is no definite, conclusive evidence. Hyperactive children seem more likely to have fathers who were hyperactive, so the condition may be partly inherited. Children with *mental retardation, cerebral palsy,* or *temporal lobe epilepsy* are also more likely to be hyperactive.

SYMPTOMS

The main feature of hyperactivity is continual overactivity, which is often worse in the classroom or in a group situation; it may not be evident during an interview by a physician. Hyperactive children are always on the go, full of energy, fidgety, and seem to sleep less than their peers. In addition, they

tend to be impulsive and reckless, with no sense of danger, and are usually irritable, emotionally immature, and aggressive. Their attention span is short and, as a result, they do not conform to orderly routine.

Hyperactivity often leads to antisocial acts and difficulty learning, although IQ is normal. It is uncertain whether this behavior is a part of the disorder or simply a result of an affected child's poor attention span and disruptive activity.

DIAGNOSIS

Overactivity in itself does not indicate that hyperactivity is present, since overactivity can be caused by a stressful home environment or physical illness. In addition, many of the behavioral problems mentioned are, to some degree, common to all young children. However, when other causes have been eliminated and the behavior continues past the age of 4 years, is intense, and is different from that of "normal" children, then it is reasonable to regard the child as being hyperactive.

TREATMENT

Paradoxically, *stimulant drugs* (amphetamine or methylphenidate) seem to be the most effective treatment. This suggests that hyperactivity results from "underarousal" of the midbrain, which causes no damping down or control of movements and sensations. Stimulant drugs seem to work by stimulating the midbrain enough to suppress the extra activity. Behavior therapy and counseling of the child and parents are also useful.

Diets that exclude certain artificial food colorings, additives, or foods are popular and heavily promoted, but research has shown that these diets benefit very few children.

Hyperactive children should have formal educational and psychological assessment; many need help at school with reading and spelling.

OUTLOOK

In many cases, hyperactivity disappears completely at puberty. In others, the overactivity subsides and is replaced by sluggishness, depression, and moodiness; these teenagers often fail at school and resort to antisocial and criminal behavior. Sometimes all the symptoms of hyperactivity continue into adult life.

Hyperacusis

An exceptionally developed sense of hearing. It may cause the sensation of pain or discomfort in the ears on exposure to loud noises.

Hyperaldosteronism

An alternative name for *aldosteronism*, or Conn's syndrome, a metabolic disorder caused by overproduction of the hormone aldosterone (secreted by the cortex of the adrenal gland).

Hyperalimentation

Administration of nutrients to patients unable to take food by mouth. (See *Feeding, artificial*.)

Hyperbaric oxygen treatment

A method of increasing the amount of oxygen in the tissues by exposing a person to oxygen at a much higher than normal atmospheric pressure.

WHY IT IS DONE

The technique is occasionally used to treat poisoning from *carbon monoxide*, in which the tissues are starved of oxygen because *hemoglobin* (the oxygen-carrying component of red blood cells) is prevented from taking up oxygen. Hyperbaric oxygen treatment is also used in cases of gas *gangrene*; the bacteria that infect gangrenous tissue cannot survive if they are oxygenated.

HOW IT IS DONE

The patient is placed in a chamber into which oxygen is pumped at up to three times normal atmospheric pressure for no more than three hours. The oxygen is inhaled and dissolves in the blood.

Hyperbilirubinemia

A raised blood level of bilirubin (a waste product formed from the destruction of red blood cells). Hyperbilirubinemia may be undetectable except by a blood test, but *jaundice* becomes apparent if the blood bilirubin level rises to two times the normal level. Both have similar causes and implications.

Hypercalcemia

An abnormally high level of calcium in the blood. Normally the blood carries (in the plasma) less than 0.1 percent of the body's total amount of calcium—the optimum amount for the efficient functioning of cells throughout the body. A raised level or a lowered one (hypocalcemia) may seriously disrupt cell function, particularly in muscles and nerves.

CAUSES

The most common cause of hypercalcemia is secondary *bone cancer*, which releases calcium from an affected bone into the blood. Other causes include *hyperparathyroidism* (overproduction of parathyroid hormone, which helps control the blood calcium level); certain inflammatory disorders, such as *sarcoidosis*; taking too much vitamin D, which helps regulate the absorption of calcium from the diet; a diet too rich in foods containing calcium; or, infrequently, taking large amounts of calcium-containing antacids.

SYMPTOMS

Mild hypercalcemia causes nausea, vomiting, lethargy, and excessive urination. Higher levels of calcium in the blood produce confusion, extreme fatigue, and muscle weakness. If the disorder is untreated and the blood calcium level continues to increase, arrhythmia (irregular heart beat), coma, and even death may result. Long-standing mild hypercalcemia may cause kidney calcifications, or stones, to form.

DIAGNOSIS

The condition is diagnosed by tests that measure the blood calcium level. If the diagnosis is confirmed, more tests are performed to discover and treat the underlying cause.

Hypercapnia

Excessive carbon dioxide in the blood. Carbon dioxide is a waste product of the metabolic processes that produce energy in body cells; dissolved in body fluids, it forms carbonic acid. The blood circulation carries the acid to the lungs, where it is eliminated from the body as carbon dioxide during exhalation. The amount of carbonic acid in the blood is normally maintained within narrow limits by mechanisms such as the breathing rate. However, if these mechanisms fail to remove enough carbon dioxide from the body (which may occur as a result of impaired breathing), carbonic acid accumulates and the blood becomes too acidic, a condition called *acidosis*.

Hyperemesis

The medical term for excessive *vomiting*, as in hyperemesis gravidarum (vomiting during pregnancy that causes dehydration and weight loss).

Hyperglycemia

An abnormally high level of glucose (sugar) in the blood. The condition occurs in people suffering from untreated or inadequately controlled *diabetes mellitus*; it may also occur in diabetics as a result of an infection, stress, or surgery.

The symptoms of hyperglycemia are the same as those of diabetes: thirst, the passing of large amounts of urine, *glycosuria* (glucose in the urine), and *ketosis* (an accumulation of ketones in the body). In severe cases, hyperglycemia may lead to confusion and coma, which require emergency medical treatment with insulin and an intravenous infusion of fluids.

Hypergonadism

Overproduction of estrogen or androgen *hormones* by the *ovaries* or *testes*, causing precocious sexual development and excessive growth.

Hyperhidrosis

A disorder marked by excessive sweating that occurs at times other than in hot conditions or during or just after exercise. It usually begins at puberty and worsens in the summer, affecting the palms, soles, armpits, or all three. Hyperhidrosis may cause the sufferer distress. The constantly moist hands that result may rule out certain occupations and activities, and excessively sweaty armpits or feet may produce an unpleasant *body odor*, which can cause social embarrassment. In many sufferers, the condition improves on its own in the middle 20s or early 30s.

TREATMENT

Treatment includes taking *anticholinergic drugs* and applying aluminum chloride paint to the affected areas to block the sweat pores. Wearing clothing and shoes made of natural, absorbent materials (such as cotton and leather) can be helpful.

Hyperkeratosis

Thickening of the outer layer of the skin due to an increased amount of *keratin* (a tough protein that is the major component of the outer layer of skin). The most common forms of hyperkeratosis are *corns* and *calluses*, caused by prolonged pressure or friction, and *plantar warts*. Hyperkeratosis also occurs in *lichen planus*.

The term is also used to describe thickening of the nails in people with a fungal nail infection or in people with *psoriasis* (a skin condition).

Hyperkinetic syndrome

Another name for *hyperactivity*.

Hyperlipidemias

A group of metabolic disorders characterized by high levels of lipids in the blood. Hyperlipidemias are the most common of the lipid disorders and are an important factor in the health disorders of middle-aged, sedentary people.

TYPES

There are six types of hyperlipidemia, differentiated principally by the extent to which the blood levels of various fatty substances are higher than normal. The characteristics of each type of hyperlipidemia, along with their symptoms and treatment, are given in the table on the next page. Many of the types produce similar symptoms; diagnosis usually depends on blood tests to measure the levels of lipids.

Lipids are carried in the blood in several forms, chiefly cholesterol, triglycerides, and lipoproteins. Lipoproteins consist of fat and cholesterol molecules linked to protein molecules. There are different types: very low-density lipoproteins (VLDLs), low-density lipoproteins (LDLs), and intermediate-density lipoproteins (IDLs). There are also high-density lipoproteins (HDLs), but they are not involved in the hyperlipidemias. Lipoproteins are differentiated according to their relative proportions of cholesterol and protein. The higher the proportion of cholesterol, the lower the density of the lipoprotein. Chylomicrons (microscopic droplets in the blood containing triglycerides, cholesterol, and protein) are usually also classed as lipoproteins.

CAUSES

Each type of hyperlipidemia may be inherited or may be secondary to another disorder. The main secondary causes for each type are: Type I—systemic lupus erythematosus (SLE); Types IIa and IIb—hypothyroidism, nephrotic syndrome, Cushing's syndrome, and corticosteroid therapy; Type III—hypothyroidism and SLE; Types IV and V—diabetes mellitus, obesity, alcoholism, nephrotic syndrome, renal failure, and corticosteroid therapy or estrogen therapy.

RISKS

There is some evidence that the hyperlipidemias are associated with a number of serious disorders, notably *atherosclerosis* and *coronary heart disease*. For this reason, if a close relative has or had either of these disorders, particularly if he or she has had a heart attack at an early age (under 50), other members of the family should be tested. Treatment is given to reduce the blood lipid levels and thus lower the risk of atherosclerosis.

Hypermetropia

See *Hyperopia*.

TYPES OF HYPERLIPIDEMIA

Type	Lipoprotein elevated	Blood cholesterol level	Blood triglyceride level	Symptoms and signs in addition to risk of heart disease	Treatment
I	Chylomicrons	Small elevation	Large elevation	Fatty nodules in skin; abdominal pain; inflammation of pancreas	Diet very low in fats
IIa	Low-density lipoproteins	Small to medium elevation	Normal	Fatty nodules around tendons (especially Achilles tendon and hand tendons) and over joints; white line around rim of cornea	Diet low in saturated fats and cholesterol; cholestyramine, colestipol, lovastatin, or clofibrate may be prescribed
IIb	Low-density and very low-density lipoproteins	Small to medium elevation	Small elevation	Fatty nodules on eyelids; white line around rim of cornea	Diet low in saturated fats, cholesterol, and carbohydrates; cholestyramine, lovastatin, or colestipol may be prescribed
III	Intermediate-density lipoproteins	Small to medium elevation	Small to medium elevation	Fat deposits in palms and sometimes over joints	Diet low in fats and carbohydrates; clofibrate, niacin, gemfibrozil, or lovastatin may be prescribed
IV	Very low-density lipoproteins	Normal	Small to medium elevation	Fatty nodules in skin; patient is often obese	Diet low in carbohydrates; weight reduction; clofibrate and sometimes niacin and gemfibrozil may be prescribed
V	Chylomicrons and very low-density lipoproteins	Small elevation	Small to medium elevation	Fatty nodules in skin; abdominal pain; inflammation of pancreas; patient may be obese	Diet low in fats and carbohydrates; weight reduction; gemfibrozil and niacin may be prescribed

Hypernephroma

An alternative name for renal cell carcinoma, a type of *kidney cancer*.

Hyperopia

Commonly called farsightedness, an error of *refraction* that initially causes difficulty in seeing near objects and then affects distance vision. Hyperopia tends to run in families.

Hyperopia is caused by the eye being too short from front to back, so that images are not clearly focused on the retina. Mild or moderate hyperopia in the young is overcome by *accommodation* (the action of the ciliary muscles to change the shape of the lens), which brings the point of focus forward to produce a clear image.

SYMPTOMS AND SIGNS

The error is present from early childhood, but symptoms generally do not appear until later life. The more severe the hyperopia, the lower the age at which the problem appears. People with hyperopia experience varying degrees of difficulty viewing close objects because the power of accommodation declines with age. In time, distant objects are also blurred.

Hyperopia may lead to *eyestrain*. Neither blurred images nor eyestrain permanently affects vision.

TREATMENT

When blurred vision occurs, an ophthalmologist may prescribe *glasses* or *contact lenses* with convex lenses to reinforce focusing power.

Hyperparathyroidism

Overactivity of the *parathyroid glands*. These pea-sized glands are embedded in the thyroid gland in the neck and produce parathyroid hormone. This hormone, together with vitamin D and calcitonin (a hormone produced by the thyroid gland), controls the level of calcium in the body. Overproduction of parathyroid hormone raises the level of calcium in the blood (a condition called *hypercalcemia*) by removing the mineral from bones, leading to *osteoporosis* and *osteomalacia* (weakening of the bones).

In an attempt to normalize the high blood calcium level, the kidneys excrete large amounts of calcium in the urine, which can result in the formation of kidney stones (see *Calculus, urinary tract*).

CAUSES AND INCIDENCE

Hyperparathyroidism is most often caused by a small benign tumor of one or more of the parathyroid glands. However, sometimes it is due to an enlargement of the glands, the cause of which is unknown.

About 40 persons per 100,000 suffer from the disorder. It usually develops after the age of 40 and is twice as common in women as men.

SYMPTOMS

Hyperparathyroidism may cause generalized aches and pains, depression, and abdominal pain. Often, the only symptoms are those of kidney stones, but if the hypercalcemia is severe, it may cause nausea, vomiting, tiredness, excessive urination, confusion, and muscle weakness.

DIAGNOSIS AND TREATMENT

The condition is diagnosed by X rays of certain bones and by tests to measure the level of calcium, phosphorus, and parathyroid hormone in the blood.

Surgical removal of all abnormal parathyroid tissue usually cures the condition; sometimes all but part of one gland requires removal. In this case, the remaining parathyroid tissue may not produce enough hormone. The affected person may then require treatment for *hypoparathyroidism* (underactivity of the glands).

Hyperplasia

Enlargement of an organ or tissue due to an increase in the number of its constituent cells. The new cells are normal, unlike those of a tumor.

Hyperplasia is usually the result of hormonal stimulation. It may be a normal occurrence (such as in the enlargement of breast tissue and uterine muscle that occurs during pregnancy) or it may indicate a disorder (such as in hyperplasia of the thyroid or adrenal glands, which may be due to oversecretion of certain pituitary hormones). See also *Hypertrophy*.

Hyperplasia, gingival

Swelling of the gums. The condition may be a feature of *gingivitis* (inflammation of the gums), especially when it occurs during pregnancy; it can also develop around the front teeth as a result of persistent breathing through the mouth. Hyperplasia can also be caused by phenytoin, the anticonvulsant drug used to treat *epilepsy*.

Ill-fitting dentures can cause rolls of fibrous tissue to form beyond the edges of the dentures. This can be irritating and may require surgical treatment. Whatever the cause, gingival hyperplasia should be checked by a dentist.

Hyperpyrexia

A medical term for extremely high body temperature; it is synonymous with hyperthermia. Heat hyperpyrexia is a term for *heat stroke*.

Hypersensitivity

An overreaction of the *immune system* (defense against infection) to an *antigen* (protein recognized as foreign). Hypersensitivity reactions occur only on second or subsequent exposures to particular antigens, after the first exposure has sensitized the immune system. Such reactions have the same mechanisms as those of protective *immunity*. However, while the latter protect against disease, hypersensitivity reactions lead to tissue damage and disease.

Hypersensitivity is closely related to *allergy*, except that only one of the four main types of hypersensitivity reaction (type I) is closely associated with allergic illnesses.

TYPES

The four main types of hypersensitivity reaction are as follows.

TYPE I This type is also called immediate or anaphylactic hypersensitivity. After a first exposure to an antigen (which may be a harmless substance such as grass pollen), *antibodies* (substances that can recognize and bind to the antigen) are formed; these antibodies coat cells called mast cells in various tissues. On second exposure, the antigen and antibodies combine, causing the mast cells to disintegrate and release various chemicals that cause the symptoms of *asthma*, allergic *rhinitis* (hay fever), *urticaria* (hives), *anaphylactic shock*, or other illnesses of an allergic nature.

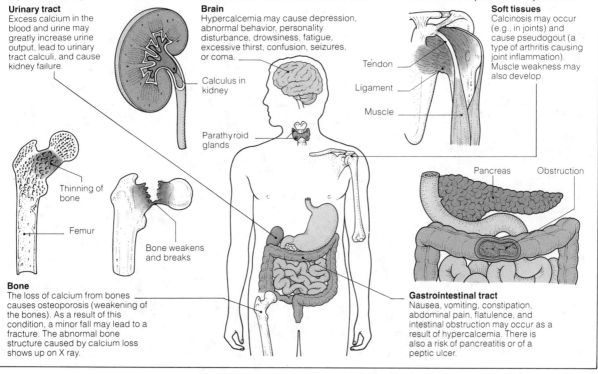

HYPERPARATHYROIDISM

In this disorder, the parathyroid glands produce too much parathyroid hormone. Symptoms, signs, and complications of the disorder occur as a result of an increased calcium level in the blood and urine, the loss of calcium from bones, and calcinosis, the formation of calcium deposits in different tissues. Surgical removal of abnormal parathyroid tissue is carried out to prevent complications.

Urinary tract
Excess calcium in the blood and urine may greatly increase urine output, lead to urinary tract calculi, and cause kidney failure.

Brain
Hypercalcemia may cause depression, abnormal behavior, personality disturbance, drowsiness, fatigue, excessive thirst, confusion, seizures, or coma.

Soft tissues
Calcinosis may occur (e.g., in joints) and cause pseudogout (a type of arthritis causing joint inflammation). Muscle weakness may also develop.

Calculus in kidney

Tendon
Ligament
Muscle

Parathyroid glands

Thinning of bone
Femur
Bone weakens and breaks

Pancreas   Obstruction

Bone
The loss of calcium from bones causes osteoporosis (weakening of the bones). As a result of this condition, a minor fall may lead to a fracture. The abnormal bone structure caused by calcium loss shows up on X ray.

Gastrointestinal tract
Nausea, vomiting, constipation, abdominal pain, flatulence, and intestinal obstruction may occur as a result of hypercalcemia. There is also a risk of pancreatitis or of a peptic ulcer.

HYPERTENSION

Hypertension is a common condition, affecting up to 10 percent of adults in the US. It is diagnosed if a person's resting blood pressure is persistently raised. Blood pressure is expressed by two values—the systolic and diastolic pressures (see bottom right) and measured in millimeters of mercury.

Although hypertension rarely causes symptoms, it is an important condition. Left untreated, it increases the risk of stroke and other disorders. In many cases, there is no obvious cause, but, in some, there is a specific cause, such as a kidney disorder, pregnancy, or use of oral contraceptives. Hypertension is linked to obesity and, in some people, to a high salt intake. Smoking appears to aggravate the effects of hypertension.

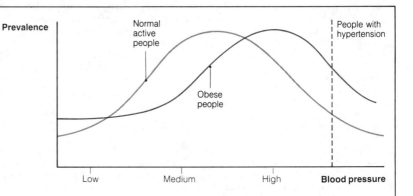

Prevalence — Normal active people — Obese people — People with hypertension — Low — Medium — High — Blood pressure

Atheroma
Hypertension and atherosclerosis, in which arteries are narrowed (left), are closely linked both to each other and to obesity.

Fatty deposits

Contracted muscle

Constriction
Factors such as nicotine in tobacco cause artery constriction (left) and a short-term rise in blood pressure that may worsen hypertension.

Artery wall

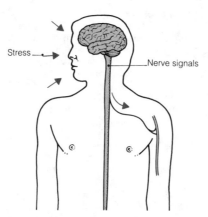

Stress — Nerve signals

Stress and hypertension
Stress acts on the nervous system, causing blood vessels to constrict and the heart to work harder. Both lead to a temporary rise in blood pressure. Hence, pressure should be measured when a person is relaxed. It is possible (but unproven) that frequent stress may eventually cause hypertension.

Variation in blood pressure
In any population, blood pressure varies over a wide range in the same way as height. Many people are considered to be hypertensive because they are at the top end of this range (see above). In obese people, the range is similarly wide but shifted toward the top end; hence, more obese people are hypertensive.

MEASURING BLOOD PRESSURE
During one heart beat, pressure varies between the (higher) systolic and the (lower) diastolic pressures.

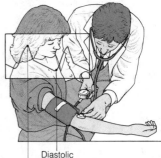

Diastolic

Systolic

Systolic pressure
The systolic pressure is the maximum pressure attained as blood surges into the arteries.

Diastolic pressure
The diastolic pressure is the lowest value to which the pressure drops.

COMMON FACTORS AND PREVENTIVE MEASURES

Factors associated with essential hypertension	Age (incidence higher in the elderly)	Family history		Race (incidence higher in blacks than in whites)	
Factors that may aggravate hypertension	Smoking	Obesity	Excess alcohol intake	Diabetes mellitus	Stress
Self-help and treatment	1. Regular screening of blood pressure is important for early diagnosis and can help prevent complications. 2. Sufferers from essential hypertension should: Reduce weight Not smoke Reduce or stop alcohol intake Reduce salt intake Learn relaxation methods to combat stress 3. Antihypertensive drugs, prescribed by a physician, can usually keep high blood pressure under control.				

TYPE II In this type, antibodies are formed that bind to antigens bound to cell surfaces, leading to possible destruction of the cells. Type II reactions may be responsible for certain *autoimmune disorders* (in which antibodies attack the body's own tissues) and for some cases of red blood cell destruction (*hemolysis*) triggered by certain drugs.

TYPE III Antibodies combine with antigens to form particles called immunocomplexes, which can lodge in various tissues and activate further immune system responses, leading to tissue damage. This type of hypersensitivity reaction is responsible for *serum sickness*, for allergic *alveolitis* (a lung disease caused by exposure to the spores of certain fungi), and for the large swellings that sometimes form after booster vaccinations.

TYPE IV This type is also called delayed hypersensitivity. In type IV, sensitized T-*lymphocytes* (a class of white blood cell and an important component of the immune system) bind to antigens and subsequently release chemicals called lymphokines, which promote an inflammatory reaction. Type IV reactions are responsible for contact *dermatitis* and the rash of *measles*; they are important in the body's defense against *tuberculosis* and may also play a part in some "allergic" reactions to drugs.

TREATMENT
Effective treatment of a hypersensitivity reaction depends on its type, cause, and severity. When possible, exposure to the offending antigen should be avoided.

Hypersplenism

Overactivity of the spleen, resulting in and associated with blood disease. One of the functions of the spleen is to break down blood cells as they age and wear out. An overactive spleen may begin to destroy cells indiscriminately, causing a deficiency of any of the types of blood cell. In most cases of hypersplenism, the spleen is also enlarged.

Hypersplenism may be primary, occurring for no known reason, but more commonly it is secondary to another disorder in which the spleen has become enlarged, such as *Hodgkin's disease* or *malaria*.

SYMPTOMS AND TREATMENT
A person with hypersplenism is likely to have the symptoms of *anemia* (due to destruction of red blood cells) or of *thrombocytopenia* (platelet deficiency), and there is sometimes a decrease in resistance to infection due to lack of white cells. There may also be symptoms of an underlying disorder, such as malaria.

Treatment of secondary hypersplenism aims to control the underlying cause. Primary hypersplenism requires *splenectomy*.

Hypertension

Abnormally high *blood pressure* (the pressure of blood in the main arteries). Blood pressure goes up as a normal response to stress and physical activity. However, a person with hypertension has a high blood pressure at rest.

Hypertension is usually defined as a resting blood pressure greater than 140 mm Hg (systolic)/90 mm Hg (diastolic). However, an elderly person normally has blood pressure readings above these values because blood pressure increases with age. Young children usually have blood pressure readings well below these values.

CAUSES
The majority of people have no obvious cause for their elevated blood pressure; in such cases it is called essential hypertension. However, in about 10 percent of patients, a definite cause can be found, including various disorders of the *kidney*, certain disorders of the *adrenal glands*, and *coarctation of the aorta*.

Tobacco smoking and *obesity* significantly increase the risk of hypertension. Hypertension sometimes develops in women who are taking the birth-control pill.

SYMPTOMS AND COMPLICATIONS
Hypertension usually causes no symptoms and generally goes undiscovered until detected by a physician during the course of a routine physical examination.

Possible complications of untreated hypertension include *stroke*, *heart failure*, kidney damage, and *retinopathy* (damage to the retina at the back of the eye). Severe hypertension may cause confusion and seizures.

TREATMENT
Mild hypertension may respond to weight reduction and a reduction in personal stress. Smokers should stop smoking and heavy drinkers should drastically reduce their consumption of alcohol. Restriction of salt intake is sometimes recommended.

If these measures have no effect, *antihypertensive drugs* may be prescribed. Occasionally, in severe cases, admission to the hospital for investigation of the cause, emergency treatment, and bed rest are required.

Hyperthermia

A medical term for extremely high body temperature. Hyperthermia has been used to treat advanced cancer. (See also *Heat stroke*.)

Hyperthermia, malignant

A rapid rise in body temperature to a dangerously high level brought on by general anesthesia. The condition is rare, occurring in only about one in 50,000 operations, and, in most cases, susceptibility to it is inherited. People suffering from certain muscle disorders may also be at risk.

The patient's temperature rises soon after the anesthetic is given. At the same time, large amounts of *lactic acid* pass from the muscles into the blood, causing *acidosis*. The muscles then stiffen and the patient turns blue; this may be followed rapidly by seizures and death if emergency treatment is not delivered.

Malignant hyperthermia may be suspected if the patient does not relax normally during the early, induction stage of anesthesia, or if he or she shows signs of abnormal muscle contractions after being given succinylcholine (a chemical used to relax muscles during operations).

TREATMENT
If malignant hyperthermia occurs, the anesthetic is stopped immediately and the patient is cooled with ice packs. Pure oxygen and intravenous injections of bicarbonate may also be given to counteract acidosis.

Hyperthyroidism

Overactivity of the *thyroid gland* and, therefore, simultaneous overproduction of thyroid hormones.

CAUSES AND INCIDENCE
The most common form of hyperthyroidism is *Graves' disease*, an *autoimmune disorder* in which the body develops antibodies that stimulate the production of excessive amounts of thyroid hormones. This condition affects about 1 percent of the adult population and is most common in young to middle-aged women. More rarely, hyperthyroidism may be associated with the development of enlarged nodules on the thyroid.

SYMPTOMS AND SIGNS
See illustration, next page.

DIAGNOSIS AND TREATMENT
The diagnosis of hyperthyroidism is confirmed by tests to measure the level of thyroid hormones in the blood. The condition may be treated with drugs that inhibit the production of thyroid hormones or by surgical

H

SYMPTOMS AND SIGNS OF HYPERTHYROIDISM

Oversecretion of thyroid hormones produces symptoms associated with overactivity of the body's metabolism. Weight loss, increased appetite, intolerance to heat, and increased sweating are early signs; there may also be tremors and a rapid heart rate. In more severe cases, the thyroid gland is often enlarged and there tends to be physical and mental hyperactivity and wasting of the muscles.

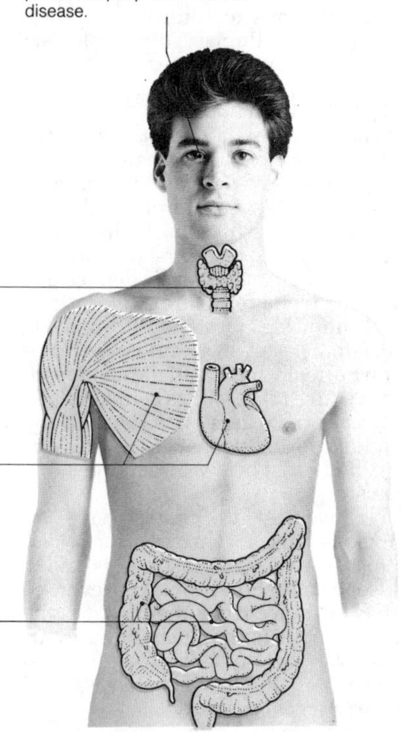

Thyroid gland enlargement
This symptom (known as goiter) may be due to hyperthyroidism. However, it may also be associated with hypothyroidism (underactivity of the thyroid).

Muscle wasting
Severe hyperthyroidism may cause wasting of both skeletal and heart muscle; the latter may lead to irregularities of heart rhythm.

Increased appetite
This symptom is a result of the metabolic overactivity that hyperthyroidism causes. Despite increased appetite, there is often weight loss.

Protruding eyes
This symptom (known as exophthalmos) affects some 30 to 50 percent of people with Graves' disease.

Hyperthyroid heart rate
Excessive thyroid hormones may result in the heart beating too rapidly or irregularly.

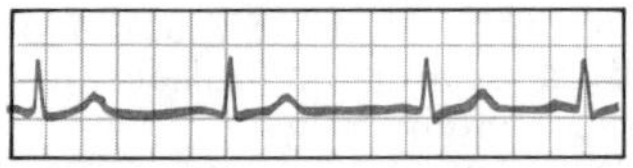

Healthy rhythm
A healthy hear beat, as shown in this ECG tracing, has a regular rhythm and a normal rate of beating.

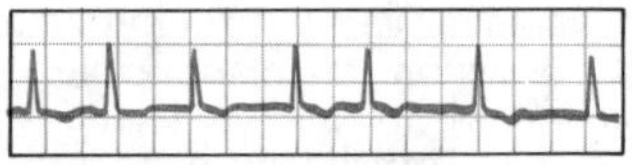

Hyperthyroid rhythm
The hyperthyroid heart beat shown in this tracing is irregular and adnormally rapid.

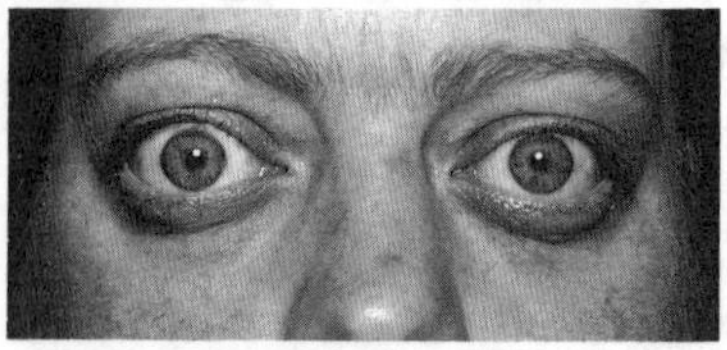

Appearance of exophthalmos
Hyperthyroidism can cause swelling of tissues around the eyes, resulting in a staring appearance.

removal of part of the thyroid gland. In older patients, an alternative is a single dose of radioactive iodine, which is taken up by the thyroid and destroys some of its tissue.

Hypertonia

Increased rigidity in a muscle. It may be caused by damage to its nerve supply or by cell changes within the muscle itself. Hypertonia causes episodes of continuous muscle spasm (e.g., in the bladder wall when the outflow of urine is being obstructed by an enlarged prostate gland).

Persistent hypertonia in limb muscles following a *stroke* or major *head injury* causes *spasticity*.

A variable increase in muscle tension associated with abnormal patterns of movement and posture is referred to as *dystonia*.

Hypertrichosis

Growth of excessive hair, often in places not normally covered with hair. Hypertrichosis is often a result of taking certain drugs (including cyclosporine, minoxidil, and diazoxide).

The disorder is not the same as *hirsutism*, which is excessive hairiness in women due to abnormal levels of male hormones.

Hypertrichosis is also the term used to describe hair growth in a colored, fleshy mole.

Hypertrophy

Enlargement of an organ or tissue due to an increase in the size, rather than number, of its constituent cells. For example, skeletal muscles increase in size in response to increased physical demands. (See also *Hyperplasia*.)

Hyperuricemia

An abnormally high level of *uric acid* in the blood. Hyperuricemia may lead to the development of *gout* due to the deposit of crystals of uric acid in the joints; it may also cause kidney stones (see *Calculus, urinary tract*) and tophi (crystals in the tissues).

CAUSES

Hyperuricemia may be caused by an inborn error of *metabolism*, by rapid destruction of cells as part of a disease such as *leukemia*, or by medication

(such as *diuretic drugs*) that reduces the excretion of uric acid by the kidneys. Increased amounts of purine in the diet may raise the level of uric acid in the blood, precipitating gout.

TREATMENT

Drugs such as allopurinol (which reduces uric acid production in cells) and probenecid or sulfinpyrazone (which increase the excretion of uric acid by the kidneys) may be prescribed for life to prevent complications. Foods high in purine (e.g., liver, poultry, and dried peas and beans) need to be avoided.

Hyperventilation

Abnormally deep or rapid breathing, usually caused by *anxiety*. Hyperventilation may also occur as a result of uncontrolled *diabetes mellitus*, oxygen deficiency, *renal failure*, and some lung disorders (such as pulmonary *edema* and *emphysema*).

Hyperventilation causes an abnormal loss of carbon dioxide from the blood, which can lead to *alkalosis* (increase in blood alkalinity). Symptoms include numbness of the extremities, faintness, and *tetany* (painful spasms and twitches of the muscles in the hands and feet), and a sense of an inability to take a full breath. The effects of alkalosis often add to the already existing feelings of anxiety, and may give rise to the "hyperventilation syndrome," in which the sufferer experiences a feeling of impending doom.

Breathing into a plastic or paper bag during an attack may help reduce the loss of carbon dioxide and avoid the risk of alkalosis.

Hyperventilation associated with uncontrolled diabetes or uremia represents a compensatory effort by the body to eliminate excess carbon dioxide in dealing with *acidosis*. In this case, the hyperventilation syndrome does not develop.

Hyphema

Blood in the front chamber of the eye, almost always caused by an injury that ruptures a small blood vessel in the iris or the ciliary body.

Vision is markedly affected while the blood remains mixed with the aqueous humor, but it clears as the red cells sink. Usually the blood disappears completely within a few days and vision is fully restored, but there is a risk of delayed bleeding three to five days after the injury. Drug treatment or surgical evacuation of the blood is sometimes necessary.

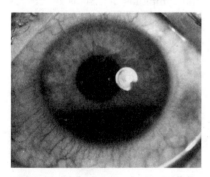

Appearance of hyphema
Blood that has collected in the front chamber of the eye is clearly visible in front of the iris; hyphema is usually caused by an injury.

Hypnosis

A trancelike state of altered awareness that is characterized by extreme suggestibility. Hypnosis was once believed to be a form of sleep. However, the *EEG* (electrical tracing of brain-wave activity) of a hypnotized person does not show any of the normal sleep patterns.

HISTORY

A form of hypnotism was first practiced by the Austrian physician Franz Mesmer in the eighteenth century. Mesmerism (renamed hypnotism after the Greek god of sleep) began to receive attention from many leading members of the medical community in the nineteenth century. The celebrated Parisian physician Charcot gave public demonstrations, and Freud used hypnosis in his early treatment of hysteria. Hypnotism continues to attract much popular interest, both theoretical and medical, but its clinical use is still much debated. Likewise, its use to stimulate the memory of witnesses for courtroom testimony is controversial. Hypnosis for this purpose is acceptable in some jurisdictions and not in others.

HOW IT IS DONE

For hypnosis to succeed, the subject must first want to be hypnotized. The second requirement is relaxation, so a comfortable chair and a quiet, dimly lit room are usually necessary. The subject is usually asked to fix his or her attention on a particular object while the therapist quietly repeats phrases such as "Be still and listen to my voice" or "Empty your mind of all thoughts." The person gradually becomes more and more relaxed, eventually losing touch with the environment and hearing only the therapist's voice. At the end of the session, the subject "wakes up" when told to do so.

With training, it is possible for people to practice autohypnosis (self-hypnosis) by repeating certain phrases to themselves or imagining relaxing scenes.

Some people are more easily hypnotized than others, usually those with an intense imaginative life. The ability seems to be related to early childhood experiences and may be partly inherited.

CHARACTERISTICS

Hypnotized subjects wait passively to be told what to do by the therapist and are very suggestible—they touch or hold imaginary objects and act out suggested roles. They do not, however, obey commands to behave in a manner they would normally regard as dangerous or improper.

Attention usually becomes highly selective, so that only one person at a time is heard. Subjects frequently will obey orders to forget everything that has happened during hypnosis, or, alternatively, to remember or repeat behavior learned while hypnotized (posthypnotic suggestion).

THERAPEUTIC USES

Some psychoanalysts use hypnosis as a means of helping patients remember and come to terms with disturbing events or feelings that have been repressed from consciousness. More often, hypnosis is used as a means of helping patients relax. It may be useful in people suffering from *anxiety*, *panic attacks*, or *phobias*, and is sometimes successful in treating addictive habits, such as smoking. Scientific studies are lacking, however, and claims of fantastic cures should be treated with skepticism.

Hypnotic drugs

Drugs that induce sleep, such as *antianxiety* and *barbiturate drugs*.

Hypo-

A prefix meaning under, below, or less than normal, as in hypodermic (under the skin), hypoglycemia (abnormally low blood sugar level), and hypotension (lower than normal blood pressure).

Hypoaldosteronism

A deficiency of *aldosterone* in the body. This hormone, along with other *corticosteroid hormones* (notably hydrocortisone), is produced by the adrenal cortex (outer part of the adrenal glands). Removal of, or damage to, the cortex results in a deficiency of these hormones, which, in turn, causes *Addison's disease*.

Hypochondriasis

The unrealistic belief or fear that one is suffering from a serious illness, despite medical reassurance.

SYMPTOMS

Hypochondriacs worry constantly about their bodily health and interpret any physical symptom, however trivial, as evidence of a serious disorder. The feared disease may involve many parts of the body or may center on a particular organ and a single disease, as in *cardiac neurosis* (fear of heart disease). Hypochondriacs constantly seek medical advice and undergo numerous tests and treatments. Rarely, an obscure physical disorder is discovered, but it does not justify the symptoms described.

CAUSES

Hypochondriasis is usually a complication of other psychological disorders, including *obsessive-compulsive behavior*, *phobia*, *generalized anxiety disorder*, *schizophrenia*, *depression*, and brain diseases, such as *dementia* and *brain tumors*.

The cause of hypochondriasis in the absence of an underlying disorder is uncertain. However, it seems to be more common in people who suffered from a true organic illness during childhood or were constantly exposed to sick relatives. The reason for this may be that the hypochondriac becomes programmed to overreact to every bodily feeling, though there may also be an inherited sensitivity to pain. Other factors that may predispose a person to hypochondriasis include social stresses and personality type (usually obstinate).

TREATMENT

When there is an underlying mental disorder, it is treated as required. Hypochondriasis alone is more difficult to treat. An understanding and patient physician can often help relieve distress.

Hypoglossal nerve

The nerve that controls movements of the tongue. The hypoglossal nerve is rarely damaged. If damage does occur (e.g., as a result of a stroke), one side of the tongue becomes paralyzed.

LOCATION OF HYPOGLOSSAL NERVE

The hypoglossal nerve arises in the medulla oblongata (part of the brain stem), passes through the base of the skull, and runs around the throat to the tongue.

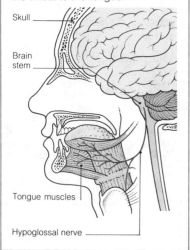

Skull

Brain stem

Tongue muscles

Hypoglossal nerve

Hypoglycemia

An abnormally low level of glucose (sugar) in the blood. Almost all cases occur in sufferers from insulin-dependent *diabetes mellitus*. In this disease, the pancreas fails to produce enough *insulin* (a hormone that regulates the level of glucose in the blood), resulting in an abnormally high level of glucose. To lower it, diabetics take either *hypoglycemic* drugs by mouth or insulin by injection. Too high a dose of either can reduce the blood sugar to too low a level, thus starving the body cells of energy. Hypoglycemia can also occur if a diabetic person misses a meal, fails to eat enough carbohydrates, or exercises too much.

Rarely, hypoglycemia can result from drinking a large amount of alcohol or from an *insulinoma* (an insulin-producing tumor of the pancreas); it also occurs for no known reason in some children, but is usually only temporary.

Hypoglycemia is a serious condition. The brain needs glucose for its metabolism and to function properly, and prolonged lack of it may lead to permanent intellectual impairment in an affected person.

SYMPTOMS

The principal symptoms include sweating, weakness, hunger, dizziness, trembling, headache, palpitations, confusion, and sometimes double vision. Behavior is often irrational and aggressive and movements are uncoordinated; this state may be mistaken for drunkenness. The victim may lapse into a coma due to extremely low blood sugar.

TREATMENT

Insulin-dependent diabetics should always carry sugar with them (in a convenient form such as sugar lumps or glucose tablets) to take at the first sign of an attack of hypoglycemia. If it is suspected that an unconscious person has suffered a hypoglycemic attack, medical help should be summoned immediately. The physician will give an injection of either glucose solution or the hormone glucagon; the latter counteracts the effects of insulin and raises the blood sugar level by stimulating the conversion of glycogen to glucose.

Hypoglycemics, oral

COMMON DRUGS

Acetohexamide Chlorpropamide Glipizide Glyburide Tolazamide Tolbutamide

WARNING

Consult your physician if you regularly experience symptoms, such as dizziness, nausea, and sweating, that are relieved only by food or a sugary drink.

A group of drugs that are used to treat non-insulin-dependent *diabetes mellitus* when *hyperglycemia* (raised blood glucose level) cannot be controlled simply by diet.

HOW THEY WORK

Oral hypoglycemics lower blood glucose levels by increasing the production by the pancreas of *insulin*, a hormone that increases the amount of glucose that is absorbed from the bloodstream into body cells. Insulin rather than oral hypoglycemics may need to be prescribed temporarily to control the blood glucose level (e.g., during surgery, pregnancy, or a severe illness). Oral hypoglycemics are of no use in treating insulin-dependent diabetes because in these cases the pancreas is unable to produce any insulin.

POSSIBLE ADVERSE EFFECTS

Oral hypoglycemic drugs may cause *hypoglycemia* (abnormally low blood glucose) if the dosage is too high or if the person has not had enough to eat.

Hypogonadism

Underactivity of the gonads (testes or ovaries). Hypogonadism may be caused by disorders of the *testis* or *ovary* or by a *pituitary gland* disorder resulting in deficient production of *gonadotropin* hormone. In affected males, hypogonadism causes the symptoms and signs of *androgen hormone* deficiency. In females, it causes the symptoms and signs of *estrogen hormone* deficiency.

Hypohidrosis

Reduced activity of the sweat glands. It is a feature of hypohidrotic ectodermal dysplasia, a rare, inherited, incurable condition characterized by reduced production of sweat usually accompanied by dry, wrinkled skin, sparse, dry hair, small, brittle nails, and conical teeth. Other causes include exfoliative *dermatitis* and some *anticholinergic drugs*.

Hypomania

A moderate form of *mania*.

Hypoparathyroidism

Insufficient production of parathyroid hormone produced by the *parathyroid glands*, which lie behind the thyroid gland in the neck. Parathyroid hormone, along with vitamin D and calcitonin (a hormone produced by the thyroid gland), regulates the level of calcium in the body. A deficiency of the hormone results in low levels of calcium in the blood and tissue fluids.

HYPOPLASTIC LEFT HEART SYNDROME

The heart defects associated with this syndrome are shown (at right) and compared with those of the normal heart (at left). Neither the left ventricle (pumping chamber) nor the aorta is properly formed.

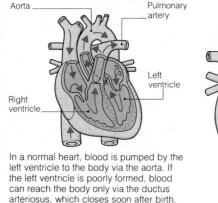

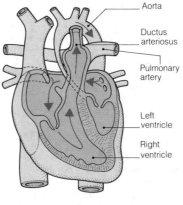

In a normal heart, blood is pumped by the left ventricle to the body via the aorta. If the left ventricle is poorly formed, blood can reach the body only via the ductus arteriosus, which closes soon after birth.

CAUSES

The most common cause of hypoparathyroidism is the accidental removal of the parathyroid glands during surgery on the thyroid gland. It may also result from surgery to remove a portion of the parathyroid glands themselves in the treatment of *hyperparathyroidism* (overproduction of parathyroid hormone). Occasionally, the parathyroid glands are absent from birth, or they may cease to function for no apparent reason.

SYMPTOMS

The main effect of a low level of calcium in the body is *tetany*, an increased excitability of the nerves that causes uncontrollable, painful, cramplike spasms of the face, hands, arms, and sometimes the feet. Rarely, general seizures similar to those of an epileptic attack may occur.

DIAGNOSIS AND TREATMENT

The condition is diagnosed by tests to measure the level of parathyroid hormone in the blood.

If the patient is suffering from an attack of tetany, calcium may be injected slowly into a vein to provide quick relief. To maintain the blood calcium at a normal level, a lifelong course of calcium and vitamin D tablets is necessary (the vitamin D is needed to increase absorption of calcium from the diet). Regular checkups are also necessary.

Hypophysectomy

Surgical removal of the pituitary gland or destruction of the gland by radioactive *implants*.

WHY IT IS DONE

Hypophysectomy is sometimes performed to remove a *pituitary tumor* that may be the cause of a number of endocrine diseases, such as *acromegaly* and *Cushing's syndrome*.

The operation may also be performed to treat some types of breast, ovary, or prostate gland cancer, the growth of which is stimulated by hormones secreted by the pituitary gland.

HOW IT IS DONE

A general anesthetic is given. Usually the gland is removed via the nose. However, if the tumor is very large, a *craniotomy* (incision into the skull) is performed just above the hairline, and a flap of bone temporarily removed to give access to the gland.

Hypoplasia

Failure of an organ or tissue to develop fully and reach its normal adult size.

Hypoplasia, enamel

A defect in tooth enamel. It is usually due to *amelogenesis imperfecta* (a hereditary condition), but may also be caused by vitamin deficiency, injury, or infection of a primary tooth that interferes with maturation of enamel.

Hypoplastic left heart syndrome

A serious and usually fatal form of congenital *heart disease* that affects about one to two newborn babies in every 10,000 live births. The baby is born with a poorly formed ventricle (pumping chamber) on the left side of the heart and other heart defects. The

aorta (main artery carrying blood from the heart to the body) is malformed and blood can reach it only via a duct (the ductus arteriosus) that links the aorta to the pulmonary artery (blood vessel that transports blood to the lungs).

At birth the baby may seem healthy, but within a day or two the ductus arteriosus closes off and the baby collapses, becoming pallid and breathless. There is no effective surgical treatment for the condition and most affected babies die within a week. The risk of parents having another affected child is small.

Hypospadias

A congenital defect, occurring in about one in 300 male babies, in which the opening of the *urethra* is situated on the underside of the glans (head) or shaft of the penis. Sometimes the penis curves downward, a condition known as *chordee*.

In an extreme form of hypospadias the urethral opening lies between the genitals and the anus, the scrotum is small, and the testes are undescended. In such cases the genitals may resemble those of a female and the true sex of the child may be in doubt.

TREATMENT

Single-stage operations to correct hypospadias are available today. The penis is straightened and a tube of skin (or occasionally bladder lining) is used to create a new urethra that extends to the tip of the penis. The operation is usually performed before the boy is two years old. Surgery is usually successful, allowing the boy to pass urine normally and, later, to have satisfactory sexual intercourse.

Hypotension

The proper medical term for low blood pressure.

Some healthy people with a normal heart and blood vessels have blood pressure well below average for their age. The term hypotension is usually used only when blood pressure has fallen to the extent that blood flow to the brain is reduced, causing dizziness and fainting.

In postural hypotension (the most common type), symptoms occur after abruptly standing or sitting up. Usually, blood pressure increases slightly with these changes in posture; in people with postural hypotension, this increase fails to occur. Postural hypotension may be an adverse effect of *antidepressant drugs* or *antihypertensive drugs* (drugs used to treat high

H

blood pressure). It also occurs in diabetics because of nerve damage disrupting the reflexes that control blood pressure.

Acute hypotension (of sudden onset) may be caused by injuries involving heavy blood loss or serious burns leading to *hypovolemia* (reduced blood volume) and physiological *shock*, or by any crisis, such as *myocardial infarction* (heart attack) or *adrenal failure*, that leads to shock.

Treatment of hypotension depends on the underlying cause (diabetes mellitus, for example). For many people with postural hypotension, adjustment of medication may resolve the condition.

Hypothalamus

A region of the brain, roughly the size of a cherry, situated behind the eyes and beneath another brain region called the thalamus. It has nerve connections to most other regions of the nervous system.

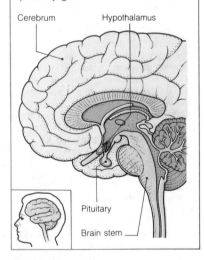

LOCATION OF HYPOTHALAMUS
This small area of the forebrain lies under the thalamus and above the pituitary gland.

Cerebrum   Hypothalamus

Pituitary

Brain stem

FUNCTION
The hypothalamus exerts overall control over the sympathetic nervous system (part of the *autonomic nervous system*, which controls the internal body organs). When we are suddenly alarmed or excited, signals are sent from higher regions of the brain to the hypothalamus, which initiates sympathetic nervous system activity. This causes a faster heart beat, increased breathing, widening of the pupils of the eyes, and increased blood flow to muscles (known as the "fight or flight" response).

Other groups of nerve cells in the hypothalamus are concerned with the control of body temperature. Some are sensitive to heat and cold so that, when blood flowing to the brain is hotter or cooler than normal, the hypothalamus switches on temperature-regulating mechanisms (among them sweating or shivering). The hypothalamus receives information from internal sense organs regarding the level of glucose in the blood and the body's water content; if they are too low, it stimulates appetite for food and drink. The hypothalamus is also involved in regulating sleep, in motivating sexual behavior, and in determining mood and the experience of emotions.

Another role of the hypothalmus is coordination of the function of the nervous and endocrine (hormonal) systems of the entire body. The hypothalamus connects with the pituitary gland through a short stalk of nerve fibers and controls hormonal secretions from this gland. It does this in two ways—through direct nerve connections and through specialized nerve cells, which secrete hormones called releasing factors into the blood to flow directly to the pituitary. In this way, the hypothalamus can convert nerve signals into hormonal signals. Thus, the hypothalamus indirectly controls many of the endocrine organs, including the pituitary, thyroid, adrenal cortex, and gonads.

DISORDERS
Disorders of the hypothalamus are usually caused by a brain hemorrhage within the hypothalamic region (see *Intracerebral hemorrhage*) or by an expanding pituitary tumor. Loss of hypothalamic function can have diverse effects, ranging from hormonal disorders (see *Endocrine system*) to disturbed temperature regulation, and increased or decreased appetite for food, sex, and sleep.

Hypothermia

A fall in body temperature to below 95°F (35°C). It causes drowsiness, lowers breathing and heart rates, and may lead to unconsciousness or death. Most victims are elderly people who are unable to keep sufficiently warm in winter.

The term hypothermia is also used to describe the deliberate lowering of body temperature during some forms of surgery (see *Hypothermia, surgical*).

CAUSES
Hypothermia can be caused by prolonged exposure to extremely cold weather, swimming in the sea, or wearing damp clothing in cold conditions. However, most cases occur in elderly people living in poorly heated homes. As the body ages, it gradually loses its sensitivity to cold; an elderly person's body temperature may drop without the individual being aware of it. In addition, the aging body also becomes increasingly less able to reverse a fall in temperature. This reduced ability is also present in the very young; aside from the elderly, babies are the most common victims of hypothermia.

The risk of hypothermia is increased if an elderly person is also suffering from a disorder that reduces the body's heat production (such as *hypothyroidism*), impairs mental function (such as senile *dementia*), or reduces mobility (such as *arthritis*).

Certain drugs may also contribute to the onset of hypothermia. For example, *tranquilizers* (such as chlorpromazine) may lower the level of consciousness and reduce the ability to shiver (shivering has a protective function against cold).

SIGNS
A person suffering from hypothermia is usually pale, puffy-faced, and listless. The heart rate is slow and the victim is often drowsy and confused. Areas of the body that are normally warm (such as the armpits and the groin) are cold.

In severe hypothermia, breathing becomes slow and shallow, the muscles are often stiff, the victim may become unconscious, and the heart may beat only faintly and irregularly or—especially if the body temperature falls below 90°F (32.2°C)—it may stop beating altogether.

DIAGNOSIS
The condition is usually obvious from the above signs and the victim's circumstances. To determine how cold the body has become, the physician takes a rectal temperature with a special low-reading thermometer. Alternatively, the temperature of the urine may be measured.

TREATMENT
Hypothermia is a medical emergency and anyone suspected of suffering from it requires immediate medical attention. Mild hypothermia usually responds to giving the victim warm drinks and covering the head (from which as much as 20 percent of the body's heat loss takes place).

FIRST AID: HYPOTHERMIA

IN BABIES

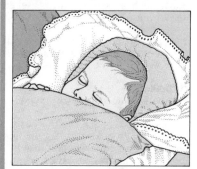

Medical help should be sought immediately. Hypothermia is often difficult to detect. The baby may look pink and healthy, but he or she may be unusually limp and drowsy. Rewarm the baby by keeping him or her well wrapped.

IN ADULTS

1 Seek medical help. If the victim is unconscious and breathing, place in the *recovery position*. If not breathing, begin *artificial respiration*.

2 Move the victim to a warm place. Take off wet clothing and replace with dry, or dry off and cover with waterproof material.

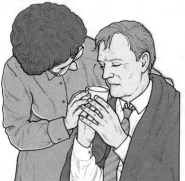

3 If the victim is conscious, give a warm (not hot) drink. Hold the mug if necessary.

4 If the victim is otherwise healthy, place in a warm (not hot) bath.

geons to perform quick (eight to 10 minutes) operations on the heart while blood circulation throughout the body was completely stopped.

Today, open heart surgery is usually performed with the general blood circulation maintained by means of a *heart-lung machine*. Nevertheless, mild hypothermia—with the body temperature reduced from 98.6°F (37°C) to about 82 to 88°F (28 to 31°C)—is still generally induced as a safety measure. It can allow heart operations to proceed for several hours. A heat exchanger, installed into the machine circuit, can be used to cool the blood before return to the body, thus inducing hypothermia.

The blood supply to the heart muscle itself is interrupted during open heart surgery, so the heart also must be vigorously cooled by continuously instilling cold saline into the open chest cavity at a temperature of about 40°F (4°C). By this method, damage to the heart muscle from lack of oxygen is minimal, even after an operation lasting several hours.

At the end of the operation, rewarming of the patient is carefully synchronized with restarting the heart and the switch back from use of the heart-lung machine.

Hypothyroidism

Underactivity of the *thyroid gland* and, therefore, underproduction of thyroid hormones.

CAUSES AND INCIDENCE

Most cases of hypothyroidism are caused by the body developing antibodies against its own thyroid gland (an example of an *autoimmune disorder*) with a resultant reduction in thyroid hormone production. *Hashimoto's thyroiditis* is an example of this phenomenon. More rarely, hypothyroidism may result from surgery to remove part of the thyroid gland as a treatment for *hyperthyroidism* (overactivity of the thyroid).

Hypothyroidism affects about 1 percent of the adult population. It is most common in elderly women, though it occurs at all ages and in both sexes.

SYMPTOMS AND SIGNS

Thyroid hormones stimulate energy production, so a deficiency of them causes generalized tiredness and lethargy. There may also be muscle weakness, cramps, a slow heart rate, dry and flaky skin, hair loss, and a deep and husky voice. In addition, the skin and other body tissues may thicken and there may be weight gain—a syndrome known as *myx-*

When the condition is more severe, treatment varies according to the age of the victim. A young person is usually warmed in a hot bath. However, this causes a rush of blood to the surface of the body, reducing the supply to the heart and brain, which could be fatal to an elderly person. For this reason, warming is carried out gradually in the elderly (at a rate of about 1°F (0.6°C per hour) by placing the person in a room with a temperature of 78°F (25°C) and covering him or her with layers of heat-reflecting material known as space blankets. Rectal temperature is monitored every half hour until the temperature and vital signs show improvement.

When hypothermia is severe enough to be life-threatening, the victim is admitted to an intensive-care unit and warmed rapidly by safe means; part of the circulating blood is bypassed outside the body, where it is warmed, or warm fluid is run into the abdominal cavity.

PREVENTION

It is recommended that an elderly person's living quarters be heated at a temperature of at least 65°F (18°C). Relatives or neighbors of elderly people living by themselves should check regularly throughout winter that these people have additional means of keeping warm, including suitable clothing, warm blankets, and nutritious food.

Elderly people should also be made aware of the need to eat hot food and drink warm fluids several times a day and wear a warm hat at all times.

People walking or climbing in cold weather should carry survival bags, lined with space blankets, which they can crawl into while waiting for help in the event of an accident.

Hypothermia, surgical

The deliberate reduction of body temperature to prolong the period for which the vital organs can safely be deprived (partially or totally) of their normal blood supply during *open heart surgery*. Cold reduces the rate of metabolism in cells and tissues; hence, lack of oxygen is better tolerated as the temperature is lowered.

In the early days of heart surgery, induced hypothermia allowed sur-

edema. In some cases, a goiter (enlargement of the thyroid gland) develops, although not all goiters are due to hypothyroidism.

The severity of the symptoms depends on the degree of thyroid deficiency. Mild deficiency may cause no symptoms; severe deficiency may produce all of the above symptoms.

If hypothyroidism occurs in childhood and remains untreated, it may retard growth, delay sexual maturation, and inhibit normal development of the brain.

DIAGNOSIS AND TREATMENT

The disorder is diagnosed by tests to measure the level of thyroid hormones in the blood.

Treatment consists of replacement therapy with the thyroid hormone thyroxine; in most cases, hormone therapy must be continued for life. Such treatment may not cure a goiter, which may require surgery.

Hypotonia

Abnormal muscle slackness. Normally, a muscle that is not being used has a certain built-in tension. In a number of disorders affecting the nervous system (such as *Huntington's chorea*) this natural tension or tone is moderately or markedly reduced.

Hypotonia in infants

Excessive limpness in infants, also called floppy infant syndrome.

FEATURES

Hypotonic babies cannot hold their limbs up against gravity and thus tend to lie flat with their arms and legs splayed. Their limbs and joints seem slack when moved by someone else. Floppy babies move around less than normal babies and their mothers may report that they did not feel the baby move much during pregnancy. When held horizontally by the trunk, face downward, they hang limply.

CAUSES

Premature infants are naturally more floppy than full-term infants, but, as they mature, their muscles attain the normal tension.

Hypotonia is often a feature of chromosomal disorders, such as *Down's syndrome*. Illnesses that affect general health (e.g., malnutrition, congenital *heart disease*, and *hypothyroidism*) may also cause hypotonia.

More specifically, disorders of the brain (particularly *cerebral palsy*) and of the spinal cord (such as *Werdnig-Hoffmann disease*) are characterized by hypotonia. Treatment depends on the cause.

Hypovolemia

An abnormally low volume of blood circulating in the body. It usually follows severe blood loss, which may occur as a result of injury, internal bleeding, or surgery. Hypovolemia also occurs in various other conditions, such as serious burns, severe dehydration, or, rarely, adrenal crisis (see *Addison's disease*).

Hypovolemia is a dangerous condition because, untreated, it can lead to *shock*, which is potentially fatal.

Hypoxia

An inadequate supply of oxygen to the tissues.

CAUSES

Temporary hypoxia may occur as a result of strenuous exercise in which the normal supply of oxygen cannot meet the additional requirements of the tissues. In such cases, the condi-

---

PERFORMING A HYSTERECTOMY

Hysterectomy may be performed through the abdomen or the vagina. For an abdominal hysterectomy, the incision is made in the lower abdomen (see below). In vaginal hysterectomy, the uterus is removed through an incision at the top of the vagina.

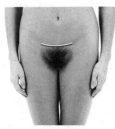

Site of incision for abdominal hysterectomy
The incision is made in the lower abdomen (in this case horizontally) level with the top of the pubic hair.

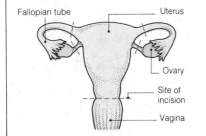

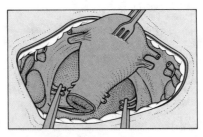

Abdominal hysterectomy
The uterine vessels are clamped. Traction is placed on the top of the uterus and the vessels are tied and then divided. In some cases, the fallopian tubes are cut and the tubes and ovaries left in place.

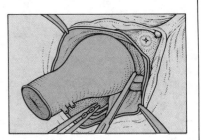

Vaginal hysterectomy
After a vaginal incision is made, the uterus and cervix are removed (the ovaries cannot be removed in a vaginal hysterectomy). The upper end of the vagina is repaired by stitching.

POSTOPERATIVE PROBLEMS

Many women worry that their sex lives will be affected by hysterectomy. Physically, there should be no noticeable change in the woman's sex life. Counseling before the procedure can help dispel any misconceptions or fears. Depression is not uncommon in women who are inadequately counseled.

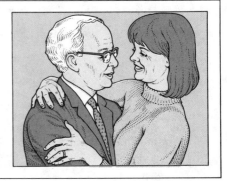

tion disappears once exercise has stopped and breathing has reoxygenated the tissues.

More serious causes include impaired breathing (see *Respiratory failure*), usually as a result of a lung disorder; *ischemia* (reduced blood flow to a tissue), which may be due to an artery disorder or a heart disorder; and severe *anemia*, in which the oxygen-carrying capacity of the blood is reduced. Another, rare, cause is *carbon monoxide* poisoning, which prevents the blood from being adequately oxygenated. In severe cases, any of these more serious causes may lead to *anoxia* (complete absence of oxygen in a tissue), which, if prolonged, may cause tissue death.

SYMPTOMS AND SIGNS
Hypoxia in muscles forces the muscle cells to produce energy by *anaerobic* metabolism, which produces lactic acid as a by-product. The accumulation of lactic acid causes cramps. Hypoxia in heart muscle may cause the chest pain of *angina pectoris*. Hypoxia of the brain initially causes confusion, dizziness, and incoordination, progressing to unconsciousness and death if the condition persists.

TREATMENT
Severe, potentially life-threatening hypoxia may require treatment by *oxygen therapy* or artificial *ventilation*. Otherwise, the treatment depends on the underlying cause.

Hysterectomy
Removal of the uterus. Hysterectomy is one of the most frequently performed operations in the US.

WHY IT IS DONE
Hysterectomy is most often performed to treat *fibroids* (benign tumors of the uterus) that are causing symptoms. It is also performed to treat cancer of the uterus or cervix (see *Uterus, cancer of*; *Cervix, cancer of*). Occasionally, a hysterectomy is performed to relieve *menorrhagia* (heavy menstrual bleeding) or *endometriosis* (a condition in which fragments of the uterine lining occur elsewhere in the pelvis) that has not responded to a *D and C* or hormone treatment. A hysterectomy may also be performed to remove a severely prolapsed uterus (see *Uterus, prolapse of*).

TYPES
The most common type of hysterectomy is a simple hysterectomy, in which the uterus and cervix only are removed. In a total hysterectomy, the fallopian tubes and ovaries are removed as well. If cancer is advanced, a radical hysterectomy (in which the pelvic lymph nodes are also removed) is necessary.

RECOVERY PERIOD
After the operation a drainage tube may be inserted at the site of the incision. For a few days there may be some vaginal bleeding and discharge and considerable tenderness and pain. The stay in the hospital depends on the age and health of the woman and whether there are postoperative problems. Full recovery requires another three to six weeks; sexual intercourse can be resumed about a month after the surgery.

OUTLOOK
After hysterectomy the woman is unable to bear children; she does not menstruate and needs no contraception. If the ovaries have also been removed from a woman before or around the *menopause, hormone replacement therapy* should be considered.

Hysteria
A term encompassing a wide range of physical or mental symptoms that are attributed to mental stress in someone who is not psychotic.

Derived from the Greek word for uterus, hysteria was originally thought to be a physical disorder confined to women. By the nineteenth century, hysteria was believed to have a psychological origin and was used to describe many seemingly bizarre states (including hallucination, sleepwalking, and trances).

Today, many psychiatrists feel that the term hysteria is no longer helpful in diagnosis. In modern classifications, therefore, the symptoms formerly grouped under this term are now included in the more specific diagnostic categories of *conversion disorder*; *dissociative disorders*; *somatization disorder*; and *factitious disorders*.

Physicians still sometimes use the term loosely to describe any difficult, unusual, or exotic behavior that does not seem consistent with the symptoms or situation of the patient. Mass hysteria describes the spread of psychologically produced symptoms (such as fainting) from person to person. It usually occurs in schools or institutions of young women in response to group tensions or worries and is often triggered by a person with a charismatic personality.

Hysterosalpingography
An X-ray procedure performed to examine the inside of the uterus and fallopian tubes.

WHY IT IS DONE
The examination is performed as part of the investigation of *infertility*. Dye injected during *laparoscopy* indicates whether the tubes are blocked, but hysterosalpingography is needed to determine the site of the blockage, which is most often due to scar tissue caused by a previous infection. Hysterosalpingography also outlines any distortion in the uterus, such as a congenital abnormality or a *fibroid*.

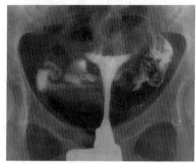

A normal hysterosalpingogram
The X-ray image shows radiopaque dye filling the uterus and passing through the fallopian tubes into the pelvic cavity.

HOW IT IS DONE
The test is an outpatient procedure performed by a radiologist and/or a gynecologist. Because the procedure may be uncomfortable (often producing a cramplike pain), the patient is usually mildly sedated.

A plastic or metal *cannula* is inserted into the cervix (neck of the uterus), a radiopaque dye (one that shows up on X-ray film) is passed through it into the uterus and the fallopian tubes, and X-ray pictures are taken to reveal any abnormalities. The procedure takes 10 to 30 minutes.

RISKS
In a woman who has just become pregnant, the dye may wash the fertilized egg out of the fallopian tube; if this does not happen, the embryo may be damaged by radiation from the X rays. To avoid these risks, the test is carried out only in the second half of the menstrual cycle, when it is certain the woman is not pregnant.

Hysterotomy
A method of late *abortion* in which the abdomen and uterus are surgically opened to remove the fetus. Hysterotomy is the most complicated method of abortion and carries the highest risk. It is rarely used today; instead, *prostaglandin drugs* are used to terminate pregnancy by inducing labor.

H